INTERNAL DERANGEMENTS
of JOINTS

Emphasis on
MR Imaging

INTERNAL DERANGEMENTS *of* JOINTS

Emphasis on MR Imaging

DONALD RESNICK, M.D.

Professor of Radiology
University of California, San Diego
Chief of Osteoradiology Section
Veterans Affairs Medical Center
San Diego, California

HEUNG SIK KANG, M.D.

Associate Professor of Radiology
Seoul National University College of Medicine
Chief, Musculoskeletal Section
Department of Diagnostic Radiology
Seoul National University Hospital
Seoul, Korea

Catherine Fix
Copy Editor

Michael Holbrook
Administrative Assistant

Debra Trudell
Technical Assistant

W.B. SAUNDERS COMPANY
A *Division of Harcourt Brace & Company*

Philadelphia   London   Toronto   Montreal   Sydney   Tokyo

W.B. SAUNDERS COMPANY
A Division of Harcourt Brace & Company

The Curtis Center
Independence Square West
Philadelphia, Pennsylvania 19106

Library of Congress Cataloging-in-Publication Data

Resnick, Donald.

Internal derangements of joints: emphasis on MR imaging / Donald Resnick, Heung Sik Kang.—1st ed.

p.   cm.

ISBN 0–7216–6760–0

1. Joints—Magnetic resonance imaging.   2. Joints—Imaging.
    3. Joints—Diseases—Diagnosis.   I. Kang, Heung Sik.   II. Title.
    [DNLM: 1. Joint Diseases—diagnosis.   2. Diagnostic Imaging—methods.
    WE 304 R434i 1997]

RC932.R465 1997   616.7′20754—dc20

DNLM/DLC   96–20546

INTERNAL DERANGEMENTS OF JOINTS—
EMPHASIS ON MR IMAGING   ISBN 0–7216–6760–0

Printed in the United States of America.

Last digit is the print number: 9   8   7   6   5   4   3   2

To my students,
whether they be in medical school, residency programs, or fellowships,
who often are my teachers.

To my colleagues,
whose opinions provide important guidance.

To my co-author, Heung Sik Kang,
who taught me the true meaning of dedication and hard work.

And to all those who have remembered their roots
and continue to shower me with their memorable cases.

D.R.

To my teachers,
Chu-Wan Kim, Man Chung Han,
and Donald Resnick,
whose teaching, guidance, advice, encouragement, and stimulation
made me what I am.

H.S.K.

Preface

Six years ago, the two authors of this book published an anatomic atlas dealing with MR imaging of the extremities (*MRI of the Extremities: An Anatomic Atlas.* Philadelphia, W.B. Saunders Company, 1991). Although at that time, we discussed the possibility of, together, also writing a text describing the applications of MR imaging to the assessment of disease processes of the musculoskeletal system, the project was put on hold. About three years ago, the issue of such a book resurfaced. We both believed that a new book must have a purpose. It must offer something that currently is not available, perhaps in the form of improved organization, more detailed information, superior illustrations with complete legends, comprehensive references to available literature, or some combination of these qualities. As we surveyed our bookshelves (and those of our colleagues), we found that many complete sources existed that described the role of MR imaging in the evaluation of the spine. It was our belief, however, that a similar detailed work dealing with MR imaging in the analysis of extraspinal sites was not available. Rather, we believed that the best of the previously published texts in this area related to the analysis of a single anatomic site or joint (e.g., knee, ankle and foot). Hence, we perceived a need for a book exploring the expanding role of MR imaging in the analysis of articular abnormalities. The purpose now in focus and the goal clearly in sight, we began work on this text.

Part of the title of this book, *Internal Derangements of Joints,* underscores our desire to concentrate on those conditions that disturb the action and function of extraspinal articulations, especially those about the shoulder, the elbow, the joints in the wrist and hand, the hip, the knee, the ankle, and the joints of the foot. What became evident early on, however, was that certain disorders leading to modification of periarticular osseous and soft tissue structures could lead to joint dysfunction as well, so that an expanded definition of internal derangements was employed in the organization of this text. The second part of the title, *Emphasis on MR Imaging,* indicates our intention to highlight the role of this most recent and challenging imaging method, one that appears to have the greatest diagnostic potential. Other complementary (not competitive) techniques are addressed, however, including CT scanning, arthrography, and ultrasonography, but emphasis is placed squarely on MR imaging.

The foundation of the book (and, indeed, its organization) parallels that in Chapter 70 of *Diagnosis of Bone and Joint Disorders,* published by W.B. Saunders Company in 1995. But the material in that single chapter has been expanded by about 300 per cent, and the vast majority of the illustrated cases are new to this work. The text is divided into three major sections. The first of these addresses technical considerations related to MR imaging, a topic covered by Dr. Richard Buxton from the Physics Division at the University of California, San Diego. Also provided are typical MR imaging protocols used to study extraspinal joints. The protocols are provided by experts in the field, all of whom (incredibly) began their careers in osteoradiology as fellows in the Department of Radiology at the University of California, San Diego. The second section addresses general concepts that govern the manner in which the disease processes of joints, muscles, tendons, and bones are displayed on MR images (or those derived from alternative imaging methods). In Chapter

7, an overview of the anatomy and pathophysiology of bone and its marrow is provided, material that in part was contributed by another expert (and previous fellow) in the field, Dr. Mini Pathria.

Clearly, however, it is the third part of the text, that dealing with individual anatomic sites, that receives the most comprehensive analysis, representing approximately 90 per cent of the text. This emphasis is planned and deserved because, after all is said and done, knowledge of function and dysfunction of these regions is what the observer brings to the viewbox when interpreting (or reviewing) MR or other advanced imaging displays. Each chapter in this part of the book considers in great depth the anatomy and pathophysiology fundamental to accurate interpretation of these studies, and each includes also a detailed assessment of MR imaging findings of disease processes. Illustrative material (with legends that include important MR imaging parameters) has been chosen carefully and deliberately, to be certain that important points of diagnosis are reinforced in both the text and the figures, and references to published articles are plentiful and up-to-date, to reinforce the concept that most of the observations did not originate with the authors of this text! To this is added a short appendix at the conclusion of the book in which some general topics (i.e., tumors and tumor-like processes of bone and soft tissue, osteomyelitis, osteochondroses) are summarized in the form of tables.

The success of any text is judged not by the good intentions of the authors but rather by the reactions of the readers and by their analyses as to whether or not the material helps them in the real-time clinical world as they interpret (or review) those imaging studies illuminated on their viewbox (or displayed on their console) each day. We are confident, however, that the most up-to-date and conclusive data related to advanced imaging of internal derangements of joints are provided here. And, further, that armed with the information contained in this text, more accurate diagnosis of these studies is possible, even likely.

DONALD RESNICK, M.D.
HEUNG SIK KANG, M.D.

Acknowledgments

The authors wish to acknowledge the considerable effort of a number of persons who contributed unselfishly with regard to their time, energy and, in some instances, case material during the production of this text. First, as is indicated in the legends aside or below the illustrative material, no fewer than 150 people provided one or more cases for inclusion in this book. They did so willingly and, often, spontaneously without request on our part, and their contributions are very much appreciated. The authors would like to mention several persons who donated innumerable cases to the cause: Dean Berthoty, Gerhard Bock, Sevil Kursunoglu Brahme, Thomas Broderick, Steven Eilenberg, Douglas Goodwin, Guerdon Greenway, Jon Jacobson, Philippe Kindynis, Josef Kramer, Vivian Lim, Mini Pathria, Mark Schweitzer, Lynne Steinbach, Marie Tartar, Phillip Tirman, and Marnix van Holsbeeck. A simple thanks hardly is sufficient.

Two persons also contributed to individual chapters in this text and we would like to acknowledge their efforts here:

Richard B. Buxton, Ph.D.   Author of Chaper 1
University of California at San Diego

Mini Pathria, M.D.   Contributor to Chapter 7
University of California at San Diego

Furthermore, the MR imaging protocols detailed in Chapter 2 were contributed by a number of experts who are acknowledged in that chapter. Also, Susan Brown was of great assistance in the coordination of the illustrative material.

The production of this text also required close cooperation between the two authors and a team of dedicated professionals at W.B. Saunders: Lisette Bralow, Lori Irvine, Annette Ferran, Walter Verbitski, and Karen O'Keefe. These persons know all too well that the road to a successful publication often is bumpy and rarely is straight; detours exist, and only through a cooperative effort between authors and publisher is the goal achieved.

Finally, as in many of our other publications, three individuals must be singled out as absolutely essential to the completion of this text. The contributions of these three, Catherine Fix (copy editor), Michael Holbrook (administrative assistant), and Debra Trudell (technical assistant), are of such magnitude that each is recognized on the title page of this text. To them and, indeed, to all of the persons cited here, we are deeply indebted.

Contents

P A R T

I

Magnetic Resonance Imaging: Techniques and Protocols

Magnetic Resonance Imaging: Technical Considerations

The phenomenon of nuclear magnetic resonance (NMR) was first investigated nearly 50 years ago.[1, 2] Since then it has become a standard tool in chemistry,[3] and in the last two decades it has served as the basis for a remarkably powerful and flexible medical imaging technique.[4] This chapter explains the basic physics that underlies the phenomenon of NMR and describes how a measurable signal is produced and used to form an image. The local NMR signal determines the intensity at each point in a magnetic resonance (MR) image, so that the contrast characteristics of MR images all follow from the physics of NMR. (In current usage the less specific term MR is used to refer to imaging applications, rather than NMR. Another related phenomenon, electron spin resonance [ESR], also falls in the category of MR, although there are not yet any medical imaging applications of ESR.)

A number of methods have been developed for creating an image of the NMR signal, and each has advantages and disadvantages in terms of imaging time and image contrast. In addition to providing anatomic images with good soft tissue contrast, MR imaging also is uniquely sensitive to blood flow, and noninvasive MR angiography techniques now are used widely.

OVERVIEW OF NUCLEAR MAGNETIC RESONANCE

The NMR Experiment

The simplest form of the pulsed NMR experiment requires just two components: a magnet and a coil. The magnet produces a uniform magnetic field with magnitude B_o. The coil is arranged so that its axis is perpendicular to the magnetic field direction (Fig. 1–1). The coil can be as simple as a loop of copper and is connected to two devices: a power circuit, which can drive an oscillating electrical current through the coil, and a sensitive detector circuit, which measures small currents in the coil. For typical MR imagers, the currents oscillate at frequencies in the range of 20 to 80 MHz, producing fields in the radiofrequency (RF) region of the electromagnetic spectrum. A sample, such as a human body, is placed in the magnet near the coil. The experiment has two parts: a transmit period and a receive period.

1. Transmit: The detector is turned off and an oscillating voltage is applied to the coil, creating in the

Transmit

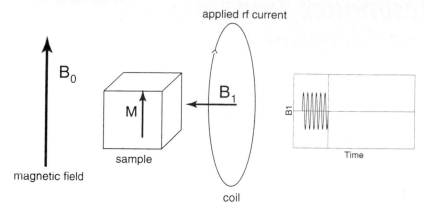

Receive

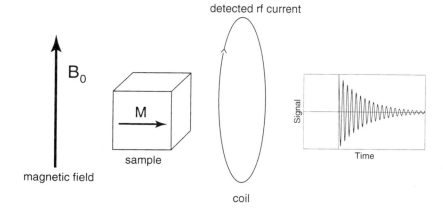

Figure 1–1
The basic NMR experiment A sample is placed in a large magnetic field B_0 with a coil nearby. During the transmit part of the experiment, an oscillating current in the coil creates an oscillating magnetic field B_1 in the sample. During the receive part of the experiment, the coil acts as a detector to measure the precessing magnetization M in the sample.

sample an additional oscillating magnetic field B_1, referred to as the *RF magnetic field*. After a few milliseconds, B_1 is turned off.

2. Receive: The detector circuit is turned on to measure any signal returned from the sample.

The NMR Phenomenon

If this experiment were performed on the human body, varying the oscillation frequency of B_1 and the magnitude of B_0, the following phenomena would be noted:

1. Resonance: For a few specific frequencies, a weak, transient signal is produced and detected with the coil. Each of these frequencies constitutes the *resonant frequency* (or *Larmor frequency*) of a particular nucleus (Table 1–1). At these frequencies, the nuclei absorb energy from the RF magnetic field and then return some of that energy to the coil during the receive part of the experiment.

2. Field Dependence: The resonant frequency is directly proportional to the magnetic field: $f_0 = \gamma B_0$, where f_0 is the resonant frequency and γ is the *gyromagnetic ratio*, which is a different constant for each nucleus. In

standard MR imaging the nucleus of interest is hydrogen (H), which has a resonant frequency of 63 MHz in a magnetic field of 1.5 Tesla (T). The linear relationship between resonant frequency and magnetic field is the physical basis for MR imaging.

3. Chemical Shift: For a particular nucleus, the resonant frequency varies by a few parts per million (ppm) depending on the chemical form of the nucleus (e.g., for H in water and lipids the difference is 3.5 ppm). This chemical shift is the basis for the use of NMR as an analytical tool in chemistry. The effect occurs because molecular electronic orbitals create additional magnetic fields that combine with B_0 to shift the magnetic field at the location of the nucleus and thus shift the resonant frequency.

Table 1–1. SOME NUCLEI THAT EXHIBIT NMR

Nucleus	Gyromagnetic Ratio (MHz/T)
^{1}H	42.6
^{19}F	40.1
^{31}P	17.2
^{23}Na	11.3
^{13}C	10.7
^{17}O	5.8

Origin of the NMR Signal

In brief, the physical picture of NMR is illustrated in Figure 1–2. Certain nuclei (such as hydrogen) have an intrinsic magnetic moment, so that they behave like small magnets when placed in a magnetic field. The nuclear magnetic moments tend to align with B_0, creating a magnetization *(M)* in the sample. *M* is essentially a weak magnetic field parallel to B_0. The oscillating field (B_1) at the resonant frequency f_0 tips *M* away from B_0. At this point *M* can be viewed as consisting of two parts: a *longitudinal* component (M_L) parallel to B_0, and a *transverse* component (M_T) perpendicular to B_0. The transverse magnetization (M_T) rotates around B_0 *(precession)* with frequency f_0, generating a signal in the detector coil that is proportional to the magnitude of M_T. Over time *M* gradually realigns with B_0 *(relaxation)* and the signal decays as M_T decays.

The precessing magnetization M_T is the source of the signal measured in all NMR experiments, from spectrometer studies in analytical chemistry to MR imaging. In MR imaging the local image intensity is proportional to the local magnitude of M_T. To understand why NMR happens, and in particular to understand the phenom-

ena of precession and relaxation, the physics of a nucleus in a magnetic field must be considered.

PRINCIPLES OF NUCLEAR MAGNETIC RESONANCE

Physics of NMR

Coils: *Electric Currents and Magnetic Fields*

Two basic principles of the physics of electricity and magnetism are involved in the generation and detection of the NMR signal[3]: (1) electric currents produce magnetic fields, and (2) changing magnetic fields produce electric currents. Electric currents in a coil (either constant or changing) produce magnetic fields in the vicinity of the coil, and these fields are strongest close to the coil. The magnetic field produced by a simple circular coil is illustrated in Figure 1–3. Changing magnetic fields in the vicinity of a coil produce currents in the coil *(induction)*, but constant magnetic fields do not. The current in the coil is strongest when the coil is near the source of the changing magnetic field.

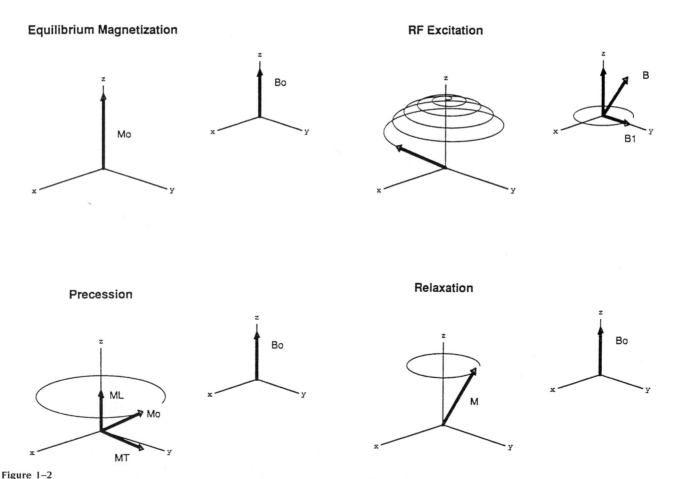

Figure 1–2
The physics of the NMR phenomenon. Hydrogen nuclei possess a magnetic dipole moment, and when placed in a constant magnetic field B_0, they tend to align with the field, creating a local magnetization *M*. When a radio frequency (RF) magnetic field B_1 oscillating at the resonant frequency is applied, the magnetization tips away from the main field direction, creating a transverse component M_T and a longitudinal component M_L. The magnetization precesses around B_0 and generates a signal proportional to M_T. Over time *M* relaxes back toward the equilibrium alignment with B_0.

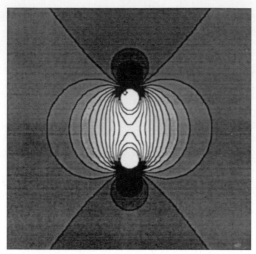

Figure I–3
The magnetic field pattern produced by a simple circular coil. The magnetic field at each point is a vector, and only the component in the horizontal direction is shown. The contour map shows the magnitude of this component of the field in a plane perpendicular to the plane of the coil. The coil intersects the plane at the two bright spots.

These principles come into play in several ways in the NMR experiment. The main magnetic field B_0 is generated by a large cylindrical coil carrying a constant current. High field (greater than 0.3 T) imagers use superconducting magnets in which the coil carrying the current is cooled to the temperature of liquid helium. At this low temperature, the electrical resistance of the conductor is zero, so the high current can be maintained without supplying any additional power to the system.

The two principles also apply to the two parts of the NMR experiment. During the transmit portion, the oscillating current in the RF coil produces an oscillating magnetic field (B_1) in the vicinity of the coil. During the receive portion, the precessing transverse magnetization (M_1) in the sample (a changing magnetic field) generates a detectable current in the coil. Often in MR imaging two separate coils are used for the transmit and receive parts of the measurement, to optimize the coils for each role. For the transmit coil the B_1 field should be as uniform as possible over the body, so that all areas are equally excited. For signal detection, however, the signal to noise ratio can be significantly improved by using a smaller receive coil. By placing the small coil closer to the location of the oscillating magnetization, a larger current is produced in the coil. In addition, because the noise in an MR imaging system arises primarily from the body itself, a small coil that is sensitive only to a small part of the body receives less noise as well.

Nuclear Spin and Magnetic Dipole Moment

Protons and neutrons possess an intrinsic angular momentum called *spin.* Like mass and charge, spin is a fundamental characteristic of subatomic particles. The concept of an intrinsic angular momentum comes from the quantum mechanical description of nature and has no analogue in the macroscopic world of everyday experience. Although we are familiar with many spinning objects, from tops to entire planets, the "spin" is not an inseparable feature of these bodies: we can stop a spinning top and we can at least imagine stopping a spinning planet. In other words, these objects could exist with zero angular momentum. But a proton always has angular momentum, and the only aspect that can be changed is the direction of the spin axis. Protons and neutrons combine to form a nucleus such that their spins mutually cancel (opposite spin axes), so that the nucleus has no net spin unless there is an odd number of protons or neutrons. Thus, the nuclei of ^{1}H (one proton) and ^{13}C (six protons and seven neutrons) have a net spin, whereas the nucleus of ^{12}C does not.

Nuclei with a net spin also possess another important physical property: a magnetic dipole moment. Each proton behaves like a magnet with the north-south axis aligned with the spin axis. The association of a magnetic moment with angular momentum of the nucleus can be understood from a simple (and naive) picture of the nucleus as a spinning charged ball. The rotational motion of the charges constitutes a current, which in turn creates a magnetic field. It is the magnetic moment of the nucleus that leads to the phenomenon of NMR, so only nuclei with a net spin exhibit NMR.

Precession in a Magnetic Field

A magnetic dipole moment has two key properties: a magnitude μ and a directional axis. When a magnetic dipole is placed in a uniform magnetic field it has an energy that is proportional to μ but also depends on its orientation. Aligned with the field is the lowest energy state, and opposite to the field is the highest energy state. A compass needle thus aligns with the earth's magnetic field because it is seeking its lowest energy state. However, when a nucleus is placed in a magnetic field, its intrinsic angular momentum prevents it from immediately aligning with the field. The field exerts a torque on the dipole, which, by itself, would rotate the dipole into alignment with the field. However, when this change in angular momentum is added to the existing angular momentum of the dipole, the net change is a *precession* of the dipole axis around the field. That is, the dipole axis rotates while keeping the same angle with the magnetic field.

This is an example of the peculiar nature of angular momentum, and it is exactly analogous to the behavior of a spinning top or bicycle wheel. A spinning top tipped at an angle to the vertical would be in a lower energy state if it simply fell over; instead, the rotation axis precesses around a vertical line. For a nucleus in a magnetic field the frequency of precession is directly proportional to the product μB_0; the stronger the field, the stronger the torque on the dipole and the faster the precession. The precession frequency (f_0) is the resonant frequency of NMR.

Relaxation

The foregoing considerations apply to a single nucleus in a magnetic field, and from the precession arguments it might be concluded that a proton would never align with the main field. In a real sample, however, B_0 is not the only source of magnetic field. The magnetic moments of other nuclei produce additional magnetic fields. For example, in a water molecule, an H nucleus feels the field produced by the other H nucleus in the molecule. Because the molecules are rapidly tumbling owing to their thermal motions, the total field felt by a particular nucleus fluctuates around the mean field B_0. These fluctuations alter both the total magnetic field magnitude and the direction. As a result, the proton's precession is more irregular, and the axis of precession fluctuates. Over time, the protons gradually tend to align more with B_0, a process called *relaxation*.

Because the energy associated with the orientation of the magnetic dipole moment of a hydrogen nucleus in a magnetic field is small compared with the thermal energy of a water molecule, the average degree of alignment with the field is small, corresponding to a difference of only about one part in 10^5 between those nuclei aligned with the field and those opposite. However, this is sufficient to produce a slight net magnetization (M) of the water. The creation of M can be understood as a relaxation toward thermal equilibrium. When a sample is first placed in a magnetic field the magnetic dipoles are oriented randomly, so that the net magnetization is zero. This means that the dipoles possess a higher energy owing to their orientation than they would if they were partly aligned with the field. (The lowest possible energy would correspond to complete alignment.) As the system relaxes, this excess energy is dissipated as heat, the dipoles align more with the field, and M grows toward its equilibrium value, M_0.

The time constant for relaxation is called T1 and varies from about 0.2 to 4.0 sec in the body.[5] In a pure water sample the main source of a fluctuating magnetic field is the field produced by the other H nucleus in the same water molecule. But the presence of other molecules in the liquid (such as protein) can alter the relaxation rate by changing either the magnitude or the frequency of the fluctuating fields. A large molecule will tumble more slowly than a water molecule, so that a water molecule that binds transiently to the large molecule will experience more slowly fluctuating fields. The magnitude of the fluctuating fields can be increased significantly in the presence of paramagnetic compounds. Paramagnetic compounds have unpaired electrons, and electrons have magnetic moments more than a thousand times larger than a proton. This is the basis for the use of paramagnetic contrast agents, such as gadopentetate dimeglumine, as a means of reducing the local relaxation time.

The fact that T1 varies by an order of magnitude between different tissues is important because this is the source of most of the contrast differences between tissues in MR images. The differences are attributable to differences in the local environment (e.g., chemical composition, biologic structures). In general, the higher the water content of a tissue, the longer the T1. The strong dependence of the relaxation time on the local environment is exactly analogous to everyday experiences of relaxation phenomena. A cup of hot coffee sitting in a cool room is not in thermal equilibrium. Over time, the coffee will cool to room temperature (thermal equilibrium), but the time constant for this relaxation depends strongly on the local environment. If the coffee is in a thin-walled open cup, it may cool in a few minutes, whereas if it is in a covered, insulated vessel, cooling may take hours. Regardless of how long it takes, however, the final equilibrium state is the same.

Generating the NMR Signal

Radio Frequency Pulse

The fact that the protons tend to align with the field, producing a net magnetization (M), does not lead to any measurable signal (a constant magnetic field produces no currents). However, if M is tipped away from the direction of B_0, it will precess; all of the nuclear dipoles will precess together if they are tipped over, so the net magnetization M also will precess at the same frequency. The transverse component of M then is a changing magnetic field and will generate a signal in a nearby detector coil.

The tipping is accomplished during the RF pulse of our basic NMR experiment by applying an oscillating magnetic field (B_1) perpendicular to B_0 and oscillating at the proton precession frequency. M then begins to precess around the net time-varying magnetic field. To see why this tips M away from B_0, imagine viewing M in a reference frame that rotates at the precession frequency f_0.[6] If M is tipped away from B_0, it will precess in the laboratory frame, but in the rotating frame it will be stationary, so that in this frame it appears as if the magnetic field is zero (Fig. 1–4). Similarly, the magnetic field B_1, which is oscillating in the laboratory frame with frequency f_0, appears to be a stationary field in the rotating frame. The complex picture of precession around a time-varying net magnetization in the laboratory frame then reduces to a simple precession around B_1 in the rotating frame.

After B_1 is turned off, M continues to precess around B_0 and generates a signal in the detector coil. Over time, M will relax until it is again aligned with B_0. Because the action of an RF pulse is to tip M away from B_0, such pulses usually are described by the *flip angle* (or *tip angle*) they produce (e.g., a 90 degree RF pulse or a 180 degree RF pulse). The flip angle is adjusted by changing either the duration or the amplitude of the RF pulse.

From the thermodynamic point of view, the process of tipping M can be interpreted as the system of magnetic dipoles absorbing energy from the RF field, because the alignment of M is changing and then dissipating this energy over time as heat as the system relaxes back to equilibrium. For this reason, the RF pulse sometimes is described as an *excitation pulse* because it raises the system to an excited (higher energy) state.

Free Induction Decay

After an RF excitation pulse (e.g., a 90 degree pulse) occurs, the signal generated in the detector coil is called

Laboratory Frame

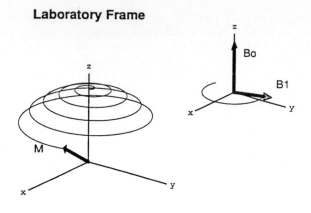

Rotating Frame

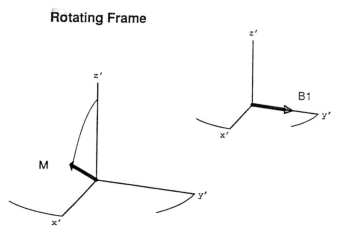

Figure 1–4

The rotating reference frame. The process of RF excitation is understood most easily by viewing the magnetization from a frame of reference that rotates at the same rate as the magnetization M precesses. In the rotating frame M appears to be stationary, and so it appears that B_0 is zero. The field B_1, which also is rotating with the same frequency in the laboratory frame, appears to be a constant field in the rotating frame. The motion of M then is a simple precession around B_1 in the rotating frame, and appears as a widening spiral when viewed in the laboratory frame.

a *free induction decay.* "Free" relates to free precession, "induction" is the physical process in which a varying magnetic field (the precessing magnetization M) produces a current in a coil, and "decay" indicates that the signal dies out over time. It might be expected that the time constant for this decay would be T1, the time constant for relaxation to equilibrium. However, the decay of the signal usually is much faster than would be expected from T1. For this reason it is necessary to introduce a second time constant, T2, to describe the signal decay.

Relaxation Times: T1, T2, and T2*

The two relaxation times T1 and T2 apply to the longitudinal and transverse components of the magnetization, respectively. At equilibrium, M is purely longitudinal (aligned with B_0), and after a 90 degree RF pulse it is purely transverse (perpendicular to B_0). Because the measured signal is proportional to the transverse

component of M, the time constant governing the decay of the signal is T2, and this process often is termed *transverse relaxation.* On the other hand, the relaxation back to thermal equilibrium is related to changes in the longitudinal component, the growth of the net magnetization. T1 thus is the time constant for *longitudinal relaxation.* In the human body at field strengths typical of MR imagers, T1 is about eight to ten times larger than T2.

In practice, experimentally the free induction decay often is found to decay much more quickly than would be expected for the T2 of the sample. This frequently is described qualitatively by saying that the decay time is T2*, with T2* less than T2. The reason for this is simply inhomogeneity of the magnetic field. If two regions of the sample feel different magnetic fields, the precession rates will differ, the local transverse magnetization vectors will quickly get out of phase with each other, and the net magnetization will decrease owing to *phase dispersion.* However, this signal decay is due to constant field offsets within the sample and not to the fluctuating fields that produce T2 decay. Because of this, the additional decay due to inhomogeneity is reversible.

Spin Echoes

Signal loss due to inhomogeneity can be reversed by applying a second RF pulse that causes the magnetization vectors to come back into phase and create an echo of the original free induction decay signal (a *spin echo*) at a time TE (the *echo time*) after the original excitation pulse.[7] To see how this remarkable effect comes about, imagine two small magnetized regions in slightly different magnetic fields. After a 90 degree excitation pulse, the magnetization vectors are tipped into the transverse plane (Fig. 1–5). As they begin to precess at slightly different frequencies, the phase difference between them grows larger. After waiting a time TE/2, an 180 degree RF pulse is applied. The action of the 180 degree pulse is to flip the transverse plane like a pancake, reversing the *sign* of the phase of each magnetization vector. In other words, the phase φ_1 of the first magnetization is changed to $-\varphi_1$, and the phase φ_2 of the second group is changed to $-\varphi_2$. After the RF pulse the phase of each magnetization continues to evolve, just as before, so that after another time delay TE/2 the first group again acquires an additional phase φ_1, and the second group again acquires an additional phase φ_2. However, the net phase of each group then is zero, meaning they are back in phase and add coherently to form a strong net signal (the echo) at time TE. In fact, the echoing process is quite general, and any RF pulse will create an echo, although with flip angles other than 180 degrees the refocusing is not complete.

Note that although an 180 degree pulse will correct for field inhomogeneities, it will *not* refocus T2 decay (Fig. 1–6). An echo forms because the phase acquired during the interval before the 180 degree pulse is exactly the same as the phase acquired during the interval after the pulse, so that by reversing the sign of the phase at the halfway point the net phase will be zero. But the phase variations associated with T2 decay are due to

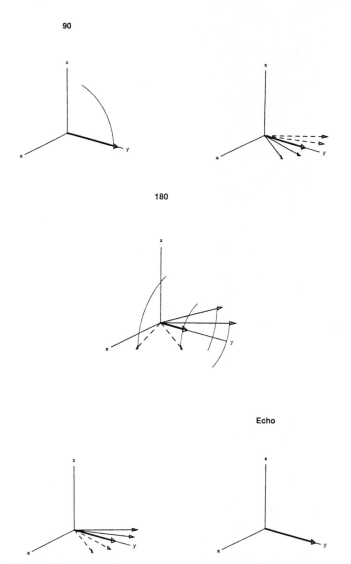

90

180

Echo

Figure 1–5
The formation of spin echoes. A 90 degree RF pulse tips over all spins to create a coherent transverse magnetization. Owing to magnetic field inhomogeneity, spins in different locations precess at different rates, leading to a spread of phase angles and a reduction in the net transverse magnetization. After a time TE/2, a 180 degree RF pulse flips the plane of magnetization vectors, reversing the phase that each spin has acquired. Continued precession for another interval TE/2 brings the spins back in phase to create an echo of the original magnetization at the echo time TE.

fluctuating fields, and the pattern of fluctuations is not repeated before and after the RF pulse. In short, a spin echo reverses the dephasing effects of static fields but not fluctuating fields. As a result, the echo signal intensity is weaker than the initial free induction decay signal owing to T2 decay during the interval TE. After the echo the signal again decays because of T2* effects, but another 180 degree RF pulse will create another echo. This can be continued indefinitely, but each echo will be weaker than the last because of T2 decay.

Spin Echo Pulse Sequence

The basic spin echo pulse sequence can be summarized as follows:

90 degree RF pulse—wait TE/2—180 degree RF pulse—wait TE/2—echo

Typically, this pulse sequence is repeated at a regular interval, called the *repetition time* (TR). In a normal MR imaging setting it is necessary to repeat the pulse sequence many times to collect all the data needed to reconstruct the image. The contrast between one tissue and another in the image will depend on the magnitude of the spin echo signal generated at each location.

Spin Echo Signal Intensity

Two pulse sequence parameters are operator controlled: the repetition time (TR) and the echo time (TE). The measured signal intensity depends strongly on both of these parameters (Fig. 1–7). The effect of TE has already been discussed. By lengthening TE (i.e., waiting a longer time after the excitation pulse before looking at the signal), more time is allowed for transverse (T2) decay. TR, on the other hand, controls how much longitudinal relaxation is allowed to happen before the magnetization is tipped over again. During the period TR, a sample with the T1 much shorter than the TR will relax nearly completely, so that the longitudinal magnetization just before the next 90 degree pulse is large, but a sample with T1 longer than TR will be relaxed only partly and the longitudinal magnetization will be smaller. After the next 90 degree pulse, this longitudinal magnetization becomes the transverse magnetization and generates a signal, so the short T1 sample will produce a stronger signal.

In addition to T1 and T2, the signal intensity also is proportional to the local density of nuclei. In MR imaging this usually is called the *hydrogen density* or *proton density*. These relationships can be summarized by the following approximate equation[8, 9]:

Spin Echoes

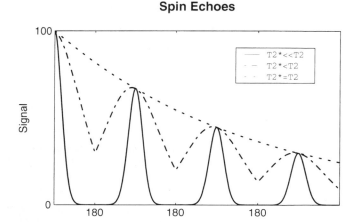

Figure 1–6
Spin echo signal decay. After an RF pulse creates a transverse magnetization, the rate of signal decay depends on T2* and T2. T2* is the apparent decay time, which includes the effects of field inhomogeneity as well as transverse relaxation (T2 decay). A series of 180 degree RF pulses will create echoes in which the inhomogeneity effects are reversed, but each echo peak still is reduced by T2 decay.

T1-Weighted SE Contrast

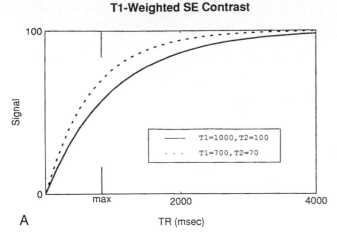

T2-Weighted SE Contrast

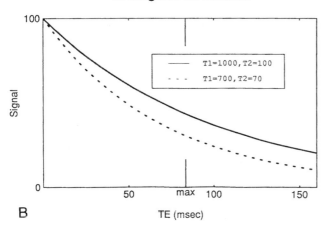

SE Contrast

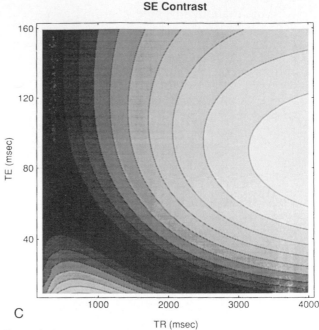

Figure 1–7

Image contrast in spin echo (SE) imaging. The plots show the effect on signal and contrast of the two operator-adjustable parameters, TR (the repetition time) and TE (the echo time). Signal curves are plotted for two hypothetical tissues with different relaxation times, and the contrast between the tissues is the difference between the two curves.

A TR dependence of the signal, assuming TE is short.

B TE dependence of the signal, assuming TR is long.

C Contour plot showing contrast for different choices of TR and TE. Note that many choices of TR and TE produce poor contrast. The two islands of high contrast are at TR≈4000 and TE≈90 (T2 weighted) and at TR≈600 with TE at the minimum possible value (T1 weighted).

$$S \cong S_0 e^{-\text{TE}/\text{T2}}\,(1 - e^{-\text{TR}/\text{T1}})$$

where S is the measured signal (e.g., the brightness of a particular pixel in an image), S_0 is proportional to the local proton density, the first exponential term describes T2 decay, and the second exponential term describes T1 relaxation. The signal thus depends on three properties of the tissue (S_0, T1, and T2) and two operator-controlled parameters (TR and TE).

Spin Echo Tissue Contrast

The proton density is always a determining factor in the signal, but in vivo the water content does not vary over as great a range as do T1 and T2. Good contrast therefore is produced by making the measured signal sensitive to the relaxation times, and the relative importance of T1 and T2 can be adjusted by changing TR and TE (Fig. 1–7). With a short TR, tissues with short T1 will relax much more than tissues with a long T1, and thus T1 will affect the signal strongly. The signal then is said to be T1 weighted. However, with long TR (several times the longest T1) all tissues will relax nearly completely and T1 will have little effect on the signal. With a long TE, differences in T2 will affect the signal strongly (T2 weighting), but with a short TE there is

little time for decay and T2 will not have an effect. These arguments lead to the following loose characterization of contrast in SE pulse sequences:

short TR: T1-weighted, short T1 tissues are bright
long TE: T2-weighted, long T2 tissues are bright

A central problem with tissue contrast in MR imaging is that the relaxation times are positively correlated: tissues with a long T1 also are likely to have a long T2. For this reason it is rarely desirable to have both substantial T1 weighting and T2 weighting in the same image. With T1 weighting a tissue with short relaxation times will tend to be bright, but with T2 weighting it will tend to be dark. As a result of this conflict, tissue contrast can be destroyed. For this reason, TR and TE should be chosen not only to emphasize sensitivity to one of the relaxation times but also to *suppress* sensitivity to the other:

"T1-weighted":	short TR, short TE
"T2-weighted":	long TR, long TE
"proton density weighted":	long TR, short TE

The terminology here is necessarily loose, and the quotation marks are meant to indicate that these terms should be used with caution. The third pulse sequence is termed proton density weighted, but in fact all three are proton density weighted; it is just that in the third one the additional sensitivity to T1 and T2 has been suppressed. Note also that "short" and "long" in this context are relative to T1 and T2, and these vary substantially in the body. For example, a spin echo image obtained with a TR of 2000 msec and a TE of 20 msec would be proton density weighted for white matter in the brain (TI $\cong$ 700 msec) but T1-weighted for cerebrospinal fluid (T1 $\cong$ 3000 msec).

Inversion Recovery Pulse Sequence

The *inversion recovery* (IR) pulse sequence typically requires three RF pulses. It begins with an 180 degree inversion pulse, and after a time delay TI (the *inversion time*) a spin echo pulse sequence is started:

180 degree RF—wait TI—90 degree RF—wait
TE/2—180 degree RF—wait TE/2—echo

The effect of the inversion pulse is to flip the longitudinal magnetization from the positive *z*-axis to the negative *z*-axis. This does not produce any signal because there is still no transverse magnetization. After the inversion pulse the magnetization begins to relax back toward equilibrium (alignment with the positive *z*-axis). However, after a time TI, before complete relaxation can occur, the 90 degree pulse tips over the longitudinal magnetization to create a transverse magnetization. The final 180 degree pulse then creates an echo of the transverse magnetization for measurement. The signal received depends on how much relaxation occurred during the interval TI, and so it is strongly T1 weighted (Fig. 1–8).

Note that as the magnetization relaxes it passes through a *null point* at which the longitudinal magnetization is zero. If the 90 degree pulse is applied at this time, no signal will be generated. This effect is exploited with a short TI inversion recovery (STIR) pulse sequence to suppress the fat signal by choosing the TI to be at the null point of fat.

PRINCIPLES OF MAGNETIC RESONANCE IMAGING

Basic Imaging Techniques

Field Gradients

MR imaging exploits the physical fact that the resonant frequency f_0 is directly proportional to the magnetic field. By altering the magnetic field in a controlled way, so that it varies linearly along a particular axis, the resonant frequency also will vary linearly with position along that axis. Such a linearly varying field is called a *gradient field* and is produced by additional coils in the scanner. An MR imager is equipped with three orthogo-

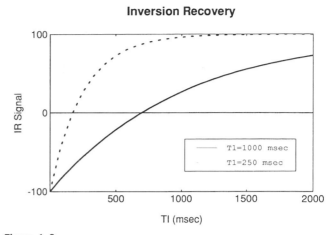

Inversion Recovery

Figure 1–8

The inversion recovery (IR) signal as a function of the inversion time (TI). The initial 180 degree inversion pulse flips the longitudinal magnetization from the positive *z*-axis to the negative *z*-axis. The magnetization is allowed to relax for a time TI and then is tipped over with a 90 degree RF pulse to create a strongly T1 weighted signal. The time TI when the longitudinal magnetization passes through zero is called the null point, and no signal is generated. By using a short TI, the signal from tissues with a short T1 (such as fat) can be suppressed substantially.

nal sets of gradient coils, allowing a field gradient to be produced along any axis. Because these gradient fields usually are turned on for only a few milliseconds at a time, they are referred to as *pulsed gradients*.

Compared to the main magnetic field (B_0), the field variations produced by the gradients are small. Typical gradient strengths used for imaging are a few milliTesla per meter (mT/m), and conventional MR imagers usually have maximum strengths of 10 mT/m. At maximum strength the magnetic field variation across a 30 cm object is 3 mT, only 0.2 per cent of a typical B_0 of 1.5 T. For the discussion of spatial encoding on the following pages it is convenient to express field gradients in units of the resonant frequency change they produce per centimeter (Hz/cm): 10 mT/m = 4258 Hz/cm for protons.

Field gradients are used in three ways to encode the spatial location of a signal: (1) *slice selection*, (2) *frequency encoding*, and (3) *phase encoding*. These three methods are used for the three spatial axes; in the following sections slice selection is used on the *z*-axis, frequency encoding on the *x*-axis, and phase encoding on the *y*-axis. This is an image-based coordinate system, with the image in the *x-y* plane, and it should not be confused with the magnet-based coordinate system in which B_0 is considered as being in the *z* direction and *x-y* is in the transverse plane. These two coordinate systems have no fixed relationship with each other; an image may be made in any orientation with respect to the main field.

Figure 1–9 illustrates how these methods are implemented in a spin echo imaging pulse sequence. Time is plotted along the horizontal axis and the rows show when different gradients or RF pulses are turned on and off. The phase encoding gradient is diagrammed as a series of gradient steps, indicating that it is changed each time the pulse sequence is repeated.

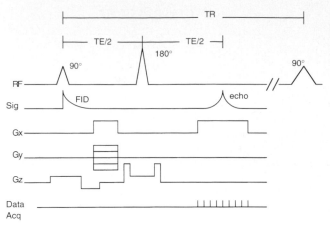

Figure 1–9
The spin echo imaging pulse sequence. The 90 degree RF pulse creates a free induction decay signal (which is not measured) and the 180 degree RF pulse creates an echo of that signal at time TE. Data acquisition is centered on the echo time. Field gradient pulses along different axes are used for slice selection in *z*, for frequency encoding in *x*, and for phase encoding in *y*. The entire pulse sequence is repeated after a repetition time TR, and with each repetition the phase encoding gradient is changed to a new value.

Slice Selection

The simplest application of a gradient field is to limit the excitation of the protons to just one desired slice. If the RF pulse with center frequency (f_0) has only a small bandwidth (Δf), turning on a *z*-gradient (G_z) will result in excitation of only a narrow band in *z* with a width $\Delta z = \Delta f / G_z$. That is, for spins above or below this slice, the resonant frequency is either too high or too low to be excited by the RF pulse, so that only the magnetization in the band Δz is tipped over to produce a signal.

Frequency Encoding

After the 90 degree excitation pulse, the *z*-gradient can be turned off, and only the selected slice will produce a signal. The *x*-axis then is frequency encoded by turning on an *x*-gradient during data collection (sometimes called a *read-out gradient*). In this way, each spin will precess with a frequency (f) that is proportional to its position along *x*. The net signal therefore is a sum of many individual signals with different frequencies, and the amplitude of each frequency can be determined from the data by the mathematical operation of a Fourier transform (discussed in more detail later). The signal at each frequency is the total signal at the corresponding position *x* summed over (or projected along) *y*.

Phase Encoding

Phase encoding is a more subtle technique. The procedure is to turn on a gradient field in *y* after the slice select gradient in *z* and before the frequency encoding gradient in *x*. The gradient is left on for a few milliseconds and then turned off. While the gradient is on, protons at a positive *y* position will precess faster than those at negative *y*, so a linear variation in phase along *y* will develop. Once the *y*-gradient is turned off, all

spins again will precess at the same rate but the linear phase variation will be locked in. When the data are read out with the *x*-gradient on, the total signal measured for each position *x* is a sum of all the signals on a line running in *y* at that value of *x*. Because of the locked-in phase variations, these signals will not add coherently; there can be some cancellation. Subsequently, the whole pulse sequence is repeated, but with a different *y*-gradient strength. Again the result of the frequency encoding will be to give a summation of all the signals along *y* at each *x* position, but because the phase variation along *y* is now different, in effect the signals are added with different weighting factors. By stepping through 128 different phase encoding gradient strengths, the signal along a *y*-projection can be separated into 128 distinct values.

In fact, the results of phase encoding and frequency encoding are mathematically identical (Fig. 1–10). With frequency encoding, data collection consists of a series of measurements that sample the total signal with an interval Δt between samples. With each successive sample, the phase difference between signals from different locations increases because the gradient is on for a longer time. With phase encoding, the sampling can be thought of as occurring every TR (instead of Δt) as the pulse sequence is repeated and the phase encoding gradient is increased to the next value. For each phase encoding sample the amplitude of the gradient pulse is increased but the duration is the same. However, increasing the amplitude with a constant duration has the same effect on the local phases as increasing the duration with constant amplitude (as in frequency encoding); the relative phase changes are determined just by the product of amplitude and duration. Thus, the samples measured every TR with different phase encode steps are exactly analogous to the samples measured

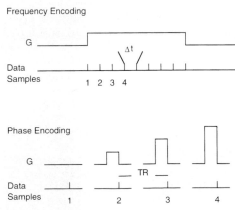

Figure 1–10
Comparison of frequency encoding and phase encoding, showing the essential similarity of the two encoding processes. In frequency encoding, successive data samples are separated by a time interval Δt, and for each sample the phase effects of the gradient are increased because the gradient has been on for a longer time. In phase encoding, data samples are separated by a time TR, and for each successive sample the phase effects are increased because the amplitude of the gradient pulse is increased. Because the phase changes produced by a field gradient pulse are proportional to the product of the gradient amplitude and duration (the area in this diagram), the signal measured in corresponding samples is the same.

every Δt with frequency encoding. Just as frequency encoding yields data that are the Fourier transform of the signal distribution in x, phase encoding yields data that are the Fourier transform of the signal distribution in y.

Spin Echo Imaging Pulse Sequence

The key features of the pulse sequence diagram in Figure 1–9 are the timings of the RF pulses and the gradient pulses used for slice selection, frequency encoding, and phase encoding. A few additional gradient pulses also are included in the diagram: (1) the x-gradient pulse between the 90 degree and 180 degree RF pulses, called the *x-compensation pulse*, (2) the negative z-gradient pulse immediately after the first slice selection gradient, called the *z-compensation pulse*, and (3) the large z-gradient pulses before and after the second slice selection pulse, sometimes called *crusher pulses*. These additional pulses are involved in producing *gradient recalled echoes* (GRE) and in *gradient spoiling*.

Gradient Spoiling and Gradient Echoes

If a gradient pulse is applied after an RF excitation pulse, spins at different positions along the gradient axis will precess at different rates. The net effect of the gradient pulse is thus to produce a large dispersion of phase angles, and the net signal is severely reduced *(spoiled)*. However, if an opposite gradient pulse is then applied for the same duration, each spin will acquire a phase angle opposite to the phase it acquired during the first pulse (Fig. 1–11). The phase dispersion therefore is removed, and all spins add coherently to produce a strong signal called a *gradient recalled echo*. If a 180 degree

RF pulse is placed between the two gradient pulses, the two gradients must have the same sign for a gradient echo to occur. The 180 degree RF pulse will reverse the phase of each spin group, and the second gradient pulse will then bring them back into phase.

x-Compensation Pulse

The x-compensation pulse is used to create a gradient echo at the center of data collection. At the middle of the read-out gradient the newly acquired phase of each group due to the read-out gradient just balances the phase acquired from the x-compensation pulse. All spins are back in phase, and the net signal again is large, creating the gradient echo. All this is done because the data samples near the time when all of the spins are in phase are critical for reconstructing the image. Without the x-compensation pulse, these samples would occur at the beginning of the read-out gradient. In practice a gradient cannot be turned on instantly; some time is required for it to ramp up and stabilize. For this reason it is desirable that these samples occur in the center of the read-gradient window. By adjusting the strength (amplitude times duration) of the x-compensation pulse the time of the gradient echo can be shifted.

Note that there are thus two echoing processes involved in an imaging spin echo pulse sequence. The x-compensation gradient is adjusted so that the gradient echo occurs at the center of data collection, and the timing of the 180 degree pulse also is adjusted so that the RF echo occurs at the same time. If the time of the RF echo is deliberately shifted from the time of the gradient echo, the resulting pulse sequence is referred to as an *asymmetric spin echo*. Asymmetric spin echo pulse sequences can be useful for chemical shift imaging, such as fat-water separation. Because the fat and water magnetizations precess at slightly different frequencies, the relative phase difference between the fat signal and the water signal is proportional to the time shift between the RF echo and the gradient echo. By adjusting the time shift so that fat and water are 180 degrees out of phase, the signals will subtract, and tissues containing both fat and water (such as vertebral marrow) will be dark in the MR image.

z-Compensation Pulse

The z-compensation pulse is necessary because spins at different z-positions within the slice are getting out of phase with each other as they precess during slice selection. Reversing the gradient and leaving it on for the right amount of time will bring all the spins back in phase; a spin that acquired a phase φ during the slice selection pulse will acquire an additional phase $-\varphi$ during the compensation pulse. In other words, another gradient echo occurs. The only difference between this gradient echo and the one formed by the x-gradient is that there is no 180 degree pulse between the two gradient pulses to reverse the first phase, so the sign of the gradient must be reversed. For the 180 degree slice selection gradient pulse, a 180 degree pulse does exist in the center, so this gradient is automatically compensated for.

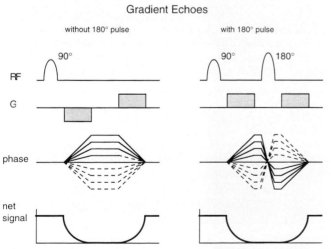

Gradient Echoes

Figure 1–11
Gradient recalled echoes (GRE). A field gradient pulse creates phase changes proportional to the spin's position, and the resulting phase dispersion spoils the signal. A second opposite gradient pulse brings the spins back into phase and creates a gradient echo. If a 180-degree RF pulse occurs after the first gradient pulse, the phase of each spin is reversed, and a second gradient pulse with the same sign as the first then will create the gradient echo.

Fourier Transforms

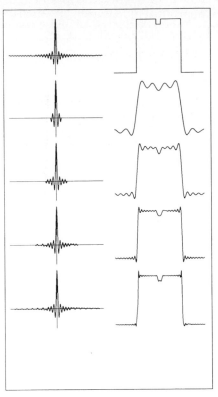

Figure 1–12

Fourier transforms. Each pair of curves is a Fourier transform pair. The curve in the top right could be a spatial distribution of signal intensity. The curve on the left then shows the contribution of different spatial frequencies. To represent the original spatial distribution curve completely, an infinite number of frequencies would be required. Successive plots show how increasing the number of spatial frequencies included provides a better approximation to the curve. Note in the bottom pair that even with a large number of frequencies a characteristic overshoot occurs at sharp edges (Gibbs phenomenon).

Crushers

The crusher gradients are designed to eliminate problems associated with imperfect 180 degree RF pulses. If the refocusing pulse is not exactly 180 degrees, some new transverse magnetization will be generated, and the signal produced will create artifacts in the image. The large gradient pulse after the 180 degree RF pulse will produce a large phase dispersion in the unwanted magnetization and thus crush (or spoil) the net signal. In order not to crush the desired transverse magnetization generated by the 90 degree RF pulse, a second large gradient pulse must be put before the 180 degree RF pulse. Then these two crusher gradients create a gradient echo of the desired magnetization and thus have no effect on the desired signal.

Fourier Transforms and *k*-Space

k-Space

At the heart of the imaging process is the concept of the Fourier transform.[10] Any signal that is a function of time can be decomposed into a sum of contributions of simple sine waves with different frequencies and amplitudes (Fig. 1–12). The signal can be specified either as a series of amplitudes at different time points (referred to as the *time domain*) or as a series of amplitudes of different frequency components (the *frequency domain*). The Fourier transform (FT) is the mathematical procedure for calculating the amplitudes in one domain given the amplitudes in the other domain. Time and frequency are called an FT pair. Figure 1–12 shows how a time domain function can be approximated by adding up the contributions of a limited range of frequencies. With only a few of the low frequencies, the approximation is poor, large ripples are apparent, and small details cannot be seen. As higher frequencies are included, however, the approximation improves and finer detail can be seen.

In a similar way, we can consider the distribution of magnetization along a spatial direction x as the sum of many sine waves with different amplitudes and spatial frequencies (k_x), where k_x is 1/wavelength. Spatial position (x) and spatial frequency (k_x) also form an FT pair. These one-dimensional arguments can be expanded to describe a two-dimensional FT between an image space with coordinates (x,y) and a k-space with coordinates (k_x, k_y), as illustrated in Figure 1–13. Because the measured

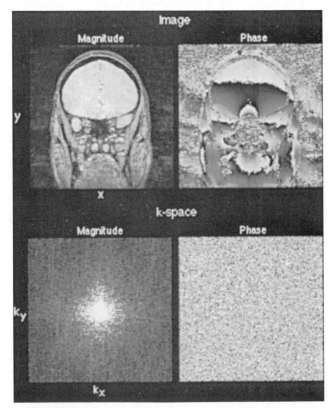

Figure 1–13

Image space and *k*-space. In MR imaging, the image domain consists of a magnitude and a phase at each point. The magnitude is proportional to the amplitude of the local transverse magnetization, and the phase is the precessional phase of the magnetization at the center of data acquisition. The two-dimensional Fourier transform of the image domain is called the *k*-space representation of the image, which consists of a magnitude and a phase for each spatial frequency. In standard MR imaging, one line in *k*-space is measured each time the pulse sequence is repeated, and the image is then calculated by computing the Fourier transform.

local magnetization is a vector quantity it is described by two numbers: a magnitude and a phase. The image space thus consists of a magnitude image and a phase image, with the phase image reflecting the local precessional phase at the center of data collection. In conventional MR imaging, only the magnitude image is displayed, but with some pulse sequences the phase image can contain information on local velocity or field offsets.

Each point in *k*-space represents the amplitude of a particular spatial pattern: the point at k_x, k_y corresponds to a spatial pattern in which intensity varies sinusoidally in the *x* direction with frequency k_x and in the *y* direction with frequency k_y across the entire image plane (Fig. 1–14). Thus, the amplitude of each point in *k*-space affects the intensity in all parts of the image.

Consider now what happens during frequency encoding in MR imaging. When the frequency encoding gradient is on, the frequency of the MR signal generated at x is proportional to *x*, so that as the data are collected the net signal as a function of time is a sum of contributions from many frequencies. The FT of the net signal will give the distribution of amplitudes at different frequencies, and thus at different *x* positions. Therefore, the net signal measured as a function of time can be interpreted directly as the spatial FT of the image. Similarly, the FT of the phase encoded data gives the spatial distribution in *y*. Imaging consists of measuring a matrix of values in *k*-space, and this matrix is then Fourier transformed to produce the reconstructed image. With each phase encoding step a new line is measured in *k*-space. The matrix of measured *k*-space values (e.g., 128 × 256) will produce the same size matrix of image pixel values.

Symmetry of *k*-Space: Partial Fourier Imaging

For an ideal situation in which all of the signals generated in the imaged volume are in phase, *k*-space is symmetric so that only the upper (positive k_y) or lower (negative k_y) halves need to be measured. This is the basis of the partial Fourier techniques, in which only 50 or 75 per cent of the k_y values are measured and the imaging time is correspondingly reduced. Similarly, the partial echo techniques measure only a fraction of the k_x values, and the others are calculated from the assumed symmetry of *k*-space. In practice perfect symmetry usually does not exist. However, by imaging somewhat more than half of the *k*-space plane (e.g., 75 per cent of the k_y lines or 60 per cent of a full echo), corrections can be made for the imperfect symmetry.

Fast Imaging: Fast Spin Echo and Echo Planar Imaging

It often is helpful in understanding novel schemes for faster imaging to examine how these methods sample (or measure) *k*-space. In conventional imaging one line in *k*-space is measured with each repetition of the pulse sequence (each phase encode step moves the sampling to a new *k*-space line). Full measurement of a *k*-space matrix with 128 k_y values then requires 128 TR periods. With the *fast spin echo* technique, several lines in *k*-space are measured in each TR interval by creating multiple echoes with 180 degree pulses and applying a different phase encoding pulse to each echo.[11] For example, if an echo train of eight echoes is used, the required imaging time is reduced by a factor of eight. In *echo planar* imaging the gradients are switched so rapidly that the entire *k*-space is sampled with the signal generated by just one RF pulse, leading to the acquisition of the full image in a few tens of milliseconds.[12] Echo planar imaging requires special hardware.

Image Properties

As described earlier, MR imaging can be viewed as measuring a matrix of values in the *k*-space (Fourier transform) of the image. This matrix usually is adjustable, but changes produce modifications in resolution, field of view, and signal to noise ratio in the reconstructed image.

Resolution

Image resolution is determined by the highest spatial frequencies that are measured and thus depends on how far out in *k*-space sampling is done (Fig. 1–15). The high spatial frequency samples are measured when the gradient effects are at their maximum: either the largest gradient amplitudes used in phase encoding or the last

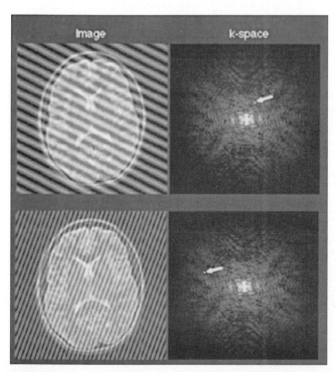

Figure 1–14
The contribution of a single point in *k*-space to the image. Examples illustrating how a single point in *k*-space represents the amplitude of a particular spatial frequency and produces a wave pattern that extends over the entire image. In each example the point marked with an arrow in the *k*-space representation was increased to create the artifactual images.

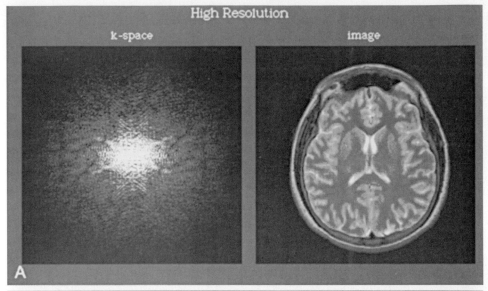

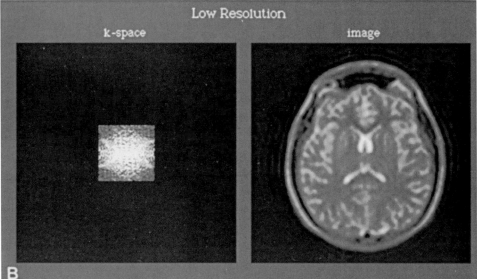

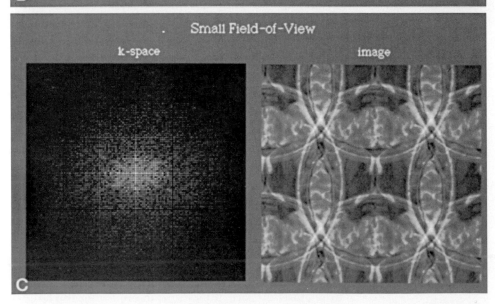

Figure 1–15
Resolution and field of view are determined by which points in *k*-space are measured (or sampled).

A A conventional high resolution image with normal *k*-space sampling.

B Only the central, low spatial frequencies are sampled, decreasing the resolution.

C Only every other point in *k*-space is sampled, decreasing the field of view and causing a wrap-around (or aliasing) artifact.

samples with the longest gradient duration in frequency encoding.

Resolution also can be understood by considering that in order to distinguish two regions that are very close together, there must be some measured data sample in which the signals from the two points have a phase difference of at least 180 degrees. Otherwise the two signals always will add approximately coherently and there will be no detectable difference in their signals. For frequency encoding, the phase difference of the signals from two nearby points is greatest in the last data sample, when the gradient has been on for the longest time. The resolution (Δx) is then the distance between two points such that their phase difference in the last data sample is 180 degrees.

Field of View

The field of view is determined by the spacing of the measurements in *k*-space (Fig. 1–15). Phase considerations also clarify this concept. Consider the data sampling that is done during frequency encoding, in which samples are separated by a short time interval Δt. For the first sample, all of the signals from different regions are in phase. For the second sample (after a delay Δt), however, phase differences will develop. If the phase of the signal at a particular point is compared with the phase at other points, the phase difference will be greater as the distance between the points increases. For a particular distance $L = 1/G_x \Delta t$ the phase difference acquired during Δt is 360 degrees. This point therefore is back in phase with the first point, and for all subsequent samples it will just go through another complete rotation. As a result, these points are indistinguishable in our data; they are never out of phase. The signals from these two points will thus be mapped to the same pixel in the image. This is the *wrap-around* artifact (or *aliasing*), and it appears as if the part of the image that continues beyond an edge were just cut off and pasted onto the other side.

Signal-to-Noise Ratio

In MR imaging, noise enters the data uniformly at all frequencies (usually) and is unrelated to the signal itself. Provided that the RF filter is matched to the data sampling interval Δt, the following equation can be used to gauge the cost of different imaging choices on signal-to-noise ratio (SNR):

$$\mathrm{SNR} \cong V\sqrt{n_s \Delta t}$$

where $V = \Delta z \Delta x \Delta y$ or the voxel volume (the product of the slice thickness and the resolutions in *x* and *y*) and $n_s = n_x n_y n_{avg}$ or the total number of data samples (the product of the number of frequency encoding samples, the number of phase encoding steps, and the number of averages). For volume imaging (discussed later), n_s also includes a factor n_z, the number of phase encoding steps in *z*.

Thus, the reason for the extreme cost of high resolution imaging becomes obvious: cutting each of the voxel dimensions by a factor of two directly decreases the signal-to-noise ratio by a factor of eight due to the factor *V*. To recover the original signal-to-noise ratio, the number of averages (and thus the imaging time) would have to be increased by a factor of 64.

Other changes in the acquisition parameters also affect the signal-to-noise ratio. Increasing the total data collection time ($T = n_x \Delta t$) increases signal-to-noise ratio. This is often done on the second echo of a double spin echo and is described as a *reduced bandwidth* acquisition. Note also that increasing the number of phase encoding steps with the same *y* resolution has the same effect as increasing the number of averages. That is, an image with 128 phase encoding steps and two averages and an image with twice the field of view (256 phase encoding steps) and one average have the same resolution, signal-to-noise ratio, and total imaging time, yet the second actually provides more information and will eliminate wrap-around problems by imaging a larger field of view. Often it is desirable to eliminate wrap-around problems along the frequency encoded axis by oversampling the data within the data collection window. For example, if n_x is doubled and Δt is halved, the field of view in *x* is doubled without changing the total data collection time, the *x* resolution, or the signal-to-noise ratio.

Other Imaging Options

Saturation Pulses

Presaturation is a useful way to suppress the signal of unwanted spins. Presaturation involves applying a selective 90 degree RF pulse followed by a strong gradient pulse before the imaging pulse sequence is started. In this way the chosen spins are tipped over and the signal is spoiled with the gradient pulse. If the imaging sequence is started (e.g., a standard spin echo) there will be very little recovery of magnetization of the presaturated spins so they will not contribute to the image. *Spatial presaturation* (e.g., above and below the desired image field of view) can be used to decrease wrap-around artifacts or prevent flow artifacts by suppressing the inflowing blood signal. *Frequency selective presaturation* can be used to suppress fat, exploiting the chemical shift difference of 3.5 ppm in resonant frequency between fat and water.

Magnetization Transfer

A recent addition to MR imaging is the use of magnetization transfer contrast, which makes use of the fact that in tissues the hydrogen being imaged consists of two exchanging pools: freely mobile water protons and restricted motion macromolecular protons. Although the center resonant frequencies of these two groups are the same, the restricted protons have a much shorter T2 and thus a much broader resonance. Consequently, the magnetization due to the restricted pool can be tipped by a much wider range of frequencies. An RF pulse applied slightly off-resonance thus will saturate the restricted protons but not affect the free protons. However, if the two pools exchange protons rapidly enough, the free protons also become saturated. As a result, additional tissue contrast is observed when imaging the free pool that depends on the rate of exchange between the two pools in different tissues.[13]

PRINCIPLES OF GRADIENT RECALLED ECHO IMAGING

Although spin echo imaging still is the standard for most clinical applications, a number of useful imaging techniques have been developed based on gradient recalled echoes.[14] In gradient recalled echo imaging there is only one RF pulse, and the flip angle may vary from 5 degrees to 90 degrees. The pulse sequence looks like the spin echo pulse sequence except that the 180 degree pulse and associated gradients are removed, and the sign of the *x*-compensation gradient is switched so that the gradient echo still will form. The term "gradient echo imaging" is somewhat unfortunate, because it suggests that this method uses gradient echoes instead of RF echoes. There is no RF echo in gradient recalled echo imaging, but as mentioned earlier, gradient echoes are an integral part of spin echo imaging as well. The difference would be better described in the following manner: spin echo imaging uses both RF and gradient echoes, whereas gradient recalled echo imaging uses only gradient echoes. The primary advantage that comes from eliminating the 180 degree pulse is that TR can be made very short (even less than 10 msec) without causing significant RF heating in the patient.

With imaging times as short as a few seconds, motion artifacts due to respiration can be reduced significantly by collecting the entire image during one breath-hold. Alternatively, three-dimensional volume acquisitions can be collected in a few minutes. Rapid sequential images make it possible to follow the kinetics of administered contrast agents, opening an area of MR imaging studies analogous to nuclear medicine studies.

In addition to the advantages of short imaging times, gradient echo images show a unique sensitivity to the relaxation times T1 and T2, to magnetic field inhomogeneities (T2* effects) and chemical shift effects, and to motion (flow and diffusion). This sensitivity sometimes is merely a source of artifacts, but when exploited in a controlled way it can provide new sources of tissue contrast or methods for rapid quantitative measurements.

Steady-State Free Precession

The bare bones of a gradient recalled echo imaging pulse sequence are simply a series of RF pulses, each with flip angle α, separated by a repetition time TR. If TR/T2, the physics of this situation is similar to that in the conventional spin echo pulse sequence, except that the 180 degree refocusing pulse has been removed: the signal is composed only of transverse magnetization generated by the most recent RF pulse. However, for fast imaging, the TR usually is shorter than T2, which

introduces a new feature. Each pulse still produces new transverse magnetization, but the transverse magnetization from previous RF pulses will not have decayed away completely. Different components of this previous transverse magnetization will have acquired different phases due to local field offsets (e.g., applied gradients, main field inhomogeneity) so that this old transverse magnetization may be incoherent. If these field offsets are the same during each TR period, however, the RF pulses will create echoes of the previous transverse magnetization at multiples of TR (Fig. 1–16). (Although 180 degree pulses produce the strongest echoes, smaller RF pulses also create echoes.) These echoes will add to the new transverse magnetization from the most recent RF pulse, creating a strong coherent signal immediately after each pulse. Also, the echoes combine to create a coherent signal just before each RF pulse.

After a number of pulses the magnetization will approach a steady state in which the signal pattern is repeated in the same way during each TR period. In this condition of *steady-state free precession*, the coherent signals after the RF pulse (M^+) and before the RF pulse (M^-) are both constant. For long TR the echoes are severely attenuated by T2 decay and M^- is not detectable, but as TR is shortened, the M^- signal becomes appreciable.

Basic Types of Fast Imaging

Several sources of signal exist that can be imaged: the most recent transverse magnetization and echoes of previous transverse magnetization. The three basic types of fast imaging pulse sequence (spoiled, steady state M^+, steady state M^-) differ in how they use or do not use these potential signals (Fig. 1–17).

Spoiled (FLASH, *Spoiled* GRASS)

Random gradient pulses are added after data collection to spoil the echoes, so the signal is produced solely by the transverse magnetization created by the most recent RF pulse. In its current standard form, FLASH is a spoiled technique, because an additional variable gradient in *z* (the slice selection axis) is added to the pulse sequence after data collection to act as a spoiler. The phase encoding gradient, which changes with each pulse, would serve to spoil the transverse magnetization over most of the image. However, because the phase encoding gradient produces only slight phase changes near the center of the image, an additional variable gradient in *z* must be added to the pulse sequence to provide spoiling over the entire image and avoid an artifactual brightening in the center where the echoes are not spoiled. To maintain uniform spoiling across the image, each phase encoding pulse is balanced by an equal but opposite pulse after data collection (a *rewinder* pulse). As an alternative to gradient spoiling, some systems use RF spoiling by varying the flip axis with each RF pulse. The magnetization then begins each TR period with a different phase angle and so ends each period with a different phase, preventing the formation

TR>T2

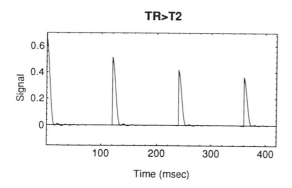

TR<T2

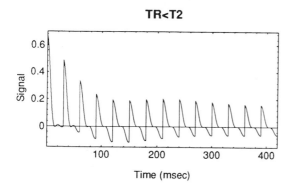

SSFP

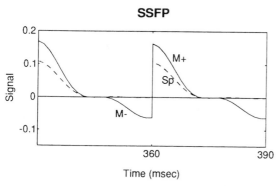

Figure 1–16
Steady-state free precession (SSFP). The development of the SSFP signal is illustrated for a series of 45 degree RF pulses applied to a sample with T2 = 60 msec for TR = 120 msec (top panel) and TR = 30 msec (middle panel). With TR > T2, each RF pulse generates a new signal, and after a number of pulses a steady-state is reached in which the signal produced after each pulse is the same. With TR < T2, each RF pulse still creates new transverse magnetization but also produces echoes of previously created transverse magnetization. The negative amplitude of the echoes means that the echo forms on the opposite axis from the initial free induction decay (e.g., if the free induction decay is on the +y axis, the echo will be on the −y axis). After a number of pulses the system approaches a steady state (bottom panel) in which a coherent signal forms both before (M⁻) and after (M⁺) each RF pulse. M⁻ consists solely of echoes, whereas M⁺ consists of echoes plus the most recent free induction decay. If the echoes are spoiled (*Sp*; dashed curve) the signal consists only of the most recent free induction decay. Fast gradient recalled echo imaging pulse sequences differ by whether the signal being imaged is the new transverse magnetization *(Sp)*, the echoes (M⁻), or both (M⁺).

of echoes. The spoiled pulse sequence will be referred to as FLASH in the sections following.

Steady-State M⁺ (GRASS, FISP, FAST)

The phase encoding gradient is balanced to prevent partial spoiling, and the coherent signal after the RF

pulse is used for imaging. This signal consists of the transverse magnetization from the most recent RF pulse plus echoes of the transverse magnetization from previous pulses. GRASS, FAST, and FISP are examples of steady-state techniques that image the M⁺ signal, and in the following sections M⁺ imaging is referred to as GRASS. When TR >> T2, the FLASH and GRASS methods produce similar images because the echoes are weak, but when TR < T2 the dependence of the signal on the tissue relaxation times is substantially different.

Steady-State M⁻ (SSFP, CE-FAST, PSIF)

The coherent signal before the RF pulse is used for imaging. The pulse sequence is structured like the

Spoiled: [FLASH, SPGR]

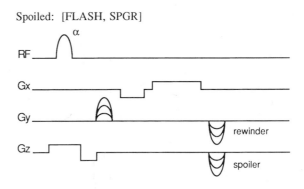

Steady-State (M⁺): [FISP, GRASS, FAST]

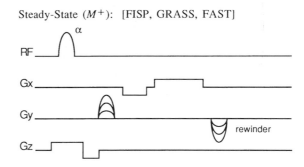

Steady-State (M⁻): [CE-FAST, PSIF, SSFP]

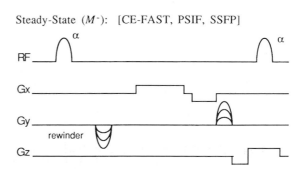

Figure 1–17
Gradient recalled echo fast imaging pulse sequences. In a spoiled sequence the echoes are spoiled and only the free induction decay from the most recent RF pulse is imaged. In a steady-state sequence designed to image the magnetization after the RF pulse (M⁺), the signal consists of both the most recent free induction decay and echoes of past free induction decays. In a steady-state sequence designed to image the magnetization before the RF pulse (M⁻) the signal consists of only the echoes from previous free induction decays (the most recent free induction decay will not contribute to the signal until after the next RF pulse forms an echo).

GRASS pulse sequence, except that it must run backward in time to image the signal before the RF pulse rather than the signal after the RF pulse. The unbalanced portion of the slice selection gradient pulse immediately after the RF pulse dephases the most recently generated transverse magnetization, so that the coherent signal before the RF pulse consists solely of the echoes of transverse magnetization from previous RF pulses. SSFP, CE-FAST, and PSIF are examples of pulse sequences that image the M^- signal, and in the following sections M^- imaging is referred to as SSFP.

Gradient Recalled Echo Imaging Signal and Contrast

Dependence on Flip Angle

In conventional spin echo imaging, the pulse sequence parameters TR and TE are adjusted to control the signal intensity and, more importantly, the contrast in the image. In gradient recalled echo imaging, the TR is kept short (typically less than 30 msec) to minimize the imaging time and is not used for altering contrast. Fortunately, with gradient echo pulse sequences an additional parameter, the flip angle (α),[14, 15] has a strong effect on the signal and contrast (Fig. 1–18).

Comparing first the two most commonly used methods, the FLASH and GRASS signals show some characteristic patterns. These two curves cross at the peak

Fast Imaging Signal Intensity

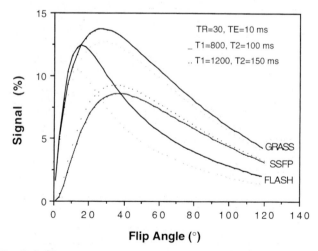

Figure 1–18
Fast gradient recalled echo imaging signal and contrast. The curves of signal versus flip angle were calculated for TR = 30 msec for the three types of gradient echo pulse sequence (FLASH, GRASS, SSFP). The signal is presented as a fraction of the fully relaxed magnetization. For each method, two curves are shown, one for a tissue with T1 = 800 msec and T2 = 100 msec, and one for T1 = 1200 msec and T2 = 150 msec, each with the same proton density. The GRASS and FLASH curves cross at the Ernst angle (α_E). Below α_E there is little sensitivity to T1, and the images are proton density weighted. Above α_E the images are more T1 weighted. Although the signal is greater with GRASS than FLASH, contrast (the difference between the two curves) is better with FLASH. With SSFP contrast is reversed and thus is more T2 weighted.

FLASH signal. This angle is called the *Ernst angle* (α_E), and is given by

$$\cos \alpha_E = e^{-TR/T1}$$

For flip angles below the Ernst angle, the FLASH and GRASS signals are nearly identical and are primarily proton density weighted. The reason the relaxation times do not affect the signal is that with small flip angles the longitudinal magnetization is disturbed only slightly, so recovery by T1 relaxation is relatively unimportant, and the echoes are weak. With larger flip angles, the GRASS signal can be substantially stronger, peaking at a larger flip angle than the FLASH signal. In this regimen, the echoes of previous pulses make more of a contribution to the GRASS signal.

The contrast is qualitatively similar but better (at least in the example in Fig. 1–18) with the FLASH signal, because for equal proton densities, contrast with FLASH is due entirely to T1 differences. T2 does not affect the steady state, because the echoes are spoiled, so the only T2 effect is in the decay between the RF pulse and the read-out period, and TE is assumed to be small. However, with the GRASS signal, echoes make an important contribution. A longer T2 leads to stronger echoes and a stronger signal, but a longer T1 leads to less recovery between RF pulses and a weaker signal. The normal positive correlation between these two relaxation times in vivo thus leads to conflicting contrast effects similar to those encountered in spin echo imaging. Therefore, although the signal with GRASS can be substantially larger than with the FLASH pulse sequence, the contrast is likely to be better with FLASH.

The SSFP signal is composed entirely of echoes from previous RF pulses (the new transverse magnetization produced by an RF pulse will not contribute to the signal until after the next RF pulse). This signal also suffers from the same conflict between T1 and T2 contrast, but the T2 weighting is much stronger than with the GRASS signal. As a result, the signal increases with increasing T1 and T2, so that the contrast pattern is more like traditional T2-weighted contrast than like T1-weighted contrast. However, the magnitude of the contrast still is much less than with the FLASH pulse sequence. Nevertheless, these curves were calculated for equal spin densities, and in practice, proton density often is correlated with T1 and T2 (higher proton density usually leads to longer relaxation times). This would tend to increase the contrast with SSFP, but decrease the contrast with GRASS and FLASH.

T2* Effects

In addition to the relaxation time effects, gradient echo imaging is more sensitive to variation in the local magnetic field. Because there is no 180 degree refocusing pulse, as there is in SE imaging, any phase changes due to differences in the resonant frequency within a voxel will not be refocused during data collection. Such differences could be attributable to inhomogeneity of the main magnetic field, but even in a perfect magnet the inhomogeneity of the human body will produce field variations owing to *magnetic susceptibility* differences. Magnetic susceptibility is a measure of the degree to which a material becomes magnetized when placed in a magnetic field. The total field inside the material is due primarily to B_0, but a small contribution comes from the magnetized material itself. For this reason, field gradients can occur at the boundaries of dissimilar tissues (e.g., bone and soft tissue).

A spread of resonant frequencies within a voxel will lead to a spread of phase angles and a resulting loss in signal. This more rapid decay often is described by a transverse decay constant T2*, which is less than T2. This terminology is convenient for characterizing these effects qualitatively, but caution should be used when interpreting T2* quantitatively. This form of the decay may not be a simple exponential, as T2 decay usually is. Also, the transverse decay rate that governs the steady-state signal discussed in the previous section is set by T2, not T2*, because the echoing processes discussed earlier refocus the effects of local field variations. T2* is operational because the signal is measured not when the echoes occur (at the time of the RF pulses) but rather at a time (TE) from the echo. In a gradient recalled echo pulse sequence, TE is the time interval between the RF pulse and the gradient echo formed by the read-out gradient pulses. To minimize T2* signal loss, TE usually is kept short. With partial echo techniques the TE can be reduced to just a few milliseconds by shifting the gradient echo toward the beginning of the data collection window.

Chemical Shift Effect

Gradient recalled echo imaging also exhibits a chemical shift effect because there is no 180 degree RF pulse to refocus phase differences due to the intrinsic difference in the resonant frequencies of water and fat. If a voxel contains both fat and water, the net signal will show oscillations in intensity as TE is changed and the fat and water come in and out of phase (Fig. 1–19). Each species will evolve at its natural resonant frequency for a time TE, so the phase difference between the two signals is $\Delta\varphi = \Delta\omega TE$, with $\Delta\omega$ being the angular frequency difference between fat and water. The chemical shift difference of fat and water is about 3.5 ppm, and the absolute frequency difference will be proportional to the field strength. For 0.5 T, the oscillation period in the signal versus TE curve is about 13.2 msec and at 1.5 T it is about 4.4 msec. In some situations, these effects will be the dominant source of image contrast, and the signal from a normal tissue with a mixture of fat and water (e.g., bone marrow) can be suppressed by choosing TE to be a time when fat and water are out of phase.

Magnetization Preparation

In recent years a new feature has been added to the more conventional gradient recalled echo fast imaging pulse sequences. In the pulse sequences described earlier the magnetization is assumed to start at equilibrium and RF pulses were assumed to be applied for a sufficiently long time that a steady state is produced. (All of

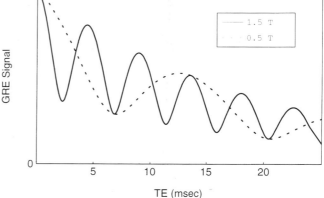

GRE Chemical Shift Effect

Figure 1–19
Chemical shift effect in gradient echo imaging. Signal decay curves for an imaging voxel that contains 30 per cent fat and 70 per cent water are shown for magnetic field strengths of 0.5 and 1.5 T. Because there is no 180 degree refocusing pulse, fat and water come in and out of phase as they precess at different frequencies for a time TE. Because the frequency difference is 3.5 ppm of the resonant frequency, the absolute difference is three times larger at the higher field.

the earlier contrast calculations were based on the steady-state assumption.) However, another possibility is to quickly image magnetization that is not in a steady state and thereby produce different contrast in the image. This is done by applying a preparation pulse (e.g., a 180 degree pulse to produce contrast like an inversion recovery sequence) before beginning a series of low flip angle, very short TR (e.g., less than 10 msec) RF pulses for imaging. This process can be broken down further with a segmented *k*-space method by collecting only one half or one quarter of the data needed for an image and then giving another preparation pulse before continuing with the data collection.[16] With schemes like this the order in which the different phase encode steps are collected can affect the resulting image contrast.

Three-Dimensional Volume Imaging

For clinical purposes it is almost always necessary to acquire images of an entire volume of tissue. Usually this is done by interleaving the pulse sequences, taking advantage of the fact that a substantial dead time exists after the pulse sequence has played out (which requires a little longer than TE) and when the pulse sequence is repeated on that slice (TR). In that dead time, the pulse sequence is started on another slice, and then another until the time TR has elapsed. Although a whole series of slices is acquired simultaneously, the pulse sequence still is essentially a single slice acquisition. An alternative method is true volume acquisition. With volume imaging no slice selection is done (or else a thick slab is excited) and the volume is divided into slices by phase-encoding along the *z*-axis as well as the *y*-axis (Fig. 1–20). The disadvantage of this approach is that many

Volume Imaging

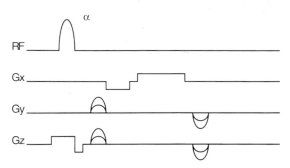

Figure 1–20
Volume imaging pulse sequence. The slice selective pulse excites a thick slab, and phase encoding is used on both the *y* and *z* axes. For each phase encode step in *y* all of the *z* phase encoding steps must be measured.

repetitions are required; for each *z*-phase encode step a full set of *y*-phase encode steps must be measured. For 64 steps in *z* and 128 steps in *y*, 8192 TR periods are required. For standard TR times used in spin echo imaging (200 to 4000 msec) the total imaging time is much too long. However, with gradient recalled echo imaging, TR can be reduced to less than 10 msec, allowing volume acquisitions in just a few minutes.

Volume imaging has two important advantages over conventional two-dimensional imaging. First, the signal-to-noise ratio is improved substantially because signal is measured from each voxel on every pulse. With a conventional multislice interleaved acquisition, only a fraction of the total number of RF pulses hit a particular slice. Second, thinner sections can be achieved. With a multislice interleaved acquisition the slice thickness is determined by the slice selective RF pulse and is limited to 2 to 3 mm with conventional gradient strengths. With volume imaging, however, the sections in *z* are determined by phase encoding, and the phase encoding pulse can be lengthened as needed to produce sections thinner than 1 mm. Signal-to-noise ratio is severely reduced because of the small voxel volumes, but the intrinsic high signal-to-noise ratio of the volume acquisition allows high resolution imaging with reasonable signal-to-noise ratio with an imaging time of 5 to 10 min.

Flow Effects and MR Angiography

Gradient recalled echo imaging pulse sequences are the basis for most of the MR angiography techniques.[17–19] Two concepts are important for understanding flow effects in fast imaging: *signal saturation*, which produces bright vessels and dark tissue; and *flow compensation*, which corrects for artifacts and phase dispersion due to flow.

Signal Saturation

With moderately large flip angles and short TR times, the steady-state signal generated is reduced substantially compared to the fully relaxed, long TR signal. To reach

this saturated state, however, may require a series of RF pulses over a period longer than T1, and with short TR this could be many pulses. With slice selective imaging, any spins that enter the imaged plane by flow will be relatively unsaturated because they have not felt as many previous pulses as the surrounding stationary tissue. The blood signal, particularly in fast flowing vessels with rapid replacement, thus can be substantially stronger than the signal from the stationary tissue. Furthermore, no flow void artifact is present as in conventional spin echo imaging. In spin echo imaging, with 90 degree and 180 degree pulses, any spins that move out of the selected slice during the interval between the two RF pulses will not contribute to the signal. With gradient echo imaging there is only one pulse, so even if spins subsequently move out of the selected slice they still will contribute to the signal. The large image contrast that can be produced between unsaturated blood and saturated stationary tissues is the basis of the time of flight MR angiography techniques.

Phase Effects Due to Flow

To make use of the potential increased signal from flowing blood, the phase dispersion effects caused by flow through pulsed gradient fields must be corrected. Consider a pair of gradient pulses such as the compensation gradient and the read-out gradient used in frequency encoding (Fig. 1–21). The initial compensating pulse is designed to balance exactly the first half of the read-out gradient, so that at the center of data collection all spins are back in phase. That is, the phase acquired by a spin during the first pulse will be exactly opposite to the phase acquired during the first half of the read-out gradient. However, if a spin moves a distance Δx in the time between the two pulses, the phases will not balance, leaving a net phase offset at the center of data collection of $\Delta\varphi = G\tau Tv$, where G is the gradient strength (Hz/cm), τ is the gradient duration, T is the

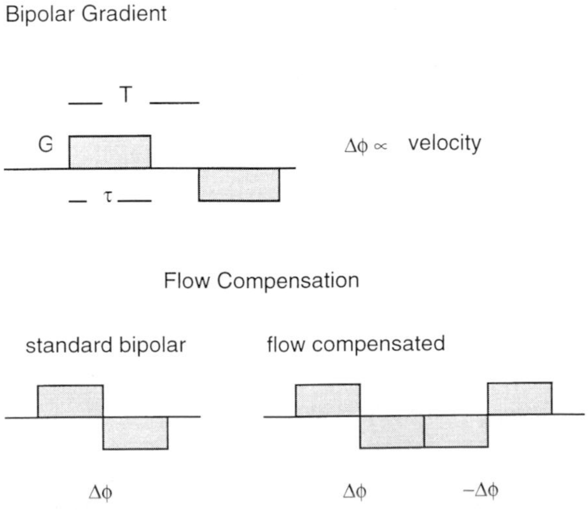

Bipolar Gradient

$$\Delta\phi \propto \text{velocity}$$

Flow Compensation

standard bipolar   flow compensated

$\Delta\phi$ $\Delta\phi$ $-\Delta\phi$

Figure 1–21
Phase changes due to flow. A bipolar pair of gradient pulses produces no net phase for stationary spins, but moving spins acquire a phase proportional to velocity. Flow-compensated gradient waveforms eliminate the phase change of spins moving with a constant velocity.

time between the start of the compensating gradient pulse and the start of the readout gradient, and v is the velocity. This is just the phase difference resulting from the gradient pulse for two spins separated by a distance $\Delta x = vT$ (the distance moved in time T).

This effect is the basis for using a bipolar gradient pulse to encode velocity information in the phase of the signal and is used in the *phase contrast* MR angiography techniques. However, this same effect due to motion during application of the imaging gradients can lead to signal loss and artifacts. If a voxel in the blood vessel contains spins with a range of velocities, as it would in normal laminar or turbulent flow, the signals generated by these spins will have a range of phases, thus reducing the net signal. With pulsatile flow, these phase offsets will vary with each RF pulse, leading to motion artifacts along the phase encoding axis.

Flow Compensation

Phase errors due to flow can be corrected in two ways. First, by minimizing the time T between the compensation gradient and the readout gradient, these effects can be reduced. If the amplitude of the compensation gradient is then reduced, the gradient echo will occur nearer to the leading edge of the readout gradient, further reducing T and thus $\Delta\varphi$. With such a *partial echo acquisition*, it often is possible to reduce the phase errors to an acceptable level, although reconstruction of images from these more limited data may require some additional processing.

The second solution to the problem is to add additional gradients to the pulse sequence that will compensate for constant velocity phase errors. *Flow compensated gradients* effectively have two pairs of gradient pulses. A moving spin acquires a phase $+\Delta\varphi$ from the first pair and a phase $-\Delta\varphi$ from the second pair. As long as the velocity is constant there will be no net phase at the peak of the gradient echo. Further gradients can be added to compensate for acceleration (and higher derivatives), but in practice velocity compensation usually is sufficient.

By combining the effects of saturation of the signal from stationary tissue with flow compensation to preserve the large, unsaturated blood signal, fast imaging can produce angiograms of acceptable quality with high contrast.

ARTIFACTS

Many image artifacts can arise when an MR imager is not working properly or is not shielded adequately from outside RF interference. A number of artifacts also can occur with a perfectly functioning MR imaging system whenever one of the two basic implicit assumptions of MR imaging is violated. These assumptions are (1) when no field gradients are turned on, all spins have the same resonant frequency, and (2) each time the pulse sequence is repeated the same local signal is generated.

The first assumption is reflected in the way gradient fields are used for spatial localization, so that both the location of a selected slice and the position along the frequency encoded axis are determined by the precession frequency. Any intrinsic variation in the resonant frequency will lead to spatial distortions. A common example is the chemical shift artifact, in which the fat appears displaced from the water image along the frequency encoded axis because of the intrinsic 3.5 ppm difference in resonant frequency. This shift typically is one or two pixels in the image and can lead to characteristic artifacts at water-fat tissue boundaries: a dark edge where fat has been shifted out of the pixel or a bright edge where fat is shifted onto the adjacent water signal.

Intrinsic differences in precession frequency also arise when the magnetic field is not uniform. This could be due to intrinsic inhomogeneity of the magnet, but current systems usually are quite homogeneous. Instead, magnetic field variations usually are due to the nonuniformity of the human body and the resulting variation in magnetic susceptibility. Metallic implants, some cosmetics, and even tattoos can produce field variations and noticeable distortions of the image.[20] The basic susceptibility differences between air, water, and bone also can produce field nonuniformity at tissue interfaces, leading to subtle image distortions. In effect, the combination of the imaging gradients with intrinsic field variations alters the shape and location of the resolved voxels. For example, an intrinsic local field gradient that adds to the slice selection gradient will shift the position and decrease the thickness of the selected slice locally.

Spatial variations in the resonant frequency will lead to distortions along both the frequency encoded axis and the slice selection axis (e.g., the excited fat and the excited water actually lie in two planes, which are slightly displaced from one another in both x and z). Phase encoding, however, is not affected by chemical shift or magnetic field variations. With phase encoding, the y-position of a local signal is encoded by the phase change from one repeat of the pulse sequence to the next, whereas with frequency encoding the x-position is determined by the phase change from one time sample to the next (i.e., by the frequency).

The second basic assumption of MR imaging is violated whenever the local MR signal changes during data acquisition. Patient motion (twisting, swallowing, and so forth), respiratory and cardiac motion, flowing blood, and cerebrospinal fluid pulsations all lead to a time-varying signal and artifacts in the image. Such motions have only a small effect on frequency encoding, because the data sampling occurs in a very short time (typically about 8 msec). However, the interval between phase encoding samples is much longer (TR), allowing time for substantial motion. Because one line in k-space is acquired with each phase encoding step, motion leads to an inconsistent set of data lines in k-space. Because each point in k-space corresponds to a simple wave pattern over the entire image plane, the image artifacts often are periodic and appear as ghosts shifted along the y-axis. It is important to remember that the spatial extent of the ghosts can be much larger than the spatial extent of the actual motion. For example, cardiac motion is limited to the vicinity of the heart, but the artifacts will propagate over the full width of the image.

SUMMARY

In this chapter the physical principles of MR imaging are reviewed. Nuclei that possess an intrinsic magnetic moment (such as hydrogen) exhibit the phenomenon of nuclear magnetic resonance (NMR). When placed in a strong magnetic field, the nuclear magnetic moments tend to align with the field, creating a local equilibrium magnetization. A second, much weaker magnetic field oscillating at the resonant frequency (the RF pulse) causes the magnetization to tip away from the main field direction and begin to precess. The precessing magnetization generates a signal in a nearby detector coil. Over time the magnetization relaxes back to equilibrium, and another RF pulse can be applied to generate another signal. The relaxation toward equilibrium is described by two time parameters: T1 is the time constant for relaxation of the longitudinal component of the magnetization, and T2 is the time constant for the transverse component.

MR imaging is based on the fact that the resonant frequency (or precession frequency) is directly proportional to the magnitude of the magnetic field. Gradient coils are used to alter the magnetic field in a controlled way so that the precession frequency varies in a linear fashion along a chosen spatial axis. The techniques of slice selection, frequency encoding, and phase encoding employ gradient pulses to encode the spatial location of the signal in the acquired NMR data. An image of the local magnetization is reconstructed from the data by a mathematical operation called the Fourier transform.

The image intensity is determined both by intrinsic properties of the tissue (e.g., proton density, relaxation times, and flow) and by the timing and amplitudes of the applied RF and gradient pulses (referred to as the pulse sequence). MR imaging is a highly flexible technique, and many pulse sequences are used to create images that differ substantially in signal-to-noise ratio, acquisition time, spatial resolution, and tissue contrast. Typical pulse sequences include spin echo, inversion recovery, and gradient recalled echo. In addition to providing high resolution anatomic images, MR imaging also is used for angiographic studies and quantitative flow measurements.

REFERENCES

1. Purcell EM, Torrey HC, Pound RV: Resonance absorption by nuclear magnetic moments in a solid. Phys Rev *69*:37, 1946.
2. Bloch F, Hansen WW, Packard M: Nuclear induction. Phys Rev *69*:127, 1946.
3. Abragam A: The Principles of Nuclear Magnetism. Oxford, Clarendon Press, 1961.
4. Lauterbur PC: Image formation by induced local interaction: Examples employing nuclear magnetic resonance. Nature *242*:190, 1973.
5. Bottomley PA, Foster TH, Argersinger RE, et al: A review of normal tissue hydrogen NMR relaxation times and relaxation mechanisms from 1–100 MHz: Dependence on tissue type, NMR frequency, temperature, species, excision and age. Med Phys *11*:425, 1984.
6. Farrar TC, Becker ED: Pulse and Fourier Transform NMR: Introduction to Theory and Methods. New York, Academic Press, 1971.
7. Hahn EL: Spin echoes. Phys Rev *80*:580, 1950.
8. Wehrli FW, MacFall JR, Glover GH, et al: The dependence of nuclear magnetic resonance (NMR) image contrast on intrinsic and pulse sequence timing parameters. Magn Reson Imaging *2*:3, 1984.
9. Hendrick RE, Nelson TR, Hendee WR: Optimizing tissue contrast in magnetic resonance imaging. Magn Reson Imaging *2*:193, 1984.
10. Bracewell RN: The Fourier Transform and Its Applications. New York, McGraw-Hill, 1986.
11. Listerud J, Einstein S, Outwater E, et al: First principles of fast spin echo. Magn Reson Q *8*:199, 1992.
12. Cohen MS, Weisskoff RM: Ultra-fast imaging. Magn Reson Imaging *9*:1, 1991.
13. Balaban RS, Ceckler TL: Magnetization transfer contrast in magnetic resonance imaging. Magn Reson Q *8*:116, 1992.
14. Wehrli FW: Fast scan magnetic resonance. Magn Reson Q *6*:165, 1990.
15. Buxton RB, Edelman RR, Rosen BR, et al: Contrast in rapid MR imaging: T1-weighted and T2-weighted imaging. J Comput Assist Tomogr *11*:7, 1987.
16. Chien D, Edelman RR: Ultrafast imaging using gradient echoes. Magn Reson Q *7*:31, 1991.
17. Finn JP, Goldmann A, Edelman RR: Magnetic resonance in the body. Magn Reson Q *8*:1, 1992.
18. Pelc NJ, Herfkens RJ, Shimakawa A, et al: Phase contrast cine magnetic resonance imaging. Magn Reson Q *7*:229, 1991.
19. Listerud J: First principles of magnetic resonance angiography. Magn Reson Q *7*:136, 1991.
20. Hendrick RE, Russ PD, Simon JH: MRI: Principles and Artifacts. New York, Raven Press, 1993.

Magnetic Resonance Imaging: Typical Protocols

Shoulder
Elbow
Wrist
Hip
Knee
Ankle and Foot
Summary

The previous chapter has described considerations, mainly technical, that are fundamental to proper assessment of the musculoskeletal system using MR imaging. It also serves to underscore the complexity of an imaging method that requires the examiner to choose a number of parameters that influence dramatically the manner in which any disease process is displayed and, for that matter, whether or not the process is detected at all. Indeed, in comparison with other imaging methods, both routine and advanced, the variety of options related to MR imaging is impressive. Considerations include, among others, the strength of the magnet itself, the position of the patient, the precise orientation of the anatomic site to be examined, the need to include one or both sides of the body, the type of imaging coil to be employed, the imaging plane or planes required, the need to employ a contrast agent and, if so, whether to deliver it to the body intravenously or with an intra-articular injection (i.e., MR arthrography), the field of view, the number of signal acquisitions or excitations, the imaging matrix, and the specific imaging sequence or sequences (each with its own parameters) that are optimal to evaluate any particular clinical problem. It is the last of these considerations, that related to the choice of a specific imaging sequence (or technique), that is most complicated, owing in part to the wide variety of such sequences and to nomenclature that often is unique to a specific manufacturer or magnet (Tables 2–1 and 2–2). Indeed, the choice of a specific imaging sequence (or sequences) often varies from one institution to another

Table 2–1. ACRONYMS USED IN GRADIENT ECHO (GRE) IMAGING

Acronym	Explanation and Manufacturer	Acronym	Explanation and Manufacturer
CE-FAST	Contrast-enhanced FAST (Picker)	GRE	Gradient echo, gradient-recalled echo
CE-FFE-T1	Contrast-enhanced fast field echo with T1 weighting (Philips)	GRECHO	Gradient recalled echo (Resonex)
		MPGR	Multiplanar GRASS (GE Medical Systems)
CE-FFE-T2	Contrast-enhanced fast field echo with T2 weighting (Philips)	MP-RAGE	Magnetization-prepared rapid GRE (Siemens)
E-SHORT	SS-GRE with SE sampling (Elscint)	PFI	Partial flip angle (Toshiba)
FAST	Fourier-acquired steady state (Picker)	PS	Partial saturation (Instrumentarium)
FE	Field echo (Otsuka, Picker, Philips, Toshiba)	PSIF	Reversed FISP (Siemens)
FEDIF	Field echo with echo time (TE) set for water/fat signals in opposition (Picker)	RAM-FAST	Rapidly acquired magnetization-prepared FAST (Picker)
FEER	Field even echo by reversal (Picker)	RF-FAST	RF-spoiled FAST (Picker)
FESUM	Field echo with TE set for water and fat signals in phase (Picker)	RS	Rapid scan (Hitachi)
		SHORT	Any fast GRE sequence (Elscint)
		SMASH	Short minimum angle shot (Shimadzu)
FFE	Fast field echo (Philips)	SPGR	Spoiled GRASS (GE Medical Systems)
FGR	Fast GRASS (GE Medical Systems)	SSFP	Steady-state free precession (GE Medical Systems, Shimadzu, Toshiba)
FISP	Fast imaging with steady-state precision (Siemens)		
FLASH	Fast low-angle shot (Siemens)	STAGE	Small tip angle GRE (Shimadzu)
FRE	Field reversal echo (Picker)	STERF	Steady-state technique with refocused FID (Shimadzu)
FS	Fast scan (GE Medical Systems)		
F-SHORT	SS-GRE with FID sampling (Elscint)	T1-FAST	FAST with T1 contrast (gradient-spoiled) (Picker)
FSPGR	Fast spoiled GRASS (GE Medical Systems)		
GFE	Gradient field echo (Hitachi)	TFE	Turbo field echo (Philips)
GFEC	Gradient field echo compensation (Hitachi)	Turbo-FE	Turbo field echo (Philips)
GRASS	Gradient recalled acquisition in the steady state (GE Medical Systems)	TurboFLASH	Turbo version of FLASH (Siemens)
		Turbo-SHORT	Turbo version of SHORT (Elscint)

Reproduced with permission from Elster AD: Radiology *186*:1, 1993.

and, at some institutions, from one day to another. In any individual patient, the choice of an imaging protocol often is influenced further by the clinical information that is supplied and the results of a review of other available imaging studies. Although not always possible in a busy radiology department, in ideal circumstances the examination also is modified according to observations made as the initial MR images are monitored.

This chapter summarizes imaging protocols used by a number of institutions for the evaluation of common problems related to six anatomic regions: shoulder, elbow, wrist, hip, knee, and ankle and foot. These protocols are supplied by experts in the field (Table 2–3) who are cognizant both of the clinical questions that require answers and of the importance of cost containment. The protocols are presented as guidelines and as a supplement to the information provided in Chapters 12 to 17 of this text. Although the data are current in terms of MR imaging in 1996, modifications of these protocols undoubtedly will occur in the years ahead as the technical aspects of MR imaging continue to evolve, presumably in a rapid fashion.

Table 2–2. SUMMARY OF FAST MR TERMS

Terminology	Abbreviation	Explanation	Example of Manufacturer	Characteristic Feature
General	EPI	Echoplanar imaging		
	ETL	Echo train length		
	FOV	Field of view		
	GRE	Gradient-recalled echo		
	IR	Inversion recovery		
	MR	Magnetic resonance		
	NEX	Number of excitations		
	NSA	Number of signals averaged		
	SE	Spin echo		
	SNR	Signal-to-noise ratio		
	TE	Echo time		
	TI	Inversion time		
	TR	Repetition time		
T1-weighted sequence	FLASH	Fast low-angle shot	Siemens, Bruker	GRE sequence with spoiling gradient
	FFE	Fast field echo	Philips	GRE sequence with spoiling gradient
	PSR	Partial saturation recovery	Picker	GRE sequence with spoiling gradient
	FE	Field echo	Elscint	GRE sequence with spoiling gradient
	MP-RAGE	Magnetization-prepared rapid gradient echo		180 degree IR pulse plus GRE sequence with spoiling gradient
	SPGR	Spoiled gradient-recalled imaging	General Electric	GRE sequence with spoiling gradient
T2-weighted sequence	SSFP	Steady-state free precession	Siemens	GRE sequence with TE>TR
	PSIF	Reversed fast imaging with steady-state precession, collection of the refocused echo	Siemens	GRE sequence with TE>TR
	CE-FAST	Contrast-enhanced Fourier-acquired steady-state technique	Picker	GRE sequence with TE>TR
	FSE	Fast spin echo		More than one echo per excitation with multiple 180 degree pulses
	FAIST	Fast-acquisition interleaved spin echo		More than one echo per excitation with multiple 180 degree pulses
	GRASE	Gradient and spin echo		Multiple 180 degree pulses and gradient recalled echoes
	GREASE	Gradient echo and spin echo		GRE with multiple 180 degree pulses
	RARE	Rapid acquisition with relaxation enhancement		More than one phase-encoding step per excitation
	RASE	Rapid acquisition spin echo	Siemens	Half Fourier imaging
	TGSE	Turbo gradient spin echo, identical to GRASE	Siemens	GRE with multiple 180 degree pulses
	turboFLASH	Turbo fast low-angle shot	Siemens, Bruker	180 degree inversion recovery pulse plus GRE sequence

Table 2–2. SUMMARY OF FAST MR TERMS (*Continued*)

Terminology	Abbreviation	Explanation	Example of Manufacturer	Characteristic Feature
	turboSE	Turbo spin echo, identical to FSE	Siemens	More than one echo per excitation with multiple 180 degree pulses
T1 + T2* weighted sequence and variable weighting	GRASS	Gradient-recalled acquisition in the steady state	General Electric	GRE without spoiling gradient
	FISP	Fast imaging with steady-state precession	Siemens	GRE without spoiling gradient
	FAST	Fourier-acquired steady-state technique	Picker	GRE without spoiling gradient
Echoplanar sequence	ABEST	Asymmetric blipped echoplanar single-pulse technique		One 90 degree pulse, rectangular scanning of K-space
	BEST	Blipped echoplanar single-pulse technique		One 90 degree pulse, rectangular scanning of K-space
	EPISTAR	Echoplanar imaging with signal targeting and alternating radiofrequency		One 90 degree pulse, rectangular scanning of K-space
	Instascan	Brand name for EPI sequence	Advanced NMR Systems	One 90 degree pulse, rectangular scanning of K-space
	MBEST	Modulus-blipped echoplanar single-pulse technique		One 90 degree pulse, rectangular scanning of K-space
	mesh	Interleaved K-space scan		Meshed scanning of K-space
Motion suppression technique	COPE	Cardiac-ordered phase encoding		Phase-encoding steps triggered by ECG
	FAT SAT	Fat saturation pulse		Presaturation pulse suppresses signal from fat
	FRODO	Flow and respiratory artifact obliteration with directed orthogonal pulses		Presaturation pulse suppresses signal from vessels and from tissue outside the area of interest
	MAST	Motion artifact suppression technique		
	ROPE	Respiratory-ordered phase encoding		Phase-encoding steps triggered by respiration
	STIR	Short inversion time inversion recovery		IR sequence with short TI

Reproduced with permission from Petersein J, Saini S: AJR *165*:1105, 1995. Copyright 1995, American Roentgen Ray Society.

Table 2–3. PROTOCOL DEVELOPERS

Developer	Institution	Magnet Type
Mini N. Pathria, M.D.	University of California San Diego, California	General Electric (1.5 Tesla)
Charles P. Ho, Ph.D., M.D.	Bayside Imaging Center Redwood City, California	General Electric (1.5 Tesla)
Mark Schweitzer, M.D.	Thomas Jefferson University Philadelphia, Pennsylvania	General Electric (1.5 Tesla)
Cooper R. Gundry, M.D.	Center for Diagnostic Imaging Minneapolis, Minnesota	General Electric (1.5 Tesla)
A. Gabrielle Bergman, M.D., and Michael Hollett, M.D.	Stanford University Medical Center Stanford, California	General Electric (1.5 Tesla)
Michael Recht, M.D.	Cleveland Clinic Foundation Cleveland, Ohio	Siemens (1.0 Tesla)
Douglas Goodwin, M.D.	Dartmouth-Hitchcock Medical Center Hanover, New Hampshire	General Electric (1.5 Tesla)
Joseph S. Yu, M.D.	Ohio State University Medical Center Columbus, Ohio	General Electric (1.5 Tesla)
Michael Zlatkin, M.D.	Radiology Associates of Hollywood Hollywood, Florida	General Electric (1.5 Tesla)

SHOULDER (Table 2–4)

The patient generally is examined in the supine position with the shoulder at his or her side in a neutral or slightly externally rotated attitude. In some instances, an abducted and externally rotated (ABER) position of the arm is used. A number of shoulder coils that vary slightly in design are available. Imaging protocols vary according to the specific clinical findings, which often fall into one of two major categories: (1) routine assessment for pain, rotator cuff disease, or the impingement syndrome, or (2) assessment of glenohumeral joint instability. For both categories, three imaging planes usually are employed (Fig. 2–1): coronal oblique (roughly parallel to the long axis of the supraspinatus tendon), sagittal oblique (at approximately 90 degrees to the coronal oblique axis and tangent to the glenoid cavity), and transaxial. In some cases, an entirely different protocol is used for each of these two major categories; in others one or two imaging sequences are used as a supplement to or replacement for one or more of the routine sequences.

No consensus exists reflecting the benefits of routine versus fast spin echo (with or without fat suppression) technique for assessment of the rotator cuff. Furthermore, for glenohumeral joint instability, disagreement exists regarding the relative benefits of standard proton density and T2-weighted spin echo versus standard or three-dimensional gradient echo technique.

The diagnostic benefit provided by the presence of fluid in the glenohumeral joint in cases of joint instability has led to the increasing popularity of some type of arthrographic method in those patients who do not have a sizcable native effusion. Several options exist:

1. Intravenous administration of a gadolinium-containing compound followed by exercise of the shoulder and delayed MR imaging, often employing fat suppression techniques.

2. Intra-articular injection of a gadolinium-containing compound followed by immediate MR imaging, often employing fat suppression techniques.

3. Intra-articular injection of saline solution followed by immediate MR imaging, including some type of T2-weighted sequence.

4. Standard glenohumeral joint arthrography employing an iodinated agent followed, when necessary, with MR imaging, including some type of T2-weighted sequence.

Additional imaging options when MR arthrographic techniques are employed include positioning of the arm in internal rotation or in the ABER position, and, when gadolinium compounds are injected, the use of a T1-weighted spin echo or some type of gradient echo sequence, or both, and of a T2-weighted spin echo sequence in order to delineate areas of accumulation of native fluid (e.g., subacromial-subdeltoid bursa).

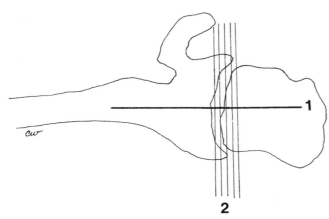

Figure 2–1
Shoulder: Imaging planes. In addition to the transaxial plane, coronal oblique (1) and sagittal oblique (2) planes are used.

Table 2–4. SHOULDER

Institution	Plane	Sequence	TR/TE (msec)	TI (msec)	FOV (cm)	Matrix	Slice Thickness (Gap) (mm)	NEX	Comments
UCSD	Coronal (localizer)	FMPIR	2500/30	150	36	256 × 128	5 (1)	1	
	Transaxial	GRE, Fat Suppression	450/15; flip angle, 30 degrees		14	256 × 192	4 (1)	1	
	Coronal (oblique)	SE, Double Echo	2000/20, 2000/80		14	256 × 192	4 (1)	1	
	Sagittal (oblique)	FSE, Fat Suppression	3000/20		14	256 × 192	4 (1)	2	
	Sagittal (oblique)	SE	600/20		14	256 × 128	4 (1)	2	
	Transaxial	SE, Double Echo	2000/20, 2000/80		14	256 × 192	4 (1)	1	Glenohumeral joint instability
BAYSIDE	Transaxial	SE, ± Fat Suppression	500/14		16	256 × 192	5 (1)	2	
	Coronal (oblique)	FSE, ± Fat Suppression, Double Echo	3000/17, 3000/102		16	256 × 192	4 (1)	2	
	Sagittal (oblique)	FSE, ± Fat Suppression, Double Echo	3000/17, 3000/102		16	256 × 192	4 (1)	2	
	Transaxial	GRE, ± Fat Suppression	600/15; flip angle, 25 degrees		16	256 × 192	4 (1)	2	Glenohumeral joint instability
T. JEFFERSON	Coronal (localizer)	SE	400/20		48	256 × 128	10 (2.5)	1	
	Transaxial	3D GRE	30/15; flip angle, 20 degrees		15	256 × 128	1.2 (0)	2	Glenohumeral joint instability
	Coronal (oblique)	FSE, Fat Suppression	3500/75		12	256 × 256	5 (1)	4	
	Coronal	SE	550/15		15	256 × 256	5 (1)	2	
	Sagittal (oblique)	FSE, Fat Suppression	3500/95		14	256 × 256	5 (1)	2	
MINNEAPOLIS	Transaxial (localizer)	SE	300/20		48	256 × 128	5 (2)	0.5	
	Coronal (oblique)	SE, Double Echo	2000/17, 2000/70		16	256 × 192	3 (1)	1	
	Sagittal (oblique)	SE, Double Echo	2000/17, 2000/70		16	256 × 192	3 (1)	1	
	Transaxial	SE, Double Echo	2000/17, 2000/70		16	256 × 192	3 (1)	1	
	Transaxial	FMPIR	3000/51	150	30	256 × 128	4 (1)	2	Glenohumeral joint instability
	Coronal (oblique)	FMPIR	3000/51	150	30	256 × 128	4 (1)	2	Rotator cuff
STANFORD	Coronal (localizer)	SE	300/min		20–24	256 × 128	5 (1)	1	
	Transaxial	FSE, Fat Suppression	4000/18		14	256 × 192	3 (1.5)	2	
	Transaxial	GRE	600/20; flip angle, 25 degrees		14	256 × 192	3 (1.5)	2	For labrum
	Coronal (oblique)	SE	600/min		14	256 × 256	3 (1.5)	2	
	Coronal (oblique)	FSE, Double Echo, Fat Suppression	4000/18, 4000/108		14	256 × 192	3 (1.5)	2	
	Coronal (oblique)	SE, Double Echo	2000/20, 2000/80		14	256 × 128	3 (1.5)	2	Optional as replacement
	Sagittal (oblique)	FSE, Fat Suppression	4000/108		14	256 × 192	3 (1.5)	2	

Table continued on following page

Table 2–4. SHOULDER (*Continued*)

Institution	Plane	Sequence	TR/TE (msec)	TI (msec)	FOV (cm)	Matrix	Slice Thickness (Gap) (mm)	NEX	Comments
CLEVELAND CLINIC	Coronal, Transaxial (localizer)	SE	200/12		50	256 × 128	5 (2.5)	1	
	Transaxial	GRE	400/10; flip angle, 25 degrees		16	256 × 192	4 (1)	4	
	Coronal (oblique)	SE	550/14		30	256 × 512	4 (1)	2	
	Coronal (oblique)	Turbo SE	3000/96		30	256 × 512	4 (1)	2	
	Sagittal (oblique)	SE	550/14		30	256 × 512	4 (1)	2	
	Sagittal	FSE	3000/96		30	256 × 512	4 (1)	2	
	Transaxial	SE, Double Echo	2000/20, 2000/80		16	256 × 128	4 (1)	2	Glenohumeral joint instability
DARTMOUTH	Coronal (localizer)	SE	200/min		48	256 × 128	5 (2)	0.5	
	Transaxial	GRE	400/14; flip angle, 18 degrees		16	256 × 256	4 (0.5)	2	
	Coronal (oblique)	SE	500/min		16	256 × 256	4 (0.5)	2	
	Coronal (oblique)	FSE	3600/96		15	256 × 256	4 (0.5)	2	
	Sagittal (oblique)	FSE	3600/96		15	256 × 256	4 (0.5)	2	
OHIO STATE	Transaxial (localizer)	3D GRE	18.9/7.4		16	256 × 192	1.5 (0)	2	
	Transaxial	SE	400/20		16	256 × 192	3 (1)	2	
	Sagittal (oblique)	SE, Double Echo	2000/11, 2000/80		16	256 × 128	3 (0.5)	2	
	Coronal (oblique)	SE, Double Echo	2000/11, 2000/80		16	256 × 128	3 (0.5)	2	
WEST HOLLYWOOD	Coronal (localizer)	FMPSPGR	100/min; flip angle, 30 degrees		20	256 × 128	8 (0.5)	2	
	Transaxial	SE, Double Echo	2500/min, 2500/70		14	256 × 192	4 (0.5)	1	
	Coronal (oblique)	SE, Double Echo	2500/min, 2500/70		14	256 × 160	3–4 (0)	1.5	Rotator cuff
	Coronal (oblique)	FSE, Fat Suppressed	2500/80		14	256 × 256	4 (0.5)	2	Rotator cuff
	Sagittal (oblique)	FSE, Separate Echoes, Fat Suppressed	2000/15, 2500/80		14	256 × 256	4 (0.5)	2	Rotator cuff
	Transaxial	GRE, Double Echo	400/15, 400/30; flip angle, 30 degrees		14	256 × 192	3 (0)	2	Rotator cuff
	Transaxial	SE, Double Echo	2500/min, 2500/70		14	256 × 192	4 (0.5)	1	Glenohumeral joint instability
	Coronal (oblique)	SE, Double Echo	2500/min, 2500/70		14	256 × 160	3–4 (0)	1	Glenohumeral joint instability

ELBOW (Table 2–5)

Positioning of the elbow joint in the MR imaging scanner can be accomplished with the patient supine or prone. With the patient supine, the arm is placed alongside the body with the elbow located as close to the isocenter of the magnet as is possible. Alternatively, the patient can be placed prone or supine with the elbow above the head, although this position may be less comfortable. A single flat surface coil, dual surface coils, or some type of extremity coil may be employed. All three imaging planes generally are required, and it is important that true coronal and sagittal images of the elbow be obtained (Fig. 2–2).

Although a standard MR imaging protocol can be designed for analysis of some problems of the elbow (e.g., tendon or ligament abnormality, osteochondritis dissecans of the capitulum), analysis of certain problems, such as the detection of intra-articular bodies, may require modifications in this protocol. In addition to standard or fast spin echo sequences, short tau inversion recovery (STIR) or fast spin echo STIR sequences of the elbow are popular owing to their sensitivity to the presence of fluid (e.g., effusion, soft tissue edema about ligaments or tendons). In the assessment of the biceps tendon, it is important that its insertion site, the radial tuberosity, is included in all imaging planes. If this tendon is completely torn and retracted, a larger field of view in the sagittal and the coronal planes is required.

The detection of intra-articular bodies in the elbow, as in other joints, may be difficult with MR imaging, particularly if the bodies are small. The presence of a native effusion aids in this detection. The value of MR arthrographic techniques, particularly in comparison to other methods such as computed arthrotomography, in the identification of such bodies is not proved.

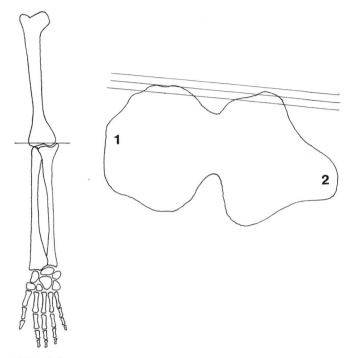

Figure 2–2
Elbow: Imaging planes. The axis of the coronal images is shown (1, capitulum; 2, medial epicondyle).

Table 2–5. ELBOW

Institution	Plane	Sequence	TR/TE (msec)	TI (msec)	FOV (cm)	Matrix	Slice Thickness (Gap) (mm)	NEX	Comments
UCSD	Transaxial (localizer)	FMPIR	2500/25	150	24	256 × 128	5 (2.5)	2	
	Transaxial	FSE, Double Echo	3000/17 3000/102			256 × 192	4 (1)	2	
	Coronal	FSE, Double Echo	3000/17 3000/102		12	256 × 192	3 (1)	2	
	Sagittal	SE	600/20		12	256 × 128	3 (1)	2	
BAYSIDE	Coronal (localizer)	SE	500/auto		15	256 × 192	4 (0.5)	2	
	Coronal	FMPIR	5000/18	150	15	256 × 192	4 (0.5)	2	
	Sagittal	FSE, Double Echo	4300/17 4300/102		15	256 × 192	4 (0.5)	2	
	Transaxial	FSE, Double Echo	4300/17 4300/102		12	256 × 192	4 (0.5)	2	
T. JEFFERSON	Coronal	SE	384/min		18	256 × 128	5 (1)	2	
	Transaxial	FSE, Fat Suppression	2500/40		13	256 × 256	5 (1)	2 or 4	
	Transaxial	FSE, Fat Suppression	8000/70		13	256 × 256	5 (1)	2	
	Sagittal	FMPIR	8000/20	150	18	256 × 256	5 (1)	2	
	Coronal	3D GRE	40/13; flip angle 20 degrees		12	256 × 128	1.2 (0)	2	
MINNEAPOLIS	Transaxial (localizer)	SE	300/20		40	256 × 128	4 (1)	0.5	
	Coronal	SE	300/20		40	256 × 128	5 (1)	0.5	
	Transaxial	SE	300/20		40	256 × 128	4 (1)	0.5	
	Sagittal	FSE, Double Echo	3000/20 3000/100		12–14	256 × 256	3 (1)	2	
	Coronal	FSE, Double Echo	3000/20 3000/100		12–14	256 × 256	3 (1)	2	

Institution	Plane	Sequence	TR/TE		Matrix1	Matrix	Thickness (gap)	NEX	Comments
	Transaxial	FSE, Double Echo	4000/20 4000/100		12–14	256 × 256	3 (1)	1	
	Coronal	FMPIR	3000/51	150	12–14	256 × 128	4 (1)	2	
STANFORD	Coronal (oblique)	SE	300/min		20	256 × 128	5 (1)	1	
	Coronal (oblique)	SE	300/min		10–14	256 × 192	3 (1.5)	2	
	Coronal (oblique)	FSE, Double Echo, Fat Suppression	4000/18 4000/108		10–14	256 × 192	3 (1.5)	4	
	Transaxial	SE	300/min		10–14	256 × 192	3 (1.5)	2	
	Transaxial	FMPIR	4000/30	150	10–14	256 × 192	3 (1.5)	2–4	
	Sagittal (oblique)	SE	300/min		10–14	256 × 192	3 (1.5)	2	Optional
CLEVELAND CLINIC	Transaxial, Sagittal, Coronal (localizer)	SE	200/15		30	256 × 128	10 (5)	1	
	Transaxial, Sagittal	SE	500/15		12	256 × 192	3–4 (1)	2–4	
	Coronal, Transaxial	SE, Double Echo	2000/20 2000/80		12	256 × 128	4 (1)	2	
	Variable	STIR	7000/22		12	256 × 180	4 (1)	2	Optional
OHIO STATE	Sagittal	SE	500/20		14–16	256 × 192	3 (1)	2	
	Transaxial	SE, Double Echo	2000/20 2000/80		12–14	256 × 128	3 (1)	2	
	Coronal	SE, Double Echo, Fat Suppression	2000/20 2000/80		12–16	256 × 128	3 (1)	2	
	Sagittal	SE, Double Echo	2000/20 2000/80		14–16	256 × 128	3 (1)	2	For intra-articular bodies
WEST HOLLYWOOD	Transaxial (localizer)	FSE	1384/17		16	256 × 128	5 (1.5)	2	
	Sagittal	SE	800/min		12–14	256 × 192	3 (0)	1	
	Coronal	SE, Double Echo	2500/min 2500/70		12–14	256 × 160	3 (0)	1.5	
	Coronal	GRE, 3D, Fat Suppressed	45/15		12–14	256 × 192	1.5 (0)	1	

WRIST (Table 2–6)

Considerable disagreement exists with regard to the optimal way to evaluate the wrist using MR imaging. The patient can be positioned supine with the arm at the side or prone with the arm extended over the head. Excessive pronation or supination of the wrist is detrimental to the quality of the examination. A dedicated wrist coil often is employed, although some examiners use two small circular coils, one placed on the dorsal and one on the volar aspect of the wrist. As with other joints, imaging in three planes often is accomplished, although the plane that is emphasized is dependent on the specific indication for the examination. Furthermore, as the wrist may lie in a slightly oblique position, the orientation of the coronal plane varies from one institution to another. One method that is useful for assessment of the triangular fibrocartilage complex and intrinsic ligaments of the wrist relies on obtaining a coronal plane that is parallel to the volar surface of the radius, allowing both the radial and ulnar styloid processes to be visualized on a single image (Fig. 2–3).

Numerous indications exist for MR imaging of the wrist, each requiring slight modifications in technique. Major indications include the following:

1. Assessment of the triangular fibrocartilage complex and intercarpal ligaments (scapholunate and lunotriquetral ligaments).
2. Assessment of the carpal tunnel (or Guyon's canal).
3. Assessment of instability of the distal radioulnar joint.
4. Detection of occult fractures (e.g., scaphoid bone or radius).

With regard to the first of these, the coronal (or coronal oblique) plane is most useful, although images obtained in the sagittal plane allow assessment of malalignment among the carpal bones (i.e., dorsal or volar intercalated carpal instability). In the coronal plane, spin echo (including images with T2 weighting) or gradient echo (standard or three-dimensional images), or both, are employed. The benefits of standard spin echo images include the identification of fluid at the site of ligamentous disruption; the advantages of three-dimensional gradient echo MR images employing thin slices include greater anatomic resolution of the triangular fibrocarti-

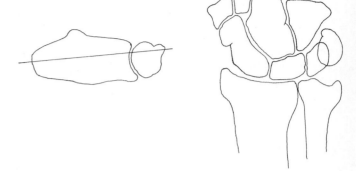

Figure 2–3
Wrist: Imaging planes. If the coronal axis is constructed roughly parallel to the volar surface of the radius, both the radial and ulnar styloid processes are visualized on a single image.

lage complex and intrinsic ligaments and, in some cases, the ability to detect abnormalities in the extrinsic ligaments (e.g., radiocarpal and ulnocarpal ligaments) of the wrist.

Assessment of the carpal tunnel syndrome requires imaging in the transverse plane, which in some institutions is coupled with dynamic imaging obtained in various positions of the wrist, such as flexion and extension and ulnar and radial deviation, or after moderate exercise of the joint, or with intravenous administration of a gadolinium compound. As the diagnosis of carpal tunnel syndrome by MR imaging often relies in part on changes in signal intensity within or around the median nerve, some type of T2-weighted imaging sequence (usually spin echo) is required.

Assessment of instability of the distal radioulnar joint requires documentation of malalignment (often subtle) between the distal ends of the radius and ulna and requires further that MR imaging of the wrist, usually in the transverse plane, be obtained in positions of supination and pronation. Including both the normal and abnormal sides in the images is advised, requiring an increase in the field of view but permitting comparison of radioulnar relationships on the two sides, thereby facilitating accurate diagnosis.

For detecting occult fractures about the wrist, STIR images or T1 weighted spin echo images, or both, appear most appropriate. The coronal plane is ideal for scaphoid and radial fractures, whereas coronal fractures of the capitate or hamate or fractures of the hook of the hamate or volar ridge of the trapezium are well demonstrated in the transverse or sagittal plane.

Table 2–6. WRIST

Institution	Plane	Sequence	TR/TE (msec)	TI (msec)	FOV (cm)	Matrix	Slice Thickness (Gap) (mm)	NEX	Comments
UCSD	Transaxial (localizer)	SE	600/20		8	256 × 128	3 (1)	2	
	Sagittal	SE	450/20		8	256 × 128	3 (1)	2	
	Coronal	SE, Double Echo	2000/20 2000/80		8	256 × 128	3 (1)	2	
	Coronal	3D GRE	45/9; flip angle, 30 degrees		8	256 × 192	0.6 to 1.2 (0)	2	
	Transaxial	SE, Double Echo	2000/20 2000/80		8	256 × 128	3 (1)	2	Carpal tunnel syndrome
BAYSIDE	Coronal (localizer)	SE	1000/20		10	256 × 192	3 (0.5)	2	
	Coronal	FMPIR	6000/18	150	10	256 × 192	3 (0.5)	2	
	Coronal	GRE	350/20; flip angle, 25 degrees		10	256 × 192	3 (0.5)	2	
	Transaxial	SE, Double Echo	2000/30 2000/80		10	256 × 192	3 (0.5)	1	
	Sagittal	FSE, Fat Suppression	4000/38		10	256 × 192	4 (0.5)	2	
T. JEFFERSON	Coronal (localizer)	SE	600/20		12	256 × 128	3 (1)	1	
	Coronal	FSE	5300/140		12	256 × 256	3 (1)	3	
	Coronal	FSE	2500/40		10	256 × 256	3 (1)	2	
	Transaxial	FSE	2500/10		10	256 × 256	3 (1)	2	
	Coronal	3D GRE	30/12; flip angle, 20 degrees		12	256 × 128	1.2 (0)	2	
MINNEAPOLIS	Coronal (localizer)	SE	300/20		48	256 × 128	5 (2)	0.5	
	Transaxial	FSE, Double Echo	3000/20 3000/100		10	256 × 192	3 (1)	1	
	Coronal	FSE, Double Echo	3000/20 3000/100		10	256 × 192	3 (1)	1	
	Sagittal	FSE, Double Echo	3000/20 3000/100		10	256 × 192	3 (1)	1	
STANFORD	Coronal	FMPIR	3000/51	150	12	256 × 128	4 (1)	1	
	Coronal (localizer)	SE	300/min		16	256 × 128	5 (1)	1	
	Coronal	SE	300/min		10	256 × 192	3 (1.5)	2	
	Coronal	FMPIR	4000/30	150	10	256 × 192	3 (1.5)	2–4	
	Transaxial	SE	300/min		10	256 × 192	3 (1.5)	2	
	Transaxial	FSE, Fat Suppression	4000/108		10	256 × 192	3 (1.5)	2	
	Coronal	GRE	600/20; flip angle, 25 degrees		10	256 × 192	3 (1.5)	2	
	Sagittal	FSE, Fat Suppression	4000/18		10	256 × 192	3 (1.5)	2	Optional

Table continued on following page

Table 2-6. WRIST (Continued)

Institution	Plane	Sequence	TR/TE (msec)	TI (msec)	FOV (cm)	Matrix	Slice Thickness (Gap) (mm)	NEX	Comments
CLEVELAND CLINIC	Transaxial Sagittal, Coronal (localizer)	SE	200/15		30	256 × 128	10 (5)	1	
	Coronal, Transaxial, Sagittal	SE	500/15		12	256 × 192	3–4 (1)	2–4	
	Coronal, Transaxial	SE, Double Echo	2000/20 2000/80		12	256 × 128	4 (1)	2	
	Variable	STIR	7000/22		12	256 × 180	4 (1)	2	Optional
DARTMOUTH	Coronal	SE	450/19		8	256 × 256	3 (1)	2	
	Coronal	FMPIR	3000/24	120	10	256 × 192	3 (1)	2	
	Transaxial	FSE	3000/99		8	256 × 256	3 (1)	2	
	Coronal	3D GRE	69/15; flip angle, 15 degrees		8	256 × 192	1.5 (0)	2	
OHIO STATE	Coronal	GRE	60/10; flip angle, 10 degrees		12 × 9	256 × 128	1 (0)	1	
	Sagittal	SE	500/15		10	256 × 128	3 (0.5)	2	
	Transaxial	SE, Double Echo	2000/20 2000/80		10	256 × 192	3 (1)	2	
	Coronal	SE	500/20		10	256 × 192	3 (0.5)	2	For fracture assessment
WEST HOLLYWOOD	Transaxial (localizer)	FSE	1667/17		14	256 × 128	5 (0.5)	1	
	Sagittal	SE	600/min		6–8	256 × 192	3 (1)	1	
	Coronal	SE, Double Echo	2500/min 2500/60		6–8	256 × 160	2 (0)	1.5	
	Coronal	GRE	400/12 400/24; flip angle, 25 degrees		6–8	256 × 192	3 (0)	2	
	Transaxial	FSE, Fat Suppressed	2500/80		6–8	256 × 256	3 (0.2)	2	Optional
	Transaxial	GRE, 3D	45/10; flip angle, 30 degrees		6–8	256 × 192	1 (0)	1	
	Transaxial	SE	600/min		8	256 × 192	3 (0)	1	Carpal tunnel syndrome
	Transaxial	SE, Double Echo	2500/min 2500/70		8	256 × 160	3 (0)	1.5	Carpal tunnel syndrome
	Coronal or Sagittal	SE, Double Echo	2500/min 2500/70		8	256 × 160	3 (0)	1.5	Carpal tunnel syndrome

HIP (Table 2–7)

Protocols used to image the hip with MR imaging vary considerably according to the specific indications for the examination. Generally, in at least one plane and sometimes in two planes (typically the coronal and transaxial planes), a body coil and large field of view with inclusion of the entire pelvis and both hips are employed. Examination of a single hip can be accomplished with a local coil or coils and a smaller field of view. Typically, the patient is in a supine position. Although standard imaging planes (coronal, transaxial, and sagittal) often suffice, some examiners prefer coronal oblique or sagittal oblique images, or both, aligned with respect to the long axis of the femoral neck, particularly for the assessment of occult femoral fractures.

Although standard MR imaging protocols can be established for assessment of hip pain, the manner in which MR imaging is performed to assess the presence and extent of osteonecrosis of the femoral head often is influenced by clinical data (whether one or both hips need to be studied) and results of preliminary sequences. As an example, establishing the presence of osteonecrosis of the femoral head in a clinically silent hip contralateral to an obviously involved femoral head may require sagittal images of the hip with a smaller field of view, allowing identification of subtle changes that otherwise might escape detection.

STIR sequences are particularly useful in the analysis of occult fractures of the hip and osseous pelvis or muscle injuries. In these situations, inclusion of the entire pelvis (including all sites of tendon attachments) becomes important. The diagnosis of injuries of the acetabular labrum may not be possible with standard MR imaging protocols, requiring MR arthrographic methods.

Table 2–7. HIP

Institution	Plane	Sequence	TR/TE (msec)	TI (msec)	FOV (cm)	Matrix	Slice Thickness (Gap) (mm)	NEX	Comments
UCSD	Coronal (localizer)	FMPIR	3000/25	150	32–36	256 × 128	4 (1)	2	
	Coronal	SE	600/20		32–36	256 × 192	4 (1)	2	
	Coronal	FSE	3000/102		32–36	256 × 192	4 (1)	2	
	Sagittal	SE	850/20		24	256 × 192	3 (1)	1	
BAYSIDE	Coronal (localizer)	FMPIR	500/14		Variable	256 × 192	4 (0.5)	2	
	Coronal	FMPIR	6000/18		Variable	256 × 192	4 (0.5)	2	
	Transaxial	FSE, Double Echo	4000/18 4000/108		Variable	256 × 192	4 (1)	2	
	Sagittal	SE	500/13		24	256 × 192	4 (1)	2	
T. JEFFERSON	Coronal (localizer)	SE	450/min		40	256 × 256	5 (1)	1	
	Sagittal	FSE, Fat Suppression	5700/50		24	256 × 256	5 (1)	2	
	Transaxial Oblique	FSE	5600/40		38	256 × 256	5 (1)	2	Angled along long axis of femoral neck
	Coronal	FMPIR	7000/45	150	38	256 × 256	5 (1)	2	
MINNEAPOLIS	Transaxial (localizer)	SE	300/20		48	256 × 128	5 (2)	0.5	
	Coronal	FSE, Double Echo	4000/20 4000/100		40	256 × 256	4 (1)	1	
	Transaxial	FSE, Double Echo	4000/20 4000/100		40	256 × 256	5 (1)	1	
	Coronal	FMPIR	3000/51	150	16	256 × 128	4 (1)	2	
	Sagittal	FSE, Double Echo	4000/20 4000/100		24	256 × 192	5 (1)	2	

Institution	Plane	Sequence	TR/TE		FOV	Matrix	Thickness (gap)	NEX
STANFORD	Coronal (localizer)	SE	300/min		20	256 × 192	5 (2.5)	2
	Transaxial	FSE, Fat Suppression	4000/108		20	256 × 192	4 (1)	2
	Transaxial	SE	300/min		20	256 × 192	4 (1)	2
	Sagittal	FSE, Fat Suppression	4000/18	150	20	256 × 192	4 (1)	2
	Coronal	FMPIR	4000/30		20	256 × 192	6 (1.5)	2–4
CLEVELAND CLINIC	Coronal, Transaxial (localizer)	SE	200/12	150	50	256 × 128	5 (2.5)	1
	Coronal	SE	700/20		42	512 × 256	5 (1)	2
	Coronal	STIR	6356/22		42	256 × 180	4 (1)	2
	Sagittal	SE	600/20		20	512 × 384	4 (1)	2
	Sagittal	Turbo SE, Fat Suppression	5250/119		20	512 × 270	4 (1)	3
	Coronal	SE	700/20		24	256 × 512	5 (1)	1
DARTMOUTH	Transaxial (localizer)	SE	200/min		40	256 × 128	5 (2)	0.5
	Coronal	SE	400/min		40	256 × 256	4 (1)	2
	Sagittal	SE	400/min		40	256 × 256	4 (1)	2
	Transaxial	FSE, Fat Suppression	4000/102		40	256 × 256	4 (1)	2
OHIO STATE	Transaxial (localizer)	SE	300/20		32	256 × 128	5 (1)	1
	Coronal	SE	400/20		32–36	256 × 256	5 (1)	1
	Coronal	SE, Double Echo	2500/30		32–36	256 × 128	4 (1)	
	Sagittal	SE	2500/80		24	256 × 128	5 (1)	2
WEST HOLLYWOOD	Transaxial (localizer)	FSE	2017/68		48	256 × 128	5 (2.5)	1
	Coronal	SE	800/min		18–20 (one hip) 30–32 (both hips)	256 × 192	4 (0)	1
	Coronal	SE, Double Echo	2500/min		18–20 (one hip) 30–32 (both hips)	256 × 160	4 (0)	1.5
	Sagittal	3D GRE (SPGR with Fat Suppression)	2500/70 45/15; flip angle, 30 degrees		18–20	256 × 192	2 (0)	1

KNEE (Table 2–8)

MR imaging protocols for the routine assessment of the knee generally agree in the following parameters: supine positioning of the patient, full extension of the knee, the use of an extremity coil, and the need to image in three planes. The sagittal plane that is chosen usually is slightly oblique to parallel the long axis of the anterior cruciate ligament (Fig. 2–4). This is accomplished either by having the patient externally rotate the involved leg about 10 degrees or by constructing a sagittal oblique axis on images obtained in another plane. One method allowing programming of the sagittal oblique images relies on construction of a line along the inner edge of the lateral femoral condyle on a transaxial image at the level of the distal portion of the femur. The coronal and sagittal (oblique) images are fundamental to analysis of the menisci and ligamentous structures about the knee; the transaxial images aid in this analysis and provide information regarding the status of the cartilage in the patellofemoral joint. The importance of filming high contrast images of the menisci (meniscal "windowing") from image data in the coronal and sagittal planes is controversial.

There is no consensus regarding the specific imaging sequences that are required as part of the routine MR imaging examination of the knee. Conventional spin echo and fast spin echo sequences (with or without fat suppression) each have their advocates. Although the value of one of these methods compared to the other in the assessment of the menisci is hotly debated, the combination of fast spin echo MR imaging and fat suppression appears to have merit in the analysis of the collateral ligaments, allowing detection of high signal intensity in involved structures in cases of acute or subacute injury and of associated trabecular microfractures (bone bruises). Owing to the sensitivity of STIR images, this technique, too, often is employed as a means to

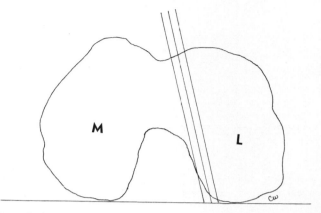

Figure 2–4
Knee: Imaging plane. Sagittal oblique images are obtained using an axis that is oriented about 10 degrees anteromedially. L, Lateral femoral condyle; M, medial femoral condyle.

allow detection of marrow and soft tissue edema or hemorrhage.

The evaluation of articular cartilage in the various compartments of the knee is accomplished in a number of ways. Transaxial images are optimal for assessment of articular cartilage in the patellofemoral joint; imaging protocols used for this assessment include standard spin echo, fat-suppressed fast spin echo, or gradient echo sequences, magnetization transfer contrast imaging, and MR arthrography. One popular technique employs transaxial spoiled gradient recalled acquisition imaging in the steady state (SPGR) combined with volumetric acquisition and fat suppression. This technique also is used in the sagittal plane to gain information regarding femoral and tibial cartilage.

Modifications in MR imaging protocols that are used to study the cruciate ligaments include dynamic imaging with various positions of knee flexion and extension and static imaging with the knee slightly flexed rather than extended. Dynamic MR imaging also is employed to evaluate instability of the patellofemoral joint.

Table 2–8. KNEE

Institution	Plane	Sequence	TR/TE (msec)	TI (msec)	FOV (cm)	Matrix	Slice Thickness (Gap) (mm)	NEX	Comments
UCSD	Sagittal (localizer)	FMPIR	2500/25	150	18	256 × 128	5 (2.5)	1	
	Transaxial	FSE, Fat Suppression	3000/20		14	256 × 256	4 (1)	2	
	Sagittal (oblique)	SE, Double Echo	2000/20 2000/80		14	256 × 192	4 (1)	1	
	Coronal	FSE, Fat Suppression	3000/20		14	256 × 192	4 (1)	2	
	Coronal (optional)	SE	600/20		14	256 × 126	4 (1)	1	
BAYSIDE	Transaxial (localizer)	SE	500/13		16	256 × 192	4 (1)	1	
	Sagittal (oblique)	SE	500/14		12	256 × 192	4 (1)	2	
	Sagittal (oblique)	FSE, Fat Suppression	4800/38		16	256 × 192	4 (1)	2	
	Coronal	FSE, Fat Suppression	3500/38		16	256 × 256	4 (1)	2	
	Coronal	SE	651/21		12	256 × 256	4 (1)	2	
	Transaxial	FSE, Fat Suppression	3500/38		16	256 × 256	4 (1)	1	
T. JEFFERSON	Transaxial	FSE, ± Fat Suppression	3600/70		14	256 × 256	4 (1)	2	
	Sagittal (oblique)	SE, ± Fat Suppression	1000/20		14	256 × 256	4 (1)	1	
	Sagittal (oblique)	FSE	4000/105		12	256 × 256	4 (1)	2	
	Coronal	SE	1000/20		14	256 × 256	4 (1)	1	
	Coronal	FSE	4000/105		11	256 × 256	4 (1)	2	
	Transaxial	3D GRE	40/13; flip angle, 20 degrees		16	256 × 198	1.2 (0)	2	
MINNEAPOLIS	Transaxial (localizer)	SE	300/20		16	256 × 192	5 (2.5)	1	
	Sagittal (oblique)	FSE, Double Echo	4000/20 4000/100		12–14	256 × 256	3 (1)	1	
	Coronal	FSE, Double Echo	4000/20 4000/100		12–14	256 × 256	3 (1)	1	
	Transaxial	FSE, Double Echo	3000/20 3000/100		12–14	256 × 256	3 (1.5)	1	
	Coronal	FMPIR	3000/51	150	16	256 × 128	4 (1)	2	
STANFORD	Coronal (localizer)	SE	600/min		14	256 × 256	4 (1)	2	
	Sagittal	FSE, Double Echo	4000/18 4000/108		14	256 × 192	3 (1)	2	
	Coronal	FSE, Fat Suppression	4000/108		14	256 × 192	4 (1)	2	Optional
	Transaxial	FSE, Fat Suppression	4000/18		14	256 × 192	4 (1)	2	Optional
	Sagittal	SE, Double Echo	2000/20 2000/80		14	256 × 128	3 (1)	2	Optional
	Coronal	FMPIR	5000/85	160	14	256 × 192	4 (1)	2	Optional
	Sagittal	3D GRE	31/15; flip angle, 30 degrees		14	256 × 256	1.5 (0)	1	Optional

Table continued on following page

Table 2–8. KNEE (*Continued*)

Institution	Plane	Sequence	TR/TE (msec)	TI (msec)	FOV (cm)	Matrix	Slice Thickness (Gap) (mm)	NEX	Comments
CLEVELAND CLINIC	Transaxial, Sagittal (localizer)	SE	200/15		20	256 × 128	10 (2)	1	
	Sagittal	SE, Double Echo	2500/20, 2500/80		14	256 × 192	3 (1)	2	
	Coronal	SE, Double Echo	2604/20, 2604/80		14	256 × 192	3 (1)	2	
	Sagittal	3D GRE, Fat Suppression	50/11; flip angle, 45 degrees		14	256 × 160	1.48 (0)	1	Reconstruct in transaxial plane
DARTMOUTH	Transaxial	SPGR	34/3.3; flip angle, 30 degrees		20	256 × 128	5 (2)	1	
	Sagittal	FMPIR	3300/38	150	20	256 × 128	5 (2)	1	
	Sagittal	SE, Double Echo	2200/32, 2200/85		15	256 × 192	4 (1)	1	
	Transaxial	MPGR	500/9; flip angle, 15 degrees		15	256 × 256	4 (1)	2	
	Coronal	FSE, Fat Suppression	1200/20		16	256 × 192	4 (1)	2	
OHIO STATE	Transaxial (localizer)	SE	500/20		14–16	256 × 128	5 (1)	2	
	Coronal	SE	600–800/20		14–16	256 × 256	5 (0)	1	
	Sagittal	SE, Double Echo	2000–2500/20, 2000–2500/80		16–18	256 × 512	3 (1)	1	
	Coronal Oblique	SE, Double Echo	2000/20, 2000/80		16	256 × 192	3 (0.5)	1	Posterolateral pain
WEST HOLLYWOOD	Transaxial (localizer)	FMPSPGR	89/min		16	256 × 256	4 (1.3)	2	
	Coronal	FSE, Separate Echoes, Fat Suppression	2000/15, 2500/80		14	256 × 256	4 (0.5)	2	
	Sagittal	SE, Double Echo	2500/min, 2500/70		14	256 × 192	4 (1)	1	
	Sagittal	3D GRE	65/12; flip angle, 30 degrees		14	256 × 192	1.5 (0)	1	

ANKLE AND FOOT (Table 2–9)

MR imaging protocols used to examine the ankle and foot are influenced by such factors as the anatomic area of interest (ankle, hindfoot, or forefoot), the clinical information that is sought (e.g., tendon or ligament abnormality, osteochondritis dissecans, tarsal coalition, osteomyelitis in the diabetic foot), and the desire to image a single extremity or both extremities. Patient positioning is not uniform: Some examiners prefer having the patient lie supine in the magnet with the knees flexed and feet flat on the examination table; others examine the patient in the prone position. Furthermore, the precise position of the ankle during the examination varies from one institution to another and, in the case of ligament injury, is chosen according to which particular ligament requires analysis. An extremity coil generally is used.

The three imaging planes used to study the ankle and foot are the coronal (tangent to the anterior surface of the tibia), sagittal (along the anteroposterior axis of the tibia), and transverse or plantar (parallel to the plantar surface of the foot). Often, images in all three planes are obtained in a single patient. Of these planes, the transverse plane usually supplies the greatest amount of anatomic information; the transverse and sagittal planes are most useful in the evaluation of the tendons about the ankle; and the transverse and coronal planes are most beneficial in the analysis of the ligaments about the ankle. Those radiologists who prefer imaging both feet at once do so in the transverse plane, indicating

the benefit of having comparison images of the opposite (and normal) side, owing to anatomic variations (e.g., bulbous insertion site of the tibialis posterior tendon or tendon striations) that make accurate diagnosis of some conditions more difficult. Obviously the precise surface coil and field of view are influenced by the decision to image one or both feet. For example, although an extremity coil and 12 cm field of view are appropriate when imaging a single extremity, a head coil and 24 cm field of view may be required when both extremities are imaged simultaneously.

Spin echo or fast spin echo MR imaging sequences usually are employed, although STIR MR imaging or MR imaging sequences obtained after the intravenous administration of a gadolinium-containing contrast agent are fundamental to assessment of infections in the foot of the diabetic patient. With fast spin echo imaging sequences, fat suppression techniques often are used. Obtaining homogeneous fat suppression in the ankle and foot is problematic, however, such that saturation pads (available commercially) wrapped about these areas may be required.

SUMMARY

The proper assessment of internal derangements of the joints of the extremity with MR imaging requires attention to imaging protocols. The choice of a specific protocol varies from one institution to another. Guidelines are offered in this chapter.

Table 2–9. ANKLE

Institution	Plane	Sequence	TR/TE (msec)	TI (msec)	FOV (cm)	Matrix	Slice Thickness (Gap) (mm)	NEX	Comments
UCSD	Transaxial (localizer)	SE, Double Echo	2000/20 2000/80		12	256 × 128	3–4 (1)	2	
	Sagittal	SE	600/20		12	256 × 128	3 (1)	2	
	Sagittal	FSE, Fat Suppression	3000/20		12	256 × 128	3 (1)	2	
	Coronal	FSE, Fat Suppression	3000/20		12	256 × 128	3–4 (1)	2	
BAYSIDE	Sagittal (localizer)	FSE	500/17		16	256 × 192	4 (0.5)	2	
	Sagittal	FMPIR	5500/18	150	16	256 × 256	4 (0.5)	2	
	Coronal	FSE, Double Echo	6000/17 6000/102		15	256 × 128	4 (0.5)	2	
	Transaxial	FSE, Double Echo	6000/17 6000/102		15	256 × 256	4 (0.5)	1	
T. JEFFERSON	Sagittal (localizer)	SE	500/min		20	256 × 192	4 (1)	1	
	Transaxial	FSE, Fat Suppression	5200/70		14	256 × 256	5 (1)	2	
	Sagittal	FMPIR	5400/48	150	16	256 × 256	4 (1)	2	
	Coronal	FMPIR	3000/38–48	150	16	256 × 256	4 (1)	2	
	Transaxial	FSE	6000/40		16	256 × 512	4 (1)	2	
MINNEAPOLIS	Coronal (localizer)	SE	300/20		24	256 × 192	5 (1)	0.5	
	Sagittal	FSE, Double Echo	4000/20 4000/100		12–14	256 × 192	3 (1)	2	
	Coronal	FSE, Double Echo	4000/20 4000/100		12–14	256 × 256	3 (1)	1	
	Transaxial	FSE, Double Echo	4000/20 4000/100		12–14	256 × 256	3 (1.5)	1	
	Sagittal	FMPIR	3000/51	150	16	256 × 128	4 (1)	2	
STANFORD	Sagittal (localizer)	SE	300/min		18	256 × 128	5 (1)	1	Skip if evaluating only Achilles tendon
	Coronal	SE	300/min		12–14	256 × 192	3 (1.5)	2	Skip if evaluating only Achilles tendon
	Coronal	FMPIR	5000/85	160	12–14	256 × 192	3 (1.5)	2–4	

Institution	Plane	Sequence	TR/TE	FOV	ETL	Matrix	Thickness (gap)	NEX	Comments
	Transaxial	SE	300/min		12–14	256 × 192	3 (1.5)	2	
	Transaxial	FSE, Fat Suppression	4000/108		12–14	256 × 192	3 (1.5)	2–4	
	Sagittal	SE	300/min		12–14	256 × 192	3 (1.5)	2	
	Sagittal	FMPIR	4000/30	160	12–14	256 × 192	3 (1.5)	2–4	Only for evaluation of Achilles tendon
CLEVELAND CLINIC	Transaxial, Sagittal, Coronal (localizer)	SE	200/12		20	256 × 128	10 (5)	1	
	Sagittal	SE	600/14		16	256 × 512	4 (1)	2	
	Coronal, Transaxial	SE	600/14		16	256 × 512	4 (1)	2	
	Transaxial	SE, Double Echo	2300/20, 2300/80		14	256 × 128	4 (1)	2	
	Variable	STIR	6356/22	150	14	256 × 180	4 (1)	2	Optional
	Variable	Turbo SE	8000/130		14	256 × 150	4 (1)	3	
DARTMOUTH	Sagittal (localizer)	SE	400/min		20	256 × 256	4 (1)	2	
	Sagittal	FMPIR	3000/38	150	16	256 × 256	4 (1)	2	
	Transaxial	SE	400/min		14	256 × 512	4 (1)	2 or 4	Plantar flexion
	Transaxial	FSE, Fat Suppression	3000/90		14	256 × 256	4 (1)	2	
OHIO STATE	Transaxial (localizer)	SE, Double Echo	2000–3000/20, 2000–3000/80		16	256 × 128	3 (1)	2	
	Coronal	SE, Double Echo	2000–3000/20, 2000–3000/80		16	256 × 192	3 (1)	1	
	Sagittal	SE	600/15		16	256 × 256	3 (1)	1	Optional for peroneal and tibialis posterior tendons
	Sagittal	SE, Double Echo	2000/20, 2000/80		16	256 × 192	3 (1)	1	
WEST HOLLYWOOD	Transaxial (localizer)	FSE	1764/17		16	256 × 160	5 (2.5)	1	
	Sagittal	SE	800/min		12–14	256 × 192	3 (0)	1	
	Coronal	SE, Double Echo	2500/min, 2500/70		12–14	256 × 160	3 (1)	1.5	
	Transaxial	FSE, Separate Echoes, Fat Suppressed	2000/15, 2500/80		12–14	256 × 256	4 (0.5)	2	
	Sagittal	3D GRE, Fat Suppression SPGR	45/15; flip angle, 30 degrees		12–14	256 × 192	1.5 (0)	1	Optional

Disorders: General Concepts

Synovial Joints: Traumatic Disorders

Traumatic Effusion and Hemarthrosis
Lipohemarthrosis
Traumatic Synovitis
Adhesive Capsulitis
Foreign Body Synovitis
Summary

Acute and chronic effects of trauma to synovial joints are well known. This chapter describes several important sequelae of injury to the synovial membrane and articular capsule, including qualitative and quantitative changes in the character of joint fluid.

TRAUMATIC EFFUSION AND HEMARTHROSIS

A joint effusion appearing within the first few hours after trauma usually is related to a hemarthrosis; non-bloody effusions usually appear 12 to 24 hours after injury.[1, 2] Experimental evidence indicates that trauma may produce a subtle increase in vascular permeability of the synovial membrane due to mechanisms other than gross disruption of vessels, suggesting that the genesis of traumatic effusions, including bloody ones, is multifactorial.[3] Pain and, occasionally, fever may be apparent in cases of hemarthrosis, and in all such cases, occult fractures or ligamentous injury must be excluded by careful clinical and radiologic examination.[4, 5] Hemarthrosis also may be associated with hemophilia and other bleeding disorders, pigmented villonodular synovitis, neuropathic osteoarthropathy, crystal deposition diseases, chronic renal failure, anticoagulant therapy, and intra-articular tumors.

Bloody or nonbloody effusions occurring after trauma are associated with radiographic findings that are related to displacement of intra-articular fat pads and edema of extra-articular fat planes.[6-12] Effusions, whether bloody or nonbloody, are detected easily with MR imaging (Fig. 3–1). The presence of 1 ml or less of fluid in the knee generally is evident on MR images, although 5 ml of fluid may be required before routine radiographs of the knee become abnormal. Nonsanguineous joint effusions are characterized by low signal intensity on T1-weighted spin echo MR images and high signal intensity on T2-weighted spin echo, short tau inversion recovery (STIR), and most gradient echo MR images. With hemarthroses, a fluid level may be evident; on T1-weighted and T2-weighted spin echo MR images, the dependent cellular layer is of low signal intensity, whereas the supernatant layer shows high signal intensity on T2-weighted images (Figs. 3–1 and 3–2).[13]

Chronic accumulation of blood in the joint, as in cases of hemophilia and pigmented villonodular synovitis, may lead to hemosiderin deposition in the synovial membrane. On spin echo and particularly on gradient echo MR images, hemosiderin accumulation is characterized by low signal intensity (Fig. 3–3). Similar low signal intensity may be apparent in the presence of intra-articular gas, calcification, or ossification and after deposition of amyloid, monosodium urate crystals, or metallic debris.

LIPOHEMARTHROSIS

Bloody synovial fluid containing fat droplets can be noted both grossly and microscopically after trauma to a joint.[14-16] The discovery of intra-articular fat, when combined with bone marrow spicules, is reliable evidence of an intra-articular fracture. Frequently, however, a hemorrhagic effusion containing fat may be observed in patients without fracture, probably related to significant cartilaginous or ligamentous injury.[17, 18]

Radiographic examination using horizontal beam technique may demonstrate a fat-blood fluid level after injury to the joint.[15, 19-23] Small amounts of fat and blood in this joint may not be sufficient to produce a fat-blood fluid level on cross-table radiography, although large amounts will reveal a typical straight line at the interface of the fat above and the blood below.

Lipohemarthroses also may be detected with CT or MR imaging (Fig. 3–4).[24] The former method allows assessment of small amounts of intra-articular fat that may escape detection with standard radiographic techniques and is useful in the diagnosis of occult fractures about the hip, shoulder, and knee. With MR imaging, the appearance of a lipohemarthrosis is more complex, as several layers and interfaces are evident with signal intensity characteristics dependent on the specific imaging sequences that are employed. The most superior zone contains floating fat, a central zone contains serum, and an inferior zone contains dependent red blood cells.[24] A signal void, representing chemical shift artifact, may be visible at the interface of fat and serum. Furthermore, in some cases, fat trapped within blood clots in the joint lead to focal changes in signal intensity

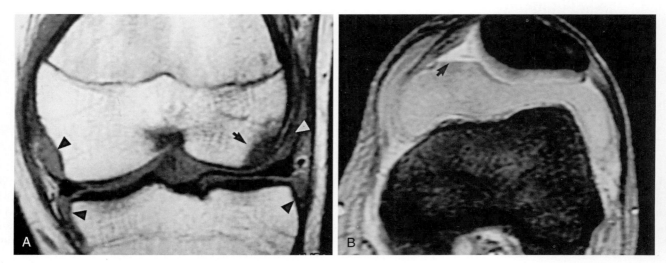

Figure 3–1
Traumatic hemarthrosis.
   A On a coronal T1-weighted (TR/TE, 500/16) spin echo MR image, note the presence of an osteochondral fracture (arrow) of the lateral femoral condyle manifested as low signal intensity in the subchondral bone marrow. A hemarthrosis is present, with blood of intermediate signal intensity filling the joint recesses (arrowheads).
   B A transaxial multiplanar gradient recalled (MPGR) MR image (TR/TE, 266/15; flip angle, 25 degrees) reveals a fluid level (arrow) with the supernatant layer showing high signal intensity.

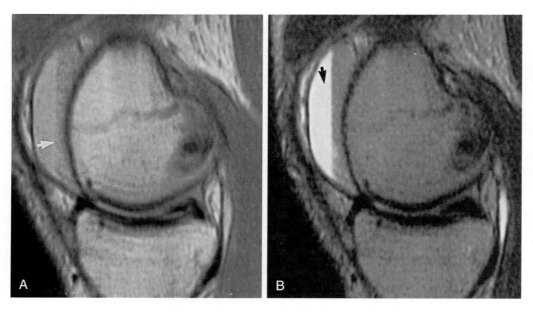

Figure 3–2
Traumatic hemarthrosis.
   A A sagittal proton density-weighted (TR/TE, 2300/30) spin echo MR image reveals a fluid level (arrow) with the supernatant layer showing higher signal intensity. A tear of the posterior horn of the medial meniscus and posterior pericapsular fluid also are evident.
   B On the sagittal T2-weighted (TR/TE, 2300/80) spin echo MR image, note the high signal intensity of the supernatant layer (arrow).

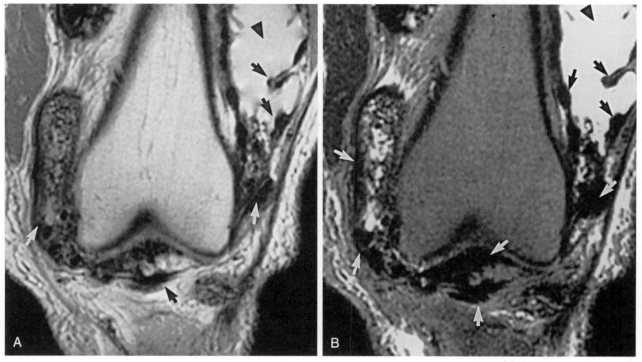

Figure 3–3
Chronic hemarthrosis with hemosiderin accumulation: Pigmented villonodular synovitis. Coronal proton density-weighted (TR/TE, 2700/19) **(A)** and T2-weighted (TR/TE, 2700/80) **(B)** spin echo MR images show joint fluid (arrowheads) of intermediate or high signal intensity and hemosiderin deposition (arrows) in the synovial membrane of persistent low signal intensity. (Courtesy of G. Greenway, M.D., Dallas, Texas.)

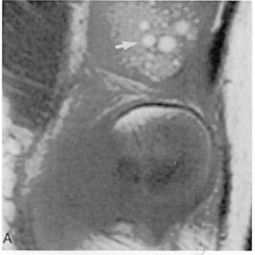

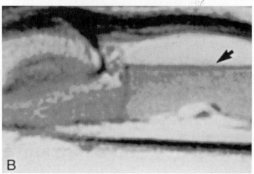

Figure 3–4
Lipohemarthrosis.

A On a coronal T1-weighted (TR/TE, 500/20) spin echo MR image of the knee, globules of fat (arrow) in the suprapatellar pouch, above the patella, are of high signal intensity. The bloody joint effusion is of intermediate signal intensity. (Courtesy of R. Reinke, M.D., Long Beach, California.)

B This sagittal T1-weighted (TR/TE, 900/30) spin echo MR image shows a dominant fluid level (arrow) at the interface of fat (above) and serum (below). The image has been rotated 90 degrees to simulate the orientation of a cross table radiograph. On a T2-weighted spin echo MR image (not shown), the top layer showed intermediate signal intensity. (Courtesy of R. Stiles, M.D., Atlanta, Georgia.)

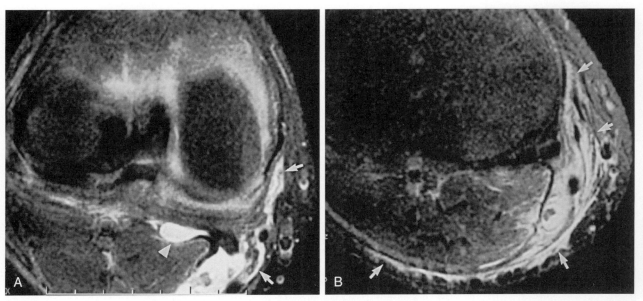

Figure 3–5
Synovial cyst with rupture. Two transaxial fast spin echo MR images of the knee (TR/TE, 2500/40; echo train, 8) obtained with fat suppression reveal a synovial cyst (arrowhead) with extravasation of synovial fluid (arrows) about the medial aspect of the joint (**A**) and, at a lower level (**B**), about the medial aspect of the tibia and adjacent musculature. (Courtesy of R. Loredo, M.D., San Antonio, Texas.)

that make even more complex the MR imaging appearance of a lipohemarthrosis.

TRAUMATIC SYNOVITIS

As an acute response to trauma, the synovial membrane may exhibit hyperemia and edema. Intermediate signal intensity on T1-weighted spin echo images and higher signal intensity on T2-weighted spin echo images of the synovial membrane may be difficult to differentiate from

the signal intensity characteristics of joint fluid.[13] Subsequently, if the response to trauma becomes chronic, thickening of the synovial membrane may be observed on MR images. Resulting synovial plicae and cysts lead to characteristic MR imaging findings (Fig. 3–5).

ADHESIVE CAPSULITIS

Post-traumatic adhesive capsulitis is encountered most frequently in the glenohumeral joint; however, adhesive

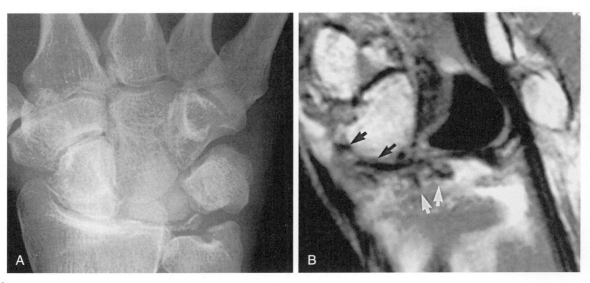

Figure 3–6
Silicone synovitis. This 46 year old man developed progressive pain and swelling of the wrist of several years' duration. More recently, symptoms and signs of a carpal tunnel syndrome had developed. Many years previously, he had had a Silastic lunate prosthesis placed in the wrist for the treatment of Kienböck's disease.
  A The plain film shows fragmentation and an abnormal tilt of the prosthesis with narrowing of the radiocarpal joint, bone fragments, and signs of ulnar impaction characterized by flattening and sclerosis of the triquetrum and styloid process of the ulna.
  B A coronal proton density-weighted (TR/TE, 2000/20) spin echo MR image reveals volar displacement and tilting of the Silastic implant, which is devoid of signal intensity. Note compression of adjacent flexor tendons and silastic fragments (arrows).

capsulitis has also been described in the ankle, hip, and wrist. Although MR imaging may reveal thickening of the articular capsule, arthrographic methods allow more precise diagnosis, and joint distention during arthrography (brisement procedure) can provide temporary relief of symptoms and signs.

FOREIGN BODY SYNOVITIS

The introduction of foreign material into a synovial joint (or into bone or soft tissue) can lead to an inflammatory reaction to the material itself in addition to contamination of the tissue with a variety of infectious agents. Plant thorns and wood splinters are two examples of such material. Others include the metal, polyethylene material, and polymethylmethacrylate cement that are employed for joint replacement, allograft implants that are placed in certain joints such as the temporomandibular joint, and silicone rubber elastomers that are used for replacement of metacarpophalangeal, metatarsophalangeal, and interphalangeal joints, the carpal bones, and the radial head. In some instances, shedding of particles occurs that results in their being embedded in the synovium with resulting synovial hypertrophy, chronic inflammatory and giant cell infiltration of the synovial membrane, and invasion of adjacent bones.

Silicone synovitis is representative of this type of phenomenon.[25] Clinically, painful synovitis occurs months or years after an otherwise uneventful course. Pathologic examination reveals intracellular and extracellular silicone particles.[26, 27] The prosthesis itself may be deformed or broken. Radiographic diagnosis usually is not difficult.[28, 29] MR imaging theoretically may play a role in the diagnosis of this condition; these prostheses and their particles are of low signal intensity on T1-weighted and T2-weighted images (Fig. 3–6).

SUMMARY

Injury to a synovial joint can lead to a variety of abnormalities, which include traumatic effusion, hemarthrosis, lipohemarthrosis, synovial membrane proliferation, and adhesive capsulitis. Although the role of routine radiography in the assessment of such abnormalities is well established, advanced imaging methods, including MR imaging, also can provide useful information.

REFERENCES

1. Davie B: The significance and treatment of haemarthrosis of the knee following trauma. Med J Aust *1*:1355, 1969.
2. Wilkinson A: Traumatic haemarthrosis of the knee. Lancet *2*:13, 1965.
3. Weinberger A, Schumacher HR: Experimental joint trauma: Synovial response to blunt trauma and inflammatory reaction to intraarticular injection of fat. J Rheumatol *8*:380, 1981.
4. Noyes FR, Bassett RW, Grood ES, et al: Arthroscopy in acute traumatic hemarthrosis of the knee. J Bone Joint Surg [Am] *62*:687, 1980
5. Eiskjaer S, Larsen ST, Schmidt MB: The significance of hemarthrosis of the knee in children. Arch Orthop Trauma Surg *107*:96, 1988.
6. Butt WP, Lederman H, Chuang S: Radiology of the suprapatellar region. Clin Radiol *34*:511, 1983.
7. MacEwan DW: Changes due to trauma in the fat plane overlying the pronator quadratus muscle: A radiologic sign. Radiology *82*:879, 1964.
8. Rogers SL, MacEwan DW: Changes due to trauma in the fat plane overlying the supinator muscle: A radiologic sign. Radiology *92*:954, 1969.
9. Bledsoe RC, Izenstark JL: Displacement of fat pads in disease and injury of the elbow: A new radiographic sign. Radiology *73*:717, 1959.
10. Bohrer SP: The fat pad sign following elbow trauma: Its usefulness and reliability in suspecting "invisible fractures." Clin Radiol *21*:90, 1970.
11. Hunter RD: Swollen elbow following trauma. JAMA *230*:1573, 1974.
12. Weston WJ: Joint space widening with intracapsular fractures in joints of the fingers and toes of children. Australas Radiol *15*:367, 1971.
13. White EM: Magnetic resonance imaging in synovial disorders and arthropathy of the knee. MRI Clin North Am *2*:451, 1994.
14. Lawrence C, Seife B: Bone marrow in joint fluid: A clue to fracture. Ann Intern Med *74*:740, 1971.
15. Kling DH: Fat in traumatic effusions of the knee joint. Am J Surg *6*:71, 1929.
16. Berk RN: Liquid fat in the knee joint after trauma. N Engl J Med *277*:1411, 1967.
17. Gregg JR, Nixon JE, DiStefano V: Neutral fat globules in traumatized knees. Clin Orthop *132*:219, 1978.
18. Graham J, Goldman JA: Fat droplets and synovial fluid leukocytes in traumatic arthritis. Arthritis Rheum *21*:76, 1978.
19. Peirce CB, Eaglesham DC: Traumatic lipohemarthrosis of the knee. Radiology *39*:655, 1942.
20. Nelson SW: Some important diagnostic and technical fundamentals in radiology of trauma, with particular emphasis on skeletal trauma. Radiol Clin North Am *4*:241, 1966.
21. Arger PH, Oberkircher PE, Miller WT: Lipohemarthrosis. AJR *121*:97, 1974.
22. Yousefzadeh DK, Jackson JH Jr: Lipohemarthrosis of the elbow joint. Radiology *128*:643, 1978.
23. Train JS, Hermann G: Lipohemarthrosis: Its occurrence with occult cortical fracture of the knee. Orthopedics *3*:416, 1980.
24. Kier R, McCarthy SM: Lipohemarthrosis of the knee: MR imaging. J Comput Assist Tomogr *14*:395, 1990.
25. Atkinson RE, Smith RJ: Silicone synovitis following silicone implant arthroplasty. Hand Clin *2*:291, 1986.
26. Gordon M, Bullough PG: Synovial and osseous inflammation in failed silicone-rubber prostheses. J Bone Joint Surg [Am] *64*:574, 1982.
27. Sammarco GJ, Tabatowski K: Silicone lymphadenopathy associated with failed prosthesis of the hallux: A case report and literature review. Foot Ankle *13*:273, 1992.
28. Rosenthal DI, Rosenberg AE, Schiller AL, et al: Destructive arthritis due to silicone: A foreign-body reaction. Radiology *149*:69, 1983.
29. Schneider HJ, Weiss MA, Stern PJ: Silicone-induced erosive arthritis: Radiologic features in seven cases. AJR *148*:923, 1987.

Synovial Joints: Inflammatory Disorders

Rheumatoid Arthritis
Summary

A variety of disorders lead to synovial inflammation. These include rheumatoid arthritis, the seronegative spondyloarthropathies, juvenile chronic arthritis, crystal deposition diseases, and septic arthritis. In this chapter, mainly rheumatoid arthritis, the prototype of these disorders, is considered. Its MR imaging features are stressed.

RHEUMATOID ARTHRITIS

Magnetic Resonance Imaging

MR imaging can be applied effectively to the evaluation of the patient with rheumatoid arthritis.[1] General applications of MR imaging include detection of articular disease, assessment of activity of such disease, determination of the nature of some of the complications of rheumatoid arthritis, and analysis of the extent of articular and para-articular changes in specific locations, such as the spine and temporomandibular joint.[2]

MR imaging is a very sensitive imaging method in the detection of articular diseases and, in some instances, the imaging abnormalities depicted are almost specific for rheumatoid arthritis.[3–5] Effusions, joint space narrowing, marginal erosions, and subchondral cystic lesions are among the described alterations (Figs. 4–1 and 4–2), and some of these findings have been detected prior to their appearance on routine radiographs.[6–9] Accompanying changes in tendons and tendon sheaths, as well as bursae and soft tissues, can assist in diagnosis (Figs. 4–3, 4–4 and 4–5).[10, 11] Synovial cysts also can be identified (Fig. 4–6). The differentiation of synovial fluid and inflammatory synovial tissue, or pannus, in the rheumatoid joint on standard spin echo and gradient echo sequences may be difficult (although possible),[12] and modification of the MR imaging technique may be required in this situation (see subsequent discussion). Furthermore, direct and accurate assessment of articular cartilage by MR imaging remains a problem, despite the multiple techniques that have been employed.[13, 14]

MR imaging has been used to assess the activity of rheumatoid arthritis and also its response to a variety of therapeutic regimens. A number of investigators have employed gadolinium-containing contrast agents in-

jected intravenously, prior to the MR imaging examination, to better assess the extent of synovial proliferation in the rheumatoid joint.[15–23] If used correctly, with the acquisition of MR images before and immediately after the injection of the gadolinium agent, differentiation of synovial inflammatory tissue and fluid is possible. On routine spin echo studies, without such injection, fluid and pannus will be of low signal intensity on T1-weighted images and high intensity signal characterizes both fluid and pannus on T2-weighted images. Comparison of proton density-weighted and T2-weighted spin echo MR images occasionally may allow the identification of inflamed synovium, thus obviating intravenous administration of a gadolinium agent,[24] but such identification may be difficult. Immediately after intravenous injection of a gadolinium-containing agent, the effusion remains of low signal intensity on T1-weighted spin echo images, and the synovium demonstrates enhancement with increased signal intensity on these images (Figs. 4–7, 4–8, 4–9, and 4–10). Delayed imaging after intravenous injection of the contrast medium is characterized by seepage of contrast material across the inflammatory pannus with an increase in the signal intensity of joint fluid on T1-weighted spin echo images. This seepage is not surprising owing to the small size of the molecules of the gadolinium contrast agents, which enables them to pass freely into the joint.[24] Exercise increases the rate, degree, and uniformity of enhancement of joint fluid.[25] The precise rate of transport of the gadolinium contrast agent depends on molecular size, the permeability of the synovium, bulk flow of fluid from the capillary bed to the joint space, and concentration gradient across the synovium.[24] The changing pattern of distribution of gadolinium-containing agent in the joint has led some investigators to employ rapid gradient echo sequences to allow quantitative assessment of the rate of gadolinium accumulation in the synovial tissue.[18] Despite the nonspecific nature of the findings,[26] the use of intravenous injection of gadolinium contrast agent as an adjunct in MR imaging of joints involved in the rheumatoid process (or in other synovial inflammatory disorders) shows promise as a means to determine the extent of the process and its response to therapy.[19] It should be recognized, however, that the gadolinium compound is costly and that the examination time is increased when images are required both before and after its

Text continued on page 61

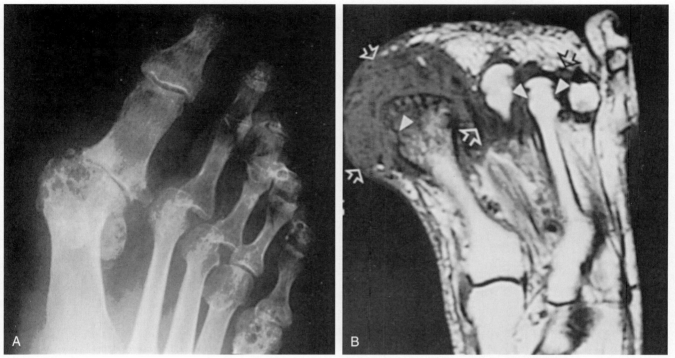

Figure 4–1

Rheumatoid arthritis: Marginal bone erosions and subchondral cysts. Routine radiograph (**A**) and transverse T1-weighted spin echo MR image (TR/TE, 600/20) (**B**) from a 69 year old man with rheumatoid arthritis. In the radiograph, extensive erosions are seen about several metatarsophalangeal joints, especially the first and fifth. Fibular deviation of the toes and dislocation of the second and third metatarsophalangeal joints are apparent. In the MR image, pannus and fluid of low signal intensity within the metatarsophalangeal joints, particularly the first, are evident (open arrows). Note erosions of multiple metatarsal heads (arrowheads).

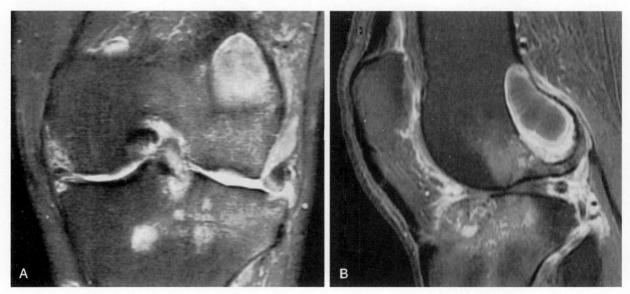

Figure 4–2

Rheumatoid arthritis: Subchondral cysts. A coronal fat-suppressed fast spin echo (TR/TE, 3000/18) MR image (**A**) shows multiple cysts of high signal intensity in the femur and tibia, erosion of articular cartilage, meniscal tears, and marginal bone erosions. Immediately after intravenous injection (**B**) of a gadolinium compound, a sagittal T1-weighted (TR/TE, 600/16) fat-suppressed spin echo MR image shows enhancement of signal intensity in the wall of the femoral cyst, in a tibial cyst, and in the synovial membrane.

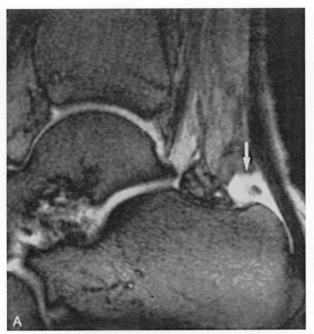

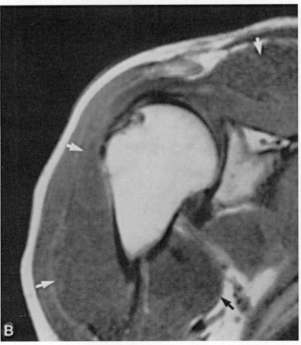

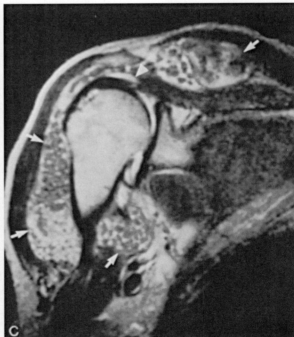

Figure 4–3

Rheumatoid arthritis: Abnormalities of bursae (MR imaging). **A** Retrocalcaneal bursitis. A sagittal gradient echo MR sequence (MPGR) (TR/TE, 500/20; flip angle, 25 degrees) reveals distention of the retrocalcaneal bursa with fluid, the latter appearing of increased signal intensity (arrow). No subjacent calcaneal erosion is apparent. Elsewhere, it is difficult to differentiate between articular cartilage and joint fluid in the ankle and intertarsal articulations.

B, C Subdeltoid-subacromial bursitis. In a 45 year old woman with rheumatoid arthritis, T1-weighted (TR/TE, 505/20) (**B**) and T2-weighted (TR/TE, 2000/80) (**C**) coronal oblique spin echo MR images reveal a markedly distended bursa (arrows). In **C**, note increase in signal intensity of fluid in the joint and in the bursa; however, regions of low signal density remain in the bursa. At surgery, these areas were found to represent small fibrous nodules, or rice bodies. Also note the tear of the supraspinatus tendon (arrowhead in **C**), which may represent a complication of rheumatoid arthritis.

(**B, C**, Courtesy of J. Hodler, M.D., Zurich, Switzerland.)

Figure 4–4

Rheumatoid arthritis: Soft tissue nodules (MR imaging). This 65 year old woman with rheumatoid arthritis had multiple subcutaneous nodules including one in the plantar aspect of the left heel.

A T1-weighted (TR/TE, 600/20) transverse MR image reveals the soft tissue nodule (arrowhead) surrounded by fat, involving the left heel.

B After the intravenous injection of gadolinium, observe diffuse enhancement of the nodule (arrowhead) in an identical T1-weighted MR image.

(Courtesy of S. Moreland, M.D., San Diego, California.)

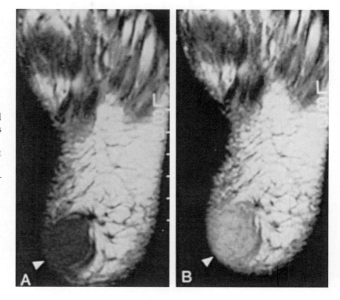

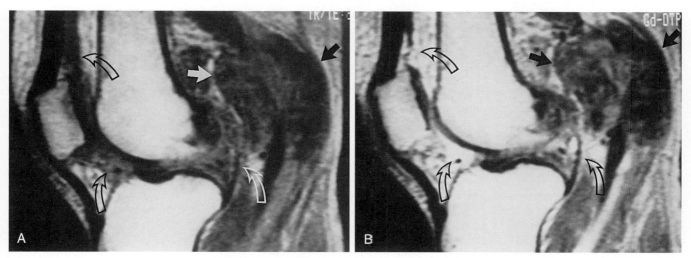

Figure 4–5

Rheumatoid arthritis: Soft tissue nodules (MR imaging). In a 59 year old woman, a sagittal T1-weighted (TR/TE, 800/30) spin echo MR image **(A)** reveals a rheumatoid soft tissue nodule (solid arrows) of low signal intensity posterior to the knee joint. The inflamed synovium (open arrows) also is of low signal intensity. After the intravenous administration of a gadolinium contrast agent **(B)**, a sagittal T1-weighted (TR/TE, 800/30) spin echo MR image reveals irregular and peripheral enhancement of signal intensity in the rheumatoid nodule (solid arrows) and diffuse enhancement of signal intensity in the inflamed synovium (open arrows).

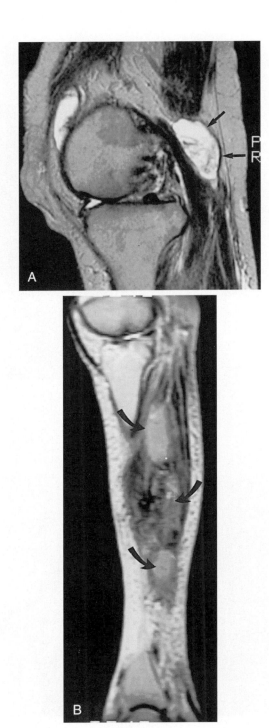

Figure 4–6
Rheumatoid arthritis: Synovial cysts, knee. Sagittal fast spin echo MR images at the level of the knee (TR/TE, 3800/120; echo train, 8) **(A)** and the lower leg (TR/TE, 3600/96; echo train, 8) **(B)** reveal a large dissecting synovial cyst (straight arrows) with intermuscular extension into the calf (curved arrows) in a 69 year old woman. Note inhomogeneity of signal intensity in the cyst and a joint effusion.

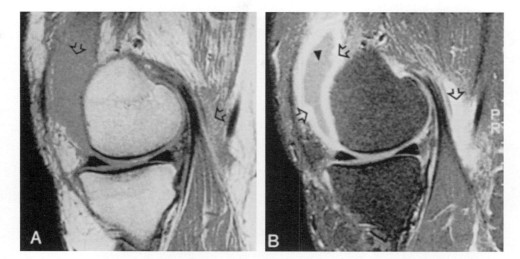

Figure 4–7
Rheumatoid arthritis (MR imaging). Differentiation of effusion and pannus using intravenous gadolinium contrast agent.

A Initial proton density-weighted parasagittal spin echo MR image (TR/TE, 1200/30) prior to intravenous injection of gadolinium compound reveals relatively low signal intensity of fluid or pannus, or both, in the knee joint and within a synovial cyst (open arrows).

B Immediately after the intravenous injection of the gadolinium agent, a proton density-weighted parasagittal spin echo MR image (TR/TE, 1600/30), obtained with fat saturation technique, reveals enhancement of the inflamed synovial membrane in the joint and bursa (open arrows). The fluid (arrowhead) remains of low signal intensity.

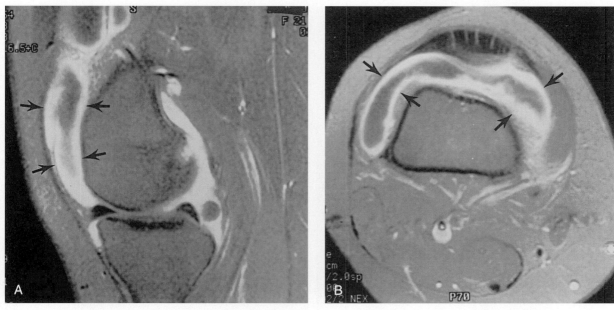

Figure 4–8
Rheumatoid arthritis (MR imaging, differentiation of effusion and pannus using intravenous contrast agent). In a 21 year old woman, sagittal (TR/TE, 549/19) **(A)** and transaxial (TR/TE, 450/17) **(B)** T1-weighted fat-suppressed spin echo MR images obtained after the intravenous administration of a gadolinium compound demonstrate intense uptake of gadolinium in the thickened synovium, particularly in the suprapatellar region (arrows). Some of the contrast agent appears to have seeped into the joint fluid. (Courtesy of S. Eilenberg, M.D., San Diego, California.)

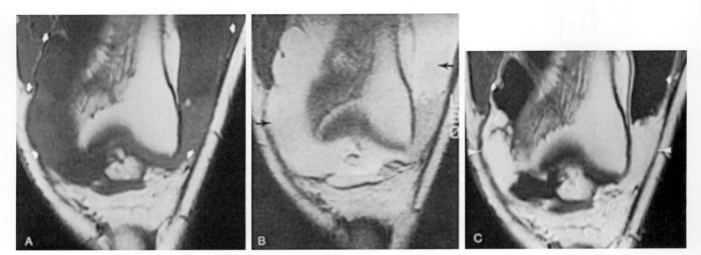

Figure 4–9
Rheumatoid arthritis (MR imaging, differentiation of effusion and pannus using intravenous gadolinium contrast agent). This patient had an acutely swollen knee.

A A coronal T1-weighted spin echo MR image (TR/TE, 800/20) demonstrates collections of low signal intensity distributed throughout the knee (arrows).

B A coronal T2-weighted spin echo MR image (TR/TE, 2000/60) shows diffuse, nearly uniform brightening of these collections (arrows).

C A coronal T1-weighted spin echo MR image (TR/TE, 800/20) after the intravenous administration of gadolinium contrast agent allows clear distinction between joint fluid, which is of low signal intensity (arrows), and inflammatory pannus, which demonstrates enhancement with an increase in signal intensity (arrowheads).

(From Kursunoglu-Brahme S, et al: Radiology *176*:831, 1990.)

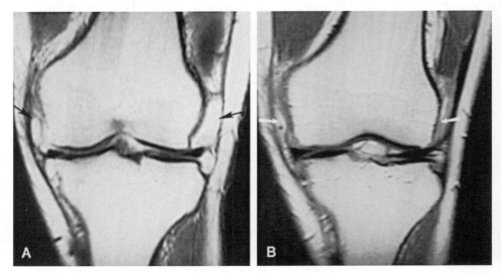

Figure 4–10
Rheumatoid arthritis (MR imaging, monitoring of response to treatment using intravenous gadolinium contrast agent).

A Prior to treatment, a coronal T1-weighted spin echo MR image (TR/TE, 800/20) obtained immediately after the intravenous injection of gadolinium contrast agent reveals collections of enhanced signal intensity (arrows), representing inflammatory pannus.

B One month after arthrocentesis and treatment with intra-articular steroids, a repeat coronal T1-weighted spin echo MR image (TR/TE, 800/20) obtained immediately after the intravenous injection of gadolinium agent shows a decrease in the amount of pannus (arrows) and a loss of signal intensity, presumably reflecting healing and fibrosis of the synovial inflammatory process.

(From Kursunoglu-Brahme S, et al: Radiology *176*:831, 1990.)

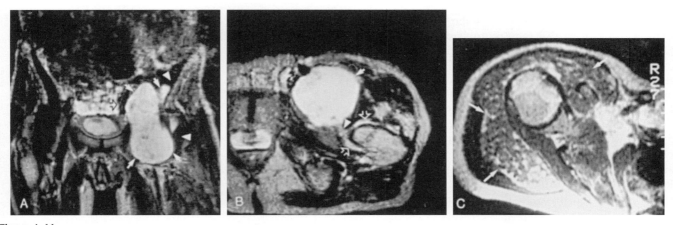

Figure 4–11

Rheumatoid arthritis (MR imaging, identification of bursitis).

A, B Iliopsoas bursitis. A 64 year old man with long-standing rheumatoid arthritis developed a progressively enlarging, painful mass in the left inguinal region. A coronal T2-weighted spin echo MR image (TR/TE, 2000/90) **(A)** shows the cyst (solid arrows) medial to the psoas muscle (arrowheads) and lateral to the external iliac vessels (open arrow). A transaxial T2-weighted spin echo MR image (TR/TE, 2000/90) **(B)** again reveals the cyst (solid arrow) with an opening (arrowhead) to a fluid-filled hip joint (open arrows). At surgery, a grossly dilated fluid-filled iliopsoas bursa, with chronically inflamed synovium, was identified.

(**A, B**, From Lupetin AR, Daffner RH: J Comput Assist Tomogr *14*:1035, 1990.)

C Subacromial bursitis. In this 34 year old woman, a transaxial T2-weighted spin echo MR image (TR/TE, 1800/70) shows the distended bursa (arrows) containing fluid of high signal intensity and areas of low signal intensity, perhaps representing fibrous synovial nodules.

(**C**, Courtesy of J. Milsap, Jr., M.D., Atlanta, Georgia.)

injection. Furthermore, some of the newer MR imaging sequences, such as three-dimensional or volumetric acquisition using gradient recalled echo techniques, including gradient recalled acquisition in the steady state (GRASS) with spoiling (SPGR) or fast low-angle shot (FLASH), when combined with fat suppression, or newer methods, such as magnetization transfer contrast sequences, may allow differentiation of inflamed syno-

vium and fluid without the requirement for the intravenous injection of gadolinium agent.[27, 28]

A variety of musculoskeletal complications of rheumatoid arthritis are well evaluated with MR imaging. These include ischemic necrosis of bone, bursitis, synovial cyst formation, tendon injury and disruption, and insufficiency fractures. Fluid collections and abnormal synovium within the iliopsoas, subdeltoid-subacromial, retro-

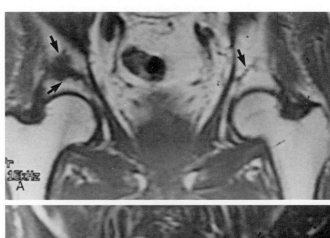
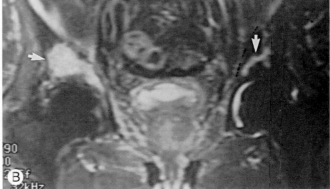

Figure 4–12

Rheumatoid arthritis (MR imaging, insufficiency type of stress fracture—innominate bone).

A A coronal T1-weighted (TR/TE, 800/11) spin echo MR image shows bilateral fractures of the ilii manifested as regions of low signal intensity (arrows).

B A coronal short tau inversion recovery (STIR) MR image (TR/TE, 5600/52; inversion time, 150 msec) shows these same fractures as regions of high signal intensity (arrows). Note the joint effusion in the left hip.

calcaneal, olecranon, and prepatellar bursae are easily demonstrated with this technique (Fig. 4–11).[29, 30] Similarly, synovial cysts about any involved joint are delineated with MR imaging.[31] In superficial joints, such as the knee, ultrasonography is equally effective in the assessment of such synovial cysts, although in deeper locations, including the hip and spine, MR imaging has distinct advantages. Tendon injury and rupture are best assessed with MR imaging. Insufficiency fractures reveal characteristic signal intensity abnormalities with MR imaging (Fig. 4–12). Indeed, MR imaging is at least equivalent and probably superior to bone scintigraphy with regard to its sensitivity in the detection of these fractures.

SUMMARY

Routine radiography remains the most important imaging technique in the assessment of rheumatoid arthritis and other synovial inflammatory processes. An occasional role exists for more advanced imaging methods in this assessment, particularly in the initial detection of disease, in the assessment of its extent, and in the identification of complications of the disease process.

REFERENCES

1. Winalski CS, Palmer WE, Rosenthal DI, et al: Magnetic resonance imaging of rheumatoid arthritis. Radiol Clin North Am 34:243, 1996.
2. Kaye JJ: Arthritis: Roles of radiography and other imaging techniques in evaluation. Radiology 177:601, 1990.
3. Foley-Nolan D, Stack JP, Ryan M, et al: Magnetic resonance imaging in the assessment of rheumatoid arthritis—a comparison with plain film radiographs. Br J Rheumatol 30:101, 1991.
4. Beltran J, Caudill JL, Herman LA, et al: Rheumatoid arthritis: MR imaging manifestations. Radiology 165:153, 1987.
5. Gilkeson G, Polisson R, Sinclair H, et al: Early detection of carpal erosions in patients with rheumatoid arthritis: A pilot study of magnetic resonance imaging. J Rheumatol 15:1361, 1988.
6. Kieft GJ, Dijkmans BAC, Bloem JL, et al: Magnetic resonance imaging of the shoulder in patients with rheumatoid arthritis. Ann Rheum Dis 49:7, 1990.
7. Moore EA, Jacoby RK, Ellis RE, et al: Demonstration of a geode by magnetic resonance imaging: A new light on the cause of juxta-articular bone cysts in rheumatoid arthritis. Ann Rheum Dis 49:785, 1990.
8. Poleksic L, Zdravkovic D, Jablanovic D, et al: Magnetic resonance imaging of bone destruction in rheumatoid arthritis: comparison with radiography. Skel Radiol 22:577, 1993.
9. Sugimoto H, Takeda A, Masuyami J, et al: Early-stage rheumatoid arthritis: Diagnostic accuracy of MR imaging. Radiology 198:185, 1996.
10. Sanchez RB, Quinn SF: MRI of inflammatory synovial processes. Magn Res Imaging 7:529, 1989.
11. Rubens DJ, Blebea JS, Totterman SMS, et al: Rheumatoid arthritis: Evaluation of wrist extensor tendons with clinical examination versus MR imaging—a preliminary report. Radiology 187:831, 1993.
12. Singson RD, Zalduondo FM: Value of unenhanced spin-echo MR imaging in distinguishing between synovitis and effusion of the knee. AJR 159:569, 1992.
13. Yao L, Sinha S, Seeger LL: MR imaging of joints: Analytic optimization of GRE techniques at 1.5T. AJR 158:339, 1992.
14. Rominger MB, Bernreuter WK, Kenney PJ, et al: MR imaging of the hands in early rheumatoid arthritis: Preliminary results. RadioGraphics 13:37, 1993.
15. Smith H-J, Larheim TA, Aspestrand F: Rheumatic and nonrheumatic disease in the temporomandibular joint: Gadolinium-enhanced MR imaging. Radiology 185:229, 1992.
16. Reiser MF, Bongartz GP, Erlemann R, et al: Gadolinium-DTPA in rheumatoid arthritis and related diseases: First results with dynamic magnetic resonance imaging. Skel Radiol 18:591, 1989.
17. Bjorkengren AG, Geborek P, Rydholm U, et al: MR imaging of the knee in acute rheumatoid arthritis: Synovial uptake of gadolinium-DOTA. AJR 155:329, 1990.
18. König H, Sieper J, Wolf K-J: Rheumatoid arthritis: Evaluation of hypervascular and fibrous pannus with dynamic MR imaging enhanced with Gd-DTPA. Radiology 176:473, 1990.
19. Kursunoglu-Brahme S, Riccio T, Weisman MH, et al: Rheumatoid knee: Role of gadopentetate-enhanced MR imaging. Radiology 176:831, 1990.
20. Yanagawa A, Takano K, Nishioka K, et al: Clinical staging and gadolinium-DTPA enhanced images of the wrist in rheumatoid arthritis. J Rheumatol 20:781, 1993.
21. Waterton JC, Rajanayagam V, Ross BD, et al: Magnetic resonance methods for measurement of disease progression in rheumatoid arthritis. Magn Res Imaging 11:1033, 1993.
22. Gubler FM, Algra PR, Dijkstra PF, et al: Gadolinium-DTPA enhanced magnetic resonance imaging of bone cysts in patients with rheumatoid arthritis. Ann Rheum Dis 52:716, 1993.
23. Ostergaard M, Gideon P, Henrikson O, et al: Synovial volume — a marker of disease activity in rheumatoid arthritis? Quantification by MRI. Scand J Rheumatol 23:197, 1994.
24. Winalski CS: Gadolinium enhancement for assessment of articular disorders. RSNA Categorical Course in Musculoskeletal Radiology 1993, p. 25.
25. Winalski CS, Aliabadi P, Wright RJ, et al: Enhancement of joint fluid with intravenously administered gadopentetate dimeglumine: Technique, rationale, and implications. Radiology 187:179, 1993.
26. Pages M, Poey C, Lassoued S, et al: MR imaging of the knee in rheumatoid arthritis and other rheumatic diseases. AJR 157:1128, 1991.
27. Peterfy CG, Majumdar S, Lang P, et al: MR imaging of the arthritic knee: Improved discrimination of cartilage, synovium, and effusion with pulsed saturation transfer and fat-suppressed T1-weighted sequences. Radiology 191:413, 1994.
28. Carpenter TA, Everett JR, Hall LD, et al: High-resolution magnetic resonance imaging of arthritic pathology in the rat knee. Skel Radiol 23:429, 1994.
29. Varma DGK, Richli WR, Charnsangavej C, et al: MR appearance of the distended iliopsoas bursa. AJR 156:1025, 1991.
30. Steinfeld R, Rock MG, Younge DA, et al: Massive subacromial bursitis with rice bodies: Report of three cases, one of which was bilateral. Clin Orthop 301:185, 1994.
31. Butler MG, Fuchigami KD, Chako A: MRI of posterior knee masses. Skeletal Radiol 25:309, 1996.

5 | Synovial Joints: Bleeding Disorders

Hemophilia
Bleeding Diatheses and Hemangiomas
Summary

Hemophilia is a term applied to a group of disorders characterized by an anomaly of blood coagulation due to a deficiency in a specific plasma clotting factor. This anomaly leads to easy bruising and prolonged and excessive bleeding. Several other vascular disorders, including the Klippel-Trenaunay and Kasabach-Merritt syndromes, may lead to osteoarticular manifestations that simulate those of hemophilia. The MR imaging features of these bleeding disorders are summarized here.

HEMOPHILIA

The remarkable ability of MR imaging to define soft tissue abnormalities and, specifically, hematomas provides an indication of its promising potential in the evaluation of intra-articular and extra-articular hemorrhagic manifestations of hemophilia.[1-3] With regard to the intra-articular abnormalities of hemophilia, MR imaging allows assessment of the extent of the process and provides information on its nature.[4-7] Histologic abnormalities in hemophilic arthropathy depend on the stage of the disease: Initial episodes of bleeding lead to mild proliferation of synovial cells, acute perivascular inflammation, and synovial accumulation of iron from sequestered red blood cells; repeated hemarthroses produce villous hypertrophy and increased vascularity of the synovial membrane, the accumulation of hemosiderin in synovial and subsynovial macrophages, and an infiltrating pannus composed of dense, avascular, acellular fibrous tissue that adheres tightly to the cartilage; with chronicity, a fibrotic synovium develops.[8] In view of this varied and changing articular environment, the MR imaging features of hemophilic arthropathy are not uniform.

Most of the reported investigations of hemophilic arthropathy using MR imaging have focused on the knee. Spin echo sequences, employed in most of these investigations, have revealed regions in the joint with low to intermediate signal intensity on T1- and T2-weighted images, with foci of increased signal intensity on T2-weighted images (Figs. 5–1 and 5–2).[5] Persistent low signal intensity in both types of images is consistent with the presence of synovial fibrosis or hemosiderin deposition, or both. The foci of high signal intensity on the T2-weighted images are consistent with areas of synovial inflammation or fluid. Owing to the changing signal characteristics of resolving hemorrhage, it may be difficult to distinguish between viscous joint fluid and fresh blood with MR imaging in this disease.[5] The role of intravenous administration of paramagnetic contrast agents, such as those containing gadolinium, in the differentiation among synovial inflammation, hemorrhage, and joint effusion in hemophilia has not yet been established.

The MR imaging characteristics of hemosiderin deposition in this disease are similar to those in other disorders accompanied by recurrent episodes of intra-articular bleeding. Such processes include pigmented villonodular synovitis, neoplasms such as synovial hemangiomas, neuropathic osteoarthropathy, and chronic renal disease. Hemosiderin collections lead to low signal intensity on all spin echo sequences and, to a greater degree, on all gradient echo sequences. The deposits of hemosiderin within the synovial membrane are accentuated, in some sequences, by the presence of adjacent fluid and synovial inflammation of high signal intensity.

As in other arthritic conditions, MR imaging may be used to assess the degree of cartilaginous and osseous destruction in hemophilia.[4, 5, 7] Subchondral cystic lesions, a prominent feature of hemophilic arthropathy, may be evaluated with MR imaging. The signal characteristics of these cysts, however, are dependent on the precise imaging sequence that is used and the contents of the lesions. Fluid, fibrotic material, hemorrhage, or hemosiderin, in various combinations, may be present in the subchondral cysts.

Hemophilic pseudotumors also may be evaluated with MR imaging (Fig. 5–3).[4, 9] The signal behavior of these pseudotumors is complex, reflecting the effects of remote and recurrent bleeding and clot organization.[9] A peripheral margin of low signal intensity on T1- and T2-weighted spin echo MR imaging sequences is consistent with the presence of fibrous tissue or hemosiderin, or both, in the wall of the pseudotumor. Less uniform, however, are the signal characteristics of the interior portions of the pseudotumor, which may reveal regions of either high or low signal intensity on one or both of these sequences.

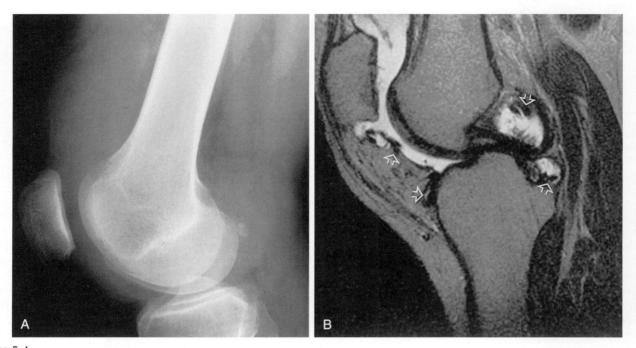

Figure 5–1
Hemophilia (MR imaging, knee).
  A Routine radiography reveals a large joint effusion.
  B A sagittal T2-weighted (TR/TE, 2000/80) spin echo MR image shows joint fluid of high signal intensity. Note regions of low signal intensity (arrows), consistent with hemosiderin deposition.
  (Courtesy of D. Goodwin, M.D., Hanover, New Hampshire.)

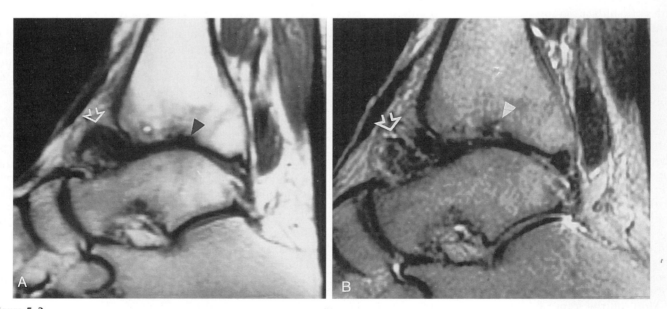

Figure 5–2
Hemophilia (MR imaging, ankle).
  A On a sagittal T1-weighted (TR/TE, 500/16) spin echo MR image, observe anterior extension of the joint (arrow). The intra-articular contents are of low signal intensity. Irregularity of the subchondral bone of the tibia is evident (arrowhead).
  B On a sagittal T2-weighted (TR/TE, 2000/80) spin echo MR image, note persistent low signal intensity anteriorly with peripheral regions of higher signal intensity (arrow). Abnormal signal intensity also is seen in the tibia (arrowhead). The articular findings indicate synovial fibrosis or hemosiderin deposition (low signal intensity) and inflammation (high signal intensity).

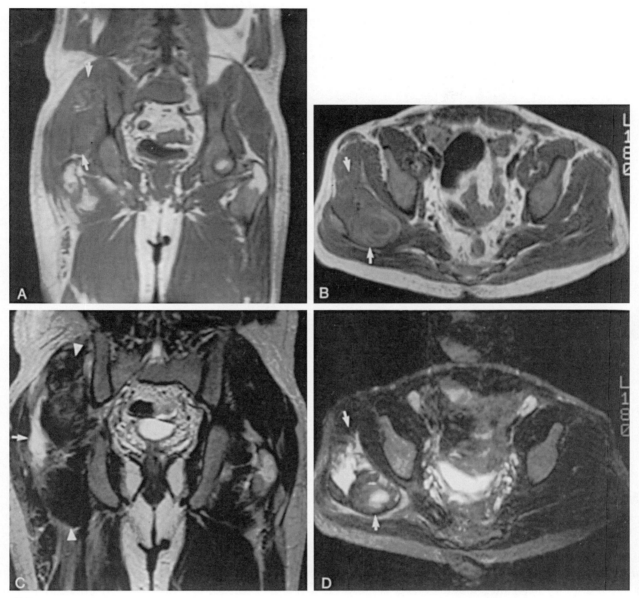

Figure 5–3

Hemophilia (MR imaging, pseudotumor).

A A T1-weighted (TR/TE, 600/10) spin echo MR image in the coronal plane reveals a large soft tissue mass (arrows), involving mainly the gluteus medius muscle. It is inhomogeneous in signal intensity, with some regions of the mass revealing signal intensity identical to that of muscle and other regions having greater signal intensity than muscle.

B A transaxial T1-weighted (TR/TE, 500/11) spin echo MR image confirms the presence of an intramuscular mass (arrows) with signal inhomogeneity.

C A coronal T2-weighted (TR/TE, 6000/102) fast spin echo MR image shows regions of low signal intensity, similar to that of muscle, and of very high signal intensity (arrow) in the mass. Note the full extent of the pseudotumor (between arrowheads).

D A transaxial T2-weighted (TR/TE, 8500/102) fast spin echo MR image, obtained with fat suppression technique (chemical presaturation), reveals the inhomogeneity of the signal intensity in the mass (arrows). Note its proximity to the ischium.

(Courtesy of M. Schweitzer, M.D., Philadelphia, Pennsylvania.)

BLEEDING DIATHESES AND HEMANGIOMAS

Hemangiomas are vascular tumors, most frequently located in the skin. They also may arise within the synovial membrane, especially that of the knee.[10, 11] Hemangiomas may be associated with unusual syndromes, some of which produce hematologic abnormality. The association of varicose veins, soft tissue and bone hypertrophy, and cutaneous hemangiomas is known as the Klippel-Trenaunay syndrome.[12] When an arteriovenous fistula occurs in this syndrome, the disorder commonly is termed the Parke-Weber syndrome.[13] The association of papillary hemangiomas and extensive purpura is designated the Kasabach-Merritt syndrome.[14–16]

Although MR imaging findings of soft tissue hemangiomas have been well described, synovial hemangiomas have received little attention.[10, 17, 18] Typically, synovial hemangiomas are of low or intermediate signal intensity on T1-weighted spin echo MR images and of high signal intensity on T2-weighted spin echo MR images (Fig. 5–4).[17] Fibrofatty septa within the synovial

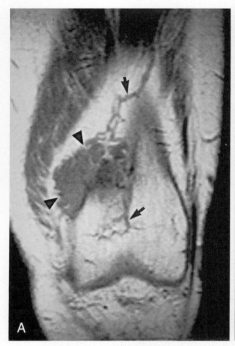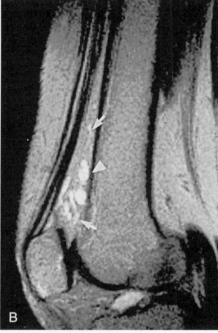

Figure 5–4
Synovial hemangioma (MR imaging, knee).

A A coronal T1-weighted (TR/TE, 677/25) spin echo MR image reveals a lobulated lesion (arrowheads) of low signal intensity applied to the anteromedial aspect of the femur. Note the presence of adjacent prominent vascular channels (arrows).

B A sagittal T2-weighted (TR/TE, 3481/120) spin echo MR image shows the lesion (arrowhead) and adjacent vessels (arrows), both of high signal intensity.

(Courtesy of T. Hughes, M.D., Christchurch, New Zealand.)

mass also may be evident. Serpentine structures, regions of signal void related to rapidly flowing blood, and fluid levels are additional findings that may be seen. Mass effect is unusual, and enhancement of signal intensity after intravenous administration of a gadolinium compound may be seen.

SUMMARY

The skeletal abnormalities associated with hemophilia and other bleeding diatheses are characteristic. Tumor-like lesions occasionally may be encountered owing to massive subperiosteal, osseous, or soft tissue hemorrhage. Hemosiderin deposition in any of these disorders leads to characteristic findings with MR imaging.

REFERENCES

1. Pettersson H, Gilbert MS: Diagnostic Imaging in Hemophilia. Berlin, Springer-Verlag, 1985.
2. Cohen MD, McGuire W, Cory DA, et al: MR appearance of blood and blood products: An in vitro study. AJR *146:*1293, 1986.
3. Kulkarni MV, Drolshagen LF, Kaye JJ, et al: MR imaging of hemophiliac arthropathy. J Comput Assist Tomogr *10:*445, 1986.
4. Hermann G, Gilbert MS, Abdelwahab IF: Hemophilia: Evaluation of musculoskeletal involvement with CT, sonography, and MR imaging. AJR *158:*119, 1992.
5. Yulish BS, Lieberman JM, Strandjord SE, et al: Hemophilic arthropathy: Assessment with MR imaging. Radiology *164:*759, 1987.
6. Armstrong SJ: Case report 661. Skel Radiol *20:*369, 1991.
7. Pettersson H, Gillespy T, Kitchens C, et al: Magnetic resonance imaging in hemophilic arthropathy of the knee. Acta Radiol *28:*621, 1987.
8. Madhok R, Bennett D, Sturrock RD, et al: Mechanisms of joint damage in an experimental model of hemophilic arthritis. Arthritis Rheum *31:*1148, 1988.
9. Wilson DA, Prince JR: MR imaging of hemophilic pseudotumors. AJR *150:*349, 1988.
10. Lenchik L, Poznanski AK, Donaldson JS, et al: Case report 681. Skel Radiol *20:*387, 1991.
11. Aalberg JR: Synovial hemangioma of the knee: A case report. Acta Orthop Scand *61:*88, 1990.
12. Klippel M, Trenaunay P: Du naevus variqueux osteo-hypertrophique. Arch Gen Med *185:*641, 1900.
13. Weber FP: Hemangiectatic hypertrophy of limbs—congenital phlebacteriectasis and so-called congenital varicose veins. Br J Child Dis *15:*13, 1918.
14. Kasabach HH, Merritt KK: Capillary hemangioma with extensive purpura: Report of a case. Am J Dis Child *59:*1063, 1940.
15. Inceman S, Tangün Y: Chronic defibrination syndrome due to a giant hemangioma associated with microangiopathic hemolytic anemia. Am J Med *46:*997, 1969.
16. Rodriguez-Erdmann F: Bleeding due to increased intravascular blood coagulation: Hemorrhagic syndromes caused by consumption of blood-clotting factors (consumption-coagulopathies). N Engl J Med *273:*1370, 1965.
17. Llauqer J, Monill JM, Palmer J, et al: Synovial hemangioma of the knee: MRI findings in two cases. Skel Radiol *24:*579, 1995.
18. Greenspan A, Azouz EM, Matthews J II, et al: Synovial hemangioma: Imaging features in eight histologically proven cases, review of the literature, and differential diagnosis. Skel Radiol *24:*583, 1995.

Pigmented Villonodular Synovitis and Idiopathic Synovial Osteochondromatosis

---

Pigmented Villonodular Synovitis
Idiopathic Synovial Osteochondromatosis
Summary

A great number of tumors and tumor-like processes may involve synovium-lined joints and surrounding tissues. Two of these processes deserve special emphasis owing to their relative frequency and distinctive MR imaging abnormalities.

PIGMENTED VILLONODULAR SYNOVITIS

This synovial proliferative disorder of unknown cause typically occurs in adults in the third or fourth decade of life but also appears less frequently in older adults, adolescents, and even children. The knee is the most common site of involvement.

With MR imaging, the deposition of hemosiderin in cases of pigmented villonodular synovitis leads to dramatic abnormalities characterized by regions of low signal intensity on both T1- and T2-weighted spin echo MR images (Figs. 6–1 to 6–3) and, especially, on gradient echo MR images.[1–9] High signal intensity on T2-weighted spin echo MR images also is observed, indicative of the presence of joint fluid, and distinctive intraosseous cystic lesions containing hemosiderin within their walls have been emphasized in some reports.[7] The presence of hemosiderin deposition on MR images is a finding consistent with the diagnosis of pigmented villonodular synovitis, but it also is evident in some cases of hemophilia and other bleeding disorders, synovial hemangioma, neuropathic osteoarthropathy, and other processes associated with chronic hemarthrosis. MR imaging also may reveal the extent of bone involvement in diffuse pigmented villonodular synovitis and may allow the diagnosis of the localized or nodular form of the disease.[10–12] The MR imaging characteristics of the localized or nodular type of lesion are varied; typically, low signal intensity is evident on both T1-weighted and T2-weighted spin echo images (Fig. 6–4), although the mass may not contain hemosiderin. Enhancement of signal intensity following the intravenous administration of gadolinium occurs in vascular portions of the lesion, a phenomenon that also occurs in portions of the synovium in cases of diffuse pigmented villonodular synovitis. The localized, nodular, intra-articular variety of the disorder shows a tendency to involve the anterior infrapatellar portion of the knee.

IDIOPATHIC SYNOVIAL OSTEOCHONDROMATOSIS

Idiopathic synovial (osteo)chondromatosis is an unusual condition involving joints with or without extension into nearby bursae. It results from metaplasia of subsynovial connective tissue into cartilage nodules that subsequently may calcify or ossify. The cause of the condition is not clear. The clinical onset of idiopathic synovial (osteo)chondromatosis varies from childhood to the seventh or eighth decade of life, although most affected patients are young and middle-aged adults.[13, 14] The two most frequent sites of involvement are the knee and the hip.

The MR imaging abnormalities depend on the stage of the disease.[15–19] In cases of synovial chondromatosis, in which intrasynovial cartilage nodules are uncalcified, the signal intensity of the process resembles that of fluid, being low on T1-weighted spin echo MR images and high on T2-weighted spin echo MR images (Fig. 6–5), and the condition may be misdiagnosed as a joint effusion. The presence of lobulated nodules of high signal intensity and fibrous septa of low signal intensity on the T2-weighted images, however, usually allows the differentiation of synovial chondromatosis from joint fluid in most cases. In cases of synovial (osteo)chondromatosis, foci of calcification appear as regions of low signal intensity on both T1- and T2-weighted images (Fig. 6–6), and with extensive calcification and ossification, ringlike structures with peripheral rims of low signal intensity and central regions of higher signal intensity identical to that of fat or cartilage are seen (Fig. 6–7). MR imaging also shows sites of bone erosion in this disorder. Enhancement of signal intensity after intravenous administration of a gadolinium compound is noted in involved synovium.

Synovial chondrosarcoma is extremely rare.[20–26] The lesion may occur as a primary process or, more commonly, secondary to idiopathic synovial (osteo)chondromatosis. Adults are affected, and the knee and the hip

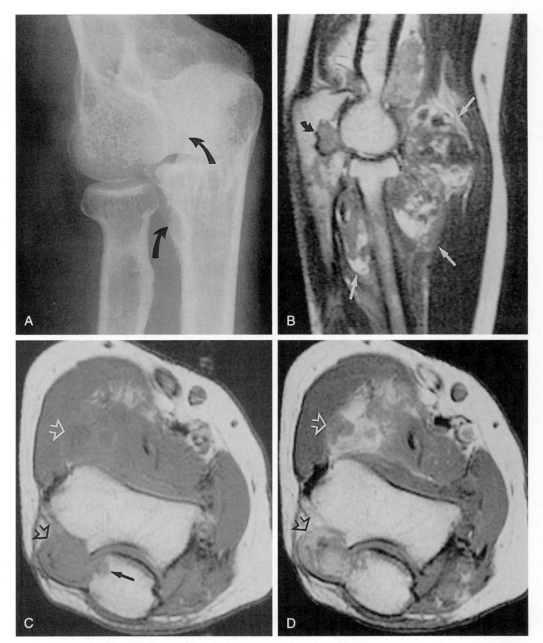

Figure 6–1

Diffuse (intra-articular) pigmented villonodular synovitis: MR imaging.

A A routine radiograph shows bone erosions of the ulna (arrows).

B A sagittal T2-weighted (TR/TE, 3000/85) spin echo MR image reveals a mass with both intra-articular and extra-articular components (straight arrows). Regions of high signal intensity may represent fluid or synovial inflammatory tissue. Note also that portions of the mass are of intermediate signal intensity and, anteriorly, of low signal intensity. The foci of low signal intensity are compatible with hemosiderin deposition. Ulnar bone erosion is seen (curved arrow).

C, D Transaxial T1-weighted (TR/TE, 650/16) spin echo MR images before (**C**) and after (**D**) the intravenous administration of a gadolinium compound show the mass (open arrows), which reveals enhancement of signal intensity in **D,** and bone erosion (solid arrow).

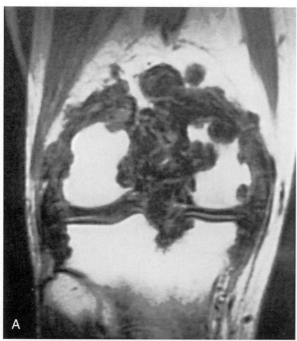

Figure 6–2

Diffuse (intra-articular) pigmented villonodular synovitis: MR imaging.

A A coronal T1-weighted (TR/TE, 650/28) spin echo MR image of the knee shows nodular soft tissue masses of low signal intensity, with joint distension and erosions of the femur and tibia.

B, C In this elbow, sagittal T1-weighted (TR/TE, 800/12) **(B)** and T2-weighted (TR/TE, 2000/80) **(C)** spin echo MR images show diffuse involvement of the joint with a process that has eroded bone (arrows) and is associated with regions of persistent low signal intensity (arrowheads). This degree of bone erosion is encountered more frequently in tight articulations such as the elbow. (Courtesy of J. Spaeth, M.D., Albuquerque, New Mexico.)

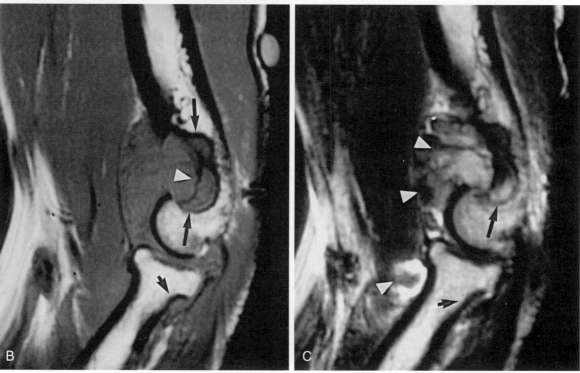

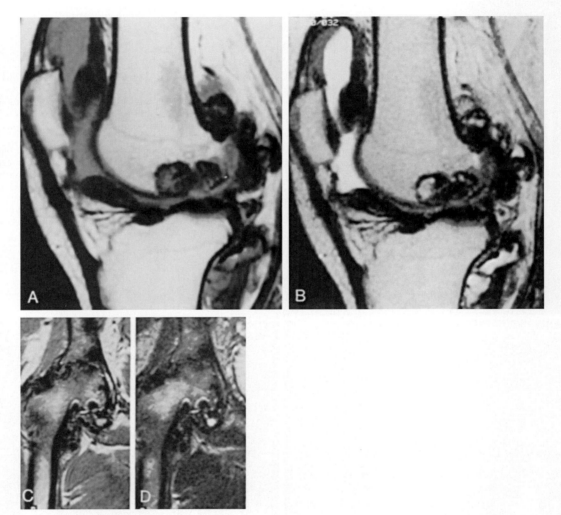

Figure 6–3

Diffuse (intra-articular) pigmented villonodular synovitis: MR imaging.

A, B Knee. Sagittal proton density (TR/TE, 2000/20) **(A)** and T2-weighted (TR/TE, 2000/80) **(B)** spin echo MR images show classic features of this disease. A joint effusion is of intermediate signal intensity in **A** and high signal intensity in **B**. Hemosiderin deposition accounts for the low signal intensity in the synovial nodules in **A** and **B**. Note the erosions of the distal end of the femur. (Courtesy of T. Broderick, M.D., Orange, California.)

C, D Hip. Coronal proton density (TR/TE, 2216/28) **(C)** and T2-weighted (TR/TE, 2216/80) **(D)** spin echo MR images reveal regions of persistent low signal intensity in the right hip. Additional findings include erosions of the femoral neck and acetabulum, joint space loss, and a small amount of articular fluid appearing of high signal intensity in **D**. (Courtesy of P. Fenton, M.D., Toronto, Ontario, Canada.)

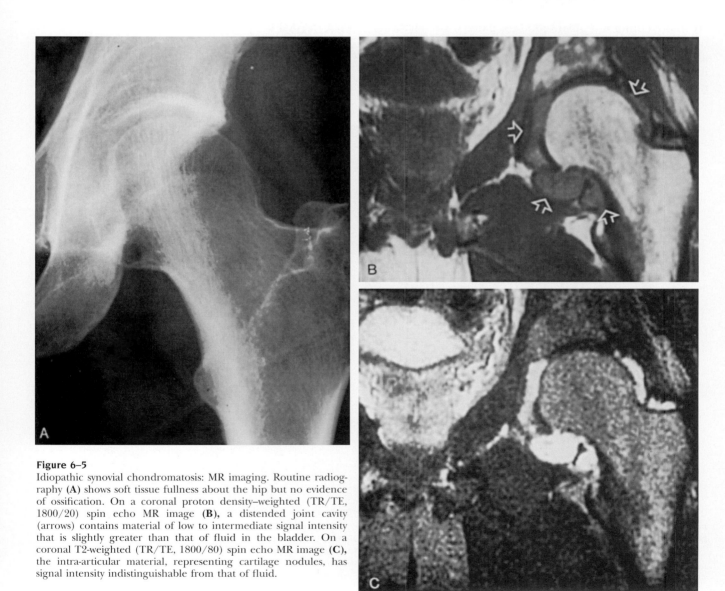

Figure 6–4
Localized nodular synovitis: MR imaging. This sagittal T2-weighted (TR/TE, 1800/80) spin echo MR image shows a mass occupying the anterior aspect of the knee and infrapatellar fat body. The mass is not homogeneous in signal intensity. Some regions reveal intermediate signal intensity; others, consistent with hemosiderin deposits, are of very low signal intensity (arrow). A small joint effusion is present. (Courtesy of G.S. Huang, M.D., Taipei, Taiwan.)

Figure 6–5
Idiopathic synovial chondromatosis: MR imaging. Routine radiography (A) shows soft tissue fullness about the hip but no evidence of ossification. On a coronal proton density–weighted (TR/TE, 1800/20) spin echo MR image (B), a distended joint cavity (arrows) contains material of low to intermediate signal intensity that is slightly greater than that of fluid in the bladder. On a coronal T2-weighted (TR/TE, 1800/80) spin echo MR image (C), the intra-articular material, representing cartilage nodules, has signal intensity indistinguishable from that of fluid.

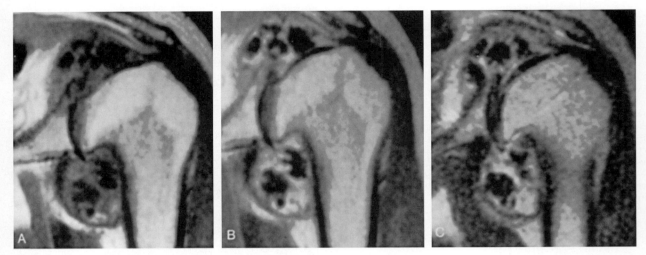

Figure 6–6
Idiopathic synovial (osteo)chondromatosis: MR imaging. Coronal oblique T1-weighted (TR/TE, 570/25) **(A)**, intravenous gadolinium-enhanced T1-weighted (TR/TE, 570/25) **(B)**, and T2-weighted (TR/TE, 1800/80) **(C)** spin echo MR images show a distended glenohumeral joint containing fluid of high signal intensity in **B** and **C** and calcified and ossified bodies of low signal intensity in all three images. (Courtesy of C. Ho, M.D., San Francisco, California.)

are most commonly involved. The pattern of calcification may be more irregular than that associated with idiopathic synovial (osteo)chondromatosis, and a poorly marginated mass with inhomogeneous signal intensity may be evident with MR imaging (Fig. 6–8).

SUMMARY

Of the tumors and tumor-like processes that involve synovium-lined joints, pigmented villonodular synovitis and idiopathic synovial osteochondromatosis are en-

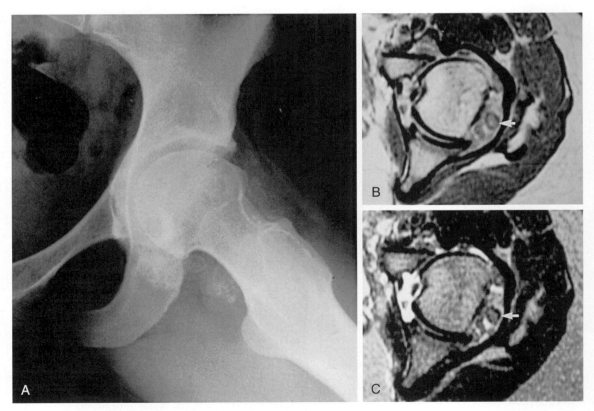

Figure 6–7
Idiopathic synovial (osteo)chondromatosis: MR imaging. This 23 year old woman had a 5 year history of increasing hip pain.
　A A routine radiograph shows ossified regions within the hip. Osteophytes about the femoral head–femoral neck junction are seen.
　B, C Transaxial proton density–weighted (TR/TE, 2200/30) **(B)** and T2-weighted (TR/TE, 2200/80) **(C)** spin echo MR images reveal ossified masses within a fluid-filled hip joint. Note the ringlike appearance (arrows) of the ossified bodies.
　(Courtesy of G. Greenway, M.D., Dallas, Texas.)

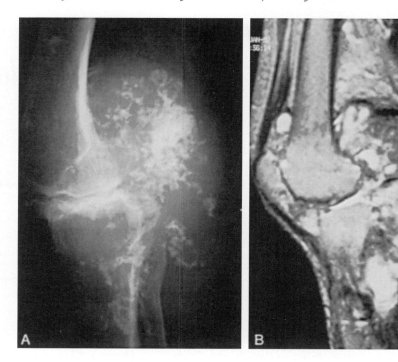

Figure 6–8
Synovial chondrosarcoma: Radiographic and MR imaging abnormalities. This 65 year old man had had knee swelling for 15 years. A synovial chondrosarcoma had been documented at surgery more than 10 years previously, although the patient refused to undergo amputation of the limb at that time.

A A lateral radiograph of the knee shows an irregularly calcified soft tissue mass behind the knee.

B A sagittal T2-weighted (TR/TE, 2500/90) spin echo MR image reveals the extra-articular and intra-articular components of the tumor. Its signal intensity is inhomogeneous, although in places it is encapsulated. A resection of the mass confirmed the diagnosis of a low grade synovial chondrosarcoma.

(Courtesy of J. Hodler, M.D., Zurich, Switzerland.)

countered most commonly. Both of these disorders produce monoarticular disease, typically in young adults. Although calcification may be evident in some patients with idiopathic synovial osteochondromatosis, routine radiographic findings are remarkably similar in both conditions. MR imaging can be used for accurate diagnosis in some cases.

REFERENCES

1. Spritzer CE, Dalinka MK, Kressel HY: Magnetic resonance imaging of pigmented villonodular synovitis: A report of two cases. Skel Radiol 16:316, 1987.
2. Kottal RA, Vogler JB III, Matamoros A, et al: Pigmented villonodular synovitis: A report of MR imaging in two cases. Radiology 163:551, 1987.
3. Weisz GM, Gal A, Kitchener PN: Magnetic resonance imaging in the diagnosis of aggressive villonodular synovitis. Clin Orthop 236:303, 1988.
4. Jelinek JS, Kransdorf MJ, Utz JA, et al: Imaging of pigmented villonodular synovitis with emphasis on MR imaging. AJR 152:337, 1989.
5. Sundaram M, Chalk D, Merenda J, et al: Case report 563. Skel Radiol 18:463, 1989.
6. Ugai K, Morimoto K: Magnetic resonance imaging of pigmented villonodular synovitis in subtalar joint: Report of a case. Clin Orthop 283:281, 1992.
7. Hughes TH, Sartoris DJ, Schweitzer ME, et al: Pigmented villonodular synovitis: MRI characteristics. Skel Radiol 24:7, 1995.
8. Frot B, Palazzo E, Zeitoun F, et al: Villonodular synovitis of the knee: Contribution of magnetic resonance imaging. Rev Rheum (Engl Ed) 61:157, 1994.
9. Cardinal E, Dussault RG, Kaplan PA: Imaging and differential diagnosis of masses within a joint. Can Assoc Radiol J 45:363, 1994.
10. Mandelbaum BR, Grant TT, Hartzman S, et al: The use of MRI to assist in diagnosis of pigmented villonodular synovitis of the knee joint. Clin Orthop 231:135, 1988.
11. Sherry CS, Harms SE: MR evaluation of giant cell tumors of the tendon sheath. Magn Reson Imaging 7:195, 1989.
12. Jelinek JS, Kransdorf MJ, Schmookler BM, et al: Giant cell tumor of the tendon sheath: MR findings in nine cases. AJR 162:919, 1994.
13. Maurice H, Crone M, Watt I: Synovial chondromatosis. J Bone Joint Surg [Br] 70:807, 1988.
14. Norman A, Steiner GC: Bone erosion in synovial chondromatosis. Radiology 161:749, 1986.
15. Blandino A, Salvi L, Chirico G, et al: Synovial osteochondromatosis of the ankle: MR findings. Clin Imaging 16:34, 1992.
16. Tuckman G, Wirth CZ: Synovial osteochondromatosis of the shoulder: MR findings. J Comput Assist Tomogr 13:360, 1989.
17. Burnstein MI, Fisher DR, Yandow DR, et al: Case report 502. Skel Radiol 17:458, 1988.
18. Kramer J, Recht M, Deely DM, et al: MR appearance of idiopathic synovial osteochondromatosis. J Comput Assist Tomogr 17:772, 1993.
19. Hermann G, Abdelwahab IF, Klein M, et al: Synovial chondromatosis. Skel Radiol 24:298, 1995.
20. Bertoni F, Unni KK, Beabout JW, et al: Chondrosarcomas of the synovium. Cancer 67:155, 1991.
21. Manivel JC, Dehner LP, Thompson R: Case report 460. Skel Radiol 17:66, 1988.
22. Ferry BE, McQueen DA, Lin JJ: Synovial chondromatosis with malignant degeneration to chondrosarcoma: Report of a case. J Bone Joint Surg [Am] 70:1259, 1988.
23. Hamilton A, Davis RI, Nixon JR: Synovial chondrosarcoma complicating synovial chondromatosis: Report of a case and review of the literature. J Bone Joint Surg [Am] 69:1084, 1987.
24. Hamilton A, Davis RI, Hayes D, et al: Chondrosarcoma developing in synovial chondromatosis: A case report. J Bone Joint Surg [Br] 69:137, 1987.
25. Kenan S, Abdelwahab IF, Klein MJ, et al: Case report 817. Skel Radiol 22:623, 1993.
26. Ontell F, Greenspan A: Chondrosarcoma complicating synovial chondromatosis: Findings with magnetic resonance imaging. Can Assoc Radiol J 45:318, 1994.

Bone and Bone Marrow: Anatomy and Pathophysiology

As a connective tissue, bone is highly specialized, differing from other connective tissues by its rigidity and hardness that relate primarily to the inorganic salts that are deposited in its matrix. These properties are fundamental to a tissue that must maintain the shape of the human body, protect its vital soft tissues, and allow locomotion, transmitting from one region of the body to another the forces generated by the contractions of various muscles. Bone also serves as a reservoir for ions, principally calcium, that are essential to normal fluid regulation and are made available as a response to stimuli produced by a number of hormones.

ANATOMY

General Structure of Bone

The prime ingredients of the mature bone are an outer shell of compact bone termed the cortex, which encloses a more loosely appearing meshwork of trabeculae, the cancellous or spongy bone, with its interconnecting spaces containing myeloid or fatty marrow, or both. The cortical bone is clothed by a periosteal membrane, which contains arterioles and capillaries that pierce the cortex, entering the medullary canal.[1] These vessels, along with larger structures that enter one or more nutrient canals, provide the blood supply to the bone. The periosteum is continuous about the bone except for that portion that is intra-articular and covered with synovial membrane or cartilage. At sites of attachment to bone, the fibers of tendons and ligaments blend with the periosteum (entheses). The structure of the periosteal membrane varies with the age of the person, being thicker, vascular, active, and loosely attached in the infant and child, and thinner, inactive, and more firmly adherent in the adult. These structural characteristics underscore the augmented ability of the infant's and child's periosteum to be lifted from the parent bone and to be stimulated to form osseous tissue.

Bone Marrow

Bone marrow is a soft pulpy tissue that lies in the spaces between the trabeculae of all bones and even in the larger haversian canals.[1] It is one of the most extensive organs of the human body, weighing between 2600 and 3000 gm in adults.[2] Its functions include the provision of a continual supply of red cells, white cells, and platelets to meet the body's demand for oxygenation, immunity, and coagulation.[2] A complex vascular supply relies mainly on a nutrient artery that, in the long tubular bones, pierces the diaphyseal cortex at an angle, penetrates the cortex, reaches the medullary bone, and extends toward the ends of the tubular bone, running parallel to its long axis.[3]

Marrow Composition. The basic composition of the bone marrow consists of mineralized osseous matrix, connective tissue, and a variety of cells. The trabeculae in the medullary space represent the osseous component of the bone marrow. The marrow itself occupies the spaces between and around the plates and struts of trabecular (cancellous or spongy) bone, and it is held in place by a network of fine fibrous tissue, called a reticulum, which is attached to the inner walls of the cortex and to the trabeculae.[2] The cancellous trabeculae, encased within the outer shell of the cortex, provide architectural support and serve as a mineral depot.[2] The interface between the marrow and the trabecular bone, the endosteal envelope, is very active metabolically.

The marrow harbors cells in all stages of erythrocytic and leukocytic development, as well as fat cells and reticulum cells. Groups of these cells are separated by the network of vascular channels, or sinusoids. The marrow microenvironment supporting the progenitor and precursor cells must provide for the normal steady state rates of renewal of the cellular elements of blood.[4]

Fat cells also are a major component of bone marrow. Although smaller than fat cells from extramedullary sites, the marrow fat cells are active metabolically and respond by changes in size to hematopoietic activity.[2] During periods of decreased hematopoiesis, the fat cells in the bone marrow increase in size and number, whereas during increased hematopoiesis, the fat cells atrophy.

Two forms of bone marrow exist, although components of both types of marrow frequently are encountered at any particular site. Red marrow is hematopoietically active marrow and consists of approximately 40 per cent water, 40 per cent fat, and 20 per cent protein; yellow marrow is hematopoietically inactive and consists of approximately 15 per cent water, 80 per cent fat, and 5 per cent protein.[2] Small nodules of lymphoid tissue also are scattered through the red marrow. The yellow marrow consists of connective tissue supporting numerous blood vessels and cells, most of which are fat cells.[1]

Marrow Conversion. The amount of red marrow versus yellow marrow at any given time depends on the age of the person, the site that is being sampled, and the health of the individual. At birth, red marrow is present throughout the skeleton, but with increasing age, owing to the normal conversion process of hematopoietic to fatty marrow, the proportion of hematopoietic marrow decreases. Fatty marrow represents approximately 15 per cent of the total marrow volume in the child but 60 per cent of this volume by the age of 80 years. A further rise in the percentage of fatty marrow versus hematopoietic marrow in advanced years of life is attributed to the additional fat cells that are necessary to replace the trabecular bone that is lost as a result of senile and postmenopausal osteoporosis.[2] Many of the factors that initiate or modulate this conversion of red to yellow marrow are not clear, although temperature, vascularity, and low oxygen tension may be important in this process.[5-7]

The conversion of red to yellow marrow that occurs during growth and development is predictable and orderly, and it has been well summarized by Vogler and Murphy.[2] In the immediate postnatal period, this conversion first becomes evident in the extremities, specifically in the terminal phalanges of the hands and feet.[8] After about the fifth year of life, the red marrow gradually is replaced in the long tubular bones (Fig. 7–1). This replacement commences earlier and is more advanced in the more distal bones of the extremities; furthermore, in each bone, the conversion to yellow marrow proceeds from the distal to the proximal end, although some authors maintain that it commences in the center of the shaft and extends in both directions but more rapidly in the distal segment.[1] Cartilaginous epiphyses and apophyses lack marrow until they ossify. Although such ossified centers initially may contain hematopoietic marrow,[9] rapid conversion to yellow marrow is the rule. Thus, as a general rule, marrow conversion in the epiphyses and apophyses as well as in the diaphyses of tubular bones occurs in the first decade of life, and that in the distal metaphyses of tubular bones occurs in the second decade of life. By the age of 20 to 25 years, marrow conversion usually is complete. At this time, the adult pattern is characterized by the presence of red marrow only in portions of the vertebrae, sternum, ribs, clavicles, scapulae, skull, and innominate bones and in the metaphyses of the femora and humeri.

Although the visualized patterns of signal intensity do not correspond precisely to anatomic sites of red and yellow marrow, MR imaging represents an effective, albeit indirect, means to determine the cellular characteristics of the bone marrow.[10-14] As is described in detail later in this chapter, the basic constituents of bone marrow that contribute individual signal intensities on MR images are fat, water, and mineral.[2] The last of these contributes in a negative fashion for two reasons: First, the mineral matrix produces little or no signal due to a lack of mobile protons; second, local field gradients are produced as a result of inhomogeneous susceptibility where mineral matrix interfaces with water or fat.[2] Although anatomic correlation with MR imaging findings of the bone marrow in normal children and adults generally is lacking,[11] the appearances of red and yellow marrow, owing to their compositional differences, are not the same. Composed predominantly of fat, yellow marrow displays the T1 and T2 relaxation patterns of adipose tissue; containing considerable amounts of water and protein as well as fat, red marrow has T1 and T2 relaxation patterns that differ from those of fatty marrow.[2] Although the major contributor to signal intensity of both types of marrow is fat, the longer T1 and T2 relaxation times of protein and water in red marrow also contribute significantly to its final signal intensity.[2]

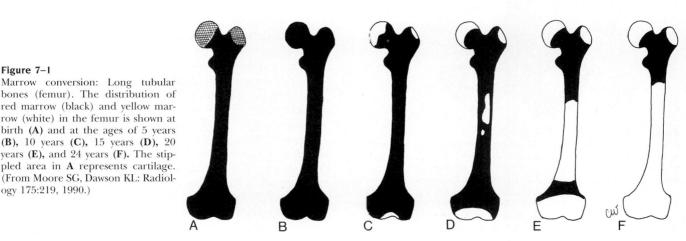

Figure 7–1
Marrow conversion: Long tubular bones (femur). The distribution of red marrow (black) and yellow marrow (white) in the femur is shown at birth (**A**) and at the ages of 5 years (**B**), 10 years (**C**), 15 years (**D**), 20 years (**E**), and 24 years (**F**). The stippled area in **A** represents cartilage. (From Moore SG, Dawson KL: Radiology 175:219, 1990.)

Therefore, on standard T1-weighted spin echo sequences, red marrow demonstrates lower signal intensity than yellow marrow.

Using such sequences, Ricci and coworkers[10] have reported in great detail the MR imaging characteristics of the normal age-related conversion of red to yellow marrow in the pelvis, proximal portion of the femur, skull, and various portions of the spine. Their findings with regard to the pelvis and femora are illustrated in Figures 7–2 and 7–3.

At times at which the body's demand for hematopoiesis increases, a reconversion of yellow marrow to red marrow occurs. The extent of reconversion depends on the severity and duration of the stimulus, and the process may be initiated or modulated by such factors as temperature, low oxygen tension, and elevated levels of erythropoietin.[2] The process of reconversion follows that of conversion but in reverse. Initial changes occur in the axial skeleton and thereafter from a proximal to distal direction in the extremities.

PATHOPHYSIOLOGY

MR imaging has been a major advance for the diagnosis and characterization of normal and abnormal marrow.

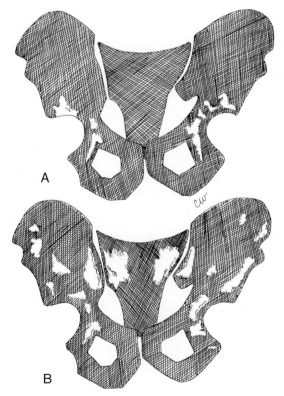

Figure 7–2
Marrow conversion: Pelvis. MR imaging appearance on T1-weighted spin echo images. Two patterns are observed. Pattern 1 (**A**) is characterized by small areas of high-signal-intensity fatty marrow in the para-acetabular region. Pattern 2 (**B**) is characterized by more widespread regions of high signal intensity, involving para-acetabular bone, ilii, and subchondral zones about the sacroiliac joints. Pattern 1 is more frequent in the first three decades of life, and pattern 2 thereafter. (From Ricci C, et al: Radiology 177:83, 1990.)

Considerable trabecular bone must be resorbed as a result of a marrow process before an area of bone lysis becomes apparent on routine radiographs. Scintigraphy using technetium-labeled phosphate compounds relies on changes in the cortical and trabecular bone that reflect marrow disease only indirectly. Direct scintigraphic imaging of marrow itself is limited to nonspecific radionuclide tracers, such as technetium-99m sulfur colloid. CT scanning is more sensitive than conventional radiography but also has limitations for marrow assessment. The Hounsfield units (HU) of normal marrow vary widely depending on the different proportions of cancellous bone, red marrow, and yellow marrow that are present in a given location.

Normal Bone Marrow

At birth, the entire marrow is hematopoietic.[15, 16] In infants, therefore, diffuse hypointense signal throughout the marrow on T1-weighted spin echo MR images does not indicate disease. Very prominent enhancement of this active marrow after the intravenous administration of a gadolinium-containing compound also is a normal finding at this stage.[17]

The cartilaginous epiphyses and apophyses lack marrow until they begin to ossify.[2, 15] As the ossification centers begin to enlarge, a marrow cavity develops. The marrow of the newly formed ossification center is initially hematopoietic, but after a few months fatty conversion takes place. On T1-weighted spin echo MR images, the epiphyseal marrow is initially hypointense and becomes hyperintense only after the secondary ossification center has been present for a few months.[9] After the first year of life, MR images typically show only fat signal within the epiphysis, and the diagnosis of epiphyseal marrow disorders with MR imaging is facilitated by the normal development of uniform hyperintensity within this region.[9, 12]

In general, MR imaging tends to underestimate the extent of hematopoietic activity within the marrow space.[12, 18] Although there are islands of red marrow histologically within the ossified epiphyses in the young child, this small amount of hematopoietic marrow is difficult to appreciate on the MR image.[12, 19] Histologically, epiphyseal red marrow is not an uncommon finding, even in the adult.[9] On MR images, normal adults show small amounts of residual epiphyseal red marrow, most commonly in the proximal humerus. Residual hematopoietic marrow, which may be curvilinear in a subcortical region, patchy, or globular, can be seen in 41 to 62 per cent of proximal humeral epiphyses.[13, 20]

Marrow conversion in the diaphyses occurs in the first decade of life and in the distal metaphyses in the second decade of life.[12, 18, 21] Hematopoietic marrow of low signal intensity in the diaphyses on T1-weighted spin echo images is normal in the first decade of life. Normally, diaphyseal conversion of marrow begins before the age of 1 year in 57 per cent of children and is complete by the age of 5 years in up to 95 per cent of normal children.[18, 21] By the age of 5 years, diaphyseal marrow is homogeneous and fatty, similar to the appearance in adults. Diaphyseal marrow in the normal young child is

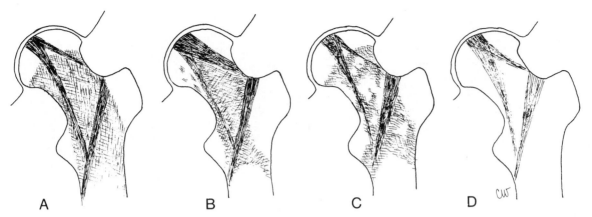

Figure 7–3

Marrow conversion: Proximal portion of the femur. MR imaging appearance on T1-weighted spin echo images. Four patterns are observed. Pattern 1 **(A)** is characterized by high-signal-intensity fatty marrow confined to the capital femoral epiphysis and greater and lesser trochanters. Pattern 2 **(B)** resembles pattern 1 with the addition of fatty marrow in the medial portion of the femoral head and in the lateral portion of the intertrochanteric region. Pattern 3 **(C)** resembles pattern 1 with the addition of many small, sometimes confluent, areas of fatty marrow in the intertrochanteric region. Pattern 4 **(D)** is characterized by uniform high-signal-intensity fatty marrow throughout the proximal portion of the femur with the exception of the regions of the major trabecular groups. Patterns 1 and 2 predominate in the first three decades of life, pattern 3 predominates in the fifth and sometimes the fourth decades of life, and pattern 4 predominates after the age of 50 or 60 years. (From Ricci C, et al: Radiology 177:83, 1990.)

more fatty than the metaphyseal marrow even prior to this age. Persistence of hematopoietic marrow in the diaphyses after the first decade is abnormal.

Conversion of marrow in the metaphyses takes place later and is less complete than in the diaphyseal regions, particularly in the femur and the proximal portion of the humerus. Large quantities of hematopoietic marrow of low signal intensity in the metaphyses on T1-weighted spin echo images is normal until the end of the second decade of life. In fact, lack of red marrow in the proximal femoral metaphyses in the young child is abnormal and raises the possibility of myeloid depletion.[19] Metaphyseal marrow conversion starts in the young child, being present in 95 per cent of normal children by the age of 5 years and complete by the age of 20 years.[18] Considerable amounts of residual marrow may be present in these regions, producing an irregular or mottled appearance to the adult metaphysis.[2, 18, 22] Prominent hematopoietic marrow is a normal finding that is seen in 15 per cent of adults imaged for knee and shoulder disorders.[22, 23] In general, the more proximal the bone, the greater the amount of hematopoietic marrow seen in the metaphysis. For example, around the knee it is normal to see greater amounts of hematopoietic marrow in the distal portion of the femur that in the proximal portion of the tibia. The proximal metaphyses of the femur and humerus often are inhomogeneous, reflecting a mixture of red and yellow marrow. Focal geographic rests or mottled irregular areas of normal hematopoietic marrow often are detected incidentally on MR imaging examinations and should not be misinterpreted as pathologic findings. These confluent areas of low signal intensity on the T1-weighted images do not increase in signal on T2-weighted sequences, spare the epiphysis, do not violate the cortex, and are less nodular than areas of tumor (Fig. 7–4).[16, 23, 24]

By the age of 25 years, marrow conversion usually is complete. The adult marrow pattern typically is characterized by confinement of the majority of red marrow

to the axial skeleton and the proximal portions of the femora and humeri.[15, 18] In the axial skeleton of the adult, considerable marrow inhomogeneity is a normal finding. Therefore, it is often more difficult to identify diffuse marrow abnormalities, particularly diffuse infiltration, in the axial skeleton than in the appendicular regions. Marrow inhomogeneity is caused by an irregular admixture of red and yellow marrow, as well as by larger nodular areas of fatty infiltration superimposed on regions of uniform hematopoietic marrow. Focal fatty infiltration has been seen at all ages in both sexes.

Magnetic Resonance Imaging. The MR imaging appearance of normal marrow reflects the relative amounts of its three basic constituents.[2, 25] Cortical and trabecular bone produce little or no signal due to the absence of mobile protons. Only the major trabecular bands can be seen on MR images, in which they appear as poorly defined linear bands of low signal intensity within the marrow space. The major trabecular bands are most evident in the proximal femora, where the compressive and tensile trabeculae result in bands of low signal intensity on the T1- and T2-weighted images.[2] Trabecular bone does produce focal field inhomogeneities that result in signal loss on gradient echo sequences, but the overall effect of bone mineral density on other pulse sequences is minimal. On spin echo imaging, the ossified elements of the marrow contribute little to the MR imaging appearance.

The MR imaging appearance of the bone marrow is determined by the relative proportions of hematopoietic and fatty marrow. In adults, fat is the primary contributor to the signal intensity of marrow. The MR imaging appearance of marrow also depends on the specific pulse sequence that is chosen. The spin echo pulse sequence is the standard technique used for bone marrow imaging. The repetition time (TR) and the echo delay (TE) can be altered to accentuate either proton density, T1, or T2. The T1-weighted sequence

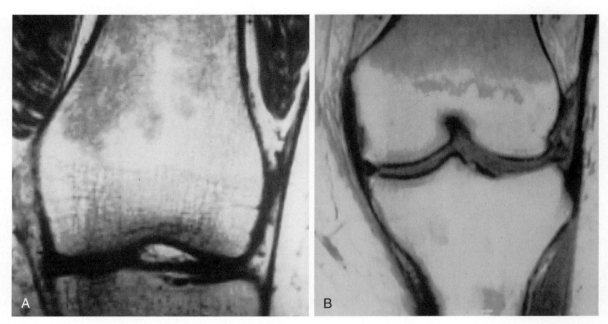

Figure 7–4

Normal adult marrow. Normal coronal T1-weighted (TR/TE, 600/20) spin echo MR images of the knees of two adults are shown. Note focal areas of residual hematopoietic marrow.

A In this example, nodular areas of low signal intensity within the metaphysis of the femur are evident. Note that the signal intensity of the nodular regions is higher than that of muscle and that small amounts of interspersed fat can be seen within these areas.

B In a second example, hematopoietic marrow is seen in the distal portion of the femur. Note the smaller amounts of hematopoietic marrow in the proximal portion of the tibia. The epiphyses show fatty signal, and the hematopoietic elements are confined to the metaphyseal regions.

has both a short TR and a short TE and optimizes the contrast between fatty marrow and red marrow and between fatty marrow and pathologic processes.[26, 27] Because fatty marrow is composed primarily of lipid, its MR imaging appearance parallels the T1 and T2 relaxation patterns of subcutaneous fat. Fatty marrow appears bright on T1-weighted images and shows intermediate signal intensity on T2-weighted images. The signal intensity of fatty marrow is slightly less than that of subcutaneous fat owing to admixed hematopoietic elements and bony trabeculae. On T2-weighted images the TR and TE are long and contrast reflects differences in T2 relaxation times. Hematopoietic marrow is of low to intermediate signal intensity on both T1- and T2-weighted images. Hematopoietic marrow still contains some fat so its signal intensity is normally higher than that of adjacent tissues, such as the intervertebral disc and muscle. Normal marrow is higher in signal intensity on the T1-weighted images than on T2-weighted images. Because the T2 relaxation values of red marrow and fatty marrow are similar, discrimination between these two normal marrow constituents is poor. However, most pathologic processes have a large quantity of slowly relaxing free water protons, resulting in a longer T2 relaxation value than that of either type of normal marrow, so they are readily identified as areas of high signal intensity.[2, 27]

Loss of the normal high signal intensity of fatty marrow on T1-weighted spin echo MR images allows accurate and early detection of marrow infiltration and replacement by abnormal tissue.[28, 29] The T1-weighted images are very sensitive for detection of marrow abnormality in the adult, although almost all lesions result in

the same type of findings.[29] Proton density-weighted images lack sufficient contrast resolution between the normal marrow and pathologic processes to be used extensively for marrow evaluation. The appearance on T2-weighted images depends upon the type of tissue replacing the normal marrow. Neoplasms, necrotic tissue, inflammatory debris, and blood typically demonstrate high signal intensity. Fibrotic tissue, sclerotic bone, and some paramagnetic substances are of low signal intensity on both the T1- and T2-weighted images.[30] Conventional spin echo imaging alone is not the optimal method for complete assessment of marrow disorders. Spin echo imaging leads to an underestimation of the proportion of hematopoietic marrow because the short T1 relaxation time of fat overwhelms the longer T1 relaxation time of the red marrow. Spin echo techniques are valuable for identifying focal lesions and advanced disease, but subtle changes in the marrow may be identified only on alternate sequences.

The alternate sequences most widely used for bone marrow assessment are fast spin echo (FSE), short tau inversion recovery (STIR), and, less commonly, gradient echo imaging. FSE imaging utilizes multiple 180 degree pulses for every 90 degree pulse. This imaging method allows more rapid imaging than conventional spin echo because more information is obtained per TR interval. On FSE sequences, normal marrow fat and subcutaneous fat appear brighter than on conventional spin echo sequences. This increased signal intensity within the fat decreases the sensitivity of the T2-weighted FSE sequence to pathologic processes of the marrow with increased water content. Fat suppression is employed routinely with FSE imaging when evaluating bone marrow

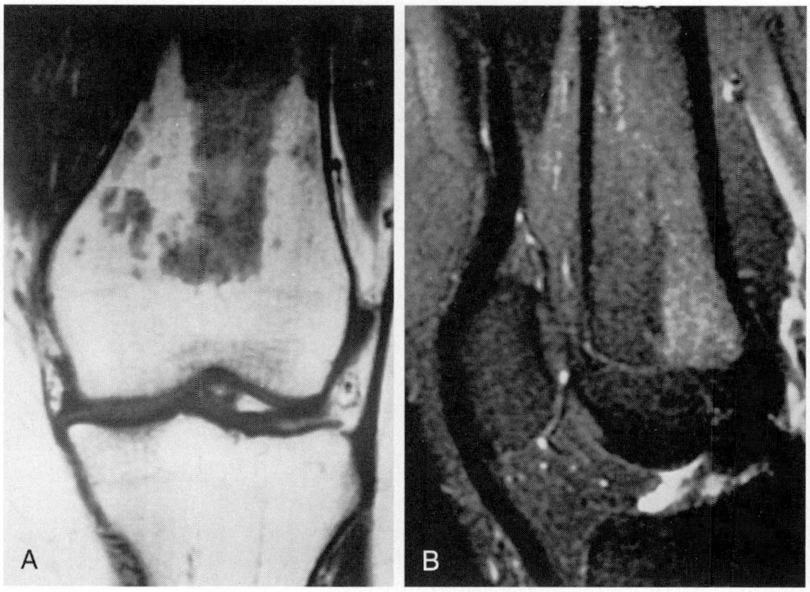

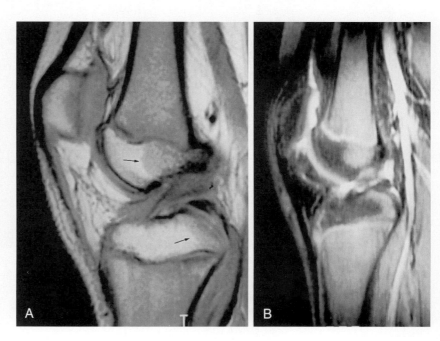

Figure 7–5
Fast spin echo (FSE) MR imaging with fat suppression to study bone marrow. In a 26 year old woman, an extended pattern of hematopoietic marrow is evident. On a coronal T1-weighted (TR/TE, 650/16) spin echo MR image **(A),** note the presence of hematopoietic marrow of low signal intensity in the distal metaphysis of the femur. A sagittal fat-suppressed FSE MR image (TR/TE, 4200/76) **(B)** shows the regions of hematopoietic marrow in the femur to be of greater signal intensity than that of the fatty marrow. (Courtesy of S.K. Brahme, M.D., San Diego, California.)

(Fig. 7–5). The addition of fat suppression to FSE results in excellent images of the bone marrow that show sensitivity equal to that of STIR images, but with a shorter imaging time and with higher tissue specificity.[31]

STIR sequences are widely used for marrow assessment because of their high sensitivity. The STIR sequence nullifies the signal from fat; therefore, the normal fatty marrow appears dark. The T1 and T2 contrast of other tissues is additive; therefore, contrast between areas with high concentrations of free water and normal tissues is greatly enhanced.[32, 33] The appearance of normal marrow on STIR images can be confusing because hematopoietic marrow shows higher signal intensity than that of the suppressed background fatty marrow (Fig. 7–6). Focal islands of nodular hematopoietic marrow often appear larger and more conspicuous on the STIR images than on T1-weighted spin echo images.

These areas of normal hematopoietic marrow typically are metaphyseal and appear isointense to muscle. On STIR images, marrow lesions that result in increased signal on T2-weighted spin echo images are of higher signal intensity than muscle and appear similar to fluid. Because most marrow lesions have abnormally increased T1 and T2 relaxation times related to their higher proportion of free water, this additive effect leads to high contrast between the lesion (which is of high signal intensity) and the suppressed fatty marrow.[31, 32] Anatomic definition may be somewhat limited owing to loss of contrast between the suppressed fatty marrow and cortical bone. The long imaging times require some sacrifice in either spatial resolution, number of slices, or signal to noise ratio. Fast STIR sequences show marrow lesions equally well as conventional STIR sequences and allow considerable savings in imaging time.[33]

Figure 7–6
STIR MR imaging to study bone marrow. In this 11 year old girl with sickle cell anemia, an extended pattern of hematopoietic marrow is evident about the knee. In a sagittal proton density-weighted (TR/TE, 2000/20) spin echo MR image **(A),** hematopoietic marrow of intermediate signal intensity (similar to that of muscle) occupies the diaphysis and metaphysis of the femur and the metaphysis of the tibia. In addition, epiphyseal foci of hematopoietic marrow can be seen (arrows). A sagittal fast spin echo STIR MR image (TR/TE, 3667/17; inversion time, 150 msec) **(B)** shows relatively high signal intensity in these regions of hematopoietic marrow.

Chemical shift imaging is a valuable supplement to the standard MR imaging techniques applied to the assessment of bone marrow.[27, 34, 35] Changes in the fat fraction of the marrow are the largest determinant of contrast on the chemical shift images of abnormal marrow.[34] Alteration in the fat fraction also is responsible for changes seen on the spin echo images, but the conspicuity of lesions is enhanced with chemical shift imaging.[34, 35] Selective fat or water suppression sequences now are standard software options on many high-field MR imaging systems. The selective fat saturation technique is particularly effective for bone marrow imaging, particularly with FSE sequences and when gadolinium compounds are being administered (Fig. 7–7).[31, 34, 36]

Gradient echo sequences offer a more rapid imaging alternative to standard spin echo imaging but are not widely used for assessment of marrow disorders. Unlike spin echo sequences, the signal on gradient echo sequences is dependent on the T2* (rather than T2) of tissues owing to the lack of a 180 degree refocusing gradient.[2, 37] Many acronyms are used for the family of gradient echo sequences, depending on the manufacturer and the specific method of signal acquisition. The major problem with the use of gradient echo imaging for bone marrow assessment is its sensitivity to local field inhomogeneities, such as those caused by trabecular bone. Contact with trabecular bone results in local shortening of the T2 relaxation time of marrow with a resultant loss in signal intensity. Regions with large amounts of trabecular bone, such as the epiphyses and metaphyses, show a greater loss of signal intensity than do regions with little or no trabecular bone, such as the diaphyses. Areas of low signal intensity on gradient echo studies may represent foci of fatty marrow with a high content of trabecular bone and should not be interpreted as hematopoietic marrow or pathologic findings.[37]

Quantitative MR imaging using both spin echo and chemical shift techniques also has been used in the evaluation of marrow disorders.[25, 35, 38] Quantitative spin echo MR imaging does not improve diagnostic accuracy for detection of diffuse marrow disorders, but it may be of value for detection of focal marrow involvement and for monitoring therapy.[35, 38]

Bone Marrow Disorders

Vogler and Murphy[2] have developed a useful classification system for bone marrow disorders and have divided these diverse entities into five major groups: reconversion or absence of normal conversion, myeloid depletion, marrow infiltration, marrow edema, and marrow ischemia. Reconversion of yellow to red marrow and failure of conversion of red to yellow marrow occur when there is an increased demand for hematopoiesis. Myeloid depletion represents an abnormal amount of regression of hematopoietic marrow with depletion of all marrow elements except fat. Marrow infiltration consists of the replacement of normal marrow by some other cellular material. Marrow edema results when there is excess water accumulation, usually as a result of hyperemia. Marrow ischemia is related to inadequate oxygenation of marrow with resultant necrosis or infarction. These categories usually can be differentiated on the basis of their distribution and signal characteristics on T1-weighted and T2-weighted images (Fig. 7–8).

Myeloid Depletion. In myeloid depletion, the normal conversion of hematopoietic to fatty marrow takes place prematurely or is abnormally accelerated. Premature

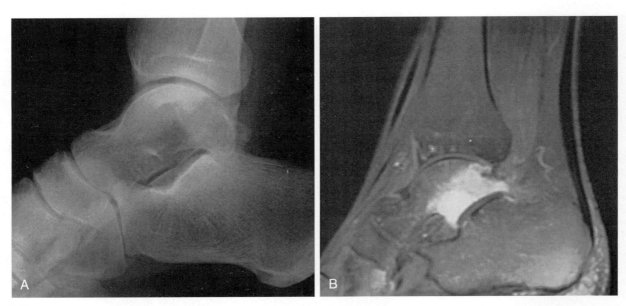

Figure 7–7
MR imaging with fat suppression and intravenous gadolinium contrast agent administration to study bone marrow. In a 55 year old man with leukemic infiltration of the marrow in the talus, a routine radiograph **(A)** reveals subtle osteolysis of the posterior portion of the bone. A sagittal T1-weighted (TR/TE, 400/11) spin echo MR image obtained with fat suppression and immediately after the intravenous administration of a gadolinium compound **(B)** shows dramatic high signal intensity in the involved portion of the talus. (Courtesy of D. Goodwin, M.D., Hanover, New Hampshire.)

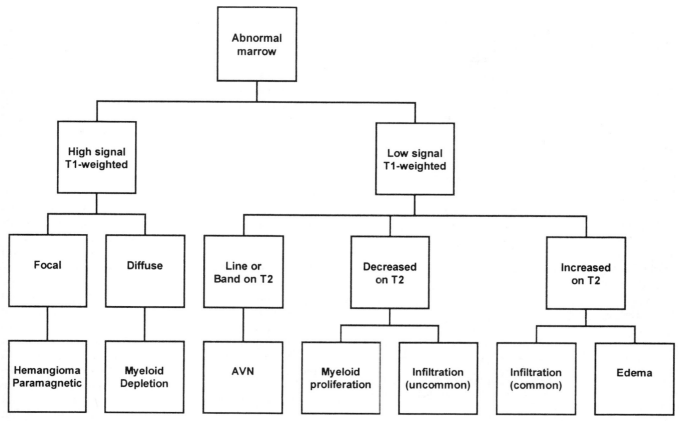

Figure 7–8

Algorithmic approach to bone marrow disorders based on pattern of altered signal intensity on T1-weighted and T2-weighted spin echo MR images. AVN, osteonecrosis.

and accelerated replacement of hematopoietic tissue by fatty marrow is seen in patients with idiopathic aplastic anemia or after numerous marrow insults, the most common of which are irradiation and chemotherapy. The marrow changes seen in aplastic anemia and after chemotherapy are diffuse, whereas irradiation produces focal myeloid depletion. This latter pattern is much easier to recognize because normal marrow is present, from which the depleted area can be differentiated. Diffuse myeloid depletion may be difficult to recognize on MR images unless prior examinations are available. This is the only category of disease that results in a widespread increase in the signal intensity of the marrow on T1-weighted spin echo images. In severe cases, the abnormal marrow shows signal intensity characteristics identical to those of subcutaneous fat (Fig. 7–9). Marrow that contains no hematopoietic elements, particularly in the axial skeleton, should be considered abnormal unless the patient is very elderly.

Aplastic anemia is an uncommon disorder of myeloid depletion in which acellular or hypocellular marrow results in pancytopenia. About 50 per cent of reported cases occur on an idiopathic basis, but the disorder can be secondary to various known etiologic factors, such as drugs, toxins, hepatitis, and viral infections.[39] With MR imaging, normal marrow, uniform fatty marrow, and inhomogeneous marrow patterns all have been described in patients with this disease.[30, 39] With treatment, the signal intensity of the marrow may change from a

diffuse fatty pattern to an inhomogeneous pattern with multiple foci of decreased signal intensity within the fatty marrow, representing islands of hematopoietic tissue.[29] Depending on the stage of treatment and the degree of response, these areas of hematopoietic elements may enlarge, coalesce, or even become diffuse.[2]

Irradiation and chemotherapy also may result in the ablation of hematopoietic marrow.[29, 40] Most reports describing these iatrogenic causes of myeloid depletion have emphasized the effect of radiation. The initial marrow response to irradiation consists of a short period of vascular congestion and edema.[36, 41] During this acute period, which peaks at approximately 9 days after radiation therapy, increased marrow signal intensity on STIR sequences may be observed.[41] Irradiated bone rapidly becomes hypocellular with progressive destruction of its vascularity. This vascular destruction prevents migration of hematopoietic cells from nonirradiated sites. After this acute phase, a rapid conversion to fatty marrow occurs in the irradiated regions. Myeloid depletion with fatty replacement can become evident within 2 weeks after the start of therapy.[2, 40] Within 6 to 8 weeks after radiation therapy, fatty replacement of the damaged marrow is present in 90 per cent of patients.[41] Fatty marrow replacement progresses rapidly during the first 6 weeks of therapy and then continues at a much slower rate. The persistence of increased signal intensity on the T1-weighted spin echo MR images appears to be permanent, suggesting that the process of fatty replace-

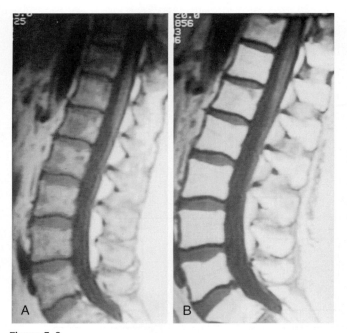

Figure 7–9
Myeloid depletion secondary to chemotherapy. This 49 year old woman underwent chemotherapy for stage IV breast cancer widely metastatic to the skeleton.
  A The pretherapy sagittal T1-weighted (TR/TE, 500/12) spin echo MR image of the lumbar spine shows multiple rounded lesions of low signal intensity within the vertebrae, consistent with metastatic disease.
  B A sagittal T1-weighted (TR/TE, 500/12) spin echo MR image obtained 8 months later, after chemotherapy, demonstrates replacement of all the marrow elements with fat of high signal intensity.

ment is irreversible, with no potential for marrow regeneration or reconversion in the adult.[40, 42]

The signal intensity of fat-replaced irradiated marrow is diffusely increased on T1-weighted spin echo MR images and coincides with the signal of fat on T2-weighted spin echo and FSE MR images.[40, 42, 43] The change is particularly evident at the edge of the radiation port with a sharp line of demarcation between the irradiated fatty marrow of high signal intensity and the normal, less intense hematopoietic marrow.[42, 43] These changes are more evident in younger patients because of their higher proportion of hematopoietic marrow.[40, 43]

Reconversion or Failure of Conversion. In the normal person, hematopoietic demands are easily met by the red marrow.[15] Failure of conversion or reconversion occurs if the demand for oxygenation exceeds the ability of the existing red marrow to meet that need.[2, 15] Failure of conversion occurs when a disorder affecting hematopoietic demands develops in childhood and the normal process of fatty conversion is arrested. Reconversion of fatty to hematopoietic marrow usually occurs when an adult's marrow is stressed but reconversion can be seen in children who have suffered premature fatty conversion, typically due to radiation or chemotherapy. Marrow composition is dynamic, and in response to hematopoietic demands, yellow marrow can be reconverted readily to red marrow.[15] MR imaging can permit detection of delayed conversion and reconversion prior to the development of any morphologic changes in the bone.

Disorders that produce an increased need for hematopoiesis include numerous causes of ineffective hematopoiesis, erythrocyte destruction, or failure of oxygenation of normal blood. Examples of these disorders include sickle cell anemia, thalassemia, chronic hemolytic anemia, congenital heart disease, and diffuse marrow replacement processes. In childhood, when most of the marrow is hematopoietic, these disorders lead to postponement of red marrow conversion. If the disorder is severe, the existing red marrow may become hyperplastic in an attempt to meet the body's need for hematopoiesis.[15] On MR images, the hyperplastic marrow shows identical signal intensity characteristics to those of normal hematopoietic marrow. Although the signal intensity characteristics of the marrow are normal, its distribution is inappropriate for the patient's age.

Sickle cell anemia and thalassemia are common causes of persistent hematopoietic marrow in an infantile distribution. In children with severe chronic hemolytic anemia, the red marrow becomes hyperplastic and normal marrow conversion is postponed. Marrow of low signal intensity in the young infant persists into childhood and adolescence in patients with severe disease. Such marrow in the diaphyses and epiphyses is typically bilateral and symmetric in uncomplicated anemia. Hemosiderin deposition leads to a further decrease in the signal intensity of the marrow in patients with sickle cell anemia.[44] Like normal hematopoietic marrow, this hyperplastic marrow remains of low signal on T2-weighted spin echo MR images and is isointense to muscle on STIR sequences (Fig. 7–10). Superimposed bone infarction in the patient with sickle cell anemia can produce asymmetric lesions that show variable behavior on T2-weighted spin echo images.[44, 45] Extramedullary hematopoiesis and osseous expansion are late features of chronic hemolytic anemias, and they are especially frequent in thalassemia major. The resultant soft tissue masses simulate tumors, particularly when they develop in a paraspinal location. Rarely, patients with extensive soft tissue hematopoietic proliferation develop symptomatic compression of adjacent structures, such as the spinal cord.[46, 47] On MR images, hematopoietic tissue in an extramedullary location appears as a mass with signal intensity slightly higher than that of the adjacent vertebrae on both T1- and T2-weighted spin echo MR images.[47]

Marrow reconversion is seen most commonly in adults who are recovering from a systemic marrow insult such as that occurring with chemotherapy. The extent of reconversion is a reflection of the severity and chronicity of the underlying disease.[15] Reconversion may be diffuse or result only in the development of a few foci or islands of hematopoietic tissue within the fatty marrow. The order of reconversion is the reverse of the sequence of normal marrow conversion, progressing centripetally from the axial to the appendicular skeleton and from proximal to distal sites.[2, 15] Variations from this pattern, with preferential reconversion of the epiphyses and apophyses, can be seen, however.[28] Reconversion of the appendicular skeleton suggests extensive replacement of the axial marrow. Reconverted marrow has the same signal intensity characteristics as normal hematopoietic

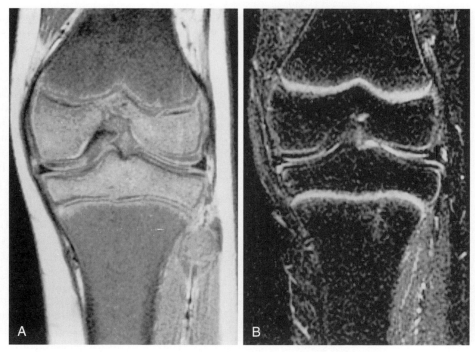

Figure 7–10
Sickle cell anemia: Coronal images of the knee in a 12 year old boy with severe sickle cell anemia.

A The T1-weighted (TR/TE, 600/20) spin echo MR image shows hematopoietic marrow of low signal intensity within the epiphyses of the distal portion of the femur and proximal portion of the tibia. The abnormal signal of the marrow approximates that of skeletal muscle.

B The T2-weighted (TR/TE, 2000/80) spin echo MR image obtained with fat suppression shows persistent low signal intensity in the hematopoietic marrow. Hemosiderosis secondary to chronic hemolysis also contributes to the low signal intensity of the marrow in this patient.

marrow, but its distribution is more extensive and more heterogeneous than normal red marrow.

Reconversion can be accelerated by administration of recombinant hematopoietic growth factors, which are being used increasingly to reduce the myelosuppression associated with chemotherapy.[48] Repopulation of depleted bone marrow also can be accomplished by bone marrow transplantation, which is being employed for the treatment of both primary and secondary osseous malignancies.[43] Large pretransplantation doses of chemotherapy and radiation therapy are given for ablation of all native hematopoietic marrow, immunosuppression, and elimination of any residual tumor.[36, 43] Hematologic engraftment of transplanted marrow typically takes place in 3 to 4 weeks.[43] On T1-weighted spin echo MR images, early hematopoietic reconstitution of marrow appears as a central zone of increased signal intensity surrounded by a peripheral zone of intermediate signal intensity (Fig. 7–11).[43] Reciprocal changes are seen on the STIR images, with a central zone of decreased signal intensity surrounded by a peripheral zone of increased signal intensity. Histologic correlation has shown that the central zone corresponds to fatty marrow and the peripheral zone to an area of regenerating hematopoietic cells.[43] The MR imaging band pattern probably is not specific for marrow transplantation and also may be seen with hematopoietic reconstitution after treatment of other disorders producing complete marrow suppression.

Marrow Edema. Bone marrow edema commonly occurs after trauma, as a reaction to adjacent neoplasm or infection, on an idiopathic basis, and, less frequently, during the early phase of marrow infarction or as part of the complex of reflex sympathetic dystrophy. It is postulated that either hypervascularity, hyperperfusion, or increased permeability produces an increase in free extracellular water but the exact histopathologic basis of marrow edema is unknown.[2, 49] MR imaging of these unrelated entities has a common appearance, demonstrating focal areas of low signal intensity on T1-weighted spin echo MR images that increase in signal intensity on T2-weighted spin echo and STIR images.

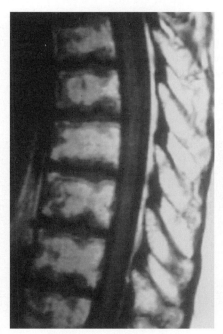

Figure 7–11
Marrow repopulation after bone marrow transplantation. A sagittal T1-weighted (TR/TE, 600/20) spin echo MR image of the spine in a 27 year man with a history of lymphoma is shown. This study was obtained 3 months after hematopoietic ablation and subsequent bone marrow transplantation and shows tissue of low signal intensity rimming the periphery of multiple vertebral bodies. Biopsy confirmed the presence of engraftment of normal hematopoietic tissue.

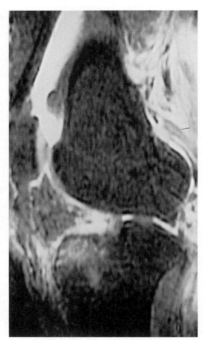

Figure 7–12
Depressed lateral tibial plateau fracture. A sagittal fast multiplanar inversion recovery (FMPIR) image (TR/TE, 3667/17; inversion time, 150 msec) shows an area of high signal intensity in the anterior portion of the lateral tibial plateau representing edema adjacent to a fracture. Note the articular incongruity secondary to a depressed tibial plateau fracture.

STIR imaging is particularly sensitive to small changes in the water content of the marrow space and is very sensitive for detecting bone marrow edema (Fig. 7–12).[50]

Traumatic edema is common after injury to the bone, even in the absence of findings on conventional radiography. MR imaging abnormalities in the marrow related to trauma typically persist for as long as 8 weeks after the injury.[50] Edema may be seen in the absence of a frank cortical or cancellous fracture or may be apparent adjacent to or surrounding a macroscopic fracture line. The "bone bruise" is a transient posttraumatic abnormality of medullary bone, presumably caused by edema and hemorrhage related to trabecular microfractures.[51, 52] These common lesions are self-limited, resolve spontaneously, and are not associated with any long-term sequelae. They may occur in isolation but frequently are associated with ligamentous rupture and meniscal pathology.[51] Edema also may be seen adjacent to stress fractures or occult fractures. In these cases, however, a dark linear band, representing the fracture line, usually is seen on both T1- and T2-weighted spin echo sequences.[51, 52] When the edema is extensive, the fracture line itself may be obscured, particularly on T1-weighted and STIR sequences (Fig. 7–13).

Three related syndromes, known as transient osteoporosis of the hip, regional migratory osteoporosis, and the "transient bone marrow edema syndrome," are associated with bone marrow edema of uncertain cause in the proximal portion of the femur.[53] All three have an identical MR imaging appearance, although they differ in their radiographic findings and clinical course. Transient osteoporosis of the hip is a self-limited process, of unknown cause, that was initially described in women in the third trimester of pregnancy, based on the radiographic demonstration of focal osteoporosis of the proximal portion of the femur. It is now known that transient osteoporosis of the hip most commonly affects the left hip of men in the third and fourth decades of life in the absence of a history of local injury.[53, 54] Regional migratory osteoporosis is a less common disorder in which multiple anatomic sites, typically the large joints of the lower extremity, are affected sequentially. The most recently described entity in this group of disorders has been designated the "transient bone marrow edema" syndrome.[53] This newly recognized pattern has no conventional radiographic findings and is diagnosed solely on the basis of clinical findings and abnormalities on MR imaging. In all three disorders, MR imaging

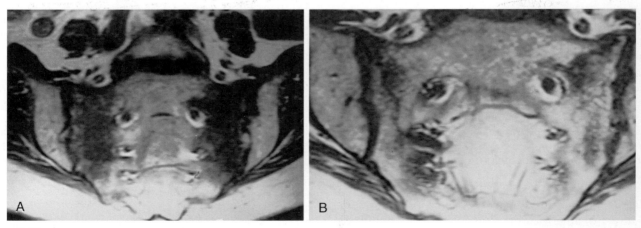

Figure 7–13
Insufficiency fractures of the sacrum. Transaxial MR images of the sacrum in a 69 year old woman with bilateral sacral insufficiency fractures secondary to a minor fall 2 months previously are shown.
 A A T1-weighted (TR/TE, 300/15) spin echo MR image shows thick bands of low signal intensity in the periphery of both sacral ala.
 B A T1-weighted (TR/TE, 350/15) spin echo MR image obtained after the intravenous administration of gadolinium compound shows enhancement of the edema, and the sacral fracture lines are now visible.

shows diffuse loss of the signal intensity of fat in the femoral head and neck on the T1-weighted spin echo images.[54] The region of low signal intensity typically extends to the intertrochanteric ridge, spares the acetabulum, and often spares the medial aspect of the femoral head. T2-weighted spin echo and STIR images show uniform high signal intensity in the area of involvement. Unlike classic osteonecrosis, no rim or band of low signal intensity is seen in the area of edema and the contour of the femoral head remains normal. Distinction between bone marrow edema and very early osteonecrosis can be problematic and follow-up MR imaging examinations may be helpful. In bone marrow edema, the abnormalities resolve spontaneously over a period of several months.

Marrow Ischemia and Osteonecrosis. Bone marrow ischemia with subsequent infarction may involve any bone and any location within that bone. Osteonecrosis usually predominates in the fatty marrow because the regional vascular supply is sparse in this region compared to that in hematopoietic marrow.[2, 15] A higher prevalence of fatty marrow in the femoral neck and intertrochanteric region of patients with established nontraumatic osteonecrosis of the femoral head has been found. Subarticular bone necrosis is common and of great clinical significance because of the potential for articular collapse and subsequent osteoarthritis (Fig. 7–14). The majority of nonepiphyseal infarcts in the long tubular bones occur in the metadiaphyses, probably due to the poor collateral circulation in this region.

The initial ischemic insult to the marrow is followed by cellular loss and the host's repair response. The most sensitive cells of the marrow are the hematopoietic cells, which die within the first 6 to 12 hours of anoxia.[43] Osteocytes, osteoblasts, and osteoclasts begin to show evidence of cellular death after 48 hours. The lipocytes are most resistant and survive for 2 to 5 days. The host's repair response begins in the viable tissue adjacent to the ischemic area and is characterized by increased vascularity, inflammation, granulation tissue, fibrosis, bone resorption, and osteoblastic reinforcement of the adjacent bone.[2] If bone resorption leads to loss of structural support, fracture of the subchondral bone can occur.

MR imaging is the most sensitive method for the detection of osteonecrosis, although it is unclear how early in the process marrow changes can first be detected.[55, 56] The MR imaging appearance of osteonecrosis varies depending on the location, duration, and stage of the disease. At a very early stage, osteonecrosis produces a nonspecific pattern of poorly defined regions of low signal intensity in the marrow on T1-weighted images that is identical to findings of bone marrow edema. In this acute stage, the T2-weighted and STIR images show high signal intensity within the infarct (Fig. 7–15). The characteristic demarcation of the necrotic zone by a band of reactive bone of low signal intensity is not present in this phase. In this very early phase, arriving at a specific diagnosis of osteonecrosis is very difficult without the use of dynamic perfusion imaging. Gadolinium-enhanced fast MR imaging has been reported to be a highly sensitive method for detecting diminution of blood flow within the femoral head.[56] Normal marrow enhances slightly after the intravenous injection of a gadolinium compound, although this enhancement may be difficult to appreciate without fat suppression. When arterial flow is compromised, a cor-

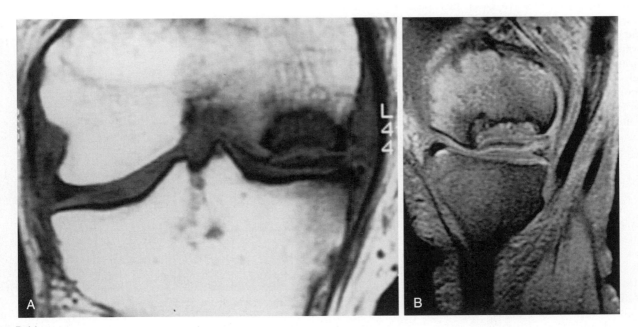

Figure 7–14

Osteonecrosis of the femoral condyle. A 90 year old woman developed spontaneous osteonecrosis of the medial femoral condyle.

A The coronal T1-weighted (TR/TE, 400/12) spin echo MR image shows a confluent area of low signal intensity abutting the subarticular surface of the medial femoral condyle.

B A sagittal proton density-weighted (TR/TE, 1200/30) spin echo MR image obtained with fat suppression shows collapse of the chondral surface and subchondral bone. An interface of low signal intensity is present between the necrotic area and the underlying normal bone.

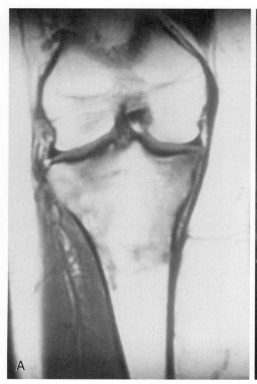
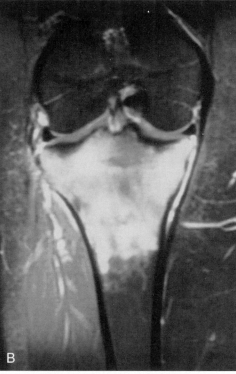

Figure 7–15
Acute bone marrow infarction. This 22 year old woman was referred with a tentative diagnosis of osteosarcoma, based on patchy sclerosis of the proximal portion of the tibia seen on a radiograph. A biopsy obtained after the MR imaging examination showed acute infarction of the marrow.

A A coronal T1-weighted (TR/TE, 600/20) spin echo MR image shows a patchy, poorly defined region of marrow hypointensity in the epiphysis and metaphysis of the proximal portion of the tibia.

B The STIR (TR/TE, 2400/40; inversion time, 160 msec) image shows high signal intensity within this area.

responding decrease is seen in the degree of enhancement of signal intensity in the marrow. The technique of gadolinium-enhanced fast MR imaging may allow detection of subtle hemodynamic compromise, which may predispose to or result in early osteonecrosis.[56] MR imaging assessment of the adequacy of marrow perfusion may allow earlier therapeutic intervention than is currently possible.

Once the ischemic process has passed the acute phase, the typical low signal intensity margins of reactive bone can be identified with MR imaging and a confident diagnosis of osteonecrosis can be established. The appearance of the these reactive lines takes place within weeks of the ischemic insult in most cases. At this stage, osteonecrosis can produce a variety of MR imaging appearances, including the ring or band pattern, the double-line sign, and patchy homogeneous or inhomogeneous areas of low signal intensity on T1-weighted images (Fig. 7–16).[55] Each of these patterns includes some component of low signal intensity on the T1-weighted images. The lines or bands of low signal intensity seen at the margins of the infarct typically abut on the cortex on at least one projection and often are wavy in contour. On T2-weighted spin echo MR images, either low or high signal intensity in the area of necrosis is seen. The double-line sign is believed to be particularly characteristic of osteonecrosis. This sign appears as a line or band of low signal intensity on the T1-weighted spin echo MR images that contains an inner margin that increases in signal intensity on the proton density-weighted and T2-weighted spin echo MR images. The inner margin of high signal intensity is thought to represent the reactive interface that separates the necrotic from the viable bone.[55]

MR imaging also has been used to evaluate bone infarcts in patients with sickle cell anemia. In patients with normal hemoglobin, infarction occurs predominantly in fatty marrow, but in patients with sickle cell anemia, infarction occurs in both red and yellow marrow.[45] Focal areas of low or intermediate signal intensity on the T1-weighted spin echo images that increase in signal intensity on the T2-weighted spin echo images

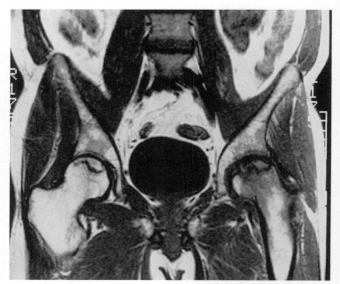

Figure 7–16
Osteonecrosis of both femoral heads. A coronal T1-weighted (TR/TE, 800/20) spin echo MR image of the pelvis in a patient with chronic renal failure shows bilateral osteonecrosis. On the right is a serpentine band of low signal intensity encircling an area of infarcted subchondral fatty marrow. On the left, material of low signal intensity is seen within the collapsed infarcted segment, presumably due to compressed bone and fibrosis.

presumably are related to edema and suggest acute marrow infarction, osteomyelitis, or liquefied cystic areas of old infarction. Focal areas that are low in signal intensity on both the T1- and T2-weighted spin echo MR images probably represent areas of remote infarction and fibrosis. Thus, MR imaging may permit differentiation of acute and chronic bone infarcts in sickle cell anemia and serve as a useful guide for monitoring the disease and selecting suitable therapy.[44]

Marrow Infiltration. The majority of cases of marrow infiltration with abnormal cellular material are secondary to tumor or infection. Other disorders associated with marrow infiltration include eosinophilic granuloma, Gaucher's disease, mucopolysaccharidoses, myelofibrosis, and osteopetrosis.[57] Numerous other disorders also are associated with abnormal cellular infiltration of the marrow and produce similar MR imaging findings, characterized by low signal intensity within the marrow on T1-weighted images. The T2-weighted spin echo and STIR images typically manifest high signal intensity within the abnormal regions, although some of these processes have more variable findings on the T2-weighted images (Fig. 7–17).

MR imaging is the procedure of choice for detection and anatomic staging of primary mesenchymal tumors of bone.[58] The extent of marrow involvement by tumor is better defined by MR imaging than by other imaging techniques.[2, 30, 58] MR imaging is useful in demonstrating areas of unsuspected neoplastic involvement such as skip lesions, characteristically seen in patients with osteosarcoma. The method also enables identification of areas of abnormal marrow toward which biopsy can be directed.[30, 58] It is the most accurate imaging method for demonstrating soft tissue extension of osseous tumors. Evaluation of the adjacent neurovascular bundles also is performed accurately and noninvasively using MR imaging.[58] Although the method is sensitive in the detection of tumor, it generally does not allow a specific histologic diagnosis.

Leukemia, lymphoma, Ewing's sarcoma, and multiple myeloma are primary malignancies arising directly from the bone marrow rather than from its supporting mesenchymal elements.[15, 29] These lesions, which arise from the hematopoietic cells, are found in sites of red marrow. Three patterns of marrow infiltration depicted with MR imaging have been described in patients with leukemia: diffuse uniform, diffuse patchy, and focal. Whereas the patchy and focal forms are easily identified on MR images, the diffuse uniform pattern may be difficult to recognize, especially with spin echo sequences, resulting in an appearance that has been termed the "flip-flop" sign.[59] On MR images, a diffuse decrease in the marrow signal intensity is seen on T1-weighted spin echo images, with an increase in signal intensity on T2-weighted spin echo images, a pattern opposite that of normal fatty marrow.

Bone metastasis almost always occurs via hematogenous spread. Because metastatic disease is most frequent after the age of 40 years, its distribution follows that of adult red marrow with axial predominance. The vertebral body, with its rich vascularity, is the most frequent site of metastatic involvement. Even though the pedicles have very little red marrow, they have a rich vascular supply, accounting for their early involvement in cases of skeletal metastasis.[15]

Scintigraphy is the traditional method for the detection of metastases owing to its ability to image the entire skeleton. Recent reports have emphasized the higher sensitivity of MR imaging for detection of metastatic disease, however. MR imaging allows detection of more lesions, presumably at an earlier stage in the disease, than conventional scintigraphy.[60, 61] For focal disease, particularly of the vertebra, MR imaging is the preferred method as it allows concurrent assessment of the spinal cord.[61] The appearance of metastatic disease on MR images is variable. Solitary, disseminated, and diffuse

Figure 7–17

Lymphoma: Coronal MR images of the distal portion of the femur in a 44 year old woman with lymphoma are shown.

A The T1-weighted (TR/TE, 800/12) spin echo MR image shows complete replacement of the fatty marrow of the distal femoral diaphysis, metaphysis, and epiphysis related to infiltration with neoplastic cells.

B The STIR (TR/TE, 2500/56; inversion time, 150 msec) image shows intense signal within the tumor. Note the thin rim of high signal intensity outside the cortex due to periostitis.

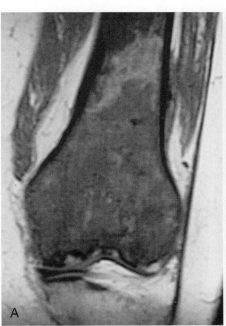
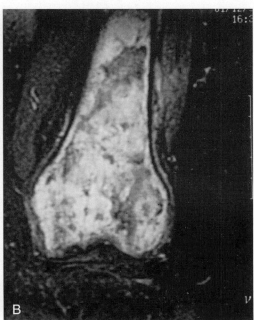

patterns may be seen. On T1-weighted spin echo images, areas of low signal intensity are seen within the normal marrow. Osteolytic lesions typically appear bright on T2-weighted spin echo and STIR images, whereas sclerotic metastases may appear hypo-, iso-, or hyperintense compared to the signal intensity of normal marrow.[61] MR imaging also is widely used for the diagnosis of osteomyelitis. Hematogenous spread of infection to bone may occur at any age but is seen most frequently in the child. The areas of greatest blood supply and most rapid growth, such as distal portion of the femur and the proximal portions of the tibia and humerus, are the most frequent sites of involvement. In the child, the metaphysis is the most common region of involvement. In adults, the prevalence of osteomyelitis in the axial skeleton increases, with the spine and pelvis being the most frequently affected site (Fig. 7–18).[15]

Bone marrow infection incites an intense inflammatory response with accumulation of marrow fluid. MR imaging and scintigraphy are both extremely sensitive for the early detection of infection and show changes when routine radiographs and CT scans are normal. MR imaging generally allows a more specific diagnosis of infection than scintigraphy and also is characterized by greater spatial resolution. MR imaging is beneficial for determining the extent of osteomyelitis and identifying adjacent soft tissue involvement. It also can aid in the identification of isolated soft tissue infection without underlying bony involvement.[2] Nonspecific adjacent edema and subperiosteal and soft tissue abscesses can be seen in acute, subacute, or chronic osteomyelitis.

Gaucher's disease is an inherited disorder in which

glucocerebroside accumulates in the reticuloendothelial system. Replacement of bone marrow by Gaucher cells produces low signal intensity lesions on both T1- and T2-weighted spin echo MR images.[57, 62] Both homogeneous and inhomogeneous patterns of altered signal intensity have been described. Marrow involvement in Gaucher's disease generally follows the distribution of red marrow and progresses from a proximal to distal direction in the appendicular skeleton. In more advanced disease, epiphyseal involvement and secondary osteonecrosis may develop.[57] A pattern of low signal intensity on both T1- and T2-weighted spin echo images, similar to that in Gaucher's disease, with loss of the signal intensity of fat within the epiphyses and apophyses, also may be seen in myelofibrosis. In advanced stages of the disease, dense fibrous tissue in the marrow and bone sclerosis both contribute to the abnormally low signal intensity.[28]

Osteopetrosis is a rare skeletal disorder characterized radiographically by a generalized increase in bone density. The infantile form of osteopetrosis is the most severe and is characterized by a complete lack of signal intensity on both the T1- and T2-weighted spin echo MR images, resulting in "black bones."[63] The intervertebral discs may have higher signal intensity than the vertebral marrow, a finding that is uniformly abnormal on T1-weighted spin echo images. Sequential MR imaging before and after bone marrow transplantation has shown promise for monitoring the response of this disease to therapy.[63] After successful therapy, an increase in the signal intensity of the bone marrow suggests repopulation with marrow elements. Hemosiderosis and diffuse marrow replacement by sclerotic metastases also can produce very low signal on both T1- and T2-weighted spin echo MR images, simulating the appearance of untreated osteopetrosis.[2]

SUMMARY

An understanding of the anatomy and physiology of bone and bone marrow is essential to the interpretation of imaging studies in patients with skeletal disorders. Owing in part to the unique signal intensity characteristics of fat, MR imaging represents an effective method in the analysis of many of these disorders. Although the resulting abnormalities often are not specific, the sensitivity of MR imaging to changes in the normal marrow, whether they relate to myeloid depletion, reconversion or failure of conversion, edema, ischemia or infiltration, is clear.

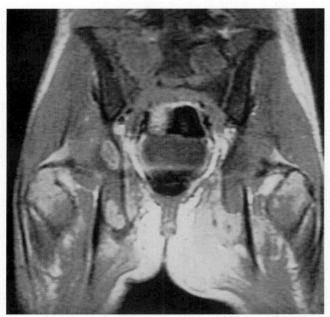

Figure 7–18
Osteomyelitis related to coccidioidomycosis. A coronal T1-weighted (TR/TE, 800/20) fat suppressed spin echo MR image of the pelvis obtained after the intravenous administration of gadolinium compound shows multiple sites of osteomyelitis in this 24 year old man with disseminated coccidiomycosis. Well-defined lesions, showing peripheral enhancement of signal intensity, are seen in both ischia and in the right acetabulum.

REFERENCES

1. Warwick R, Williams PL: Gray's Anatomy. 35th British ed. Philadelphia, WB Saunders CO, 1973, p. 49.
2. Vogler JB III, Murphy WA: Bone marrow imaging. Radiology *168*:679, 1988.
3. De Bruyn PH, Breen PC, Thomas TB: The microcirculation of the bone marrow. Anat Rec *168*:55, 1970.
4. Nathan DG: Introduction. Hematologic and hematopoietic diseases. *In* JB Wyngaarden, LH Smith Jr (Eds): Cecil Textbook of Medicine. 16th Ed. Philadelphia, WB Saunders Co, 1982, p 824.
5. Piney A: The anatomy of the bone marrow. Br Med J *2*:792, 1922.
6. Tribukait B: Experimental studies on the regulation of erythropoiesis with

special reference to the importance of oxygen. Acta Physiol Scand *58*:1, 1963.

7. Huggins C, Blocksom BH Jr: Changes in outlying bone marrow accompanying a local increase of temperature within physiologic limits. J Exp Med *64*:253, 1936.

8. Emery JL, Follett GF: Regression of bone-marrow haematopoiesis from the terminal digits in the foetus and infant. Br J Haematol *10*:485, 1964.

9. Jaramillo D, Laor T, Hoffer FA, et al: Epiphyseal marrow in infancy: MR imaging. Radiology *180*:809, 1991.

10. Ricci C, Cova M, Kang YS, et al: Normal age-related patterns of cellular and fatty bone marrow distribution in the axial skeleton: MR imaging study. Radiology *177*:83, 1990.

11. Dawson KL, Moore SG, Rowland JM: Age-related changes in the pelvis: MR and anatomic findings. Radiology *183*:47, 1992.

12. Moore SG, Bisset GS III, Siegel MJ, et al: Pediatric musculoskeletal MR imaging. Radiology *179*:345, 1991.

13. Richardson ML, Patten RM: Age-related changes in marrow distribution in the shoulder: MR imaging findings. Radiology *192*:209, 1994.

14. Duda SH, Laniado M, Schick F, et al: Normal bone marrow in the sacrum of young adults: Differences between the sexes seen on chemical-shift MR imaging. AJR *164*:935, 1995.

15. Kricun ME: Red-yellow marrow conversion: Its effect on the location of some solitary bone lesions. Skel Radiol *14*:10, 1985.

16. Pathria MN, Isaac P: Magnetic resonance imaging of bone marrow. Curr Opin Radiol *4*:21, 1992.

17. Sze G, Bravo S, Baierl P, et al: Developing spinal column: Gadolinium-enhanced MR imaging. Radiology *180*:497, 1991.

18. Zawin JK, Jaramillo D: Conversion of bone marrow in the humerus, sternum, and clavicle: Changes with age on MR images. Radiology *188*:159, 1993.

19. Moore SG, Dawson KL: Red and yellow marrow in the femur: Age-related changes in appearance at MR imaging. Radiology *175*:219, 1990.

20. Mirowitz SA: Hematopoietic bone marrow within the proximal humeral epiphysis in normal adults: Investigation with MR imaging. Radiology *188*:689, 1993.

21. Waitches G, Zawin JK, Poznanski AK: Sequence and rate of bone marrow conversion in the femora of children as seen on MR imaging: Are accepted standards accurate? AJR *162*:1399, 1992.

22. Richardson ML, Patten RM: Age-related changes in marrow distribution in the shoulder: MR imaging findings. Radiology *192*:209, 1994.

23. Shellock FG, Morris E, Deutsch AL, et al: Hematopoietic bone marrow hyperplasia: High prevalence on MR images of the knee in asymptomatic marathon runners. AJR *158*:335, 1992.

24. Deutsch AL, Mink HJ, Rosenfelt FP, et al: Incidental detection of hematopoietic hyperplasia on routine knee MR imaging. AJR *152*:333, 1989.

25. Sugimura K, Yamasaki K, Kitagaki H, et al: Bone marrow diseases of the spine: Differentiation with T1 and T2 relaxation times in MR imaging. Radiology *165*:541, 1987.

26. Dooms GC, Fisher MR, Hricak H, et al: Bone marrow imaging: Magnetic resonance studies related to age and sex. Radiology *155*:429, 1985.

27. Schick F, Bongers H, Aicher K, et al: Subtle bone marrow edema assessed by frequency selective chemical shift MRI. J Comput Assist Tomogr *16*:454, 1992.

28. Kaplan KR, Mitchell DG, Steiner RM, et al: Polycythemia vera and myelofibrosis: Correlation of MR imaging, clinical, and laboratory findings. Radiology *183*:329, 1992.

29. Cohen MD, Klatte EC, Baehner R, et al: Magnetic resonance imaging of bone marrow disease in children. Radiology *151*:715, 1984.

30. Daffner RH, Lupetin AR, Dash N, et al: MR in the detection of malignant infiltration of bone marrow. AJR *146*:353, 1986.

31. Mirowitz SA, Apicella P, Reinus WR, et al: MR imaging of bone marrow lesions: Relative conspicuousness on T1-weighted, fat-suppressed T2-weighted, and STIR images. AJR *162*:215, 1994.

32. Shuman WP, Patten RM, Baron RL, et al: Comparison of STIR and spin-echo MR imaging at 1.5 T in 45 suspected extremity tumors: Lesion conspicuity and extent. Radiology *179*:247, 1991.

33. Weinberger E, Shaw DWW, White KS, et al: Nontraumatic pediatric musculoskeletal MR imaging: Comparison of conventional and fast-spin-echo short inversion time inversion-recovery technique. Radiology *194*:721, 1995.

34. Wismer GL, Rosen BR, Buxton R, et al: Chemical shift imaging of bone marrow: Preliminary experience. AJR *145*:1031, 1985.

35. Rosen BR, Fleming DM, Kushner DC, et al: Hematologic bone marrow disorders: Quantitative chemical shift MR imaging. Radiology *169*:799, 1988.

36. McKinstry CS, Steiner RE, Young AT, et al: Bone marrow in leukemia and aplastic anemia: MR imaging before, during, and after treatment. Radiology *162*:701, 1987.

37. Sebag GH, Moore SG: Effect of trabecular bone on the appearance of marrow in gradient-echo imaging of the appendicular skeleton. Radiology *174*:855, 1990.

38. Smith SR, Williams CE, Davies JM, et al: Bone marrow disorders: Characterization with quantitative MR imaging. Radiology *172*:805, 1989.

39. Kaplan PA, Asleson RJ, Klassen, LW, et al: Bone marrow patterns in aplastic anemia: Observations with 1.5-T MR imaging. Radiology *164*:441, 1987.

40. Yankelevitz DF, Henschke CI, Knapp PH, et al: Effect of radiation therapy on thoracic and lumbar bone marrow: Evaluation with MR imaging. AJR *157*:87, 1991.

41. Blomlie V, Rofstad EK, Skjonsberg A, et al: Female pelvic bone marrow: Serial MR imaging before, during and after radiation therapy. Radiology *194*:537, 1995.

42. Ramsey R, Zacharias CE: MR imaging of the spine after radiation therapy: Easily recognizable effects. AJR *144*:1131, 1985.

43. Stevens SK, Moore SG, Amylon MD: Repopulation of marrow after transplantation: MR imaging with pathologic correlation. Radiology *175*:213, 1990.

44. Rao VM, Fishman M, Mitchell DG, et al: Painful sickle cell crisis: Bone marrow patterns observed with MR imaging. Radiology *161*:211, 1986.

45. Rao VM, Mitchell DG, Rifkin MD, et al: Marrow infarction in sickle cell anemia: Correlation with marrow type and distribution by MRI. Magn Res Imaging *7*:39, 1989.

46. Gouliamos A, Dardoufas C, Papiliou I, et al: Low back pain due to extramedullary hemopoiesis. Neuroradiology *33*:284, 1991.

47. Papavasiliou C, Gouliamos A, Vlahos L, et al: CT and MRI of symptomatic spinal involvement by extramedullary hematopoiesis. Clin Radiol *42*:91, 1990.

48. Fletcher BD, Wall JE, Hanna SL: Effect of hematopoietic growth factors on MR images of bone marrow in children undergoing chemotherapy. Radiology *189*:745, 1993.

49. Steen RG: Edema and tumor perfusion: Characterization by quantitative ^{1}H MR imaging. AJR *158*:259, 1992.

50. Meyers SP, Wiener SN: Magnetic resonance imaging of fractures using the short tau inversion recovery (STIR) sequence: Correlation with radiographic findings. Skel Radiol *20*:499, 1991.

51. Mink JH, Deutsch AL: Occult cartilage and bone injuries of the knee: Detection, classification, and assessment with MR imaging. Radiology *170*:823, 1989.

52. Yao L, Lee JK: Occult intraosseous fracture: Detection with MR imaging. Radiology *167*:749, 1988.

53. Hayes CW, Conway WF, Daniel WW: MR imaging of bone marrow edema pattern: Transient osteoporosis, transient bone marrow edema syndrome, or osteonecrosis. RadioGraphics *13*:1001, 1993.

54. Bloem HL: Transient osteoporosis of the hip: MR imaging. Radiology *167*:753, 1988.

55. Mitchell DG, Rao VM, Dalinka MK, et al: Femoral head avascular necrosis: Correlation of MR imaging, radiographic staging, radionuclide imaging, and clinical findings. Radiology *162*:709, 1987.

56. Cova M, Kang YS, Tsukamoto H, et al: Bone marrow perfusion evaluated with gadolinium-enhanced dynamic fast MR imaging in a dog model. Radiology *179*:535, 1991.

57. Lanir A, Hadar H, Cohen I, et al: Gaucher disease: Assessment with MR imaging. Radiology *161*:239, 1986.

58. Sundaram M, McLeod RA: MR imaging of tumor and tumorlike lesions of bone and soft tissue. AJR *155*:817, 1990.

59. Ruzal-Shapiro C, Berdon WE, Cohen MD, et al: MR imaging of diffuse bone marrow replacement in pediatric patients with cancer. Radiology *181*:587, 1991.

60. Frank JA, Ling A, Patronas NJ, et al: Detection of malignant bone tumors: MR imaging vs scintigraphy. AJR:155, 1990.

61. Algra PR, Bloem JL, Tissing H, et al: Detection of vertebral metastases: Comparison between MR imaging and bone scintigraphy. Radiographics *11*:219, 1991.

62. Rosenthal DI, Barton NW, McKusick KA, et al: Quantitative imaging of Gaucher disease. Radiology *185*:841, 1992.

63. Rao VM, Dalinka MK, Mitchell DG, et al: Osteopetrosis: MR characteristics at 1.5 T. Radiology *161*:217, 1986.

8 | *Traumatic Disorders of Bone*

Physical injury contributes to a wide variety of alterations in the bones, joints, and soft tissues. In addition to fractures, dislocations, subluxations, and capsular, tendinous, muscular, and ligamentous tears, trauma can affect the growth plate of the immature skeleton as well as the hyaline cartilaginous and fibrocartilaginous joint structures. Additional complications of trauma include reflex sympathetic dystrophy, osteolysis, osteonecrosis, many of the osteochondroses, neuropathic osteoarthropathy, infection, and heterotopic bone formation. Nonmechanical trauma to the musculoskeletal system can result from thermal and electrical injury, irradiation, and chemical substances.

This chapter represents an overview of the subject of skeletal trauma. Emphasis is placed on the general principles governing the analysis of fractures and dislocations in both the adult and the child, the consequences of injuries to synchondroses (growth plates) in the immature skeleton, and special types of injury.

ADVANCED DIAGNOSTIC TECHNIQUES

Although routine radiography is adequate as an imaging technique in the assessment of most skeletal injuries, CT is able to define the presence and extent of certain fractures or dislocations, to detect intra-articular abnormalities, including cartilage damage and osteocartilaginous bodies (Fig. 8–1), and to assess the nearby soft tissues. Its application to traumatic abnormalities in regions of complicated anatomy, such as the spine, the bones in the face and pelvis, the glenohumeral and sternoclavicular joints, the wrist (Fig. 8–2), and the midfoot and hindfoot, is especially noteworthy. The facts that the examination with CT is accomplished with a greater degree of patient comfort than with routine radiography and that plaster casts do not create significant deterioration of the image quality also are important.

After trauma to the musculoskeletal system, the important indication for arteriography is the identification of vascular abnormalities, including disruption and occlusion of major vessels, arteriovenous fistulae, and aneurysms, in patients whose physical examination indicates signs such as ischemia, pulse deficit, or bleeding that are compatible with a significant injury to the blood vessels. With regard to the extremities, the vessels that are injured most commonly are in close proximity to a bone and held in a relatively fixed position by fascial or muscular attachment. The subclavian artery may be injured by the distal fragment of a clavicular fracture; the axillary artery may be damaged in shoulder dislocations owing to the injury itself or to attempts at reduction of the humeral head; the brachial artery may be injured by a fracture of the humerus or a dislocation of the elbow; the radial or ulnar artery may be lacerated

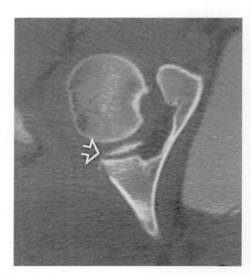

Figure 8–1
Physical injury (CT scanning). Transaxial CT scans are useful in the detection of intra-articular bodies (arrow), as in this patient who had had a fracture-dislocation of the hip.

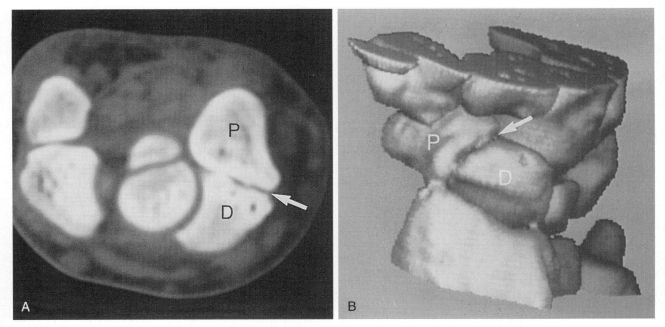

Figure 8–2
Physical injury (CT scanning). A transaxial CT scan **(A)** and a three-dimensional CT display **(B)** of the wrist show a subacute fracture of the midportion of the scaphoid bone (arrows), with bone sclerosis at the fracture site indicative of a fracture nonunion. The proximal (P) and distal (D) portions of the scaphoid bone are indicated.

by fractures of the radius and ulna; the femoral artery in the adductor canal and the popliteal artery throughout its course are vulnerable in fractures or dislocations of contiguous bones; the anterior tibial artery or, less commonly, the posterior tibial artery may be compromised by fractures of the tibia; and the posterior tibial and dorsalis pedis arteries may be affected in fractures or dislocations of the ankle or foot.[1] With regard to injuries of the bony pelvis, bleeding may result from laceration or tearing of one or more vessels and may be massive; the identification of the site of arterial compromise can be accomplished with arteriography.[2]

Scintigraphy also is useful in the evaluation of patients with skeletal trauma. This role is perhaps best exemplified in the diagnosis of stress fractures (see later discussion), although scintigraphy may be helpful in detecting subtle acute fractures when radiographs are normal (e.g., in the carpal bones, the ribs, the foot, and the bones of the pelvis and the hip) (Fig. 8–3) or in excluding fractures in the presence of significant clinical findings. It also can be used to evaluate the healing response.[3]

Although ultrasonography is extremely useful in the assessment of soft tissue injuries, such as those involving muscles and tendons, its role in the evaluation of bone and cartilage injuries is limited, and this method compares poorly with MR imaging in this regard.[4]

MR imaging is assuming ever-increasing importance in the analysis of many musculoskeletal disorders, including injury. The unique signal intensity characteristics of marrow allow MR imaging to provide a valuable perspective with regard to abnormalities, including traumatic ones, that involve the interior of a bone and, indeed, new terms such as bone marrow edema and bone bruise have been developed to describe some of

the alterations visible on MR images (see later discussion). Furthermore, in an indirect fashion, MR imaging provides information regarding the bone cortex. Although compact cortical bone is devoid of signal on MR

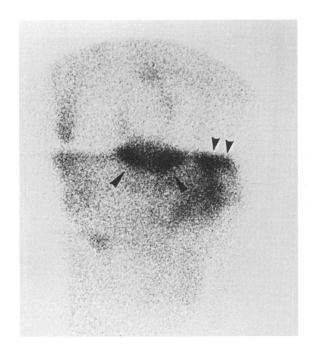

Figure 8–3
Physical injury (bone scintigraphy). Anterior pinhole scintigram shows intense tracer uptake at the site of fractures of the tibial spines (larger arrowheads) and fibular neck and similar uptake at the site of a radiographically inapparent fracture of the lateral tibial plateau (smaller arrowheads). (Reproduced with permission of YW Bahk: Combined Scintigraphic and Radiographic Diagnosis of Bone and Joint Disorders. New York, Springer-Verlag, 1994.)

images, its interruption or violation by tumor, infection, or fracture may be evident during the MR imaging examination, and the accompanying response of the periosteal membrane also may be visible. The physician should understand, however, that it is the ancillary findings such as marrow and soft tissue edema and hemorrhage accompanying the fracture that are displayed more dramatically than the fracture line itself on the MR images.

The extreme sensitivity of MR imaging to bone (and cartilage) injury makes it an indispensable supplementary technique in some patients whose initial routine radiographs after acute trauma either are negative or equivocal (Fig. 8–4).[5] In this regard, MR imaging competes favorably with bone scintigraphy, even single photon emission computed tomography (SPECT). MR imaging examination also enjoys far greater specificity. An abbreviated MR imaging study whose cost is not unlike that of scintigraphy may be sufficient for diagnosis of occult fractures of the femoral neck, about the knee, or elsewhere.[6–8] Additionally, modifications in MR imaging technique such as fat suppression, intravenous administration of gadolinium contrast agent, and short tau inversion recovery (STIR) imaging,[9] while increasing the duration and the expense of the examination, may provide even greater sensitivity for fracture detection. MR imaging is far better when employed to evaluate a single region of the body, whereas bone scintigraphy is more effective as a general surveyor of the skeleton, which assumes clinical importance in cases of multiple injuries or of child abuse.

As is noted later in this chapter, various types of occult fractures have been identified using MR imaging techniques. In many instances, it is not the fracture itself but the reaction of the neighboring bone marrow that is the dominant MR imaging abnormality. This reaction often is designated marrow edema, although histologic data confirming the existence of such edema are meager. The sensitivity of the MR imaging examination to the detection of these important marrow abnormalities depends on the sequences employed. Owing to the frequent occurrence of occult fractures in areas of the peripheral skeleton that contain abundant marrow fat, standard T2-weighted spin echo MR images, in which both fat and edema are of relative high signal intensity, may not be adequate for detection of the injury. Although standard T1-weighted spin echo MR images may be positive in cases of occult fracture, they too are not extremely sensitive. To overcome this problem, modifications in MR imaging technique have been employed. The major and most popular modifications include spin echo or fast spin echo images obtained with fat suppression, short tau inversion recovery (STIR) or fast spin echo STIR images, and T1-weighted fat-suppressed spin echo MR images obtained after the intravenous administration of a gadolinium contrast agent (Figs. 8–5 and 8–6).[10, 11] Although practical considerations prevent the use of all of these methods in a single patient, the choice of which one (or ones) to employ is not agreed on. Indeed, each of these methods, although sensitive in the detection of marrow edema, has both advantages and disadvantages. In general, STIR sequences, because of the combined effect of fat suppression and the addi-

tive T1 and T2 effects of water-containing substances,[12] represent an effective screening method for a variety of pathologic conditions, and their combination with fast spin echo pulse sequences allows image acquisition in a shorter period of time.[13] In some studies, fast spin echo STIR images have been found to be preferable to fat-suppressed fast spin echo MR images because of better image homogeneity and lesion conspicuity.[11] In other studies, both fast spin echo STIR and fat-suppressed fast spin echo sequences have been preferred over conventional STIR sequences in assessing bone injuries.[13] The use of gadolinium-enhanced T1-weighted spin echo images combined with fat suppression also provides a sensitive method when applied to marrow abnormalities. This technique, however, requires an intravenous injection and is better applied to evaluation of infectious and neoplastic disorders of bone rather than traumatic ones. The advantages of intra-articular injection of a gadolinium compound (MR arthrography) when combined with spin echo or gradient echo MR images lie not in the detection of posttraumatic marrow edema but rather in the assessment of cartilage integrity, as in patients with osteochondritis dissecans.

FRACTURES

Fracture Healing

After a bone is fractured (Fig. 8–7), three indistinctly separated phases of healing are recognized: an inflammatory phase, representing approximately 10 per cent of the entire time of fracture healing; a reparative phase, representing about 40 per cent of this time; and a remodeling phase, the longest phase, representing as much as 70 per cent of the time.[14, 15] The orderly sequence of events terminating in complete healing of a fracture does not invariably take place as described, however. In some instances, the healing process is markedly slowed (*delayed union*) or arrested altogether (*nonunion*). Nonunion generally indicates that the fracture site has failed to heal completely during a period of approximately 6 to 9 months after the injury and that a typical *pseudarthrosis* (consisting of a synovium-lined cavity and synovial fluid typically related to persistent motion at the nonunion site) or a fibrous union has developed, in which the ends of the bone are either osteoporotic and atrophic or sclerotic.[16] Nonunion of a scaphoid, tibial, or femoral fracture is encountered most commonly, whereas nonunion occurring after a fracture of the humerus, radius, ulna, and clavicle is somewhat less frequent (Fig. 8–8). Ancillary imaging techniques such as bone scintigraphy, CT, and MR imaging may be used in the assessment of fracture healing and in the diagnosis of delayed union, nonunion, or pseudarthroses, although data regarding the efficacy of these techniques are incomplete.[17]

Special Types of Fractures

Pathologic Fractures

A pathologic fracture is one in which the bone is disrupted at a site of preexisting abnormality, frequently

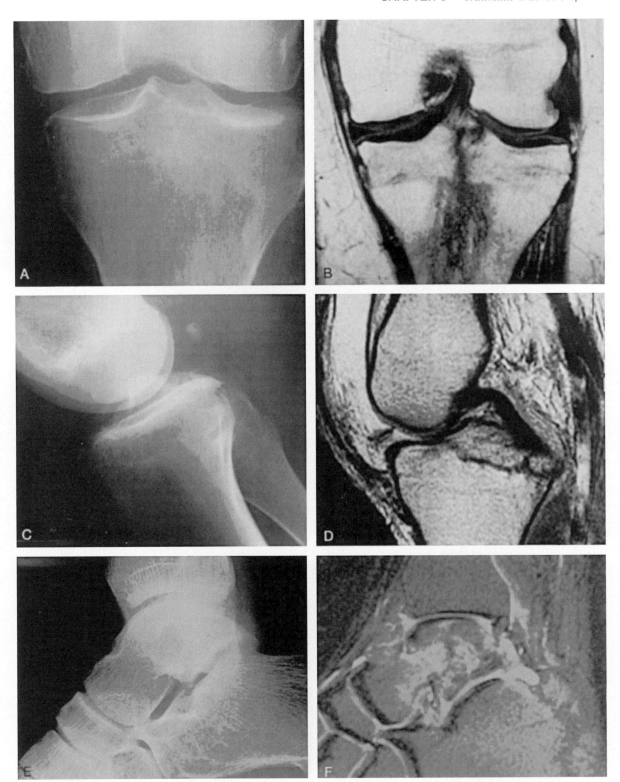

Figure 8–4

Physical injury (MR imaging).

A, B Proximal portion of the tibia. The initial radiograph **(A)** reveals minimal sclerosis beneath the tibial eminences but was interpreted as normal. A coronal T1-weighted (TR/TE, 750/20) spin echo MR image **(B)** vividly displays the fracture.

C, D Proximal portion of the tibia. With routine radiography **(C),** a subtle fracture line is evident. A sagittal proton density (TR/TE, 2000/30) spin echo MR image **(D)** displays the fracture of the posterior portion of the tibial plateau as a region of low signal intensity. Note subtle surrounding marrow edema of higher signal intensity and the attachment of an intact posterior cruciate ligament to the fragment. A joint effusion is present.

E, F Talus. A fracture is not seen on the plain film **(E),** nor was it detected with conventional tomography (not shown). A sagittal T2-weighted (TR/TE, 2050/80) spin echo MR image **(F)** clearly shows the fracture of the body of the talus with bone marrow edema and joint effusions.

(**E, F,** Courtesy of G. Greenway, M.D., Dallas, Texas.)

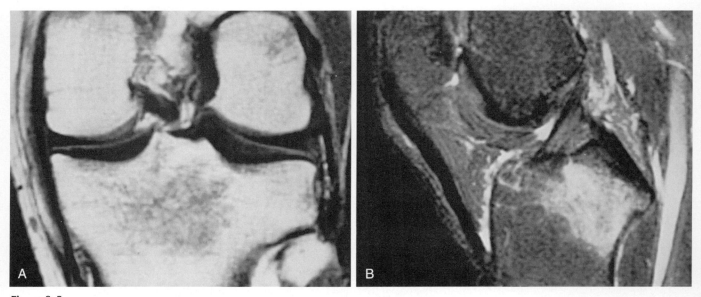

Figure 8–5
Physical injury (MR imaging, bone marrow edema).

A A coronal T1-weighted (TR/TE, 650/16) spin echo MR image reveals an area of decreased signal intensity involving the posterior aspect of the proximal portion of the tibia. A reticulated appearance is evident, typical of a bone bruise.

B A sagittal fat-suppressed fast spin echo MR image (TR/TE, 4200/76) more dramatically displays the region of bone marrow edema, manifested as a geographic pattern of high signal intensity.

(Courtesy of S.K. Brahme, M.D., San Diego, California)

by a stress that would not have fractured a normal bone. The most common underlying abnormalities are tumors and osteoporosis. Although the size of the lesion and, more important, the extent of cortical destruction generally are believed to be fundamental in influencing the likelihood of pathologic fracture, routine radiography represents an inadequate technique in evaluating such factors.[18] Conventional tomography and, particularly, CT with its transaxial image display are superior methods in this evaluation. The value of MR imaging in the identification of lesions at risk for fracture is not yet clear.

Trabecular Microfractures (Bone Bruises)

With the application of MR imaging to the evaluation of musculoskeletal injuries has come the identification

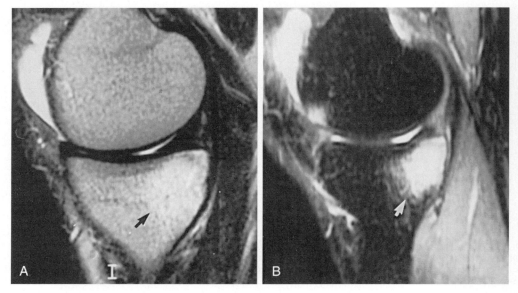

Figure 8–6
Physical injury (MR imaging, bone marrow edema).

A A sagittal fast spin echo MR image (TR/TE 4000/105) obtained without fat suppression does not optimally show the site of abnormality (arrow) in the posteromedial portion of the tibia, owing to the surrounding high signal intensity of normal fatty marrow.

B A sagittal fast spin echo STIR MR image (TR/TE, 3667/17; inversion time, 150 msec) dramatically reveals the site of marrow edema (arrow).

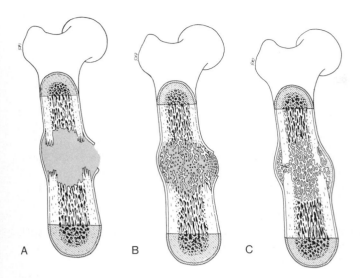

Figure 8–7
Normal fracture healing.

A After the injury, bleeding is related to osseous and soft tissue damage. A hematoma followed by clot formation develops within the medullary canal between the fracture ends and beneath the periosteal membrane, which itself may have been torn.

B Callus formation takes place, consisting of external bridging callus at the periosteal surface, intramedullary callus, and primary callus at the ends of the fracture fragments.

C The callus envelops the bone ends rapidly, producing increasing stability at the fracture site.

of intraosseous regions of altered signal intensity that have been designated occult intraosseous fractures[19, 20] or bone bruises.[21] These injuries, which typically are located close to a joint surface, are believed to result from compression or impaction forces, although no correlative histologic data exist to confirm this belief.

Their frequent association with other traumatic abnormalities such as cruciate and collateral ligament injuries of the knee[8, 21] is consistent with the occurrence of trabecular microfractures with resultant hyperemia, hemorrhage, and edema in the bone marrow. Arthroscopy in cases in which bone bruises are evident on MR examination fails to reveal corresponding lesions, documenting that the adjacent articular surface is grossly normal.[7] The presence of similar changes in the signal intensity of the bone marrow on MR images in patients with osteochondral lesions supports the concept of injury in the pathogenesis of bone bruises, and histologic data that indicate marrow edema in cases of transient osteoporosis of periarticular bone (in which these same signal intensity changes are observed) are further evidence that intraosseous fluid accumulation accompanies these bone bruises. It appears likely that the trabecular alterations that characterize bone bruises are very similar if not identical to those associated with stress fractures, although in the former situation an acute episode of trauma rather than chronic repetitive stress is the initiating event. Indeed, in one study typical MR imaging findings of bone bruises in the feet were observed in volunteers after a 2 week period of altered weight-bearing.[22] Whether bone bruises themselves are symptomatic is not clear, although their occurrence as an isolated finding in patients with local pain supports the possibility. Resolution of the MR imaging abnormalities associated with bone bruises generally occurs over a period of 1 month to several months and may coincide with decrease or disappearance of the patient's symptoms.[7] Such resolution, however, is not uniformly present (see later discussion).

Many descriptions exist of subchondral and intraosseous foci of altered signal intensity, especially about the

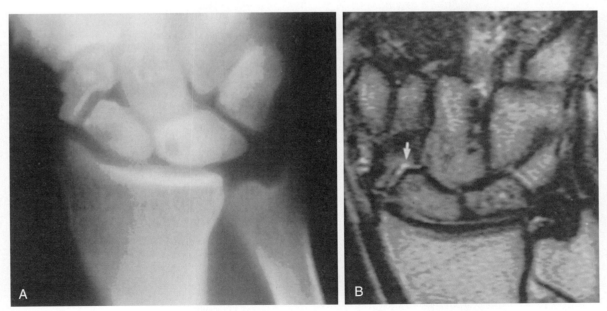

Figure 8–8
Abnormal fracture healing: Nonunion with pseudarthrosis. Scaphoid bone of the wrist. The conventional tomogram (**A**) reveals sclerotic fracture lines with smooth margins in the scaphoid bone. Cystic and sclerotic changes in the lunate bone are consistent with Kienböck's disease. A coronal T2-weighted (TR/TE, 2500/60) spin echo MR image (**B**) shows fluid of high signal intensity (arrow) in the fracture gap as well as increased signal intensity in the lunate bone.

knee. However, during MR imaging examinations of patients with a history of injury, frequently acute, the terminology applied to these lesions and the methods used to classify them have not been consistent.[19–21, 23–25] Some of the lesions are located at a distance from the chondral surface and are consistent with trabecular microfractures, whereas others, on the basis of clinical or imaging data, appear to represent stress fractures or avulsion injuries (e.g., the Segond fracture of the lateral portion of the tibia[26]). What remains in these descriptions are a number of subchondral abnormalities, frequently extending to the joint surface. Whether these latter abnormalities represent microfractures of subchondral trabeculae alone or whether they are part of a more extensive injury involving the adjacent articular cartilage (i.e., osteochondral fracture) is not always clear. Numerous investigators have tried to clarify this issue, often by introducing classification systems based on the appearance of the MR imaging abnormalities.

In 1989, Mink and Deutsch,[7] in a retrospective analysis of 66 patients who had MR imaging findings consistent with fractures about the knee, identified four types of injury: bone bruise, stress fracture, femoral and tibial fracture, and osteochondral fracture. Bone bruises (Fig. 8–9), representing 30 lesions in 27 knees, were defined as posttraumatic, subchondral, geographic, and nonlinear areas of signal loss on T1-weighted spin echo MR images, with increased signal intensity observed on T2-weighted spin echo MR images. These involved the epiphysis and usually a portion of the metaphysis, were associated with normal-appearing articular cartilage, and were evident in the femur, the tibia, and the fibula, in decreasing order of frequency. The mechanism of injury commonly involved twisting of the knee, and associated ligamentous abnormalities (e.g., of the collateral ligaments and anterior cruciate ligament) were frequent. Arthroscopy confirmed the existence of these ligamentous tears wherever it was employed, and the bone bruises were not apparent at the time of arthroscopic surgery. These investigators regarded this lesion as one associated with a benign clinical course. Stress fractures, observed in six patients, were associated with two patterns of abnormality on the MR images: a linear zone of decreased signal intensity surrounded by a broader, poorly defined zone of less decreased signal intensity on T1-weighted spin echo MR images, the latter zone showing increased signal intensity on T2-weighted spin echo MR images; and an amorphous lesion without a linear component but with similar signal intensity characteristics. The MR imaging appearance of the amorphous lesion was virtually identical to that of the bone bruise, the differentiation being made on the basis of history (no single traumatic event in cases of stress fracture) and information provided by

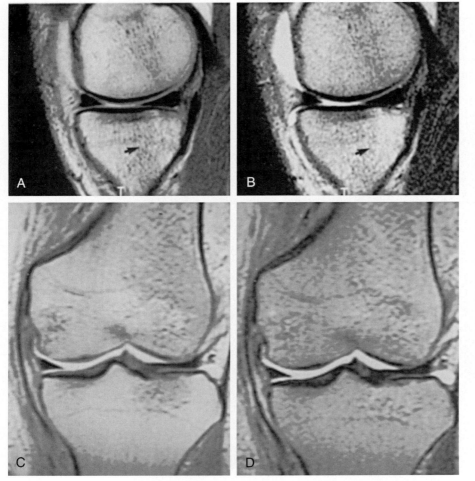

Figure 8–9
Physical injury: Trabecular microfractures (bone bruises).

A, B Sagittal proton density (TR/TE, 2200/30) (**A**) and T2-weighted (TR/TE, 2200/80) spin echo MR images show the characteristic finding of a bone bruise (arrows), which in this case involves mainly the posterior portion of the medial tibial plateau. The lesion is of high signal intensity in **B.** Note the joint effusion.

C, D Similar abnormalities of signal intensity in a different patient are evident on coronal proton density (TR/TE, 2500/20) (**C**) and T2-weighted (TR/TE, 2500/60) (**D**) spin echo MR images. The bone bruises are located in the lateral portions of the distal end of the femur and proximal tibia and, to a lesser extent, in the medial femoral condyle. They are of higher signal intensity in **D** and are associated with a partial tear of the medial collateral ligament and a joint effusion.

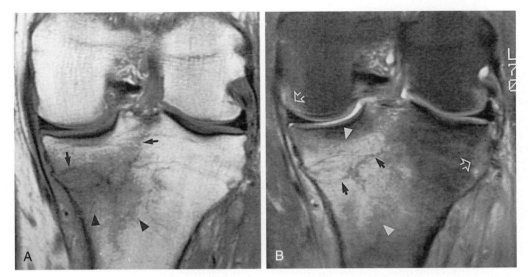

Figure 8–10

Physical injury: Tibial plateau fracture. This 50 year old man suffered an acute injury to the knee. Routine radiographs (not shown) revealed an avulsion fracture of the fibular head and a joint effusion.

A A coronal T1-weighted (TR/TE, 800/13) spin echo MR image shows an irregular, linear region of low signal intensity (arrows) extending to the surface of the intercondylar eminence of the tibia, indicative of a nondisplaced tibial plateau fracture (which was confirmed on subsequent radiographs). Surrounding the fracture line, a broader region of slightly higher (but still low) signal intensity (arrowheads) represents marrow edema.

B A coronal fat-suppressed fast spin echo MR image (TR/TE, 4000/18) shows the fracture (solid arrows), still of low signal intensity, and the tibial marrow edema (arrowheads), of high signal intensity. Note bone bruises of high signal intensity in the medial femoral condyle and lateral tibial plateau (open arrows).

follow-up radiographic examinations. Femoral and tibial fractures were characterized by single or multiple areas of decreased signal intensity that extended vertically to involve the articular surfaces on both T1- and T2-weighted images (Fig. 8–10). Osteochondral fractures were described as either displaced (in which the cartilage and often a small underlying segment of bone were fractured and at least partially displaced from their site of origin) or impacted (in which the overlying cartilage and the subchondral bone were impacted into the medullary cavity, and no large, free fragments were generated) (Fig. 8–11). Displaced osteochondral fractures arose from the patella or from either the medial or the lateral femoral condyle, and all were confirmed at arthroscopy; impacted osteochondral fractures were encountered almost invariably in the lateral femoral condyle. The impacted fractures were characterized by a very marked decrease in signal intensity at the site of injury on T1- and T2-weighted MR images and by surrounding marrow edema, with an increase in signal intensity on T2-weighted MR images.

In 1989, Lynch and associates,[27] in a retrospective study of 434 patients who had undergone MR imaging examinations of the knee, divided signal intensity loss in the marrow on short echo time (20 or 25 msec) images into three types: a type 1 pattern was characterized by a diffuse, often reticulated signal intensity loss in the metaphyseal and epiphyseal regions of the bone; a type 2 pattern was associated with an interruption in the smooth flat subchondral bone plate; and a type 3 pattern was characterized by a profound loss of signal intensity presumably restricted to the subchondral bone located immediately adjacent to the bone plate. The type 1 pattern, which often was associated with an in-

crease in signal intensity on T2-weighted spin echo MR images, was believed to be related to microfractures of the subchondral trabeculae that led to a local increase in fluid content (e.g., hemorrhage or nonhemorrhagic edema) in cancellous marrow. This pattern was observed commonly in patients with additional evidence of ligamentous injury, was almost uniformly accompanied by normal findings on routine radiographs, and, in more than 70 per cent of cases, was not associated

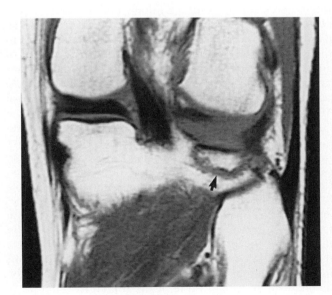

Figure 8–11

Physical injury: Osteochondral fracture. On this coronal T1-weighted (TR/TE, 800/13) spin echo MR image, a slightly depressed osteochondral fracture (arrow) of the lateral tibial plateau is evident. A bucket-handle tear of the lateral meniscus also is evident.

Table 8–1. PERIARTICULAR BONE LESIONS

	Cartilage	Ligaments	Radiography	Arthroscopy	Epiphysis	Metaphysis	MR Imaging Appearance		
							T1	*T2*	*Pattern*
Bone bruise	—	±	—	—	±	±	↓	↑	Reticular
Osteochondral Fracture	±	±	±	±	+	—	↓	↑	Curvilinear
Stress fracture	—	—	±	—	±	±	↓	↑	Linear
Osteonecrosis	±	—	±	±	+	—	↓	↑↓	Broad
Osteoarthritis: Sclerosis	+	—	±	+	+	—	↓	↓	Broad
Osteoarthritis: Cysts	+	—	±	+	+	—	↓	↑	Circular

+ Abnormal; — Normal; ± Possibly abnormal; ↓ Decreased signal intensity; ↑ Increased signal intensity.

with arthroscopically evident abnormalities of the articular cartilage. The type 1 pattern of abnormality disappeared over a period of weeks to several months. The type 2 pattern, usually also accompanied by increased signal intensity on the T2-weighted spin echo MR images, was believed to be related to frank fractures of the subchondral bone plate, although such fractures often were not evident on routine radiographs or even at the time of arthroscopic surgery (i.e., the articular cartilage was judged to be grossly normal). The type 3 pattern, which was not associated with increased signal intensity on T2-weighted spin echo MR images, was believed to be indicative of degenerative changes within the bone, some of which were apparent on routine radiographs.

In 1991, Vellet and associates,[24] in a study of patients with acute posttraumatic hemarthrosis of the knee, detected occult subcortical femoral and tibial fractures in 72 per cent of patients. Lesions were divided into two types, depending on their appearance on T1-weighted spin echo MR images: occult, including reticular, geographic, linear, impaction, and osteochondral fractures; and overt, including osteochondral and frank fractures. Occult fractures predominated in the lateral compartment of the knee, consistent with the occurrence of valgus forces at the time of injury. On the basis of the observation that occult fractures in the lateral femoral condyle often were accompanied by similar fractures in the posterolateral portion of the tibia, a mechanism of anterior dislocation of the tibia relative to the femur was proposed. Significant osteochondral sequelae of these occult fractures frequently were observed at the time of MR imaging 6 to 12 months later.

On the basis of the results of these and other investigations, MR imaging appears to be extremely sensitive in the detection of a heterogeneous group of acute posttraumatic lesions of the knee (and of other sites) that escape detection with routine radiography (Table 8–1). Some of these clearly involve the articular surfaces and are best considered various forms of osteochondral fractures, whereas others appear to be located at a distance from these surfaces. They may represent a spectrum of injury whose precise MR imaging manifestations in any individual patient are dictated primarily by the mechanism and magnitude of the injury. At one end of the spectrum is the bone bruise, a self-limited benign abnormality with no osteochondral sequelae[28]; at the other end of the spectrum is the overt, or frank, fracture that may or may not involve the osteochondral surface.

In between these two are a number of other traumatic lesions, varying in location with respect to the articular surface, frequently occult without routine radiographic abnormality. The fact that arthroscopy also may fail to document the presence of an abnormality of the joint surface serves only to underscore the limitations of the arthroscopic examination, as histologic evidence of abnormality may exist.[29]

The classification of occult injuries to bone not on the basis of their MR imaging patterns but rather on their anatomic distribution also can be attempted (Table 8–2). Acutely, such fractures can involve the articular cartilage alone (chondral fracture), the articular cartilage and subchondral bone plate together (osteochondral fracture), the subchondral trabeculae or those in the spongiosa at a distance from the articular cartilage (trabecular microfractures or infractions), the cortical bone (major fractures and stress fractures), or the periosteal membrane (traumatic periostitis). Sequelae of chronic injuries of the articular cartilage and subchondral bone plate (osteochondritis dissecans), the trabecular bone (stress reaction), the cortical bone (stress reaction), or the periosteal membrane (florid reactive periostitis and bizarre parosteal osteochondromatous proliferation, or BPOP) also can be recognized. This system, too, has its disadvantages owing to such factors as the inability to define the true extent of the injury in the acute state and the further anatomic extension of an injury during its subacute and chronic stages (e.g., the extension of a trabecular microfracture to the articular surface).

Although no ideal classification system of occult injuries to bone currently exists, clearly MR imaging represents the most sensitive and specific of presently

Table 8–2. OCCULT INJURIES OF BONE

Site	Acute	Chronic
Osteochondral surface	(Osteo)chondral fracture	Osteochondritis dissecans
Periosteal membrane	Traumatic periostitis	Florid reactive periostitis
		Bizarre parosteal osteochondromatous proliferation
Cortex	Fracture	Stress reaction
Spongiosa	Bone bruise	Stress reaction

available imaging methods in their assessment. The described characteristics of trabecular microfractures (i.e., bone bruises) on MR images are remarkably constant. The findings are those of marrow fluid, with low signal intensity regions on T1-weighted spin echo MR images and high signal intensity regions on T2-weighted spin echo and short tau inversion recovery (STIR) images. The bone bruises are displayed most prominently on the STIR images,[30] which even may lead to overestimation of their size, and they also may be vividly apparent when fat suppression techniques with or without the use of intravenous administration of gadolinium contrast agent are employed.[31] Bone bruises typically are poorly defined and speckled in appearance, although linear areas of altered signal intensity also may be observed. Such linear areas, however, are more characteristic of stress fractures. As amorphous regions of low signal intensity on T1-weighted spin echo MR images that characterize bone bruises may be difficult to differentiate from similar regions of low signal intensity resulting from normal trabeculae, the increased signal intensity seen with bone bruises on T2-weighted spin echo and STIR images assumes diagnostic importance. Furthermore, the detection of bone bruises at specific anatomic sites provides secondary evidence that other injuries may be present. Examples of this include the occurrence of bone bruises in the lateral femoral condyle and posterolateral portion of the tibia in patients with injuries of the anterior cruciate ligament (Fig. 8–12),[8, 21, 32, 33] in the anterior aspect of the tibia in patients with injuries of the poste-

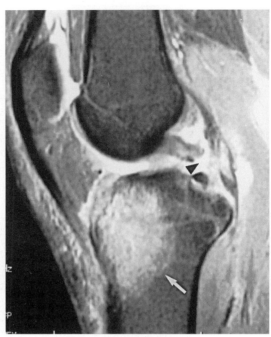

Figure 8–13

Physical injury: Trabecular microfractures (bone bruises). Posterior cruciate ligament injury. This sagittal fat-suppressed fast spin echo MR image (TR/TE, 2700/18) shows the anterior tibial bone bruise (arrow) that is characteristic of an injury to the posterior cruciate ligament (arrowhead). (Courtesy of R. Loredo, M.D., San Antonio, Texas.)

rior cruciate ligament (Fig. 8–13), in the lateral or medial femoral condyle in persons with injuries of the medial collateral ligament of the knee (Fig. 8–14),[34] and in the lateral femoral condyle and medial portion of the patella in patients with lateral patellar dislocation (Fig. 8–15). Indeed, as the pathogenesis of bone bruises appears to include compression or impaction forces, their sites of occurrence about the knee or elsewhere are entirely predictable on the basis of the mechanisms of subluxation or dislocation of joints or other injuries.

Stress Fractures

Stress fractures can occur in normal or abnormal bone that is subjected to repeated cyclic loading, with the load being less than that which causes acute fracture of bone.[35, 36] Two types of stress fractures can be recognized: a *fatigue fracture*, resulting from the application of abnormal stress or torque to a bone with normal elastic resistance; and an *insufficiency fracture*, occurring when normal stress is placed on a bone with deficient elastic resistance. Both fatigue and insufficiency fractures can occur in the same person if an abnormal stress is placed on an abnormal bone.

Fatigue fractures frequently share the following features: The activity is new or different for the person; the activity is strenuous; and the activity is repeated with a frequency that ultimately produces symptoms and signs. The causes of insufficiency fractures are diverse[35] and include rheumatoid arthritis, osteoporosis, Paget's disease, osteomalacia or rickets, hyperparathyroidism, renal osteodystrophy, osteogenesis imperfecta,

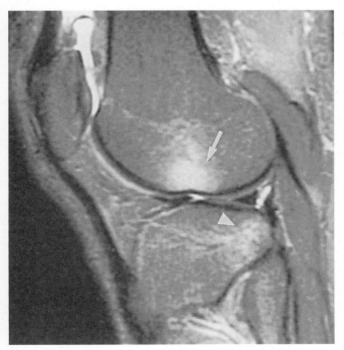

Figure 8–12

Physical injury: Trabecular microfractures (bone bruises). Anterior cruciate ligament injury. On a sagittal fast spin echo STIR MR image (TR/TE, 3200/38; inversion time, 110 msec), bone bruises in the midportion of the lateral femoral condyle (arrow) and posterolateral aspect of the tibia (arrowhead) are virtually diagnostic of an injury to the anterior cruciate ligament. (Courtesy of D. Goodwin, M.D., Hanover, New Hampshire.)

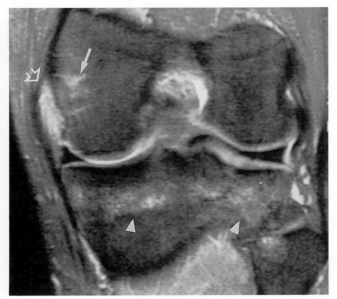

Figure 8–14
Physical injury: Trabecular microfractures (bone bruises). Medial collateral and anterior cruciate ligament injury. This patient had a partial tear of the medial collateral ligament (open arrow) and a complete tear of the anterior cruciate ligament, as well as a tear of the posterior horn of the medial meniscus. The coronal fat-suppressed fast spin echo MR image (TR/TE, 2000/18) shows a bone bruise in the medial femoral condyle (solid arrow) and in medial and lateral portions of the proximal region of the tibia (arrowheads).

osteopetrosis, fibrous dysplasia, and irradiation. Indeed, any process leading to infiltration of trabecular and cortical bone can lead to an insufficiency fracture (Fig. 8–16).

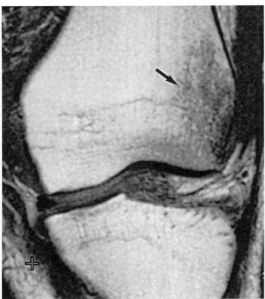

Figure 8–15
Physical injury: Trabecular microfractures (bone bruises). Lateral patellar dislocation. The location of the bone bruise (arrow) in the anterior portion of the lateral femoral condyle, as shown on this coronal T1-weighted (TR/TE, 416/18) spin echo MR image, is characteristic in cases of lateral patellar subluxation or dislocation. (Courtesy of D. Goodwin, M.D., Hanover, New Hampshire.)

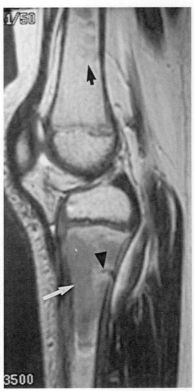

Figure 8–16
Stress fractures: MR imaging abnormalities. A sagittal fast spin echo (TR/TE, 3500/108) MR image of the knee in a patient with acute lymphoblastic leukemia shows tumor infiltration of low signal intensity (arrows) in the femur and tibia and an insufficiency fracture (arrowhead) of the tibia. Note that the fracture line is of low signal intensity and is surrounded by a small zone of edema of higher signal intensity. (Courtesy of E. Bosch, M.D., Santiago, Chile.)

Although routine radiography plays an essential role in the diagnosis of stress fractures (see following discussion), it is the radionuclide examination that provides not only a means of early detection but also a visual account of the biomechanical properties of bone that are fundamental to the pathogenesis of stress fractures. The stressed and "painful" bone undergoing accelerated remodeling produces an abnormal radionuclide image in which nondescript, poorly defined areas of increased accumulation of bone-seeking pharmaceutical agents are observed in the absence of radiographic findings. Appropriate modification of the physical activity may allow osseous "healing" without the appearance of cortical infraction. If the strenuous activity continues, the painful bone may reveal focal fusiform, sharply marginated areas of increased radionuclide activity that can be associated with radiolucent cortical areas and periosteal and endosteal thickening on the roentgenogram, and a diagnosis of a true stress fracture is substantiated (Fig. 8–17). Thus, a stress fracture appears to represent one end of the spectrum of bone response to stress.

The identification of abnormal scintigraphic patterns in athletic persons who subsequently do not develop stress fractures has led to a redefinition of some of the conditions that had formerly been considered together as osseous stress injuries. Shin splints represents one of these conditions, in which a specific abnormality has

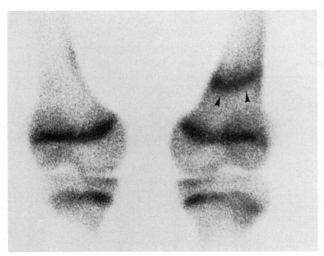

Figure 8–17
Stress fractures: Radionuclide abnormalities. Anterior pinhole bone scan of both femora in a 16 year old girl reveals transverse, bandlike tracer uptake across the distal portion of the left femoral shaft (arrowheads). (Reproduced with permission from Bahk YW: Combined Scintigraphic and Radiographic Diagnosis of Bone and Joint Disorders. New York, Springer-Verlag, 1994.)

been identified during bone scintigraphy, especially if three-phase studies (angiographic, blood pool, and delayed phases) are performed.[37, 38] In patients with shin splints, radionuclide angiograms and blood pool images are normal, whereas on delayed images, a longitudinally oriented area of increased radionuclide accumulation is seen most often in the posteromedial cortex of the tibia (Fig. 8–18). This pattern of abnormality differs from that typically seen in an acute stress fracture (in which all phases of the radionuclide examination are abnormal and a more fusiform area of augmented activity is apparent) and is consistent with the belief that shin splints represent periosteal disruptions of varying length, possibly caused by rupture of the Sharpey's fibers that extend from the muscle through the periosteum into the cortical structure of bone.[38] The location of the scintigraphic abnormality suggests that abnormal excursion of the soleus muscle and, perhaps, other muscle-tendon complexes, such as that related to the tibialis posterior muscle or the flexor digitorum longus muscle, is responsible for the clinical manifestations. Although the posteromedial aspect of the tibia is involved most commonly, the anterolateral aspect of the bone also may be affected.[39] An equivalent lesion occurring in the anteromedial portion of the cortex in the upper or middle region of the femur, corresponding in location to the insertion site or sites of one or more adductor muscle groups, has been designated thigh splints.[40] At each of these anatomic sites, a spectrum of injury that includes acute tendinitis, traction periostitis, and stress fracture may occur, depending on the magnitude and duration of exaggerated forces.[39] Together, the tibial findings often are designated chronic medial tibial stress syndrome,[41, 42] and their severity can be determined not only by bone scintigraphy but also by MR imaging.

MR imaging represents a diagnostic method with comparable sensitivity and superior specificity with re-

spect to bone scintigraphy in the assessment of stress fractures.[43–46] As with bone scintigraphy, a spectrum of abnormalities characterizes the MR imaging appearance of stress injury. Classic stress fractures appear most typically as a linear zone of low signal intensity surrounded by a broader, poorly defined area of slightly higher (although still low) signal intensity on T1-weighted spin echo MR images and as a linear area of low signal intensity surrounded by a broader region of high signal intensity on T2-weighted spin echo images. High signal intensity on STIR images and after the intravenous administration of gadolinium contrast agent also may be observed (Fig. 8–19). Less typically, the MR imaging abnormalities of a stress fracture are identical to those of a bone bruise. Indeed, in such cases, diffuse patchy abnormalities, characterized by low signal intensity on T1-weighted spin echo MR images and high signal intensity on T2-weighted spin echo, fat-suppressed long repetition time fast spin echo, and STIR images, are evident. These may involve any segment of a tubular bone (especially the tibia) or a flat or irregular bone (particularly those in the feet) and may be considered evidence of an overuse syndrome (Fig. 8–20). Although similar cases have been designated painful (idiopathic) transient edema of bone,[47] most often such abnormalities are stress-related. In some stress injuries, periosteal inflammation and edema are the main MR imaging find-

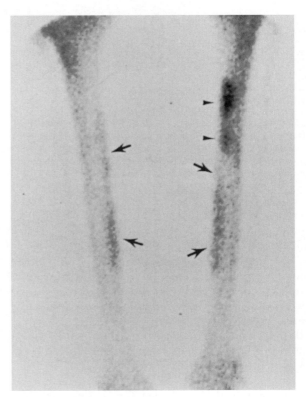

Figure 8–18
Stress changes: Shin splints (radionuclide abnormalities). A 19 year old female athlete who was running 3 miles each day for 3 months developed pain in both calves. On a frontal view of the lower legs during the delayed portion of a bone scan, longitudinally oriented areas of increased tracer accumulation are apparent in the medial cortex of the midportion of the tibiae (arrows). Two localized areas of increased radionuclide activity in the left tibia (arrowheads) may represent stress fractures.

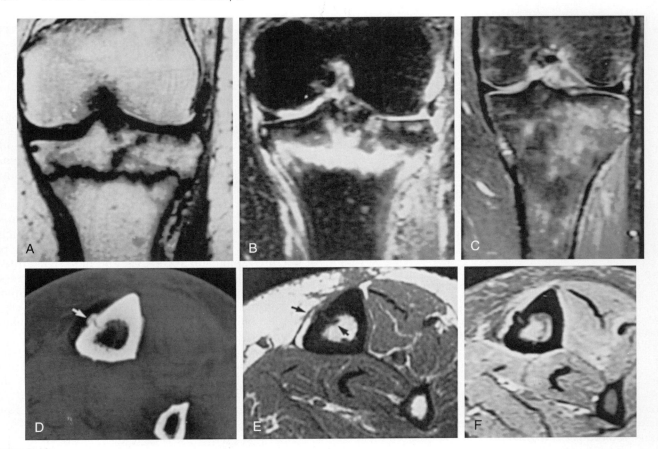

Figure 8–19

Stress fractures: MR imaging abnormalities.

A, B Insufficiency fracture of tibia. In this 72 year old woman, coronal T1-weighted (TR/TE, 500/20) **(A)** and short tau inversion recovery (STIR) (TR/TE, 2500/40; inversion time, 160 msec) **(B)** MR images reveal the horizontal and vertical fracture lines in the proximal portion of the tibia. In **B,** note high signal intensity in and about the fracture. A joint effusion is present.

C Fatigue fracture of tibia. This 42 year old woman developed left knee pain after starting a new jogging program. A coronal T1-weighted (TR/TE, 550/20) spin echo MR image obtained with chemical presaturation of fat (ChemSat) and after intravenous administration of a gadolinium contrast agent shows a broad area of high signal intensity in the lateral tibial plateau and lateral portion of the tibial metaphysis. The findings are consistent with a stress fracture.

D–F Insufficiency fracture of tibia. In a 73 year old woman, transaxial CT **(D)** and T1-weighted (TR/TE, 683/17) spin echo MR image **(E)** reveal the site of cortical violation (arrows). This finding as well as adjacent marrow and soft tissue edema, of high signal intensity, is better seen in a transaxial T1-weighted (TR/TE, 683/17) spin echo image obtained with fat suppression and after intravenous administration of a gadolinium contrast agent **(F).**

(**D–F,** Courtesy of D. Levey, M.D., Corpus Christi, Texas.)

ings, as would be expected in the chronic medial tibial stress syndrome (see previous discussion). In other cases, involvement of bone, periosteum, and soft tissue (including muscle) is documented on MR images. The extent of soft tissue abnormality may be profound, with MR imaging findings simulating those of infection or tumor (Fig. 8–21).[48]

Biomechanical principles can be applied to the explanation of stress fractures in various sites of the body.[35] A few specific examples are included in Table 8–3.

Calcaneal or Other Tarsal Stress Fracture. Fatigue fracture of the calcaneus is not uncommon in military recruits, and insufficiency fractures in this site can accompany rheumatoid arthritis, neurologic disorders, and other diseases (Fig. 8–22). Stress fractures in the tarsal navicular bone have been observed in physically active persons, especially in basketball players and runners. Characteristically, the stress fracture is oriented in

the sagittal plane and is located dorsally and in the central one third of the bone (Fig. 8–23).

Fibular Stress Fracture. In the act of running, the calf musculature is active in flexion and extension of the ankle and in closer approximation of the tibia and fibula. The magnitude of the muscular activity is influenced by the type of ground surface, increasing in the presence of hard turf. Changing muscular stresses can result in the "runner's fracture." Jumping also can produce fibular stress fractures.

Tibial Stress Fracture. Stress fracture of the proximal diaphysis of the tibia can occur during running and stress fracture of the middle and distal tibial diaphysis can take place during long-distance running, marching, and ballet dancing.[49] The posteromedial portion of the cortex is affected more frequently than the anterolateral portion (Figs. 8–24 and 8–25). Stress fractures involving

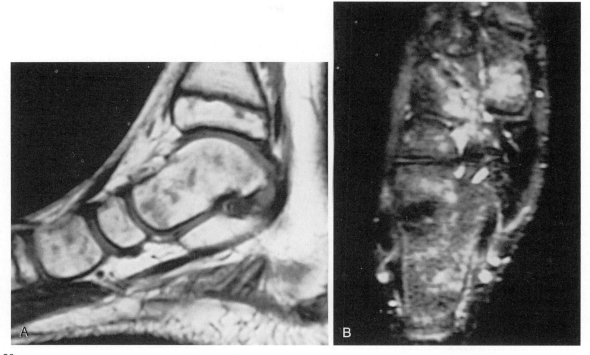

Figure 8–20
Stress changes: Overuse syndrome (MR imaging abnormalities). This 9 year old athletic girl developed diffuse foot pain.

A A sagittal T1-weighted (TR/TE, 600/16) spin echo MR image shows diffuse, patchy regions of low signal intensity in the talus and navicular and medial cuneiform bones.

B On a transverse (plantar) fast spin echo STIR MR image (TR/TE, 4000/51; inversion time, 130 msec), patchy areas of high signal intensity are observed in the tarsal bones.

(Courtesy of S.K. Brahme, M.D., San Diego, California)

Figure 8–21
Stress fractures: MR imaging abnormalities. A transverse fat-suppressed fast spin echo (TR/TE, 4600/108) MR image shows a fatigue fracture of the third metatarsal bone in this track star. Note callus and periosteal new bone appearing as low signal intensity along the medial aspect of the shaft and neck of the bone and edematous changes of high signal intensity in the medullary cavity and soft tissues. (Courtesy of D. Goodwin, M.D., Hanover, New Hampshire.)

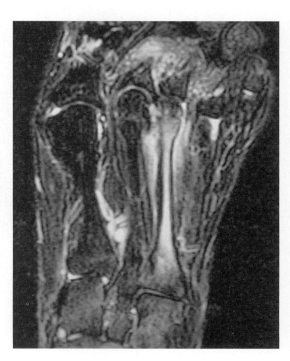

Table 8–3. LOCATIONS OF STRESS FRACTURE BY ACTIVITY

Location	Activity or Event
Sesamoids of metatarsal bones	Prolonged standing
Metatarsal shaft	Marching; stamping on ground; prolonged standing; ballet; postoperative bunionectomy
Navicular	Stamping on ground; marching; long distance running
Calcaneus	Jumping; parachuting; prolonged standing; recent immobilization
Tibia: Midshaft and distal shaft	Long distance running
Proximal shaft (children)	Running
Fibula: Distal shaft	Long distance running
Proximal shaft	Jumping; parachuting
Patella	Hurdling
Femur: Shaft	Ballet; long distance running
Neck	Ballet; marching; long distance running; gymnastics
Pelvis: Obturator ring	Stooping; bowling; gymnastics
Lumbar vertebra (pars interarticularis)	Ballet; lifting heavy objects; scrubbing floors
Lower cervical, upper thoracic spinous process	Clay shoveling
Ribs	Carrying heavy pack; golf; coughing
Clavicle	Postoperative radical neck
Coracoid of scapula	Trapshooting
Humerus: Distal shaft	Throwing a ball
Ulna: Coronoid	Pitching a ball
Shaft	Pitchfork work; propelling wheelchair
Hook of hamate	Holding golf club, tennis racquet, baseball bat

Modified from Daffner RH: Skel Radiol 2:221, 1978.

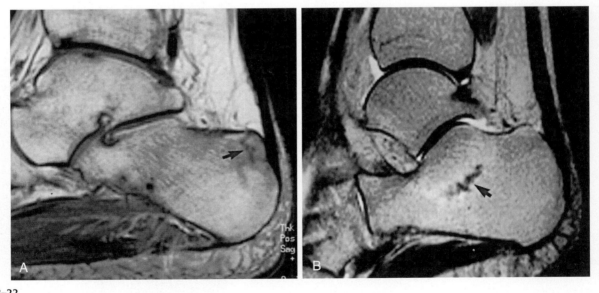

Figure 8–22
Calcaneal stress fractures.
   A On a T1-weighted (TR/TE, 700/16) spin echo MR image, observe a linear area of low signal intensity (arrow), representing an insufficiency fracture of the calcaneus in this patient receiving corticosteroid medication.
   B In this 27 year old woman who was receiving corticosteroid therapy following renal transplantation, a sagittal T2-weighted (TR/TE, 4168/140) spin echo MR image shows an insufficiency fracture (arrow) of the calcaneus with surrounding marrow edema. (Courtesy of T. Hughes, M.D., Christchurch, New Zealand.)

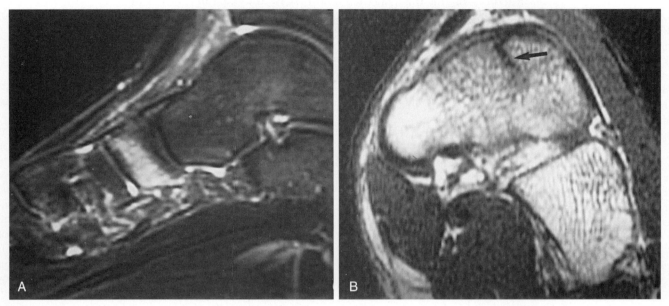

Figure 8-23
Tarsal navicular stress fractures. In a 25 year old man, a sagittal fat-suppressed fast spin echo MR image (TR/TE, 3500/102) **(A)** shows high signal intensity in the tarsal navicular bone. The coronal T1-weighted (TR/TE, 300/16) spin echo MR image **(B)** shows more specific abnormalities, as the fracture line (arrow) can be identified. (Courtesy of P. Kindynis, M.D., Geneva, Switzerland.)

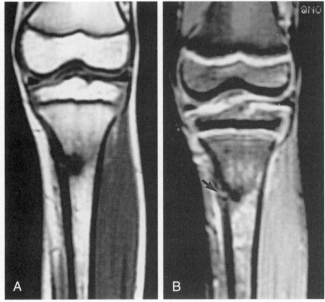

Figure 8-24
Tibial stress fractures. In an 8 year old boy, coronal T1-weighted (TR/TE, 600/25) **(A)** and multiplanar gradient recalled (MPGR) (TR/TE, 620/25; flip angle, 30 degrees) **(B)** MR images demonstrate a fatigue fracture of the medial cortex of the proximal portion of the tibia. The fracture (arrow) of the cortex and the soft tissue, subperiosteal, and marrow edema are more easily seen in **B.** (Courtesy of E. Bosch, M.D., Santiago, Chile.)

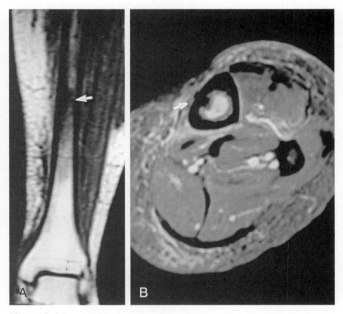

Figure 8-25
Tibial stress fractures. In this 69 year old physically active woman, a fatigue fracture of the midportion of the tibia is evident on a T1-weighted (TR/TE, 333/16) spin echo **(A)** and a fat-suppressed fast spin echo (TR/TE, 4000/17) MR image **(B).** The coronal image **(A)** shows a focal region of low signal intensity (arrow) surrounded by a more diffuse region of slightly decreased signal intensity. The transaxial image **(B)** reveals endosteal and periosteal callus (arrow) and soft tissue and marrow edema, of high signal intensity.

the medial malleolus also may be encountered in young athletes (Fig. 8–26).[50]

On MR images, stress fractures of the tibia may be seen to involve long segments of the shaft of the bone (Fig. 8–27). This is particularly true in cases in which the fracture is oriented in a vertical or longitudinal direction (Fig. 8–28). Such longitudinal stress fractures lead to widespread marrow edema that simulates the appearance of osteomyelitis or a malignant bone tumor. Transaxial images are of diagnostic importance, allowing the identification of endosteal and periosteal callus.[51]

Femoral Stress Fracture. Stress fracture of the shaft or neck of the femur (Fig. 8–29) can result from long-distance running, ballet dancing, and marching. The propensity for some femoral stress fractures to become complete and even displaced deserves emphasis.[52]

Metatarsal Stress Fracture. The metatarsal bones are very frequent sites of stress fracture. The middle and distal portions of the shafts of the second and third metatarsal bones are affected most often (see Fig. 8–21), but any metatarsal bone, including the first, may be involved. Occasionally, stress fractures involve the metatarsal heads, leading to sclerosis and flattening of the subchondral bone (Fig. 8–30).[53]

Other Lower Extremity Stress Fractures. Stress fractures of the patella are either transverse or longitudinal, occur in both children and adults, and are associated with physical activities that include hurdling, running, walking, soccer, and fencing.[54, 55]

Pubic Rami and Symphysis Stress Fracture. Stress fractures of the pubic arch and parasymphyseal bone are encountered in pregnant women, joggers, military recruits, long-distance runners, or marathoners,[56] although similar fractures occur in patients with osteoarthritis of the hip, in those who have undergone hip arthroplasty, and in association with osteoporosis (Fig. 8–31) and rheumatoid arthritis.

Other Pelvic Stress Fractures. Although fatigue fractures of the sacrum have been described in children and athletes and in pregnant women, far more emphasis has been given to insufficiency fractures of the sacrum and other pelvic sites in patients with postmenopausal or senile osteoporosis or rheumatoid arthritis, and in those who have received corticosteroid medications or radiation therapy.[57] Sacral insufficiency fractures involve one or both sides of the bone with vertical fracture lines typically located close to the sacroiliac joint or joints. Gas may collect within the fracture gaps.[58, 59] Bone scintigraphy reveals accumulation of the radionuclide at the fracture sites, sometimes producing an "H" pattern of increased radiotracer uptake in the sacrum (Fig. 8–32). The transaxial displays provided by CT and MR imaging are well suited to the detection of sacral insufficiency fractures (Fig. 8–32). MR images usually reveal low signal intensity in the involved marrow on T1-weighted spin echo images, high signal intensity in this marrow on T2-weighted spin echo images,[60] and enhancement of signal intensity after intravenous administration of gadolinium contrast agent,[61] and they can be used to monitor fracture healing and a decrease in adjacent bone marrow edema.[62]

Upper Extremity Stress Fracture. These fractures are far less frequent than stress fractures in the bones of the lower extremity. Typical sites include the ribs in golfers, rowers, and tennis players; the coracoid process of the scapula in trapshooters; the ulnae of rodeo riders, tennis players,[63] baseball pitchers, volleyball players,

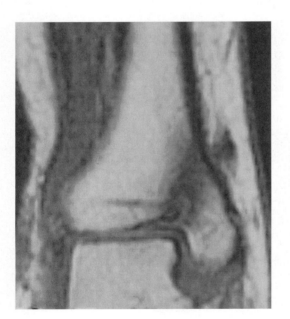

Figure 8–26
Stress fracture of the medial malleolus. A T1-weighted spin echo MR image in a 54 year old woman with ankle pain exacerbated during prolonged walking shows a fatigue fracture of the medial malleolus that only later became obvious on radiographs. (Reproduced with permission from K. Okada et al: Foot Ankle *16*:49, 1995.)

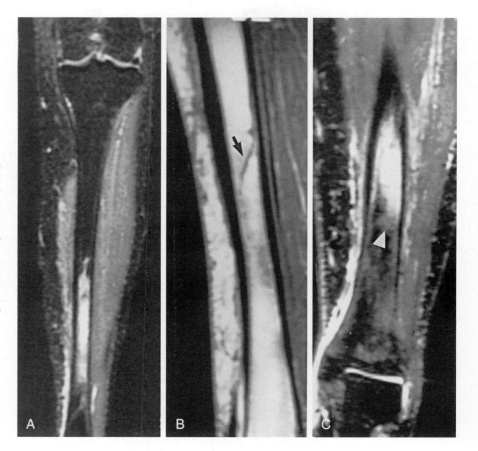

Figure 8–27
Tibial stress fractures.

A This coronal fast spin echo STIR MR image (TR/TE, 3000/16; inversion time, 150 msec) shows high signal intensity involving a long segment of the tibial shaft in an elderly woman with leg pain. (Courtesy of D. Goodwin, M.D., Hanover, New Hampshire.)

B, C In a second elderly woman, a longitudinally oriented insufficiency fracture (arrow) and surrounding edema (arrowhead) are shown on a sagittal T1-weighted (TR/TE, 600/12) spin echo MR image **(B)** and a coronal STIR (TR/TE, 6100/24; inversion time, 140 msec) MR image **(C)**. (Courtesy of J. Schils, M.D., Cleveland, Ohio.)

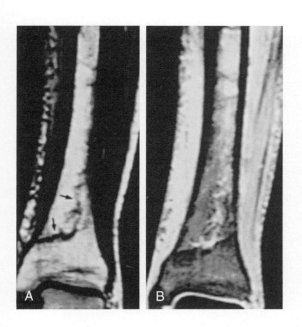

Figure 8–28
Tibial stress fractures. Fatigue fracture (longitudinal type) of the tibia. In a 58 year old man who jogged regularly, a coronal proton density (TR/TE, 1800/22) spin echo MR image **(A)** shows a stress fracture of the distal end of the tibia with both horizontal and vertical limbs (arrows). A coronal STIR MR image (TR/TE, 2000/20; inversion time, 140 msec) **(B)** reveals high signal intensity in the tibial metaphysis and diaphysis. Soft tissue edema also is present.

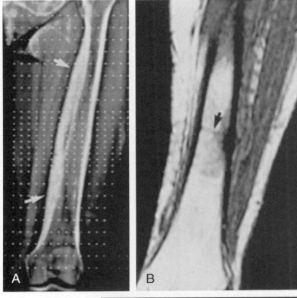

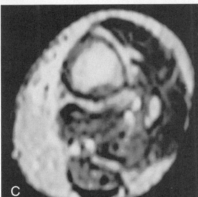

Figure 8–29
Femoral stress fractures: Femoral shaft.

A A scout CT scan of the femur in a 56 year old woman with a 10 year history of thigh pain shows diffuse, mature periosteal bone formation (arrows) along the medial portion of the entire diaphysis. The findings are consistent with a stress reaction. (Courtesy of A. Newberg, M.D., Boston, Massachussetts.)

B, C In a 76 year old woman with exercise-related thigh and leg pain, a coronal T1-weighted (TR/TE, 550/25) spin echo MR image **(B)** shows a linear region of low signal intensity (arrow) compatible with a stress fracture, a broader region of diminished signal intensity consistent with marrow edema, and cortical thickening. On a transaxial T2-weighted (TR/TE, 2100/70) spin echo MR image **(C),** observe high signal intensity in the edematous bone marrow of the femur and adjacent soft tissues. (Courtesy of T. Broderick, M.D., Orange, California.)

D, E In a 19 year old military recruit, a bone scan **(D)** shows evidence of fatigue fractures (arrows) in both femora. A coronal fat-suppressed T1-weighted (TR/TE, 715/15) spin echo MR image obtained following intravenous gadolinium administration **(E)** confirms these fractures manifest as marrow and soft tissue edema (arrows).

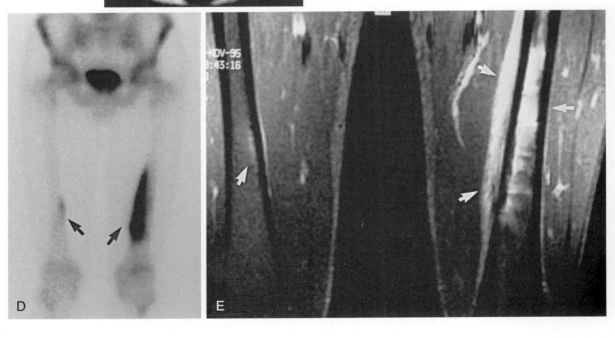

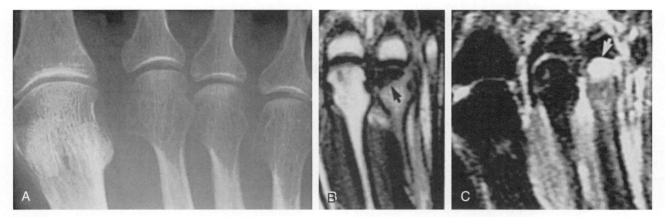

Figure 8–30
Metatarsal stress fractures: Metatarsal heads.
   A In this 56 year old female jogger, note subtle sclerosis of the subchondral bone in the second, third, and fourth metatarsal heads.
   B, C In a 46 year old man with a 6 month history of foot pain during running, a transverse T1-weighted (TR/TE, 500/17) spin echo MR image **(B)** shows an area of low signal intensity (arrow) in the head of the third metatarsal bone. A transverse short tau inversion recovery (STIR) image (TR/TE, 2000/43; inversion time, 140 msec) **(C)** reveals high signal intensity in this region (arrow) and fluid in the first and second metatarsophalangeal joints.

weightlifters, and patients using wheelchairs (Fig. 8–33); the hook of the hamate in tennis players, golfers, and baseball players (Fig. 8–34); the olecranon process in baseball pitchers and javelin throwers; the phalangeal tufts in guitar players; the phalanges of the hand in bowlers; and the inferior edge of the glenoid fossa in baseball pitchers.

Greenstick, Torus, and Bowing Fractures

In the immature skeleton, fractures that do not completely penetrate the entire shaft of a bone are not infrequent. The main types of incomplete fractures, in addition to stress fractures, are greenstick, torus, and bowing fractures.

A *greenstick (hickory stick, willow) fracture* is one that perforates one cortex and ramifies within the medullary bone. Greenstick fractures result from angular force and commonly become converted to complete fractures because of the exaggeration of the deformity as the bone continues to grow. Typical locations of greenstick

fractures are the proximal metaphysis or diaphysis of the tibia and the middle third of the radius and ulna. In the healing stage of these fractures, well-defined subperiosteal defects containing fat may be observed (Fig. 8–35).[64] These defects may result from the inclusion of medullary fat drops in the subperiosteal hematoma.[65]

A *torus (buckling) fracture* results from an injury insufficient in force to create a complete discontinuity of bone but sufficient to produce a buckling of the cortex. A longitudinal compression force generally is involved.

Bowing fractures are a plastic response, usually to longitudinal stress in a bone. They are virtually confined to children and occur most typically in the radius and the ulna.

Toddler's Fractures

Infants and toddlers frequently show a limp of acute onset without a clear history of specific injury. The classic toddler's fracture is a nondisplaced, oblique fracture of the distal diaphysis of the tibia. Other causes for these clinical manifestations are occult fractures of the fibula, femur, metatarsal bones, and less commonly the

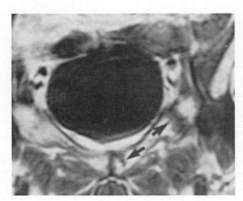

Figure 8–31
Pubic rami stress fractures. In this 80 year old man, a coronal T1-weighted (TR/TE, 600/11) spin echo MR image shows two fractures (arrows) appearing as linear regions of low signal intensity in the iliopubic bone column of the pelvis. (Courtesy of S. K. Brahme, M.D., La Jolla, California.)

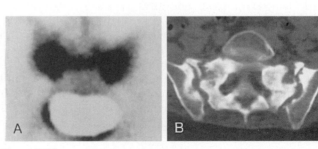

Figure 8–32
Sacral stress fractures. The typical imaging features of insufficiency fractures of the sacrum, as shown in a 65 year old woman, include an "H" pattern of radionuclide uptake on a bone scan **(A)** and comminuted fracture lines with sclerosis on transaxial CT **(B).** In this case, the ilium adjacent to both sacroiliac joints also is involved. (Courtesy of G. Greenway, M.D., Dallas, Texas.)

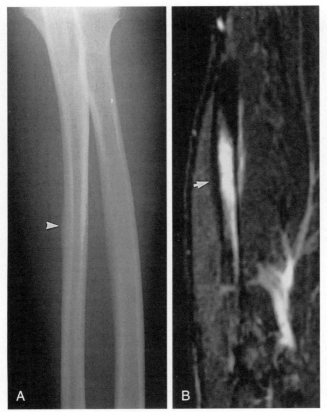

Figure 8–33
Stress fractures of the ulna. This 19 year old weightlifter developed progressive pain in the forearm. The routine radiograph **(A)** shows subtle cortical thickening (arrowhead) in the shaft of the ulna. On a coronal fat-suppressed fast spin echo MR image (TR/TE, 5000/51) **(B),** with the elbow at the top of the image, high signal intensity (arrow) is seen in the corresponding marrow.

calcaneus, the cuboid bone, the pubic rami, or the patella.[66] Scintigraphy represents a sensitive test for the diagnosis of toddler's fractures.

Acute Chondral and Osteochondral Fractures

Shearing, rotational, or tangentially aligned impaction forces generated by abnormal joint motion may produce fractures of one or both of the two apposing joint surfaces. Acute injuries can produce fragments consisting of cartilage alone (chondral fractures) or cartilage and underlying bone (osteochondral fractures).[67] In general, the fracture line parallels the joint surface, and it is the depth of the lesion that defines the cartilaginous and osseous components of the fragment. A purely cartilaginous fragment creates no direct radiographic abnormalities, whereas one containing calcified cartilage and bone becomes apparent as a result of its varying degrees of radiodensity. Fluoroscopy and arthrography with or without conventional tomography or CT scanning may be used to define the nature and location of the fracture more accurately.

After the injury, the detached portion of the articular surface can remain in situ, be slightly displaced, or become loose, or free, within the joint cavity. Common sites of localization of such bodies include the olecranon fossa in the elbow, the axillary and subscapular recesses

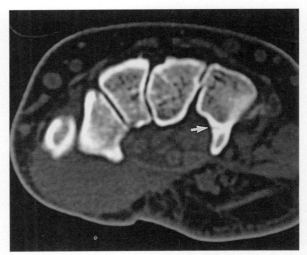

Figure 8–34
Stress fractures of the hook of the hamate bone. In a 50 year old male golfer, a transaxial CT scan shows a fatigue fracture of the hook of the hamate bone manifested as a radiolucent line and adjacent bone sclerosis (arrow). (Courtesy of D. Wilcox, M.D., Kansas City, Missouri.)

in the glenohumeral joint, and the posterior regions in the knee. Purely chondral bodies require arthrography often combined with CT scanning for detection. Although MR imaging[68] or MR arthrography also may be used for this purpose (Fig. 8–36), CT arthrography appears to be superior.

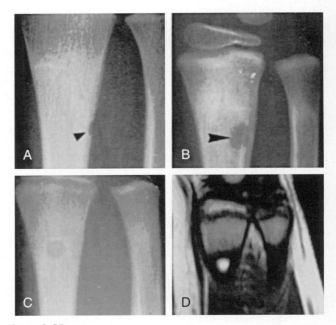

Figure 8–35
Greenstick fractures: Posttraumatic cysts.
  A Three months after a greenstick fracture of the radius, a small subperiosteal cyst (arrowhead) can be identified in this 7 year old girl.
  B Two months after a similar type of fracture of the radius (and ulna) in a different child, a larger cyst (arrowhead) is seen. (Courtesy of A. Newberg, M.D., Boston, Massachusetts.)
  C, D Routine radiography **(C)** and a coronal T1-weighted (TR/TE, 650/25) spin echo MR image **(D)** show a fat-containing posttraumatic cyst of the radius in a 7 year old girl. Note its high signal intensity in **D.** The ulna also had been fractured. (Courtesy of S. K. Brahme, M.D., La Jolla, California.)

Figure 8–36
Acute chondral and osteochondral fractures: Intra-articular bodies.

A On a lateral radiograph, large intra-articular bodies are identified in the suprapatellar bursa, and an osteochondral defect is evident in the weight-bearing aspect of the medial femoral condyle.

B In a sagittal T2-weighted spin echo MR image (TR/TE, 2000/80) an osteochondral defect (arrow) is present in the weight-bearing aspect of the medial femoral condyle and is defined by the presence of a large joint effusion.

C In a more lateral T2-weighted (TR/TE, 2000/80) image, an intra-articular body (arrow) is outlined by the joint fluid anterior to the femoral condyle.

(A, From Pavlov H, Torg JS: The Running Athlete. Chicago, Year Book, 1987.)

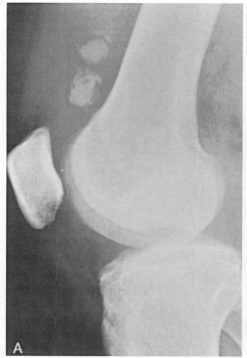
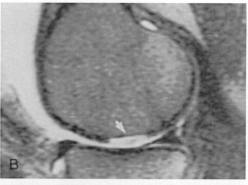
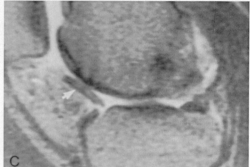

Osteochondral injuries are a well-recognized component of a variety of momentary or persistent subluxations and dislocations. Classic examples include injuries of the glenoid region of the scapula and humeral head with dislocations of the glenohumeral joint; of the patella and lateral femoral condyle with dislocations of the patella (Fig. 8–37); and of the femoral head with dislocations of the hip.

MR imaging has provided direct evidence of the frequency of these osteochondral injuries (Fig. 8–38). The location of osteochondral and subchondral lesions, as detected by MR imaging, in patients with acute trauma provides important information with regard to mechanism of injury and associated abnormalities. Occult injuries of the posterolateral portion of the tibia and midportion of the lateral femoral condyle, frequently occurring together, are associated with complete disruption of the anterior cruciate ligament and appear to represent a response to impaction of these two regions during anterior translation of the tibia and relative external rotation of the femur.[21] A deep lateral femoral notch identifiable on routine lateral projections of the knee appears to represent the radiographic counterpart of these MR imaging abnormalities.[69] Occult injuries of the lateral femoral condyle and patella, including osteochondral fractures, may accompany transient lateral dislocations of the patella.[70] Numerous other patterns of bone injury (e.g., bone bruise, osteochondral fracture) are encountered regularly in the assessment of the knee, the shoulder, the hip, the ankle, and other locations in which signal intensity changes in the marrow not only confirm a structural cause of the patient's pain but also delineate precisely the impaction forces accompanying abnormal joint motion.

Osteochondritis Dissecans

Osteochondritis dissecans indicates fragmentation and possible separation of a portion of the articular surface.

Patients may be entirely asymptomatic; however, pain aggravated by movement, limitation of motion, clicking, locking, and swelling may be apparent. Although the role of trauma is undeniable in most locations, a familial history has been evident in some cases, especially in osteochondritis of the knee. It is also possible that a separate variety of osteochondritis dissecans occurs in the juvenile patient due to irregularities of ossification. Indeed, based on analysis of age of onset, two distinct populations have been identified[71]: children and adolescents between the ages of 5 and approximately 15 years, who have open physes, are considered to have the juvenile form of the disease; older adolescents with closed physes and adults are considered to have the adult form of the disease. It has been suggested that the juvenile form of the disease often is self-limited owing to healing of the lesion, whereas the adult form of the disease generally relates to the presence of an incompletely healed lesion that had originally developed in adolescence. Osteochondritis dissecans is believed by most investigators to be the eventual result of an osteochondral fracture that initially was caused by shearing, rotatory, or tangentially aligned impaction forces.

The natural history of osteochondritis dissecans is variable. As indicated previously, juvenile lesions are more likely to heal spontaneously than adult lesions. In both age groups, however, softening of articular cartilage may occur with loss of support of subchondral bone.[71] In such cases, if the disease process is not arrested, separation of a chondral or osteochondral fragment may occur, diminishing the likelihood of spontaneous healing. In weight-bearing regions, resulting incongruity of joint surfaces predisposes to the development of osteoarthritis.

A uniformly accepted classification system for the morphologic changes of osteochondritis dissecans does not exist. Arthroscopic findings confirm the existence

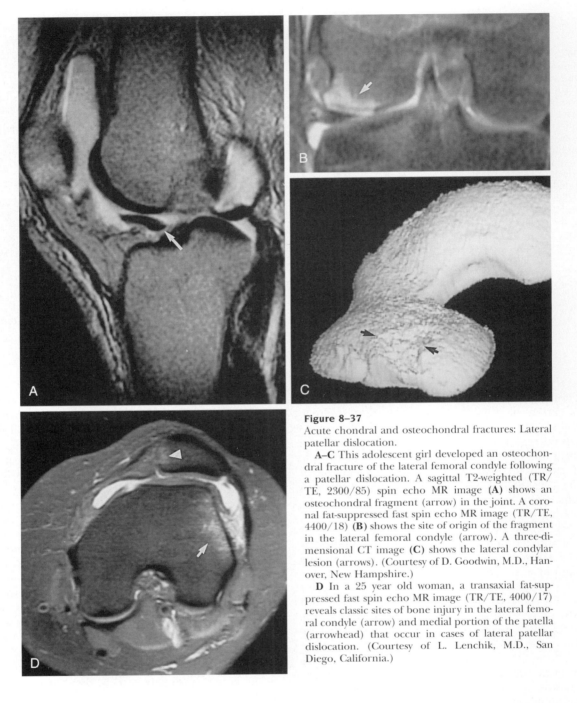

Figure 8–37
Acute chondral and osteochondral fractures: Lateral patellar dislocation.

A–C This adolescent girl developed an osteochondral fracture of the lateral femoral condyle following a patellar dislocation. A sagittal T2-weighted (TR/TE, 2300/85) spin echo MR image **(A)** shows an osteochondral fragment (arrow) in the joint. A coronal fat-suppressed fast spin echo MR image (TR/TE, 4400/18) **(B)** shows the site of origin of the fragment in the lateral femoral condyle (arrow). A three-dimensional CT image **(C)** shows the lateral condylar lesion (arrows). (Courtesy of D. Goodwin, M.D., Hanover, New Hampshire.)

D In a 25 year old woman, a transaxial fat-suppressed fast spin echo MR image (TR/TE, 4000/17) reveals classic sites of bone injury in the lateral femoral condyle (arrow) and medial portion of the patella (arrowhead) that occur in cases of lateral patellar dislocation. (Courtesy of L. Lenchik, M.D., San Diego, California.)

of a spectrum of abnormalities ranging from intact overlying cartilage to cartilage disruption with a displaced fragment. The precise management of osteochondritis dissecans likewise is not agreed on, and the patient's age, clinical manifestations, and level of physical activity, as well as the specific anatomic location of the lesion and the experience and preference of the orthopedic surgeon, all influence the choice of therapy. The basic tenets of operative treatment include restoration of the congruity of the joint surfaces, enhancement of local blood supply to the fragment or crater, rigid fixation of unstable fragments, and protected weight-bearing with early postoperative joint motion.[71] Considerable interest, therefore, has developed concerning the determination of the stability of the fragment (i.e., stable or unstable

[or loose]). Those fragments that are ballottable but are associated with intact overlying cartilage, sometimes referred to as loose in situ fragments, may be fixed surgically; those that are grossly loose may be removed. With this in mind, orthopedic surgeons have attempted to identify noninvasive or minimally invasive imaging examinations that would provide information about the lesion similar to that apparent on arthroscopic assessment. There are many such examinations from which to choose, including routine radiography, conventional tomography or CT scanning with or without arthrography, standard arthrography, scintigraphy, MR imaging, and MR arthrography. None is ideal.

Mesgarzadeh and colleagues[72] used conventional radiography, bone scintigraphy, and MR imaging to assess

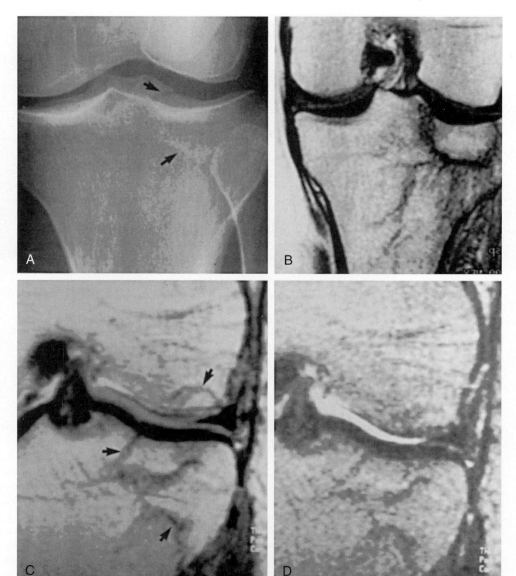

Figure 8–38

Acute chondral and osteochondral fractures: Various types.

A, B Lateral tibial plateau. A routine radiograph **(A)** shows a subtle fracture (arrows) of the lateral tibial plateau. A coronal T1-weighted (TR/TE, 450/19) spin echo MR image **(B)** reveals a curvilinear fracture line in the lateral tibial plateau with radiating fracture lines in the adjacent tibial metaphysis.

C, D Lateral tibial plateau and lateral femoral condyle. A coronal proton density (TR/TE, 1800/20) spin echo MR image **(C)** reveals fractures (arrows) in both the lateral femoral condyle and the lateral tibial plateau. With T2 weighting (TR/TE, 1800/90) **(D)**, hyperintensity in the affected bone marrow is seen. A tear of the medial collateral ligament of the knee also was present.

mechanical stability of osteochondritis dissecans, mainly in the femoral condyles, and employed arthroscopy as a means of verification of the findings. Lesions that were large (particularly when greater than 0.8 cm^2 in area) or associated with a broad sclerotic margin (especially when greater than 3 mm thick) on routine radiographic examination tended to be loose grossly. Significant accumulation of the bone-seeking radionuclide during the flow, blood-pool, and late phases of the radionuclide examination generally indicated the presence of a loose fragment. MR imaging findings of loose fragments included displacement from its bed of origin and the presence of fluid at the interface of the fragment and its parent bone (Fig. 8–39). The signal intensity of the fragment itself, which usually increased on T2-weighted MR images, was not a useful indicator of the stable or unstable nature of the lesion.

Although subsequent studies using MR imaging to evaluate osteochondritis dissecans noted its value in delineating the status of the overlying cartilage,[73, 74] it was the investigations of De Smet and coworkers on osteo-

chondritis dissecans of the femoral condyles[75] and talus[76] that next focused mainly on the signal intensity characteristics of the zone between the lesion and the parent bone. High signal intensity, indicative of fluid or granulation tissue, in this zone on T2-weighted MR images proved to be strong but not infallible evidence of an unstable lesion, whereas the presence of fluid encircling the fragment or focal cystic areas beneath the fragment were the best indicators of such instability (Fig. 8–40). Similarly, the absence of a zone of high signal intensity at the interface of the fragment and the parent bone was a reliable sign of lesion stability.

The intravenous[77, 78] or intra-articular[79] administration of a gadolinium contrast agent has been used as a supplementary MR imaging method in the assessment of osteochondritis dissecans. Intravenous administration of the gadolinium agent has led to enhancement of signal intensity in the zone between the fragment and the parent bone, which corresponded to histologic evidence of a loose fragment and subjacent granulation tissue; absence of such enhancement corresponded to

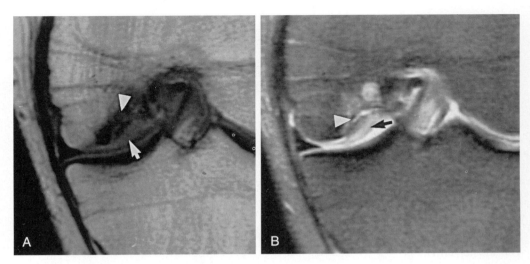

Figure 8-39

Osteochondritis dissecans (MR imaging, femoral condyles, unstable lesion).

A A coronal T1-weighted (TR/TE, 800/13) spin echo MR image shows osteochondritis dissecans of the inner portion of the medial femoral condyle. The cartilage (arrow) appears swollen, and low signal intensity is evident in the adjacent bone marrow (arrowhead).

B The coronal fat-suppressed fast spin echo MR image (TR/TE, 3400/18) provides more useful information. Displacement of the cartilage fragment (arrow) is evident, and fluid (arrowhead) of high signal intensity (derived from the joint effusion) is located between the fragment and the parent bone, clear evidence of an unstable lesion. Regions of high signal intensity are present in the femoral condyle.

histologic findings of a stable fragment with subjacent trabeculae and without granulation tissue.[77] When compared to standard T1-weighted spin echo and gradient echo MR imaging techniques, the administration of intra-articular gadolinium contrast agent (MR arthrography) prior to using such techniques resulted in an improvement in accurate assessment of the overlying articular cartilage.[79]

Although the available data would appear to indicate a role for MR imaging in the analysis of lesion stability in cases of osteochondritis dissecans, further analysis is required to determine its advantages over those of other methods, particularly arthroscopy. The finding of fluid at the base of the osteochondral fragment represents indirect but reliable evidence that the overlying cartilage is not intact, and this is a finding that corresponds to the presence of radiopaque contrast material or air that collects in this region when arthrographic methods are used to study osteochondritis dissecans. The likelihood of fluid extending through the cartilaginous defect and into the base of the fragment depends not only on the extent of the chondral damage but also on the amount of joint fluid that is present. In this regard, the use of MR arthrography appears to have merit owing to the large amounts of fluid that may be introduced into the joint (Fig. 8-41). In addition, the sensitivity of MR imaging in detecting fluid at the interface between the fragment and the parent bone varies according to the precise methods that are employed and may be greater when volumetric acquisition and thin sections are used. Furthermore, the differentiation of fluid and granulation tissue in this interface with MR imaging techniques may be challenging. A theoretical value exists with respect to the direct analysis of the cartilage surface with MR imaging, but specific imaging parameters that are most suited to this analysis still are evolving.

With regard to the role of MR imaging in establishing the diagnosis of osteochondritis dissecans, the technique clearly is sensitive and relatively specific, although diagnostic pitfalls may be encountered. False diagnosis of this condition may relate to misinterpretation of the sometimes irregular pattern of epiphyseal ossification that can be observed normally in the distal portion of a child's femur (Fig. 8-42); of normal grooves in the articular surfaces (such as those of the femoral condyles) that are seen in both children and adults; and of partial volume effects that are encountered in the assessment of round or angulated bone surfaces. Furthermore, other lesions, such as osteonecrosis (Fig. 8-43), osteoarthritis, and stress fractures, can lead to MR imaging abnormalities that are similar to those of osteochondritis dissecans. This technique, however, is useful in defining the extent of the lesion and, sometimes, in assessing its response to operative intervention.[80]

Ultimately, the choice of an appropriate diagnostic method may depend on the specific anatomic site involved. Consequently, a survey of the most typical locations of osteochondritis dissecans is appropriate.

Femoral Condyles. The most typical location of osteochondritis dissecans is the condylar surfaces of the distal portion of the femur. The inner aspect of the medial femoral condyle is involved most frequently. Purely chondral lesions require arthrography, CT arthrography, MR imaging, or arthroscopy for accurate diagnosis. The osseous component of an osteochondral lesion is detectable with routine radiography or standard CT. Disruption and displacement of the osteochondral fragment, which can be detected with MR imaging (Fig. 8-44), produce a loose or synovium-embedded intra-articular osseous body.

Patella. In comparison to osteochondritis dissecans of the femoral condyles, involvement of the patella is rare. Unilateral involvement predominates. The age of clinical onset usually is between 15 and 20 years. The

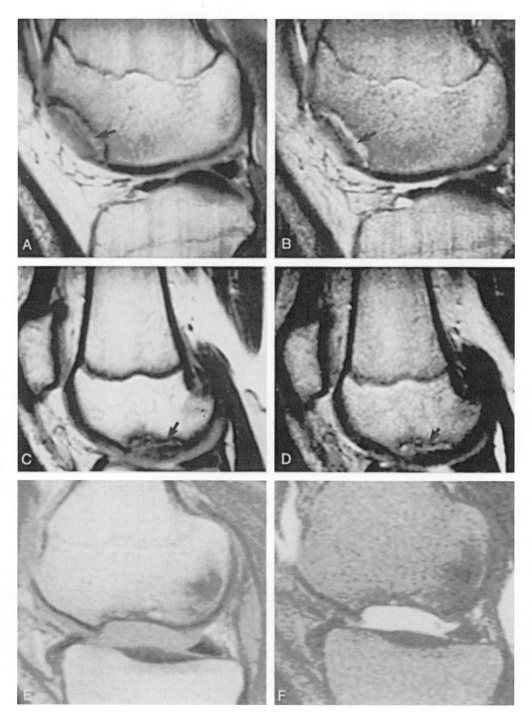

Figure 8–40

Osteochondritis dissecans (MR imaging, femoral condyles, various stages of disease).

A, B Lateral femoral condyle. In this 17 year old man, sagittal proton density (TR/TE, 2200/30) **(A)** and T2-weighted (TR/TE, 2200/80) **(B)** spin echo MR images reveal the lesion involving the anterior surface of the lateral condyle. The fragment is ossified, and the junction between it and the parent bone (arrows) demonstrates intermediate signal intensity in **A** and high signal intensity in **B.** The abnormalities are consistent with granulation tissue or fluid in this junctional area. Although the overlying cartilage is not seen well, the MR imaging findings suggest the presence of an unstable lesion. (Courtesy of J. Blassinghame, M.D., San Diego, California.)

C, D Medial femoral condyle. In this 12 year old boy, sagittal proton density (TR/TE, 2000/20) **(C)** and T2-weighted (TR/TE, 2000/80) **(D)** spin echo MR images show features similar to those in **A** and **B.** The junctional tissue (arrows) shows higher signal intensity in **D** than in **C.** A small joint effusion is present. Although the findings are consistent with the presence of an unstable fragment, the patient responded well to conservative therapy. (Courtesy of D. Gershuni, M.D., San Diego, California.)

E, F Lateral femoral condyle. Sagittal proton density (TR/TE, 3000/20) **(E)** and T2-weighted (TR/TE, 3000/80) **(F)** spin echo MR images in this 35 year old man show a large condylar defect containing fluid in continuity with the joint effusion. No fragment is evident within this osseous bed, and the overlying cartilage is absent. An intra-articular osteochondral fragment was present elsewhere in the joint.

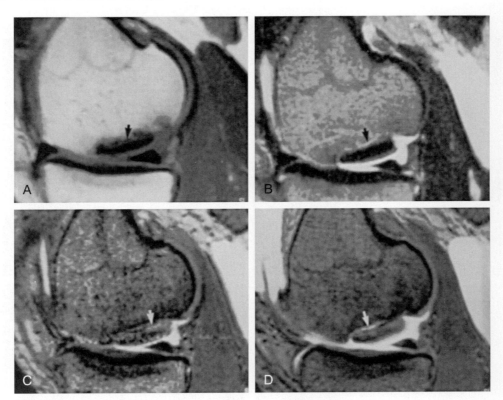

Figure 8–41

Osteochondritis dissecans (MR imaging, femoral condyles, various MR imaging techniques). This patient developed osteochondritis dissecans in the medial femoral condyle. A posterior synovial cyst (popliteal cyst) was palpable.

A On a sagittal T1-weighted (TR/TE, 700/15) spin echo MR image, a large osteochondral lesion is present. The junctional tissue (arrow) between the fragment and parent bone is of the same signal intensity as that of muscle. The cartilaginous surface is seen poorly. A synovial cyst is present posteriorly.

B On a sagittal T2-weighted (TR/TE, 2500/90) spin echo MR image, a large joint effusion is apparent. The junctional tissue (arrow) shows slight hyperintensity, consistent with fluid or granulation tissue. Disruption of the articular cartilage posteriorly is evident.

C On a sagittal gradient echo (fast imaging steady precession [FISP] image (TR/TE, 40/10; flip angle, 40 degrees) MR image obtained with volumetric acquisition, the posterior defect in the articular cartilage again is evident. No fluid is apparent in the junctional zone (arrow).

D After the intra-articular administration of a gadolinium contrast agent, a sagittal FISP gradient echo volumetric image with the same imaging parameters as in **C** shows fluid in the junctional zone (arrow) and disruption of articular cartilage. This method provides the most complete information in this case.

(Courtesy of J. Kramer, M.D., Vienna, Austria.)

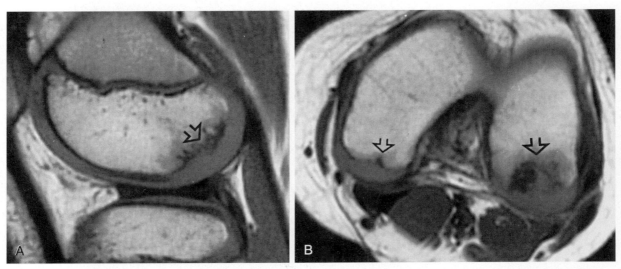

Figure 8–42

Normal epiphyseal ossification simulating osteochondritis dissecans. Femoral condyles. As shown on these T1-weighted (TR/TE, 600/13) sagittal (**A**) and T1-weighted (TR/TE, 400/20) transaxial (**B**) spin echo MR images, irregular ossification (arrows) of the femoral condyles (more evident in the lateral femoral condyle in this case) can simulate the appearance of osteochondritis dissecans. Note the normal, smooth articular and epiphyseal cartilage overlying the condylar surfaces. (Courtesy of D. Witte, M.D., and B. Edwards, M.D., Memphis, Tennessee.)

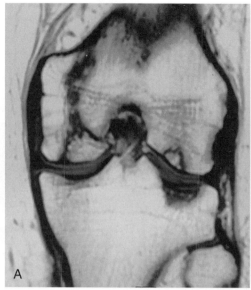
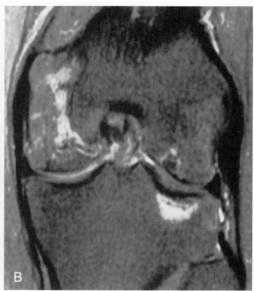

Figure 8–43
Osteonecrosis simulating osteochondritis dissecans. Coronal T1-weighted (TR/TE, 600/12) spin echo (**A**) and coronal fat-suppressed fast spin echo (TR/TE, 3500/14) (**B**) MR images show classic features of osteonecrosis involving both femoral condyles and lateral tibial plateau. In **A,** note the arc-like configuration of the subchondral lesions and vertical lesion of the medial femoral condyle. In **B,** high signal intensity is evident in certain regions, and the findings simulate those of osteochondral fractures or osteochondritis dissecans. (Courtesy of D. Witte, Memphis, Tennessee.)

typical site of the lesion is the medial facet of the patella. Involvement of the lateral facet occurs in approximately 30 per cent of cases, and the most medial or "odd" facet generally is spared. The middle or lower portion of the bone is affected almost universally. The lesions are identified optimally on lateral and axial radiographs of the patella. Arthrography can identify the chondral component of the injury. CT rarely is necessary in the evaluation of this lesion.[81] MR imaging may provide information regarding the viability and stability of the osteochondritic fragment (Fig. 8–45).[82]

Talus. Osteochondritis dissecans also is recognized in the talar dome. The middle third of the lateral border of the talus and the posterior third of the medial border are the two most common sites of injury, and they are involved with approximately equal frequency.[83] Patients usually are in the second to fourth decades of life. The

lateral talar lesion appears to relate to an inversion injury of the ankle. As the foot is inverted, the lateral border of the talar dome is compressed against the fibula. Further inversion ruptures the lateral collateral ligament and results in an avulsion of a small piece of the dome. This osteochondral fragment may remain in place or be displaced by continued inversion. The fragment may invert or rotate or lodge in the inferior tibiofibular joint. The medial talar dome lesion, which generally but not invariably is considered to be traumatic in pathogenesis, may be related to plantar flexion of the foot with inversion, followed by rotation of the tibia on the talus.[83] The medial talar fracture frequently is cup-shaped, deeper, and larger than the lateral talar lesion, which may be shallow and wafer-shaped.[84]

Carefully obtained radiographs usually can delineate the site of injury. These views may be supplemented by radiographs taken with the ankle in stress and with

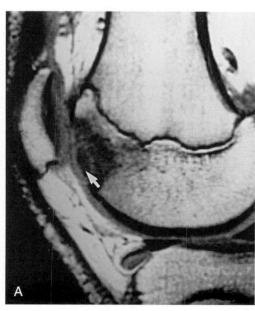
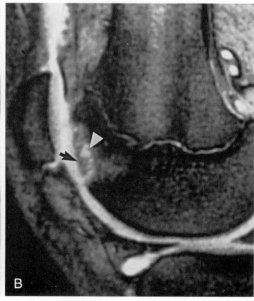

Figure 8–44
Osteochondritis dissecans of the femoral condyles: MR imaging. Sagittal proton density-weighted (TR/TE, 2000/20) spin echo (**A**) and multiplanar gradient recalled (MPGR) (TR/TE, 500/11; flip angle, 20 degrees) (**B**) MR images reveal osteochondritis dissecans involving the anterior aspect of the lateral femoral condyle. The osseous crater in the condyle contains a fragment (arrows). Fluid between the fragment and parent bone, better shown in **B** (arrowhead), indicates the presence of an unstable lesion. (Courtesy of S.K. Brahme, M.D., San Diego, California.)

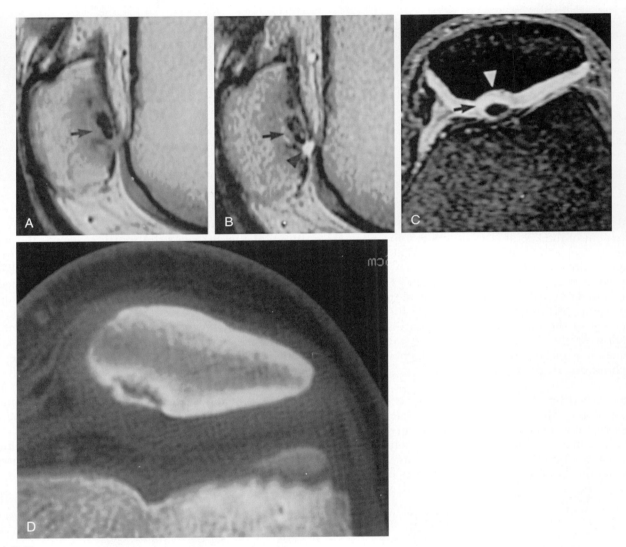

Figure 8–45

Osteochondritis dissecans of the patella.

A–C In this 30 year old man, a sagittal proton density (TR/TE, 2200/20) spin echo MR image **(A)** shows the patellar defect containing a bone fragment of low signal intensity. The junctional region (arrow) is of intermediate signal intensity. The patellar articular cartilage is not well evaluated. A sagittal T2-weighted (TR/TE, 2200/80) spin echo MR image **(B)** reveals higher signal intensity of the junctional region (arrow). Fluid arising from the joint has collected in a defect (arrowhead) in the patellar articular cartilage. A transaxial spoiled gradient recalled acquisition in the steady state (SPGR) MR image (TR/TE, 58/10; flip angle, 60 degrees), obtained with volumetric acquisition and chemical presaturation of fat (ChemSat) **(C),** shows the bone fragment, adjacent high signal intensity (arrow) in the junctional zone, and the osseous bed (arrowhead) in the patella. The articular cartilage of the patella is thinned or absent at the site of the bone fragment.

D In a second patient, transaxial CT shows the classic appearance of osteochondritis dissecans of the patella. The appearance of the lateral femoral condyle is normal in this adolescent patient. (Courtesy of P. Kindynis, M.D., Geneva, Switzerland.)

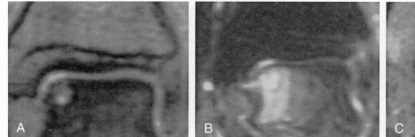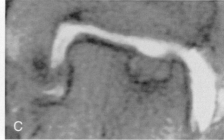

Figure 8–46

Osteochondritis dissecans of the talus (MR imaging).

A, B In a 19 year old woman, a coronal multiplanar gradient recalled (MPGR) MR image (TR/TE, 267/15; flip angle, 25 degrees) **(A)** shows a medial talar lesion of high signal intensity. This finding is compatible with fluid in the lesion. No alterations in signal intensity in the remainder of the talus can be seen. A coronal short tau inversion recovery (STIR) MR image (TR/TE, 2500/40; inversion time, 160 msec) **(B)** reveals the hyperintense lesion. Also note increased signal intensity around the lesion, consistent with marrow edema, and a small amount of joint fluid.

C In a second patient, a coronal T1-weighted (TR/TE, 500/20) spin echo MR image, obtained with chemical presaturation of fat (ChemSat) and after the intra-articular injection of a gadolinium contrast agent, shows a lateral talar lesion with loss of the overlying articular cartilage.

varying degrees of plantar flexion and dorsiflexion of the ankle, and by fluoroscopy and conventional tomography or CT scanning. Arthrography and conventional or computed arthrotomography are indicated in some cases to delineate the fracture site better, to define the condition of the overlying chondral coat, and to detect intra-articular osseous and cartilaginous bodies. MR imaging (Fig. 8–46) also has been used to define the extent of the lesion,[74, 76, 85] although its precise role is not yet clear.[86] Precise identification of the location and the extent of injury is important in determining the need for surgery and the specific surgical approach that must be used. Arthroscopy has been used successfully to treat both lateral and medial talar lesions, although the arthroscopic access to the posteromedial portion of the talar dome is more difficult. In some cases, arthrotomy rather than arthroscopy may be required.

Capitulum of Humerus. Osteochondritis dissecans about the elbow usually involves the capitulum,[87, 88] although the trochlear region of the humerus also may

be affected.[89] A history of acute injury or chronic stress, as occurs in gymnastics, is frequent. As in other sites, CT scanning, CT arthrography,[90] and MR imaging[91–93] (Fig. 8–47) have been used to evaluate the lesion. A normal groove that occurs between the capitulum and the lateral epicondyle of the humerus may create diagnostic difficulty, especially on MR images.[94] Lesions of the capitulum, in common with those of the talus, often are treated surgically with débridement and subchondral curettage or drilling.

DISLOCATIONS

Subluxations and *dislocations* usually are caused by physical trauma. Dislocations of the glenohumeral joint and other sites such as the hip may occur during seizures. Many dislocations and subluxations related to trauma are associated with fractures of a neighboring bone. Although the radiographic diagnosis of a dislocation or a subluxation is not difficult when the bones remain

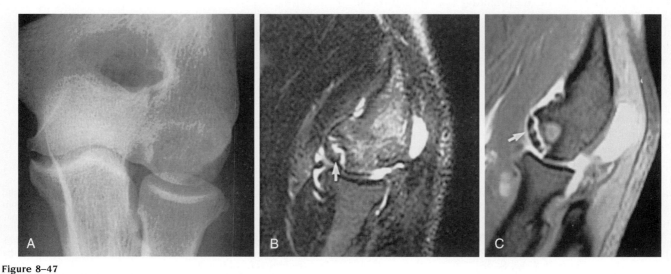

Figure 8–47

Osteochondritis dissecans of the capitulum of the humerus.

A Routine radiography reveals a large subchondral radiolucent lesion of the capitulum.

B, C In a sagittal fat-suppressed fast spin echo MR image (TR/TE, 3000/120) **(B)** and a sagittal fat-suppressed T1-weighted (TR/TE, 800/20) spin echo MR image obtained after the intra-articular injection of a gadolinium compound **(C)**, an osseous fragment (arrows) is seen. In both images, fluid is present between the fragment and the parent bone. High signal intensity in the bone marrow of the humerus is seen in **B**, and a cystlike area in the capitulum is seen in **C**. An unstable lesion was confirmed at the time of arthroscopy.

malaligned after the injury, spontaneous reduction can occur. In these cases, characteristic fractures in periarticular bone can confirm the presence of a previous dislocation. Furthermore, these fractures may predispose the joint to future dislocations. A third type of joint derangement is termed a *diastasis*. This term refers to abnormal separation of a joint that normally is only slightly moveable (e.g., the distal tibiofibular syndesmosis, the symphysis pubis, or the sacroiliac joint).

Traumatic dislocation of a joint implies that the joint capsule and protective ligaments have been damaged. A tear in these tissues may permit the extrusion of the articular end of the bone. Alternatively, the capsule may be stripped from one of its osseous sites of attachment, or a stretched ligament may lead to avulsion of a bone fragment. Although trauma may produce a dislocation of any joint, the most commonly involved sites are the glenohumeral joint, the elbow, the ankle, the hip, and the interphalangeal joints (see Chapters 12–17).

TRAUMA TO SYNCHONDROSES (GROWTH PLATES)

Mechanisms and Classification

The growth plate of the immature skeleton is especially vulnerable to injury; approximately 6 to 15 per cent of fractures of the tubular bones in children under the age of 16 years involve the growth plate and neighboring bone.[95–97] Forces that produce ligamentous tear or joint dislocation in the adult may lead to growth plate injury in the child and adolescent, as the joint capsule and ligamentous structures are approximately two to five times stronger than the cartilaginous plate. Four types of stress may produce growth plate injury; shearing or avulsive forces account for approximately 80 per cent of injuries, and splitting or compressive stresses account for the remainder.[98] Sites that are affected most typically are the growth plates of the phalanges of the hand, the distal tibial, fibular, ulnar, and radial growth plates, and the proximal humeral growth plate.[99] Growth plate injuries may occur acutely as a result of a single episode of trauma or chronically as a consequence of prolonged stress, particularly that associated with athletics (e.g., gymnastics).

Avulsion injury to the growth plate commonly is observed at sites of apophyses. Examples include the lesser trochanter, the medial epicondyle of the distal portion of the humerus, the tibial tubercle, the spinous process of a vertebra, and the base of the fifth metatarsal bone. The vulnerability of any specific apophysis to avulsion injury is governed by its development and maturation and, specifically, depends on the time of appearance and fusion of the apophysis.

Although several classification systems of growth plate injuries have been proposed, that of Salter and Harris is accepted most widely (Fig. 8–48).[97]

Approximately 25 to 30 per cent of patients with growth plate injuries develop some degree of growth deformity, and in 10 per cent of patients, this deformity is quite significant.[98] The prognosis is related to the age of the patient, the anatomy of the vascular supply to the region, the type of injury, and the immediacy and adequacy of the reduction. In general, the younger the patient at the time of injury, the poorer the prognosis for residual deformity. Types I, II, and III injuries have a relatively good prognosis, whereas type IV injuries carry a guarded prognosis, and for type V injuries the outlook is poor. Late sequelae include growth impairment, premature growth plate fusion, epiphyseal malposition and rotation, and osteonecrosis.[98]

MR imaging has been used clinically and experimentally to investigate traumatic abnormalities of the growth plate.[99–107] Both spin echo and gradient echo MR imaging techniques have been employed. Some investigators regard the latter technique as being superior for delineation of the cartilage of the growth plate,[100] whereas others indicate that although gradient echo methods are optimal for differentiating between cartilage and bone, they are suboptimal for distinguishing among the zones of the cartilaginous epiphysis.[101] With either method, the appearance of the growth plate varies with its stage of development and, hence, the age of the patient, and regional factors dependent on the specific anatomic site that is studied are encountered.[108]

In a study of the normal knee, Harcke and col-

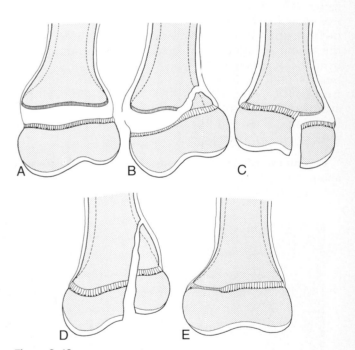

Figure 8–48

Growth plate injuries: Classification system.

A Type I: A split in the growth plate occurs through the zone of hypertrophic cells. The periosteum is intact.

B Type II: The growth plate is split and the fracture enters the metaphyseal bone, creating a triangular fragment. The periosteum about the fragment is intact, whereas that on the opposite side may be torn.

C Type III: A vertical fracture line extends through the epiphysis to enter the growth plate. It then extends transversely across the hypertrophic zone of the plate.

D Type IV: A fracture extends across the epiphysis, growth plate, and metaphysis. Note the incongruity of the articular surface and the violation of the germinal cells of the growth plate.

E Type V: Compression of portion of the growth plate may be unassociated with immediate radiographic abnormalities.

leagues[100] divided the MR imaging characteristics into four stages, based primarily on the extent of physeal development. MR imaging findings in children less than 2 years of age, in whom the distal femoral and proximal tibial epiphyses were composed primarily of cartilage, represented the first of these stages. The cartilage of the physes had intermediate signal intensity on T1-weighted spin echo MR images and high signal intensity on gradient echo images. The developing ossification centers initially were of low signal intensity on both types of images, owing to the presence of calcification, and subsequently revealed fat-containing bone marrow with high signal intensity on these MR images. MR imaging findings in children between the ages of 2 and 12 years, representing stage II, were characterized by thinning of the physes owing to enlargement of the ossifying epiphyses. The signal intensity of the cartilage in the growth plates varied according to the type of imaging sequence that was employed in a fashion similar to that

in stage I. After children had reached the age of 12 years (stage III), MR imaging findings were characterized by incomplete visualization of the cartilaginous physeal plates, particularly their central portion, designated the drop-out sign, which was more apparent on spin echo than on gradient echo MR images. As physeal closure commenced, spin echo images failed to demonstrate intermediate signal intensity cartilage in larger portions of the physis, although gradient echo images often depicted a thin, hyperintense band of cartilage. Finally, at the time of complete closure of the physes, MR imaging findings (stage IV) consisted of a single hypointense band between the metaphysis and epiphysis, representing the thick physeal ghost comprising dense osseous metaphyseal and epiphyseal plates. The authors concluded that the drop-out sign, which may relate to technical or anatomic factors, could simulate the appearance of premature closure of the physis. Furthermore, its central location was similar to that of traumatically

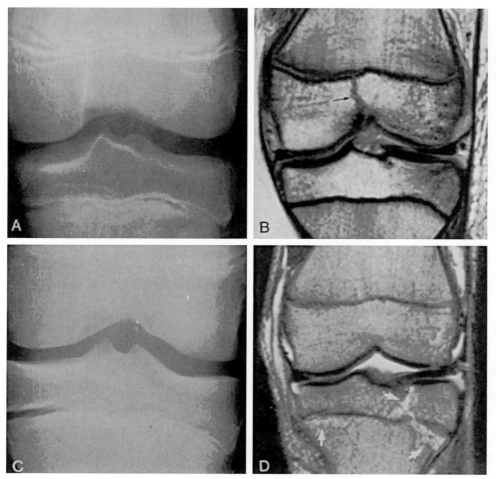

Figure 8–49

Growth plate injuries: MR imaging.

   A, B In a 13 year old boy, a frontal radiograph **(A)** reveals no significant abnormalities. A coronal T1-weighted (TR/TE, 800/20) spin echo MR image **(B)** shows a vertical fracture line (arrow) in the distal femoral epiphysis, indicative of a Salter-Harris type III physeal injury. Bone bruises appear as regions of diminished signal intensity in the metaphysis and epiphysis of the distal part of the femur and in the epiphysis of the proximal end of the tibia. (Courtesy of S. K. Brahme, M.D., La Jolla, California.)

   C, D This young boy suffered an injury to the knee while playing soccer. A routine radiograph **(C)** shows widening of the medial portion of the proximal tibial physis, suggesting a Salter-Harris type I injury. A coronal T2-weighted (TR/TE, 2000/80) spin echo MR image **(D)** reveals high signal intensity (arrows) in the tibia, consistent with a Salter-Harris type IV injury, in a bone bruise of the lateral portion of the distal femoral epiphysis, and in and about the medial collateral ligament, indicating ligamentous disruption and soft tissue edema. An effusion is present. (Courtesy of A. Newberg, M.D., Boston, Massachusetts.)

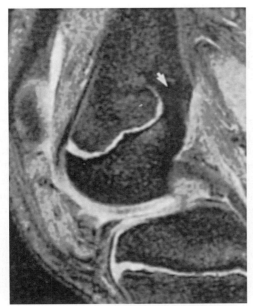

Figure 8–50

Growth plate injuries: Premature partial arrest of growth. This 9 year old boy had had an injury involving the distal femoral metaphysis 2 years previously that had been treated surgically. A local infection then developed and, subsequently, progressive deformity of the bone occurred. In a sagittal multiplanar gradient recalled (MPGR) MR image (TR/TE, 700/20; flip angle, 40 degrees) a physeal bar (arrow) is evident, accounting for the deformity. (Courtesy of D. Witte, M.D., Memphis, Tennessee.)

induced closure of the physis, creating further diagnostic difficulty. Comparison MR imaging studies of the opposite extremity might be helpful.

Despite these potential diagnostic pitfalls, MR imaging may prove useful in the analysis of acute physeal injury or delayed posttraumatic complications of such injury. Such imaging may allow definition of the plane or planes of acute injury to physeal cartilage and neighboring bone and, in so doing, provide more accurate information than that displayed on routine radiographs

(Fig. 8–49), particularly in infants and young children, in whom large portions of the epiphyses are unossified. MR imaging data in such instances may lead to a change in the classification of the physeal injury (e.g., type II injury to type IV injury) and indicate the coexistence of ligamentous or other soft tissue damage.[101, 108] Horizontal tears of the physeal cartilage may appear as regions of low signal intensity on MR images,[101] and increased vascularity and edema of marrow in areas of injury (or physeal bar formation) typically are demonstrated as regions of high signal intensity on T2-weighted spin echo and certain gradient echo MR images and of enhanced signal intensity after the intravenous administration of a gadolinium contrast agent.[102] In experimental investigations, MR imaging also has provided information regarding disturbances of physeal growth after epiphyseal and metaphyseal injury.[103] Injury to the epiphyseal vessels produces ischemic damage to the proliferative zone of the growth plate, and resulting bone bridges or focal curving of the growth plate may be observed on MR images; injury to the metaphyseal vessels blocks normal endochondral ossification, and thickening of the growth plate and tonguelike extensions of physeal cartilage into the metaphysis may be evident on such images.[103]

Although much of the data related to the delineation of growth disturbances after physeal injury using MR imaging have been derived from experimental studies in animals, results of preliminary investigations in humans also have been encouraging with regard to the detection with MR imaging of premature partial growth arrest after such injury (Figs. 8–50 and 8–51).[104, 105] This detection may be easier when peripheral rather than central portions of the physis are involved, and the failure to demonstrate a physeal bar by MR imaging in cases in which a bridge is suspected radiographically may be of prognostic significance[101] and has a dramatic effect on therapeutic planning.

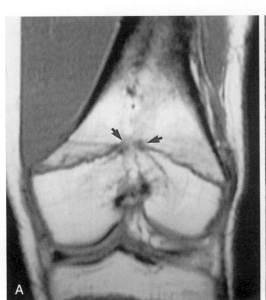

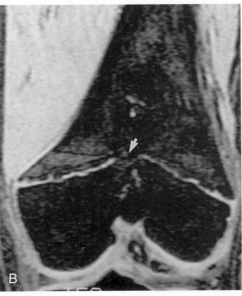

Figure 8–51

Growth plate injuries: Premature partial arrest of growth. This 13 year old boy suffered a Salter-Harris type IV injury to the growth plate of the distal portion of the femur at the age of 11 years.

A A coronal T1-weighted (TR/TE, 600/12) spin echo MR image shows a bone bar (arrows) of the femoral physis that has resulted in a tentlike configuration of the growth plate.

B The coronal spoiled GRASS (SPGR) MR image (TR/TE, 46/10; flip angle, 40 degrees) obtained with volumetric acquisition and fat suppression confirms the presence of a bone bar (arrow).

Chronic Stress Injuries

A variety of musculoskeletal manifestations occur in professional and recreational athletes that are related to the chronic application of stress. Although similar manifestations may be observed in children and adolescents, the open physes of the developing skeleton provide an additional anatomic site at which stress-related abnormalities may appear. The growth plates in the distal portions of the radius and ulna, the proximal portion of the humerus, the distal aspect of the femur, and the distal aspect of the tibia are affected most commonly in a variety of athletic endeavors that include gymnastics, soccer, baseball, basketball, American football, and swimming.

The imaging abnormalities occurring about the physes of the distal part of the radius and the distal end of the ulna in gymnasts serve as an appropriate prototype of this type of injury.[109–113] Unlike the case with most other sports, in gymnastics the upper extremities are used as weight-bearing limbs. In many of the specific gymnastic events, both compression and rotational forces are applied to the wrist and are borne mainly by the distal end of the radius. The resulting physeal changes usually occur first and are more prominent in the radius than in the ulna, but both bones commonly are involved. The injury appears to represent a Salter-Harris type I or type II lesion, but repetitive forces may result in subtle but permanent sequelae. MR imaging findings include horizontal fractures of the metaphysis of the radius, with metaphyseal extension of physeal cartilage, and premature closure of the growth plate of the radius (Fig. 8–52).[112, 113] Complications include symmetric or asymmetric retardation of or halted

growth at the affected site or sites, positive ulnar variance, and abnormalities of the distal radioulnar joint.

SUMMARY

This chapter emphasizes major types of traumatic disorders of bone and the application of advanced imaging methods, particularly MR imaging, to their analysis. Further discussion of these topics is contained in Chapters 12 to 17.

REFERENCES

1. Pradhan DJ, Juanteguy JM, Wilder RJ, et al: Arterial injuries of the extremities associated with fractures. Arch Surg *105*:582, 1972.
2. Ring EJ, Athanasoulis C, Waltman AC, et al: Arteriographic management of hemorrhage following pelvic fracture. Radiology *109*:65, 1973.
3. Matin P: Bone scintigraphy in the diagnosis and management of traumatic injury. Semin Nucl Med *13*:104, 1983.
4. Chhem RK, Kaplan PA, Dussault RG: Ultrasonography of the musculoskeletal system. Radiol Clin North Am *32*:275, 1994.
5. Feldman F, Staron R, Zwass A, et al: MR imaging: Its role in detecting occult fractures. Skel Radiol *23*:439, 1994.
6. Quinn SF, McCarthy JL: Prospective evaluation of patients with suspected hip fracture and indeterminate radiographs: Use of T1-weighted MR images. Radiology *187*:469, 1993.
7. Mink JH, Deutsch AL: Occult cartilage and bone injuries of the knee: Detection, classification, and assessment with MR imaging. Radiology *170*:823, 1989.
8. Berger PE, Ofstein RA, Jackson DW, et al: MRI demonstration of radiographically occult fractures: What have we been missing? Radiographics *9*:407, 1989.
9. Meyers SP, Wiener SN: Magnetic resonance imaging features of fractures using the short tau inversion recovery (STIR) sequence: Correlation with radiographic findings. Skel Radiol *20*:499, 1991.
10. Vahlensieck M, Lang PH, Seelos K, et al: Musculoskeletal MR imaging: Turbo (fast) spin-echo versus conventional spin-echo and gradient-echo imaging at 0.5 Tesla. Skel Radiol *23*:607, 1994.
11. Hilfiker P, Zanetti M, DeBatin JF, et al: Fast spin-echo inversion-recovery imaging versus fast T2-weighted spin-echo imaging in bone marrow abnormalities. Invest Radiol *30*:110, 1995.
12. Dwyer AJ, Frank JA, Sank VJ, et al: Short-T1 inversion-recovery pulse sequence: Analysis and initial experience in cancer imaging. Radiology *168*:827, 1988.
13. Arndt WF III, Truax AL, Barnett FM, et al: MR diagnosis of bone contusions of the knee: Comparison of coronal T2-weighted fast spin-echo with fat suppression and fast spin-echo STIR images with conventional STIR images. AJR *166*:119, 1996.
14. Cruess RL, Dumont J: Healing of bone, tendon and ligament. *In* CA Rockwood Jr, DP Green (Eds): Fractures. Philadelphia, JB Lippincott, 1975, p 97.
15. McKibbin B: The biology of fracture healing in long bones. J Bone Joint Surg [Br] *60*:150, 1978.
16. Milgram JW: Radiologic and Histologic Pathology of Nontumorous Diseases of Bones and Joints. Northbrook, IL, Northbrook Publishing Co, 1990, p. 385.
17. Wallace AL, Strachan RK, Best JJK, et al: Quantitative early phase scintigraphy in the prediction of healing of tibial fractures. Skel Radiol *21*:241, 1992.
18. Keene JS, Sellinger DS, McBeath AA, et al: Metastatic breast cancer in the femur: A search for the lesion at risk of fracture. Clin Orthop *203*:282, 1986.
19. Lee JK, Yao L: Occult intraosseous fracture: Magnetic resonance appearance versus age of injury. Am J Sports Med *17*:620, 1989.
20. Yao L, Lee JK: Occult intraosseous fracture: Detection with MR imaging. Radiology *167*:749, 1988.
21. Murphy BJ, Smith RL, Uribe JW, et al: Bone signal abnormalities in the posterolateral tibia and lateral femoral condyle in complete tears of the anterior cruciate ligament: A specific sign? Radiology *182*:221, 1992.
22. Schweitzer ME, White LM: Does altered biomechanics cause marrow edema? Radiology *198*:851, 1996.
23. Kirsch MD, Fitzgerald SW, Friedman H, et al: Transient lateral patellar dislocation: Diagnosis with MR imaging. AJR *161*:109, 1993.
24. Vellet AD, Marks PH, Fowler PJ, et al: Occult posttraumatic osteochondral lesions of the knee: Prevalence, classification, and short-term sequelae evaluated with MR imaging. Radiology *178*:271, 1991.
25. Stallenberg B, Gevenois PA, Sintzoff SA Jr, et al: Fracture of the posterior aspect of the lateral tibial plateau: Radiographic sign of anterior cruciate ligament tear. Radiology *187*:821, 1993.

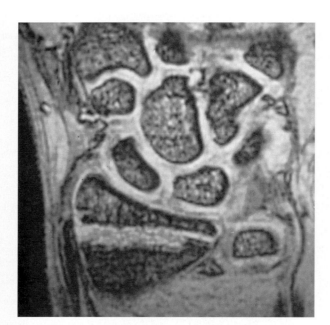

Figure 8–52
Growth plate injury: Chronic stress in athletics. In this 13 year old male gymnast, a coronal three-dimensional GRASS MR image (TR/TE, 70/11; flip angle, 20 degrees) shows widening and irregularity of the radial physis. (Courtesy of C. Shih, M.D., Taipei, Taiwan.)

26. Weber WN, Neumann CH, Barakos JA, et al: Lateral tibial rim (Segond) fractures: MR imaging characteristics. Radiology *180*:731, 1991.

27. Lynch TCP, Crues JV III, Morgan FW, et al: Bone abnormalities of the knee: Prevalence and significance at MR imaging. Radiology *171*:761, 1989.

28. Deutsch AL, Mink JH: Magnetic resonance imaging of musculoskeletal injuries. Radiol Clin North Am *27*:983, 1989.

29. Thompson RC Jr, Vener MJ, Griffiths HJ, et al: Scanning electron-microscopic and magnetic resonance-imaging studies of injuries to the patello-femoral joint after acute transarticular loading. J Bone Joint Surg [Am] *75*:704, 1993.

30. Lance E, Deutsch AL, Mink JH: Prior lateral patellar dislocation: MR imaging findings. Radiology *189*:905, 1993.

31. Kapelov SR, Teresi LM, Bradley WG, et al: Bone contusions of the knee: Increased lesion detection with fast spin-echo MR imaging with spectroscopic fat saturation. Radiology *189*:901, 1993.

32. Fowler PJ: Bone injuries associated with anterior cruciate ligament disruption. J Arthrosc Rel Surg *10*:453, 1994.

33. Stein LN, Fischer DA, Fritts HM, et al: Occult osseous lesions associated with anterior cruciate ligament tears. Clin Orthop *313*:187, 1995.

34. Schweitzer ME, Tran D, Deely DM, et al: Medial collateral ligament injuries: Evaluation of multiple signs, prevalence, and location of associated bone bruises, and assessment with MR imaging. Radiology *192*:825, 1995.

35. Daffner RH: Stress fractures: Current concepts. Skel Radiol *2*:221, 1978.

36. Anderson MW, Greenspan A: Stress fractures. Radiology *199*:1, 1996.

37. Holder LE, Michael RH: The specific scintigraphic pattern of "shin splints in the lower leg": Concise communication. J Nucl Med *25*:865, 1984.

38. Rupani HD, Holder LE, Espinola DA, et al: Three-phase radionuclide bone imaging in sports medicine. Radiology *156*:187, 1985.

39. Batt ME: Shinsplints: A review of terminology. Clin J Sport Med *5*:53, 1995.

40. Charkes ND, Siddhivarn N, Schneck CD: Bone scanning in the adductor insertion avulsion syndrome ("thigh splints"). J Nucl Med *28*:1835, 1987.

41. Detmer DE: Chronic shin splints — classification and management of medial tibial stress syndrome. Sports Med *3*:436, 1986.

42. Beck BR, Osternig LR: Medial tibial stress syndrome: The location of muscles in the leg in relation to symptoms. J Bone Joint Surg [Am] *76*:1056, 1994.

43. Stafford SA, Rosenthal DI, Gebhardt MC, et al: MRI in stress fracture. AJR *147*:553, 1986.

44. Froelich JW: Imaging of fractures: Stress and occult. J Rheumatol *18*:4, 1991.

45. Lee JK, Yao L: Stress fractures: MR imaging. Radiology *169*:217, 1988.

46. Martin SD, Healey JH, Horowitz S: Stress fracture: MRI. Orthopedics *16*:75, 1993.

47. Reinus WR, Fischer KC, Ritter JH: Painful transient tibial edema. Radiology *192*:195, 1994.

48. Tuite MJ, DeSmet AA, Gaynor PS: Tibial stress fracture mimicking neuroblastoma metastasis in two young children. Skel Radiol *24*:287, 1995.

49. Mulligan ME, Shanley DJ: Supramalleolar fatigue fractures of the tibia. Skeletal Radiol *25*:325, 1996.

50. Schils JP, Andrish JT, Piraino DW, et al: Medial malleolar stress fractures in seven patients: Review of the clinical and imaging features. Radiology *185*:219, 1992.

51. Umans HR, Kaye JJ: Longitudinal stress fractures of the tibia: diagnosis by magnetic resonance imaging. Skeletal Radiol *25*:319, 1996.

52. Tountas AA, Waddell JP: Stress fractures of the femoral neck: A report of seven cases. Clin Orthop *210*:160, 1986.

53. LeChevalier D, Fournier B, LeLeu T, et al: Stress fractures of the heads of the metatarsals: A new cause of metatarsal pain. Rev Rhum [Eng] *62*:255, 1995.

54. Pietu G, Hauet P: Stress fracture of the patella. A case report. Acta Orthop Scand *66*:481, 1995.

55. Mason RW, Moore TE, Walker CW, et al: Patellar fatigue fractures. Skeletal Radiol *25*:329, 1996.

56. Hill PF, Chatterji S, Chambers D, et al: Stress fracture of the pubic ramus in female recruits. J Bone Joint Surg [Br] *78*:383, 1996.

57. Peh WCG, Khong P-L, Yin Y, et al: Imaging of pelvic insufficiency fractures. RadioGraphics *16*:335, 1996.

58. Arafat QW, Davies AM: Sacral insufficiency fracture with intraosseous gas. Eur J Radiol *18*:232, 1994.

59. Stäbler A, Beck R, Bartl R, et al: Vacuum phenomena in insufficiency fractures of the sacrum. Skel Radiol *24*:31, 1995.

60. Brahme SK, Cervilla V, Vint V, et al: Magnetic resonance appearance of sacral insufficiency fractures. Skel Radiol *19*:489, 1990.

61. Mammone JF, Schweitzer ME: MRI of occult sacral insufficiency fractures following radiotherapy. Skel Radiol *24*:101, 1995.

62. Lien HH, Blomlie V, Talle K, et al: Radiation-induced fracture of the sacrum: Findings on MR. AJR *159*:227, 1992.

63. Bollen SR, Robinson DG, Crichton KJ, et al: Stress fractures of the ulna in tennis players using a double-handed backhand stroke. Am J Sports Med *21*:751, 1993.

64. Pfister-Goedek L, Braune M: Cyst-like cortical defects following fractures in children. Pediatr Radiol *11*:93, 1981.

65. Malghem J, Maldague B: Transient fatty cortical defects following fractures in children. Skel Radiol *15*:368, 1986.

66. Moss EH, Carty H: Scintigraphy in the diagnosis of occult fractures of the calcaneus. Skel Radiol *19*:575, 1990.

67. Milgram JW, Rogers LF, Miller JW: Osteochondral fractures: Mechanisms of injury and fate of fragments. AJR *130*:651, 1978.

68. Quinn SF, Haberman JJ, Fitzgerald SW, et al: Evaluation of loose bodies in the elbow with MR imaging. J MRI *4*:169, 1994.

69. Cobby MJ, Schweitzer ME, Resnick D: The deep lateral femoral notch: An indirect sign of a torn anterior cruciate ligament. Radiology *184*:855, 1992.

70. Virolainen H, Visuri T, Kuusela T: Acute dislocation of the patella: MR findings. Radiology *189*:243, 1993.

71. Schenck RC Jr, Goodnight JM: Osteochondritis dissecans. J Bone Joint Surg [Am] *78*:439, 1996.

72. Mesgarzadeh M, Sapega AA, Bonakdarpour A, et al: Osteochondritis dissecans: Analysis of mechanical stability with radiography, scintigraphy, and MR imaging. Radiology *165*:775, 1987.

73. Lehner K, Heuck A, Rodammer G, et al: MRI bei der Osteochondrosis dissecans. ROFO *147*:191, 1987.

74. Yulish BS, Mulopulos GP, Goodfellow DB, et al: MR imaging of osteochondral lesions of the talus. J Comput Assist Tomogr *11*:296, 1987.

75. De Smet AA, Fisher DR, Graf BK, et al: Osteochondritis dissecans of the knee: Value of MR imaging in determining lesion stability and the presence of articular cartilage defects. AJR *155*:549, 1990.

76. De Smet AA, Fisher DR, Burnstein MI, et al: Value of MR imaging in staging osteochondral lesions of the talus (osteochondritis dissecans): Results in 14 patients. AJR *154*:555, 1990.

77. Adam G, Bühne M, Prescher A, et al: Stability of osteochondral fragments of the femoral condyle: Magnetic resonance imaging with histopathologic correlation in an animal model. Skel Radiol *20*:601, 1991.

78. Adam G, Neuerburg J, Peib J, et al: Magnetresonanztomographie der Osteochondrosis dissecans des Kniegelenkes nach intravenöser Gadolinium–DTPA-Gabe. ROFO *160*:459, 1994.

79. Kramer J, Stiglbauer R, Engel A, et al: MR contrast arthrography (MRA) in osteochondrosis dissecans. J Comput Assist Tomogr *16*:254, 1992.

80. Smith DS, Sharp DC, Resendes M: MRI of healing osteochondritis dissecans fragment with absorbable pins. J Comput Assist Tomogr *18*:832, 1994.

81. Howie JL: Computed tomography in osteochondritis dissecans of the patella. J Comput Assist Tomogr *36*:197, 1985.

82. Pfeiffer WH, Gross ML, Seeger LL: Osteochondritis dissecans of the patella: MRI evaluation and a case report. Clin Orthop *271*:207, 1991.

83. Berndt AL, Harty M: Transchondral fracture (osteochondritis dissecans) of the talus. J Bone Joint Surg [Am] *41*:988, 1959.

84. Canale ST, Belding RH: Osteochondral lesions of the talus. J Bone Joint Surg [Am] *62*:97, 1980.

85. Nelson DW, DiPaola J, Colville M, et al: Osteochondritis dissecans of the talus and knee: Prospective comparison of MR and arthroscopic classifications. J Comput Assist Tomogr *14*:804, 1990.

86. Anderson IF, Crichton KJ, Grattan-Smith T, et al: Osteochondral fractures of the dome of the talus. J Bone Joint Surg [Am] *71*:1143, 1989.

87. Bauer M, Jonsson K, Josefsson PO, et al: Osteochondritis dissecans of the elbow: A long-term follow-up study. Clin Orthop *284*:156, 1992.

88. Maffulli N, Chan D, Aldridge J: Derangement of the articular surfaces of the elbow in young gymnasts. J Pediatr Orthop *12*:344, 1992.

89. Vanthournout I, Rudelli A, Valenti PH, et al: Osteochondritis dissecans of the trochlea of the humerus. Pediatr Radiol *21*:600, 1991.

90. Holland P, Davies AM, Cassar-Pullicino VN: Computed tomographic arthrography in the assessment of osteochondritis dissecans of the elbow. Clin Radiol *49*:231, 1994.

91. Murphy BJ: MR imaging of the elbow. Radiology *184*:525, 1992.

92. Jawish R, Rigault P, Padovani JP, et al: Osteochondritis dissecans of the humeral capitellum in children. Eur J Pediatr Surg *3*:97, 1993.

93. Peiss J, Adam G, Casser R, et al: Gadopentetate-dimeglumine-enhanced MR imaging of osteonecrosis and osteochondritis dissecans of the elbow: Initial experience. Skel Radiol *24*:17, 1995.

94. Rosenberg ZS, Beltran J, Cheung YY: Pseudodefect of the capitellum: Potential MR imaging pitfall. Radiology *191*:821, 1994.

95. Rogers LF: The radiography of epiphyseal injuries. Radiology *96*:289, 1970.

96. Siffert RS: The effect of trauma to the epiphysis and growth plate. Skel Radiol *2*:21, 1977.

97. Salter RB, Harris WR: Injuries involving the epiphyseal plate. J Bone Joint Surg [Am] *45*:587, 1963.

98. Ozonoff MB: Pediatric Orthopedic Radiology. Philadelphia, WB Saunders Co, 1979.

99. Snyder M, Harcke HT, Bowen JR, et al: Evaluation of physeal behavior in response to epiphyseodesis with the use of serial magnetic resonance imaging. J Bone Joint Surg [Am] *76*:224, 1994.

100. Harcke HT, Snyder M, Caro PA, et al: Growth plate of the normal knee: Evaluation with MR imaging. Radiology *183*:119, 1992.

101. Jaramillo D, Hoffer FA: Cartilaginous epiphysis and growth plate: Normal and abnormal MR imaging findings. AJR *158*:1105, 1992.

102. Jaramillo D, Shapiro F, Hoffer FA, et al: Post-traumatic growth-plate abnormalities: MR imaging of bony-bridge formation in rabbits. Radiology *175*:767, 1990.

103. Jaramillo D, Laor T, Zaleske DJ: Indirect trauma to the growth plate: Results of MR imaging after epiphyseal and metaphyseal injury in rabbits. Radiology *187*:171, 1993.

104. Havránek P, Lizler J: Magnetic resonance imaging in the evaluation of partial growth arrest after physeal injuries in children. J Bone Joint Surg [Am] *73*:1234, 1991.

105. Gabel GT, Peterson HA, Berquist TH: Premature partial physeal arrest: Diagnosis by magnetic resonance imaging in two cases. Clin Orthop *272*:242, 1991.

106. White PG, Mah JY, Friedman L: Magnetic resonance imaging in acute physeal injuries. Skel Radiol *23*:627, 1994.

107. Smith BG, Rand F, Jaramillo D, et al: Early MR imaging of lower-extremity physeal fracture-separations: A preliminary report. J Pediatr Orthop *14*:526, 1994.

108. Chung T, Jaramillo D: Normal maturing distal tibia and fibula: Changes with age at MR imaging. Radiology *194*:227, 1995.

109. Carter SR, Aldridge MJ: Stress injury of the distal radial growth plate. J Bone Joint Surg [Br] *70*:834, 1988.

110. Caine D, Roy S, Singer KM, et al: Stress changes of the distal radial growth plate: A radiographic survey and review of the literature. Am J Sports Med *20*:290, 1992.

111. Chang C-Y, Shih C, Penn I-W, et al: Wrist injuries in adolescent gymnasts of a Chinese opera school: Radiographic survey. Radiology *195*:861, 1995.

112. Shih C, Chang C-Y, Penn I-W, et al: Chronically stressed wrists in adolescent gymnasts: MR imaging appearance. Radiology *195*:855, 1995.

113. Liebling MS, Berdon WE, Ruzal-Shapiro C, et al: Gymnast's wrist (pseudorickets growth plate abnormality) in adolescent athletes: Findings on plain films and MR imaging. AJR *164*:157, 1995.

Paget's Disease

Magnetic Resonance Imaging
Summary

Paget's disease (osteitis deformans) is a condition of unknown cause affecting approximately 3 per cent of the population over the age of 40 years. The disease is characterized by excessive and abnormal remodeling of bone leading to a diagnostic pathologic and radiographic appearance in which irregular bone fragments with a thickened and disorganized trabecular (mosaic) pattern are visualized as coarsened and enlarged osseous trabeculae on radiographs. The MR imaging features are summarized in this chapter.

MAGNETIC RESONANCE IMAGING

MR imaging is not required for the diagnosis of Paget's disease of bone, which is better accomplished with routine radiography. Furthermore, owing to the variability in the MR imaging appearance of Paget's disease, diagnostic difficulty may arise when the MR images are interpreted in the absence of routine radiographs.

MR imaging alterations are most characteristic in those patients who have long-standing inactive phases of Paget's disease (Fig. 9–1). In this situation, the morphologic features observed during the MR imaging examination are identical to those evident with routine radiography and include cortical thickening, coarse trabeculation, enlargement of the bone, reduction in the size of the medullary cavity, and, in tubular bones, bowing. Typically but not invariably, the cortex remains devoid of signal on all imaging sequences. Thickened trabeculae in the medullary cavity also reveal a signal void. In the tubular bones of the extremities, the trabeculae reveal a criss-crossing appearance and are separated by normal-appearing fatty bone marrow with its typical signal characteristics.[1–3] Indeed, Kaufman and coworkers[3] emphasized the persistence of signal from normal fat as a potential way of differentiating osteosclerotic Paget's disease alone from that associated with fracture or tumor in symptomatic patients. Obliteration of areas of normal fatty marrow would be expected in the presence of edematous or neoplastic tissue. In some instances of long-standing, uncomplicated Paget's disease, the signal intensity of the bone marrow in involved regions is similar to that of fat but even more intense and more homogeneous.[2] Cystlike areas, representing fat-filled marrow spaces, are surrounded by thickened

and somewhat distorted trabeculae, resulting in a characteristic MR imaging appearance.[2]

The active stage of Paget's disease leads to variability in the MR imaging findings, making diagnostic difficulty more likely (Fig. 9–2). In this stage, the hematopoietic marrow is replaced by fibrous connective tissue with numerous large vascular channels. These histologic characteristics resemble those of granulation tissue and account for the MR imaging features that may resemble findings in tumor or infection.[2] With spin echo imaging, the signal intensity of the involved bone marrow may be decreased on the T1-weighted sequences and increased on the T2-weighted sequences.[4, 5] These signal character-

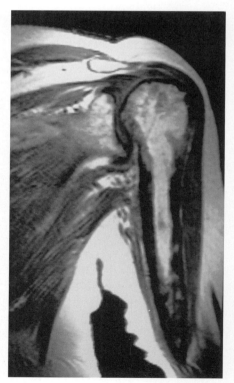

Figure 9–1

Paget's disease: MR imaging—inactive disease. This T1-weighted (TR/TE, 660/22) coronal oblique spin echo MR image shows a coarsened trabecular pattern manifested as regions of low signal intensity in the humerus and scapula. The marrow otherwise appears normal. The cortex of the humerus is thickened. (Courtesy of T. Claudice-Engle, M.D., Stanford, California.)

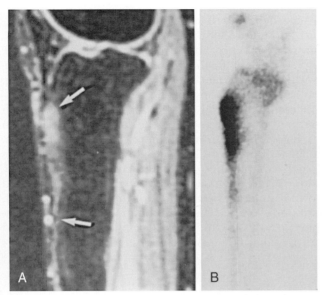

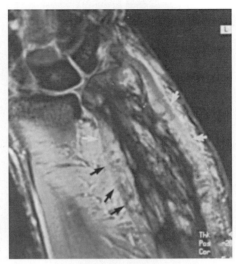

Figure 9–2

Paget's disease: MR imaging abnormalities. Active disease. In an elderly woman with Paget's disease of the tibial tuberosity, STIR imaging (TR/TE, 2800/20; inversion time, 150 msec) in the sagittal plane **(A)** shows high signal intensity (between arrows) in the anterior portion of the tibia. With bone scintigraphy **(B),** increased radionuclide accumulation is evident. (Courtesy of W. Glenn, M.D., Los Angeles, California.)

Figure 9–3

Paget's disease: MR imaging abnormalities. Soft tissue osteoid formation. This 44 year old man with known Paget's disease had pain and swelling of the forearm. A coronal multiplanar gradient recalled (MPGR) MR image (TR/TE, 578/18; flip angle, 30 degrees) shows pagetic involvement of the ulna and surrounding osteoid (arrows). Biopsy confirmed the absence of a pagetic sarcoma. (Courtesy of P. Kaplan, M.D., Charlottesville, Virginia.)

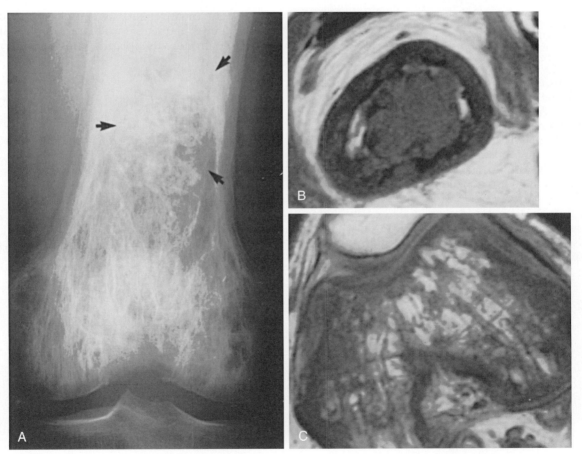

Figure 9–4

Paget's disease: MR imaging abnormalities—associated benign tumor of bone. In this patient, a frontal radiograph **(A)** shows typical features of Paget's disease of the femur as well as an osteolytic region (arrows) containing calcification. A transaxial T1-weighted (TR)TE, 690/15) spin echo MR image through the osteolytic region **(B)** reveals a lesion of low signal intensity in the marrow, which histologically proved to be an enchondroma. A transaxial T1-weighted (TR/TE, 690/15) spin echo MR image through the distal end of the femur **(C)** shows thickened trabeculae of Paget's disease with intertrabecular islands of fat. (Courtesy of M. Recht, M.D., Cleveland, Ohio.)

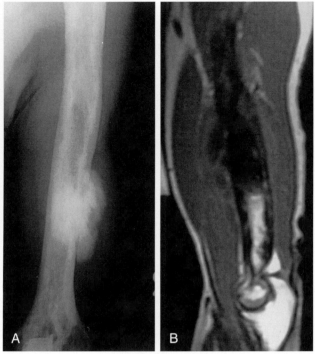

Figure 9–5

Paget's disease: MR imaging abnormalities, pagetic sarcoma. An os-
teogenic sarcoma complicating Paget's disease is evident on a routine
radiograph of the humerus (**A**). It is of low signal intensity on a
coronal T1-weighted (TR/TE, 433/10) spin echo MR image (**B**).
(Courtesy of L. White, M.D., Toronto, Ontario, Canada.)

gressive behavior of the lesion (e.g., cortical destruction) also are evident. Indeed, soft tissue extension is a
known occurrence in uncomplicated Paget's disease
(Fig. 9–3), and, furthermore, benign tumors may appear in areas of skeletal involvement in this disease (Fig.
9–4). Ultimately, biopsy of the lesion often is required.

In common with CT, MR imaging in patients with
Paget's disease may be employed for effective evaluation
of some of the neurologic complications of the disease.
Basilar impression and spinal stenosis, two of the causes
of such complications, are studied well with both CT
scanning and MR imaging, although the latter method
provides superior visualization of the brain, spinal cord,
and cauda equina. Also, in common with CT, MR imaging provides useful information about the extent and
neurovascular compromise of pagetic sarcomas (Fig. 9–
5).[8]

SUMMARY

Paget's disease is a common disorder of middle-aged
and elderly patients, characterized by excessive and abnormal remodeling of bone. Its radiographic features
are virtually diagnostic. Other imaging techniques, such
as scintigraphy, CT scanning, and MR imaging, are best
reserved for study of atypical features of the disease, its
response to therapy, and its complications, including
insufficiency fractures, neurologic symptoms and signs,
skeletal deformities, neoplasms, and joint alterations.

REFERENCES

1. Neuerburg J, Bohndorf K, Krasny RM: Paget des Skeletts: MR-Charakteristika
   bei 1,5 T. ROFO *149*:609, 1988.
2. Roberts MC, Kressel HY, Fallon MD, et al: Paget disease: MR imaging findings. Radiology *173*:341, 1989.
3. Kaufmann GA, Sundaram M, McDonald DJ: Magnetic resonance imaging in
   symptomatic Paget's disease. Skel Radiol *20*:413, 1991.
4. Mirra JM, Brien EW, Tehranzadeh J: Paget's disease of bone: Review with
   emphasis on radiologic features, part II. Skel Radiol *24*:173, 1995.
5. Steinbach LS, Johnston JO: Case report 777. Skel Radiol *22*:203, 1993.
6. Tjon-A-Tham RTO, Bloem JL, Falke THM, et al: Magnetic resonance imaging
   in Paget disease of bone. AJNR *6*:879, 1985.
7. Kelly JK, Denier JE, Wilner HI, et al: MR imaging of lytic changes in Paget
   disease of the calvarium. J Comput Assist Tomogr *13*:27, 1989.
8. Som PM, Hermann G, Sacher M, et al: Paget disease of the calvaria and
   facial bones with an osteosarcoma of the maxilla: CT and MR findings. J
   Comput Assist Tomogr *11*:887, 1987.

istics differ from those of fibrosis alone, which would be
expected to be of low signal intensity on both types of
sequences.[6, 7] Although prominent trabeculae that are
not destroyed about such regions of marrow may allow
a correct MR imaging diagnosis of Paget's disease alone,
elimination of the possibility of secondary tumor or
fracture may be impossible in some cases. The likelihood of a sarcoma in a patient with Paget's disease
increases when MR images show a solitary focus of at
least 2 or 3 cm in diameter whose signal intensity characteristics are unlike those of fat, particularly when an
adjacent soft tissue mass is present.[4] The findings appear
to lack specificity, however, unless obvious signs of ag-

Muscles and Tendons: Anatomy and Pathophysiology

Muscles and tendons are intimately related both anatomically and functionally. To consider one without the other is not appropriate, nor is it possible. The musculoskeletal system comprises more than 400 muscles. Allowing for some regional variations, such muscles arise either directly from a bone or from dense connective tissue or indirectly by way of a tendon. The muscle then passes distally, or rarely, proximally, to insert as a tendon into bone. The length of the muscle-tendon unit is variable; it may span only a single joint or may extend across two or more joints. The anatomic relationship of the muscle-tendon unit to bone also varies. Some such units are located close to the surface of the bone, whereas others, particularly those that cross multiple joints, are found more superficially at some distance from this surface. Any of the individual muscles with their accompanying tendons may be injured, although certain ones are more vulnerable than others. Injuries are classified using terms that indicate the pattern of injury and the specific type of soft tissue structure that is affected (Table 10–1).

Correct diagnosis and early treatment of musculotendinous injuries rely heavily on careful physical examination. The value of imaging techniques is greatest in those cases in which the nature of the injury is more obscure, particularly when its extent is not certain. Of the available techniques, MR imaging is most useful, owing to its excellent contrast resolution and its ability to allow assessment of injured tissue in multiple planes. The integrity of tendons and muscles can be deter-

mined directly with MR imaging and, when attention is given to signal intensity characteristics, the extent of musculotendinous injury can be defined.

TENDONS

Anatomy

Tendons represent a portion of a muscle and are of constant length, consisting of interlacing bundles of collagen fibers that transmit muscle tension to a mobile part of the body. They are flexible cords, white in color, smooth in texture, that can be angulated about bony protuberances, changing the direction of pull of the muscle. In comparison to ligaments, tendons contain fibers that are arranged in a more parallel fashion along their long axis.[1] On the surface of the tendon and enveloping it, a membrane structurally similar to a synovial membrane is found, designated an epitenon. On its inner surface, the epitenon is continuous with a thin layer of connective tissue, the endotenon, that serves to bind together individual collagen fibers and that contains nerves, lymphatics, and blood vessels.[2] In certain locations, a paratenon, consisting of loose areolar tissue, surrounds the epitenon, functioning as a sheath that promotes free movement of the tendon.[1] The epitenon and paratenon together are designated a peritenon. When the paratenon is replaced by a true synovial sheath, the structure is designated tenosynovium. A mesotenon refers to an elongated mesentery that connects the visceral and parietal layers of the tendon synovial sheaths. Although anatomic variations exist in the precise structure of the tendon and its coverings, these various layers and types of connective tissue are of fundamental importance in such mechanical properties as free movement and elongation.

At one end of the tendon, the perimysium about the muscle becomes continuous with the endotenon, compressing the musculotendinous junction[1] (see later discussion). At the other end of the tendon is the tendo-osseous junction (i.e., an enthesis), which may be classi-

Table 10–1. DEFINITIONS OF SOFT TISSUE INJURIES

Contusion	Bruised skin and underlying soft tissues secondary to edema and bleeding
Hemorrhage	Poorly defined soft tissue bleeding
Hematoma	Well-defined and restricted blood collection
Strain	Inflammation or rupture at the musculotendinous junction or muscle
Sprain	Inflammation or rupture of a ligament

Courtesy of H. Pavlov, M.D., New York, New York.

fied into two types: direct insertion and indirect insertion.[3, 4]

The vascular supply to tendons, although adequate, is not as abundant as that to muscles, and in certain tendons, such as the Achilles and supraspinatus tendons, regions of relatively low vascularity may be identified normally, coinciding in location to areas of the tendon that are vulnerable to degeneration and disruption.[5]

Injury and Repair

In an intact musculotendinous system, complete with its bony attachment, the muscle belly itself is the weakest point; in a tendon-bone preparation, the bone-tendon junction is the weakest point.[6, 7] The ultimate strength of such a system depends on many factors, including the rate of loading. Most tendons are subject to axial loads, although in certain sites, such as the flexor surface of the hand, where tendons wrap about articular surfaces, compressive loading also occurs.[1]

Tears of tendons most typically occur at their insertion sites into bone, with or without avulsion of a small osseous fragment. Tears also may develop at the musculotendinous junction and, rarely, within the substance of the tendon.[8] Intrasubstance tendon tears are encountered, however. After injury, tendon healing is related to fibroblastic infiltration from surrounding soft tissues.[9, 10] Proliferating connective tissue penetrates between the ends of sutured tendons and deposits collagen fibers that reveal progressive orientation, finally forming tendon fibers identical to those in normal tendons.[6, 11] An effective healing process requires close approximation of the ends of the divided tendons; complete tendon ruptures leading to separation of tendon ends will not heal unless they are closely applied to each other, so that collagenous tissue from the periphery can proliferate and penetrate the injured areas.

Tendon tears or ruptures can appear at virtually any site in the body. Typical examples are injuries of the tendons in the hands and feet and of the patellar, triceps, peroneal, quadriceps, rotator cuff, and Achilles tendons.[12–17] In most cases, the tendon injury results from significant trauma, although spontaneous ruptures have been documented,[18] especially in patients with rheumatoid arthritis and systemic lupus erythematosus and in those receiving local corticosteroid injection. Radiographic diagnosis of a purely soft tissue injury can be difficult. The gold standard for the imaging of tendons is MR imaging (Fig. 10–1).

Repetitive submaximal loading of tendons, as occurs in sports, may lead to an "overuse injury" that differs from tendinous injuries resulting from acute trauma.[1] Fatigue changes in tendon fibers or inflammation in surrounding tissues, or both, appear to characterize these overuse injuries, which involve preferentially the musculotendinous unit (see later discussion).[1, 19] Overuse syndromes may develop in either the upper or lower extremity, related most often to changes affecting the supraspinatus tendon, biceps brachii tendons, flexor or pronator tendons about the elbow, extensor tendons of the wrist, patellar tendon, Achilles tendon, or tibialis posterior or flexor hallucis longus tendons about the ankle. They are frequent in certain sports, such as swimming, weightlifting, golf, tennis, running, basketball, and ballet dancing. Histologically, the primary abnormality within the involved tendon is degeneration, not inflammation, occurring mainly in vulnerable regions of the tendon that normally exhibit diminished blood flow.[1] Because of the absence of accumulation of cells indicative of an acute inflammatory response, the term tendinitis would appear incorrect, as the suffix -itis is indicative of inflammation. Rather, fibroblasts and vascular connective tissue may be apparent,[20] histologic features that have been interpreted as evidence of angiofibroblastic hyperplasia.[1] The entire process may be referred to more accurately as tendinosis or tendinopathy.

Avulsion Injuries

Abnormal stress on tendons may lead to characteristic avulsions at their sites of attachment to bone.[21, 22] For example, avulsion of a portion of the calcaneus, the patella, or the ulnar olecranon may accompany exaggerated pull of the Achilles, quadriceps, or triceps tendon.[23, 24] Avulsion injuries of the proximal portion of the humerus, occurring generally during a dislocation of the glenohumeral joint, may involve either of the tuberosities and are related to tendinous traction provided by the various components of the rotator cuff. Indeed, virtually any skeletal site of attachment of a tendon (or ligament) may be affected by an avulsion injury, occurring either as an isolated phenomenon or as part of a more complex fracture or dislocation. Cartilaginous or cartilaginous and bony fragments may be avulsed (Fig. 10–2). The size of the avulsed fragment is quite variable; in the adult, only small osseous flecks may be pulled from the parent bone, whereas in the child or adolescent, an entire apophysis may undergo avulsion. The degree of displacement of the fragment also is variable.

Although the detection of avulsion injuries in adults may be difficult as a result of the small size or minimal displacement of the bone fragment, such injuries in children provide even greater diagnostic challenges owing primarily to the presence of unossified portions of the immature skeleton. Because the tendinous, ligamentous, and capsular tissue is much stronger than the physeal cartilage, forces that might produce a ligamentous or tendinous injury or dislocation in an adult may lead to physeal avulsion in a child. Such injuries commonly involve the apophyses of the skeleton. The apophyses are not involved in longitudinal growth but are responsible for the development of bone protuberances to which a tendon is attached or from which muscles arise or insert.[8] What appears to be a minor injury in the young child with a small avulsed piece of bone in reality may represent an avulsion of the entire apophysis. Apophyseal avulsions may occur at many different skeletal sites, although those of the pelvis and hips are encountered most frequently.

Several avulsion injuries about the pelvis and the hips

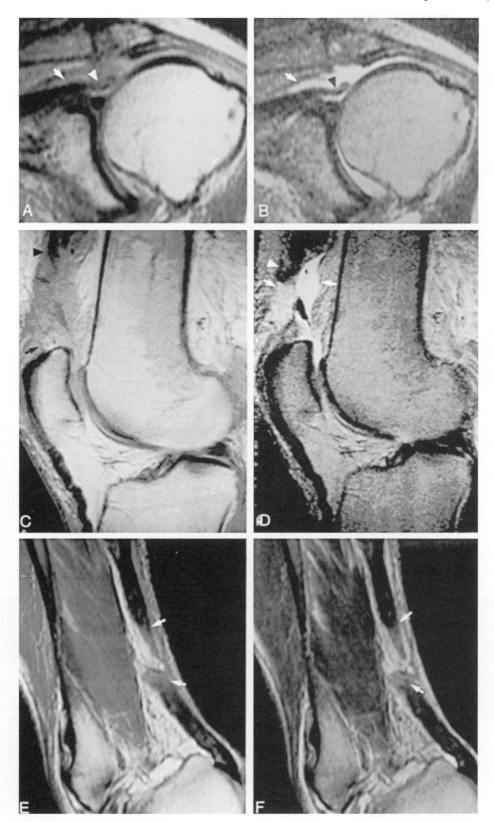

Figure 10–1

Tendon injuries (MR imaging, various sites).

A, B Supraspinatus tendon of the rotator cuff. Coronal proton density (TR/TE, 2000/30) **(A)** and T2-weighted (TR/TE, 2000/80) **(B)** spin echo MR images reveal a massive tear of the supraspinatus tendon. The tendon is retracted medially (arrowheads), fluid is present both in the glenohumeral joint and in the subacromial portion (arrows) of the subacromial-subdeltoid bursa, and the humeral head is elevated.

C, D Quadriceps tendon. On sagittal proton density (TR/TE, 1800/20) **(C)** and T2-weighted (TR/TE, 1800/80) **(D)** spin echo MR images, note disruption of the quadriceps tendon (arrowheads) with fluid in the tendinous gap (arrows). The patella is low in position (patella baja), and the patellar tendon has a wrinkled appearance. (Courtesy of R. Kerr, M.D., Los Angeles, California.)

E, F Achilles tendon. Sagittal proton density (TR/TE, 2000/20) **(E)** and T2-weighted (TR/TE, 2000/60) **(F)** spin echo MR images show complete disruption (between arrows) of the Achilles tendon.

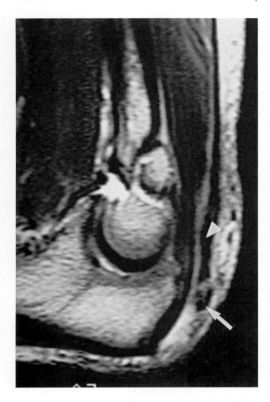

Figure 10–2
Avulsion injuries of the elbow: Olecranon process of ulna. On a sagittal T2-weighted (TR/TE, 1800/70) spin echo MR image, an avulsion injury of the olecranon process is evident. An enthesophyte (arrow) has been pulled away from the olecranon process by a portion of the triceps tendon (arrowhead). Abnormally high signal intensity is seen at the site of injury and in the nearby soft tissues. (Courtesy of S. Eilenberg, M.D., San Diego, California.)

in young athletes have characteristic imaging features.[25–30] These include (1) avulsion injuries of the anterior superior iliac spine, which occur in sprinters as the result of stress at the origin of the tensor fasciae femoris or the sartorius muscle (Fig. 10–3); (2) avulsion injuries of the anterior inferior iliac spine and of a groove just above the superior aspect of the acetabular rim, which relate to stress at the origins of the straight and reflected heads of the rectus femoris muscle (Fig. 10–4); (3) avulsion injuries of the apophysis of the lesser trochanter owing to stress of the psoas major during strenuous hip flexion; (4) avulsion injuries of the apophysis of the ischial tuberosity due to violent contraction of the hamstring muscles (Fig. 10–5), often occurring in hurdlers; (5) avulsion injuries of the greater trochanter of the femur produced by gluteal muscle contraction; (6) avulsion of the apophysis of the iliac crest due to severe contraction of the abdominal muscles associated with abrupt directional change during running; and (7) avulsion injuries near the symphysis pubis related to adduc-

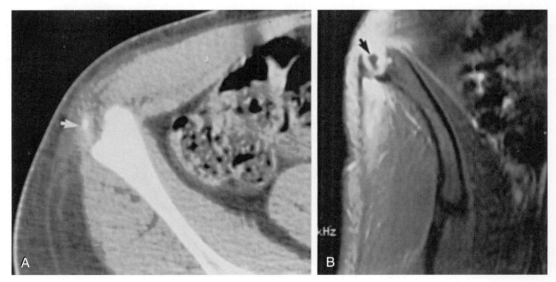

Figure 10–3
Avulsion injuries of the pelvis: Anterior superior iliac spine. Transaxial CT (**A**) and a coronal T1-weighted (TR/TE, 816/11) spin echo MR image obtained with fat suppression and after the intravenous injection of a gadolinium compound (**B**) show the site of avulsion (arrows). Note associated high signal intensity in **B**.
(Courtesy of D. Levey, M.D., Corpus Christi, Texas.)

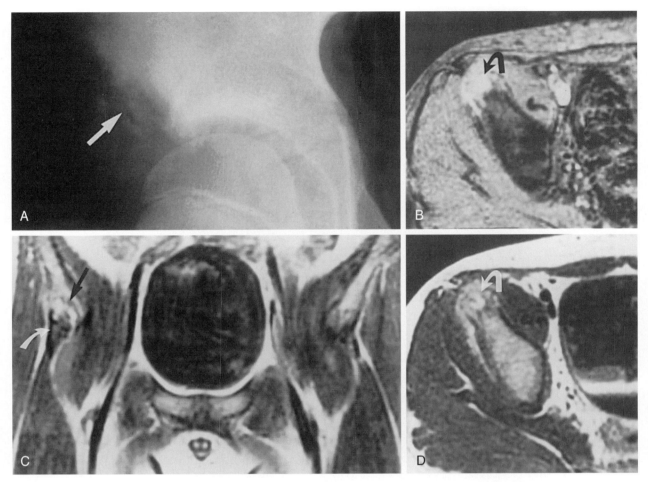

Figure 10–4

Avulsion injuries of the pelvis: Anterior inferior iliac spine.

  A The avulsed bone fragment (arrow) and subjacent irregular parent bone are evident.

  B A transaxial multiplanar gradient recalled (MPGR) MR image (TR/TE, 750/20; flip angle, 30 degrees) shows the bone defect with adjacent high signal intensity (arrow).

  C On a coronal T1-weighted (TR/TE, 600/25) spin echo MR image obtained after the intravenous injection of a gadolinium compound, the bone defect (straight arrow) of the ilium and the enhancement of signal intensity at the site of injury are observed. Note the position of the rectus femoris muscle and tendon (curved arrow).

  D The transaxial gadolinium-enhanced T1-weighted (TR/TE, 600/25) spin echo MR image shows findings similar to those in **B,** with enhancement of signal intensity at the site of injury (arrow).

Illustration continued on following page

tor muscle (adductor longus, adductor brevis, gracilis) insertion sites.[31–34] The fracture line may extend directly through the physeal cartilage or extend into the subjacent bone or ossifying apophysis, or both.

Another type of avulsion injury that is confined to the immature skeleton is the sleeve fracture. This injury has been described with respect to the patella,[35–37] although similar injuries conceivably may occur at other skeletal sites. The chondrosseous junction of the developing patella is affected in this avulsion injury. Although avulsion injuries of the tibial tuberosity have been observed in children and adolescents,[38, 39] those involving the site of attachment of the patellar tendon to the inferior margin of the patella are more typical (Fig. 10–6). An extensive sleeve of cartilage may be pulled away from the main portion of the patella, together with an osseous fragment from its distal pole.[37] A similar lesion may affect the superior portion of the patella or the medial margin of the bone (owing to acute lateral

dislocation of the patella). Indeed, the bipartite patella or dorsal defect of the patella (both involving the lateral side of the bone) and the Sinding-Larsen-Johansson lesion (affecting the inferior portion of the patella) may represent chronic sequelae of this type of injury.[37]

SKELETAL MUSCLES

Any discussion of physical injury would be incomplete if injury to skeletal muscle was not given consideration. Such injury can occur as an isolated abnormality or as part of a more complex situation in which fractures, dislocations, and other soft tissue abnormalities are present. Trauma to skeletal muscle may result from any type of accidental injury, but it is encountered most often in the setting of physical exertion, particularly that of athletic endeavors. Intense and prolonged exercise, espe-

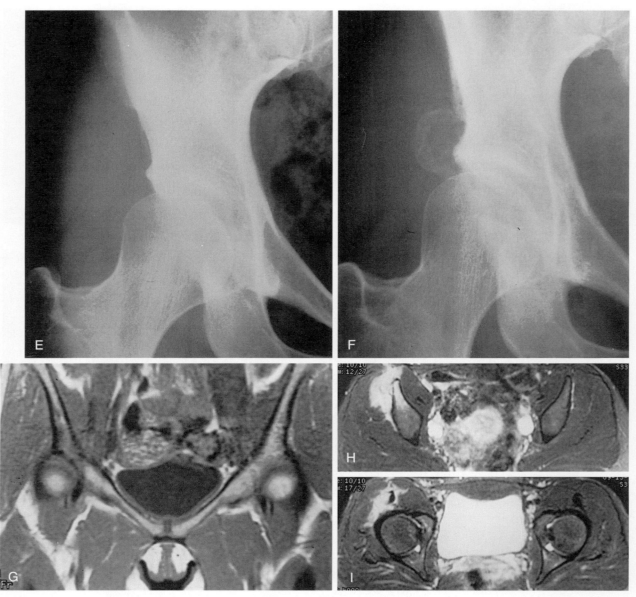

Figure 10–4 *Continued*

E–I In a second patient with an avulsion injury at the same site, a routine radiograph at the time of injury **(E)** shows no abnormality. Eight weeks later **(F)**, ossification is evident. MR imaging was performed approximately 1 week after the injury. A coronal T1-weighted (TR/TE, 550/11) spin echo MR image **(G)** shows little abnormality. Transaxial fat-suppressed fast spin echo (TR/TE, 4000/68) MR images at the level of the acetabulum **(H)** and femoral head **(I)** reveal high signal intensity about the avulsed tendon of the rectus femoris muscle and within the muscle itself. (Courtesy of J. Taylor, D.C., Portland, Oregon.)

cially in a person who is not properly trained or conditioned, can produce a muscle strain or pull, related to rapid and violent contraction of the muscle, but this is but one of a spectrum of injuries that affect skeletal muscle. Accurate assessment of the type and extent of injury previously had been the sole responsibility of the examining physician who, on the basis of clinical history and careful physical examination, arrived at his or her conclusion on the nature and significance of the muscle abnormalities. With the introduction and refinement of MR imaging as a diagnostic technique that can be applied effectively to the analysis of skeletal muscle, the examining physician, should he or she choose, has an additional method to judge the severity of the injury.

Skeletal muscles do not act independently. Rather, they transmit their contractile forces to adjacent structures through tendinous attachments. The muscle serves as the active element in this action, and the tendon is the passive element. The junctional region between the muscle fibers and the tendinous attachment is termed the myotendinal, or musculotendinous, junction. At this junction, muscle fibers of variable shape thicken and become continuous with the fibrous bundles of the tendon. Many, if not most, of the injuries to muscle in fact occur at the myotendinal junction. In the discussion that follows, physical injury to skeletal muscle, including the myotendinal junction, is addressed. Excellent reviews of this subject are provided by Mink,[40] Gross,[41] and Best and Garrett,[1] many of whose observations are included here.

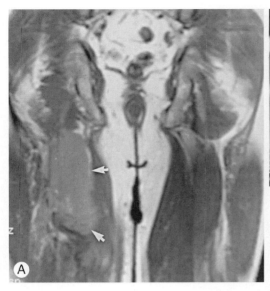

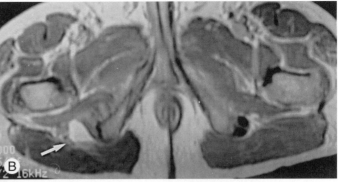

Figure 10–5
Avulsion injuries of the pelvis: Ischial tuberosity. In this 48 year old man who had heard a popping noise while tripping on the stairs, an avulsion of the right hamstring muscles from the ischial tuberosity is shown (arrows) on a coronal T1-weighted (TR/TE, 650/17) spin echo MR image **(A)** and a transaxial fast spin echo (TR/TE, 5000/15) MR image **(B)**. (Courtesy of J. Spaeth, M.D., Albuquerque, New Mexico.)

Anatomy

The basic units of skeletal muscle are the fibers themselves, each of which is a single cell containing many hundreds of nuclei.[42] These fibers are arranged in bundles, or fasciculi, of various sizes within the muscle. Connective tissue located between muscle fibers, around a fasciculus, or about the entire muscle is designated endomysium, perimysium, or epimysium, respectively. Each fiber is elongated, stretching either from one end of the muscle to the other or through part of the length of the muscle (and ending in tendinous or other connective tissue insertions that penetrate the body of

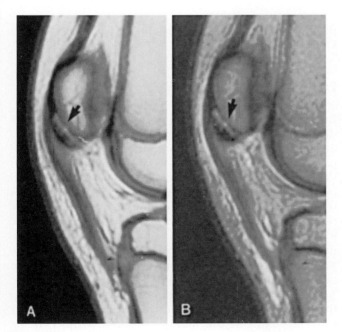

Figure 10–6
Avulsion injuries of the patella: Sleeve fracture. In this 9 year old girl, sagittal proton density (TR/TE, 2000/30) **(A)** and T2-weighted (TR/TE, 2000/80) **(B)** spin echo MR images show avulsion (arrows) of the inferior portion of the developing chondro-osseous patella with adjacent edema.

the muscle).[42] The cytoplasm, or sarcoplasm, of the muscle cell is divided into longitudinal threads, or myofibrils. The myofibrils, in longitudinal section, are traversed by striations that differ in their chemical and optical properties and are termed the I (isotropic), A (anisotropic), Z (Krause's membrane), and H (Hensen's line) bands.[42] Myofilaments are smaller structures within each myofibril. Two types of myofilaments exist: fine filaments consisting of actin, and thicker ones composed of myosin. Each of the myofilaments is crossed by Z bands, creating regions known as sarcomeres. During muscle contraction, the actin filaments slide toward the center of the sarcomere, bringing Z bands closer together, and producing shortening of the entire muscle unit.[40]

Most muscles show a mixture of two types of fibers, known as type I, or slow twitch, fibers and type II, or fast twitch, fibers. Histochemical differences differentiate between these types of fibers. Type I fibers are better suited to a relatively slow but repetitive type of contraction, such as the tonic forces characteristic of postural muscles, and are more resistant to fatigue than type II fibers. Hence, type I fibers are more involved in endurance activities than those requiring speed and strength of short duration. Type II fibers, in contrast, are adapted to produce rapid phasic forces that are operational in large-scale movements of the human body.[42]

Injury and Repair

The vast majority of sports-related injuries involving muscle are either strains or contusions.[41, 43] As indicated later, the two types of injury involve different parts of the muscle, although the local reaction to the injury and the repair processes are similar for both lesions. Typically, skeletal muscle contracts as a response to injury. Such contraction leads to an increase of pressure in the muscle. The sheath that encloses the muscle, the epimysium, and the overlying fascia serve as a relatively rigid tissue and give counterpressure to the forces of muscular contraction.[44, 45] As a consequence, large intracompartmental hematomas can develop within the muscle tissue before the transmural pressure is high enough to prevent further intramuscular fluid expansion.[44] The anatomic arrangement of muscle tissue within surrounding sheaths contributes to the frequent development of compartment syndromes after trauma (see later discussion).

Skeletal muscle is capable of limited regeneration. Fibers on each side of a damaged zone break up into nucleated cylinders of cytoplasm, macrophages enter the necrotic area, and they engulf dead materials but leave the basement membrane intact.[42] The muscle fiber cylinders then fuse and grow inside the original basement membrane to form a myotube. Eventual fusion of the two undamaged ends and hypertrophy and maturation lead to a creation of the new intact fiber.[42] With extensive muscle damage, however, such regeneration is not possible, and connective tissue is formed to replace the injured muscle, with resultant loss of function. In certain situations, such as after laceration, healing of skeletal muscle is associated with extensive scarring and ossification.[43]

Direct Muscle Injury

Muscle Laceration

Muscle lacerations result from penetrating injuries. The typical healing response results in the formation of a scar composed of dense connective tissue.[40] Owing to limited muscle regeneration and the absence of extensive reinnervation of the distal portion of the muscle, restoration of function of the muscle is not complete. MR imaging in cases of lacerated muscle is characterized by a defect, often transverse, with interruption of the continuity of the muscle and changes in signal intensity reflecting the presence of blood and edema (Fig. 10–7).[40]

Muscle Contusion

Compression of a muscle from direct trauma leads to a contusion. The force necessary to produce a contusion is not infrequent in certain contact sports, such as American football, and the term "charleyhorse" sometimes is used to describe the injury, particularly when the quadriceps muscles are involved. The blow results in capillary rupture and interstitial hemorrhage (bleeding between the fibers of the damaged connective tissue) followed by development of edema and an inflammatory mass.[40] Contusions vary in severity, although the muscle still is able to function, even in severe cases.

Four basic MR imaging features characterize a muscle contusion[40]: (1) The affected muscle usually is slightly increased in girth; (2) edema leads to an increase in signal intensity on T2-weighted spin echo and short tau inversion recovery (STIR) MR images and, owing to its isointensity with muscle, is not well seen on T1-weighted spin echo images; (3) a feathery, interstitial pattern is evident that relates to the dispersion of inflammatory fluid within and between the muscle fibers; and (4)

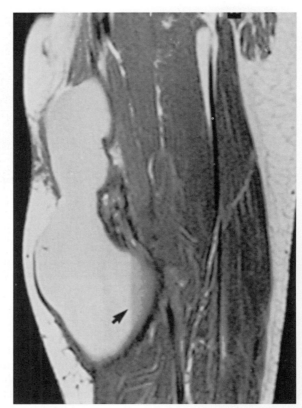

Figure 10–7
Skeletal muscle injury: Laceration. This young man lacerated his thigh while on a motorcycle. A soft tissue mass developed and enlarged quickly. It followed the course of the sartorius muscle. A sagittal T1-weighted (TR/TE, 650/20) spin echo MR image shows high signal intensity within the superficial intramuscular mass, with a fluid-debris level (arrow), findings consistent with a recently formed hematoma. (Courtesy of S. Eilenberg, M.D., San Diego, California.)

there is no evidence of disruption of muscle fibers (Fig. 10–8).

Indirect Muscle Injury

Indirect injuries to muscle occur from overzealous use during physical exercise. Certain muscles are prone to develop exercise-related, or exertional, muscle injury, in part because of the specific type of muscle contraction that they exhibit. Such muscle contractions are divided into two basic types: Isometric contraction produces tension without a change in muscle length; isotonic contraction produces tension associated with a change in muscle length.[40] Isotonic contraction is divided further into two types: Concentric action occurs when the muscle shortens during contraction; eccentric action occurs when the muscle lengthens during contraction. As muscles produce greater tension during stretching than when shortening, eccentric contractions, as occur when a weight in the hand is lowered parallel to the thorax, lead to greater tension than concentric contractions and are considered the primary cause of exertional muscle injury.[40] Injury-prone muscles show several typical characteristics.[40] First, such muscles commonly perform eccentric actions (e.g., hamstring muscles). Higher

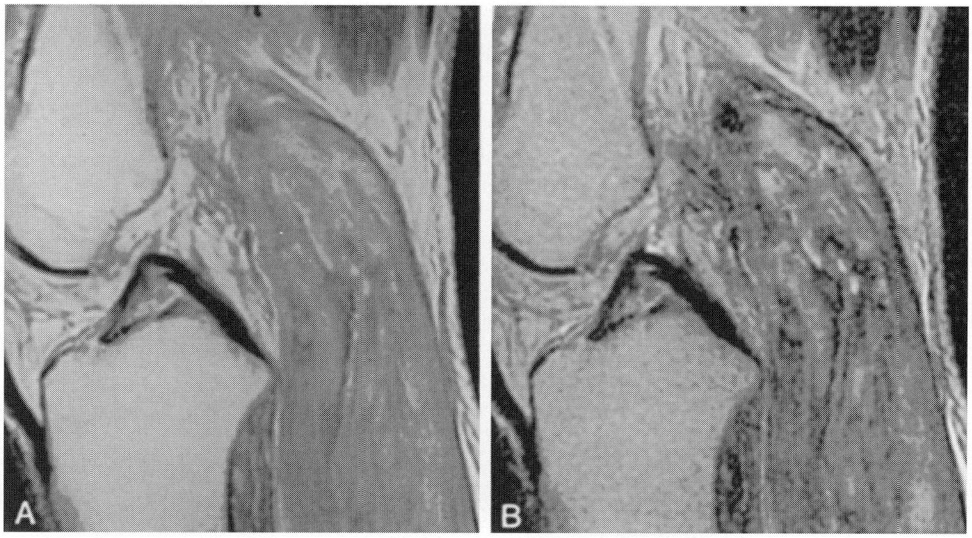

Figure 10–8
Skeletal muscle injury: Contusion. This 29 year old man suffered a direct blow to the back of the knee and calf. Sagittal proton density (TR/TE, 2000/30) **(A)** and T2-weighted (TR/TE, 2000/80) **(B)** spin echo MR images show enlargement of the medial head of the gastrocnemius muscle. The muscle is inhomogeneous in signal intensity in both images and generally is of higher signal intensity than normal.

forces are generated in the muscle-tendon unit after injury to muscles performing eccentric actions.[1] Second, the muscles commonly act across two joints (e.g., biceps brachii and gastrocnemius muscles). Third, muscles having type II or fast fibers and involved in activities requiring sudden acceleration or deceleration typically are affected (e.g., hip flexors and adductors, rectus femoris muscle).

MR imaging has been employed to evaluate physiologic and pathologic alterations in skeletal muscle after physical exertion.[46–53] After moderate exercise, T2 relaxation times increase regardless of the type of exercise performed, although the T2 values are significantly higher in those muscles performing concentric actions than in those performing eccentric actions.[40] Resulting increases in signal intensity within muscles on T2-weighted spin echo MR images and STIR images correlate strongly with the mean force exerted during the exercise.

Similar alterations in signal intensity are observed after acute muscle strains.[54–57] Such strains are defined as painful stress-induced injuries resulting from the application of a single violent force.[40] Whereas contusions produce injury at the point of impact, strains lead to injury at or near the musculotendinous junction.[1] This location has been confirmed during surgical exploration of injuries involving the medial head of the gastrocnemius muscle, the rectus femoris muscle, the triceps brachii muscle, the adductor longus muscle, the pectoralis major muscle, the semimembranosus muscle, and other muscles.[1, 58–62] The precise MR imaging findings are influenced by the severity of the strain and its duration (Figs. 10–9, 10–10, 10–11, 10–12, and 10–13).[63, 64] Minor, or grade 1, strains produce MR imaging findings similar to those of a muscle contusion. With moderate, or grade 2, muscle strains, a focal masslike lesion or a stellate defect, or both, can be observed on the MR images.[40] The signal intensity of the involved muscle or muscles reflects the presence of edema or blood. Serial MR imaging in cases of grade 1 or 2 muscle strain reveals initial alterations in the center of the affected muscle, subsequent involvement of the entire muscle,

and, finally, resolution of the abnormalities.[40] With severe, or grade 3, muscle strains, discontinuity of the muscle is evident, and blood collects between the torn edges. A true hematoma may form.

Delayed onset muscle soreness (DOMS) represents another response to physical exertion.[65] It is especially marked after the initiation or resumption of training by athletes after a period of time without training.[1] Clinical findings, consisting of muscle soreness and tenderness to palpation, occur within one to several days after muscle exertion. There is restricted range of motion of nearby joints. Neurovascular signs are absent. MR imaging findings in DOMS resemble those of grade 1 muscle strains, and the conspicuity of these findings generally follows the clinical course and correlates with histologic and ultrastructural changes in the involved musculature.[50] Imaging studies, however, are rarely required for diagnosis, owing to the presence of characteristic clinical findings.

The precise pathogenesis of DOMS is not clear, although an inflammatory response to muscle injury is likely. It is a self-limiting condition that responds to topical application of ice, ultrasound, oral analgesics, and anti-inflammatory medication.

Muscle Herniation

Focal herniation of muscle through a defect in its enclosing fascia may occur as a complication of local blunt trauma or as a result of muscle hypertrophy.[66, 67] Typically, the lower leg, especially its anterior tibial compartment, is involved, the tibialis anterior muscle being affected most frequently. A soft tissue mass that becomes tense and decreases in size during muscle contraction is a common clinical finding. MR imaging represents an effective diagnostic technique when such herniation is suspected.[67] Surgical repair with closure of the fascial defect may lead to an anterior compartment syndrome.

Muscle Contracture

Contracture of a muscle may relate to a number of factors. Congenital contractures are well recognized, in-

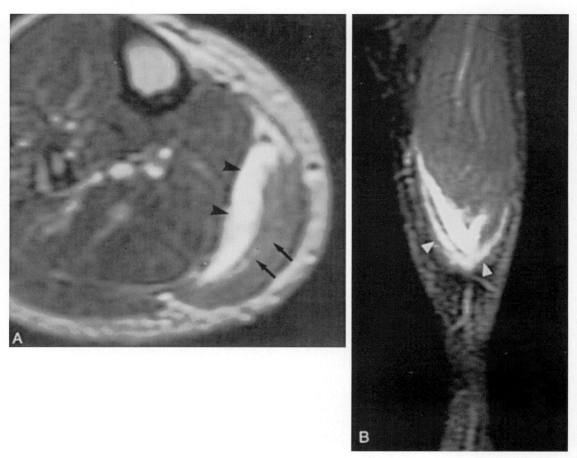

Figure 10–9
Skeletal muscle injury: Grade 1 strain. A transaxial T2-weighted (TR/TE, 2000/80) spin echo MR image **(A)** reveals an increase in signal intensity of the gastrocnemius muscle (arrows) and a perifascial fluid collection (arrowheads). A coronal short tau inversion recovery (STIR) MR image (TR/TE, 2200/35; inversion time, 160 msec) **(B)** defines the fluid collection (arrowheads) just deep and distal to the gastrocnemius muscle. (From Deutsch AL, Mink JH, Kerr R: MRI of the Foot and Ankle. New York, Raven Press, 1992.)

volving particularly the gastrocnemius and sternocleidomastoid muscles.[68–70] Muscle contracture also can result from contusion,[71] and it may follow intramuscular injections (Fig. 10–14).[69, 72, 73] Indeed, MR imaging performed after such injections, especially of corticosteroid medications, may reveal abnormalities of signal intensity that simulate findings in other conditions (Fig. 10–15).

Rhabdomyolysis

Rhabdomyolysis is a relatively common syndrome of muscle injury that alters the integrity of the cell membrane, allowing the escape of cellular contents into the general circulation.[74, 75] Causative factors include burns, crush injuries, prolonged muscular compression, exposure to toxins, seizures, and extremely intense exercise, especially in hot climates.[40] Although multiple intracellular enzymes may be released, creatine kinase is the most sensitive to muscle injury.[75] Myoglobulin can be detected in the urine. Clinical findings include fever and intense pain and weakness; among the complications that may be encountered are tetany, acute renal failure, compartment syndrome, and disseminated intravascular coagulation. Ultrasonography,[76] CT,[75, 77, 78] scin-

tigraphy,[79] and MR imaging[51, 80] may be used to investigate this condition and its complications. Swelling and regions of low attenuation in muscles are typical CT findings of rhabdomyolysis.[75] MR imaging reveals increased intramuscular signal intensity on T2-weighted spin echo and STIR images.[40, 80]

Compartment Syndrome and Myonecrosis

Compartment syndrome is a condition characterized by elevated pressure within an anatomically confined space leading to irreversible damage to the contents (i.e., muscle and neurovascular components) of the closed space.[81] Any condition that increases the contents of a compartment or that reduces the volume of a compartment may lead to a compartment syndrome. Common causes are trauma with hemorrhage, fractures, increased capillary permeability after thermal burns, and intense physical activity. Regardless of the precise cause, elevation of intracompartmental pressure leads to some degree of venous obstruction; pressure within the involved compartment may continue to rise until the low intramuscular arteriolar pressure is exceeded.[81] With further increase in the intracompartmental pressure, muscle

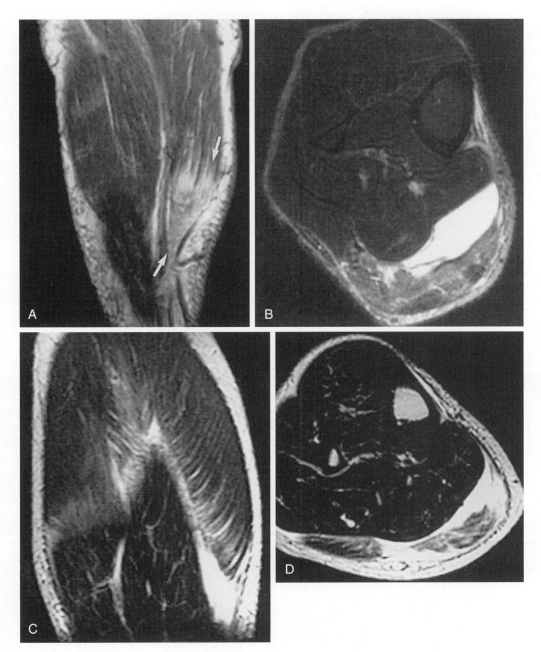

Figure 10–10

Skeletal muscle injury: Grade 1 or 2 strain.

   A A coronal T1-weighted (TR/TE, 600/11) spin echo MR image shows blood of high signal intensity accumulating in the lower portion of the medial head of the gastrocnemius muscle and the musculotendinous junction (arrows). Some muscle fibers appear to be disrupted.

   B A transaxial fat-suppressed fast spin echo MR image (TR/TE, 5000/85) shows a perifascial collection of blood.

   (**A, B** Courtesy of S.K. Brahme, M.D., San Diego, California.)

   C, D Very similar findings are evident in this radiologist who injured himself on a skiing vacation during his bone fellowship. Note high signal intensity in and about the medial head of the gastrocnemius muscle as shown in coronal (TR/TE, 4000/128) (**C**) and transaxial (TR/TE, 4000/119) (**D**) fast spin echo MR images. (Courtesy of A. Brossmann, M.D., San Diego, California.)

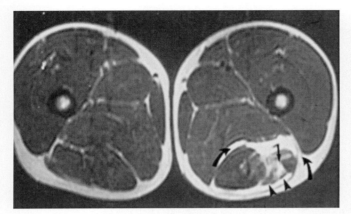

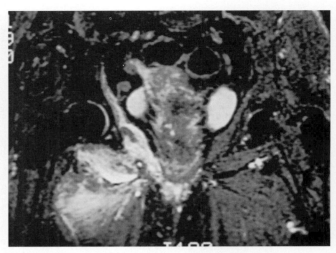

Figure 10–11

Skeletal muscle injury: Grade 2 strain. This professional football player suffered an acute hamstring strain during pushoff from the line of scrimmage. On a transaxial T2-weighted (TR/TE, 2000/80) spin echo MR image, note that the biceps femoris muscle demonstrates edema throughout its substance (arrowheads) with several small focal areas perhaps representing limited interruption of muscle fibers (small arrow). Perifascial edema (large arrows) is striking. (From Deutsch AL, Mink JH, Kerr R: MRI of the Foot and Ankle. New York, Raven Press, 1992.)

Figure 10–12

Skeletal muscle injury: Grade 2 strain. This coronal STIR MR image (TR/TE, 3700/36; inversion time, 150 msec) shows high signal intensity in the obturator externus and internus muscles and several adductor muscles about the right hip. (Courtesy of J. Kirkham, M.D., Minneapolis, Minnesota.)

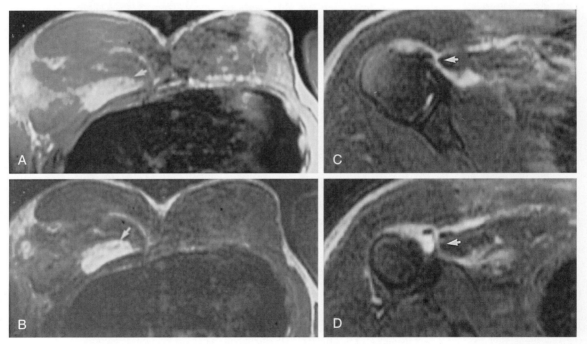

Figure 10–13

Skeletal muscle injury: Rupture and retraction. **A, B** During bench pressing, this weightlifter ruptured his right pectoralis muscle. On transaxial T1-weighted (TR/TE, 600/20) **(A)** and T2-weighted (TR/TE, 2000/80) **(B)** spin echo MR images, note distortion of muscle anatomy with localized edema and a focal hematoma (arrows) of high signal intensity in both images. (From Fleckenstein JL, Shellock FG: Top Magn Reson Imaging *3*:50, 1991.)

C, D In a 23 year old man, fat-suppressed transaxial fast spin echo (TR/TE, 3500/68) MR images, with **C** at a higher level than **D**, show avulsion (arrows) of the pectoralis muscle from the humerus. (Courtesy of R. Loredo, M.D., San Antonio, Texas.)

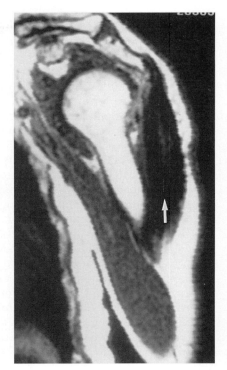

Figure 10–14
Skeletal muscle injury: Muscle contracture. After repeated injections of medication into the deltoid muscle, fibrosis and contracture of the muscle (arrow) developed, as shown in this sagittal oblique T1-weighted (TR/TE, 350/16) spin echo MR image. Note the low signal intensity of the muscle and abduction of the arm. (Courtesy of C. Chen, M.D., Kaohsiung, Taiwan.)

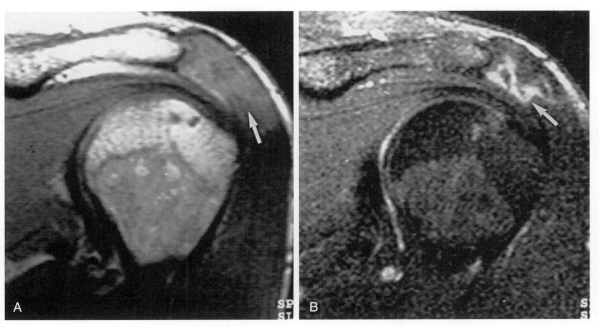

Figure 10–15
Skeletal muscle injury: Muscle inflammation. This 36 year old male pilot had multiple injections of corticosteroid medication into the deltoid muscle.

A A coronal oblique proton density-weighted (TR/TE, 1500/25) spin echo MR image shows a slight increase in signal intensity in the proximal portion of the deltoid muscle (arrow).

B After intravenous administration of a gadolinium agent, a coronal oblique T1-weighted (TR/TE, 688/15) spin echo MR image obtained with fat suppression confirms high signal intensity in this region (arrow). It is difficult to determine the extent of muscle injury and inflammation at sites of such injection.

(Courtesy of M. Lin, M.D., Hong Kong.)

and nerve ischemia develops, and the changes become irreversible. The current explanation for the development of a compartment syndrome is the theory of the arteriovenous gradient; an increase in tissue pressure reduces the local arteriovenous gradient and therefore local perfusion.[44] If perfusion is reduced to the degree that metabolic needs are not met, a compartment syndrome will result. In cases of acute compartment syndrome, pressure within the compartment never rises sufficiently to totally counter the systolic or diastolic pressure in the major artery traversing the compartment.[82]

The list of potential causes of this syndrome is impressive indeed. A decrease in the size of the compartment, which may lead to the compartment syndrome, may result from the application of a tight cast, constrictive dressings, or pneumatic antishock garments.[81] An increase in the contents of the compartment, which likewise may lead to this syndrome, may be related to hemorrhage (fractures of the tibia, femur, bones of the forearm, or those about the elbow) or to edema (postischemic swelling after arterial injury or restoration of arterial flow after arterial thrombosis).[81] Additional causes are bleeding disorders, anticoagulant therapy, excessive skeletal traction, and osteotomy. Compartment syndromes also can relate to physical exertion in athletes.[83]

The clinical manifestations of a compartment syndrome may be acute or chronic. Typical acute findings are pain out of proportion to the extent of the injury, weakness and pain on passive stretching of the extremity, hypesthesia in the distribution of the nerves traversing the compartment, and the presence of a tense, swollen compartment.[40] Pulses always are palpable in cases of acute compartment syndrome. Chronic compartment syndromes are associated with prolonged and repetitive physical exertion, and they can lead to exercise-related pain in recreational or professional athletes. Techniques allowing direct measurement of intracompartmental pressure provide evidence of elevated pressure and permit accurate diagnosis, particularly in acute cases. If not diagnosed and treated early, an acute compartment syndrome subsequently may be associated with muscle necrosis and permanent neurologic damage with fibrous contracture (e.g., Volkmann's contracture).

MR imaging findings in patients with an acute compartment syndrome include swelling of the affected extremity and abnormalities of signal intensity in the muscles of the involved compartment and, less commonly, other compartments.[40] Similar and often transient abnormalities on MR images may accompany chronic compartment syndromes. Complications such as myonecrosis may be delineated with MR imaging, and even routine radiography may reveal diagnostic findings in cases of long-standing compartment syndrome (Fig. 10–16).[84]

Although myonecrosis is a recognized complication of the ischemia that results from a compartment syndrome, it occurs in other situations as well. Infectious myonecrosis may relate to a variety of microorganisms. Additional causes of myonecrosis are vascular disease or occlusion (as in sickle cell anemia and diabetes mellitus) and coma or prolonged sleep from drug overdose, in which prolonged compression of a tissue compartment may be the responsible factor. Although gas formation in involved muscles and other soft tissues in instances

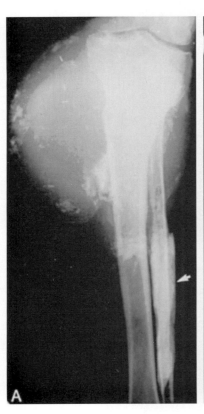
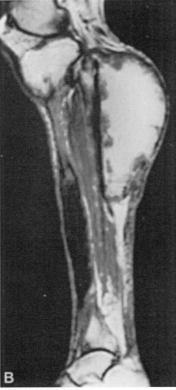

Figure 10–16
Skeletal muscle injury: Compartment syndrome and myonecrosis. In this patient, a chronic compartment syndrome in the lower leg that occurred after a tibial fracture has led to enlargement and calcification of the gastrocnemius muscle, evident with routine radiography **(A).** Also note sheetlike calcification (arrow) in the anterolateral compartment of the leg. A sagittal proton density (TR/TE, 2000/15) spin echo MR image **(B)** shows the enlarged muscle with central high signal intensity. Cystic degeneration of the gastrocnemius muscle had produced these findings. The calcification with its signal void is seen in the anterior soft tissues and periphery of the gastrocnemius muscle. (Courtesy of J. Spaeth, M.D., Albuquerque, New Mexico.)

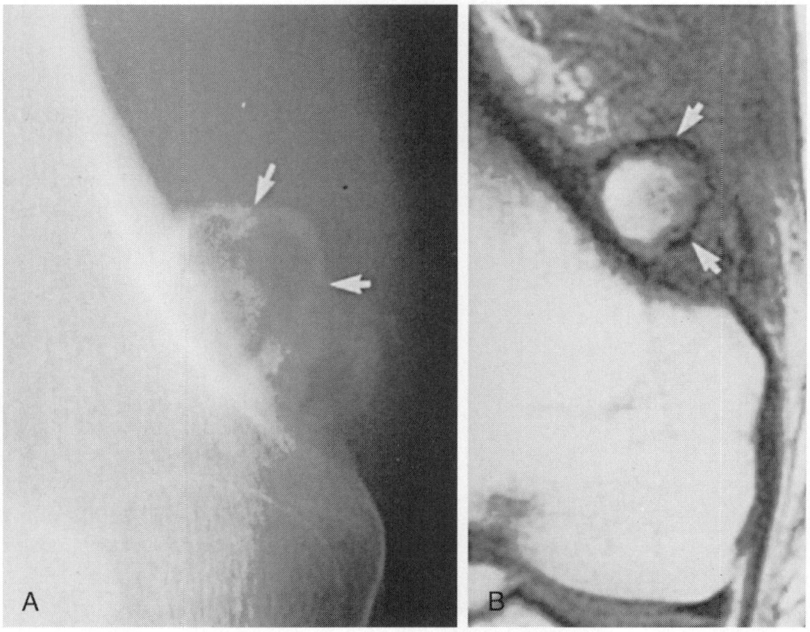

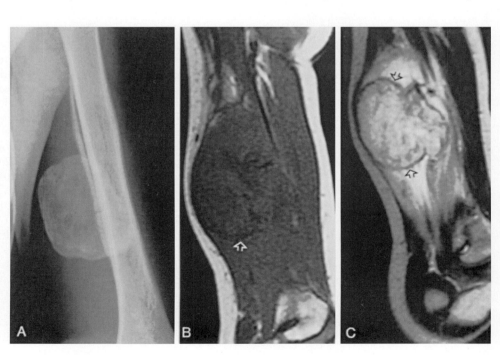

Figure 10–17

Myositis ossificans traumatica: Peripheral rim of calcification and ossification.

A A frontal radiograph shows a lesion applied to the medial cortex of the distal end of the femur. Adjacent mature periosteal reaction is seen. Note the rimlike pattern of ossification (arrows).

B A coronal T1-weighted (TR/TE, 600/20) spin echo MR image reveals low signal intensity at the margin of the lesion (arrows) and central higher signal intensity identical to that of fat or blood.

(Courtesy of M. Zlatkin, M.D., North Hollywood, Florida.)

of infective myonecrosis may be noted on routine radiographs, more subtle findings of myonecrosis are detected with bone scintigraphy, CT, and MR imaging.[85, 86]

Myositis Ossificans Traumatica

Sixty[87] to 75 per cent[88] of patients with localized soft tissue ossifications (myositis ossificans circumscripta) relate a clear history of trauma; the other patients either suffer from one of the systemic problems associated with soft tissue ossification, such as neurologic conditions, burns, and tetanus, or develop the lesions spontaneously. The spontaneous cases are termed myositis ossificans nontraumatica or pseudomalignant osseous tumor of soft tissue. The accuracy of the designation "myositis ossificans" for this lesion has been challenged on numerous occasions. Indeed, the absence of inflammation as well as muscular involvement in some cases would indicate the inappropriateness of this name.[89] It has been postulated that the soft tissue ossification results from damage to the interstitium, not to the muscle.[89, 90]

Myositis ossificans traumatica usually appears in adolescents or young adults; rarely, infants or children are affected. The sites of localization are areas susceptible to injury, such as the elbow, the thigh, the buttocks, and, less often, the shoulder and the calf. The appearance of ossification after elbow injuries or about the region

Figure 10–18

Myositis ossificans traumatica: MR imaging abnormalities. This 4 year old boy fell on his arm.

A A radiograph obtained 4 weeks later shows classic features of myositis ossificans. Note the well-defined ossific mass and mature periosteal new bone formation in the humeral diaphysis.

B A sagittal oblique T1-weighted (TR/TE, 600/14) spin echo MR image shows a poorly defined intramuscular mass with signal intensity similar to that of muscle. Some foci of very low signal intensity are seen (arrow).

C A sagittal oblique T2-weighted (TR/TE, 3000/95) fast spin echo MR image reveals high signal intensity in the mass and surrounding tissues. Note the peripheral rim of low signal intensity (arrows), representing ossification.

(Courtesy of D. Witte, M.D., Memphis, Tennessee.)

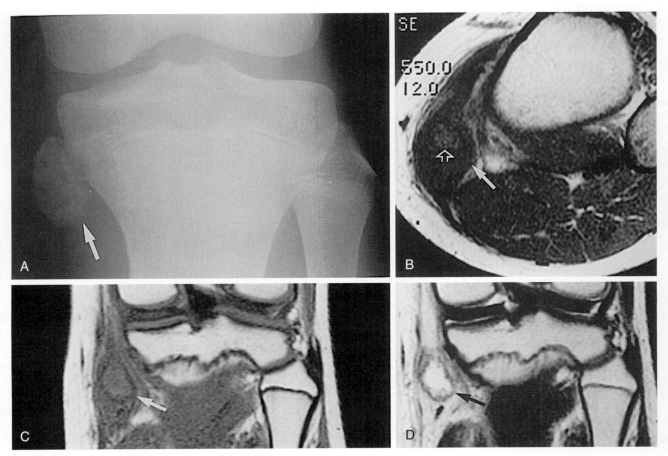

Figure 10–19

Myositis ossificans traumatica: MR imaging abnormalities. After an injury, this 13 year old boy developed a mass in the medial aspect of the knee.

A Routine radiography shows an ossified mass (arrow) with more extensive ossification occurring in its periphery.

B A transverse T1-weighted (TR/TE, 550/12) spin echo MR image demonstrates the mass (solid arrow) of low signal intensity, which contains a fluid level (open arrow).

C, D Coronal T1-weighted (TR/TE, 500/11) **(C)** and T2-weighted (TR/TE, 3000/85) **(D)** spin echo MR images show the mass (arrows). Its periphery is of low signal intensity in both **C** and **D**; centrally, low signal intensity is seen in **C** and high signal intensity in **D**. Surgery confirmed the presence of ossification in the medial head of the gastrocnemius muscle.

of the quadriceps is well recognized. In general, the frequency of myositis ossificans traumatica is greater in the proximal than the distal portion of an extremity.[91]

Shortly after injury, a soft tissue mass becomes apparent, which may be associated with periosteal reaction in 7 to 10 days. Flocculent dense lesions arise in the mass from 11 days to 6 weeks after the trauma. The calcific dense areas gradually enlarge, and at 6 to 8 weeks a lacy pattern of new bone is sharply circumscribed about the periphery of the mass.[87] An enlarging central cavity combined with peripheral calcification and ossification resembles an eggshell. Maturity is reached in 5 to 6 months, and the mass then shrinks.

The recognition of a peripheral rim of calcification and ossification about a more lucent center cannot be overemphasized as an important radiographic manifestation of myositis ossificans (Fig. 10–17). Although other diagnostic techniques, such as arteriography,[92] ultrasonography,[93–95] scintigraphy,[96–98] and CT,[99–102] occasionally may aid in the evaluation of this condition, they usually are not required for correct diagnosis but may be helpful in identifying the maturity of the lesion. MR imaging

also has been employed to study myositis ossificans.[103–108] The MR imaging appearance of the ossifying lesions varies according to the stage of development and, in some cases, may simulate that of a soft tissue neoplasm.[107] Less diagnostic difficulty is encountered in chronic lesions (see Fig. 10–17), which tend to be well defined, possess a border of low signal intensity, and contain fat (with its characteristic signal intensity), although occasional chronic lesions reveal regions of high signal intensity on T2-weighted images.[105] In acute or subacute stages of myositis ossificans, signal intensity inhomogeneity may be evident; high signal intensity on T2-weighted images may be seen (Figs. 10–18 to 10–20), particularly centrally in a proliferating core of fibroblasts and myofibroblasts.[104] In these early stages, enhancement of signal intensity in the rim of the lesion following intravenous administration of a gadolinium contrast agent may lead to an appearance simulating that of an abscess or necrotic tumor.[107] Fluid levels also may be apparent (see Fig. 10–19). When results of routine radiography or of other imaging methods are not diagnostic, histologic documentation may be necessary to establish a

Figure 10–20

Myositis ossificans traumatica: MR imaging abnormalities. A mass in the vastus lateralis muscle with associated edema is evident in a coronal fat-suppressed fast spin echo (TR/TE, 4000/108) MR image **(A)**. Enhancement of signal intensity in a portion of the mass occurred after intravenous gadolinium administration, as shown in a coronal T1-weighted (TR/TE, 300/17) spin echo MR image **(B)**. (Courtesy of P. Kindynis, M.D., Geneva, Switzerland.)

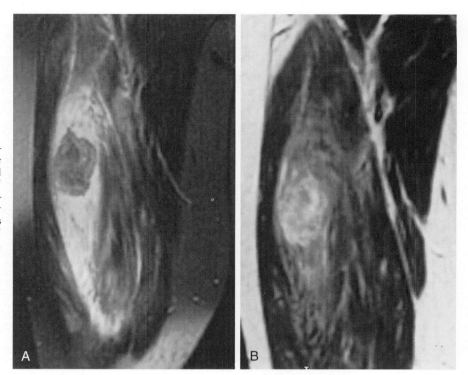

definite diagnosis; however, the pathologist must be wary of the "pseudomalignant" nature of the central portion of the lesion.

SUMMARY

Injuries to muscles and tendons are encountered commonly, especially in athletes. Clinical assessment generally is adequate for accurate diagnosis, although characteristic findings are detected when MR imaging is applied to assessment of these injuries. An overview of anatomic and pathophysiologic principles fundamental to interpretation of the MR images is provided in this chapter.

REFERENCES

1. Best TM, Garrett WE Jr: Muscle and tendon. *In* JC DeLee, D Drez Jr (Eds): Orthopaedic Sports Medicine: Principles and Practice. Philadelphia, WB Saunders, 1994, p 1.
2. Edwards DAW: The blood supply and lymphatic drainage of tendons. J Anat *80:*147, 1946.
3. Cooper RR, Misol S: Tendon and ligament insertion. J Bone Joint Surg [Am] *52:*1, 1970.
4. Canoso JJ: Bursae, tendons, and ligaments. Clin Rheum Dis *7:*189, 1981.
5. Lundborg G, Rank F: Experimental intrinsic healing of flexor tendons based upon synovial fluid nutrition. J Hand Surg *3:*21, 1978.
6. Cruess RL, Dumont J: Healing of bone, tendon and ligament. *In* CA Rockwood Jr, DP Green (Eds): Fractures. Philadelphia, JB Lippincott, 1975, p 97.
7. Welsh RP, MacNab I, Riley V: Biomechanical studies of rabbit tendon. Clin Orthop *81:*171, 1971.
8. Rogers LF: Radiology of Skeletal Trauma. 2nd Ed. New York, Churchill Livingstone, 1992.
9. Peacock EE: Biological principles in the healing of long tendons. Surg Clin North Am *45:*461, 1965.
10. Peacock EE: A study of the circulation in normal tendons and healing grafts. Ann Surg *149:*415, 1959.
11. Minns RJ, Stevens FS: Local denaturation of collagen fibers during the mechanical rupture of collagenous fibrous tissue. Ann Rheum Dis *39:*164, 1980.
12. Reveno PM, Kittleson AC: Spontaneous Achilles tendon rupture. Radiology *93:*1341, 1969.
13. Margles SW, Lewis MM: Bilateral spontaneous concurrent rupture of the patellar tendon without apparent associated systemic disease: A case report. Clin Orthop *136:*186, 1978.
14. Newberg A, Wales L: Radiographic diagnosis of quadriceps tendon rupture. Radiology *125:*367, 1977.
15. Kamali M: Bilateral traumatic rupture of the infrapatellar tendon. Clin Orthop *142:*131, 1979.
16. Donati RB, Cox S, Echo BS, et al: Bilateral simultaneous patellar tendon rupture in a female collegiate gymnast: A case report. Am J Sports Med *14:*237, 1986.
17. Andersen E: Triceps tendon avulsion. Injury *17:*279, 1986.
18. Stern RE, Harwin SF: Spontaneous and simultaneous rupture of both quadriceps tendons. Clin Orthop *147:*188, 1980.
19. Herring S, Nilson K: Introduction to overuse injuries. Clin Sports Med *6:*225, 1987.
20. Nirschl RP: Rotator cuff tendinitis: Basic concepts of pathoetiology. Instr Course Lect 38, 1989.
21. Tehranzadeh J, Serafini AN, Pais MJ: Avulsion and Stress Injuries of the Musculoskeletal System. Basel, Karger Press, 1989.
22. Tehranzadeh J: The spectrum of avulsion and avulsion-like injuries of the musculoskeletal system. Radiographics *7:*945, 1987.
23. Farrar EL III, Lippert FG III: Avulsion of the triceps tendon. Clin Orthop *161:*242, 1981.
24. Tiger E, Mayer DP, Glazer R: Complete avulsion of the triceps tendon: MRI diagnosis. Computer Med Imaging Graphics *17:*51, 1993.
25. Metzmaker JN, Pappas AM: Avulsion fractures of the pelvis. Am J Sports Med *13:*349, 1985.
26. Fernbach SK, Wilkinson RH: Avulsion injuries of the pelvis and proximal femur. AJR *137:*581, 1984.
27. Vazelle F, Rochcongar P, Lejeune JJ, et al: Le syndrome d'algie pubienne du sportif (pubialgie). J Radiol *63:*423, 1982.
28. Tehranzadeh J, Kurth LA, Elyaderani MK, et al: Combined pelvic stress fracture and avulsion of the adductor longus in a middle-distance runner: A case report. Am J Sports Med *10:*108, 1982.
29. Schneider R, Kaye JJ, Ghelman B: Adductor avulsive injuries near the symphysis pubis. Radiology *120:*567, 1976.
30. Sundar M, Carty H: Avulsion fractures of the pelvis in children: A report of 32 fractures and their outcome. Skel Radiol *23:*85, 1994.
31. Stayton CA: Ischial epiphysiolysis. AJR *76:*1161, 1956.
32. Symeonides P: Isolated traumatic rupture of the adductor longus muscle of the thigh. Clin Orthop *88:*64, 1972.
33. Ellis R, Greene A: Ischial apophyseolysis. Radiology *87:*646, 1966.
34. Lombardo SJ, Retting AC, Kerlan RK: Radiographic abnormalities of the iliac apophysis in adolescent athletes. J Bone Joint Surg [Am] *65:*444, 1983.
35. Houghton GR, Ackroyd CE: Sleeve fracture of the patella in children. J Bone Joint Surg [Br] *61:*165, 1979.
36. Bishay M: Sleeve fracture of upper pole of patella. J Bone Joint Surg [Br] *73:*339, 1991.
37. Grogan DP, Carey TP, Leffers D, et al: Avulsion fractures of the patella. J Pediatr Orthop *10:*721, 1990.

38. Lepse PS, McCarthy RE, McCullough FL: Simultaneous bilateral avulsion fracture of the tibial tuberosity: A case report. Clin Orthop 229:232, 1987.

39. Frankl U, Waisilewski SA, Healy WL: Avulsion fracture of the tibial tubercle with avulsion of the patellar ligament: Report of two cases. J Bone Joint Surg [Am] 72:1411, 1990.

40. Mink JH: Muscle injuries. In AL Deutsch, JH Mink, R Kerr (Eds): MRI of the Foot and Ankle. New York, Raven Press, 1992, p 281.

41. Gross RH: Acute musculotendinous injuries. In CL Stanitski, JC DeLee, D Drez Jr (Eds): Pediatric and Adolescent Sports Medicine. Philadelphia, WB Saunders, 1994, p 131.

42. Warwick R, Williams PL: Gray's Anatomy. 35th British Ed. Philadelphia, WB Saunders Co, 1973, p 474.

43. Best TM: Muscle-tendon injuries in young athletes. Clin Sports Med 14:669, 1995.

44. Nerlich ML, Tscherne H: Biology of soft tissue injuries. In BD Browner, JB Jupiter, AM Levine, et al (Eds): Skeletal Trauma: Fractures, Dislocations, Ligamentous Injuries. Philadelphia, WB Saunders Co, 1992, p 77.

45. Letho M, Alanen A: Healing of muscle trauma: Correlation of sonographical and histological findings in an experimental study in rats. J Ultrasound Med 6:425, 1987.

46. Fleckenstein JL, Canby RC, Parkey RW, et al: Acute effects of exercise on MR imaging of skeletal muscle in normal volunteers. AJR 151:231, 1988.

47. Fleckenstein JL, Weatherall PT, Parkey RW, et al: Sports-related muscle injuries: Evaluation with MR imaging. Radiology 172:793, 1989.

48. Shellock FG, Fukunaga T, Mink JH, et al: Exertional muscle injury: Evaluation of concentric versus eccentric actions with serial MR imaging. Radiology 179:659, 1991.

49. Shellock FG, Fukunaga T, Mink JH, et al: Acute effects of exercise on MR imaging of skeletal muscle: Concentric vs eccentric actions. AJR 156:765, 1991.

50. Nurenberg P, Giddings CJ, Stray-Gundersen J, et al: MR imaging–guided muscle biopsy for correlation of increased signal intensity with ultrastructural change and delayed-onset muscle soreness after exercise. Radiology 184:865, 1992.

51. Fleckenstein JL, Shellock FG: Exertional muscle injuries: Magnetic resonance imaging evaluation. Top Magn Res Imaging 3:50, 1991.

52. Drace JE, Pelc NJ: Measurement of skeletal muscle motion in vivo with phase-contrast MR imaging. JMRI 4:157, 1994.

53. Drace JE, Pelc NJ: Skeletal muscle contraction: Analysis with use of velocity distributions from phase-contrast MR imaging. Radiology 193:423, 1994.

54. El-Khoury GY, Brandser EA, Kathol MH, et al: Imaging of muscle injuries. Skeletal Radiol 25:3, 1996.

55. Rubin SJ, Feldman F, Staron RB, et al: Magnetic resonance imaging of muscle injury. Clinical Imag 19:263, 1995.

56. Steinbach LS, Fleckenstein JL, Mink JH: Magnetic resonance imaging of muscle injuries. Orthopedics 17:991, 1994.

57. Weatherall PT, Cruess JV III: Musculotendinous injury. MRI Clin North Am 3:753, 1995.

58. Durig M, Schuppisser JP, Gauer EF, et al: Spontaneous rupture of the gastrocnemius muscle. Injury 9:143, 1977.

59. Miller WA: Rupture of the musculotendinous junction of the medial head of the gastrocnemius muscle. Am J Sports Med 5:191, 1977.

60. Rask MR, Lattig GJ: Traumatic fibrosis of the rectus femoris muscle. JAMA 221:368, 1972.

61. Bach BR, Warren RF, Wickiewicz TL: Triceps rupture: A case report and literature review. Am J Sports Med 15:285, 1987.

62. Peterson L, Stener B: Old rupture of the adductor longus muscle. Acta Orthop Scand 47:653, 1976.

63. De Smet AA: Magnetic resonance findings in skeletal muscle tears. Skel Radiol 22:479, 1993.

64. Yoshioka H, Anno I, Niitsu M, et al: MRI of muscle strain injuries. J Comput Assist Tomogr 18:454, 1994.

65. MacIntyre DL, Reid WD, McKenzie DC: Delayed muscle soreness. The inflammatory response to muscle injury and its clinical implications. Sports Med 20:24, 1995.

66. Wolfort FG, Mogelvang LC, Filtzer HS: Anterior tibial compartment syndrome following muscle hernia repair. Arch Surg 106:97, 1993.

67. Zeiss J, Ebraheim NA, Woldenberg LS: Magnetic resonance imaging in the diagnosis of anterior tibialis muscle herniation. Clin Orthop 244:249, 1989.

68. Chiu SS, Furuya K, Arai T, et al: Congenital contracture of the quadriceps muscle: Four case reports in identical twins. J Bone Joint Surg [Am] 56:1054, 1974.

69. Lloyd-Roberts GC, Thomas TG: The etiology of quadriceps contracture in children. J Bone Joint Surg [Br] 46:498, 1964.

70. Shen Y-S: Abduction contracture of the hip in children. J Bone Joint Surg [Br] 57:463, 1975.

71. Matsusue Y, Yamamuro T, Ohta H, et al: Fibrotic contracture of the gastrocnemius muscle: A case report. J Bone Joint Surg [Am] 76:739, 1994.

72. Peiro A, Fernandez CI, Gomar E: Gluteal fibrosis. J Bone Joint Surg [Am] 57:987, 1975.

73. Euliano JJ: Fibrosis of the quadriceps mechanism in children. Clin Orthop 70:181, 1970.

74. Gabow PA, Kaehy WD, Kelleher SP: The spectrum of rhabdomyolysis. Medicine 61:141, 1982.

75. Barloon TJ, Zachar CK, Harkens KL, et al: Rhabdomyolysis: Computed tomography findings. CT 12:193, 1988.

76. Kaplan GN: Ultrasonic appearance of rhabdomyolysis. AJR 134:375, 1980.

77. Mangano FA, Zaontz M, Pahira JJ, et al: Computed tomography of acute renal failure secondary to rhabdomyolysis. J Comput Assist Tomogr 9:777, 1985.

78. Messing ML, Feinzimer ET, Brosman JJ, et al: CT of rhabdomyolysis associated with malignant hyperthermia and seizures. Clin Imaging 17:258, 1993.

79. Ludmer LM, Chandeysson P, Barth WF: Diphosphonate bone scan in an unusual case of rhabdomyolysis: A report and literature review. J Rheumatol 20:382, 1993.

80. Lamminen AE, Hekali PE, Tiula E, et al: Acute rhabdomyolysis: Evaluation with magnetic resonance imaging compared with computed tomography and ultrasonography. Br J Radiol 62:326, 1989.

81. Rorabeck CH: Compartment syndromes. In BD Browner, JB Jupiter, AM Levine, et al (Eds): Skeletal Trauma: Fractures, Dislocations, Ligamentous Injuries. Philadelphia, WB Saunders Co, 1992, p 285.

82. Rorabeck CH: The treatment of compartment syndromes in the leg. J Bone Joint Surg [Br] 66:93, 1984.

83. Hutchinson MR, Ireland ML: Common compartment syndromes in athletes: Treatment and rehabilitation. Sports Med 17:200, 1994.

84. Hyder N, Shaw DL, Bollen SR: Myositis ossificans: Calcification of the entire tibialis anterior after ischaemic injury (compartment syndrome). J Bone Joint Surg [Br] 78:318, 1996.

85. Farmlett EJ, Fishman EK, Magid D, et al: Computed tomography in the assessment of myonecrosis. J Can Assoc Radiol 38:278, 1987.

86. Timmons JH, Hartshorne MF, Peters VJ, et al: Muscle necrosis in the extremities: Evaluation with Tc-99m pyrophosphate scanning—a retrospective review. Radiology 167:173, 1988.

87. Norman A, Dorfman HD: Juxtacortical circumscribed myositis ossificans: Evolution and radiographic features. Radiology 96:301, 1970.

88. Paterson DC: Myositis ossificans circumscripta: Report of four cases without history of injury. J Bone Joint Surg [Br] 52:296, 1970.

89. Ackerman LV: Extra-osseous localized non-neoplastic bone and cartilage formation (so-called myositis ossificans): Clinical and pathological confusion with malignant neoplasms. J Bone Joint Surg [Am] 40:279, 1958.

90. Adams RD, Denny-Brown D, Pearson CM: Diseases of Muscle: A Study in Pathology. 2nd Ed. New York, Harper & Row, 1962.

91. Puzas JE, Miller MD, Rosier RN: Pathologic bone formation. Clin Orthop 245:269, 1989.

92. Yaghmai I: Myositis ossificans: Diagnostic value of arteriography. AJR 128:811, 1977.

93. Kramer FL, Kurtz AB, Rubin C, Goldberg BB: Ultrasound appearance of myositis ossificans. Skel Radiol 4:19, 1979.

94. Kirkpatrick JS, Koman LA, Rovere GD: The role of ultrasound in the early diagnosis of myositis ossificans: A case report. Amer J Sports Med 15:179, 1987.

95. Peck RJ, Metreweli C: Early myositis ossificans: A new echographic sign. Clin Radiol 39:586, 1988.

96. Drane WE: Myositis ossificans and the three-phase bone scan. AJR 142:179, 1984.

97. Orzel JA, Rudd TG: Heterotopic bone formation: Clinical, laboratory, and imaging correlation. J Nucl Med 26:125, 1985.

98. Moreno AJ, Yedinak MA, Spicer MJ, et al: Myositis ossificans with Ga-67 citrate positivity. Clin Nucl Med 10:40, 1985.

99. Amendola MA, Glazer GM, Agha FP, et al: Myositis ossificans circumscripta: Computed tomographic diagnosis. Radiology 149:775, 1983.

100. Zeanah WR, Hudson TM: Myositis ossificans: Radiologic evaluation of two cases with diagnostic computed tomograms. Clin Orthop 168:187, 1982.

101. Bressler EL, Marn CS, Gore RM, et al: Evaluation of ectopic bone by CT. AJR 148:931, 1987.

102. Laurin NR, Powe JE, Pavlosky WF, et al: Multimodality imaging of early heterotopic bone formation. J Can Assoc Radiol 41:93, 1990.

103. Ehara S, Nakasato T, Tamakawa Y, et al: MRI of myositis ossificans circumscripta. Clin Imaging 15:130, 1991.

104. Kransdorf MJ, Meis JM, Jelinek JS: Myositis ossificans: MR appearance with radiologic-pathologic correlation. AJR 157:1243, 1991.

105. DeSmet AA, Norris MA, Fisher DR: Magnetic resonance imaging of myositis ossificans: Analysis of seven cases. Skel Radiol 21:503, 1992.

106. Cvitanic O, Sedlak J: Acute myositis ossificans. Skel Radiol 24:139, 1995.

107. Shirkhoda A, Armin A-R, Bis KG, et al: MR imaging of myositis ossificans: Variable patterns at different stages. J Magn Res Imaging 5:287, 1995.

108. Bouchardy L, Garcia J: Apport de l'imagerie par resonance magnetique (IRM) dans le diagnostic de la myosite ossifiante circonscrite (MOC). J Radiol 75:101, 1994.

11 | *Entrapment Neuropathies*

Peripheral nerve entrapment syndromes involve the compression of a short segment of a single nerve at a specific site, frequently as a result of the vulnerability of that nerve as it passes through a fibro-osseous tunnel or an opening in fibrous or muscular tissue. The clinical manifestations of entrapment neuropathies vary with the specific site or sites of involvement. In addition, in some cases the manifestations are persistent and in others they occur only with certain maneuvers of the extremity. The latter situation often is referred to as dynamic compression neuropathy.[1] One example of this is the occurrence of the carpal tunnel syndrome when the wrist is placed in an extended or flexed position and the absence of nerve compression when the wrist is in a neutral position. Various provocative clinical tests have been described during which gentle pressure on the nerve at the site of entrapment is accompanied by paresthesias in the distribution of that nerve. These provocative tests, when applied carefully and combined with data derived from the clinical history and routine physical examination, aid in the assessment of entrapment neuropathies. Imaging studies, particularly MR imaging, provide supplementary information in some cases that delineate a specific and sometimes treatable cause of the compression neuropathy.[2] In this chapter, the MR imaging findings in a number of entrapment neuropathies (Table 11–1) are reviewed.

MEDIAN NERVE

Entrapment of the median nerve occurs most frequently in the wrist as the carpal tunnel syndrome, but it also may develop in the region of the distal portion of the humerus or proximal portion of the forearm.[3–5]

Ligament of Struthers

In approximately 1 per cent of limbs, the ligament of Struthers connects an anomalous bony excrescence (the supracondylar process), arising from the anterior sur-

face of the distal portion of the humerus, to the medial epicondyle of the humerus. Although a supracondylar process usually is an incidental finding on radiographs and is unassociated with symptoms and signs, compromise of the median nerve is a possible complication, especially in patients who have had trauma to the area.[4]

Pronator Syndrome

An entrapment neuropathy of the median nerve can occur in the antecubital area where the nerve passes between the two heads of the pronator teres muscle and then under the edge of the flexor digitorum sublimis muscle (Fig. 11–1). Clinical manifestations include an aching pain in the forearm, often initiated by repetitive movements of the elbow, as occurs in weightlifting, tennis, needlework, and writing.[6] The anatomic basis of this syndrome includes hypertrophy of the pronator muscle, trapping by the lacertus fibrosus (bicipital aponeurosis) from the biceps tendon, or an aberrant median artery or a fibrous component of the flexor carpi radialis muscle originating from the ulna.[2, 3, 7, 8]

Anterior Interosseous Nerve Syndrome (Kiloh-Nevin Syndrome)

The anterior interosseous nerve is the largest branch of the median nerve and is purely motor, supplying the flexor pollicis longus, the pronator quadratus, and the radial part of the flexor digitorum profundus muscles.[3] Its compression leads to weakness of the thumb and index finger and occurs on an idiopathic basis, after radial or supracondylar humeral fractures, in association with thrombosed vessels or enlarged bursae or, most commonly, as a result of aberrant fibrous bands.[9] Such entrapment also is seen sporadically in athletes owing to muscle contractures associated with aggressive forearm exercises. A variation of this syndrome related to isolated compression of the nerve branch to the flexor pollicis longus muscle is seen in baseball pitchers, weightlifters, gymnasts, tennis players, and swimmers.[5]

Table 11–1. SOME NERVE ENTRAPMENT SYNDROMES

Nerve	Site (Syndrome)	Causes or Findings
Median	Distal end of humerus	Supracondylar spur, ligament of Struthers
	Elbow (pronator syndrome)	Abnormality of pronator teres, flexor digitorum sublimis, or biceps
	Elbow (anterior interosseous nerve syndrome, Kiloh-Nevin syndrome)	Fracture of humerus or radius, fibrous band, or idiopathic
	Wrist (carpal tunnel syndrome)	Systemic and local factors or idiopathic
	Wrist (sublimis syndrome, pseudo-carpal tunnel syndrome)	Sublimis muscle belly
Ulnar	Elbow (cubital tunnel syndrome, tardy ulnar palsy)	Fracture, arthritis, cubitus valgus, trochlear hypoplasia
	Wrist (ulnar tunnel syndrome, Guyon's canal syndrome)	Fracture, ganglion, arthritis, ulnar artery abnormalities
Radial	Axilla (Saturday night palsy, sleep palsy)	Alcoholism, drug addiction, prolonged sleep with abnormal position of arm
	Distal end of humerus	Fracture involving spiral groove
	Elbow (posterior interosseous nerve syndrome)	Fracture, dislocation, rheumatoid arthritis, tumor, fibrous band
Suprascapular	Shoulder	Scapular fracture, glenohumeral joint dislocation, ganglion, tumor
Plantar and interdigital	Foot (Morton's metatarsalgia)	Digital nerve compression and ischemia, digital neuroma
Posterior tibial	Ankle (tarsal tunnel syndrome)	Sprain, fracture, arthritis, tumor, ganglion, venous tortuosity
Common peroneal	Knee	Sprain, fracture, use of casts, surgery, ganglion, fabella, popliteal cyst
Lateral femoral cutaneous	Anterior superior iliac spine (meralgia paresthetica)	Trauma, pelvic fracture, pelvic tilt
Femoral	Inguinal region	Trauma, tumor, abscess, aneurysm, bleeding
Obturator	Obturator canal	Hernia, inflammation
Sciatic	Sciatic foramen (including piriformis syndrome)	Hip surgery, gluteal injection, tumor
	Knee	Popliteal cyst
Brachial plexus	Neck and shoulder (thoracic outlet syndrome, scalenus anticus syndrome)	Fracture, dislocation, tumor, infection, surgery, injection, cervical rib

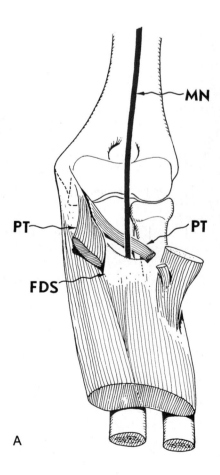

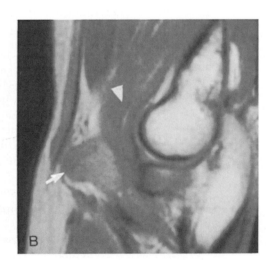

Figure 11–1

Entrapment of the median nerve: Pronator syndrome.

A The median nerve (MN) normally passes between the two heads of the pronator teres muscle (PT) and then under the edge of the flexor digitorum sublimis muscle (FDS). It may be compromised in this region. (Reprinted by permission of the New England Journal of Medicine. From Thompson WAL, Kopell HP: N Engl J Med 260:1261. Copyright 1959, Massachusetts Medical Society.)

B In this 42 year old woman with signs of compression of the median nerve, a sagittal proton density (TR/TE, 1800/20) spin echo MR image reveals a ganglion (arrow) arising from the proximal radioulnar joint located, in part, in front of the brachialis muscle (arrowhead). (Courtesy of S. K. Brahme, M.D., La Jolla, California.)

Carpal Tunnel Syndrome

The most frequent entrapment syndrome of the median nerve occurs where the nerve passes through the narrow fibro-osseous tunnel that exists between the carpal bones and a roof consisting of the inelastic transverse carpal ligament. Although specific radiologic projections, such as the carpal tunnel view, allow analysis of the osseous components of this passageway, delineation of the fibrous roof and the structures within the canal requires ultrasonography, CT, or MR imaging.[10–19]

Causes of the carpal tunnel syndrome are many (Fig. 11–2; Table 11–2). Many of the cases occur on an idiopathic basis, however. Most patients are between the ages of 35 and 65 years. Although bilateral involvement is common, the dominant hand usually is involved first and more severely. Aggravating factors include occupations or sporting activities that require a great deal of repetitive hand and wrist motion, pregnancy, and use of oral contraceptive agents. In athletes, repetitive flexion and extension of the wrist, as seen in lacrosse and gymnastics, and grip-intensive activities, such as cycling, are known to aggravate the condition.[5] In weightlifters, hypertrophy of the lumbrical muscles also may cause the carpal tunnel syndrome. Clinical findings include sensory and motor deficits with numbness and paresthesias of the thumb, index, middle, and one half of the ring finger and atrophy and weakness of the thenar

Table 11–2. SOME CAUSES OF THE CARPAL TUNNEL SYNDROME

Synovitis	**Anatomic Factors**
Rheumatoid arthritis	Small carpal canal
Scleroderma	Thick transverse carpal
Systemic lupus erythematosus	ligament
Dermatomyositis	Anomalous nerves, muscles,
Seronegative spondyloarthropathies	bursae
Granulomatous and	**Medical and Surgical**
nongranulomatous infections	**Procedures**
Hemophilia	Arteriovenous fistulae
Crystal deposition diseases	Artery punctures,
Infiltrative Diseases	catheterizations
Amyloidosis	**Miscellaneous**
Myxedema	Diabetes mellitus
Acromegaly	Polymyalgia rheumatica
Mucopolysaccharidoses	Hemorrhage
Trauma	Hypoparathyroidism
Fractures and dislocations	Pregnancy
Repetitive and prolonged stress	Use of oral contraceptives
Tumors and Tumor-Like Lesions	Gynecologic surgery
Neuromas	Osteoarthritis
Lipomas	Pyridoxine deficiency
Synovial cysts	Paget's disease
Ganglia	Idiopathic
Multiple myeloma	

muscles.[20] Physical examination documents a positive Tinel's sign (paresthesias after percussion of the nerve in the volar aspect of the wrist) and reproduction of pain and paresthesias with the Phalen maneuver, accom-

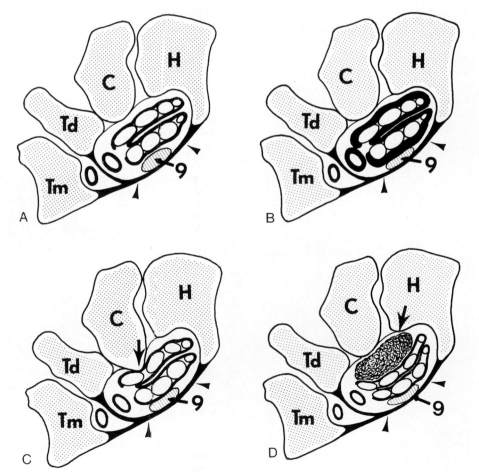

Figure 11–2
Entrapment of the median nerve: Carpal tunnel syndrome—potential causes.
  A Normal. The median nerve (9) and transverse carpal ligament (arrowheads) are indicated. H, Hamate; C, capitate; Td, trapezoid; Tm, trapezium.
  B Tenosynovitis.
  C Osseous spur (arrow).
  D Mass (arrow).
  (From Lipscomb TR: J Musculoskel Med *1*(8):35, 1984. Original artwork by Robert Margulies.)

plished by flexing the patient's hand at the wrist for longer than 1 minute. Nerve conduction tests reveal typical motor or sensory impairment, or both.

The analysis of carpal tunnel syndrome using MR imaging deserves emphasis. Proper interpretation of MR images requires knowledge of the osseous and soft tissue components of the carpal tunnel. This tunnel represents a narrow channel approximately 6 cm long extending from the wrist to the midportion of the palm, through which pass the nine extrinsic finger flexor tendons and the median nerve. The dorsal portion of the carpal tunnel is formed by a concave arch of carpal bones covered by the intrinsic and extrinsic wrist ligaments; the volar portion of the canal is formed by the transverse carpal ligament.[20] This ligament, which is 2.5 to 3.5 mm thick and 3 to 4 cm wide, is attached to the tuberosity of the scaphoid and the crest of the trapezium on the radial side and to the pisiform and the hook of the hamate on the ulnar side.[20] The median nerve normally becomes superficial to the flexor digitorum superficialis muscle bellies approximately 5 cm proximal to the transverse carpal ligament and ordinarily lies superficial in the carpal tunnel and volar to the flexor digitorum superficialis tendons of the index and long fingers.[20] In the palm, the median nerve divides into five branches. The first, and most radial, is the motor branch that supplies the thenar muscles; the remaining four branches supply sensation to the thumb, index, and middle fingers and the radial half of the ring finger.

The narrowest part of the carpal canal is located 2 to 4 cm distal to the wrist crease.[21] At this site, which corresponds to the palmar oriented prominence of the capitate bone, the width of the carpal canal is approximately 10 mm. Variations occur in the carpal canal width and area in asymptomatic men and women, however, although the cross-sectional area and width tend to be decreased in patients with the carpal tunnel syndrome, findings that may be more prominent in the proximal portion of the canal.[22] Compression of the median nerve in the carpal tunnel occurs when too little space or too much tissue, or both, exists within the tunnel. Patients with the carpal tunnel syndrome have elevated intracarpal tunnel pressure, which increases further with flexion or extension of the wrist.

In 1989, Mesgarzadeh and coworkers[14, 15] provided a detailed description of MR imaging findings of the carpal tunnel in normal persons and in those with the carpal tunnel syndrome. The MR imaging appearance of the structures in the normal carpal tunnel in the neutral position and with flexion and extension of the wrist was further delineated by Zeiss and associates[16] in the same year. Both studies emphasized the value of the transaxial plane in the assessment of the median nerve, although supplementary data were provided by coronal and sagittal imaging. In the neutral position, the normal median nerve typically is situated in one of two standard positions: either anterior to the superficial flexor tendon of the index finger or interposed more posterolaterally between this tendon and the flexor pollicis longus tendon.[16] During wrist extension, the nerve always maintains or assumes an anterior position between the superficial index finger flexor and the flexor retinaculum, while the flexor tendons move posteriorly; during wrist flexion, the tendons shift anteriorly toward the retinaculum, and the median nerve either remains in its anterior position between the superficial index finger flexor and retinaculum or becomes interposed between the superficial flexor tendons of the index finger and thumb or middle and ring fingers.[16, 17] When positioned anteriorly, the median nerve may appear flattened in an anteroposterior plane between the tendon and the flexor retinaculum, a finding that is most evident in wrist flexion and least evident in wrist extension; interposed median nerves may be either round or flattened in a mediolateral plane.[16] In general, however, the size of the normal median nerve is fairly constant within the carpal tunnel, although it may appear slightly smaller at the level of the pisiform bone.[14]

As defined by Mesgarzadeh and colleagues,[15] four general findings characterize the MR imaging appear-

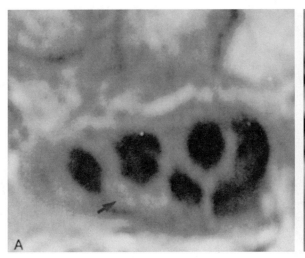
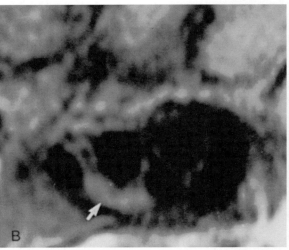

Figure 11–3
Entrapment of the median nerve: Carpal tunnel syndrome. Transverse proton density (TR/TE, 1800/20) **(A)** and T2-weighted (TR/TE, 1800/70) **(B)** spin echo MR images at the level of the metacarpal bases reveal enlargement and flattening of the median nerve (arrows) with subtle increased signal intensity in **B**. (Courtesy of C. Sebrechts, M.D., San Diego, California.)

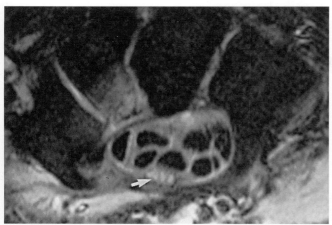

Figure 11–4

Entrapment of the median nerve: Carpal tunnel syndrome. A transverse multiplanar gradient recalled (MPGR) MR image (TR/TE, 733/15; flip angle, 30 degrees) obtained with fat suppression shows that the median nerve (arrow) at the level of the hook of the hamate has a slightly increased signal intensity and that tenosynovitis is present. (Courtesy of S. Eilenberg, M.D., San Diego, California.)

ance of the carpal tunnel syndrome: swelling of the medial nerve, best evaluated at the level of the pisiform bone; flattening of the median nerve, judged most reliably at the level of the hamate bone; palmar bowing of the flexor retinaculum, best visualized at the level of the hamate bone; and increased signal intensity of the median nerve on T2-weighted spin echo MR images (Fig. 11–3) or on certain gradient echo images (Fig. 11–4). Additional MR imaging findings of the carpal tunnel syndrome that were noted in this investigation were cause-specific and included evidence of tenosynovitis, synovial hypertrophy in rheumatoid arthritis, ganglion cysts (Fig. 11–5), a persistent median artery, an increased amount of fatty tissue, and a large adductor pollicis muscle. Other investigators have confirmed the general and cause-specific MR imaging abnormalities of the carpal tunnel syndrome (Fig. 11–6),[18, 23] although the alterations may be subtle and changes in size and configuration of the median nerve may require quantitative assessment. Furthermore, the clinical impact of

MR imaging in cases of carpal tunnel syndrome needs additional study.[24]

Supplementary techniques may aid in the diagnosis of the carpal tunnel syndrome by MR imaging. These techniques include assessment of the carpal tunnel during flexion and extension of the wrist,[25] imaging with or without the intravenous injection of a gadolinium compound,[19] and MR imaging after provocative movement of the wrist. MR imaging after exercise of the wrist may accentuate bowing of the flexor retinaculum, abnormalities in size of the median nerve, and abnormal fluid collections in adjacent tendon sheaths.

Incision of the flexor retinaculum, the carpal tunnel release, commonly is used to treat carpal tunnel syndrome. This can be accomplished with open surgery or endoscopic control.[26] It is an operation not without complications, including residual or recurrent compression of the median nerve, although the reported frequency of such complications has varied.[27, 28] These complications may reflect the presence of fibrous fixation of the nerve leading to traction neuropathy or of congenital variation or anomalies of the median nerve, tendons, and adjacent muscles.[29] The role of MR imaging in the assessment of postoperative residual or recurrent carpal tunnel syndrome is not clear, although reports indicate that the technique may outline incomplete incision of the flexor retinaculum, persistent neuritis of the median nerve, excessive fat within the carpal tunnel, and the development of neuromas (Fig. 11–7).[15, 30] After carpal tunnel release, a change in shape and an increase in volume of the carpal tunnel occur, which must be taken into account when assessing postoperative MR images. Furthermore, volar descent of the contents of the carpal tunnel and soft tissue scarring may be observed after carpal tunnel release. The diagnostic benefit of supplementary MR imaging techniques, including dynamic studies and the intravenous administration of gadolinium contrast agent, in the postoperative period is not defined.

ULNAR NERVE

Entrapment of the ulnar nerve occurs most commonly near the elbow or wrist[31] and rarely in the forearm.[32]

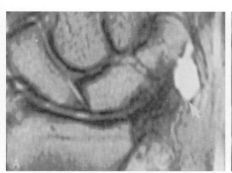
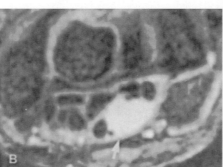
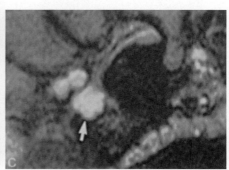

Figure 11–5

Entrapment of the median nerve: Carpal tunnel syndrome—ganglia.

A, B A coronal T2-weighted (TR/TE, 2000/80) spin echo MR image **(A)** and a transverse multiplanar gradient recalled (MPGR) MR image (TR/TE, 550/17; flip angle, 20 degrees) **(B)** show high signal intensity in a synovial cyst (arrows) that arose from the pisiform-triquetral joint and extended into the carpal tunnel.

C In this patient, a transverse T2-weighted (TR/TE, 2200/80) spin echo MR image shows a recurrent ganglion (arrow) adjacent to the median nerve.

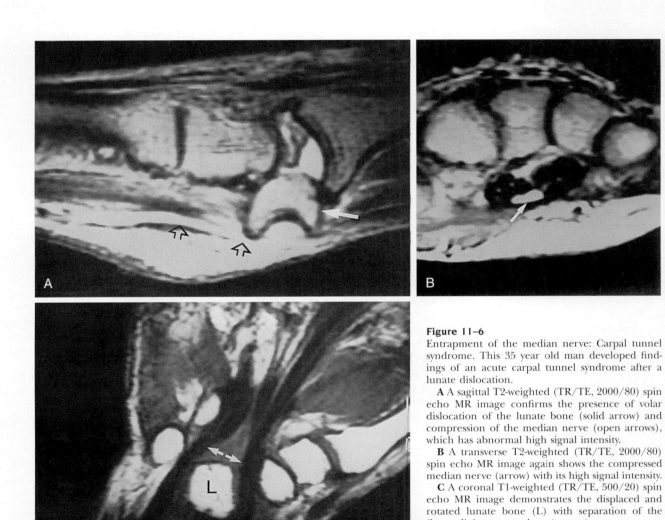

Figure 11–6

Entrapment of the median nerve: Carpal tunnel syndrome. This 35 year old man developed findings of an acute carpal tunnel syndrome after a lunate dislocation.

A A sagittal T2-weighted (TR/TE, 2000/80) spin echo MR image confirms the presence of volar dislocation of the lunate bone (solid arrow) and compression of the median nerve (open arrows), which has abnormal high signal intensity.

B A transverse T2-weighted (TR/TE, 2000/80) spin echo MR image again shows the compressed median nerve (arrow) with its high signal intensity.

C A coronal T1-weighted (TR/TE, 500/20) spin echo MR image demonstrates the displaced and rotated lunate bone (L) with separation of the flexor digitorum tendons (arrows).

(Courtesy of M. J. Shin, M.D., Seoul, Korea.)

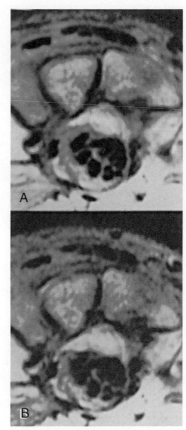

Figure 11–7
Entrapment of the median nerve: Recurrent carpal tunnel syndrome. Transverse proton density (TR/TE, 1800/20) **(A)** and T2-weighted (TR/TE, 1800/70) **(B)** spin echo MR images show evidence of prior incision of the flexor retinaculum with volar migration of the contents of the carpal tunnel, a vertically oriented median nerve, and subtle evidence of proliferative synovitis. This 43 year old woman had persistent symptoms of median nerve compression after the operative procedure. (Courtesy of S. K. Brahme, M.D., La Jolla, California.)

Cubital Tunnel Syndrome

Ulnar nerve entrapment is seen most frequently at the level of the cubital tunnel. In this location, the ulnar

nerve extends through a fibro-osseous canal formed by the medial epicondyle and an aponeurotic band bridging the dual origin of the flexor carpi ulnaris muscle.[33] This condition probably is the second most common compressive neuropathy of the upper extremity (after the carpal tunnel syndrome).[34] Typical causes of compression of the ulnar nerve in the cubital tunnel are trauma and progressive cubitus valgus deformity (tardy ulnar nerve palsy), although additional causes include nerve subluxation, osteoarthritis, rheumatoid arthritis, synovial cysts, prolonged bedrest, flexion deformity of the elbow, anomalous muscles, trochlear hypoplasia, aneurysms, and masses as well as idiopathic entrapment (Fig. 11–8). Axial radiographs may reveal medial trochlear osteophytes or medial incongruity of the elbow joint, or both.[35] MR images, particularly those in the transaxial and sagittal planes, may reveal evidence of compression and inflammation, the latter appearing as thickening and alterations in signal intensity of the ulnar nerve.[2] Conservative measures may be used to treat this condition, although operative intervention with either local decompression or anterior transposition of the nerve may be required (Fig. 11–9).

Clinical manifestations simulating those of the cubital tunnel syndrome may accompany subluxation of the ulnar nerve related to a tear or laxity of the arcuate ligament, shallow epicondylar groove, or cubitus valgus.[2] Such subluxation may be seen in asymptomatic persons, however.[2] It is demonstrated optimally when the MR imaging examination is obtained with flexion of the elbow.[2]

Guyon's Canal Syndrome (Ulnar Tunnel Syndrome)

An entrapment neuropathy of the ulnar nerve may occur in the wrist where the nerve enters the palm through the canal of Guyon, the ulnar tunnel (Fig. 11–10). The walls of the canal consist of the pisiform bone medially and the hook of the hamate laterally.[4] The floor of the canal is composed of the flexor retinaculum and the origin of the hypothenar muscles, and the roof is com-

Figure 11–8
Entrapment of the ulnar nerve: Cubital tunnel syndrome. A lipoma (arrows) adjacent to the ulnar nerve (arrowheads) is well shown in these transverse proton density (TR/TE, 2000/20) spin echo MR images. It led to clinical findings of ulnar nerve entrapment in this 36 year old man. (Courtesy of Z. Rosenberg, M.D., New York, New York.)

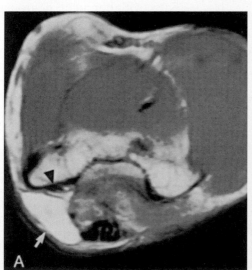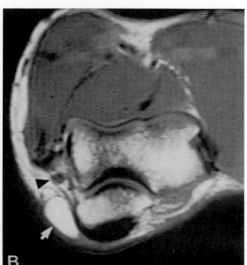

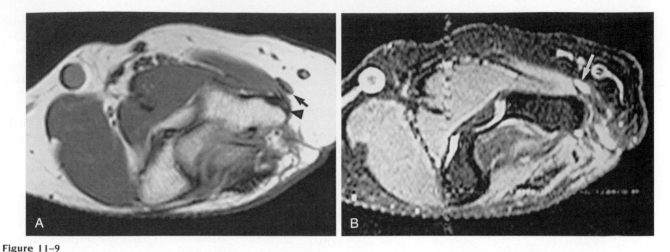

Figure 11–9

Entrapment of the ulnar nerve: Cubital tunnel syndrome—recurrent neuropathy after anterior transposition of the nerve.

A A transverse T1-weighted (TR/TE, 750/20) spin echo MR image at the level of the tip of the olecranon process and trochlea shows the ulnar nerve (arrow) located anterior to the site of origin of the common flexor tendons (arrowhead) and medial to the pronator teres muscle.

B On a transverse STIR MR image (TR/TE, 2000/30; inversion time, 140 msec), high signal intensity of the ulnar nerve (arrow) is seen. (Courtesy of S. Eilenberg, M.D., San Diego, California.)

posed of the volar carpal ligament, palmaris brevis muscle, and fibers from the palmar fascia.[36] The contents of the canal are the ulnar nerve, ulnar artery, and fatty tissue; no flexor tendons pass through the canal.[37]

MR imaging can be used to study the normal Guyon's canal and its abnormalities.[2, 38] In one study, the normal ulnar nerve had a mean diameter of 3 mm and bifurcated an average distance of 12 mm from the proximal margin of the pisiform bone.[38] The precise role of this imaging technique in the evaluation of the ulnar tunnel syndrome is not established, however.

SUPRASCAPULAR NERVE

Entrapment of the suprascapular nerve occurs most commonly as it passes through the suprascapular notch.

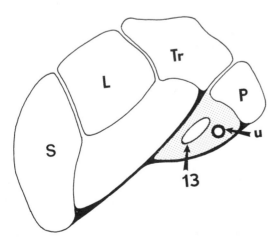

Figure 11–10

Entrapment of the ulnar nerve: Guyon's canal syndrome (ulnar tunnel syndrome)—normal sectional anatomy. Observe the ulnar nerve (13) and ulnar artery (u). S, scaphoid; L, lunate; Tr, triquetrum; P, pisiform. (From Grundberg AB: J Hand Surg [Br] 9.72, 1984.)

This nerve, which contains motor and sensory fibers, arises from the upper trunk of the brachial plexus, runs deep to the trapezius and omohyoid muscles, and enters the supraspinous fossa through the suprascapular notch, passing below the superior transverse scapular ligament.[39, 40] After the suprascapular nerve passes through the notch, it supplies the supraspinatus and infraspinatus muscles and the articular branches to both the glenohumeral and acromioclavicular joints. The most frequent site of nerve encroachment is at the point where the suprascapular nerve traverses the suprascapular notch adjacent to the suprascapular ligament; variability of the size and shape of the notch and ligament, together with the angulation of the nerve as it crosses the superior portion of the notch, predisposes the nerve to injury at this point.[41] As the nerve continues over the lateral part of the scapular spine and spinoglenoid notch and under the inferior transverse ligament and the spinoglenoid ligament to the infraspinatus fossa, other sites of entrapment are possible but rare.[41, 42]

Entrapment neuropathy of the suprascapular nerve by a ganglion deserves special emphasis.[43–47] Most affected patients are young men involved in jobs requiring manual labor or weightlifters. Such ganglia arising at the scapular notch compress both motor branches of the suprascapular nerve, resulting in weakness or atrophy of both the supraspinatus and the infraspinatus muscles; ganglia arising near the spinoglenoid notch affect a more distal segment of the nerve, resulting in selective involvement of the infraspinatus muscle. Ultrasonography, CT, and MR imaging can be used to diagnose such ganglia.[48] On MR images, a fluid-filled mass communicating with the joint, muscle atrophy, and in some cases a rotator cuff tear are evident (Fig. 11–11). Associated tears of the glenoid labrum and posterior portion of the glenohumeral joint capsule also are observed, suggesting that the pathogenesis of some of these ganglion cysts is similar to that of meniscal cysts about the knee.

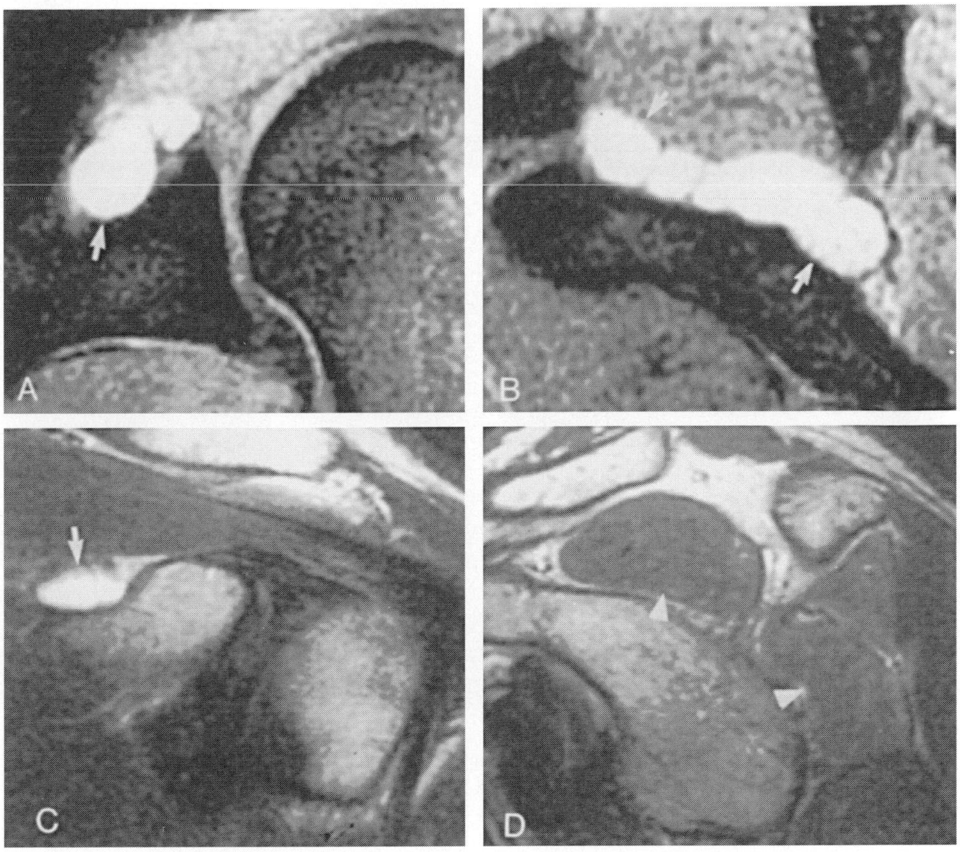

Figure 11-11
Entrapment of the suprascapular nerve: Ganglia.

A, B Coronal oblique multiplanar gradient recalled (MPGR) (TR/TE, 540/15; flip angle, 25 degrees) **(A)** and sagittal oblique multiplanar gradient recalled (MPGR) (TR/TE, 580/18; flip angle, 20 degrees) **(B)** MR images show the ganglion (arrows) located deep to the supraspinatus and infraspinatus muscles. (Courtesy of P. Kindynis, M.D., Geneva, Switzerland.)

C, D Coronal oblique T2-weighted (TR/TE, 2500/96) **(C)** and sagittal oblique T2-weighted (TR/TE, 2500/96) **(D)** spin echo MR images reveal the ganglion (arrow) and subtle changes in signal intensity in the supraspinatus and infraspinatus muscles (arrowheads). (Courtesy of S. Eilenberg, M.D., San Diego, California.)

AXILLARY NERVE

The axillary nerve arises from the posterior cord of the brachial plexus, its fibers being derived from the fifth and sixth cervical nerves. It is located behind the axillary artery and anterior to the subscapularis muscle. At the lower margin of this muscle, the axillary nerve extends backward and, in company with the posterior circumflex humeral vessels, enters the quadrilateral space, which is bounded above by the teres minor muscle, below by the teres major muscle, medially by the long head of the triceps muscle, and laterally by the surgical neck of the humerus. Although rare, a quadrilateral space syndrome produced by compression of the posterior circumflex humeral artery and the axillary nerve or one or more of its major branches has been described.[40, 49] The syndrome predominates in young men and women, usually being seen in the third or fourth decade of life, and is more common in the dominant upper extremity. Symptoms include paresthesias in the upper extremity and anterior shoulder pain that may interfere with daily physical activity. Asymmetry in peripheral pulses in the arm may be encountered. Subclavian arteriography usually is diagnostic.[49] MR imaging also allows accurate diagnosis (Fig. 11–12).[2]

MEDIAL OR LATERAL PLANTAR NERVES

Entrapment of the medial or lateral plantar nerves of the foot as a result of injury to these nerves near the transverse intertarsal ligament leads to local weakness and burning sensation. In this location, a neuroma may develop. This is especially common between the third and fourth toes, where it is termed a Morton's neuroma[50]; the second most common location is between the second and third toes. Resulting symptoms and signs are known as Morton's metatarsalgia.[51] The precise cause of Morton's neuralgia is not clear; nerve ischemia or entrapment has been implicated. The taut transverse metatarsal ligament appears to play a critical role in the compression of the interdigital nerve, and the compressive effect may be augmented by an enlarged forefoot bursa that may occur in such diseases as rheumatoid arthritis.[52]

Ultrasonography[53] and MR imaging[54] may be used in the diagnosis of a Morton's neuroma. The MR imaging characteristics include a mass with decreased signal intensity, well demarcated from adjacent fat tissue, on T1-weighted spin echo MR images, a mass that is isointense or slightly hypointense to fat tissue on T2-weighted spin echo images, and evidence of intermetatarsal bursitis (Fig. 11–13).[54] The relatively low signal intensity of the lesions on T2-weighted images, which differs from the high signal intensity of true neuromas on such images, is consistent with their fibrous composition.[55] MR imaging accomplished with fat suppression techniques after the intravenous administration of gadolinium-based contrast agents may lead to improved detection of Morton's neuromas.[56]

POSTERIOR TIBIAL NERVE

Compression of the posterior tibial nerve at the medial aspect of the ankle results in the tarsal tunnel syn-

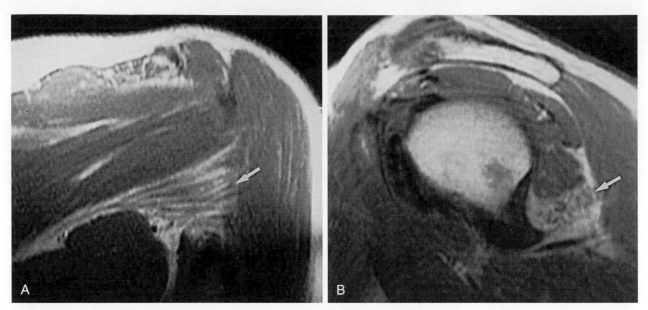

Figure 11–12
Entrapment of the axillary nerve: Quadrilateral space syndrome. T1-weighted (TR/TE, 800/12) coronal oblique **(A)** and proton density-weighted (TR/TE, 2000/20) sagittal oblique **(B)** MR images show selective atrophy and fatty infiltration of the teres minor muscle (arrows).

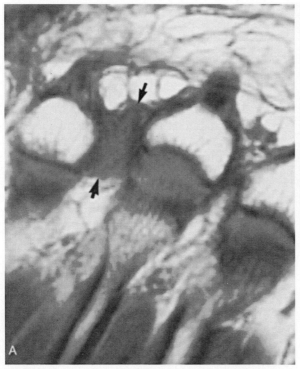

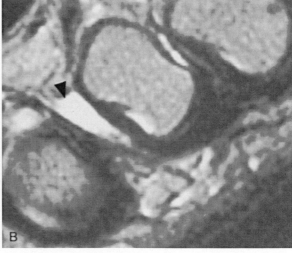

Figure 11–13
Morton's neuroma.

A An oblique transverse T1-weighted (TR/TE, 500/27) spin echo MR image shows the neuroma (arrows), of low signal intensity, in the web space between the third and fourth toes.

B An oblique coronal T2-weighted (TR/TE, 2500/80) spin echo MR image reveals a fluid-filled intermetatarsal bursa (arrowhead) at a level just proximal to the neuroma.

(From Erickson SJ, et al: Radiology *181*:833, 1991.)

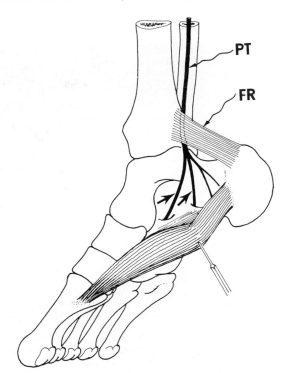

Figure 11–14
Entrapment of the posterior tibial nerve: Tarsal tunnel syndrome—normal anatomy. The posterior tibial nerve (PT) passes beneath the flexor retinaculum (FR), and then divides into various nerves including the medial and lateral plantar nerves (arrows). (Reprinted by permission of the New England Journal of Medicine. From Kopell HP, Thompson WAL: N Engl J Med *262*:56. Copyright 1960, Massachusetts Medical Society.)

drome.[57, 58] The tarsal tunnel is located behind and below the medial malleolus; its floor is bony and its roof is formed by the flexor retinaculum.[57] The resulting fibro-osseous channel allows passage of the tibialis posterior, flexor digitorum longus and flexor hallucis longus tendons, and the posterior tibial artery and vein, in addition to the posterior tibial nerve (Fig. 11–14). Trauma is the leading cause of this compression neuropathy.

MR imaging represents an effective technique in the assessment of the tarsal tunnel syndrome. The complex normal anatomy of the tarsal tunnel as delineated with MR imaging has been the subject of several investigations, to which the interested reader should refer.[59, 60] Coronal, transaxial, and oblique transaxial imaging planes are most useful, allowing identification of the flexor retinaculum, the fine septa deep to the retinaculum, the contents of the tunnel, the separating septum between the medial and lateral plantar nerves distal to the retinaculum, and the three terminal branches of the posterior tibial nerve (Fig. 11–15). In instances of the tarsal tunnel syndrome, MR imaging can provide information regarding its cause, including the documentation of the presence and nature of an extrinsic mass (Fig. 11–16).[60–62] MR imaging also can be used to document causes of ineffectual operative treatment of the tarsal tunnel syndrome.[63]

COMMON PERONEAL NERVE

Compression of the common peroneal nerve or its branches (deep, superficial, recurrent) occurs near the knee (Fig. 11–17). Entrapment of the common peroneal nerve, although relatively infrequent, typically occurs as it winds around the neck of the fibula (Fig. 11–18).

FEMORAL NERVE

Entrapment of the femoral nerve is rare but occurs in the inguinal region of the pelvis. Causes include an inguinal hernia, surgical scar, psoas abscess, pelvic tumor, lymphoma, iliopsoas bursitis, bleeding (hemophilia and anticoagulant therapy), aneurysms of the external iliac and femoral arteries, and trauma.

SCIATIC NERVE

The sciatic nerve exits the pelvis by traversing the greater sciatic foramen, below the piriformis muscle, and then descends between the greater trochanter of the femur and the ischial tuberosity, deep to the gluteus maximus muscle. The course of the sciatic nerve and its major branches is well shown with CT, ultrasonography, and MR imaging.[64, 65] Although a prolapsed intervertebral disc is the most common cause of sciatica, entrapment neuropathies of the sciatic nerve also relate to Paget's disease of the ischium, avulsion of the ischial tuberosity, fractures about and dislocations of the hip, posttraumatic ossification in the biceps femoris muscle, intramuscular injections, and hip surgery. Below the sciatic foramen, a piriformis syndrome represents a distinct pattern of nerve compression caused by enlargement, inflammation, or anatomic variations of the piriformis muscle.

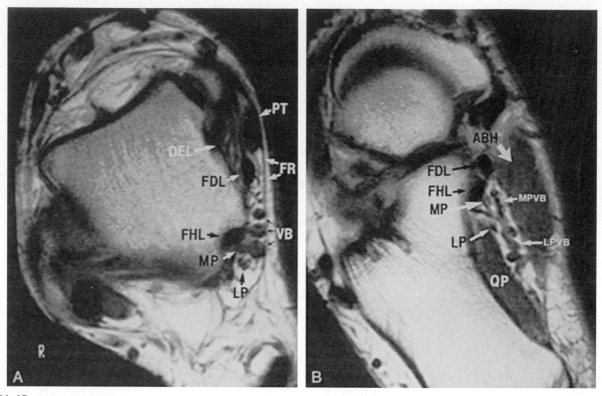

Figure 11–15
Entrapment of the posterior tibial nerve: Tarsal tunnel syndrome—normal anatomy. Transverse T1-weighted (TR/TE, 600/20) spin echo MR images through the tibiotalar **(A)** and talocalcaneal **(B)** portions of the tarsal tunnel are shown. In **A,** note the position of the posterior tibial tendon (PT) and flexor retinaculum (FR). The medial plantar (MP) and lateral plantar (LP) nerves lie deep to the vascular bundles (VB). The medial plantar nerve is in close proximity to the flexor hallucis longus tendon (FHL). The deltoid ligament (DEL) and flexor digitorum longus tendon (FDL) are seen. In **B,** the lateral plantar neurovascular bundle (LPVB) and medial plantar neurovascular bundle (MPVB) lie deep to the abductor hallucis muscle (ABH), and beneath these bundles lie the medial plantar (MP) and lateral plantar (LP) nerves. Other identified structures are the quadratus plantae muscle (QP), the flexor hallucis longus tendon (FHL), and the flexor digitorum longus tendon (FDL). The roof of the tarsal tunnel is formed in **A** by the flexor retinaculum and in **B** by the abductor hallucis muscle. (From Kerr R, et al: J Comput Assist Tomogr *15*:280, 1991.)

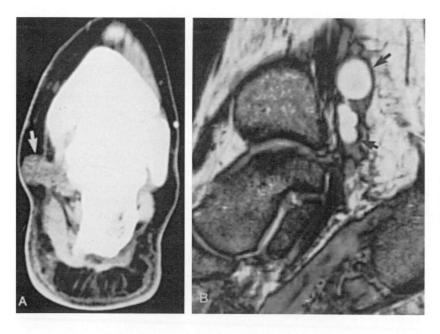

Figure 11–16
Entrapment of the posterior tibial nerve: Tarsal tunnel syndrome—ganglion. A ganglion (arrows) occurring on the medial and posterior portions of the ankle in this 48 year old man is shown on a soft tissue image of a coronal CT scan **(A)** and on a sagittal gradient re-called acquisition in the steady state (GRASS) image obtained with volumetric acquisition (TR/TE, 30/12; flip angle, 40 degrees) **(B).** (Courtesy of G. Bock, M.D., Winnipeg, Manitoba, Canada.)

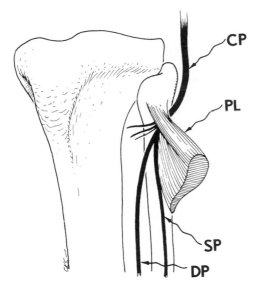

Figure 11–17

Entrapment of the common peroneal nerve and its branches: Normal anatomy. On this posterior view, observe that the common peroneal nerve (CP) winds around the back of the fibula in intimate association with the peroneus longus muscle (PL) and then divides into the deep peroneal nerve (DP) and the superficial peroneal nerve (SP). (Reprinted by permission of the New England Journal of Medicine. From Kopell HP, Thompson WAL: N Engl J Med *262*:56. Copyright 1960, Massachusetts Medical Society.)

SUMMARY

Entrapment neuropathies occur at specific anatomic regions along the course of many peripheral nerves. MR imaging is well suited to the assessment of many of these neuropathies.

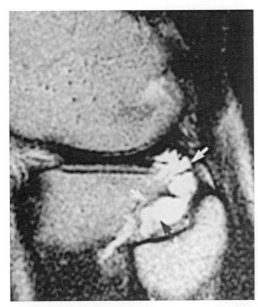

Figure 11–18

Entrapment of the common peroneal nerve and its branches: Ganglion. A sagittal T2-weighted (TR/TE, 2200/80) spin echo MR image shows the ganglion (arrows), of high signal intensity, in close proximity to the proximal tibiofibular joint.

REFERENCES

1. Mackinnon SE: Double and multiple "crush" syndromes: Double and multiple entrapment neuropathies. Hand Clin *8*:369, 1992.
2. Beltran J, Rosenberg ZS: Diagnosis of compressive and entrapment neuropathies of the upper extremity: Value of MR imaging. AJR *163*:525, 1994.
3. Wertsch JJ, Melvin J: Median nerve anatomy and entrapment syndromes: A review. Arch Phys Med Rehabil *63*:623, 1982.
4. Thompson WAL, Kopell HP: Peripheral entrapment neuropathies of the upper extremities. N Engl J Med *260*:1261, 1959.
5. Plancher KD, Peterson RK, Steichen JB: Compressive neuropathies and tedinopathies in the athletic elbow and wrist. Clin Sports Med *15*:331, 1996.
6. Gerstner DL, Omer GE Jr: Peripheral entrapment neuropathies in the upper extremity. I. Key differential findings, median nerve syndromes. J Musculoskel Med *5*:14, 1988.
7. Johnson RK, Spinner M, Shrewsbury MM: Median nerve entrapment syndrome in the proximal forearm. J Hand Surg *4*:48, 1979.
8. Jones NF, Ming NL: Persistent median artery as a cause of pronator syndrome. J Hand Surg [Am] *13*:728, 1988.
9. Stern MB: The anterior interosseous nerve syndrome (the Kiloh-Nevin syndrome). Clin Orthop *187*:223, 1984.
10. Weiss KL, Betran J, Shamam OM, et al: High-field MR surface-coil imaging of the hand and wrist. I. Normal anatomy. Radiology *160*:160, 1986.
11. Weiss KL, Betran J, Lubbers LM: High-field MR surface-coil imaging of the hand and wrist. II. Pathologic correlations and clinical relevance. Radiology *160*:147, 1986.
12. Middleton WD, Kneeland JB, Kellman GM, et al: MR imaging of the carpal tunnel: Normal anatomy and preliminary findings in the carpal tunnel syndrome. AJR *148*:307, 1987.
13. Richman JA, Gelberman RH, Rydevik BL, et al: Carpal tunnel volume determination by magnetic resonance imaging three-dimensional reconstruction. J Hand Surg [Am] *12*:712, 1987.
14. Mesgarzadeh M, Schneck CD, Bonakdarpour A: Carpal tunnel: MR imaging. I. Normal anatomy. Radiology *171*:743, 1989.
15. Mesgarzadeh M, Schneck CD, Bonakdarpour A, et al: Carpal tunnel: MR imaging. II. Carpal tunnel syndrome. Radiology *171*:749, 1989.
16. Zeiss J, Skie M, Ebraheim N, et al: Anatomic relations between the median nerve and flexor tendons in the carpal tunnel: MR evaluation in normal volunteers. AJR *153*:533, 1989.
17. Skie M, Zeiss J, Ebraheim NA, et al: Carpal tunnel changes and median nerve compression during wrist flexion and extension seen by magnetic resonance imaging. J Hand Surg [Am] *15*:934, 1990.
18. Healy C, Watson JD, Longstaff A, et al: Magnetic resonance imaging of the carpal tunnel. J Hand Surg [Br] *15*:243, 1990.
19. Sugimoto H, Miyaji N, Ohsawa T: Carpal tunnel syndrome: Evaluation of median nerve circulation with dynamic contrast-enhanced MR imaging. Radiology *190*:459, 1994.
20. Omer GE Jr: Median nerve compression at the wrist. Hand Clin *8*:317, 1992.
21. Shuman S, Osterman L, Bora FW: Compression neuropathies. Semin Neurol *7*:76, 1987.
22. Papaioannou T, Rushworth G, Atar D, et al: Carpal canal stenosis in men with idiopathic carpal tunnel syndrome. Clin Orthop *285*:210, 1992.
23. Buchberger W, Judmaier W, Birbamer G, et al: Carpal tunnel syndrome: Diagnosis with high-resolution sonography. AJR *159*:793, 1992.
24. Rosenbaum RB: The role of imaging in the diagnosis of carpal tunnel syndrome. Invest Radiol *28*:1059, 1993.
25. Yoshioka S, Okuda Y, Tamai K, et al: Changes in carpal tunnel shape during wrist joint motion: MRI evaluation of normal volunteers. J Hand Surg [Br] *18*:620, 1993.
26. Rowland EB, Kleinert JM: Endoscopic carpal-tunnel release in cadavers. J Bone Joint Surg [Am] *76*:266, 1994.
27. Agee JM, Peimer CA, Pyrek JD, et al: Endoscopic carpal tunnel release: A prospective study of complications and surgical experience. J Hand Surg [Am] *20*:165, 1995.
28. Bozentka DJ, Osterman AL: Complications of endoscopic carpal tunnel release. Hand Clinics *11*:91, 1995.
29. Hunter JM: Recurrent carpal tunnel syndrome, epineural fibrous fixation, and traction neuropathy. Hand Clin *7*:491, 1991.
30. Murphy RX Jr, Chernofsky MA, Osborne MA, et al: Magnetic resonance imaging in the evaluation of persistent carpal tunnel syndrome. J Hand Surg [Am] *18*:113, 1993.
31. Norkus SA, Meyers MC: Ulnar neuropathy of the elbow. Sports Med *17*:189, 1994.
32. Holtzman RNN, Mark MH, Patel MR, et al: Ulnar entrapment neuropathy in the forearm. J Hand Surg [Am] *9*:576, 1984.
33. O'Driscoll SW, Horii E, Carmichael SW, et al: The cubital tunnel and ulnar neuropathy. J Bone Joint Surg [Br] *73*:613, 1991.
34. Rayan GM: Proximal ulnar nerve compression: Cubital tunnel syndrome. Hand Clin *8*:325, 1992.
35. St John JN, Palmaz JC: The cubital tunnel in ulnar entrapment neuropathy. Radiology *158*:119, 1986.
36. Grundberg AB: Ulnar tunnel syndrome. Hand [Br] *9*:72, 1984.
37. Konig PSA, Hage JJ, Bloem JAM, et al: Variations of the ulnar nerve and ulnar artery in Guyon's canal: A cadaveric study. J Hand Surg (Am) *19*:617, 1994.

38. Zeiss J, Jakab E, Khimji T, et al: The ulnar tunnel at the wrist (Guyon's canal): Normal MR anatomy and variants. AJR *158*:1081, 1992.

39. Garcia G, McQueen D: Bilateral suprascapular-nerve entrapment syndrome: Case report and review of the literature. J Bone Joint Surg [Am] *63*:491, 1981.

40. Post M, Grinblat E: Nerve entrapment about the shoulder girdle. Hand Clin *8*:299, 1992.

41. Kaspi A, Yanai J, Pick CG, et al: Entrapment of the distal suprascapular nerve: An anatomical study. Int Orthop (SICOT) *12*:273, 1988.

42. Demaio M, Drez D Jr, Mullins RC: The inferior transverse scapular ligament as a possible cause of entrapment neuropathy of the nerve to the infraspinatus: A brief note. J Bone Joint Surg [Am] *73*:1061, 1991.

43. Ogino T, Minami A, Kato H, et al: Entrapment neuropathy of the suprascapular nerve by a ganglion: A report of three cases. J Bone Joint Surg [Am] *73*:141, 1991.

44. Takagishi K, Maeda K, Ikeda T, et al: Ganglion causing paralysis of the suprascapular nerve: Diagnosis by MRI and ultrasonography. Acta Orthop Scand *62*:391, 1991.

45. Skirving AP, Kozak TKW, Davis SJ: Infraspinatus paralysis due to spinoglenoid notch ganglion. J Bone Joint Surg [Br] *76*:588, 1994.

46. Takagishi K, Saitoh A, Tonegawa M, et al: Isolated paralysis of the infraspinatus muscle. J Bone Joint Surg [Br] *76*:584, 1994.

47. Fehrman DA, Orwin JF, Jennings RM: Suprascapular nerve entrapment by ganglion cysts: A report of six cases with arthroscopic findings and review of the literature. Arthroscopy *11*:727, 1995.

48. Fritz RC, Helms CA, Steinbach LS, et al: Suprascapular nerve entrapment: Evaluation with MR imaging. Radiology *182*:437, 1992.

49. Cormier PJ, Matalon TAS, Wolin PM: Quadrilateral space syndrome: A rare cause of shoulder pain. Radiology *167*:797, 1988.

50. Koppell HP, Thompson WAL: Peripheral entrapment neuropathies of the lower extremity. N Engl J Med *262*:56, 1960.

51. Guiloff RJ, Scadding JW, Klenerman L: Morton's metatarsalgia: Clinical, electrophysiological and histological observations. J Bone Joint Surg [Br] *66*:586, 1984.

52. Alexander IJ, Johnson KA, Parr JW: Morton's neuroma: A review of recent concepts. Orthopedics *10*:103, 1987.

53. Redd RA, Peters VJ, Emery SF, et al: Morton neuroma: Sonographic evaluation. Radiology *171*:415, 1989.

54. Erickson SJ, Canale PB, Carrera GF, et al: Interdigital (Morton) neuroma: High-resolution MR imaging with a solenoid coil. Radiology *181*:833, 1991.

55. Sartoris DJ, Brozinsky S, Resnick D: Magnetic resonance images: Interdigital or Morton's neuroma. J Foot Surg *28*:78, 1989.

56. Terk MR, Kwong PK, Suthar M, et al: Morton neuroma: Evaluation with MR imaging performed with contrast enhancement and fat suppression. Radiology *189*:239, 1993.

57. Radin EL: Tarsal tunnel syndrome. Clin Orthop *181*:167, 1983.

58. Takakura Y, Kitada C, Sugimoto K, et al: Tarsal tunnel syndrome: Causes and results of operative intervention. J Bone Joint Surg [Br] *73*:125, 1991.

59. Zeiss J, Fenton P, Ebraheim N, et al: Normal magnetic resonance anatomy of the tarsal tunnel. Foot Ankle *10*:214, 1990.

60. Erickson SJ, Quinn SF, Kneeland JB, et al: MR imaging of the tarsal tunnel and related spaces: Normal and abnormal findings with anatomic correlation. AJR *155*:323, 1990.

61. Zeiss J, Ebraheim N, Rusin J: Magnetic resonance imaging in the diagnosis of tarsal tunnel syndrome: Case report. Clin Imaging *14*:123, 1990.

62. Kerr R, Frey C: MR imaging in tarsal tunnel syndrome. J Comput Assist Tomogr *15*:280, 1991.

63. Zeiss J, Fenton P, Ebraheim N, et al: Magnetic resonance imaging for ineffectual tarsal tunnel surgical treatment. Clin Orthop *264*:264, 1991.

64. Lanzieri CF, Hilal SK: Computed tomography of the sacral plexus and sciatic nerve in the greater sciatic foramen. AJR *143*:165, 1984.

65. Graif M, Seton A, Nerubai J, et al: Sciatic nerve: Sonographic evaluation and anatomic-pathologic considerations. Radiology *181*:405, 1991.

Disorders: Specific Joints

In the last 10 years, imaging of the shoulder has received more attention than that of any other peripheral joint with the exception of the knee. Although emphasis has been given to abnormalities of the rotator cuff and glenohumeral joint instability, the diverse nature of shoulder disorders may involve not only the glenohumeral joint but also the acromioclavicular and sternoclavicular joints. Often, as a supplement to clinical evaluation, the examining physician relies on information provided by routine radiography. Increasingly, however, additional imaging methods also are employed to assess shoulder problems. In this regard, arthrography, CT scanning and CT arthrography, ultrasonography, and MR imaging deserve special attention. Such emphasis forms the foundation of the current chapter.

ANATOMY

Osseous Anatomy

Glenohumeral Joint

The glenohumeral joint lies between the roughly hemispherical head of the humerus and the shallow cavity of the glenoid region of the scapula. Stability of this joint is limited, for two reasons: the scapular "socket" is small compared to the size of the adjacent humeral head, so that apposing osseous surfaces provide little inherent stability; the joint capsule is quite redundant, providing little additional support. Stability of the glenohumeral joint is supplied by surrounding structures (see later discussion).

The upper end of the humerus consists of the head and the greater and lesser tuberosities (tubercles) (Fig. 12–1). With the arm at the side of the body, the humeral head is directed medially, upward, and slightly backward to contact the glenoid cavity of the scapula. The head is inclined 130 to 150 degrees with respect to the humeral shaft and has an average retrotorsion angle of 20 to 30 degrees.[1] Beneath the head is the anatomic neck of the humerus, a slightly constricted area that encircles the bone, separating the head from the tuberosities. The anatomic neck is the site of attachment of the capsular ligaments of the glenohumeral joint. The greater tuberosity is located on the lateral aspect of the proximal humerus. The tendons of the supraspinatus and infraspinatus muscles insert on its superior portion, whereas

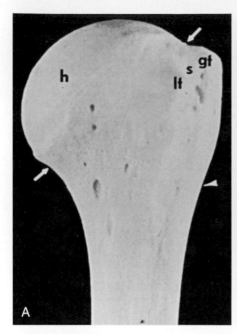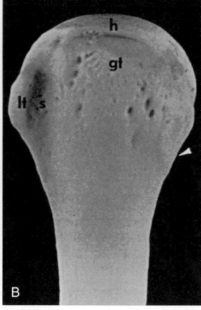

Figure 12–1
Proximal portion of the humerus: Osseous anatomy.

A Anterior aspect, external rotation. Observe the articular surface of the humeral head (h), greater tuberosity (gt), lesser tuberosity (lt), intertubercular sulcus (s), anatomic neck (arrows), and surgical neck (arrowhead).

B Anterior aspect, internal rotation. The same structures as in **A** are indicated. The lesser tuberosity is seen in profile on the medial aspect of the humeral head and the greater tuberosity is seen en face.

the tendon of the teres minor muscle inserts on its posterior aspect. The lesser tuberosity is located on the anterior portion of the proximal humerus, immediately below the anatomic neck. The subscapularis tendon attaches to the medial aspect of this structure. Between the greater and lesser tuberosities is located the intertubercular sulcus or groove (bicipital groove) through which passes the tendon of the long head of the biceps brachii muscle, surrounded by a synovial sheath and fixed by a transverse ligament extending between the tuberosities.[2] The bicipital groove is 30 degrees medial to a line passing from the shaft through the center of the humeral head.[1] The rough lateral lip of the groove is the site of attachment of the tendon of the pectoralis major muscle; the floor of the groove gives rise to the attachment of the tendon of the latissimus dorsi muscle; and the medial lip of the groove is the site of attachment of the tendon of the teres major muscle.

The shallow glenoid cavity is located on the lateral margin of the scapula (Fig. 12–2). Although variation occurs in the osseous depth of the glenoid region,[3] a fibrocartilaginous labrum encircles and slightly deepens the glenoid cavity.[4] The glenoid contour may be almost flat or slightly curved, or it may possess a deep, socket-like appearance. The average vertical dimension of the glenoid cavity is 35 mm, and the transverse diameter is 25 mm.[1] The glenoid cavity may be either anteverted or retroverted with respect to the plane of the scapula; retroversion (which averages about 7 degrees) is more common than anteversion (which varies from 2 to 10 degrees).[3, 5] Retroversion of the glenoid cavity has been associated with osteoarthritis of the glenohumeral joint.[6] The curvature of the glenoid cavity may be smaller than, larger than, or identical to the curvature of the humeral head.[1] A supraglenoid tubercle is located above the glenoid cavity, to which is attached the tendon of the long head of the biceps brachii muscle. Below the cavity is a thickened ridge of bone, the infraglenoid tubercle,

which is a site of attachment for the tendon of the long head of the triceps muscle.

The width of the glenohumeral joint surface at the central portion of the glenoid, as defined on radiographs, generally is less than 6 mm.[7] The subacromial space, defined as the distance between the head of the humerus and the inferior aspect of the acromion, in adults is approximately 9 or 10 mm; a measurement less than 6 mm in a middle-aged person suggests rotator cuff atrophy or tear.[8]

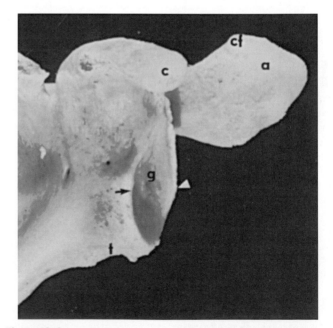

Figure 12–2
Lateral portion of the scapula: Osseous anatomy. Note the glenoid cavity (g), coracoid process (c), acromion process (a), clavicular facet (cf), and infraglenoid tubercle (t). Also note the anterior (arrow) and posterior (arrowhead) rims of the glenoid region.

Acromioclavicular Joint

The lateral or acromial end of the clavicle is a flattened structure with a small, oval articular facet that faces laterally and slightly downward. This facet articulates with the acromial facet of the scapula and is the site of attachment of the joint capsule of the acromioclavicular joint. The inferior surface of the acromial end of the clavicle possesses a rough osseous ridge, termed the trapezoid line. A conoid tubercle is located at the posterior aspect of the lateral clavicle. The trapezoid line and conoid tubercle are the sites of attachment of the trapezoid and conoid parts of the coracoclavicular ligament, respectively.

The acromion is a forward protuberance of the lateral aspect of the scapula. An articular facet, the acromial facet, is located on the medial border of the acromion and is small and oval, directed medially and superiorly.

A joint may be noted between the clavicle and coracoid process in 0.1 to 1.2 per cent of people.[9–13] In these cases, a triangular outgrowth from the undersurface of the clavicle approaches the dorsomedial surface of the coracoid process. On dissection, the joint may be found to contain a capsule and synovial membrane as well as a cartilaginous disc.[13]

Sternoclavicular Joint

At the sternoclavicular joint, the medial end of the clavicle articulates with the clavicular notch of the manubrium sterni and with the cartilage of the first rib. The enlarged medial or sternal end of the clavicle projects above the upper margin of the manubrium and is directed medially, inferiorly, and anteriorly. The articular surface is smooth except on its superior portion, where a roughened area allows attachment of an articular disc. The inferior portion of the articular surface is extended to allow articulation with the first costal cartilage. The medial portion of the inferior surface of the clavicle has a rough impression for attachment of the costoclavicular ligament.

The superolateral portions of the manubrium contain oval articular surfaces, the clavicular facets or notches, which are directed superiorly, posteriorly, and laterally. Below each clavicular notch is a rough projection, which receives the first costal cartilage.

Articular Anatomy

Glenohumeral Joint

The articular surfaces of the glenoid and the humerus are covered with hyaline cartilage (Fig. 12–3). The cartilage on the humeral head is thickest at its center and thinner peripherally, whereas the reverse is true on the glenoid portion of the joint. A fibrocartilaginous structure, the labrum, attaches to the glenoid rim and adds an element of stability to the glenohumeral joint (see later discussion).

A loose fibrous capsule arises medially from the circumference of the glenoid labrum or, anteriorly, the

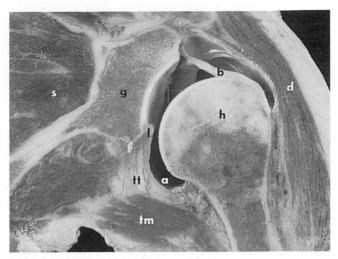

Figure 12–3
Glenohumeral joint: Articular anatomy. A coronal section of an air-distended articular cavity reveals the glenoid region (g) of the scapula, humeral head (h), axillary pouch (a), inferior portion of the labrum (l), tendon (b) of the long head of the biceps brachii muscle, portions of the subscapularis (s), deltoid (d), and teres major (tm) muscles, and the tendon (tt) of the long head of the triceps muscle. Note the hyaline cartilage covering both the glenoid cavity and the humeral head. The size of the articular surface of the humerus is much larger than that of the glenoid cavity.

neck of the scapula.[14] It inserts distally into the anatomic neck of the humerus and periosteum of the humeral diaphysis. In certain areas the fibrous capsule is strengthened by its intimate association with surrounding ligaments and tendons; with regard to tendons, the capsule is reinforced above by the supraspinatus, below by the long head of the triceps, anteriorly by the subscapularis, and posteriorly by the infraspinatus and teres minor. The tendons of the supraspinatus, infraspinatus, teres minor, and subscapularis form a cuff—the rotator cuff—which blends with and reinforces the fibrous capsule (see later discussion). The coracohumeral ligament strengthens the upper part of the capsule. It arises from the lateral edge of the coracoid process, extends over the humeral head, and attaches to the greater tuberosity. Anteriorly, the capsule may thicken to form the superior, middle, and inferior glenohumeral ligaments. These ligaments and the recesses formed between them are variable in configuration (see later discussion). The fibrous capsule is strengthened additionally by extensions from the tendons of the pectoralis major and teres major muscles.

Three openings may be found in the fibrous capsule (Figs. 12–4 and 12–5). An anterior perforation below the coracoid process establishes joint communication with the bursa behind the subscapularis tendon, the subscapular "recess." A second opening between the greater and lesser tuberosities allows passage of the tendon and synovial sheath of the long head of the biceps brachii muscle. A third, inconstant perforation may exist posteriorly, allowing communication of the articular cavity and a bursa under the infraspinatus tendon.

A synovial membrane lines the inner aspect of the fibrous capsule. It covers the anatomic neck of the hu-

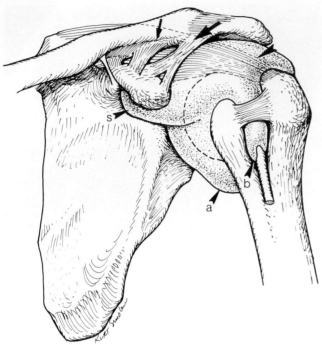

Figure 12–4
Glenohumeral joint: Normal articular extensions. A drawing of the anterior aspect of the distended glenohumeral joint depicts axillary pouch (a), subscapular recess (s), and synovial extension over the bicipital tendon (b). Note the rotator cuff (arrowhead), coracoacromial ligament (heavy arrow), and coracoclavicular ligament (light arrow).

merus and extends to the articular cartilage on the humeral head. The synovium passes distally to line the bicipital groove and is reflected over the biceps tendon.

Several bursae occur about the glenohumeral joint.

1. *Subscapular bursa.* This bursa lies between the subscapularis tendon and the scapula, communicating with the joint via an opening between the superior and middle glenohumeral ligaments or between the middle and inferior glenohumeral ligaments, or in both locations (see later discussion). This bursa is readily apparent on arthrograms of the glenohumeral joint as a tongue-shaped collection of contrast material extending medially from the glenohumeral space underneath the coracoid process.[15] It is prominent in internal rotation but is less obvious in external rotation, as the taut subscapularis muscle compresses the bursa.

2. *Bursa about the infraspinatus tendon.* This inconstant bursa separates the infraspinatus tendon and joint capsule and may communicate with the joint cavity.

3. *Subacromial (subdeltoid) bursa.* This important bursa lies between the deltoid muscle and joint capsule (Fig. 12–6).[16] It extends underneath the acromion and the coracoacromial ligament. It also may extend beneath the coracoid process as the subcoracoid portion of the subacromial (subdeltoid) bursa, although the subcoracoid bursa also may exist as a distinct or independent structure. The subacromial (subdeltoid) bursa is separated from the articular cavity by the rotator cuff and does not communicate with the joint unless the cuff has been perforated. Layers of fat tissue about this bursa

have been identified on radiographs of the normal shoulder[17]; a thin, crescentic radiolucent area passes from the inferior aspect of the acromion process and distal end of the clavicle along the outer margin of the upper humerus. Obliteration of the peribursal fat plane is an important sign of shoulder disease and can be recognized not only on routine radiographs[18] but on CT and MR images as well (see later discussion).

4. *Bursa above the acromion.* This bursa is located on the superior surface of the acromion process of the scapula.

5. *Additional bursae.* Additional bursae may be found between the coracoid process and the capsule, behind the coracobrachialis, between the teres major and the long head of the triceps, and about the latissimus dorsi.

Acromioclavicular Joint

The articular surfaces about the acromioclavicular joint are covered with fibrocartilage (Fig. 12–7). In the central portion of the joint is an articular disc[19] that divides the joint cavity partially or, more rarely, completely. The fibrous capsule surrounds the articular margin and is reinforced on its superior and inferior surfaces. Surrounding ligaments include the acromioclavicular and coracoclavicular ligaments (Fig. 12–8). The former ligament, which is located at the superior portion of the joint, extends between the clavicle and acromion and controls horizontal stability of the joint. The coracoclavicular ligament, which attaches to the coracoid process of the scapula and clavicle, controls vertical stability of the joint and is composed of a trapezoid part and a conoid part. The trapezoid portion extends from the upper surface of the coracoid process to the trapezoid line on the inferior aspect of the clavicle; the conoid portion extends from the coracoid process to the conoid

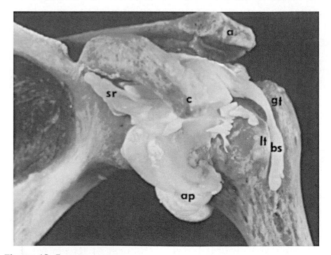

Figure 12–5
Glenohumeral joint: Normal articular extensions. A photograph of the anterior portion of a joint that has been distended with methylmethacrylate reveals the acromion (a), coracoid process (c), and greater tuberosity (gt) and lesser tuberosity (lt) of the humerus. Note the finger-like medial extension of the joint, designated the subscapular recess (sr), the axillary pouch (ap), and the synovial sheath (bs) about the tendon of the long head of the biceps brachii muscle. This sheath is located within the intertubercular sulcus.

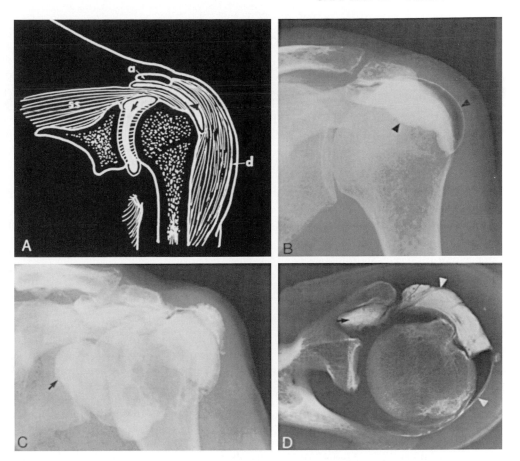

Figure 12–6
Subacromial (subdeltoid) bursa: Normal anatomy.

A A diagram of a coronal section of the shoulder shows the glenohumeral joint (arrow) and subacromial (subdeltoid) bursa (arrowhead), separated by a portion of the rotator cuff (i.e., supraspinatus tendon). The supraspinatus (ss) and deltoid (d) muscles and the acromion (a) are indicated.

B A subdeltoid-subacromial bursogram, accomplished with the injection of both radiopaque contrast material and air, shows the bursa (arrowheads) sitting like a cap on the humeral head and greater tuberosity of the humerus. Note that the joint is not opacified, indicating an intact rotator cuff.

C In a different cadaver, a subacromial-subdeltoid bursogram shows a much more extensive structure owing to opacification of the subacromial, subdeltoid, and subcoracoid (arrow) portions of the bursa.

D A radiograph of a transverse section of the specimen illustrated in **C** shows both the subdeltoid (arrowheads) and subcoracoid (arrow) portions of the bursa. The glenohumeral joint is not opacified.

tubercle on the inferior clavicular surface. The trapezoid and conoid parts of the coracoclavicular ligament may be separated by fat or a bursa.

Normal anteroposterior radiographs of the acromioclavicular joint may reveal a soft tissue plane about the joint related to the aponeurosis associated with the trapezius and deltoid muscles. Contrast opacification of the joint reveals an L-shaped articular cavity with a horizontal limb extending under the inferior surface of the distal clavicle.[20]

The acromioclavicular joint allows the acromion to glide in a forward and backward direction and to rotate on the clavicle. These movements depend on additional movements at the sternoclavicular joint.

Sternoclavicular Joint

The articular end of the clavicle is covered with a layer of fibrocartilage that is thicker than the cartilage on the sternum (Fig. 12–9). A flat, circular disc is located between the articulating surfaces of the clavicle and sternum; it is attached superiorly to the posterior border of the clavicle, inferiorly to the cartilage of the first rib, and, at other sites, to the fibrous capsule, and it divides

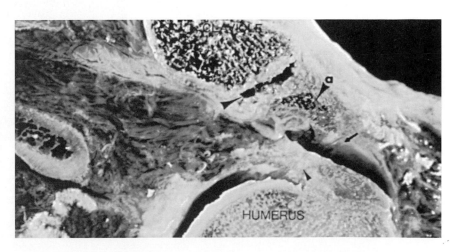

Figure 12–7
Acromioclavicular joint: Normal articular anatomy. Visualized structures on this coronal section are the articular space (large arrowhead) between the distal clavicle and acromion (a) (an articular disc is not visible), rotator cuff (small arrowhead), and subacromial (subdeltoid) bursa (arrow).

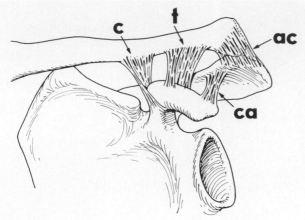

Figure 12–8
Acromioclavicular joint: Normal ligamentous anatomy. Important structures are the fibrous capsule of the joint, which is strengthened by the acromioclavicular ligament (ac), the coracoacromial ligament (ca), and the conoid (c) and trapezoid (t) portions of the coracoclavicular ligament.

the joint into two articular cavities.[21] The disc acts as a checkrein against medial displacement of the inner clavicle. Perforations in the disc are frequent in older persons. A fibrous capsule surrounds the joint[22] and is attached to the clavicular and sternomanubrial articular surfaces. The inferior portion of the capsule is weak as it passes between the clavicle and superior surface of the first costal cartilage. Elsewhere the capsule is strong, reinforced by the anterior and posterior sternoclavicular ligaments and the interclavicular ligament. Nearby, the costoclavicular ligament attaches below to the upper surface of the first rib and adjacent cartilage and above

to the inferior surface of the medial end of the clavicle. This ligament consists of anterior and posterior portions, between which is located a bursa.[23] This ligament resists forces that attempt to displace the medial clavicle anteriorly, posteriorly, upward, or laterally.

The sternoclavicular joint is freely mobile. It participates in movements of the upper extremity, including elevation, depression, protraction, retraction, and circumduction.[24]

Soft Tissue Anatomy

Glenohumeral Ligaments

The glenohumeral ligaments represent thickenings, or reinforcements, of the joint capsule (Fig. 12–10). They are not visible on the external surface of the glenohumeral joint but are identifiable from within the glenohumeral joint, as can be appreciated during arthroscopy. Their function depends on (1) their collagenous integrity, (2) their sites of attachment, and (3) the position of the arm.[1] Three glenohumeral ligaments exist: superior, middle, and inferior. In any individual person, the number of ligaments present varies and, even when present, the glenohumeral ligaments vary considerably in size. Anatomic studies have indicated the presence of a superior glenohumeral ligament in 90 to 97 per cent of cases, of a middle glenohumeral ligament in 73 to 92 per cent of cases, and of an inferior glenohumeral ligament in almost 100 per cent of cases.[1, 25, 26] Each extends from the anterior aspect of the glenoid cavity, near the glenoid labrum, to the proximal portion of the humerus. Apertures between these ligaments provide areas

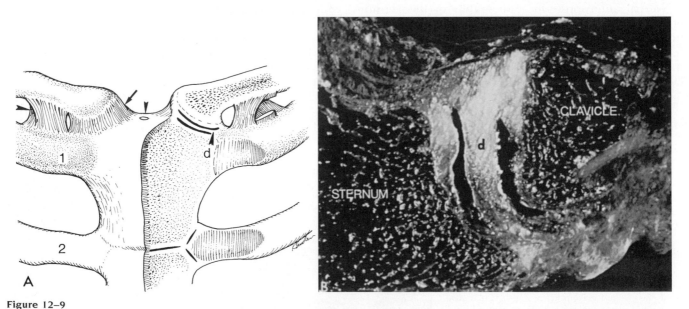

Figure 12–9
Sternoclavicular joint: Normal articular anatomy.
  A A diagrammatic depiction of the anterior aspect of the upper sternum and medial clavicles. On the right-hand side, the superficial bone has been removed, exposing the sternoclavicular, manubriosternal, and second sternocostal joints. Identified structures are the anterior sternoclavicular ligament (arrow), costoclavicular ligament (arrowhead on left), interclavicular ligament (arrowhead in center), and articular disc (d). Note the first (1) and second (2) costal cartilages. (From Warwick R, Williams P: Gray's Anatomy. 35th British Ed. Philadelphia, WB Saunders Co, 1973.)
  B Photograph of a coronal section through the sternoclavicular joint reveals characteristics of the normal intra-articular disc (d).

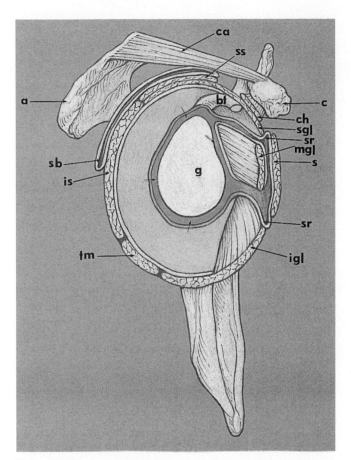

Figure 12–10

Glenohumeral joint: Ligamentous and capsular anatomy. A lateral view of an opened glenohumeral joint is shown in which the humeral head has been removed. Identified structures (beginning superiorly and continuing in a clockwise direction) are the coracoacromial ligament (ca), the supraspinatus tendon (ss), the tendon of the long head of the biceps brachii muscle (bt), the coracoid process (c), the coracohumeral ligament (ch), the superior glenohumeral ligament (sgl), an opening into the subscapular recess (sr), the middle glenohumeral ligament (mgl), the subscapularis tendon (s), a second opening into the subscapular recess (sr), the inferior glenohumeral ligament (igl), the teres minor tendon (tm), the infraspinatus tendon (is), the subacromial-subdeltoid bursa (sb), and the acromion (a). Also identified is the cartilage-covered glenoid cavity (g) surrounded by the glenoid labrum (arrows).

of communication between the glenohumeral joint and the subscapular bursa; some variability exists in the size of these apertures as well as that of the bursa itself (see later discussion).[25, 27] The bursa extends medially from the joint, along the superior tendinous border of the subscapularis muscle, toward the inferior surface of the coracoid process.[27]

DePalma and colleagues[25] described six common variations in the opening of the subscapular bursa (Fig. 12–11): type 1 pattern is characterized by one synovial recess above the middle glenohumeral ligament; type 2 pattern is accompanied by one synovial recess below the middle glenohumeral ligament; type 3 pattern is characterized by one recess above and one recess below the middle glenohumeral ligament; type 4 pattern is indicative of the presence of a large recess above the inferior glenohumeral ligament with the absence of the

middle glenohumeral ligament; type 5 pattern is characterized by two synovial recesses about the middle glenohumeral ligament; and type 6 pattern is indicative of absence of all synovial recesses with well defined glenohumeral ligaments.[1] In general, the closer the anterior portion of the joint capsule attaches to the labrum or glenoid margin, the less prominent are the synovial recesses.[25]

The detailed anatomy of the glenohumeral ligaments has been summarized by O'Brien and coworkers,[1] whose observations are included here. When present, the superior glenohumeral ligament varies in size from a thin wisp of capsular tissue to a prominent bandlike region within the joint capsule. It arises either from a common origin with the tendon of the long head of the biceps brachii muscle, from the anterior portion of the labrum just anterior to this tendon, or from the middle glenohumeral ligament (Fig. 12–12).[25] It inserts into the fovea capitis just superior to the lesser tuberosity.[28] In this latter region, it is intimate with the coracohumeral ligament.[27] The functional importance of the superior glenohumeral ligament is debated; however, owing to its small size in some persons, its vulnerability for tearing during forceful abduction of the glenohumeral joint, and its protection from excessive tension by the other glenohumeral ligaments, the superior glenohumeral ligament probably contributes very little to static stability of the glenohumeral joint.[1, 27, 29]

The middle glenohumeral ligament is the least constant of the glenohumeral ligaments and shows the most

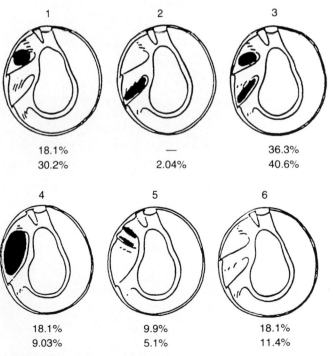

1	2	3
18.1%	—	36.3%
30.2%	2.04%	40.6%

4	5	6
18.1%	9.9%	18.1%
9.03%	5.1%	11.4%

Figure 12–11

Variations in the types of anterior recesses in the capsule. The original percentages of DePalma are listed (top lines) along with percentages from more recent anatomic studies (bottom lines). (From O'Brien SJ, Amoczky SP, Warren RF, et al [Eds]: Developmental anatomy of the shoulder and anatomy of the glenohumeral joint. *In* CA Rockwood Jr, FA Matsen III [Eds]: The Shoulder. Philadelphia, WB Saunders Co, 1990, p 27.)

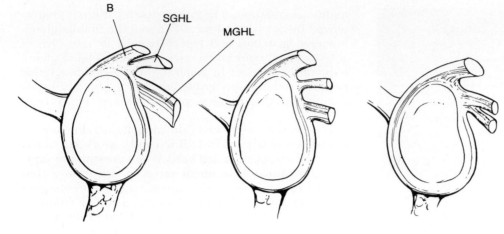

B

SGHL

MGHL

Figure 12–12

Superior glenohumeral ligament. Three common variations of the origin of the superior glenohumeral ligament (SGHL). B, Biceps tendon; MGHL, middle glenohumeral ligament. (From O'Brien SJ, Amoczky SP, Warren RF, et al [Eds]: Developmental anatomy of the shoulder and anatomy of the gleno-humeral joint. *In* CA Rockwood Jr, FA Matsen III [Eds]: The Shoulder. Philadelphia, WB Saunders Co, 1990, p 18.)

variability in size. It usually arises from the anterior portion of the labrum below the superior glenohumeral ligament or from the adjacent neck of the glenoid region, and it inserts just medial to the lesser tuberosity of the humerus, under the tendon of the subscapularis muscle, to which it attaches.[1, 28] When thick, the middle glenohumeral ligament can act as an important secondary restraint to anterior translation of the humeral head if the anterior portion of the inferior glenohumeral ligament is damaged.[1]

The inferior glenohumeral ligament is the main stabilizer of the abducted glenohumeral joint. Turkel and colleagues[28] described three portions of this ligament (Fig. 12–13): the superior band of the inferior glenohumeral ligament, representing the thick anterosuperior edge of the ligament; the anterior axillary pouch, representing the region between the superior band and the middle glenohumeral ligament; and the axillary pouch, representing the remainder of the capsule posterior to the superior band. O'Brien and collaborators[1, 26] introduced the term inferior glenohumeral ligament complex, consisting of an anterior band, a posterior band, and an intervening axillary pouch. This complex is a hammock-like structure originating from the glenoid

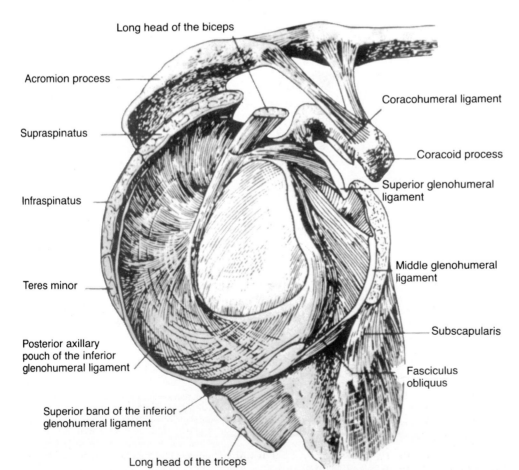

Long head of the biceps

Acromion process

Supraspinatus

Infraspinatus

Teres minor

Posterior axillary pouch of the inferior glenohumeral ligament

Superior band of the inferior glenohumeral ligament

Long head of the triceps

Coracohumeral ligament

Coracoid process

Superior glenohumeral ligament

Middle glenohumeral ligament

Subscapularis

Fasciculus obliquus

Figure 12–13

Inferior glenohumeral ligament. The anatomic description by Turkel and colleagues of the inferior glenohumeral ligament called attention to the anterior-superior edge of this ligament, which was especially thickened; they called this the superior band of the inferior glenohumeral ligament. However, there are no posterior structures defined. (Reproduced from Turkel SJ, et al: J Bone Joint Surg [Am] *63*:1208, 1981.)

labrum and inserting into the anatomic neck of the humerus.[1] The anterior band extends from the inferior aspect of the lesser tuberosity of the humerus, courses along the humeral neck, and inserts in the midanterior and inferior portions of the labrum.[656] It is seen consistently during arthroscopy, whereas the posterior band is less prominent and far more difficult to visualize on arthroscopic examination. The components of the inferior glenohumeral complex change in configuration with changes in position of the arm (Fig. 12–14): with abduction and external rotation of the arm, the anterior band fans out to support the humeral head, and the posterior band becomes cordlike; with internal rotation of the arm, the opposite occurs.[1] The anterior and posterior bands often are of equal thickness, although occasionally the posterior band is thicker than the anterior band.[1] Both contain well-organized collagen bundles, signifying their ligamentous function, whereas the

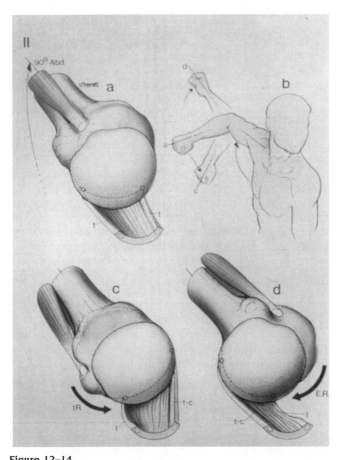

Figure 12–14
Inferior glenohumeral ligament. The inferior glenohumeral complex is tightened during abduction **(A)**. During abduction and internal or external rotation different parts of the band are tightened **(B)**. With internal rotation the posterior band fans out to support the head and the anterior band becomes cordlike or relaxed, depending on the degree of horizontal flexion or extension **(C)**. On abduction and external rotation, the anterior band fans out to support the head and the posterior band becomes cordlike or relaxed, depending on the degree of horizontal flexion or extension. **(D)**. (From O'Brien SJ, Amoczky SP, Warren RF, et al [Eds]: Developmental anatomy of the shoulder and anatomy of the glenohumeral joint. *In* CA Rockwood Jr, FA Matsen III [Eds]: The Shoulder. Philadelphia, WB Saunders Co, 1990, p 20.)

collagen in the thick axillary pouch is randomly organized.[656]

Coracohumeral Ligament

The coracohumeral ligament is the most constant area of thickening of the capsule of the glenohumeral joint. Edelson and colleagues[30] found a coracohumeral ligament in 100 per cent of 20 cadaveric shoulders, and Neer and coworkers[31] detected this ligament in 94 per cent of 63 cadaveric shoulders. The coracohumeral ligament is of variable thickness and generally is trapezoidal in shape. It arises from the lateral aspect of the coracoid process, either at its base[31] or over much of its surface.[30] The coracohumeral ligament then passes over the top of the glenohumeral joint, joining the capsule, and inserts into the greater and lesser tuberosities of the humerus, on either side of the bicipital groove.[30] It is intimate with the rotator interval between the subscapularis and supraspinatus tendons (see later discussion) and with the tendon of the long head of the biceps brachii muscle.

The function of the coracohumeral ligament is not clear. It has been regarded as a central element in the suspension of the humerus, a stabilizer of the tendon of the long head of the biceps brachii muscle, and a structure restraining external rotation of the arm (especially with the arm at the side of the torso).[30, 31] The coracohumeral ligament may prevent inferior displacement of the humeral head,[32, 33] and shortening of this ligament has been noted in cases of adhesive capsulitis of the shoulder (see later discussion).[31]

Glenoid Labrum

The glenoid labrum is a cuff of fibrous and fibrocartilaginous tissue that surrounds the glenoid cavity, serving to deepen the glenoid fossa and to allow attachment of the tendon of the long head of the biceps brachii muscle and the glenohumeral ligaments (Figs. 12–10 and 12–15). According to some investigators, most of the labrum consists of fibrous tissue with fibrocartilage present only in a small and narrow transitional zone where the capsule, the periosteum of the scapular neck, and the hyaline articular cartilage of the glenoid fossa meet.[27, 34] Other investigators, however, have emphasized the fibrocartilaginous nature of the labrum, indicating that the structure modulates from undifferentiated mesenchymal tissue to fibrocartilage during postnatal development in the first decade of life.[35]

The morphology and the capsular relationships of the glenoid labrum vary according to which portion of the structure is being studied. The inferior part of the labrum generally appears as a rounded and elevated structure that is continuous with the articular cartilage; loosening of the inferior half of the labrum is considered an abnormal finding.[34] In contrast, the superior part of the labrum tends to be meniscal and normally is more loosely attached and more mobile.[34] This normal laxity leads to diagnostic difficulty in the identification of superior labrum, anterior and posterior (SLAP) lesions (see later discussion). Posteriorly, the capsule of the

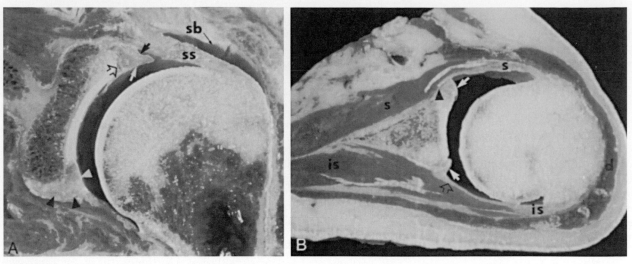

Figure 12–15

Glenohumeral joint: Labral anatomy. Coronal **(A)** and transverse **(B)** sections of an air-distended glenohumeral joint show portions of the glenoid labrum. In **A,** note the meniscus-like shape of the superior portion of the labrum (solid arrows) and the rounded appearance of the lower portion of the labrum (arrowheads). The superior portion of the labrum is separated from the adjacent articular cartilage of the glenoid cavity by a small joint recess (open arrow). No such recess is identified inferiorly. Other indicated structures in **A** are the supraspinatus tendon (ss) and a portion of the subacromial-subdeltoid bursa (sb). In **B,** the anterior and posterior portions of the labrum are seen (solid arrows). The posterior part of the joint capsule (open arrow) attaches to the labrum. Anteriorly, a type 1 capsular insertion (arrowhead) is evident (see text for details). In this midglenoid level, other indicated structures are the subscapularis muscle and tendon (s), infraspinatus muscle and tendon (is). and deltoid muscle (d).

glenohumeral joint is intimately related to the glenoid labrum along the entire posterior margin of the glenoid cavity. Anteriorly, however, variations in the relationship of the joint capsule and glenoid labrum are encountered. The anterior capsular insertions have been classified into two or three types on the basis of the proximity of the insertion site to the anterior portion of the labrum.[14, 36] In the three-part classification system, which is used throughout this chapter, a type I capsular insertion occurs close to or into the labrum, a type II capsular insertion occurs more medially, and a type III capsular insertion occurs into the scapular neck; in the two-part classification system, a type I capsular insertion occurs into the labrum, and a type II capsular insertion occurs into the scapular neck. Medial insertions of the anterior portion of the capsule (i.e., type III in the first classification system and type II in the second classification system) generally are considered less stable, perhaps causing or resulting from anterior glenohumeral joint instability. A type I capsular insertion in either classification system usually is considered more stable. The documentation of anterior capsular redundancy as a common finding in fetal glenohumeral joints, however, raises the possibility that such redundancy is a developmental variation rather than a consequence of trauma.[14] Nonetheless, categorizing the type of anterior capsular insertion on the basis of transaxial data supplied by CT and MR imaging remains popular (see later discussion).

The assessment of glenohumeral joint instability using CT and MR imaging requires analysis of the shape of the glenoid labrum in transverse sections. Complicating this assessment is the documented variability of the labral-capsular complex in the presumed normal shoulders of asymptomatic persons. Although a triangular shape of the anterior and posterior portions of the labrum often is considered evidence of a normal structure, imaging studies have confirmed normal variations in labral shape.[37, 38] In one very detailed study employing MR images of 52 shoulders in 30 asymptomatic volunteers, the anterior and posterior parts of the labra varied in shape but showed several dominant features: the anterior part of the labrum was triangular (45 per cent), round (19 per cent), cleaved (15 per cent), notched (8 per cent), flat (7 per cent), or absent (6 per cent); and the posterior part of the labrum was triangular (73 per cent), round (12 per cent), flat (6 per cent), or absent (8 per cent).[38] These findings suggest far more variability in the anterior than in the posterior portion of the glenoid labrum. Further complicating the imaging analysis of the glenoid labrum are known variations in its shape that relate to rotation of the humeral head[27] and variability in its histologic composition[35] that may lead to modifications in its signal intensity (as seen with MR imaging).

The precise role of the glenoid labrum in providing stability to the glenohumeral joint is not clear. Although a portion of the labrum frequently is detached in cases of anterior glenohumeral joint instability, leading to the designation of a detached glenoid labrum as the essential lesion responsible for the high prevalence of recurrent glenohumeral joint dislocations,[39, 40] the labrum enhances only slightly the depth of the glenoid cavity and, further, is intimately associated with other soft tissue structures (such as the inferior glenohumeral ligament complex) that appear to influence the degree of stability of the glenohumeral joint. As it is difficult to define the role of each of these structures in this regard, the designation of the anterior and posterior soft tissue structures of the glenohumeral joint as pillars, supports, or capsular mechanisms seems wise.[27, 41] The anterior capsular mechanism of the glenohumeral joint comprises the synovial membrane, anterior portion of the joint capsule including the glenohumeral ligaments, anterior portion of the glenoid labrum, scapular periosteum, subscapular recess, and subscapularis muscle and tendon; the posterior capsular mechanism consists of the posterior portion of the joint capsule, synovial membrane, posterior portion of the glenoid labrum, scapular periosteum, and posterosuperior structures of the rotator cuff (supraspinatus, infraspinatus, and teres minor muscles and tendons).[27] The anterior and posterior capsular mechanisms are separated superiorly by the coracohumeral ligament and the tendon of the long head of the biceps brachii muscle and inferiorly by the long head of the triceps muscle. A further discussion of these mechanisms is presented later in this chapter.

Rotator Cuff

The tendons of four muscles contribute to the rotator cuff of the shoulder: the supraspinatus muscle, the infraspinatus muscle, the teres minor muscle, and the subscapularis muscle (Fig. 12–16).

The supraspinatus muscle arises from the supraspinatus fossa (i.e., above the spine of the scapula) and overlying fascia, and it extends laterally over the humeral head. It ends as a tendon that inserts into the

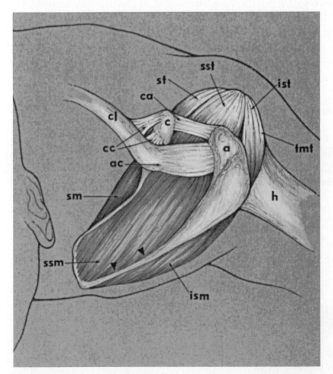

Figure 12–16
Rotator cuff: Normal anatomy—Superior view of the rotator cuff and related structures. Identified structures (beginning at the top and continuing in a clockwise direction) are the supraspinatus tendon (sst), infraspinatus tendon (ist), teres minor tendon (tmt), infraspinatus muscle (ism), supraspinatus muscle (ssm), subscapularis muscle (sm), acromioclavicular ligament (ac), coracoclavicular ligament (cc), coracoacromial ligament (ca), and subscapularis tendon (st). Also identified are the clavicle (cl), coracoid process (c), acromion (a), humerus (h), and spine of the scapula (arrowheads).

uppermost facet in the greater tuberosity in common with the infraspinatus tendon posteriorly and the coracohumeral ligament anteriorly.[42] The tendon forms centrally within the muscle belly and, as it extends laterally, assumes a more anterior position with respect to the muscle fibers (see later discussion). The thick, triangular infraspinatus muscle originates from the infraspinatus fossa (i.e., below the spine of the scapula), overlying fascia, and spine of the scapula. The muscle fibers converge to form a single tendon or multiple tendons, which pass across the posterior aspect of the capsule of the glenohumeral joint to insert on the middle facet in the greater tuberosity of the humerus. A bursa may exist between the tendon and the joint capsule. The teres minor muscle is narrow and elongated, and it arises from the middle portion of the lateral border of the scapula and the dense fascia of the infraspinatus muscle. Its tendon is united with the inferior, posterior surface of the capsule of the glenohumeral joint, and it inserts into the lowest of the three facets in the greater tuberosity of the humerus and directly into the humerus just below this facet. More medially, the quadrilateral space is evident between the teres minor and teres major muscles; the posterior humeral circumflex artery and axillary nerve pass through this space. The subscapularis muscle is large and triangular, and it arises from the medial portion of the subscapular fossa on the anterior surface of the scapula. The subscapularis muscle extends laterally, and its muscle fibers are converted into a tendon that attaches to the lesser tuberosity of the humerus. Close to this site of attachment, the transverse humeral ligament extends between the greater and lesser tuberosities of the humerus. The tendon of the subscapularis muscle is separated from the neck of the scapula by the large subscapular bursa, which communicates with the glenohumeral joint through apertures in the joint capsule (see previous discussion).

These four components of the rotator cuff—the supraspinatus, infraspinatus, teres minor, and subscapularis muscles—are important stabilizers of the glenohumeral joint, channeling the motion of the joint and preventing excessive sliding at the joint. These muscles are involved in the initial phases of abduction of the arm.[43] When intact, the rotator cuff muscles also counteract the superior translational force produced by the action of the deltoid muscle. Furthermore, these muscles reinforce the superior (supraspinatus and infraspinatus muscles), posterior (infraspinatus and teres minor muscles), and anterior (subscapularis muscle) portions of the capsule of the glenohumeral joint. The infraspinatus muscle prevents posterior subluxation of the humeral head with internal rotation of the arm and anterior subluxation of the humeral head with external rotation and abduction of the arm; the teres minor muscle is an external rotator of the humerus and is important in controlling glenohumeral joint stability in an anterior direction; and the subscapularis muscle functions as an internal rotator of the humerus, as a stabilizer preventing anterior subluxation of the humeral head, and as a depressor of the humeral head.[42]

Although the rotator cuff consists of four muscles and their tendons with individual functions, the coordinated

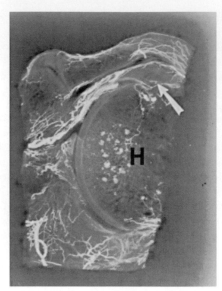

Figure 12–17

Rotator cuff: Normal hypovascular zone of the supraspinatus tendon. A radiograph of a coronal section of a cadaveric shoulder, obtained after the use of a modified Spalteholz technique to delineate the blood supply of the rotator cuff, reveals a critical zone of relative avascularity in the outer portion of the supraspinatus tendon (arrow) in which tears usually occur. H, Humeral head.

action of these structures is required to maintain joint stability. Electromyographic studies have documented that all four muscles of the rotator cuff are active during movement of the glenohumeral joint but with varying force.[44] One cadaveric investigation has shown that, of the four, the subscapularis muscle is the most powerful, followed, in order of decreasing strength, by the infraspinatus, supraspinatus, and teres minor muscles.[45] Although results from other studies have provided similar data,[46] information derived from a limited number of cadaveric specimens may not be applicable to living patients. Furthermore, age-dependent changes in tendons, including those of the rotator cuff, which include mucoid degeneration tendolipomatosis, hypoxic tendinopathy, and even calcification,[47, 48] may alter the relative strengths of the rotator cuff muscles. These changes may predispose the tendon to tear and, furthermore, as described later, alter the signal intensity characteristics of the tendon when examined with MR imaging.

Although the tendons of the rotator cuff pass in front of, over, and behind the humeral head, a normal space in the cuff exists anterosuperiorly where the cuff is perforated by the coracoid process. This space has been designated the rotator interval or rotator interval capsule.[49, 50] It is triangular and located between the anterior border of the supraspinatus tendon and the superior border of the subscapularis tendon. The base of the interval is the coracoid process, and the apex of the interval is the transverse humeral ligament at the intertubercular sulcus of the humerus.[50] Capsular tissue bridges this space. The coracohumeral and superior glenohumeral ligaments are important structures within the rotator interval. The fibers of the joint capsule and superior glenohumeral ligament blend together and insert into the borders of the supraspinatus and subscapularis tendons, the transverse humeral ligament, and the greater and lesser tuberosities of the humerus.[50] The tendon of the long head of the biceps brachii muscle also is intimate with this interval. The rotator interval, with its supporting structures, appears to play an important role in providing stability to and channeling the motion in the glenohumeral joint.[49, 50]

Six arteries contribute regularly to the vascular supply of the tendons of the rotator cuff: the suprascapular, anterior circumflex humeral, posterior circumflex humeral, thoracoacromial, suprahumeral, and subscapular arteries.[1, 51] Approximately two thirds of shoulders reveal a hypovascular zone in the supraspinatus tendon just proximal to its insertion (Fig. 12–17); less commonly, the infraspinatus and the subscapularis tendons reveal similar zones of hypovascularity.[1] A deficiency of blood flow to the supraspinatus tendon has commonly but not uniformly[52] been regarded as important in the pathogenesis of its rupture.

Coracoacromial Arch

The coracoacromial arch is intimate with portions of the rotator cuff, with the tendon of the long head of the biceps brachii muscle, and with the subacromial bursa. It consists of the coracoacromial ligament, the coracoid process, and the acromion (Fig. 12–18). Abnormalities of any of the structures of the arch and of the acromioclavicular joint can lead to impingement on the adjacent soft tissue structures, particularly the rotator cuff, a situation designated the shoulder impingement syndrome.

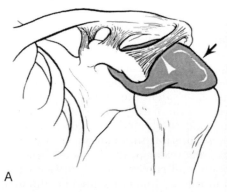

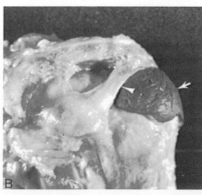

Figure 12–18

Coracoacromial arch: Normal anatomy.

A Drawing shows the coracoacromial arch, consisting of the coracoid process anteriorly, the acromion posteriorly, and the intervening coracoacromial ligament (arrowhead). Note the intimate relationship between this arch and the subacromial-subdeltoid bursa (arrow).

B An anterior view of a dissected shoulder reveals the coracoacromial ligament (arrowhead) and a latex-filled subacromial-subdeltoid bursa (arrow).

The coracoacromial ligament is a strong and triangular band that forms part of the roof of the glenohumeral joint. It extends from the edge of the acromion, anterior to the articular surface of the acromioclavicular joint, to the lateral border of the coracoid process of the scapula. The coracoacromial ligament may be uniform in composition or consist of two marginal bands and less dense intervening tissue. In some instances, prominent separate bands of tissue create a distinctive bipartite appearance to the ligament.[657] A tendon of the pectoralis minor muscle occasionally may pass between the marginal bands of this ligament. The coracoacromial ligament is firm and unyielding,[53] and it generally is regarded as an important cause of the shoulder impingement syndrome (see later discussion).

The coracoid process of the scapula projects from the head of the scapula in an anterior and lateral direction. It serves as a site of origin of the tendons of the short head of the biceps brachii muscle and of the coracobrachialis muscle and as the site of insertion of the tendon of the pectoralis minor muscle and the coracoacromial and coracoclavicular ligaments. The space between the coracoid process and the humeral head varies somewhat in size, although the coracohumeral interval is smallest in internal rotation and forward flexion of the arm.[42] One form of the shoulder impingement syndrome appears to relate to encroachment of the lesser tuberosity of the humerus on the coracoid process, a situation that can be aggravated by developmental or acquired conditions (e.g., coracoid fractures, fractures of the lesser tuberosity of the humerus, calcification within the subscapularis tendon, glenoid osteotomy, and surgical procedures in which transfer of the coracoid process is accomplished).[54] Transaxial CT has been employed as a means of measurement of the lateral extent of the coracoid process and may be a useful technique in the assessment of coracohumeral impingement.[54]

The acromion projects forward from the lateral end of the scapular spine. The lateral border and tip of the acromion are the sites of origin of the middle fibers of the deltoid muscle; the acromial tip also serves as the attachment site of the coracoacromial ligament. Behind the clavicular facet of the acromion, horizontal fibers of the tendon of the trapezius muscle arise. An accessory bone, the os acromiale, may be apparent at the tip of the acromion in 1 to 15 per cent of shoulders.[55] Its relationship to the shoulder impingement syndrome and disruption of the rotator cuff is not clear (see later discussion).

Variations in the morphology of the acromion, in both the sagittal and coronal planes, have received a great deal of attention owing to their possible association with rotator cuff pathologic processes.[56, 57] Bigliani and coworkers[58] divided the profile shape (i.e., in the sagittal plane) of the acromion into three types; the undersurface of the bone was categorized as flat (type I), curved (type II), or hooked (type III) (Fig. 12–19). Reported data regarding these shapes have indicated a flat undersurface in 17 to 22 per cent of shoulders, a curved undersurface in 43 to 62 per cent of shoulders, and a hooked undersurface in 16 to 40 per cent of shoulders.[57, 58] This variation in the reported data may

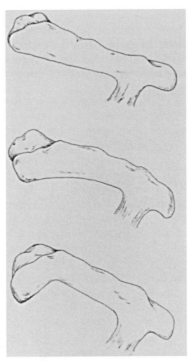

Figure 12–19
Acromion: Variations in morphology in the sagittal plane. Three variations are illustrated. The upper drawing depicts a flat undersurface; the middle drawing depicts a curved undersurface; and the lower drawing depicts a hooked undersurface of the acromion.

relate to changes in the shape of the undersurface of the acromion in its medial and lateral portions, varying degrees of angulation of the x-ray beam, or mislabeling of acromial shape when osteophytes or enthesophytes are present.[59–61] More accurate assessment of the frequency of various types of acromial morphology is provided by inspection of cadaveric scapular specimens. In one such study of 394 scapulae, type I acromions were found in 22.8 per cent, type II acromions in 68.5 per cent, and type III acromions in 8.6 per cent of specimens.[668] In this investigation, acromial morphology was symmetric (i.e., right versus left sides) in about 70 per cent of cadavers, and subacromial enthesophytes, a finding generally associated with the shoulder impingement syndrome, were encountered most commonly when a type III acromion was present. Type I acromions appear to have the lowest association with the impingement syndrome, and type III acromions appear to have the highest association with this syndrome.[58] In one study, the presence of a type III acromion also allowed identification of patients with shoulder impingement syndrome and distinguishing such patients from those with shoulder instability.[62] The slope of the acromion, a different parameter, relates to its coronal inclination as determined by an angle related to the intersection of two lines, one constructed along the inferior portion of the very anterior and posterior parts of the acromion, and the second line representing the horizontal. The importance of the slope of the acromion, as distinct from a hooked undersurface, in the pathogenesis of the shoulder impingement syndrome has been emphasized.[57] A horizontal acromion (i.e., one with a decreased slope) together with an increased length of the acromion, as well as a diminished height of the arch of the bone, leads to increased cover of the humeral head and a diminished space between the humeral head and acromion.

This interest in acromial morphology has led to the definition of the supraspinatus outlet space between the acromion and the humerus.[63] Frontal radiographs of the shoulder provide some information regarding the capaciousness of this outlet; calculations of the space between the humeral head and acromion indicate an

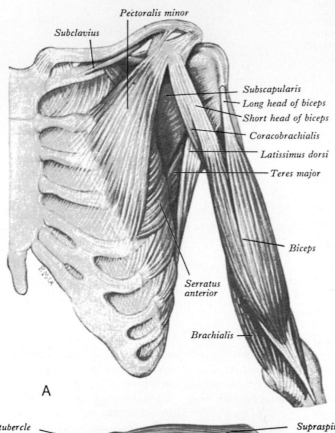

A

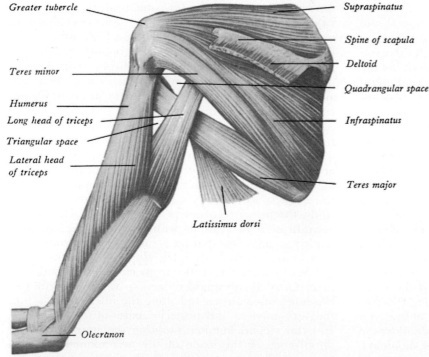

B

Figure 12–20
Deep muscles of the shoulder and upper arm: Normal anatomy.
A Anterior aspect of the shoulder.
B Posterior aspect of the shoulder.
(From Williams PL, Warwick R [Eds]: Gray's Anatomy. 36th British Ed. Edinburgh, Churchill Livingstone, 1980, pp. 537, 539.)

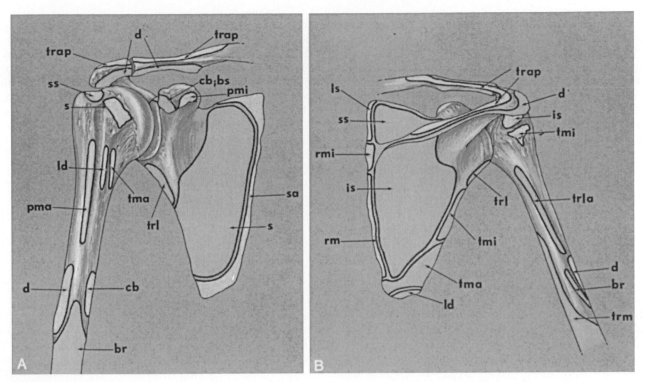

Figure 12–21
Muscles of the shoulder: Normal sites of origin and insertion. Sites of origin are depicted in darker gray, and sites of insertion in lighter gray.

A Anterior aspect of the shoulder. Identified structures (starting at the top and proceeding in a clockwise direction) are the deltoid muscle (d), trapezius muscle (trap), coracobrachialis muscle (cb), short head of the biceps brachii muscle (bs), pectoralis minor muscle (pmi), serratus anterior muscle (sa), subscapularis muscle (s), long head of the triceps muscle (trl), teres major muscle (tma), coracobrachialis muscle (cb), brachialis muscle (br), deltoid muscle (d), pectoralis major muscle (pma), latissimus dorsi muscle (ld), subscapularis muscle (s), supraspinatus muscle (ss), and trapezius muscle (trap).

B Posterior aspect of the shoulder. Identified structures (starting at the top and proceeding in a clockwise direction) are the trapezius muscle (trap), deltoid muscle (d), infraspinatus muscle (is), teres minor muscle (tmi), lateral head of the triceps muscle (tria), deltoid muscle (d), brachialis muscle (br), medial head of the triceps muscle (trm), long head of the triceps muscle (trl), teres minor muscle (tmi), teres major muscle (tma), latissimus dorsi muscle (ld), rhomboideus major muscle (rm), infraspinatus muscle (is), rhomboideus minor muscle (rmi), supraspinatus muscle (ss), and levator scapulae muscle (ls).

average measurement of 9 or 10 mm (6.6 to 13.8 mm in men and 7.1 to 11.9 mm in women).[7] An anteroposterior radiograph of the shoulder made with the patient erect and with a 30 degree caudal tilt of the x-ray beam has been found helpful in assessment of the supraspinatus outlet.[64, 65] Lateral radiographs of the scapula obtained with approximately 10 degrees of caudal angulation of the x-ray tube in a medial to lateral direction (the supraspinatus outlet view) also are useful in the analysis of this space.[58, 63]

Muscles

The muscles about the shoulder are numerous and complex, and their anatomy has been well described by Jobe.[42] A brief summary of this anatomy follows. These muscles can be divided into scapulothoracic muscles, glenohumeral (or scapulohumeral) muscles, and multiple joint muscles[42] (Figs. 12–20 and 12–21).

The scapulothoracic muscles include the trapezius, the rhomboideus major and minor, the levator scapulae, the serratus anterior, the pectoralis minor, and the subclavius muscles. The trapezius muscle is superficial and large. It arises from the spinous processes of the seventh cervical through twelfth thoracic vertebrae (with some

anatomic variations) and from the ligamentum nuchae and the external occipital protuberance, and this muscle inserts in the clavicle and acromion and in the spine of the scapula.[66] In combination with other muscles attaching to the scapula, the trapezius muscle elevates the lateral angle of the scapula. The rhomboid muscles arise from the spines of the second through fifth thoracic vertebrae (rhomboideus major) and those of the seventh cervical and first thoracic vertebrae (rhomboideus minor). They insert on the medial border of the scapula. The levator scapulae arises from the posterior tubercles of the transverse processes of the third and fourth cervical vertebrae and from the transverse processes of the atlas and axis. It inserts distally in the upper medial border of the scapula. Either alone or in combination with other scapular muscles, the rhomboids and the levator scapulae muscles control the position of the scapula during active movements of the arm. The serratus anterior muscle takes origin from the upper eight or nine ribs and passes laterally to attach to the superior and inferior angles and medial border of the scapula. The serratus anterior muscle protracts the scapula and participates in upward rotation of this bone.[42] The pectoralis minor muscle arises from the anterior surface of the second through fifth ribs (with some anatomic variations), and it inserts into the base of the coracoid process of the scapula. Aberrant slips of this muscle also may attach to the clavicle, humerus, and glenoid cavity and other portions of the scapula. Working with other scapular muscles, the pectoralis minor aids in forward movement and rotation of this bone. Finally, the subclavius muscle usually does not attach to the scapula but is involved indirectly in assisting scapulothoracic motion.[42] It arises from the first rib and its costal cartilage and attaches to the inferior surface of the medial third of the clavicle. Rarely, an attachment of this muscle to the coracoid process of the scapula is evident. The subclavius muscle stabilizes the sternoclavicular joint.

The glenohumeral (or scapulohumeral) muscles are the deltoid, teres major, coracobrachialis, and the components of the rotator cuff (supraspinatus, infraspinatus, teres minor, and subscapularis) described earlier in this chapter. The deltoid muscle is large and consists of three major portions: the anterior portion arises from the lateral third of the clavicle; the middle portion arises from the acromion; and the posterior portion arises from the spine of the scapula.[42] All portions of the deltoid muscle insert as a prominent tendon in the deltoid tuberosity on the lateral surface of the humerus. Individual portions of the deltoid muscle or the entire muscle are involved in most movements of the arm with the exception, perhaps, of medial and lateral rotation. The deltoid muscle accounts for 60 per cent of strength in horizontal abduction of the arm, but this muscle has limited leverage in the first 30 degrees of abduction,[42] during which its action is mainly one of upward traction (which is counteracted by various components of the rotator cuff). The teres major muscle arises from the posterolateral surface of the scapula, and it inserts along with the tendon of the latissimus dorsi muscle adjacent to the medial margin of the intertubercular sulcus of the humerus. The function of this muscle is to internally rotate, adduct, and extend the arm. The coracobrachialis muscle arises from the apex of the coracoid process, in common with the origin of the short head of the biceps brachii muscle, and it inserts on the anteromedial surface of the midportion of the humerus. The coracobrachialis muscle is involved in flexion and adduction of the arm.

The last category of muscles, multiple joint muscles, performs action on the glenohumeral joint and one other joint, most commonly the scapulothoracic joint.[42] The pectoralis major, latissimus dorsi, biceps brachii, and triceps brachii muscles fall in this category. The pectoralis major muscle arises from the anterior surface of the medial margin of the clavicle and the anterior surface of the sternum, the upper costal cartilages, and the aponeurosis of the obliquus externus abdominis muscle. The pectoralis major muscle attaches to the lateral edge of the intertubercular groove of the humerus. Its various components, or the muscle as a whole, are involved in adduction and internal rotation of the humerus. The latissimus dorsi muscle originates from the dorsal spines of the seventh thoracic through fifth lumbar vertebrae, iliac crest, and sacrum. It inserts into the medial margin and floor of the intertubercular sul-

cus. Actions of this muscle are internal rotation and adduction of the humerus and extension of the shoulder. The biceps brachii muscle is actively involved in elbow motion. Its long head arises from the supraglenoid tubercle atop the glenoid cavity where it is continuous with the superior portion of the glenoid labrum; its short head arises from the tip of the coracoid process of the scapula. Anatomic studies have indicated some variability in the attachment site of the tendon of the long head of the biceps brachii muscle, however.[67] In approximately 50 per cent of cadavers, this tendon arises directly from the superoposterior portion of the labrum or, less commonly, the superoanterior and superoposterior portions of the labrum, and in the remainder of cadavers, it arises from the supraglenoid tubercle.[67] The tendon of the long head of the biceps brachii muscle extends laterally above the head of the humerus, enclosed in a synovial sheath, passes behind the transverse humeral ligament, and exits the joint in the intertubercular sulcus. The bicipital tendon is kept within this sulcus by the transverse humeral ligament. This tendon acts as a stabilizer of the humeral head during abduction of the shoulder in the plane of the scapula.[68] The biceps muscle also is involved in flexion and supination at the elbow. The long head of the triceps muscle originates from the infraglenoid tubercle of the scapula, where it is intimately related to the inferior portion of the glenoid labrum and the joint capsule, and the lateral and medial heads of the triceps muscle arise from the posterior surface of the humeral shaft. The distal attachment site and action at the elbow of the triceps muscle are discussed in Chapter 13.

FUNCTION

Proper shoulder function requires the coordinated activity of numerous and complex structures. Unlike the hip and knee, the shoulder is a non–weight-bearing joint, but it is one that is load bearing owing to the significant forces that traverse it. For example, when the arm is held in 90 degrees of abduction, the joint reaction force equals about 90 per cent of body weight, and such force increases with overhead lifting, with throwing, and when weight is added to the hand.[69] Shoulder motion occurs at four separate sites: sternoclavicular joint, acromioclavicular joint, glenohumeral joint, and scapulothoracic "joint."[70] Of these sites, the glenohumeral joint represents the central core of shoulder motion, the great three-dimensional mobility exhibited by this joint being the product of the relatively incongruous articular surfaces and a surrounding soft tissue envelope that provides both dynamic active and varying degrees of passive stability without restricting joint motion.[70] The static (or passive) stabilizers of the joint are the articular surfaces and the capsular complexes (which include the labrum and ligaments); the dynamic (or active) stabilizers of the joint are the muscles, particularly those of the rotator cuff and the scapular rotators (trapezius, serratus anterior, rhomboids, and levator scapulae).[70] The existence of a reflex arc from mechanoreceptors within the glenohumeral joint capsule to muscles crossing the joint underscores the presence of a synergism between these passive and active stabilizers.[71]

The three basic patterns of shoulder motion are elevation, internal and external rotation, and horizontal flexion and extension.[72] Shoulder elevation can be defined in three planes: sagittal (flexion), scapular (neutral), and coronal (abduction).[70, 72] Elevation of the shoulder is limited to about 60 degrees.[70] Sagittal plane elevation is restricted by capsular torsion and coronal plane elevation by impingement of the greater tuberosity of the humerus on the acromion. Internal and external rotation of the shoulder occurs mainly at the glenohumeral joint, and the extent of such rotation depends on the degree of elevation of the arm.[70] With the arm at the side, the maximum arc of rotation is about 180 degrees (with external rotation being greater than internal rotation); at 90 degrees of abduction of the arm, this maximum arc is about 120 degrees (with internal rotation being greater than external rotation). Horizontal flexion and extension also occur mainly at the glenohumeral joint. The maximum arc of flexion-extension is about 180 degrees, motion being limited by the humeral articular surface.[70]

The scapulothoracic joint is not a true joint but rather represents the movement of the scapula on the posterior surface of the thoracic cage. Although scapular motion can occur independently, it normally occurs as an integral component of overall shoulder motion.[70] Approximately two thirds of full overhead shoulder motion occurs at the glenohumeral joint and one third at the scapulothoracic joint.[69] Scapular movement during shoulder elevation is complex, however, and depends (in part) on elevation of the clavicle at the sternoclavicular joint and rotation of the clavicle at the acromioclavicular joint.

IMAGING TECHNIQUES

Routine Radiography

Although advanced imaging methods often are applied to the assessment of internal derangements of the shoulder region, routine radiography plays a fundamental role in this assessment. Unfortunately, however, disagreement exists regarding the specific radiographic projections that should be employed for studying the shoulder.

With regard to the glenohumeral joint, anteroposterior radiographs of the upper part of the humerus usually are obtained in external and internal rotation of the arm. Neither of these projections is a true anteroposterior radiograph of the scapula. A true anteroposterior radiograph of the scapula is obtained with the patient in a 40 degree posterior oblique position. In evaluating the shoulder after trauma, an additional radiograph at approximately right angles to the frontal radiographs is mandatory to determine the relative positions of the humeral head and glenoid. An axillary projection is particularly useful, although it may be difficult to acquire in patients with fractures and disloca-

tions about the shoulder. A transthoracic projection has been used in some patients, but it may be difficult to interpret. The most favorable view makes use of a true lateral projection of the scapula which is acquired with the patient in a 60 degree anterior oblique position.

Several different radiographic projections have been described to evaluate patients with previous anterior dislocations of the glenohumeral joint. These radiographs are used to delineate a typical compression fracture of the posterolateral aspect of the humeral head, the Hill-Sachs lesion, which is associated with such dislocations, and include an angulated internal rotation projection, Hermodsson's tangential projection, the "notch" view of Stryker, and the Didiee view. A West Point projection also is described.

With regard to the acromioclavicular joint, radiographs obtained in the frontal projection with cephalad tilt of the incident beam of approximately 15 degrees are employed. Stress radiographs frequently are necessary to diagnose acromioclavicular joint subluxation and dislocation. Adequate radiographs of the sternoclavicular joints are difficult to obtain. Many special views have been recommended. The Hobbs view, a superoinferior projection of the sternoclavicular joint, and lordotic projection may both be helpful, particularly in evaluating a patient with a possible dislocation of the sternoclavicular joint. One additional view, the Heinig view, also can document dislocation of this joint.

Arthrography

Two basic techniques have been advocated for glenohumeral joint arthrography: single contrast and double contrast examinations.[73–87] Modifications of these techniques, including digital arthrography and conventional and computed arthrotomography, are necessary in certain situations (see later discussion). The proponents of the double contrast technique observe that, with this technique, the width of the rotator cuff tear and the integrity of cuff tendons can be assessed, allowing the surgeon to plan the operative technique more accurately. Furthermore, the internal structures of the joint, including the glenoid labrum, are better identified.

With either technique, contrast material normally is identified between the humeral head and the glenoid (Fig. 12–22). In external rotation, the contrast substance ends abruptly laterally at the anatomic neck of the humerus. In this view, an axillary pouch may be opacified on the undersurface of the humeral head. In internal rotation, a prominent subscapular recess is observed overlying the glenoid and lateral scapular region. The axillary and subscapular recesses are not a continuous sac, as a definite indentation is observed between them. The tendon of the long head of the biceps muscle is visible as a radiolucent filling defect within the articular cavity and can be traced for a variable distance within the contrast-filled tendon sheath into the bicipital groove and along the metaphysis of the humerus.

In the axillary view, contrast material is identified between the glenoid cavity and humeral head, anterior to the scapula (subscapular recess), and within the bicip-

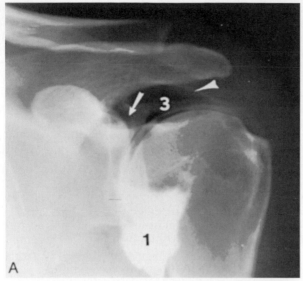

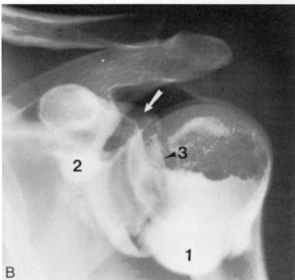

Figure 12–22
Glenohumeral joint arthrography: Normal double contrast arthrogram (upright projections).

A Normal arthrogram: External rotation. Visualized structures include the axillary pouch (1), bicipital tendon (3), glenoid fibrocartilage (arrow), and articular cartilage of the humeral head. The distended articular cavity (arrowhead) above the bicipital tendon should not be misinterpreted as filling of the subacromial (subdeltoid) bursa.

B Normal arthrogram: Internal rotation. Visualized structures include the subscapular recess (2), axillary pouch (1), bicipital tendon (3), glenoid fibrocartilage (arrow), and articular cartilage of the humeral head.

ital tendon sheath. The cartilaginous surfaces of the glenoid and humerus, as well as the glenoid labrum, are seen. In this projection, contrast material should not overlie the surgical neck of the humerus. The tangential view of the bicipital groove demonstrates an oval filling defect within the contrast-filled sheath, representing the biceps tendon.

Ultrasonography

Ultrasonography has been used successfully in the diagnosis of a number of shoulder disorders, including par-

tial and complete tears of the rotator cuff, bicipital tendon abnormalities, muscle tears, bursitis, and soft tissue masses.[88] The method is technically difficult but, once mastered, provides a relatively direct and inexpensive diagnostic test. Some of the specific applications of diagnostic ultrasonography are illustrated in appropriate sections of this chapter.

Magnetic Resonance Imaging
(Plates 12–1 through 12–10)

Although the three most common indications for MR imaging of the shoulder are related to evaluation of the rotator cuff tendons, glenohumeral joint instability, and the impingement syndrome, this method also can be employed for assessment of many other shoulder problems as well. As indicated throughout this chapter, the specific MR imaging techniques that are used are dependent on the precise indication for the examination. Generally, however, the patient is positioned supine in the magnet with the upper extremity alongside the torso in order to minimize the deleterious effects of respiratory motion transmitted to the shoulder. Typically, the arm is placed in a neutral position or is in slight external rotation, and the elbow is extended.[89] Positioning the arm in abduction and external rotation (ABER position) has been recommended as a useful technique, when combined with MR arthrography, in depicting some tears of the rotator cuff.[90] Off-center field-of-view capability is necessary because the shoulder is not easily positioned in the center of the magnetic field. Local or surface coils are necessary to obtain the signal-to-noise ratio that is required for high resolution, small field-of-view imaging.[91] Commonly used local coil designs include paired flat coils placed above and below the shoulder in a Helmholtz arrangement, a single loop coil curved to fit the contour of the shoulder, or a quadrature configuration.[91] In most cases, three imaging planes are used to study the shoulder: transaxial, coronal oblique, and sagittal oblique (Fig. 12–23). The last two are particularly helpful in assessing the rotator cuff tendons and the shoulder impingement syndrome; the transaxial plane is the best for evaluation of glenohumeral joint instability. One imaging protocol begins with a series of transaxial images from the level of the acromion to that of the inferior margin of the glenoid cavity below. This plane allows identification of a number of structures, including the glenoid labrum, glenohumeral ligaments, tendon of the long head of the biceps brachii muscle, and bony contour of the glenoid cavity and humeral head. Supplements to the transaxial images include, in some cases, filming in positions of internal and external rotation of the humerus and oblique transaxial scanning in the ABER postion.[91] From the transaxial MR images, the proper orientations of the coronal oblique images (i.e., approximately parallel to the long axis of the supraspinatus tendon, along the coronal axis of the scapula) and the sagittal oblique images (i.e., perpendicular to the long axis of the supraspinatus tendon and to the coronal axis of the scapula) can be ascertained. The coronal oblique MR images

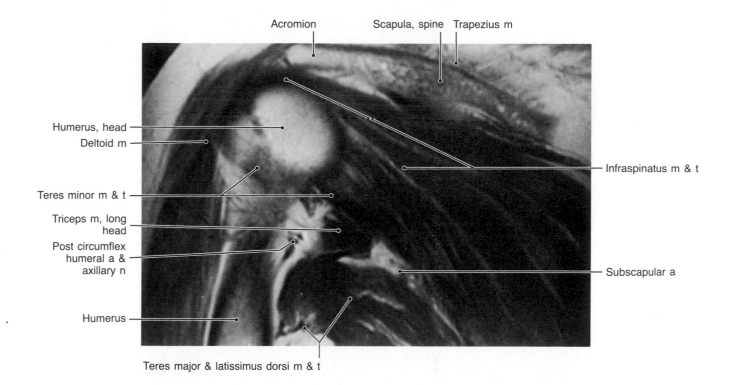

Acromion   Scapula, spine   Trapezius m

Humerus, head —

Deltoid m —

Teres minor m & t —

Triceps m, long
head —

Post circumflex
humeral a &
axillary n —

Humerus —

Infraspinatus m & t

Subscapular a

Teres major & latissimus dorsi m & t

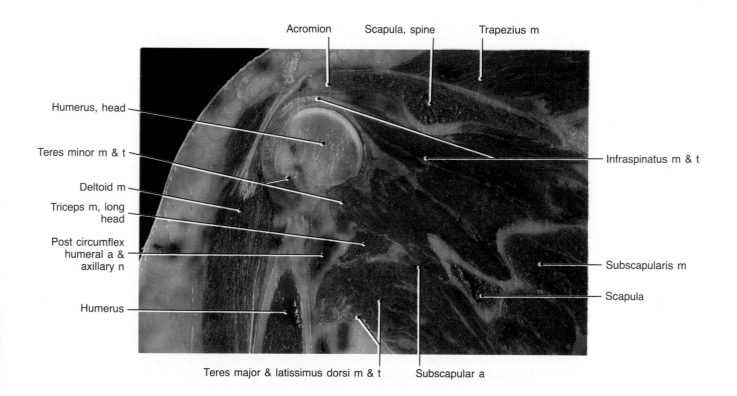

Acromion   Scapula, spine   Trapezius m

Humerus, head —

Teres minor m & t —

Deltoid m —

Triceps m, long
head —

Post circumflex
humeral a &
axillary n —

Humerus —

Infraspinatus m & t

Subscapularis m

Scapula

Teres major & latissimus dorsi m & t   Subscapular a

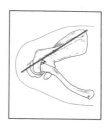

PLATE 12–1

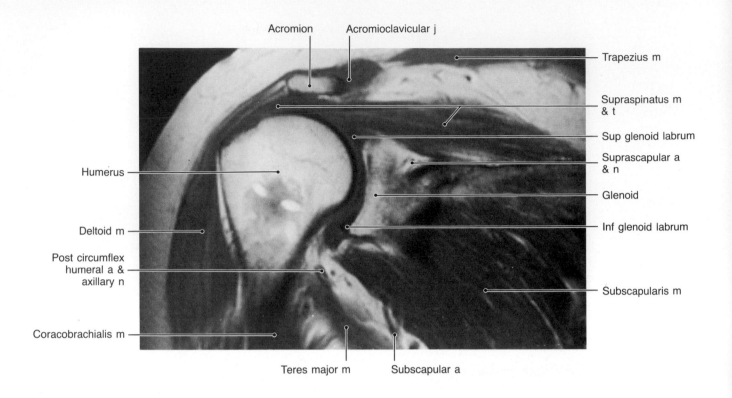

Acromion   Acromioclavicular j

Trapezius m

Supraspinatus m & t

Sup glenoid labrum

Suprascapular a & n

Glenoid

Inf glenoid labrum

Humerus

Deltoid m

Post circumflex humeral a & axillary n

Coracobrachialis m

Subscapularis m

Teres major m   Subscapular a

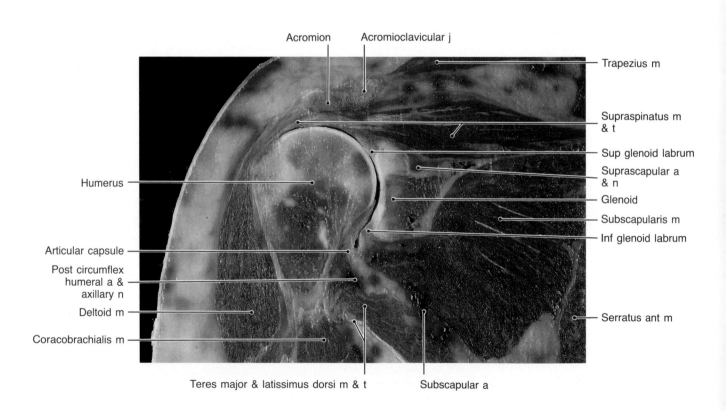

Acromion   Acromioclavicular j

Trapezius m

Supraspinatus m & t

Sup glenoid labrum

Suprascapular a & n

Glenoid

Subscapularis m

Inf glenoid labrum

Humerus

Articular capsule

Post circumflex humeral a & axillary n

Deltoid m

Coracobrachialis m

Serratus ant m

Teres major & latissimus dorsi m & t   Subscapular a

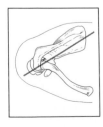

PLATE 12–2

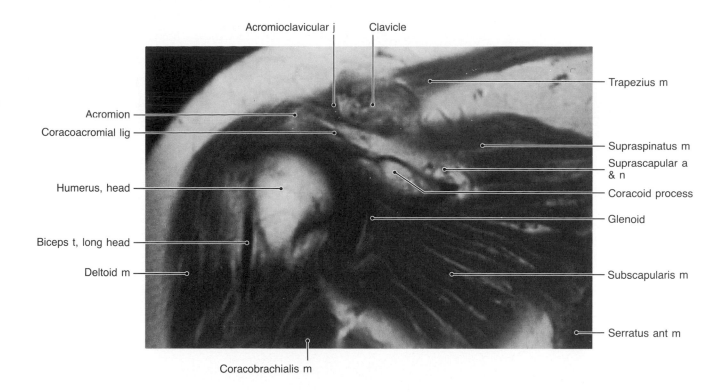

Acromioclavicular j | Clavicle | Trapezius m | Acromion | Coracoacromial lig | Supraspinatus m | Suprascapular a & n | Coracoid process | Humerus, head | Glenoid | Biceps t, long head | Deltoid m | Subscapularis m | Serratus ant m | Coracobrachialis m

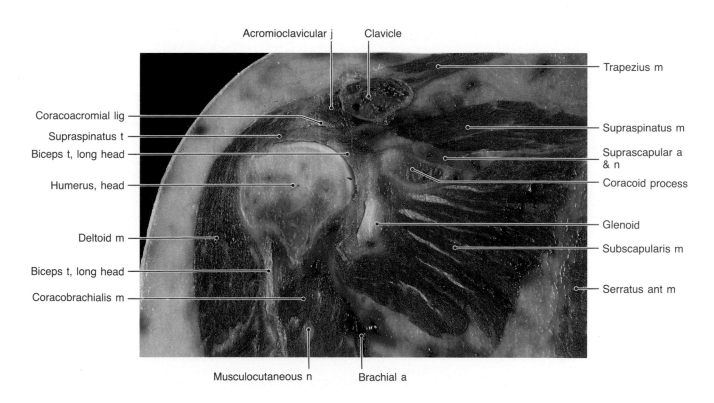

Acromioclavicular j | Clavicle | Trapezius m | Coracoacromial lig | Supraspinatus t | Supraspinatus m | Biceps t, long head | Suprascapular a & n | Humerus, head | Coracoid process | Deltoid m | Glenoid | Biceps t, long head | Subscapularis m | Coracobrachialis m | Serratus ant m | Musculocutaneous n | Brachial a

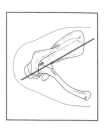

PLATE 12–3

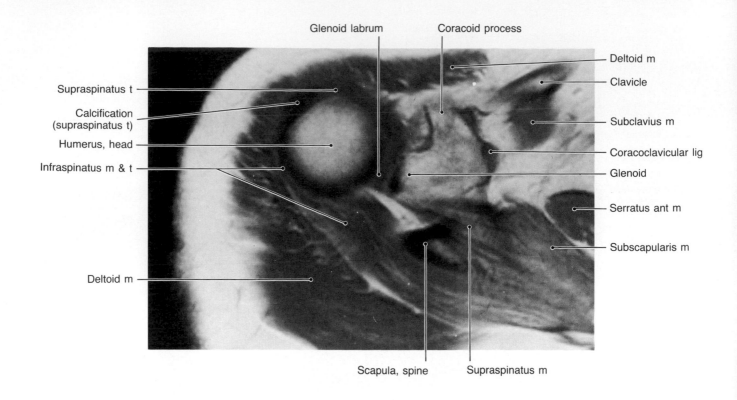

Glenoid labrum   Coracoid process

Supraspinatus t

Calcification
(supraspinatus t)

Humerus, head

Infraspinatus m & t

Deltoid m

Deltoid m

Clavicle

Subclavius m

Coracoclavicular lig

Glenoid

Serratus ant m

Subscapularis m

Scapula, spine   Supraspinatus m

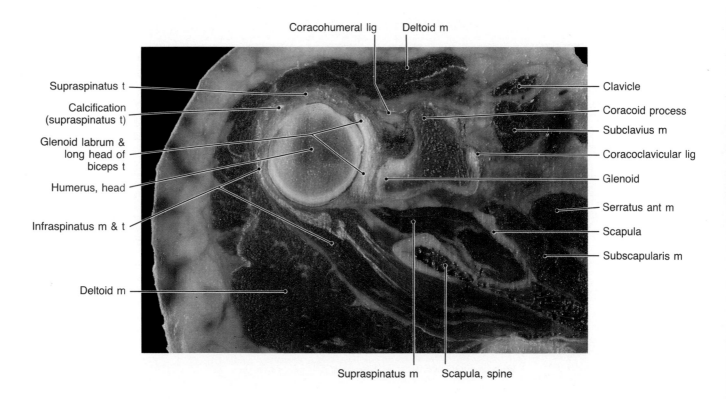

Coracohumeral lig   Deltoid m

Supraspinatus t

Calcification
(supraspinatus t)

Glenoid labrum &
long head of
biceps t

Humerus, head

Infraspinatus m & t

Deltoid m

Clavicle

Coracoid process

Subclavius m

Coracoclavicular lig

Glenoid

Serratus ant m

Scapula

Subscapularis m

Supraspinatus m   Scapula, spine

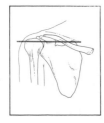

PLATE 12-4

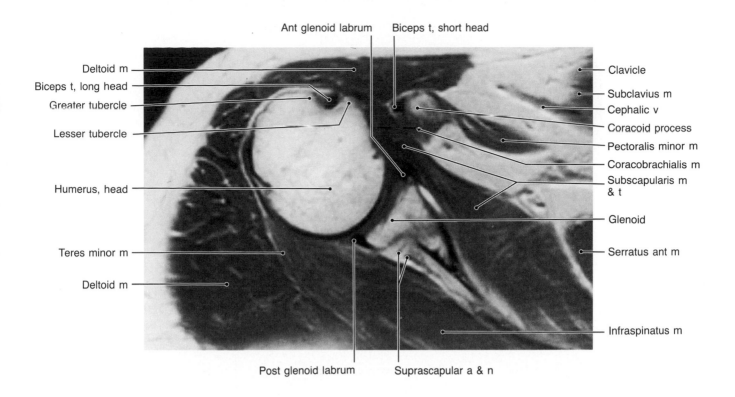

Ant glenoid labrum Biceps t, short head

Deltoid m

Biceps t, long head

Greater tubercle

Lesser tubercle

Humerus, head

Teres minor m

Deltoid m

Clavicle

Subclavius m

Cephalic v

Coracoid process

Pectoralis minor m

Coracobrachialis m

Subscapularis m & t

Glenoid

Serratus ant m

Infraspinatus m

Post glenoid labrum Suprascapular a & n

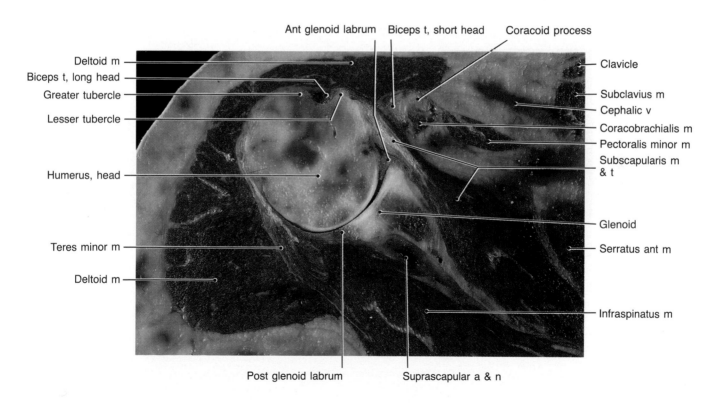

Ant glenoid labrum Biceps t, short head Coracoid process

Deltoid m

Biceps t, long head

Greater tubercle

Lesser tubercle

Humerus, head

Teres minor m

Deltoid m

Clavicle

Subclavius m

Cephalic v

Coracobrachialis m

Pectoralis minor m

Subscapularis m & t

Glenoid

Serratus ant m

Infraspinatus m

Post glenoid labrum Suprascapular a & n

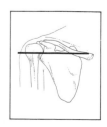

PLATE 12–5

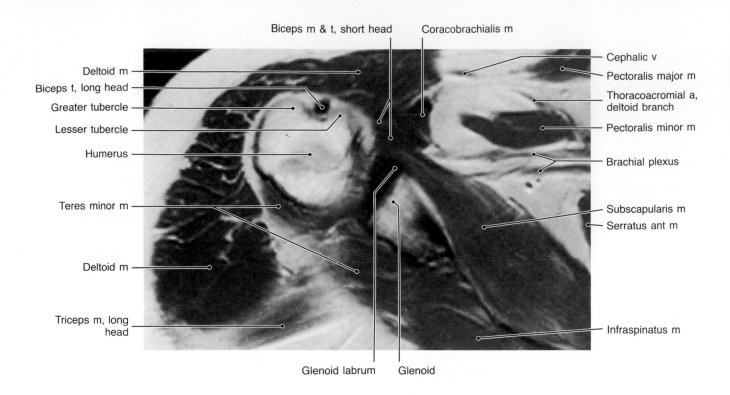

Biceps m & t, short head — Coracobrachialis m

Deltoid m

Biceps t, long head

Greater tubercle

Lesser tubercle

Humerus

Teres minor m

Deltoid m

Triceps m, long head

Cephalic v

Pectoralis major m

Thoracoacromial a, deltoid branch

Pectoralis minor m

Brachial plexus

Subscapularis m

Serratus ant m

Infraspinatus m

Glenoid labrum — Glenoid

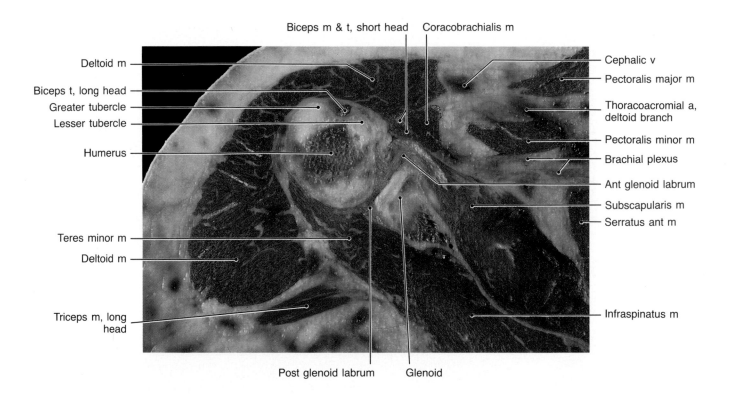

Biceps m & t, short head — Coracobrachialis m

Deltoid m

Biceps t, long head

Greater tubercle

Lesser tubercle

Humerus

Teres minor m

Deltoid m

Triceps m, long head

Cephalic v

Pectoralis major m

Thoracoacromial a, deltoid branch

Pectoralis minor m

Brachial plexus

Ant glenoid labrum

Subscapularis m

Serratus ant m

Infraspinatus m

Post glenoid labrum — Glenoid

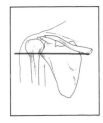

PLATE 12–6

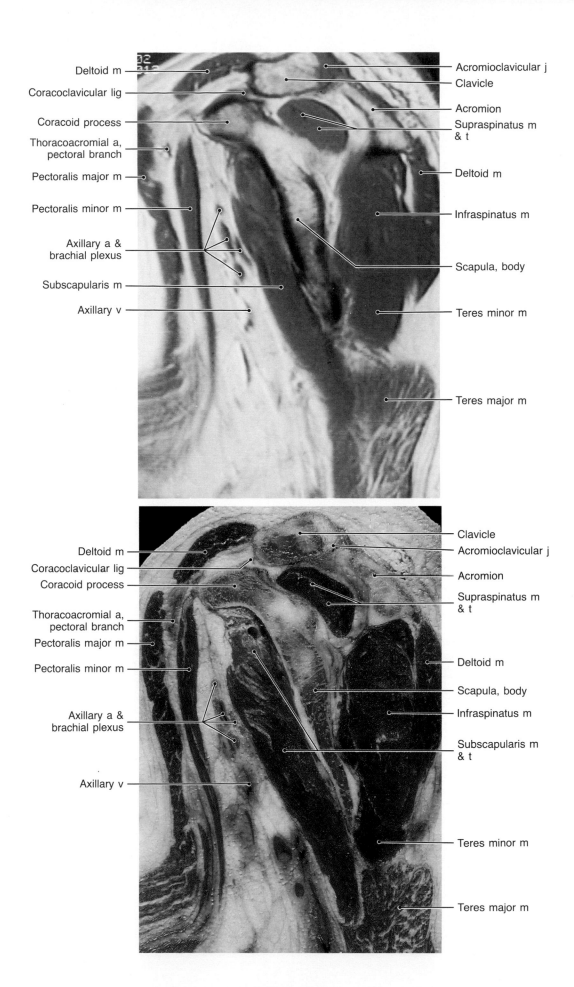

Deltoid m
Coracoclavicular lig
Coracoid process
Thoracoacromial a, pectoral branch
Pectoralis major m
Pectoralis minor m
Axillary a & brachial plexus
Subscapularis m
Axillary v

Acromioclavicular j
Clavicle
Acromion
Supraspinatus m & t
Deltoid m
Infraspinatus m
Scapula, body
Teres minor m
Teres major m

Deltoid m
Coracoclavicular lig
Coracoid process
Thoracoacromial a, pectoral branch
Pectoralis major m
Pectoralis minor m
Axillary a & brachial plexus
Axillary v

Clavicle
Acromioclavicular j
Acromion
Supraspinatus m & t
Deltoid m
Scapula, body
Infraspinatus m
Subscapularis m & t
Teres minor m
Teres major m

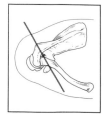

PLATE 12–7

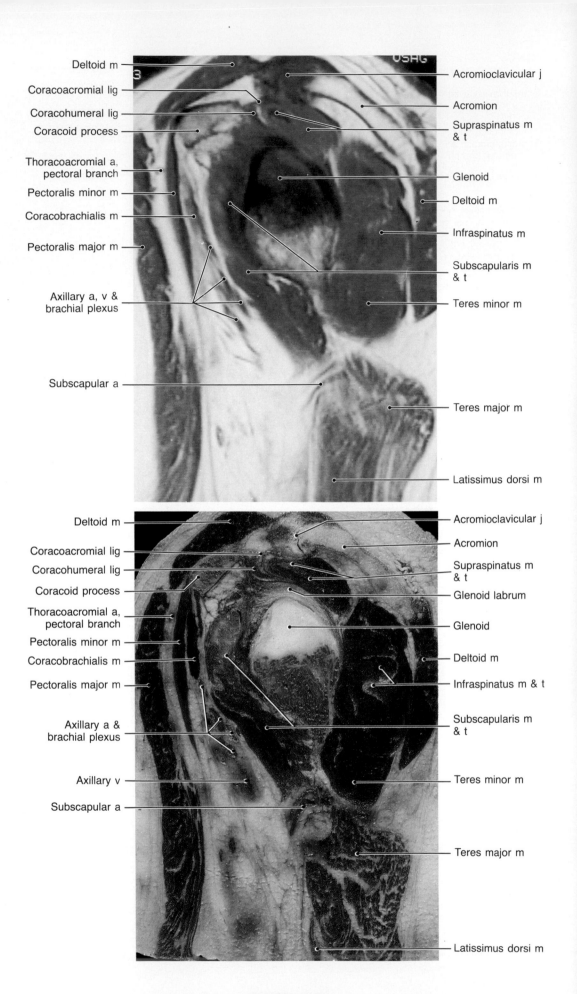

Deltoid m

Coracoacromial lig

Coracohumeral lig

Coracoid process

Thoracoacromial a,
pectoral branch

Pectoralis minor m

Coracobrachialis m

Pectoralis major m

Axillary a, v &
brachial plexus

Subscapular a

Acromioclavicular j

Acromion

Supraspinatus m
& t

Glenoid

Deltoid m

Infraspinatus m

Subscapularis m
& t

Teres minor m

Teres major m

Latissimus dorsi m

Deltoid m

Coracoacromial lig

Coracohumeral lig

Coracoid process

Thoracoacromial a,
pectoral branch

Pectoralis minor m

Coracobrachialis m

Pectoralis major m

Axillary a &
brachial plexus

Axillary v

Subscapular a

Acromioclavicular j

Acromion

Supraspinatus m
& t

Glenoid labrum

Glenoid

Deltoid m

Infraspinatus m & t

Subscapularis m
& t

Teres minor m

Teres major m

Latissimus dorsi m

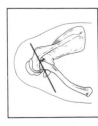

PLATE 12–8

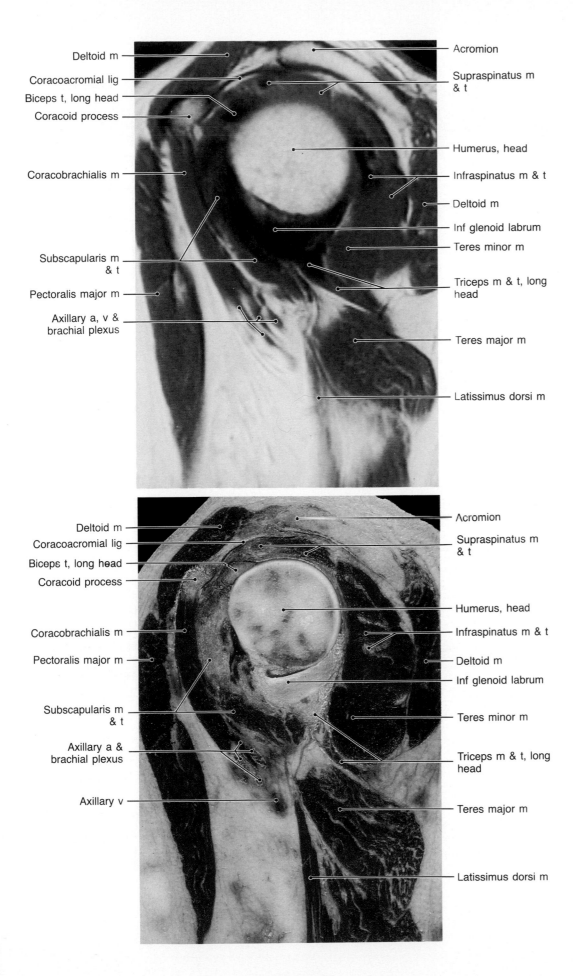

Deltoid m — Acromion

Coracoacromial lig — Supraspinatus m & t

Biceps t, long head —

Coracoid process —

Humerus, head —

Coracobrachialis m — Infraspinatus m & t

Deltoid m —

Inf glenoid labrum —

Subscapularis m & t — Teres minor m

Pectoralis major m — Triceps m & t, long head

Axillary a, v & brachial plexus —

Teres major m —

Latissimus dorsi m —

Deltoid m — Acromion

Coracoacromial lig — Supraspinatus m & t

Biceps t, long head —

Coracoid process —

Humerus, head —

Coracobrachialis m — Infraspinatus m & t

Pectoralis major m — Deltoid m

Inf glenoid labrum —

Subscapularis m & t — Teres minor m

Axillary a & brachial plexus —

Triceps m & t, long head —

Axillary v — Teres major m —

Latissimus dorsi m —

PLATE 12–9

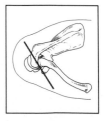

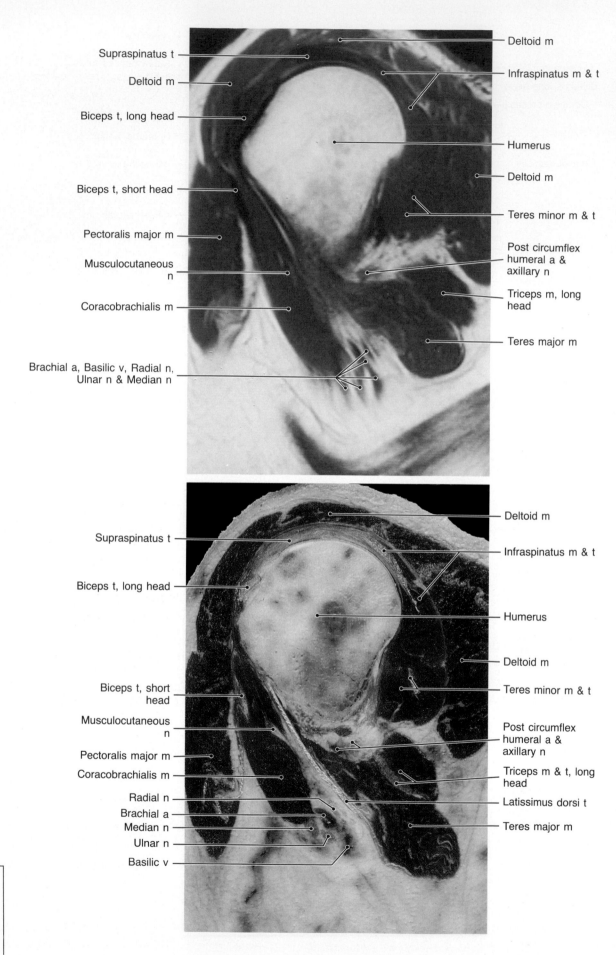

Supraspinatus t

Deltoid m

Biceps t, long head

Biceps t, short head

Pectoralis major m

Musculocutaneous n

Coracobrachialis m

Brachial a, Basilic v, Radial n, Ulnar n & Median n

Deltoid m

Infraspinatus m & t

Humerus

Deltoid m

Teres minor m & t

Post circumflex humeral a & axillary n

Triceps m, long head

Teres major m

Supraspinatus t

Biceps t, long head

Biceps t, short head

Musculocutaneous n

Pectoralis major m

Coracobrachialis m

Radial n

Brachial a

Median n

Ulnar n

Basilic v

Deltoid m

Infraspinatus m & t

Humerus

Deltoid m

Teres minor m & t

Post circumflex humeral a & axillary n

Triceps m & t, long head

Latissimus dorsi t

Teres major m

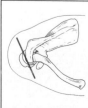

PLATE 12–10

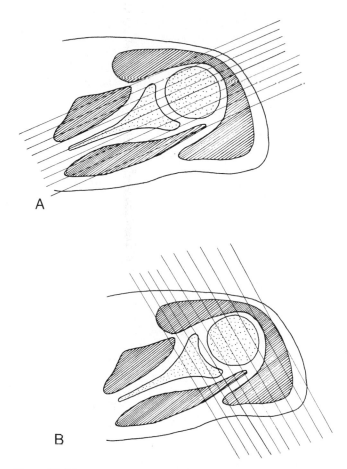

Figure 12–23

Shoulder: MR imaging—imaging planes. Three MR imaging planes usually are used to study the shoulder. The first plane is the transaxial plane from which the orientations of the coronal oblique plane (**A**) and the sagittal oblique plane (**B**) are determined. The coronal oblique plane is parallel to the long axis of the scapula and, with the arm in a neutral position, is approximately parallel to the long axis of the supraspinatus tendon. The sagittal oblique plane is perpendicular to the long axis of the scapula.

should begin anteriorly at the level of the subscapularis muscle and tendon and continue posteriorly to the level of the infraspinatus and teres minor muscles and of the quadrilateral space. The sagittal oblique MR images should extend medially from the region of the body of the scapula to a lateral location that includes the entire humeral head and its tuberosities. Together, these oblique imaging planes allow assessment of all of the components of the rotator cuff, the coracoacromial arch, the acromioclavicular joint, portions of the glenoid labrum, and the tendon of the long head of the biceps brachii muscle.[92]

The choice of pulse sequences varies according to the indications for the examination. With standard spin echo imaging, variable echo sequences with long repetition times (TR), providing proton density–weighted and T2-weighted images, usually are obtained in at least two of the imaging planes. T1-weighted spin echo MR images also are helpful, providing anatomic information about both the bone (and marrow) and soft tissues. Despite reports that indicate the benefits of using fast

spin echo MR imaging sequences (with or without fat suppression) to study the shoulder,[93] the use of these sequences remains controversial. The advantages of the fast spin echo technique include a shorter examination time (as heavily T2-weighted images can be obtained rapidly by acquiring multiple lines of k space during each TR interval), fewer artifacts related to patient motion, and greater spatial resolution (when compared to standard spin echo technique) because high-order phase encodings (which provide the majority of the spatial information in the image) are gathered earlier in the sequence, before substantial T2 decay has occurred.[94] In contrast to conventional spin echo images, fast spin echo dual-echo MR images require additional imaging time because multiple echoes are necessary to generate each set of images.[94] Furthermore, short echo time fast spin echo MR images are accompanied by blurring of anatomic structures because of underrepresentation of the high-order phase encodings, which must now be acquired later in the sequence, only after greater T2 decay.[94] Magnetization transfer effects are more pronounced with fast spin echo imaging.[91] Also, the signal intensity derived from fat remains relatively high, even on heavily T2-weighted fast spin echo MR images, which leads to diagnostic problems in the differentiation of fluid in the subacromial-subdeltoid bursa (a finding that may indicate bursitis or a full-thickness tear of the rotator cuff) and the peribursal fat plane (a normal finding); or in the identification of marrow edema, tumor, or infection. The combination of fast spin echo MR imaging and frequency-selective fat saturation based on the chemical-shift phenomenon may overcome these problems, although inhomogeneous fat suppression and loss of well-defined interfaces between muscle and fat may create new difficulties.

Gradient refocused echo (GRE) imaging sequences also have been used to study the shoulder. These sequences usually are employed in the transaxial plane in patients in whom labral abnormalities are suspected. Either two-dimensional or three-dimensional GRE MR images are obtained, the benefits of the three-dimensional imaging techniques including acquisition of very thin MR images (on the order of 1 to 1.5 mm).[95] GRE sequences, which do not employ the 180 degree radiofrequency refocusing pulse that is used with spin echo sequences, are subject to increased magnetic susceptibility effects, however. Intra-articular collections of gas (i.e., the vacuum phenomenon) may appear as circular or linear regions of low signal intensity on GRE MR images that simulate the appearance of calcification (e.g., chondrocalcinosis) or intra-articular bodies.[96] Susceptibility-induced signal loss in these images also occurs at the interface between trabecular bone and marrow, which leads to decreased sensitivity to the detection of marrow abnormalities.[91]

Short tau inversion time recovery (STIR) MR images can be used as a screening examination for the shoulder (or other regions) owing to their sensitivity in the delineation of sites of abnormality. Such abnormalities appear as areas of high signal intensity, made more obvious because of the suppression of signal intensity from adjacent fatty tissues. STIR imaging can be combined with fast spin echo techniques (i.e., fast STIR), although many of the problems associated with fast spin echo MR images (see previous discussion) may be encountered. With STIR or fast STIR imaging, anatomic detail is poor, leading to difficulty in identifying osseous and soft tissue landmarks. Slight modification in the choice of the inversion time employed for STIR imaging results in less than ideal suppression of signal intensity from fat but, also, facilitates identification of important anatomic landmarks.

As in other skeletal sites, gadolinium-containing contrast agents may be used for evaluation of disorders of the shoulder.[669] Intravenous administration of such agents is most beneficial in cases of musculoskeletal infections and tumors, although this method also provides information regarding the presence and extent of synovial inflammation. Furthermore, delayed imaging after such administration is characterized by an arthrogram-like effect, as the contrast agent leaks into the joint space. The quality of the resulting arthrogram depends on many factors, including the amount of contrast agent that is injected, the timing of the MR images, and the permeability of the synovial membrane. Movement of the shoulder facilitates intra-articular extension of the contrast agent. A superior and far more predictable arthrogram is accomplished by direct intra-articular administration of the gadolinium compound, a technique that may have value in the assessment of glenohumeral joint instability and of small full-thickness and partial-thickness (i.e., articular surface) tears of the tendons of the rotator cuff (see later discussion). Ten to 15 ml of contrast material injected into the glenohumeral joint appears to be optimal for MR arthrography.[97] Suggested modifications in technique for MR arthrography include the use of saline solution, iodinated contrast agents, or iodinated contrast agents and a gadolinium compound.[98] In general, when gadolinium compounds are employed, T1-weighted spin echo MR images combined with fat suppression are chosen. GRE MR images, however, also may be used in this situation.

Other Techniques

Radionuclide imaging, CT scanning, CT arthrography, and angiography represent additional methods that may be applied to the analysis of shoulder abnormalities.

SPECIFIC ABNORMALITIES

Shoulder Impingement Syndrome

Although he was not the first to suggest a relationship between subacromial impingement and chronic shoulder disability, Neer clarified and popularized the concept of the shoulder impingement syndrome in 1972 and is recognized as its main advocate.[99] Based on observations in scapular specimens, Neer described a characteristic bone excrescence that arose from the undersurface of the anterior portion of the acromion that he believed was caused by repeated impingement of the

rotator cuff and the humeral head with traction of the coracoacromial ligament. He emphasized the dynamic relationship between (1) the intertubercular sulcus (bicipital groove) and the insertion site of the supraspinatus tendon in the greater tuberosity, and (2) the coracoacromial arch. Neer noted that although the bicipital groove and supraspinatus tendon were located anterior to the coracoacromial arch when the arm was in the neutral position, these structures passed beneath this arch during forward flexion of the arm (Fig. 12–24). He believed that this dynamic relationship explained the occurrence of impingement of portions of the rotator cuff during movements of the arm that eventually could result in complete disruption of the rotator cuff as well as of rupture of the tendon of the long head of the biceps brachii muscle.[99–102] Three progressive stages of the shoulder impingement syndrome were described by Neer: stage 1, consisting of reversible edema and hemorrhage about the rotator cuff, typically seen in patients below the age of 25 years; stage 2, consisting of fibrosis and tendinitis in the rotator cuff, usually seen in patients between the ages of 25 and 40 years; and stage 3, consisting of tendon rupture and subacromial spurs (enthesophytes), generally evident in patients over the age of 40 years.

The basis of the shoulder impingement syndrome is the restricted space that exists between the coracohumeral arch above and the humeral head and tuberosities below. Through this space pass the tendons of the rotator cuff and, within the rotator interval, the tendon of the long head of the biceps brachii muscle and the coracohumeral ligament. The subacromial-subdeltoid bursa, consisting of two serosal surfaces lubricated by synovial fluid and surrounded by a layer of fat (peribursal fat), aids in the passage of these structures.[103] Compression of these structures also is minimized by a normal acromioclavicular joint, a shape of the coracoacromial arch that allows free passage of the subjacent cuff mechanism, and normal capsular laxity.[103] Contributing to the vulnerability of the supraspinatus tendon are the following:

1. A relatively avascular critical zone near the site of attachment of the tendon to the greater tuberosity. Compromise of blood flow to the tendon has been shown experimentally with adduction[104] and flexion[105] at the glenohumeral joint.

2. Anatomic variations in the anterior excursion and slope of the acromion and the shape of its inferior margin (see previous discussion).

3. Abnormal laxity of the capsule of the glenohumeral joint.

The large number of factors that potentially could cause shoulder impingement syndrome have led to several attempts at classification. As one example (Table 12–1), Matsen and Arntz[103] divided the causative factors into two groups: structural factors and functional factors. Structural factors relate to the acromioclavicular joint (congenital anomalies or osteophytes), acromion (alterations in shape, fractures with malunion or nonunion, os acromiale, or osteophytes), coracoid process (congenital anomalies or posttraumatic or postsurgical

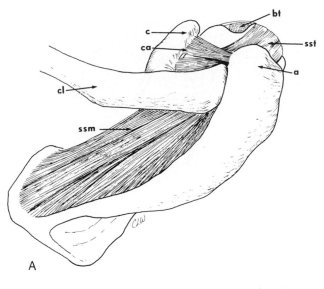

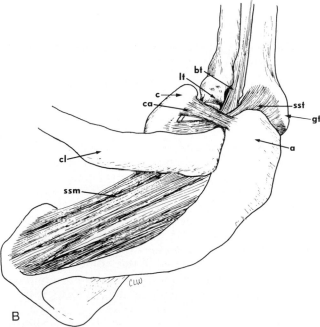

Figure 12–24

Shoulder impingement syndrome: Pathogenesis.

A Superior view of the shoulder with the arm in a neutral position. The supraspinatus tendon (sst) and the tendon of the long head of the biceps brachii muscle (bt) lie anterior to the acromion (a), acromioclavicular joint, and coracoacromial ligament (ca). The supraspinatus muscle (ssm), clavicle (cl), and coracoid process (c) also are indicated.

B Superior view of the shoulder with forward flexion of the arm. The supraspinatus tendon (sst), greater tuberosity of the humerus (gt), and tendon of the long head of the biceps brachii muscle (bt) become more intimate with the acromion (a), the acromioclavicular joint, and the coracoacromial ligament (ca). The supraspinatus muscle (ssm), coracoid process (c), clavicle (cl), and lesser tuberosity of the humerus (lt) also are indicated.

(Modified from Rockwood CA Jr: J Bone Joint Surg [Am] 75:409, 1993.)

changes), subacromial-subdeltoid bursa (inflammation, thickening, or surgical or nonsurgical foreign bodies), rotator cuff (calcification, thickening, or irregularity related to tendon tears, or postoperative or posttraumatic

scars), or humerus (congenital anomalies, fractures with malunions, or altered position of a humeral head prosthesis). Functional factors include abnormalities in position or motion of the scapula, disruption of the mechanism leading to normal depression of the humeral head, capsular laxity, and capsular stiffness (Fig. 12–25). Fu and associates[106] divided impingement syndromes into

Table 12–1. FACTORS POTENTIALLY INCREASING ROTATOR CUFF IMPINGEMENT

Structural

Acromioclavicular joint
   Congenital abnormality
   Degenerative spurs

Acromion
   Unfused (bipartite acromion)
   Abnormal shape (flat or overhanging)
   Degenerative spur
   Nonunion of fracture
   Malunion of fracture

Coracoid
   Congenital abnormality
   Posttraumatic or postsurgical change in shape or location

Bursa
   Primary inflammatory bursitis (e.g., rheumatoid arthritis)
   Chronic thickening from previous injury or inflammation or injection
   Pins, wires, sutures, and other foreign materials projecting into the bursal space

Rotator cuff
   Thickening related to chronic calcium deposits
   Thickening from retraction of partial-thickness tears
   Flaps and other irregularities of upper surface due to partial or complete tearing
   Postoperative or posttraumatic scarring

Humerus
   Congenital abnormalities or fracture malunions producing relative or absolute prominence of the greater tuberosity
   Abnormally inferior position of a humeral head prosthesis producing relative prominence of the greater tuberosity

Functional

Scapula
   Abnormal position
      Thoracic kyphosis
      Acromioclavicular separation
   Abnormal motion
      Paralysis (e.g., of trapezius)
      Fascioscapulohumeral muscular dystrophy
      Restriction of motion at the scapulothoracic joint

Loss of normal humeral head depression mechanism
   Rotator cuff weakness (e.g., suprascapular nerve palsy or C5–C6 radiculopathy)
   Rotator cuff tear (partial- or full-thickness)
   Constitutional or posttraumatic rotator cuff laxity
   Rupture of long head of biceps

Tightness of posterior shoulder capsule forcing the humeral head to rise up against the acromion during shoulder flexion

Capsular laxity

From O'Brien SJ, Amoczky SP, Warren RF, et al: Developmental anatomy of the shoulder and anatomy of the glenohumeral joint. *In* CA Rockwood Jr, FA Matsen III (Eds): The Shoulder. Philadelphia, WB Saunders Co, 1990, p. 627.)

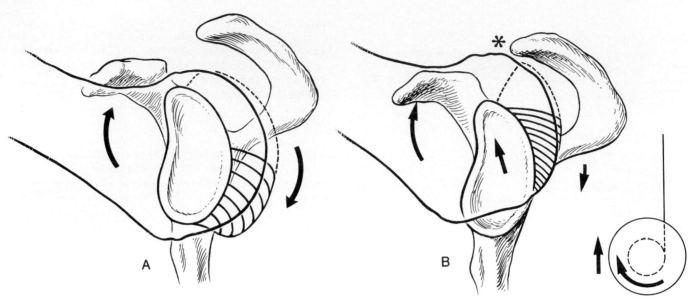

Figure 12–25
Shoulder impingement syndrome: Stiffness of the posterior glenohumeral capsule is commonly associated with signs of impingement.
A A normally lax posterior capsule allows the humeral head to remain centered in the glenoid with shoulder flexion.
B Stiffness of the posterior glenohumeral capsule will aggravate the impingement process by forcing the humeral head upward against the anteroinferior portion of the acromion as the shoulder is flexed. This upward translation in association with rotation is analogous to the action of a spinning yo-yo climbing a string.
(From Matsen FA III, Arntz CT: Subacromial impingement. *In* CA Rockwood Jr, FA Matsen III [Eds]: The Shoulder. Philadelphia, WB Saunders Co, 1990, p 628.)

two major categories: primary impingement occurring mainly in nonathletic persons and related to alterations in the coracoacromial arch; and secondary impingement occurring mainly in athletes involved in sports requiring overhead movement of the arm, and related to either glenohumeral or scapular instability. The relationship of anterior instability of the glenohumeral joint and rotator cuff impingement has been emphasized repeatedly.[107–110] Such instability results in fatigue of the components of the rotator cuff, allowing the humeral head to translate anteriorly, and mechanical impingement of the supraspinatus tendon on the coracoacromial arch may be seen. As the occurrence of the shoulder impingement syndrome implies a diminution of the space between the coracohumeral arch and the humeral head and its tuberosities, its causes are predictable, related to alterations in any of the components of the arch or humerus that serve to narrow this space or to transient malposition of the humeral head and glenoid cavity that also leads to diminution of this space. Additional factors intrinsic to the rotator cuff such as ischemia and inflammation make it more vulnerable to the impingement syndrome.

As knowledge regarding the functional anatomy of the shoulder continues to grow, the identification of additional factors important in the causation of the shoulder impingement syndrome is not surprising. As examples of this, reports have emphasized the critical role assumed by the tendon of the long head of the biceps brachii muscle as a stabilizer of the humeral head in the glenoid fossa during abduction of the shoulder in the scapular plane.[68] Not surprising, then, is the implication of lesions of this tendon as a potential cause

of the impingement syndrome.[68] Anterior (i.e., subcoracoid) and posterior subgroups of such impingement also have been emphasized. One example of the latter subgroup is the occurrence of impingement of the rotator cuff on the posterosuperior portion of the glenoid labrum in throwing athletes,[658] leading to posterior shoulder pain, associated with anterior glenohumeral joint instability, and sometimes requiring for diagnosis MR arthrography performed in the ABER position.[111–113]

The clinical manifestations of the shoulder impingement syndrome are well documented and vary with the severity of the process. Certain occupations such as tree pruning, fruit picking, grocery clerking, longshoring, carpentry, and painting or certain types of athletic activity such as throwing a ball, swimming, tennis, and skiing are common among affected patients.[103] Such patients complain of chronic shoulder pain, stiffness, and weakness, and the findings may be accentuated when the arm is flexed or internally rotated. A limited range of motion usually restricts internal rotation and adduction of the arm. Pain may be provoked by elevation of the shoulder. Matsen and Arntz[103] emphasized the clinical importance of differentiation among signs of subacromial impingement (subacromial crepitus on flexion and rotation), signs of tightness (limited range of motion), and signs of tendon involvement (atrophy, weakness, and pain or restricted motion of the shoulder). Clinical tests for mechanical impingement of the shoulder have been described.[99, 108, 114, 115] Most of these relate to patterns of subacromial contact influenced by the excursion of the rotator cuff under the acromion that takes place during movement of the arm[116] and to the occurrence of pain during forward flexion and internal rotation of the arm. A painful arc exists between 60 degrees and 120 degrees of shoulder abduction. In general, these various clinical manifestations increase as the stage of the process increases.[114] Injection of local anesthetic agents into the subacromial space may lead to relief of pain in patients with the impingement syndrome.

Routine radiography plays a minor diagnostic role in the evaluation of patients with early clinical stages of shoulder impingement. Nonspecific sclerosis and cyst formation in the greater tuberosity or osteoarthritis of the acromioclavicular joint may be seen. This last finding, although of value in defining a possible cause of the shoulder impingement syndrome, is not diagnostic of this syndrome. Similarly, evidence of calcific tendinitis and loss of the peribursal fat plane does not allow a specific diagnosis of the shoulder impingement syndrome. Evaluation of the subacromial space may require angulated frontal and lateral radiographs of the shoulder (see earlier discussion).

A highly specific but late radiographic manifestation of the shoulder impingement syndrome is an anterior acromial enthesophyte (Fig. 12–26).[117–119] This enthesophyte may be apparent on routine anteroposterior radiographs of the shoulder (Fig. 12–27) or on those obtained with 30 degrees of caudal angulation of the x-ray beam.[65] Lateral radiographs of the scapula (scapular "Y" view) and fluoroscopy represent additional useful techniques for its identification. The enthesophyte extends from the anteroinferior surface of the acromion in a medial and slightly inferior direction toward the coracoid process. It arises at the acromial attachment site of the coracoacromial ligament and differs in location and morphology from a "pseudospur" associated with prominence of the acromial angle (Fig. 12–28). In some instances, the tip of the acromion simulates the radiographic appearance of a subacromial enthesophyte.

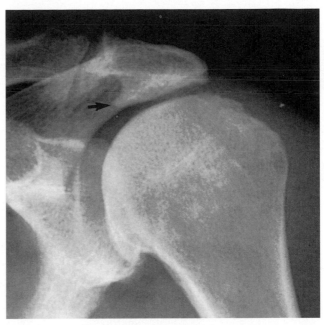

Figure 12–27
Shoulder impingement syndrome: Routine radiographic abnormalities. A frontal radiograph of the shoulder shows a large enthesophyte (arrow) extending from the anteroinferior portion of the acromion, associated with osteophytes at the acromioclavicular joint and in the inferior portion of the humeral head.

More advanced imaging methods, such as standard arthrography, computed arthrotomography, ultrasonography, subacromial bursography, and MR imaging, may be employed in patients with the shoulder impingement syndrome (Fig. 12–29), but their role primarily is one of defining the extent and precise cause of the shoulder impingement syndrome and not one of establishing the diagnosis. Each of these techniques can be used to determine the status of the rotator cuff, which may be disrupted in persons with the shoulder impingement syndrome (see later discussion).

The value of MR imaging in the assessment of the shoulder impingement syndrome has been the subject of a number of investigations.[119–123] Without question, this imaging method allows detection of abnormalities of the rotator cuff (such as changes in its signal intensity or frank disruption), the acromioclavicular joint (such as osteoarthritis with inferiorly protruding osteophytes or capsular hypertrophy), and the subacromial bursa (such as bursitis with the accumulation of bursal fluid).[124] None of these findings, however, is specific for the shoulder impingement syndrome, being seen in asymptomatic persons[125, 670] and in those with shoulder pain from other causes. Part of the difficulty in using MR imaging as a means to diagnose the shoulder impingement syndrome relates to the fact that, owing to constraints on patient positioning mandated by the configuration of the MR gantry, the patient typically is examined with the arm at his or her side and not in the position of impingement. The relationships of the coracoacromial arch and the components of the rotator cuff change during movement of the arm; the absence of depression of the supraspinatus tendon by the cor-

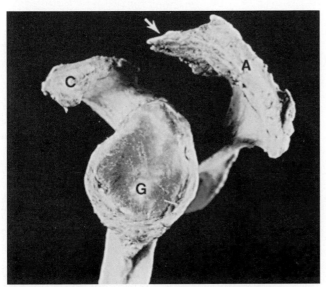

Figure 12–26
Shoulder impingement syndrome: Subacromial enthesophyte—pathologic correlation. A photograph of the medial aspect of a macerated scapula reveals a bony excrescence (arrow) arising from the anteroinferior aspect of the acromion (A) and extending toward the coracoid process (C). G, Glenoid cavity.

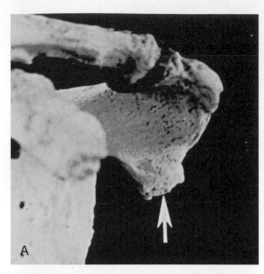

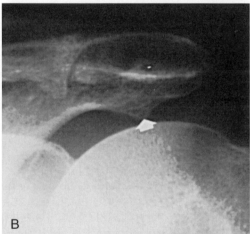

Figure 12–28
Pseudoenthesophyte of the acromion.

A A photograph of this specimen demonstrates a prominent acromial angle (arrow), which projects from the posterior aspect of the acromion.

B Such a pseudoenthesophyte (arrow) is seen in this patient. Observe that it is continuous with the posterior margin of the acromion, a feature that helps to differentiate it from a true enthesophyte.

(From Cone RO, et al: Radiology *150*:29, 1984.)

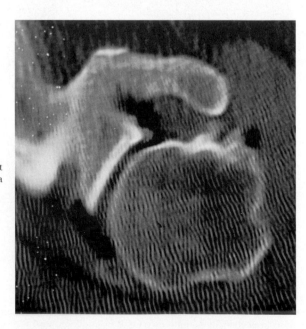

Figure 12–29
Shoulder impingement syndrome: CT arthrography. Subcoracoid impingement related to the presence of an elongated coracoid process is well shown on a transverse CT arthrographic image.

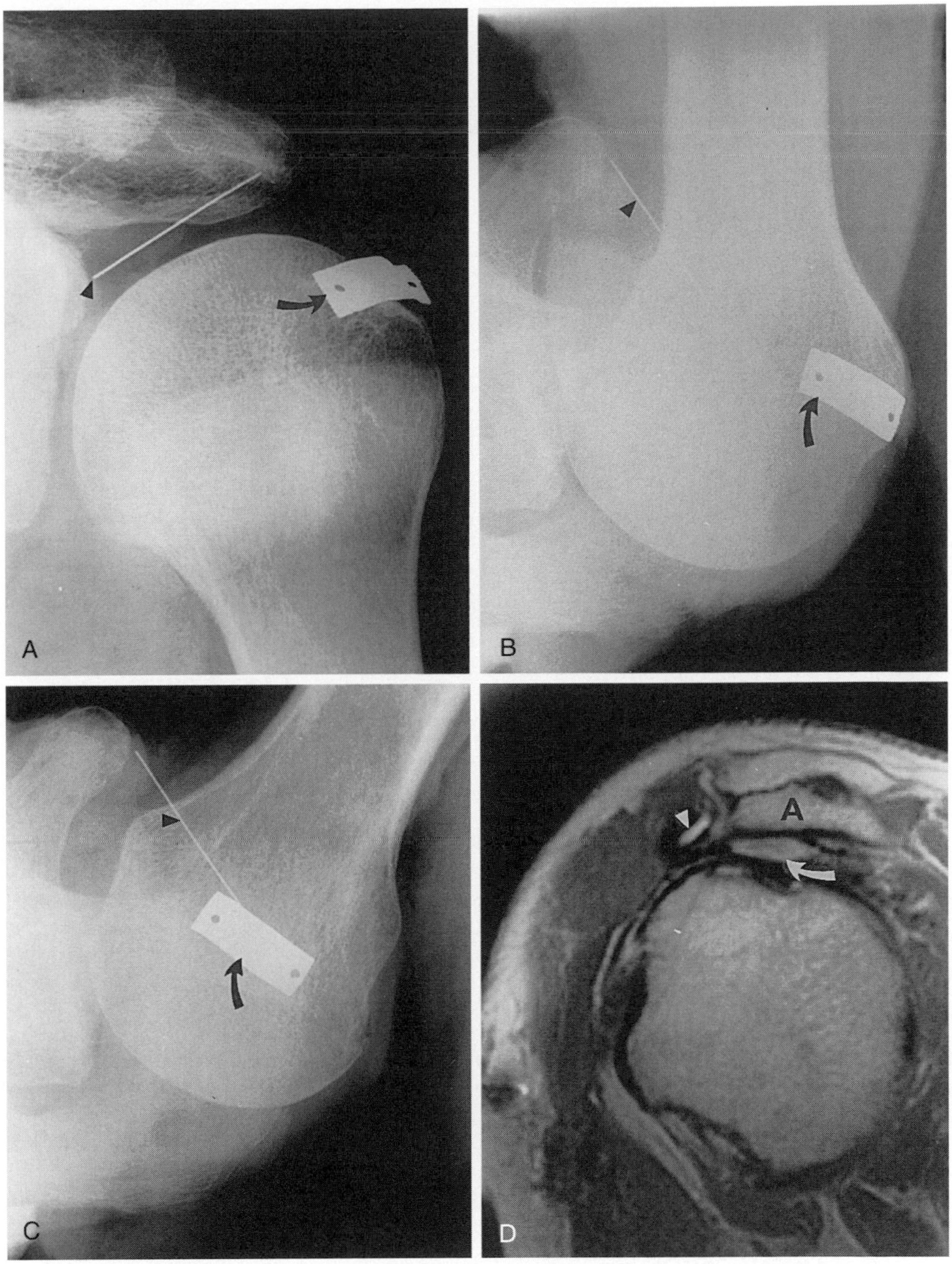

Figure 12–30

Shoulder impingement syndrome: Importance of shoulder position. Cadaveric preparation in which a metal marker is attached to the distal aspect of the supraspinatus tendon (critical zone) and a straight wire is inserted in the coracoacromial ligament for routine radiographs; a gadolinium-impregnated marker and a gadolinium-filled tube are attached to these same structures for MR imaging.

A Anteroposterior radiograph with arm at zero degrees of forward flexion, zero degrees of abduction, and neutral position. The critical zone of the supraspinatus tendon (arrow) is remote from the coracoacromial ligament (arrowhead).

B Axillary radiograph with the arm at 60 degrees of forward flexion, zero degrees of abduction, and internally rotated. The two structures (arrow, arrowhead) approach each other.

C, D Classic impingement position. Axillary radiograph (**C**) with the arm at 60 degrees of abduction, and internally rotated. The critical zone of the supraspinatus tendon (arrow) is directly beneath the junction of the coracoacromial ligament (arrowhead) and the acromion. Sagittal MR image (**D**) with the arm in this same position shows intimate relationship of the distal portion of the supraspinatus tendon (arrow) and the coracoacromial ligament (arrowhead).

acoacromial arch when the arm is alongside the torso does not exclude the diagnosis of shoulder impingement and, conversely, the presence of such depression with the arm in this position may occur in patients who do not have symptoms and signs of shoulder impingement (Fig. 12–30). Although MR imaging may provide information regarding anatomic features such as acromial morphology that have been associated with shoulder impingement and rotator cuff abnormalities,[59–62, 123, 126] MR imaging also may reveal thickening (>2 mm) of the coracoacromial ligament or an os acromiale (Fig. 12–31), although the specificity of these findings likewise is not clear[127] and, further, an os acromiale can be identified with routine radiography. These features are

not diagnostic of the shoulder impingement syndrome. Rather, as with routine radiography, the only MR imaging finding that is almost specific for this syndrome is a subacromial enthesophyte (Fig. 12–32). Such enthesophytes are observed on coronal oblique and sagittal oblique MR images as bone outgrowths, often containing marrow, extending from the anteroinferior portion of the acromion. When a region of persistently low signal intensity is detected at the tip of the acromion, caution must be exercised in the interpretation of this MR imaging finding, as this appearance may relate to the normal inferior tendon slip of the deltoid muscle rather than to a subacromial enthesophyte.[128]

The diagnostic value of MR imaging in cases of im-

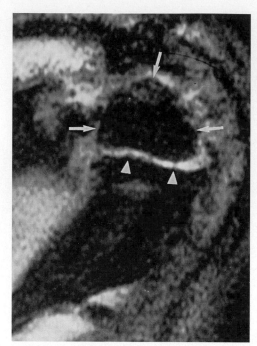

Figure 12–31
Os acromiale: MR imaging. In a 38 year old man with the shoulder impingement syndrome and rotator cuff tear, a transaxial MPGR (TR/TE, 783/15; flip angle, 60 degrees) MR image shows an os acromiale (arrows), separated from the remaining portion of the acromion (arrowheads). (Courtesy of D. Levey, M.D., Corpus Christi, Texas.)

pingement syndrome would be enhanced if the examination could be performed in shoulder positions known to provoke symptoms. The recent development of open-type magnets makes this feasible. Short of this, however, documentation of the typical impingement syndrome with MR imaging is problematic. Use of the ABER position of the shoulder combined with MR imaging (and MR arthrography) has shown promise as a means to diagnose posterosuperior glenoid impingement (see previous discussion).[113, 129] This peculiar variety of impingement occurs during the late cocking phase of throwing, with abnormal contact between the posterosuperior portion of the glenoid rim and the undersurface of the rotator cuff (see Fig. 12–32D). A classic triad of findings results: posterosuperior labral tears, impaction of the posterosuperior portion of the humeral head, and abnormalities of the posterosuperior portion of the rotator cuff.

The severity of the shoulder impingement syndrome guides the orthopedic surgeon with regard to the choice of appropriate therapy. Most patients with stages I and II impingement respond well to conservative care (rest, avoidance of activities requiring overhead movements of the arm, and physical therapy), whereas some with stage II impingement and many with stages III and IV impingement do not respond to such conservative measures and become candidates for surgery. Some form of anterior acromioplasty generally is employed.[65, 99] This can be accomplished arthroscopically or with an open surgical procedure.[130–132] Acromioplasty usually involves the resection of the anterior third of the undersurface

of the acromion and the coracoacromial ligament, although the amount of bone removed may vary. The distal portion of the clavicle also is resected (i.e., Mumford procedure) in some cases. Surprisingly, routine radiographs may reveal little evidence that an acromioplasty has been performed, although the radiodense line normally seen along the undersurface of the acromion and the distal portion of the clavicle may be absent. Heterotopic ossification at the site of surgery, a potential cause of failure of subacromial decompression, also may be identified on routine radiographs.[133] MR images commonly reveal artifacts, especially with gradient echo sequences, presumably related to small metal fragments that break off from the burring instruments used during surgery.[134] The signal intensity within the remaining portions of the acromion may be altered, with regions of decreased signal intensity in both T1- and T2-weighted spin echo images.[134] MR findings related to surgical repairs of the rotator cuff also may be evident (see later discussion).

Rotator Cuff Tears

Classification

A variety of methods have been used to classify failure of the rotator cuff. One simple method is to divide tears of the rotator cuff into those that are acute and those that are chronic. Acute tears occur suddenly or as a result of a definite injury; chronic tears have existed for a long time, generally for months or even years.[135] Acute tears have been reported to represent less than 10 per cent of all tears of the rotator cuff.[136] A chronic tear is at risk for acute extension, with the sudden failure of additional fibers and the onset of new clinical manifestations.[135]

A second method of classification relates to the depth of the rotator cuff tear (Fig. 12–33). Full-thickness (or complete) tears extend from the articular surface to the bursal surface of the cuff, and partial-thickness (or incomplete) tears involve only the articular surface or the bursal surface of the cuff. A tear within the substance of the rotator cuff (intrasubstance tear) represents a special type of incomplete tear.

Patte[137] has provided an extensive classification system in which lesions are divided according to their extent, their topography in the sagittal and coronal planes, the quality of the involved muscle, and the status of the tendon of the long head of the biceps brachii muscle. In this system, the extent of the lesion is measured in centimeters at the level of the bone insertion and is judged as grade I (partial-thickness and full-thickness tears measuring less than 1 cm in their sagittal diameter), grade II (full-thickness tears that measure approximately 2 cm in their sagittal diameter and that usually are confined to the supraspinatus tendon), grade III (full-thickness tears that measure 4 cm or more in their sagittal diameter and that involve not only the supraspinatus tendon but also other tendons such as the infraspinatus and subscapularis tendons), and grade IV (massive full-thickness tears with secondary osteoarthritis of the

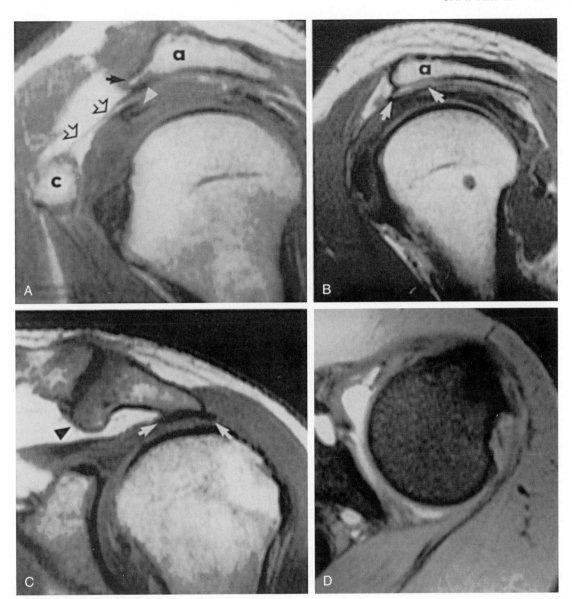

Figure 12–32

Shoulder impingement syndrome: MR imaging abnormalities.

A In a sagittal oblique T1-weighted (TR/TE, 800/20) spin echo MR image, a subacromial enthesophyte (solid arrow) containing marrow projects from the anterior surface of the acromion (a) toward the coracoid process (c). Note its relationship to the coracoacromial ligament (open arrows) and supraspinatus tendon (arrowhead).

B In a second patient, a sagittal oblique T1-weighted (TR/TE, 800/12) spin echo MR image shows a large subacromial enthesophyte (arrows). The acromion (a) is indicated.

C In a third patient, a coronal oblique proton density–weighted (TR/TE, 2000/30) spin echo MR image reveals the flattened contour and low signal intensity characteristic of a subacromial enthesophyte (arrows). Also observe osteoarthritis of the acromioclavicular joint manifest as osteophytosis (arrowhead) and an elevated position of the humeral head, indicative of a rotator cuff tear. The tear was demonstrated better in other MR images (not shown).

D In a professional baseball pitcher, a transaxial MPGR (TR/TE, 450/15; flip angle, 25 degrees) MR image shows erosion of the posterior surface of the humeral head beneath the infraspinatus tendon. Note abnormality of the posterior portion of the labrum.

glenohumeral joint). The topography of the tears in the sagittal plane relates to their extent with respect to specific components of the rotator cuff, which, from anterior to posterior, are subscapularis tendon, coracohumeral ligament, supraspinatus tendon, and infraspinatus (as well as teres minor) tendon. Segment 1 lesions are isolated to the subscapularis tendon, usually resulting from a traumatic evolution rather than a degenerative lesion. Segment 2 lesions are isolated to the coracohumeral ligament and, again, typically are trau-

matic. Segment 3 lesions generally are isolated to the supraspinatus tendon, although additional involvement of other segments also may be seen. Segments 4 and 5 lesions involve the supraspinatus tendon and the superior half (segment 4) or all (segment 5) of the infraspinatus tendon. Segment 6 lesions involve all the components of the rotator cuff. Anterosuperior lesions of the rotator cuff involve segments 1, 2, and 3; superior lesions of the cuff involve segments 2 and 3; and posterosuperior lesions of the cuff involve segments 4 and 5.

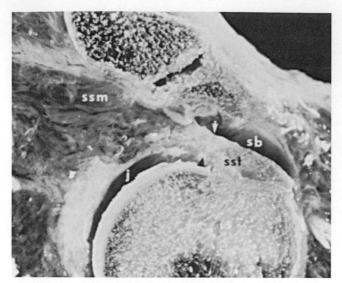

Figure 12–33

Rotator cuff tears: Classification system based on depth of the tear. A coronal section of the glenohumeral joint shows portions of the supraspinatus muscle (ssm) and tendon (sst), subacromial bursa (sb), and glenohumeral joint (j). Partial-thickness tears of the rotator cuff may involve either the bursal (arrow) or articular (arrowhead) side of the cuff, or they may occur within its substance. Those on the bursal side of the cuff may be detected by subacromial-subdeltoid bursography, but they are invisible on glenohumeral joint arthrograms. Partial-thickness tears involving the articular side of the cuff may be detected by glenohumeral joint arthrography but not by subacromial-subdeltoid bursography. Full-thickness tears allow communication of the glenohumeral joint and the subacromial-subdeltoid bursa and may be detected with injection of contrast material into either structure.

This classification system also considers the topography of the tear in the coronal plane. Three stages are described in relation to the degree of retraction of the tendon proximal to the tear. Finally, the system also is based on the extent of fatty degeneration of the involved muscle (as determined by CT) and on the status of the tendon of the long head of the biceps brachii muscle (i.e., normal, displaced, or torn).

The value of this comprehensive classification system is not proved, but it does emphasize the importance of determining not only the depth of the lesion (i.e., partial-thickness versus full-thickness) but also its coronal and sagittal extent. Although lesions of the rotator cuff generally begin in the supraspinatus tendon, their extension into other components of the rotator cuff is well established, and such extension influences the therapeutic options available and, ultimately, the likelihood of partial or complete recovery of shoulder function.

Prevalence

Much of the data regarding the prevalence of rotator cuff tears is based on studies of cadaveric shoulders. In these shoulders, derived mainly from persons who were elderly at the time of death, the reported prevalence of full-thickness tears of the rotator cuff has varied from about 5 to 25 per cent,[99, 100, 138–140] and that of partial-thickness tears of the rotator cuff has varied from about 12 to 35 per cent.[135, 136, 138, 140, 141] Data regarding the prevalence of rotator cuff tears in living patients are

more limited. Such tears appear to be common in patients who have sustained one or more dislocations of the glenohumeral joint, particularly those older than 50 years of age. In one study, Pettersson[142] noted arthrographic evidence of a partial-thickness or full-thickness tear of the rotator cuff in 30 per cent of patients in the fourth decade of life who had had an anteroinferior dislocation of the glenohumeral joint and in 60 per cent of patients in the sixth decade of life who had had such a dislocation.[135]

The general consensus indicates that partial-thickness tears of the rotator cuff are more common than full-thickness tears and that those of the articular side of the rotator cuff probably are slightly more common than those of the bursal side of the rotator cuff. Intratendinous tears appear to be less frequent than those involving the articular or bursal portion of the rotator cuff. As no standard exists that allows detection of all intrasubstance tears, their true prevalence is difficult to ascertain.

The prevalence of rotator cuff disruption increases in the later decades of life. The discovery of chronic tears of the rotator cuff as incidental findings on chest radiographs obtained for unrelated reasons is well known. The strength of human tendons decreases in older persons; as an example, it has been shown that the strength of the anterior cruciate ligament in a person in the eighth decade of life is only about 25 per cent of that in a person in the third decade of life.[135]

Etiology and Pathogenesis

Proposed causes of rotator cuff failure have included trauma, attrition, ischemia, and impingement.[135] An association of rotator cuff tears and acute traumatic episodes is well known. One example of this is an isolated rupture of the subscapularis tendon that may result from an anterior dislocation of the glenohumeral joint.[143, 144] This type of rupture predominates in men and in persons over the age of 40 years. It differs from an avulsion fracture of the lesser tuberosity at the site of insertion of the subscapularis tendon, which occurs in elderly women and men,[145] and from tears of the subscapularis tendon that accompany disruptions of most or all of the components of the rotator cuff. Superior dislocations of the glenohumeral joint also are accompanied by disruption of the rotator cuff, as the humeral head is driven upward acutely through the cuff.

Most rotator cuff tears are unrelated to an acute injury. Rather, rupture of the rotator cuff occurs during movements and activities that should not—and usually do not—damage the involved musculotendinous units.[47] This occurrence can be designated a spontaneous rupture. Furthermore, the general consensus is that normal tendons do not rupture spontaneously. Although evidence to the contrary may be provided by arthroscopic evidence corroborating partial-thickness tears of the rotator cuff tendons in the "normal" shoulders of athletes,[135] these lesions may represent minor tendinous avulsion injuries rather than intratendinous tears. Most full-thickness tears of the rotator cuff appear to occur in a tendon that is weakened by some combination of age, repetitive stress, corticosteroid injection, hypovascularity, or damage produced by impingement.[135] A variety of histopathologic changes are observed in tendons prior to their rupture; these include hypoxic tendinopathy, mucinous change, tendolipomatosis, alterations in collagen composition, and calcifying tendinopathy, occurring either alone or in combination.[47, 146, 147] The manner in which these histologic abnormalities are interpreted has led to the concepts of an ischemic, degenerative, and mechanical (i.e., impingement) cause for rotator cuff disruption.

The school that emphasizes the importance of ischemic events in failure of the rotator cuff is based, in part, on anatomic studies that confirm the presence of a critical zone of hypovascularity in the distal portion of the central region of the supraspinatus tendon.[104, 148] As the supraspinatus tendon is the component of the rotator cuff that tears most often, and its site of failure corresponds closely to the location of this critical zone, hypovascularity has been implicated in the pathogenesis of rotator cuff failure. Brooks and coworkers,[52] however, did not support this concept, indicating that results of perfusion studies (in which the critical zone has been identified) do not represent proof of hypovascularity, and showing that the vascular patterns of the distal portions of both the supraspinatus and infraspinatus tendons are similar.

A second school emphasizes the importance of age-related degeneration of the tendon manifest by changes in cell arrangement, calcium deposition, fibrinoid thickening, fatty infiltration, necrosis, and rents, in the pathogenesis of failure of the rotator cuff.[135, 142, 149] The changes usually are apparent histologically in the tendons of persons in the third or fourth decade of life, and they increase in frequency and severity in the later decades.[47] The alterations may be prominent at the site of attachment of the cuff tendons to the tuberosities of the humerus, leading to tearing away of the tendinous fibers from the bone.[142, 150] The relationship of such degenerative alterations to clinical manifestations that may be interpreted as evidence of tendinitis or to complete failure of the tendon is not clear.[135] These degenerative abnormalities, however, can lead to alterations of the signal intensity in the rotator cuff on MR images that may simulate the signal intensity changes of a tendon tear (see later discussion).

A third theory regarding the pathogenesis of rotator cuff disruption emphasizes extrinsic factors rather than intrinsic factors (i.e., ischemia, degeneration). It is this school that holds to the belief that cuff impingement related to the coracoacromial arch is the most important cause of rotator cuff tears. Although, as indicated earlier, data exist that support this theory,[151] other data tend to refute it. A relationship exists between morphologic changes in the anterior portion of the undersurface of the acromion and in the rotator cuff, supporting the concept that shoulder impingement produces cuff tears, but this relationship is not constant, and partial-thickness (or even complete) tears of the rotator cuff occur in the absence of morphologic abnormalities of the acromion.[152] Furthermore, although results of cadaveric studies, including those using scanning electron microscopy, support the detrimental effects of friction and rubbing (related to the adjacent coracoacromial arch) on the surface of the cuff, these results also confirm the occurrence of intrinsic degeneration of the cuff at a time when the coracoacromial arch is normal.[153, 154] Cadaveric studies also document isolated histologic abnormalities on the articular side of the rotator cuff, whereas the bursal side of the cuff would be expected to be more severely affected in instances of shoulder impingement.[155]

It appears likely that no single factor is responsible for most failures of the rotator cuff and that several working in concert are important in causing rotator cuff tears. Abnormalities intrinsic to the cuff, such as ischemia, contusion, and degeneration, place its fibers at risk. With the application of loads (whether repetitive or abrupt, compressive or tensile), each fiber fails when the applied force exceeds its strength.[135] This may occur a few fibers at a time or en masse (an acute tear or an acute extension of a chronic tear).[135] The typical initial site of cuff failure is within the critical zone in the distal portion of the central region of the supraspinatus tendon; the very anterior region of this tendon is less vulnerable owing to its relative strength.[156] Once ruptured, the tendons of the cuff show little evidence of healing, perhaps related to their being bathed by the synovial fluid of the glenohumeral joint and subacromial-subdeltoid bursa. Extension of the tear in the central, distal portion of the supraspinatus tendon occurs more often in the posterior direction (and then may expand to involve the infraspinatus tendon). Less commonly, anterior extension of the tear occurs (with eventual involvement of the subscapularis tendon) or extension of the tear occurs in both anterior and posterior directions.[156] With loss of function of the rotator cuff, progressive elevation of the humeral head occurs (Fig. 12–34), leading to deterioration of the glenohumeral joint, contact of the humeral head and acromion, and subacromial enthesophytes, eventually resulting in disorganization, designated cuff arthropathy or the Milwaukee shoulder syndrome (see later discussion).

Clinical Abnormalities

Tears of the rotator cuff predominate in patients over the age of 40 years, in men, and in the dominant arm. Shoulder pain, stiffness, and weakening are common clinical manifestations, although patients may be entirely asymptomatic. On physical examination, shoulder crepitus may be elicited when the arm is internally rotated, abducted, and flexed. Weakness of flexion, abduction, and external rotation of the arm may be apparent. Such weakness is greater in patients with large tears and, in such patients, a defect in the rotator cuff may be palpable.

The clinical manifestations of rotator cuff disease may allow accurate diagnosis; however, in some cases, they simulate the findings of other disorders of the shoulder, such as adhesive capsulitis and calcific or noncalcific tendinitis. When the clinical diagnosis is not clear, imaging studies may provide diagnostic help.

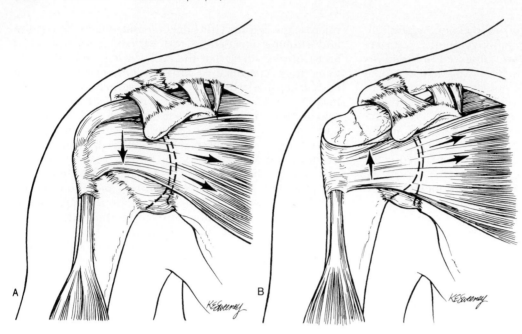

Figure 12–34
Rotator cuff tears: Pathogenesis.
  A In addition to the supraspinatus muscles, the anterior and posterior rotator cuff muscles and the long head of the biceps tendon depress the humeral head and balance the upward-directed forces applied by the deltoid muscle.
  B Major cuff fiber failure and retraction allow the humeral head to protrude upward through the cuff defect, creating a type of boutonniere lesion. When the remaining cuff tendons slip below the equator of the head, their action is converted from humeral head depression to humeral head elevation.
  (From Matsen FA III, Arntz CT: Rotator cuff tendon failure. *In* CA Rockwood Jr, FA Matsen III [Eds]: The Shoulder. Philadelphia, WB Saunders Co, 1990, p 649.)

Routine Radiographic Abnormalities

No routine radiographic findings are diagnostic of an acute rotator cuff tear that has occurred in the absence of glenohumeral joint dislocation. The peribursal fat plane, which normally is seen as a curvilinear radiolucent region about the lateral margin of the humerus on internal rotation views of the shoulder, may be obliterated in patients with acute tears of the rotator cuff, but such loss also is evident in inflammatory processes of adjacent tissues, including rheumatoid arthritis and calcific tendinitis.[18] The presence of calcification in the tendon of the supraspinatus muscle has been regarded as a finding that rarely coexists with rotator cuff disruption, although a recent arthrographic study in patients with calcific tendinitis has indicated the frequent occurrence of incomplete or complete tears of the rotator cuff.[157] Radiographs obtained during active abduction

of the shoulder to 90 degrees from the horizontal or to the maximum extent that is possible may reveal narrowing of the coracoacromial distance in patients with rotator cuff disruption (Fig. 12–35).[158, 159]

With chronic tears of the rotator cuff, a number of radiographic abnormalities may become apparent (Fig. 12–36)[160–162]:

1. *Narrowing of the acromiohumeral space.* This interosseous space may measure less than the lower limit of normal, 0.6 to 0.7 cm. The narrowing should be evident in both internal and external rotation radiographs, as some diminution of the acromiohumeral space can be seen in external rotation projections in normal persons.

2. *Reversal of the normal inferior acromial convexity.* Elevation of the humeral head leads to closer apposition of the humerus and the acromion and repeated traumatic insult to the acromion. Straightening and concavity of

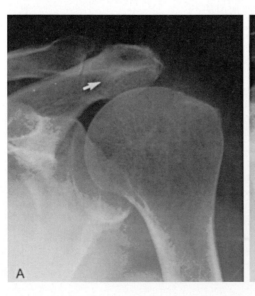

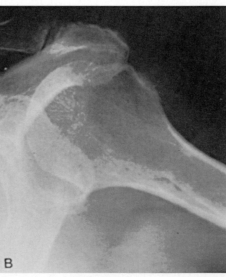

Figure 12–35
Rotator cuff tears: Routine radiographic abnormalities. In a 70 year old man with clinical manifestations of the shoulder impingement syndrome and a recent fall with acute exacerbation of shoulder pain, an initial anteroposterior radiograph of the shoulder **(A)** shows mild elevation of the humeral head with respect to the glenoid cavity, leading to narrowing of the acromiohumeral space, and a subacromial enthesophyte (arrow). With abduction of the arm **(B)**, note further narrowing of the acromiohumeral space.

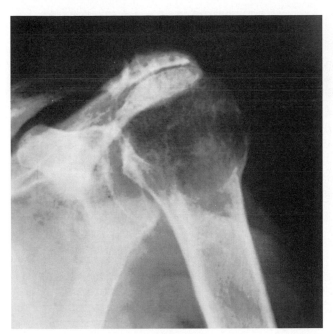

Figure 12–36
Rotator cuff tears: Routine radiographic abnormalities. This patient with a chronic rotator cuff tear reveals elevation of the humeral head with respect to the glenoid, contact of the humeral head and the acromion, concavity of the inferior surface of the acromion, and sclerosis and cyst formation on apposing surfaces of acromion and humeral head.

the undersurface of the acromion may then become evident. This finding must be evident on both internal rotation and external rotation projections, as a pseudo-concavity can be seen in normal persons on a single view owing to the anatomic characteristics of the acromion process.

3. *Cystic lesions and sclerosis of the acromion and humeral head.* Small cystic lesions surrounded by a thin rim of sclerosis can be noted along the inferior aspect of the acromion. Similarly, cysts appear within the greater tuberosity in areas of bone sclerosis and contour irregularity. These latter cystic lesions may develop by the process of synovial intrusion, in which synovial fluid is forced into the subchondral bone because of repeated stress.[163] The loss of soft tissue and the elevation of the humeral head may allow abutment of the acromion and greater tuberosity in full abduction. Notching of the superior aspect of the humeral neck also may be seen.[163]

Several limitations of these radiographic findings as diagnostic aids in rotator cuff tears must be noted. First, apparent elevation of the humeral head with malalignment of the humerus and glenoid and narrowing of the acromiohumeral space can be an artifact of the x-ray technique related to incident beam angulation. Second, severe degeneration and atrophy of the rotator cuff without tear can lead to many of the same abnormalities that are noted in association with chronic tears of the rotator cuff. Third, many of the radiographic changes also can appear in patients with other disorders, particularly those with "frozen" shoulders.

Rotator cuff atrophy and tear can complicate a variety

of articular diseases, such as rheumatoid arthritis, ankylosing spondylitis, and septic arthritis (Fig. 12–37A). In these processes, synovial inflammation may lead to erosion of the undersurface of the cuff and subsequent disruption. Radiographs reveal the typical signs that are listed earlier and, additionally, changes of the glenohumeral joint consistent with the underlying disease (e.g., joint space narrowing, osseous erosion). In rotator cuff disruption uncomplicated by the presence of an underlying disorder, the glenohumeral joint may appear surprisingly normal, although secondary degenerative joint disease (cuff arthropathy) can develop later. In some cases, severe articular abnormalities, with disorganization of the glenohumeral joint, accompany disruption of the rotator cuff. This arthropathy, which has been designated the Milwaukee shoulder syndrome, may relate to intra-articular deposition of calcium hydroxyapatite crystals (Fig. 12–37B). Other causes of glenohumeral joint disruption that may simulate cuff arthropathy and the Milwaukee shoulder syndrome are included in Table 12–2.

Arthrographic Abnormalities

Standard arthrography remains a popular technique in the diagnosis of some tears of the rotator cuff. In one recent study of full-thickness tears of the rotator cuff, glenohumeral joint arthrography revealed a sensitivity of 93 per cent, an accuracy of 94 per cent, a positive predictive value of 96 per cent, and a negative predictive value of 91 per cent.[164] Double contrast shoulder arthrography is the preferred technique. Suggested arthrographic modifications include the application of stress,[165] the supplementary use of conventional or computed tomography,[166–168] the use of digital radiographic technique,[169] and the monitoring of intra-articular pressure.[170, 171] Complete tears of the rotator cuff are associated with abnormal communication between the glenohumeral joint cavity and the subacromial (subdeltoid) bursa (Fig. 12–38). Contrast material can be identified within the bursa as a large collection superior and lateral to the greater tuberosity and adjacent to the undersurface of the acromion. The contrast material in the bursa is separated from the articular cavity by a lucent area of varying size, representing the rotator cuff itself. If the musculature is thick, this lucent region is quite large, whereas if the musculature is atrophic, it is small

Table 12–2. SOME CAUSES OF SEVERE DESTRUCTION OF THE GLENOHUMERAL JOINT

Milwaukee shoulder syndrome*
Cuff-tear arthropathy*
CPPD crystal deposition disease
Neuropathic osteoarthropathy
Alkaptonuria
Infection
Idiopathic chondrolysis*
Senile hemorrhagic shoulder syndrome*
Ischemic necrosis
Rheumatoid arthritis

*These may represent four names for a single disease.

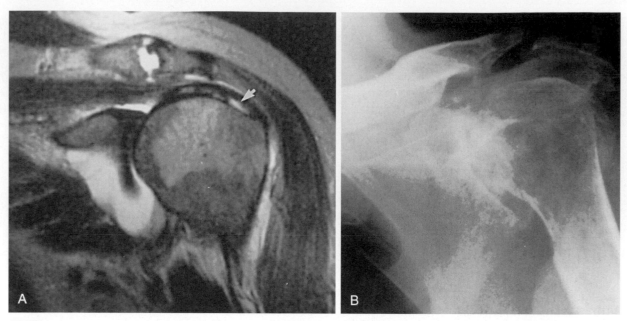

Figure 12–37
Rotator cuff tears: Associated articular abnormalities.
   A Septic arthritis. In a 58 year old woman with chronic lymphocytic leukemia, a coronal oblique fast spin echo (TR/TE, 4000/115) MR image shows fluid distending the glenohumeral joint, disruption of the supraspinatus tendon (arrow), which was shown to be complete on other images, and fluid in the subacromial-subdeltoid bursa and acromioclavicular joint. (Courtesy of D. Goodwin, M.D., Hanover, New Hampshire.)
   B Milwaukee shoulder syndrome. The radiographic characteristics of this syndrome are well delineated in this 75 year old man. Note joint space narrowing, subchondral sclerosis, and erosion of the undersurface of the clavicle and acromion.

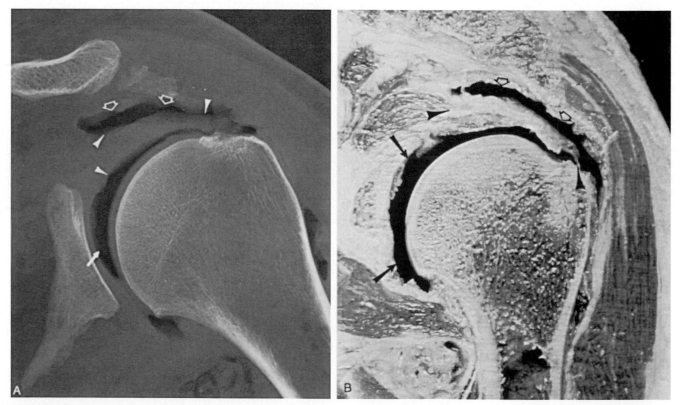

Figure 12–38
Full-thickness rotator cuff tears: Glenohumeral joint arthrography. This coronal section was prepared following air arthrography of the glenohumeral joint in a cadaver. On a corresponding sectional radiograph **(A)** and photograph **(B)** note the irregular and torn rotator cuff (arrowheads), allowing communication of the glenohumeral joint (solid arrows) and subacromial (subdeltoid) bursa (open arrows).

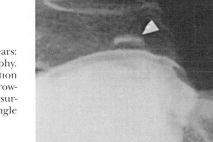
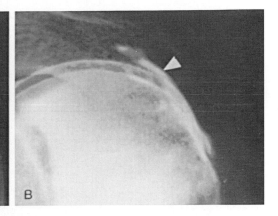

Figure 12–39
Partial-thickness rotator cuff tears: Glenohumeral joint arthrography. External (**A**) and internal (**B**) rotation views show contrast material (arrowheads) extending into the undersurface of the rotator cuff in this single contrast arthrogram.

or even absent. In the presence of a complete rotator cuff tear, contrast material is identified as a "saddle-bag" radiodense area across the surgical neck of the humerus on the axillary view. In some patients with complete tears, the contrast material will pass from the subacromial bursa into the acromioclavicular joint.[172, 173]

Using double contrast shoulder arthrography, the degree of degeneration of the torn rotator cuff can be recognized.[87, 174] Furthermore, the width of the tear itself is identified. The location of the disrupted tendons is apparent as the tendinous ends are coated by positive contrast material. In some patients, the torn rotator cuff tendons are either absent or consist of only a few small pieces.

Killoran and associates[73] have emphasized three potential sources of error in the diagnosis of a complete rotator cuff tear: Inadequate distribution of opaque material within the joint may prevent adequate visualization of the subacromial bursa; the contrast-filled sheath of the biceps tendon may project slightly lateral to the greater tuberosity on external rotation, simulating filling of the subacromial bursa; and inadvertent bursal injection may simulate a complete tear unless it is recognized that the articular cavity is not opacified. Inadvertent injection of the subcoracoid bursa, rather than the glenohumeral joint, results in opacification of a well-defined circular or oval sac.

Tears within the substance of the cuff generally will escape arthrographic detection. Tears involving the superior surface of the cuff also will not be demonstrated on glenohumeral joint arthrography, although they rarely may be seen with direct subacromial bursography.[175] Tears on the inferior surface of the rotator cuff can be diagnosed on arthrography. In these cases, an irregular circular or linear collection of contrast material may be identified above the opacified joint cavity, near the anatomic neck of the humerus (Fig. 12–39).[73, 176, 177] The intact superficial fibers of the rotator cuff prevent opacification of the subacromial bursa.[83] A false-negative arthrogram in the presence of a partial tear of the rotator cuff can indicate that the tear is too small for recognition or that a fibrous nodule has occluded the defect.

The combination of arthrography and CT scanning (i.e., CT arthrography) employing intra-articular injection of air alone or of air and a small amount of iodinated contrast material has been used effectively in the assessment of glenohumeral joint instability (see later discussion). This technique is not applied commonly to the evaluation of the rotator cuff, although it has important advantages in documenting disruption of the subscapularis tendon (Figs. 12–40 and 12–41). Furthermore, CT arthrography or CT scanning alone may reveal fatty infiltration in the muscles of the rotator cuff when chronic tendon tears are present.[178, 179] The infraspinatus and subscapularis muscles are involved most frequently. Although such infiltration often occurs in muscles whose tendons are torn, this is not invariable. For example, tears of the supraspinatus tendon may be accompanied by fatty infiltration of the infraspinatus muscle. Fat accumulation may occur within 6 months of the tendon rupture. Regression of intramuscular fatty infiltration may be observed after repair of the tendon tear, but this too is not invariable.

Ultrasonographic Abnormalities

The value of ultrasonography in the assessment of the rotator cuff is well established This technique can be

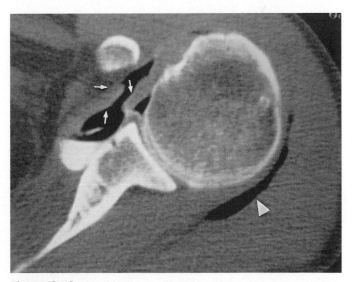

Figure 12–40
Tears of the subscapularis tendon: CT arthrography. A transverse CT scan at the midglenoid level obtained after the introduction of both air and iodinated contrast material into the glenohumeral joint shows disruption of the subscapularis tendon (arrows) with air in the subdeltoid bursa (arrowhead). (Courtesy of G. Greenway, M.D., Dallas, Texas.)

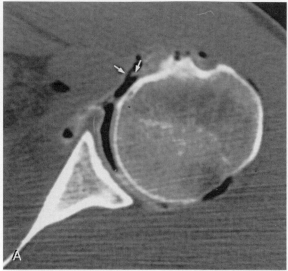

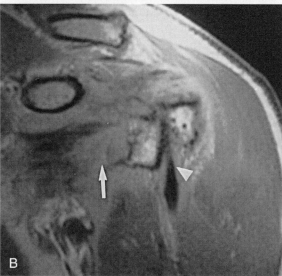

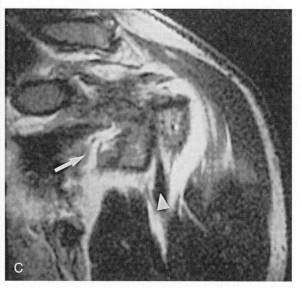

Figure 12–41

Tears of the subscapularis tendon: CT arthrography and MR imaging. A transverse CT scan (**A**) at the midglenoid level obtained after the introduction of both air and iodinated contrast material into the glenohumeral joint shows disruption of the subscapularis tendon (arrows). The tendon tear (arrows) also is evident in coronal oblique T1-weighted (TR/TE, 700/20) (**B**) and T2-weighted (TR/TE, 2000/80) (**C**) spin echo MR images. The biceps tendon (arrowheads) is not displaced.

applied to the evaluation of acute or chronic tears of the rotator cuff and of full-thickness or partial-thickness tendon disruptions (Fig. 12–42).[180, 181] Discontinuity of the tendon is direct evidence of its disruption. Fluid in the subacromial-subdeltoid bursa alone or in both the bursa and the glenohumeral joint is an important secondary sonographic sign of rotator cuff tear.[182] Furthermore, sonographic detection of fluid in the biceps tendon sheath should prompt careful evaluation of the rotator cuff.

Magnetic Resonance Imaging Abnormalities

General Considerations. MR imaging has been applied to the analysis of shoulder disorders, including tears of the rotator cuff, for approximately 10 years. Although its sensitivity and specificity in such analysis still are debated, it is clear that technical advances such as those related to the design of surface coils have led to a gradual improvement in the quality and diagnostic accuracy of MR examinations of the shoulder. Currently, MR imaging generally is considered superior to ultrasonography and conventional arthrography in the

assessment of the rotator cuff. Most MR imaging protocols used for this purpose rely heavily on standard or fast spin echo sequences, although additional methods such as routine and volumetric gradient echo sequences, STIR imaging, fat suppression techniques, and MR arthrography may be useful (see later discussion).

As indicated previously, MR imaging examination of the shoulder generally emphasizes three imaging planes: a coronal oblique plane that is parallel to the long axis of the scapula and roughly parallel to the long axis of the supraspinatus tendon; a sagittal oblique plane that is perpendicular to the long axis of the scapula and roughly tangent to the glenoid cavity; and a transaxial plane (see Fig. 12–23). For rotator cuff disorders, both the coronal oblique and sagittal oblique planes are useful (Figs. 12–43 and 12–44), although whether both are required for accurate diagnosis is debated.[183] The coronal oblique plane displays much of the entire length of the supraspinatus tendon, and the sagittal oblique plane displays the coracoacromial arch (including the acromion, coracoid process, and coracoacromial ligament) and all of the components of the rotator cuff.

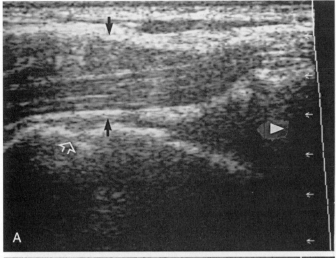

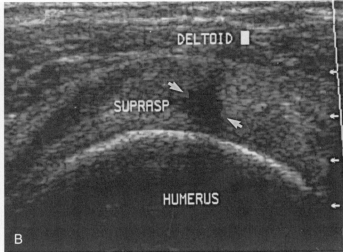

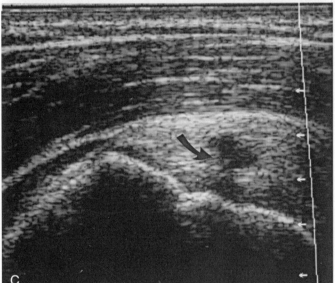

Figure 12–42

Rotator cuff tears: Ultrasonography.

A Large full-thickness tear. A sonogram in the coronal oblique plane demonstrates the deltoid muscle (black arrows) contacting the irregular greater tuberosity (open arrow) of an elevated humeral head, with retraction of the supraspinatus tendon (arrowhead).

B Small full-thickness tear. A sonogram in the sagittal oblique plane demonstrates the hypoechogenic tear (arrows) in the supraspinatus tendon.

C Partial-thickness tear. A sonogram in the coronal oblique plane shows a hypoechoic tear (arrow) involving the inferior surface of the supraspinatus tendon near its attachment to the greater tuberosity with anechoic subdeltoid bursal fluid.

(Courtesy of M. van Holsbeeck, M.D., Detroit, Michigan, and J. Jacobson, San Diego, California.)

In the transaxial plane, the subscapularis muscle and tendon are well seen, and the location of the tendon of the long head of the biceps brachii muscle can be defined.

The position of the arm during the MR imaging examination is critical to the assessment of the rotator cuff.[184] Generally, the patient is in a supine position with the arm placed alongside his or her body. A neutral position of the arm (i.e., with the thumb up) is preferred.[185] Although some investigators favor a position of internal rotation of the arm,[120] internal rotation produces overlap of the supraspinatus and infraspinatus tendons and apparent tendon discontinuities, factors that make analysis of the rotator cuff more difficult.[186] With exaggerated external rotation of the shoulder, the tendon of the long head of the biceps brachii muscle is projected close to the critical area of the supraspinatus tendon, and fluid within the bicipital tendon sheath may simulate the appearance of a cuff tear.[186] Therefore, the neutral position of the arm is optimal. As discussed earlier in this chapter, recent modifications of MR imaging technique in the assessment of the rotator cuff

have included the development of dedicated shoulder surface coils, the use of small fields of view (14 to 18 cm), the employment of fast spin echo sequences with or without fat suppression, and the use of combined spin echo and gradient echo imaging protocols (Fig. 12–45).[187–189, 671, 672]

Normal Rotator Cuff. The normal tendons of the supraspinatus, infraspinatus, teres minor, and subscapularis muscles usually have been reported as regions of low signal intensity on all MR imaging sequences, contrasting with areas of high signal intensity in these tendons on some MR imaging sequences that are characteristic of tears.[190–196] Although these differences in signal intensity in the normal and torn tendons of the rotator cuff are fundamental to the diagnosis of cuff disruption, regions of intermediate signal intensity and signal inhomogeneity in intact tendons of the rotator cuff are encountered regularly,[197] creating some diagnostic difficulty. Specifically, regions of intermediate and, sometimes, high signal intensity within the outer portion of the supraspinatus tendon on T1-weighted and proton

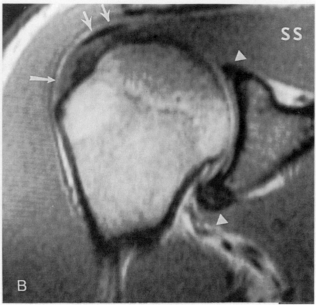

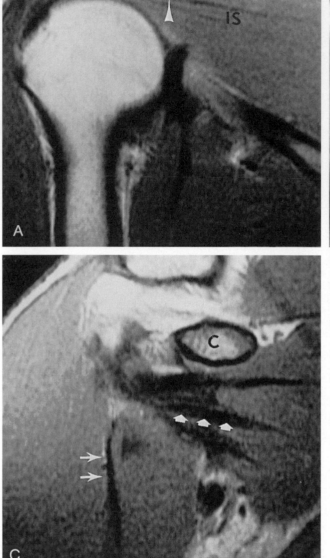

Figure 12–43

Normal rotator cuff: MR imaging. Coronal oblique plane. T1-weighted (TR/TE, 800/20) spin echo MR images.

A Posterior MR image. Note the infraspinatus muscle (IS) and its tendon (arrowhead). In this image, the infraspinatus tendon passes over the humeral head.

B Middle MR image. The supraspinatus muscle (SS) and its tendon (upper arrows) are evident. The tendon is inhomogeneous in signal intensity but contains regions of very low signal intensity. The peribursal fat plane (lower arrow) is of high signal intensity, located beneath the deltoid muscle. Superior and inferior portions of the glenoid labrum (arrowheads) are seen as triangular structures of low signal intensity.

C Anterior MR image. Note the subscapularis muscle and its tendinous fibers (short arrows) attaching to the lesser tuberosity of the humerus. A portion of the tendon of the long head of the biceps brachii muscle (long arrows) and the coracoid process (c) are seen.

(From Kursunoglu-Brahme S, et al: Radiol Clin North Am *28*: 941, 1990.)

density–weighted spin echo MR images have been documented both in cadavers with grossly intact tendons and in asymptomatic living persons.[155, 198, 199] These regions may be more conspicuous and more clearly defined with fat suppression MR imaging.[93, 200] The pathogenesis of such regions of intermediate or high signal intensity is not agreed on, resulting in the emergence of several different theories.

1. *Magic angle phenomenon.* The spin-spin relaxation for poorly hydrated tissues such as tendons depends on the orientation of the tissues in the magnetic field because of the effects of anisotropy of water molecule motion.[201–204] Higher signal intensity within normal tendons oriented obliquely to the direction of the main magnetic field, rather than parallel or perpendicular to it, may occur and could account for the regions of

intermediate and high signal intensity in the supraspinatus tendon that are seen on MR images employing short echo times (TE).

2. *Partial volume averaging.* As the distal portion of the supraspinatus tendon may contain fat and muscle fibers in addition to tendon fibers, averaging of signal intensity of these various components theoretically could occur if the imaging plane were not strictly parallel to the supraspinatus tendon.[197] The persistence of regions of intermediate signal intensity within the supraspinatus tendon on fat-suppressed MR images[200, 203] does not support the importance of volume averaging as a causative factor, however. Furthermore, inability to detect TE-dependent signal oscillation (i.e., in-phase and opposed phases of protons of different bindings) typical of fat within these regions on gradient echo images also suggests that partial volume averaging with peritendinous

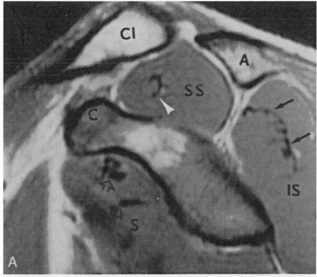

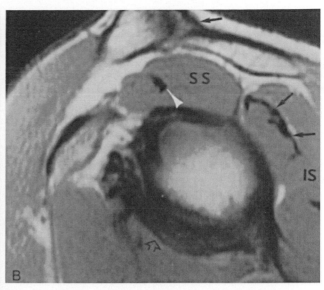

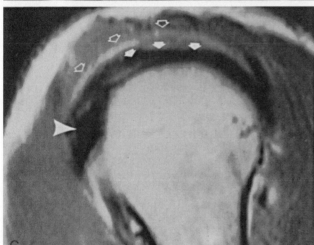

Figure 12–44

Normal rotator cuff: MR imaging—sagittal oblique plane, T1-weighted (TR/TE, 800/20) spin echo MR images.

A Medial MR image. Note the acromion (A), clavicle (Cl), and coracoid process (C). The supraspinatus muscle (SS) and its tendon (arrowhead), the infraspinatus muscle (IS) and its tendon (solid arrows), and the subscapularis muscle (S) and its tendon (open arrows) are shown.

B Middle MR image. Note the region of the acromioclavicular joint (solid arrow), the supraspinatus muscle (SS) and its tendon (arrowhead), the infraspinatus muscle (IS) and its tendon (solid arrows), and the subscapularis tendon (open arrow). A fat plane is seen above and in front of the supraspinatus muscle.

C Lateral MR image. The tendons of the supraspinatus and infraspinatus muscles are seen as a curvilinear region of low signal intensity (solid arrows). The subscapularis tendon (arrowhead) at its site of insertion in the lesser tuberosity is identified. The peribursal fat plane (open arrows) can be seen.

(From Kursunoglu-Brahme S, et al: Radiol Clin North Am *28*:941, 1990.)

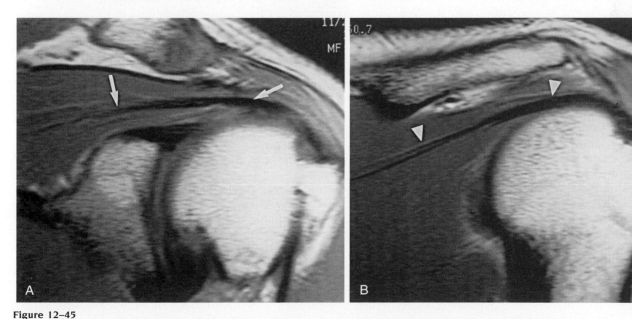

Figure 12–45

Normal rotator cuff: MR imaging. Coronal oblique plane. Proton density–weighted (TR/TE, 2000/20) spin echo MR images with quadrature coil, 14 cm field of view, 512 × 128 matrix, 2 excitations, and 4 mm thick sections. The supraspinatus (arrow, **A**) and infraspinatus (arrowheads, **B**) tendons are well shown. (Courtesy of D. Bates, M.D., San Diego, California.)

adipose tissue is not a likely cause of areas of increased signal intensity.

3. *Tendon and muscle anatomy.* The supraspinatus muscle has been reported to consist of two distinct portions: A fusiform portion originates from the anterior supraspinous fossa and inserts via a dominant tendon anteriorly on the greater tuberosity; a second portion of the supraspinatus muscle is located posteriorly with muscle fibers originating from the posterior aspect of the supraspinous fossa and the scapular spine.[203] Several distinct tendinous slips originate from this second portion of the supraspinatus muscle and attach to the greater tuberosity. The orientation of the dominant tendon differs from that of the main muscle by approximately 10 degrees.[203] This anatomic complexity of the distal few centimeters of the supraspinatus tendon may explain its inhomogeneous signal intensity.

4. *Histologic changes in the tendon.* The occurrence of eosinophilic, fibrillar, and mucoid changes in the tendinous fibers of the supraspinatus muscle, which has been confirmed in cadavers,[155] may account for the regions of inhomogeneous and intermediate signal intensity. Such changes, interpreted as evidence of tendon degeneration (i.e., tendinosis, tendinopathy), are discussed later in this chapter.

Although the cause of altered signal intensity within the supraspinatus tendon remains unclear, these changes should not be interpreted as evidence of tendon disruption.[128, 205] As a general rule, the signal intensity of nondisrupted tendons of the rotator cuff, including the supraspinatus tendon, on T2-weighted spin echo MR images is equal to or less than that on T1-weighted and proton density–weighted spin echo MR images. When the signal intensity of the rotator cuff tendons on T2-weighted spin echo images is higher than that on T1-weighted and proton density–weighted spin echo MR images, a tendon disruption usually is present. Unfortunately, however, there are exceptions to this rule (see later discussion).

The musculotendinous junction of the supraspinatus muscle generally is apparent over the center of the humeral head (i.e., at the 12 o'clock position) on coronal oblique MR images with the arm held in neutral position. Some variation in this position can be normal, however. Neumann and coworkers,[198] in a study of 55 shoulders in 32 asymptomatic volunteers, observed that the musculotendinous junction was located 15 degrees lateral to the 12 o'clock position in 18 shoulders (33 per cent), 30 degrees lateral to the 12 o'clock position in 4 shoulders (7 per cent), and 15 degrees medial to this 12 o'clock position in 3 shoulders (6 per cent). Some 93 per cent of all musculotendinous junctions in these volunteers were found in a 30 degree radius (i.e., 15 degrees medial to 15 degrees lateral to the 12 o'clock position).

The fat that surrounds the subacromial-subdeltoid bursa generally can be identified on MR images. Although failure to visualize this fat plane has been emphasized as a finding consistent with rotator cuff disruption (see later discussion), portions of it, particularly the subacromial portion, may not be visualized on MR

images of asymptomatic persons.[128, 198, 200, 205] Furthermore, small amounts of fluid normally may be present in the subacromial-subdeltoid bursa or in the glenohumeral joint, or in both locations; the detection of such fluid collections during MR imaging of the shoulder is not diagnostic of a tear of the rotator cuff.

Full-Thickness Tears of the Rotator Cuff. The MR imaging features of full-thickness tears of the rotator cuff have been detailed in a number of publications.[90, 91, 93, 129, 185, 193–195, 206–214] The most definite and direct feature of such tears is a tendinous defect that is filled with fluid or granulation tissue, or both (Figs. 12–46, 12–47, 12–48, and 12–49). A second direct feature is retraction of the musculotendinous junction beyond the limits of normal (see previous discussion) (Fig. 12–50). When the first of these two signs is present alone or when the first and second signs are present together, the diagnosis of a full-thickness tear of the rotator cuff can be made with confidence. When the second finding alone is present, such a tear is likely, although as previously indicated, the location of the musculotendinous junction of the supraspinatus muscle varies in asymptomatic persons, and this location is influenced by the precise position of the arm during the MR imaging examination. The absence of either of these two direct signs does not exclude the presence of a tear. Small full-thickness tears or those accompanied by scar formation may not reveal obvious regions of tendinous discontinuity on MR images (Fig. 12–51). In these cases, morphologic alterations (e.g., poor definition, attenuation, or thickening) of the involved segment of the tendon may be evident. Furthermore, small full-thickness tears of the rotator cuff may not be associated with retraction of the musculotendinous junction.

A number of secondary signs of a full-thickness tear of the rotator cuff have been described (see Fig. 12–51), but none of these occurring in isolation is diagnostic of such a tear. These signs include fluid in the subacromial-subdeltoid bursa, fluid in the glenohumeral joint, loss of the peribursal fat plane, and muscle atrophy. The first of these findings, fluid in the subacromial-subdeltoid bursa, may occur in asymptomatic persons or in those with bursitis. Similarly, fluid in the glenohumeral joint also is encountered in asymptomatic persons and may occur in association with arthritis. Although fluid in both the bursa and the joint may be more specific for the diagnosis of rotator cuff disruption than fluid in either of these locations, this pattern likewise is not diagnostic of a tendon tear and may be evident in patients with inflammatory articular and bursal processes (e.g., rheumatoid arthritis). The loss of the peribursal fat plane is a documented feature of rotator cuff disruption, related to bursal fluid, granulation tissue, or scar formation, but it also is a finding seen in asymptomatic persons. Chronic rotator cuff tears are associated with muscle atrophy,[690] but such atrophy also is apparent in patients with neurologic compromise, adhesive capsulitis, and other conditions in which shoulder movement is restricted or absent.

The accumulation of fluid or granulation tissue, or both, in a site of tendon discontinuity leads to a charac-

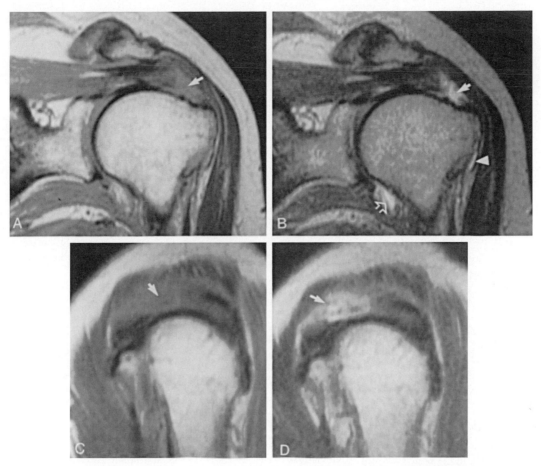

Figure 12–46
Full-thickness rotator cuff tears: MR imaging.

   A, B In the coronal oblique plane, proton density–weighted (TR/TE, 2000/20) **(A)** and T2-weighted (TR/TE, 2000/60) **(B)** spin echo MR images show fluid in a gap (solid arrows) in the supraspinatus tendon, the fluid being of increased signal intensity in **B.** Also in **B,** note increased signal intensity related to fluid in the glenohumeral joint (open arrow) and subdeltoid bursa (arrowhead). Osteoarthritis of the acromioclavicular joint is evident.

   C, D In the same patient, sagittal oblique proton density–weighted (TR/TE, 2000/20) **(C)** and T2-weighted (TR/TE, 2000/60) **(D)** spin echo MR images show the site (arrows) of disruption of the supraspinatus tendon, which is of high signal intensity in **D.**

teristic change in signal intensity evident in about 80 per cent of rotator cuff tears: high signal intensity on T2-weighted spin echo MR images.[208] In about 20 per cent of rotator cuff tears, no such increased signal intensity is evident. In these cases, the diagnosis of a tear is based on other MR imaging findings related to altered tendon morphology (Fig. 12–52). Extreme caution should be exercised, however, in diagnosing a rotator cuff tear solely on the basis of morphologic alterations, as similar alterations of the tendon may be observed in patients with degenerative abnormalities (tendinosis or tendinopathy) or calcific tendinitis. Analysis of coronal oblique and sagittal oblique images provides information regarding the extent of the full-thickness rotator cuff tear. As indicated earlier, initial tears in the supraspinatus tendon may extend (1) anteriorly to involve the coracohumeral ligament and subscapularis tendon, (2) posteriorly to involve the infraspinatus tendon and, rarely, the teres minor tendon, or (3) anteriorly and posteriorly to involve the entire cuff. The width of the tendon gap also can be gauged by the size of the high signal intensity region and the presence of tendon re-

traction. The retracted margin may be of normal size or thickened, the latter related to hemorrhage, edema, fibrosis, or reparative tissue. With massive tears that extend anteriorly to involve the subscapularis tendon (Fig. 12–53) or in those that are isolated to the subscapularis tendon,[215] the bicipital tendon may dislocate medially and, in some cases, may become entrapped within the joint (see later discussion).

   The published reports of the accuracy of MR imaging in the diagnosis of rotator cuff tears have varied. Zlatkin and collaborators[206] were able to diagnose all 17 surgically confirmed full-thickness tears on the basis of MR imaging abnormalities. These authors diagnosed small full-thickness tears of the rotator cuff after analysis of MR images in two patients who had partial-thickness tears confirmed at surgery. Rafii and colleagues,[208] using MR imaging in the assessment of 31 full-thickness tears that subsequently were confirmed surgically, reported a sensitivity of 0.97, a specificity of 0.94, an accuracy of 0.95, a positive predictive value of 0.94, and a negative predictive value of 0.97. Iannotti and coworkers,[210] in an analysis of MR imaging in 33 surgically confirmed full-

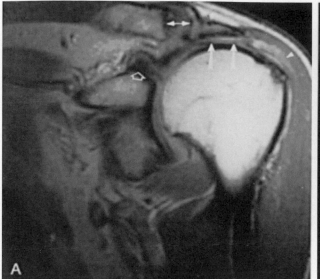
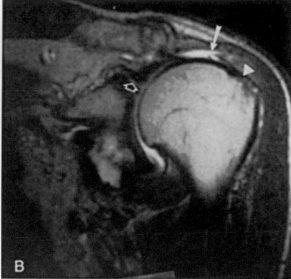

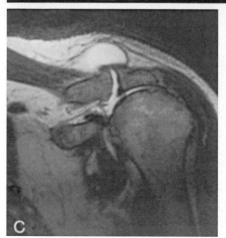

Figure 12–47

Full-thickness rotator cuff tears: MR imaging.

A A coronal oblique proton density–weighted (TR/TE, 2000/20) spin echo MR image reveals discontinuity of the supraspinatus tendon (solid arrows), an elevated humeral head with narrowing of the acromiohumeral space, obliteration of the peribursal fat plane (arrowhead), osteoarthritis of the acromioclavicular joint (double-headed arrow), and an ovoid region of low signal intensity (open arrow) which, at arthroscopy, proved to be an intra-articular body.

B A coronal oblique T2-weighted (TR/TE, 2000/70) spin echo MR image reveals fluid within the subacromial bursa (closed arrow) and within a full-thickness tear of the supraspinatus tendon, the intra-articular body (open arrow), and irregularity of the greater tuberosity of the humerus (arrowhead) related to the shoulder impingement syndrome.

(**A, B,** From Kursunoglu-Brahme S, et al: Radiol Clin North Am 28:941, 1990.)

C In a different patient, a coronal oblique T2-weighted (TR/TE, 4100/96) fast spin echo MR image reveals a chronic and massive tear of the rotator cuff. The humeral head contacts the acromion. Fluid of high signal intensity is seen in the glenohumeral and acromioclavicular joints and in a mass (synovial cyst) above the acromioclavicular joint.

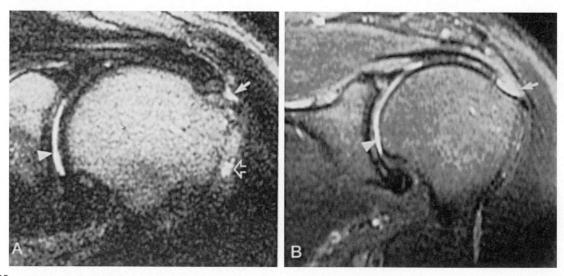

Figure 12–48

Full-thickness rotator cuff tears: MR imaging.

A A coronal oblique T2-weighted (TR/TE, 4000/92) fast spin echo MR image shows fluid of high signal intensity in the glenohumeral joint (arrowhead), in a small gap in the supraspinatus tendon (solid arrow), and in the subdeltoid bursa (open arrow). The findings suggest the presence of a partial-thickness bursal-sided tear of the tendon.

B In the same patient, a coronal oblique T2-weighted (TR/TE, 5000/76) fast spin echo MR image obtained with chemical presaturation of fat (ChemSat) better defines the extent of this full-thickness tear of the supraspinatus tendon. Note fluid of high signal intensity in the joint (arrowhead) and in the tendinous gap (solid arrow).

(Courtesy of S. K. Brahme, M.D., La Jolla, California.)

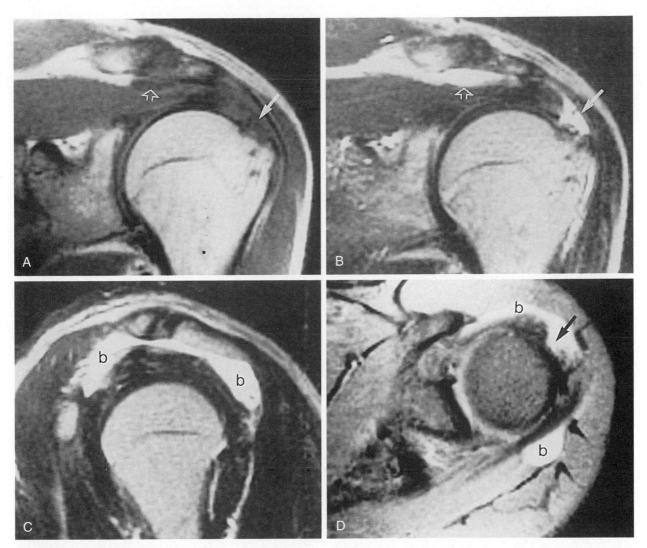

Figure 12–49

Full-thickness rotator cuff tears: MR imaging.

A A coronal oblique T1-weighted (TR/TE, 500/20) spin echo MR image shows a tear (solid arrow) of the supraspinatus tendon and fluid (open arrow) in the subacromial bursa.

B On a coronal oblique T2-weighted (TR/TE, 2000/90) spin echo MR image, these same findings (solid and open arrows) are more evident owing to the high signal intensity of fluid.

C A sagittal oblique T2-weighted (TR/TE, 2000/90) spin echo MR image shows fluid of high signal intensity in the subacromial-subdeltoid bursa (b).

D The transaxial MPGR (TR/TE, 850/25; flip angle, 30 degrees) MR image reveals the tendon tear (arrow) and bursal (b) fluid.

thickness tears of the rotator cuff, indicated 100 per cent sensitivity and 95 per cent specificity in the assessment of these tears with MR imaging. Nelson and collaborators[211] also reported high accuracy regarding the diagnosis of full-thickness tears of the rotator cuff using MR imaging. Sonin and coworkers[671] reported a sensitivity of 0.89, a specificity of 0.94, and an accuracy of 0.92 in the MR diagnosis of full-thickness tears of the rotator cuff. They also found no differences in these results when comparing conventional with fast spin echo sequences. Singson and colleagues[672] found a sensitivity of 100 per cent in the diagnosis of such full-thickness tears using fast spin echo sequences with or without fat suppression. Based on these results, it appears that experienced observers interpreting carefully performed MR imaging examinations will provide an accurate diag-

nosis of a full-thickness rotator cuff tear in more than 90 per cent of patients with such tears,[216] although occasionally they will provide an incorrect diagnosis of a full-thickness tear when a partial-thickness tear or degenerative tendinopathy is present. Less experienced observers will not do as well, and both experienced and inexperienced observers will be less successful in diagnosing partial-thickness tears of the rotator cuff correctly. Diagnostic pitfalls that cause the most difficulty are the normal alterations in signal intensity that occur at the attachment site of the supraspinatus tendon and at the rotator interval, the presence of articular cartilage of the humeral head beneath the distal portion of the supraspinatus tendon, and the occurrence of muscle fibers between the supraspinatus and infraspinatus tendons.[214] Furthermore, it should be apparent that the

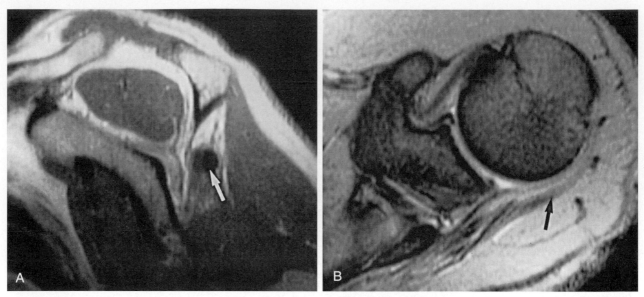

Figure 12–50

Full-thickness rotator cuff tears: MR imaging. A chronic tear of the infraspinatus tendon is associated with tendon retraction (arrows), as shown on a sagittal oblique fast spin echo (TR/TE, 3800/18) MR image (**A**) and transaxial MPGR (TR/TE, 450/15; flip angle, 20 degrees) MR image (**B**).

discovery of a full-thickness rotator cuff tear on MR images in older persons does not indicate with certainty that it is the cause of the shoulder symptoms.[217]

In an attempt to improve diagnostic accuracy in cases of full-thickness (and partial-thickness) rotator cuff tears, some investigators have employed MR arthrography, accomplished by the injection of gadolinium compounds (or iodinated contrast material or saline solu-

tion) into the glenohumeral joint.[218, 219] This technique combines the advantages of both MR imaging and standard arthrography. The injection of gadolinium compounds rather than saline solution allows the use of T1-weighted spin echo MR images in which the gadolinium compounds have high signal intensity (Fig. 12–54). The main advantage of MR arthrography is direct opacification of full-thickness rotator cuff tears and partial-thick-

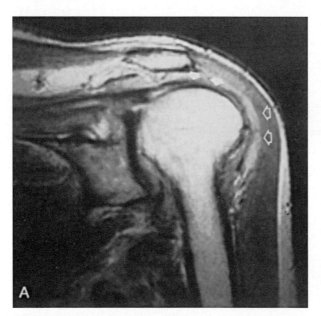
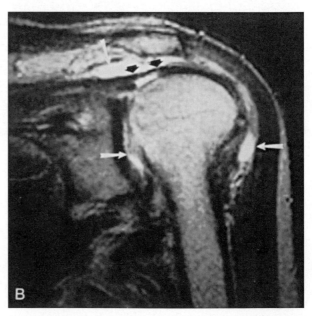

Figure 12–51

Full-thickness rotator cuff tears: MR imaging.

A A coronal oblique proton density–weighted (TR/TE, 2000/20) spin echo MR image, obtained with the arm in internal rotation, shows diffuse thinning of the supraspinatus tendon (solid arrows), atrophy of the supraspinatus muscle, and distention of the subdeltoid bursa (open arrows).

B A coronal oblique T2-weighted (TR/TE, 2000/70) spin echo MR image confirms the presence of an attenuated supraspinatus tendon (small arrows) and reveals fluid of increased signal intensity in the glenohumeral joint and subacromial-subdeltoid bursa (large arrows).

(From Kursunoglu-Brahme S, et al: Radiol Clin North Am 28:941, 1990.)

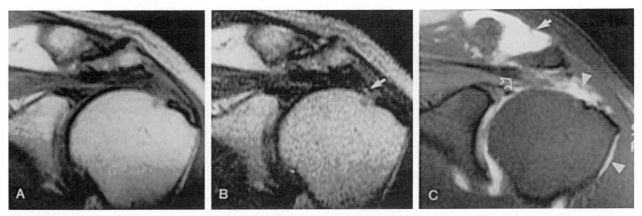

Figure 12–52

Full-thickness rotator cuff tears: MR imaging and MR arthrography. Coronal oblique proton density–weighted (TR/TE, 2000/20) **(A)** and T2-weighted (TR/TE, 2000/80) **(B)** spin echo MR images show osteoarthritis of the acromioclavicular joint and an enlarged and irregular distal portion of the supraspinatus tendon. Only one region of the tendon, however, reveals increased signal intensity in **B** (arrow). A coronal oblique T1-weighted (TR/TE, 650/20) spin echo MR image obtained with chemical presaturation of fat (ChemSat) after the intra-articular administration of a gadolinium compound **(C)** reveals the high signal intensity of the contrast agent in the glenohumeral joint, subacromial-subdeltoid bursa (arrowheads), and acromioclavicular joint (solid arrow). Note the completely torn and retracted supraspinatus tendon (open arrow).

ness tears involving the articular side of the cuff (see later discussion). Its disadvantages include a longer examination time, higher cost, and invasive nature. Furthermore, the technique is not useful in the assessment of partial-thickness tears confined to the bursal side of the cuff or intratendinous tears. Hodler and coworkers[218] reported no added accuracy in the diagnosis of full-thickness tears when results of MR arthrography were compared with those of standard MR imaging. These investigators emphasized the value of MR arthrography in the assessment of partial-thickness tears of the rotator cuff, however. One diagnostic pitfall encoun-

tered with MR arthrography that may lead to a false-positive diagnosis of a full-thickness tear relates to misinterpretation of the peribursal fat plane as evidence of contrast medium that has leaked into the subacromial-subdeltoid bursa. This pitfall can be eliminated if fat-suppression methods are used in combination with the MR arthrogram.[220, 221] The resulting suppression of the signal from the peribursal fat allows detection of even

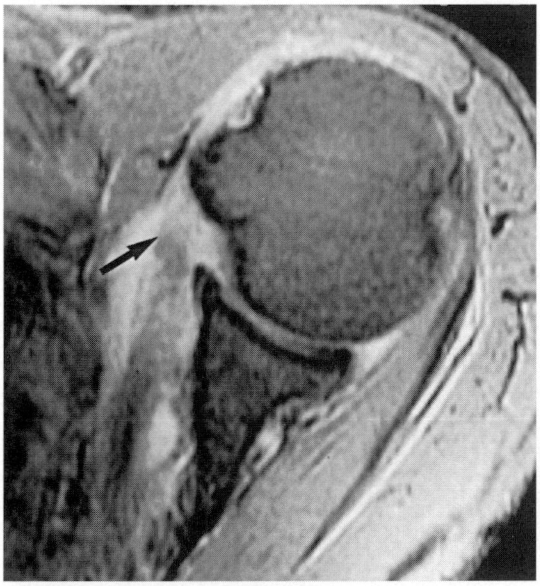

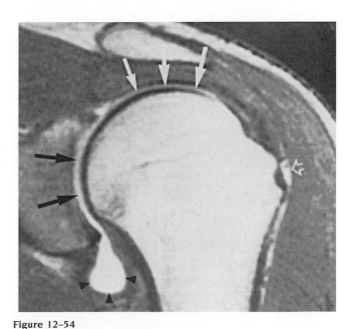

Figure 12–54

Normal rotator cuff: MR arthrography. A coronal oblique T1-weighted (TR/TE, 600/20) spin echo MR image after the intra-articular injection of a gadolinium compound reveals that all the contrast material remains in the glenohumeral joint. The high signal intensity fluid coats the undersurface of the supraspinatus tendon (white arrows), fills the space between the humeral head and glenoid cavity (black arrows), and distends the axillary recess (arrowheads). A source of diagnostic error with MR arthrography relates to the high signal intensity of peribursal fat (open arrow) that may be misinterpreted as evidence of fluid escaping from the joint through a full-thickness tear of the rotator cuff. (From Hodler J, et al: Radiology *182*:431, 1992.)

Figure 12–53

Full-thickness rotator cuff tears: MR imaging. In this 71 year old man with a massive tear of the rotator cuff, a transverse MPGR (TR/TE, 450/15; flip angle, 20 degrees) MR image shows disruption of the subscapularis tendon (arrows) and fluid in the subdeltoid bursa. At surgery, the tendon of the long head of the biceps brachii muscle was found to be torn.

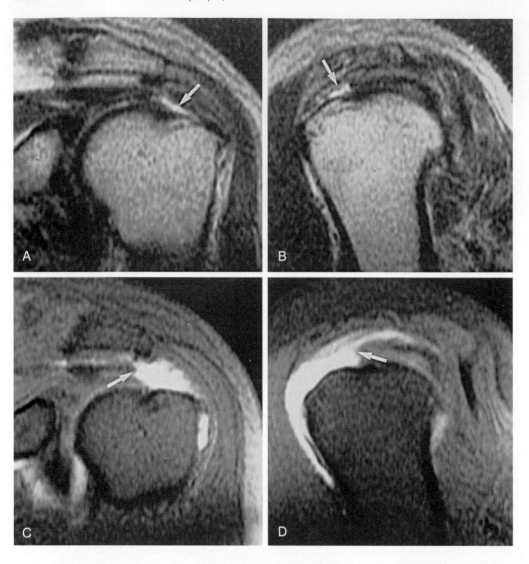

Figure 12–55
Full-thickness rotator cuff tears: MR arthrography. When compared to the coronal oblique (**A**) and sagittal oblique (**B**) T2-weighted (TR/TE, 2000/80) spin echo MR images, in which a rotator cuff tear appears as a region of high signal intensity (arrows), fat-suppressed T1-weighted (TR/TE, 650/14) coronal oblique (**C**) and T1-weighted (TR/TE, 700/14) sagittal oblique (**D**) MR images obtained after intra-articular administration of a gadolinium compound show the extent of the tear (arrows) and subacromial-subdeltoid accumulation of the contrast material more vividly.

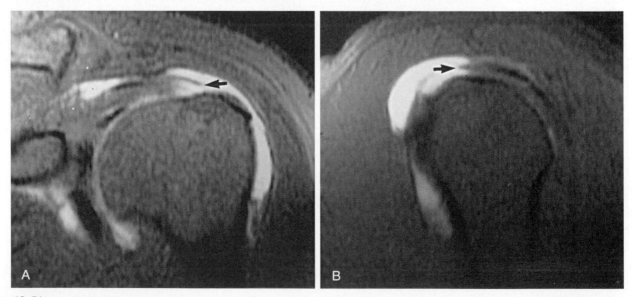

Figure 12–56
Full-thickness rotator cuff tears: MR arthrography. Coronal oblique (TR/TE, 766/14) (**A**) and sagittal oblique (TR/TE, 800/14) (**B**) fat-suppressed T1-weighted spin echo MR images obtained after intra-articular administration of a gadolinium contrast agent show a large tear (arrows) of the supraspinatus tendon with the contrast agent in both the joint and the subacromial-subdeltoid bursa.

small amounts of contrast material within the subacromial-subdeltoid bursa (Figs. 12–52, 12–55, and 12–56). The main value of MR arthrography of the shoulder performed with or without fat suppression is related to the detection of partial-thickness tears involving the articular side of the rotator cuff and to the differentiation of partial-thickness and small full-thickness tears of the rotator cuff. The use of an abducted and externally rotated position (ABER position) of the arm during MR arthrography may improve the diagnostic value of the study.[90] Furthermore, the addition of a T2-weighted spin echo sequence during MR arthrography allows identification of fluid collections about the shoulder that are not related to the gadolinium-containing compound, and the inclusion of at least one fat-suppressed sequence before the intra-articular injection of the gadolinium-containing compound may be useful for comparison purposes.

The benefit of MR arthrography using saline solution instead of a gadolinium compound relates to safety issues. The long-term effects of gadolinium compounds on articular cartilage and synovial tissue are not known. Saline arthrography employing T2-weighted fast spin echo MR imaging sequences may be an effective procedure in some patients with rotator cuff tears (Fig. 12–57). One additional imaging method involves the use of an iodinated contrast agent (either alone or in combination with a small amount of gadolinium compound) for the arthrographic procedure.[98] With this method, a routine arthrogram of the glenohumeral joint can be obtained first. If this arthrogram does not provide the necessary information, the patient can then be transported to the MR imaging suite.

The intravenous administration of gadolinium compounds has also been used to investigate rotator cuff disease, including tears (Fig. 12–58). Enhancement of signal intensity in the synovial membrane and in the rotator cuff immediately after the injection is a constant finding, but preliminary data have indicated that patterns of enhancement of signal intensity in the rotator cuff do not allow reliable differentiation of rotator cuff tears and degenerative disease (tendinopathy or tendinosis). If the shoulder is exercised after the intravenous injection and imaging is delayed about 15 or 20 minutes, the gadolinium compound extends into the joint fluid and an arthrographic effect is apparent. Studies comparing the effectiveness of such indirect MR arthrography and that related to direct intra-articular instillation of the gadolinium-containing compound in the diagnosis of tears of the rotator cuff are not available.

Partial-Thickness Tears of the Rotator Cuff. Recent years have witnessed an increased interest in the occurrence of partial-thickness tears of the rotator cuff. In large part, this has related to the increased popularity of shoulder arthroscopy that may be used to diagnose and, in some cases, treat these tears.[222] Minor lesions of the rotator cuff may be decompressed and debrided successfully using arthroscopy, whereas incomplete tears that extend into or exist within the substance of the cuff generally are treated by open surgical technique.[223] Among partial-thickness tears, deep (articular-sided) tears appear to be most frequent, followed by superficial (bursal-sided) tears and those occurring within the substance of the tendon.[223] Incomplete tears of the rotator

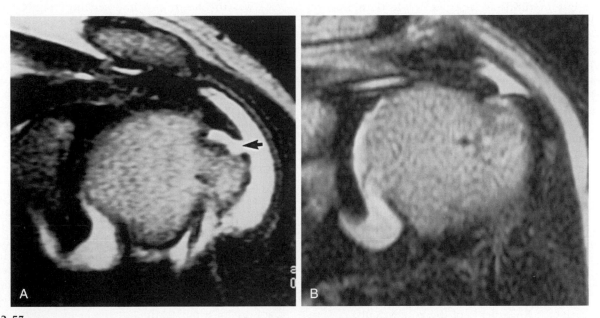

Figure 12–57
Full-thickness rotator cuff tears: MR arthrography.
   A A coronal oblique T2-weighted (TR/TE, 2000/80) spin echo MR image obtained after intra-articular injection of a saline solution shows a tear (arrow) of the supraspinatus tendon. (Courtesy of D. Levey, M.D., Corpus Christi, Texas.)
   B In a second patient in whom a saline solution was instilled in the joint, a coronal oblique T2-weighted (TR/TE, 2000/80) spin echo MR image shows fluid of high signal intensity in both the joint and subacromial-subdeltoid bursa, compatible with the presence of a full-thickness tear of the rotator cuff. Occasionally, however, similar findings are seen in patients with an intact rotator cuff and subacromial-subdeltoid bursitis. (Courtesy of D. Levey, M.D., Corpus Christi, Texas.)

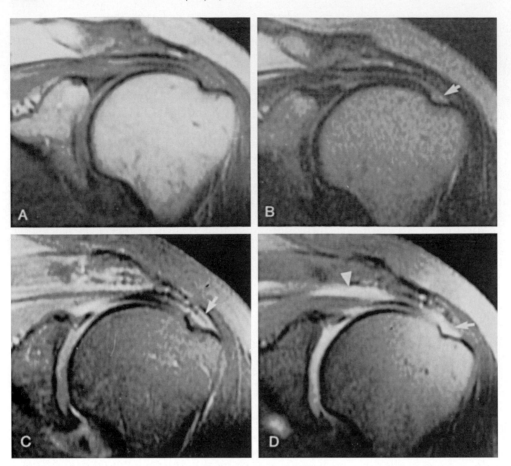

Figure 12–58

Full-thickness rotator cuff tears: MR imaging with and without intravenous administration of a gadolinium compound and MR arthrography. Coronal oblique proton density–weighted (TR/TE, 2000/20) (**A**) and T2-weighted (TR/TE, 2000/80) (**B**) spin echo MR images reveal altered signal intensity in the distal portion of the supraspinatus tendon with high signal intensity in this region in **B** (arrow). The findings are consistent with a small full-thickness tendon tear. A coronal oblique T1-weighted (TR/TE, 600/20) spin echo MR image obtained with chemical presaturation of fat (ChemSat) and immediately after intravenous administration of a gadolinium compound (**C**) shows enhancement of signal intensity in the region of the tendon tear (arrow) and in several areas of the glenohumeral joint itself. A coronal oblique T1-weighted (TR/TE, 600/15) spin echo MR image obtained with chemical presaturation of fat (ChemSat) and after intra-articular injection of a gadolinium compound (**D**) confirms a full-thickness tear of the supraspinatus tendon with the contrast agent of high signal intensity located in the tendinous gap (arrow) and in the subacromial bursa (arrowhead), as well as within the joint.

cuff may be twice as common as full-thickness tears. The detection of partial-thickness tears of the rotator cuff with imaging methods is more difficult than that of full-thickness tears. Arthrography, bursography, and MR imaging are techniques that have diagnostic potential in the assessment of partial-thickness tears of the rotator cuff. Arthrography is useful only in instances of articular-sided defects, and accurate detection of these defects may require filming after exercise of the patient's shoulder or arthrotomographic methods. Bursography, with opacification of the subacromial-subdeltoid bursa, is technically difficult and time consuming, and it, too, may necessitate tomographic techniques.

MR imaging in cases of partial-thickness tears of the rotator cuff requires careful analysis of patterns of signal intensity and of morphologic alterations in the distal portion of the tendons, particularly the supraspinatus tendon. The value of secondary MR imaging signs of cuff abnormalities in these cases has been emphasized,[206] but these signs lack specificity. Even with such analysis, the results of the MR imaging examinations are not as good diagnostically as in cases of full-thickness tears of the rotator cuff. In five cases of surgically confirmed partial-thickness tears of the rotator cuff, Zlatkin and coworkers,[206] on the basis of MR imaging abnormalities, reported an accurate interpretation in one patient and inaccurate interpretations in four patients (two partial-thickness tears of the inferior surface of the cuff were interpreted as small full-thickness tears and two such tears were interpreted as abnormal but intact ten-

dons). Rafii and collaborators[208] indicated that in only 7 of 16 patients with surgically confirmed partial-thickness tears was the tendinous abnormality manifested as intense increased signal intensity on the T2-weighted spin echo MR images. In the remaining nine patients, focal areas of tendon interruption or depression, marked by regions of moderate to marked increased signal intensity on proton density–weighted and T2-weighted spin echo MR images, were seen. Nelson and colleagues[211] were successful in identifying partial-thickness tears of the rotator cuff with MR imaging in five of seven patients who had such tears confirmed surgically. Traughber and Goodwin[224] were unable to detect four of nine partial-thickness tears of the rotator cuff (confirmed with arthroscopy and bursography) using MR imaging.

Careful evaluation of the pattern of increased signal intensity within the rotator cuff on T2-weighted spin echo MR images provides important information regarding the presence and the type of tear of the rotator cuff (Fig. 12–59). A region of increased signal intensity in the superficial portion of the tendon, perpendicular to the long axis of the tendon, on coronal oblique T2-weighted spin echo images is most consistent with the diagnosis of a partial-thickness tear involving the bursal side of the tendon; a similar region in the deep portion of the tendon, again perpendicular to the long axis of the tendon, on these images is most consistent with the diagnosis of a partial-thickness tear involving the articular side of the tendon; a region of increased signal intensity on T2-weighted spin echo MR images that

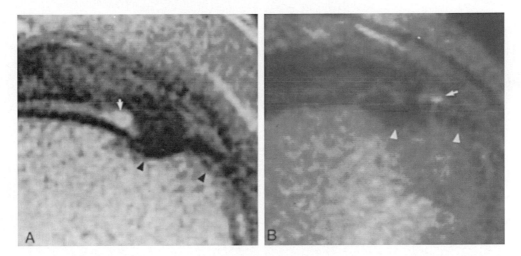

Figure 12–59
Partial-thickness rotator cuff tears: MR imaging.

A Partial-thickness tear of the articular side of the supraspinatus tendon. A coronal oblique T2-weighted (TR/TE, 2000/75) spin echo MR image shows a region of high signal intensity (arrow) involving the inferior or articular surface of the supraspinatus tendon. The supraspinatus tendon attaches to the flat portion of the greater tuberosity of the humerus (between arrowheads), allowing the physician to judge which portion of the tendon is abnormal.

B Partial-thickness tear of the bursal side of the supraspinatus tendon. A coronal oblique T2-weighted (TR/TE, 2000/75) spin echo MR image shows a linear region of high signal intensity (arrow), extending in a horizontal fashion and located in the superior or bursal portion of the tendon. The site of attachment of the supraspinatus tendon to the greater tuberosity of the humerus again is indicated (between arrowheads).

extends in a linear fashion through the entire cuff, without retraction of the tendon, is most consistent with the diagnosis of a small full-thickness tear of the tendon; and a region of increased signal intensity on these images that is parallel to the long axis of the tendon is most consistent with the diagnosis of an intrasubstance tear of the tendon or, perhaps, acute tendinitis. These patterns of altered signal intensity are helpful clues to correct diagnosis (Figs. 12–60, 12–61, and 12–62), but they are not foolproof (Fig. 12–63). Partial-thickness tears of the rotator cuff may be associated with changes in tendon morphology (attenuated or thickened tendon) and unassociated with changes in signal intensity.

Some reported studies have indicated that standard spin echo images are not sufficient for the diagnosis of partial-thickness tears of the rotator cuff.[224, 225] STIR imaging sequences may lead to increased diagnostic accuracy in such cases (Fig. 12–64).[224] Studies employing chemical presaturation of fat also may improve diagnostic accuracy,[224, 659, 672] but increased signal intensity in the distal portion of the tendons of the rotator cuff, even in normal tendons, is encountered with this method.[200] MR arthrography, employing the intra-articular administration of gadolinium compounds, represents an ancillary method that may increase diagnostic accuracy in patients with articular-sided partial-thickness tears of the rotator cuff (Fig. 12–65).[218, 219] Hodler and collaborators,[218] using MR arthrography, were able to correctly diagnose 6 of 13 arthroscopically proved partial-thickness tears of the articular side of the cuff. In 5 of these 13 cases, the results of the MR arthrographic study were interpreted as normal and in two, they were interpreted as evidence of a full-thickness tear.

Surgically Repaired Rotator Cuff Tears. Full-thickness and partial-thickness rotator cuff tears may be entirely asymptomatic and require no therapy. Symptomatic

tears of the rotator cuff can be treated conservatively or surgically. Nonoperative methods of treatment include rest, physical therapy, anti-inflammatory medications, and corticosteroid injections. In cases of full-thickness tears that do not respond to these conservative measures, some type of operative repair, which may include tendon-to-tendon repair or tendon advancement to bone with or without an anterior acromioplasty, may be required.[226, 227] Release of the coracoacromial ligament and resection of the outer end of the clavicle also may be done.[228] Occasionally, biologic and prosthetic grafts are used to repair large cuff defects.[135] Partial-thickness tears of the rotator cuff also may be treated surgically in accordance with principles identical to those used in the treatment of full-thickness tears. Arthroscopic management of incomplete tears (and some complete tears) with débridement, acromioplasty, and even suture placement also is possible, and an approach combining arthroscopic and open techniques can be employed.[229-231] The mechanical strength of the repaired rotator cuff, whether the repair is accomplished with either open or arthroscopic technique, varies considerably.[232] Clinical manifestations after any type of surgical repair may relate to persistent or recurrent rotator cuff tear, persistent shoulder impingement, subdeltoid adhesions, tendinitis, deltoid muscle detachment, and nerve injury.[135, 673] Predisposing factors for recurrent rotator cuff tear include advancing age of the patient, larger size of the initial tendon tear, and increased levels of physical activity.[233] Poorer postoperative results occur when muscle atrophy is present at the time of cuff repair.

Imaging of the postoperative shoulder presents a diagnostic challenge. Even after a clinically adequate repair, glenohumeral joint arthrography may reveal communication of the joint and the subacromial-subdeltoid bursa.[234] Furthermore, owing to the presence of adhe-

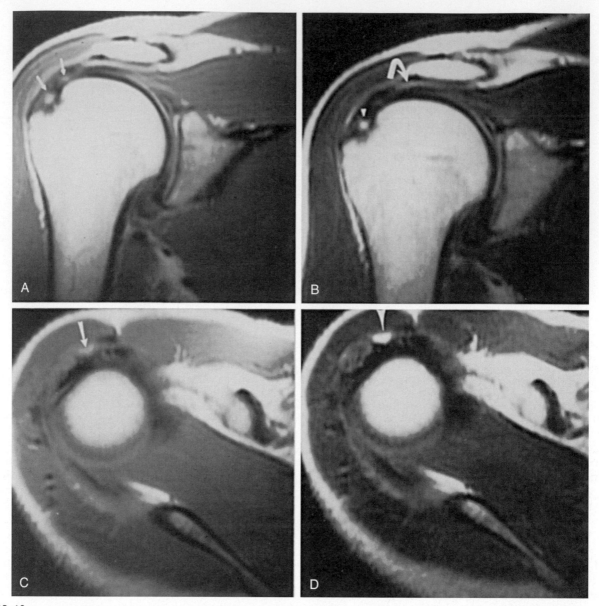

Figure 12–60
Partial-thickness rotator cuff tears: MR imaging—articular side of the supraspinatus tendon. Coronal oblique proton density–weighted (TR/TE, 2000/20) **(A)** and T2-weighted (TR/TE, 2000/70) **(B)** spin echo MR images show two small regions of altered signal intensity (arrows in **A**) in the distal portion of the supraspinatus tendon. One of these regions shows a further increase in signal intensity (arrowhead) in **B**. There is no fluid in the subacromial-subdeltoid bursa (curved arrow in **B**). Transaxial proton density–weighted (TR/TE, 2000/20) **(C)** and T2-weighted (TR/TE, 2000/60) **(D)** spin echo MR images confirm a region of altered signal intensity in the leading edge of the supraspinatus tendon which is of intermediate signal intensity (arrow) in **C** and of high signal intensity (arrowhead) in **D**. (From Kursunoglu-Brahme S, et al: Radiol Clin North Am *28*:941, 1990.)

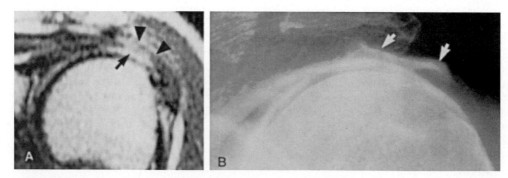

Figure 12–61
Partial-thickness rotator cuff tears: MR imaging and arthrography—articular side of the supraspinatus tendon. A coronal oblique T2-weighted (TR/TE, 2500/60) spin echo MR image **(A)** shows a region of high signal intensity (arrow) involving the articular portion of the supraspinatus tendon. Some intact tendinous fibers (arrowheads) appear to extend over the region of high signal intensity. Glenohumeral joint arthrography **(B)** confirms a partial-thickness tear (arrows) of the supraspinatus tendon.

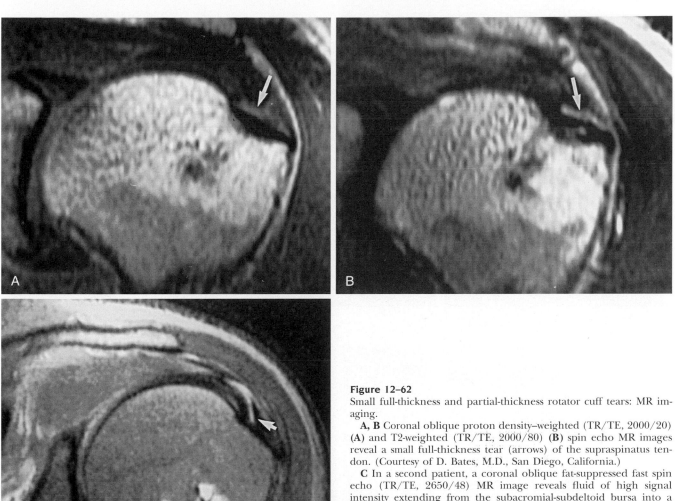

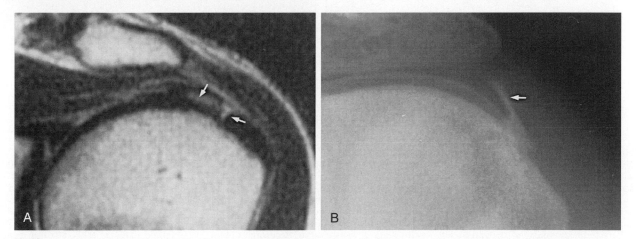

Figure 12–62

Small full-thickness and partial-thickness rotator cuff tears: MR imaging.

A, B Coronal oblique proton density–weighted (TR/TE, 2000/20) **(A)** and T2-weighted (TR/TE, 2000/80) **(B)** spin echo MR images reveal a small full-thickness tear (arrows) of the supraspinatus tendon. (Courtesy of D. Bates, M.D., San Diego, California.)

C In a second patient, a coronal oblique fat-suppressed fast spin echo (TR/TE, 2650/48) MR image reveals fluid of high signal intensity extending from the subacromial-subdeltoid bursa into a partial tear (arrow) in the outer substance of the infraspinatus tendon. A small bone infarct is present in the proximal portion of the humerus. (Courtesy of V. Lim, M.D., San Diego, California.)

Figure 12–63

Partial-thickness versus full-thickness rotator cuff tears: MR imaging.

A A coronal oblique T2-weighted (TR/TE, 3000/105) fast spin echo MR image shows regions of high signal intensity (arrows) in the distal portion of the supraspinatus tendon that were interpreted as evidence of a bursal-sided or intrasubstance tendon tear.

B An arthrogram reveals a partial-thickness tear (arrow) involving the articular side of the tendon. Several weeks later, arthroscopy revealed a small full-thickness tear of the supraspinatus tendon. In this case, it is possible that a partial-thickness tendon tear at the time of arthrography and MR imaging had progressed to a full-thickness tear evident at arthroscopy.

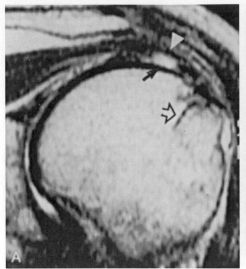
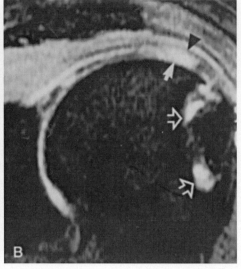

Figure 12–64
Partial-thickness rotator cuff tears: MR imaging including STIR images—articular side of the supraspinatus tendon. A coronal oblique T2-weighted (TR/TE, 2000/80) spin echo MR image **(A)** reveals a region of high signal intensity (solid arrow) involving the articular side of the supraspinatus tendon, with overlying intact tendinous fibers (arrowhead). Note the presence of a fracture (open arrow) of the greater tuberosity of the humerus and a joint effusion. A coronal oblique STIR (TR/TE, 2000/20; inversion time, 160 msec) MR image **(B)** confirms the partial-thickness tear of the tendon (solid arrow), overlying intact tendinous fibers (arrowhead), and the fracture (open arrows) of the greater tuberosity of the humerus.

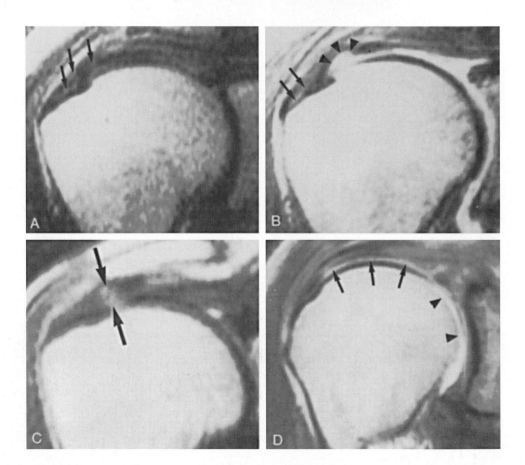

Figure 12–65
Partial-thickness rotator cuff tears: MR imaging and MR arthrography.

A, B Partial-thickness tears of the articular and bursal sides of the supraspinatus tendon. A coronal oblique T2-weighted (TR/TE, 2000/80) spin echo MR image **(A)** reveals minor irregularities of signal intensity (arrows) in the supraspinatus tendon, although regions of high signal intensity are not evident. A coronal oblique T1-weighted (TR/TE, 600/20) spin echo MR image after the intra-articular injection of a gadolinium compound **(B)** reveals a partial-thickness tear (arrowheads) of the articular side of the supraspinatus tendon and additional sites (arrows) of intermediate signal intensity of questionable significance. The diagnosis of a partial-thickness tear of the bursal side of the supraspinatus tendon, which was confirmed during bursoscopy, is not possible on the basis of the MR arthrographic findings.

C, D Partial-thickness tear of the bursal side of the supraspinatus tendon. A coronal oblique T2-weighted (TR/TE, 2000/80) spin echo MR image **(C)** shows a region of high signal intensity (arrows) in the supraspinatus tendon, although it is not clear if this indicates a partial-thickness or full-thickness tear. A coronal oblique T1-weighted (TR/TE, 600/20) spin echo MR image after the intra-articular administration of a gadolinium compound **(D)** confirms that the articular side of the supraspinatus tendon is normal (arrows). Note the contrast material within the joint (arrowheads). No information is provided regarding the integrity of the bursal side of the tendon, which was found to be torn during bursoscopy.

(From Hodler J, et al: Radiology *182*:431, 1992.)

sions at the site of repair, failure to reveal such communication during arthrography does not eliminate the possibility of a persistent or recurrent rotator cuff tear. At ultrasonographic examination, defects in the rotator cuff may be detected,[233, 235] although anatomic landmarks are distorted, making sonography less useful here. MR imaging also may be used to evaluate the surgically repaired rotator cuff.[214, 691] As reported by Owen and coworkers,[134] acromioplasty frequently results in alteration of the normal signal intensity of the fatty marrow within the remaining portion of the acromion with persistently decreased signal intensity on both T1-weighted and T2-weighted spin echo MR images. The MR imaging criteria for full-thickness rotator cuff tears in the shoulder after surgery are the presence of fluid-like signal intensity on T2-weighted spin echo MR images that extends through an area of the rotator cuff and the nonvisualization of a portion of the rotator cuff.[134, 214] Although accurately identifying 90 per cent of such tears, Owen and collaborators[134] were unable to differentiate partial-thickness cuff tears and repaired tendons. The presence of fluid in the glenohumeral joint or in the subacromial-subdeltoid bursa does not necessarily indicate a recurrent cuff tear.[214] A potential diagnostic role may exist for MR arthrography in the evaluation of complete and incomplete tears after shoulder surgery (Figs. 12–66 and 12–67).

Rotator Cuff Tendinitis, Tendinosis, and Tendinopathy

The designation of tendinitis often is applied loosely to a variety of shoulder problems that lead to focal pain and tenderness and subacromial crepitation. These complaints are common in persons involved in occupations requiring heavy manual labor, frequent arm elevation, and the use of hand tools.[236] Similar symptoms and signs are encountered in persons involved in sporting activities that require considerable shoulder movement. As histologic data supporting the occurrence of true tendon inflammation generally are lacking in these persons, it appears likely that a number of different disorders, such as avulsion or disruption of rotator cuff tendons and shoulder impingement, are responsible for these clinical manifestations. The vulnerability of components of the rotator cuff to ischemia and extrinsic compression during arm elevation has been addressed earlier.

Histologic abnormalities similar to those observed in ligamentous tissue about the elbow in cases of overuse syndrome[237] have been documented in some instances of rotator cuff tendinitis. Initial alterations include fibroblastic invasion and vascular granulation-like tissue that has been described as angiofibroblastic hyperplasia.[146, 237] Subsequent alterations include similar hyperplasia, fibrosis, and vacuolar, mucoid, eosinophilic, and fibrillary degeneration with or without calcification.[155] In neither the acute nor chronic stages, however, are abundant inflammatory cells evident. When chronic inflammatory cells are detected, they are seen more commonly in the supporting tissues and not in the tendon. The histologic findings are more compatible with an ischemic or degenerative process than an inflammatory one. A more appropriate term for this process is tendinosis or tendinopathy rather than tendinitis.

The reported MR imaging characteristics of rotator cuff tendinosis or tendinopathy (i.e., tendinitis) have included increased signal intensity in a tendon with normal or abnormal morphology and an intact peribursal fat plane.[206] The increase in signal intensity generally

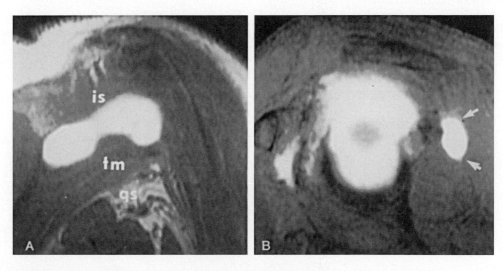

Figure 12–66

Full-thickness rotator cuff tears after surgical repair of the rotator cuff: MR arthrography. This patient had had tendon-to-tendon repair of a full-thickness tear of the supraspinatus and infraspinatus tendons, prior to developing recurrent shoulder pain and limitation of motion.

A A coronal oblique proton density (TR/TE, 2200/30) spin echo MR image after the intra-articular injection of a gadolinium compound shows the contrast material of high signal intensity, extending posteriorly, between the infraspinatus muscle (is) and teres minor muscle (tm). Note the quadrilateral space (qs).

B A sagittal oblique T1-weighted (TR/TE, 900/20) spin echo MR image obtained with chemical presaturation of fat (ChemSat) after the intra-articular injection of a gadolinium compound confirms the posterior leakage of contrast material (arrows).

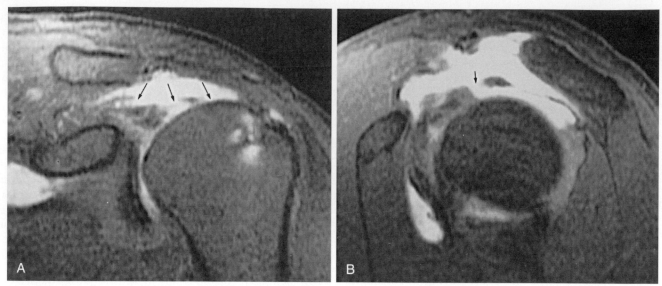

Figure 12–67

Full-thickness rotator cuff tears after surgical repair of the rotator cuff: MR arthrography. Fat-suppressed T1-weighted coronal oblique (TR/TE, 700/20) **(A)** and sagittal oblique (TR/TE, 850/20) **(B)** spin echo MR images after the intra-articular injection of a gadolinium compound show disruption (arrows) of the surgically repaired rotator cuff, which appears attenuated, free communication between the joint and the subacromial bursa, and resection of a portion of the acromion and clavicle. High signal intensity in the humeral head relates to the previous surgery.

is moderate and not extreme, creating an inhomogeneous appearance to the tendon (Fig. 12–68). It is apparent on T1-weighted and proton density–weighted spin echo MR images and is less evident on T2-weighted spin echo MR images.[208] Regions of intense signal within the cuff tendons on T2-weighted spin echo MR images that is similar to the signal intensity of fluid are not compatible with the diagnosis of tendinosis or tendinopathy. Such regions suggest the presence of a full-thickness or partial-thickness tear of the rotator cuff or, perhaps, even a posttraumatic strain.[674] The MR imaging findings of tendinosis or tendinopathy can be identified in asymptomatic persons, suggesting that in most cases they lack clinical importance. Similar MR imaging findings are associated with tendon scars, perhaps related to healing of a previous tendon tear (Fig. 12–69).

Histopathologic observations using cadaveric shoulders have confirmed the presence of tendon degeneration in regions of increased signal intensity on the T1-weighted and proton density–weighted spin echo MR images (see Fig. 12–68).[155, 208] Increased internal signal intensity has been shown to have several different distributions; in general, these reflect the extent of the eosinophilic, fibrillary, and mucoid changes.[155]

Calcific Tendinitis and Bursitis

The capsular, tendinous, ligamentous, and bursal tissues about the shoulder are the most common sites of articular and periarticular calcific deposits.[238–241] The frequency of these collections has been studied by Bos-

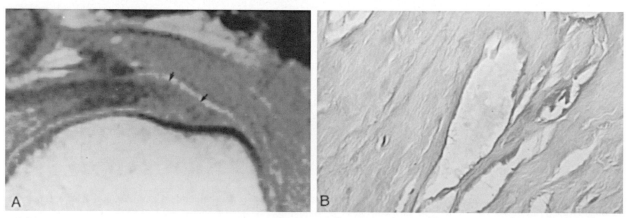

Figure 12–68

Tendinosis or tendinopathy of the rotator cuff: MR imaging and histopathology. A coronal oblique proton density–weighted (TR/TE, 2000/25) spin echo MR image **(A)** reveals increased signal intensity in the distal part of the supraspinatus tendon (arrows). There was no further increase in signal intensity in T2-weighted spin echo MR images. The peribursal fat plane is intact. A photomicrograph (H & E stain, ×100) **(B)** reveals mucoid and vacuolar degeneration in the affected portion of the supraspinatus tendon. No inflammatory cells are evident. (From Kjellin I, et al: Radiology *181*:837, 1991.)

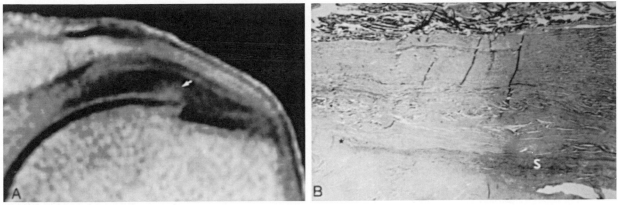

Figure 12–69

Tendon scar of the rotator cuff: MR imaging and histopathology. A coronal oblique proton density–weighted (TR/TE, 2000/25) spin echo MR image **(A)** shows increased signal intensity in the articular side of the distal portion of the supraspinatus tendon (arrow). There was no further increase in signal intensity in the T2-weighted spin echo MR images. A photomicrograph (H & E stain, ×16) **(B)** demonstrates a linear scar (s) in the articular side of the supraspinatus tendon. The lateral end of the scar is indicated by an asterisk. (From Kjellin I, et al: Radiology *181*:837, 1991.)

worth,[242] who reported that 2.7 per cent of 6061 employees with sedentary occupations revealed calcium deposits on shoulder fluoroscopy. These deposits, which were more common on the right side and were bilateral in almost 50 per cent of persons, were located most frequently in the supraspinatus tendon (52 per cent). Clinical findings were apparent in 34 per cent of patients who revealed calcification. Other investigators have observed that calcification may be present in 40 to 45 per cent of patients with painful shoulders.[243, 244] The frequency of bilateral shoulder calcification has been further substantiated by Arner and associates,[245] who, in a 3½ year follow-up investigation of 85 patients with unilateral calcific tendinitis, observed that greater than 50 per cent developed calcification in the opposite shoulder. These calcifications frequently were asymptomatic, although Sandstrom[246] noted that 12 of 20 patients with asymptomatic calcium deposits developed symptoms within a 5 year period. Calcific collections about the shoulder, as at other sites, may produce significant symptoms and signs, including pain, tenderness, swelling, and restricted motion.

Routine Radiographic Abnormalities

The radiographic appearance of shoulder calcification will depend on the exact location of the abnormal deposits; they commonly are encountered in the tendons of the rotator cuff, adjacent tendons, and bursae (Fig. 12–70). In fact, calcification may appear in one site initially, such as the supraspinatus tendon, and migrate to another location subsequently, such as the subacromial bursa. Moseley[247] has suggested that the following sequence may be observed (Fig. 12–71):

1. *Silent phase.* Calcium salts are first deposited in the substance of the tendons of the rotator cuff at the critical zone in the area of arterial anastomosis between tendinous vessels arising from muscular and osseous vasculature. In this location, the tendinous calcification may cause no significant clinical findings.

2. *Mechanical phase.* The tendinous collections in-

crease in size and produce elevation of the floor of the subacromial bursa. At this stage, increased tension produces pain of varying severity, and bursitis may appear, related to hyperemia of the subbursal vessels.

a. *Subbursal rupture.* The deposits may be extruded partially from the tendon under the floor of the bursa. This process of subbursal rupture may be repeated several times, and eventually the complete deposit may be expelled from the tendon.

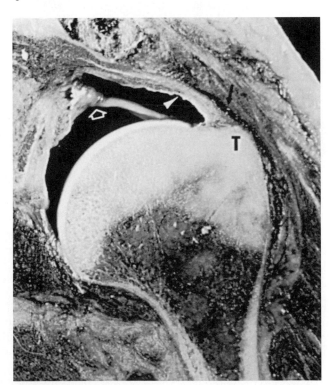

Figure 12–70

Tendon calcification about the shoulder: Sites of involvement—coronal section of the glenohumeral joint. Calcific deposits may be located in the tendons of the rotator cuff (arrowhead), particularly near the site of their attachment to the greater tuberosity (T), bicipital tendon at the site of its attachment to the superior rim of the glenoid (open arrow), and subdeltoid (subacromial) bursa (solid arrow).

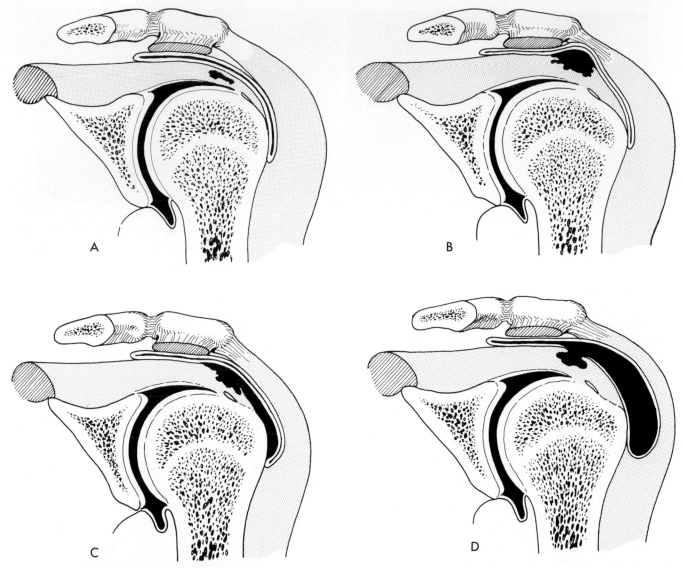

Figure 12–71
Calcification of the rotator cuff: Phases of the disease.
   A Silent phase. Subclinical deposition of calcium occurs in the substance of the rotator cuff tendons.
   B Mechanical phase—elevation of bursal floor. As the deposits increase in size, the floor of the subdeltoid (subacromial) bursa is raised.
   C Mechanical phase—subbursal rupture. Observe that rupture of the calcific deposits has occurred beneath the floor of the bursa.
   D Mechanical phase—intrabursal rupture. The entire deposit is being expelled into the subdeltoid bursa.

b. *Intrabursal rupture.* Complete intrabursal rupture of the tendinous or subbursal calcific material may be associated with severe pain and tenderness.

3. *Adhesive periarthritis phase.* In this stage, calcific deposits within the tendon are accompanied by adhesive bursitis.

4. *Intraosseous loculation.* In some patients, extension of calcific collections into the adjacent greater tuberosity may be observed, producing intraosseous cystic lesions of varying size.

5. *Dumbbell loculation.* A rare occurrence is dumbbell deformity of the subbursal deposit related to pressure from the adjacent coracoacromial ligament.

Although this sequence may not always be apparent, it does underscore the fact that tendinous and bursal calcification in the shoulder may have a variable appearance. Furthermore, the position of the calcification on shoulder radiographs depends on the specific tendon in which it is located.[248]

Supraspinatus Tendon Calcification. The supraspinatus tendon is the most frequent site of calcification. The deposits are located at the tendinous insertion on the promontory of the greater tuberosity (Fig. 12–72). Radiodense lesions at this site may be seen in profile on external rotation of the shoulder. They may remain in profile on internal rotation, although as the calcification moves medially in this projection, it may overlie the humeral head.[249]

Infraspinatus Tendon Calcification. Calcification within the substance of the infraspinatus tendon may be projected over the lateral aspect of the humeral head

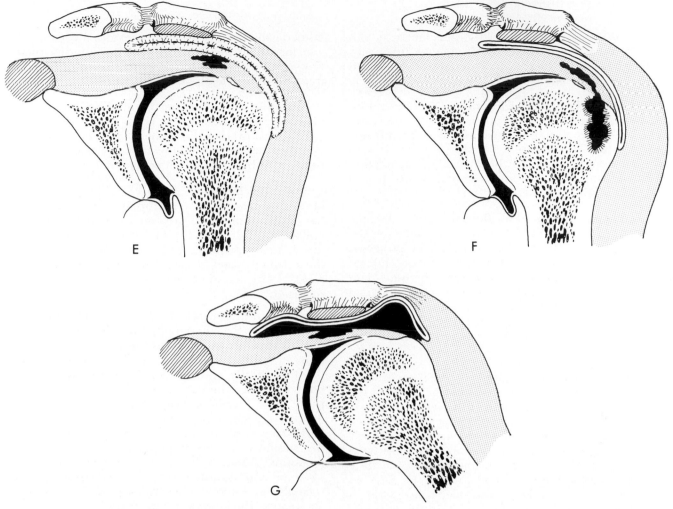

Figure 12–71 *Continued*

E Adhesive periarthritis stage. Note adduction of shoulder with adhesive bursitis.

F Intraosseous loculation. The calcific deposit has extended into the bone.

G Dumbbell loculation. Rarely, a biloculated deposit may be seen related to pressure from the adjacent coracoacromial ligament. (Redrawn after Moseley HF: Shoulder Lesions. 3rd Ed. Edinburgh, E & S Livingstone, 1969.)

Figure 12–72
Calcification of the rotator cuff: Supraspinatus tendon calcification. In external rotation, calcification is apparent above the greater tuberosity (arrow).

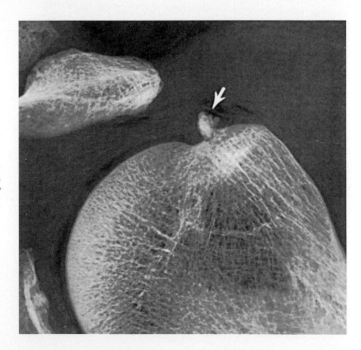

in external rotation because of the attachment of this tendon to the posterior aspect of the greater tuberosity. In internal rotation, the calcification moves laterally and may be seen in profile (Fig. 12–73).

Teres Minor Tendon Calcification. The teres minor tendon attaches to the posterior aspect of the greater tuberosity below the site of attachment of the infraspinatus tendon. Calcification within this tendon is projected over the humeral head in external rotation and moves laterally in internal rotation, where it may be seen in profile (see Fig. 12–73).

Subscapularis Tendon Calcification. The subscapularis tendon attaches to the lesser tuberosity of the humerus. Subscapularis tendon calcification is projected over the humeral head in external rotation, related to the anterior position of the lesser tuberosity. This calcification moves medially on internal rotation and can be seen near the inner surface of the humeral head in this position (see Fig. 12–73). Calcification is seen tangentially adjacent to the lesser tuberosity in an axillary projection.

Bicipital Tendon Calcification. As the long head of the biceps tendon attaches to the superior aspect of the glenoid fossa after passing through the bicipital groove, calcific tendinitis of this structure appears as a radiodense area in this location, which does not move appreciably on external or internal rotation. The short head of the biceps attaches to the coracoid process. Calcification in this tendon is apparent adjacent to the coracoid tip. Calcification in the long head of the biceps also is seen along the shaft of the humerus.[250] In this location, calcification occurs at the junction of the tendon and muscle.[251] The calcification is apparent lateral to the

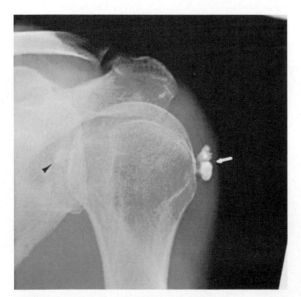

Figure 12–73
Calcification of the rotator cuff: Infraspinatus, teres minor, and subscapularis tendon calcification. In internal rotation, calcific deposits in the infraspinatus and teres minor tendons appear lateral to the humeral head (arrow), and those in the subscapularis tendon are located near the lesser tuberosity, overlying the joint space (arrowhead).

humeral shaft or overlying it on external rotation views and medial to the humeral shaft on internal rotation views. Its appearance simulates that of an osseous body trapped in the sheath of the tendon.

Pectoralis Major Tendon Calcification. Calcific tendinitis of this structure rarely is recorded.[252, 253] The calcification overlies the humeral shaft in external rotation and lies medial to the humeral shaft in internal rotation. Subjacent cortical erosion may be observed.

Bursal Calcification. Calcification in the subacromial bursa appears as a teardrop-shaped, ulcerated, or "skullcap" radiodense area adjacent to the superolateral aspect of the joint capsule, which may extend under the greater tuberosity. Fluid levels due to layering of the calcified material have been identified in unusual cases.[254] Calcific supracoracoid bursitis also has been reported.[255]

Although, in general, there is no significant correlation between the radiographic appearance and size of the calcification and the clinical features of the condition,[245, 256] some reports have indicated that poorly defined or "fluffy" calcification is associated with acute flares of pain, whereas sharply defined calcification is not.[238] The former is accompanied by histologic evidence of calcium resorption and the latter is not.[238] Furthermore, obliteration of the peribursal fat plane of the shoulder has been identified in cases of calcific tendinitis, although the finding lacks specificity, being observed also in cases of rotator cuff disruption, and its reliability in differentiating symptomatic and asymptomatic tendon calcification is not defined.

In the past, many techniques have been used to treat calcific tendinitis and bursitis of the shoulder, with varying success. These techniques have included heat and cold therapy, ultrasonic and diathermic procedures, needle insertion and aspiration, steroid injections, surgery, and radiotherapy. In certain instances, calcific collections may diminish in size and even disappear; at other times, calcification may become more extensive or the deposits may remain unchanged in size.[246, 257–259]

Ultrasonographic Abnormalities

Calcifications within the tendons of the rotator cuff can be detected with ultrasonography.[260–262, 675] An intratendinous hyperechoic mass is seen. Similar hyperechoic patterns, however, can relate to normal inhomogeneity of the cuff, to abnormalities such as fibrosis, blood, and granulation tissue, and even to technical variables such as the use of too much gain and reverberation. Indeed, the presence of calcific tendinitis can lead to diagnostic difficulty when ultrasonography is used to detect rotator cuff tears. Some reports indicate superiority of ultrasonography over fluoroscopy as a means to monitor needle punctures, aspiration, and lavage used to treat calcific tendinitis.[261, 676]

Magnetic Resonance Imaging Abnormalities

Calcific tendinitis is diagnosed far more easily on plain films than on MR images (Figs. 12–74 and 12–75).

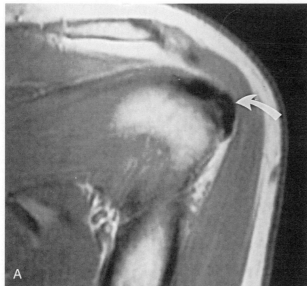

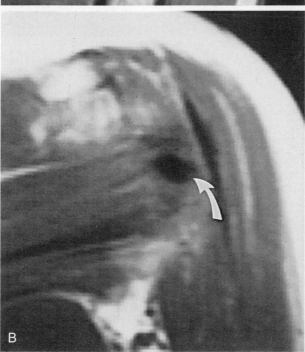

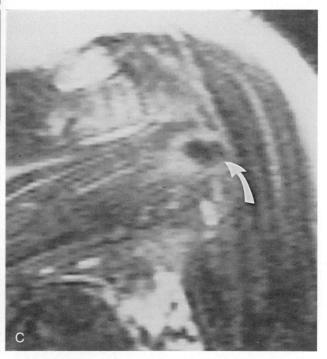

Figure 12–74

Calcific tendinitis: MR imaging—Infraspinatus tendon.

A In a 34 year old woman, a coronal oblique proton density–weighted (TR/TE, 2200/21) spin echo MR image reveals the calcification (arrow) as a region of low signal intensity. (Courtesy of S. K. Brahme, M.D., La Jolla, California.)

B, C In a 51 year old woman, coronal oblique T1-weighted (TR/TE, 600/15) **(B)** and T2-weighted (TR/TE, 2000/90) **(C)** spin echo MR images show the tendon calcification (arrows) of low signal intensity surrounded by a zone of high signal intensity in **C.**

Regions of low signal intensity on all imaging sequences (but particularly on gradient echo sequences) are typical of intratendinous (and intrabursal) calcification (Fig. 12–76), but these regions may be difficult to differentiate from a thickened tendon without calcification.[263] Although areas of high signal intensity may be observed about foci of calcification in tendons and bursae on T2-weighted spin echo MR images and after the intravenous administration of a gadolinium compound (Figs. 12–77 and 12–78), the correlation of such findings to symptomatic calcific tendinitis and bursitis has not been proved.

Adhesive Capsulitis

Adhesive capsulitis is one of several terms applied to a clinical condition in which there is severe restriction of active and passive motion of the glenohumeral joint and in which no other cause can be documented. Additional designations for this disorder are capsulitis, periarthritis, and frozen shoulder. Although some investigators prefer the term frozen shoulder to describe this disorder,[264] abnormalities in the capsule of the glenohumeral joint generally are considered fundamental to its pathogenesis; therefore, the designation adhesive capsulitis is used in this chapter. A similar condition may involve the ankle, wrist, and hip.

Several different systems have been introduced to classify adhesive capsulitis of the shoulder. Lundberg[265] divided the condition into two categories: primary disease, in which no predisposing cause or event can be documented; and secondary disease, in which a traumatic injury has occurred previously. Other investigators use classification systems based on the degree of restric-

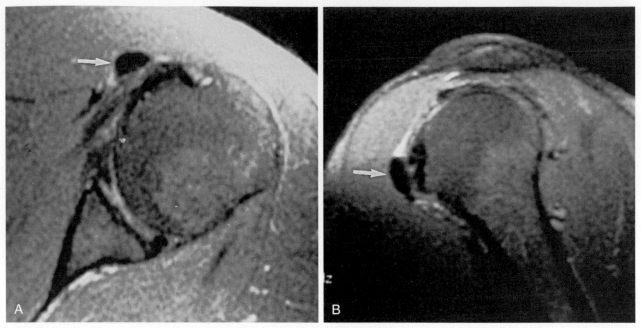

Figure 12–75
Calcific tendinitis: MR imaging. Subscapularis tendon. Fat-suppressed transaxial (TR/TE, 1600/17) **(A)** and sagittal oblique (TR/TE, 4800/22) **(B)** fast spin echo MR images show tendon calcification (arrows) of low signal intensity. (Courtesy of R. Loredo, M.D., San Antonio, Texas.)

tion of the joint capsule,[266] the results of physical examination done with the patient under anesthesia,[267] or the arthrographic findings.[268]

Most patients with adhesive capsulitis are between the ages of 40 and 70 years. Predisposing factors include trauma, hemiplegia, cerebral hemorrhage, diabetes mellitus, hyperthyroidism, and cervical disc disease. Many patients report a period during which the shoulder

has been immobile because of pain, injury, cervical spondylosis, or other causes.[264] Unilateral involvement of the shoulder predominates, although subsequent involvement of the opposite shoulder may occur in as many as 20 per cent of patients. Three stages, or phases, of the disease are recognized[264]: the painful phase, characterized by progressive pain, usually worse at night, over a period of weeks to months; the stiffening phase,

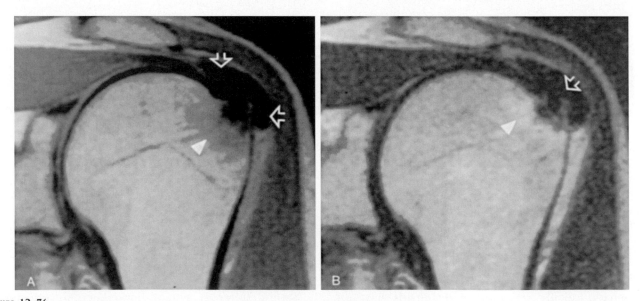

Figure 12–76
Calcific tendinitis: MR imaging—Tendon calcification with intraosseous penetration.

A On a coronal oblique proton density (TR/TE, 1800/20) spin echo MR image, calcification in the supraspinatus tendon (arrows) appears as a region of low signal intensity. The calcific collection has extended into the greater tuberosity, and low signal intensity in the bone marrow (arrowhead) is indicative of edema.

B On a coronal oblique T2-weighted (TR/TE, 1800/90) spin echo MR image, the calcification remains of low signal intensity (arrow). Edema in the bone marrow appears bright (arrowhead).

(Courtesy of C. Ho, M.D., San Francisco, California.)

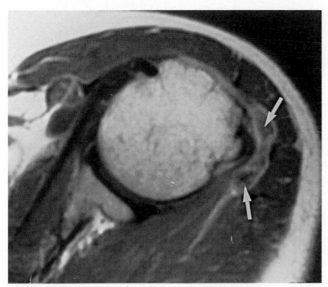

Figure 12–77
Calcific bursitis: MR imaging. A transaxial T1-weighted (TR/TE, 666/17) spin echo MR image obtained after intravenous administration of a gadolinium contrast agent shows the calcific focus (arrows) of relatively low signal intensity with a surrounding zone of enhanced signal intensity. (Courtesy of B. Y. Yang, M.D., Taipei, Taiwan.)

of 4 to 12 months, characterized by slowly progressive loss of shoulder motion; and the thawing phase, usually weeks to months in duration, during which shoulder motion is regained gradually. Although adhesive capsulitis commonly is a self-limited condition that lasts about 12 to 18 months, its outcome is variable and, in some cases, full recovery of shoulder motion never occurs.

The pathogenesis and gross morphologic abnormalities of adhesive capsulitis have been investigated extensively. These investigations have been summarized by Murnaghan.[264] Fifty years ago, Neviaser[269] described the capsular changes that characterize this condition, which consisted of thickening and contraction, and he introduced the term adhesive capsulitis. Approximately 6 years later, McLaughlin[270] confirmed the capsular alterations and indicated also that a proliferative synovitis was evident and that the tendon sheath of the long head of the biceps brachii muscle was involved frequently. At about the same time, Simmonds[271] implicated a chronic inflammatory process of the supraspinatus tendon in the pathogenesis of adhesive capsulitis, and Macnab[272] expanded on this theory, suggesting that an autoimmune response to alterations of the supraspinatus tendon resulted in this condition. Although capsular thickening[265] and adhesions either between the capsule and bicipital tendon[273] or in the subacromial-subdeltoid bursa and beneath the coracoid process[274] have been emphasized in many reports of adhesive capsulitis, they are not confirmed uniformly.[265] Recent studies have implicated changes in the rotator interval and, specifically, the coracohumeral ligament in the pathogenesis of this condition.[275, 276] Tissue samples derived from biopsies of this ligament and the area of the rotator interval confirm the presence of vascular collagenous tissue containing fibroblasts and myofibroblasts, similar to tissue occurring in cases of Dupuytren's contracture.[276] Con-

ceivably, thickening and contracture of the coracohumeral ligament and rotator interval act as a tight checkrein that prevents external rotation of the arm.[276]

Routine radiography rarely contributes to the diagnosis of adhesive capsulitis. Rather, it serves mainly to eliminate other conditions, such as a chronic rotator cuff tear or calcific tendinitis, that may lead to similar clinical manifestations. In adhesive capsulitis, nonspecific periarticular osteoporosis and sclerotic and cystic changes in the greater tuberosity of the humerus are encountered. Rarely, thickening or buttressing of the cortex of the proximal and medial portion of the humeral neck is apparent.

Glenohumeral joint arthrography has been used in the diagnosis and treatment of adhesive capsulitis.[277, 278] Indeed, arthrography is considered by most investigators, although not all,[279] as a reliable means of detecting adhesive capsulitis. Single contrast (radiopaque contrast agent) technique is preferable,[280] and simultaneous determination of the intra-articular pressure has been described.[281] The main arthrographic abnormality in adhesive capsulitis of the glenohumeral joint is a joint of low capacity, evidenced by increased resistance to injection and a "tight" feel (Fig. 12–79). Only a small amount of fluid (5 to 8 ml) may be injected successfully, and when the hand is released from the plunger, the fluid may quickly return to the syringe. The subscapular and axillary recesses are small or absent. Filling of the bicipital tendon sheath is variable; in some cases it appears normal, whereas in others it fills poorly or not at all, or contrast agent may leak from the sheath. Contrast material also commonly leaks elsewhere in the joint, particu-

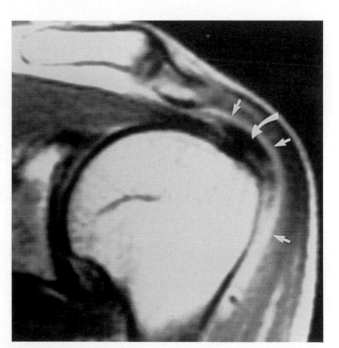

Figure 12–78
Calcific bursitis: MR imaging. A coronal oblique T1-weighted (TR/TE, 430/21) spin echo MR image obtained after intravenous administration of a gadolinium contrast agent shows bursal calcification (curved arrow) of low signal intensity, with diffuse enhancement of signal intensity in the subdeltoid bursa (straight arrows).

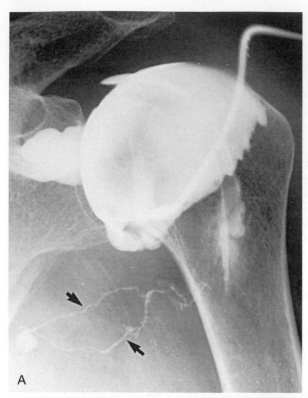

A

Figure 12–79
Adhesive capsulitis: Arthrography.

A After the introduction of 10 ml of contrast material, the patient complained of pain and it was difficult to inject any additional amount of the solution. Note the "tight-looking" joint with a small axillary recess and opacification of lymphatic channels (arrows).

B, C In a second patient, findings after the introduction of 10 ml of contrast material (**B**) confirm the presence of adhesive capsulitis. Note opacification of lymphatic channels: A brisement procedure then was performed, with joint distention. After the introduction of 30 ml of contrast agent (**C**), note medial extravasation of the solution.

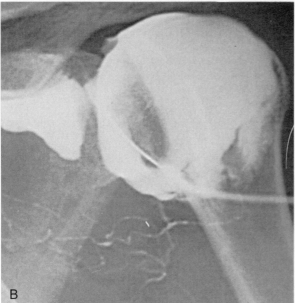

B

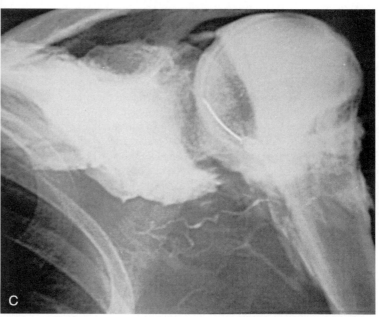

C

larly from the subscapular recess. An additional finding is irregularity of the capsular insertion.

Joint distention during arthrography, the "brisement" procedure,[282] may aid in treatment of this condition.[278] This technique requires slow, intermittent injection of larger and larger volumes of contrast material (mixed with saline solution and lidocaine), allowing some of the fluid to return into the syringe after each injection (see Fig. 12–79). The patient is instructed to move the arm carefully during the procedure. In some patients, 100 ml of fluid eventually may be injected, although free extravasation, particularly at the subscapular recess

or the bicipital tendon sheath, frequently occurs with extensive distention, and the procedure is halted. Post-procedural physical therapy is advised. With severe capsular restriction, the brisement procedure is less beneficial, and in all patients, symptoms may return, requiring repeated examinations. The technique also has been applied to the treatment of adhesive capsulitis in other locations, such as the hip, with inconstant therapeutic results.

There is yet no proven diagnostic role for MR imaging in the assessment of adhesive capsulitis of the shoulder. In one report, thickening of the joint capsule (and

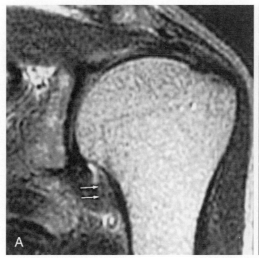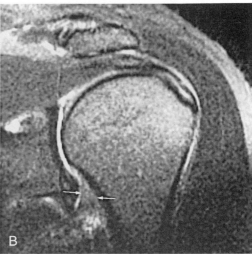

Figure 12–80

Adhesive capsulitis: MR imaging.

A A coronal oblique T2-weighted (TR/TE, 1800/80) spin echo MR image shows thickening of the joint capsule (arrows) adjacent to the medial aspect of the humeral neck. (Courtesy of B. Y. Yang, M.D., Taipei, Taiwan.)

B In a second patient, a coronal oblique fast spin echo MR image shows a similar finding (arrows). (Courtesy of M. Schweitzer, M.D., Philadelphia, Pennsylvania.)

synovial membrane) was evident in patients with adhesive capsulitis (Fig. 12–80).[283] When the joint capsule was measured as the width of tissue located between the axillary pouch and medial cortex of the adjacent humerus, a value greater than 4 mm (representing the thickness of the capsule) was a specific (95 per cent) and sensitive (70 per cent) criterion for the diagnosis of adhesive capsulitis.[283] The volume of articular fluid and the thickness of the coracohumeral ligament were not found to be helpful parameters in establishing this diagnosis. The role of MR arthrography in patients with adhesive capsulitis is not clear.

The role of ultrasonography as a diagnostic technique in cases of adhesive capsulitis likewise is not clear[284] but probably is limited. Limitation of movement of the supraspinatus tendon with respect to the acromion was found to be a useful sonographic sign in the diagnosis of adhesive capsulitis in one study.[285]

Bone scintigraphy in patients with adhesive capsulitis of the shoulder reveals nonspecific uptake of the radiopharmaceutical agent.[279, 286] In general, no association exists between the abnormalities depicted on bone scans and the severity or prognosis of the disease or the arthrographic findings.[279]

Arthroscopy has been used to define the extent of synovial and capsular abnormalities in adhesive capsulitis, both before and after manipulation of the shoulder under anesthesia, but the role of shoulder arthroscopy in the diagnosis of adhesive capsulitis is not established.[264, 287, 288] Arthroscopy has been used effectively as a therapeutic modality, however, allowing capsular release and sectioning of the coracohumeral ligament.[289, 290]

Synovial Abnormalities

Involvement of the glenohumeral joint in a variety of synovial inflammatory disorders, such as rheumatoid arthritis, the seronegative spondyloarthropathies, crystal deposition diseases, infection, amyloidosis, pigmented villonodular synovitis, and idiopathic synovial (osteo)-chondromatosis, is well recognized. Similar involvement of the subacromial-subdeltoid bursa, either alone or in combination with glenohumeral joint involvement, also is well documented.[692] The arthrographic and bursographic findings accompanying these conditions include a corrugated, enlarged synovial space, nodular filling defects, lymphatic filling, adhesive capsulitis with a restricted joint cavity, adhesive bursitis with a contracted bursal cavity, and rotator cuff disruption (Figs. 12–81 and 12–82). In cases of rheumatoid arthritis, para-articular synovial cysts may be encountered, and in cases of septic arthritis, soft tissue abscesses may be evident.

Ultrasonography provides a rapid and inexpensive technique for detection of abnormal amounts of fluid and synovial inflammatory tissue in the glenohumeral joint (Fig. 12–83) and subacromial-subdeltoid bursa (Fig. 12–84).

MR imaging is extremely sensitive to the presence of joint fluid. The detection of an effusion in the acro-

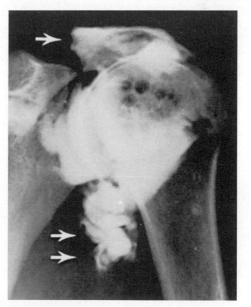

Figure 12–81

Septic arthritis: Glenohumeral joint arthrography. Note opacification of a soft tissue abscess (lower arrows) and, owing to a rotator cuff tear, the subacromial-subdeltoid bursa (upper arrow).

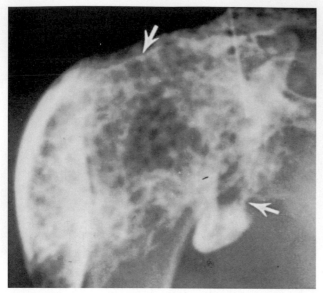

Figure 12–82
Rheumatoid arthritis: Subacromial bursography. A frontal radiograph reveals an enlarged subacromial bursa with innumerable nodular filling defects (arrows). (Courtesy of W. J. Weston, M.D., Lower Hutt, New Zealand.)

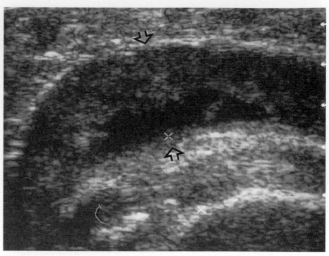

Figure 12–84
Rheumatoid bursitis: Ultrasonography. A transverse sonogram of the upper arm demonstrates anechoic fluid and adjacent hypoechoic synovial thickening within the subdeltoid bursa (arrows). (Courtesy of M. van Holsbeeck, M.D., Detroit, Michigan, and J. Jacobson, M.D., San Diego, California.)

mioclavicular joint with this method generally is considered an abnormal finding, indicative of articular disease, usually osteoarthritis.[291] Similarly, the detection of more than 2 or 3 ml of fluid in the glenohumeral joint with MR imaging usually indicates an abnormal situation.[97, 292] Most commonly, such fluid is indicative of a rotator cuff tear or osteoarthritis.[292]

MR imaging in cases of synovitis within the glenohumeral joint or subacromial-subdeltoid bursa shows a

variety of findings, including an increased amount of synovial fluid, intrasynovial regions of low signal intensity representing fibrous (or rice) bodies, synovial cysts, and enhancement of the synovial membrane after the intravenous administration of gadolinium compounds (Figs. 12–85 and 12–86).[693] The extent of cartilaginous and osseous destruction may be identifiable (Fig. 12–87). In cases of pigmented villonodular synovitis or idio-

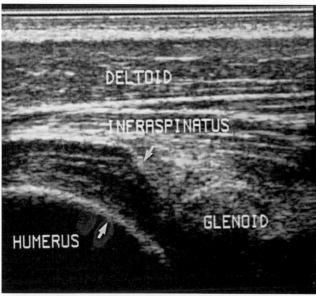

Figure 12–83
Septic arthritis: Ultrasonography. A transverse sonogram of the posterior aspect of the shoulder shows joint fluid of mixed echogenicity (arrows) separating the humeral head and infraspinatus tendon. (Courtesy of M. van Holsbeeck, M.D., Detroit, Michigan, and J. Jacobson, M.D., San Diego, California.)

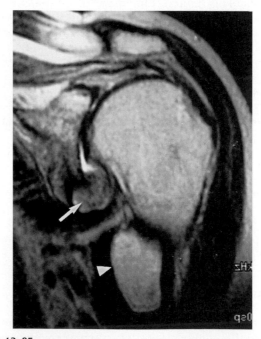

Figure 12–85
Rheumatoid arthritis: MR imaging. In a coronal oblique fast spin echo (TR/TE, 2683/105) MR image, note disruption of the supraspinatus tendon with elevation of the humeral head, intra-articular fluid, synovial inflammation and fibrosis (arrow), erosion of the humeral head, cartilage loss, and a synovial cyst (arrowhead) arising from the bicipital tendon sheath.

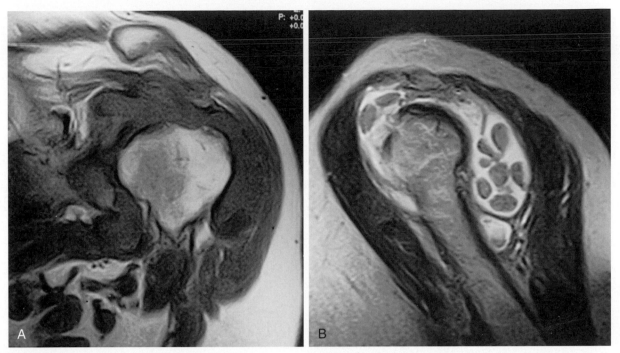

Figure 12–86
Rheumatoid arthritis: MR imaging. In a coronal oblique T1-weighted (TR/TE, 500/20) spin echo MR image **(A),** findings include a massive tear of the rotator cuff, erosions of the humeral head, and fluid and rice bodies in a distended subacromial-subdeltoid bursa. In a sagittal oblique T2-weighted (TR/TE, 2000/80) spin echo MR image **(B),** the distended bursa is seen to contain fluid of high signal intensity and rice bodies of low signal intensity. (Courtesy of J. Dillard, M.D., San Diego, California.)

pathic synovial (osteo)chondromatosis, diagnostic MR imaging abnormalities may be seen, owing to the presence of hemosiderin deposition (in pigmented villonodular synovitis) or cartilage nodules (in idiopathic synovial [osteo]chondromatosis) (Figs. 12–88, 12–89, and 12–90). In amyloidosis, particularly that related to long-term hemodialysis, nodular masses, often with persistent low signal intensity, may be evident. Ultrasonography also can be used in the detection of amyloidosis involving the shoulder.[660]

Ganglion cysts (Fig. 12–91) about the glenohumeral joint are not uncommon. Many of these cysts are incidental findings, although they may be associated with shoulder impingement,[293] labral tears, or nerve entrapment syndromes (see later discussion).

Cartilage Abnormalities

Despite the relative frequency of minor degrees of cartilage fibrillation that has been observed in autopsy stud-

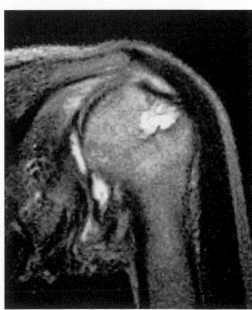

Figure 12–87
Chronic synovitis of the glenohumeral joint: MR imaging. This coronal oblique T2-weighted (TR/TE, 1800/90) spin echo MR image shows disruption and retraction of the rotator cuff tendons, elevation of the humeral head, joint and bursal fluid, and a large erosion of the humeral head.

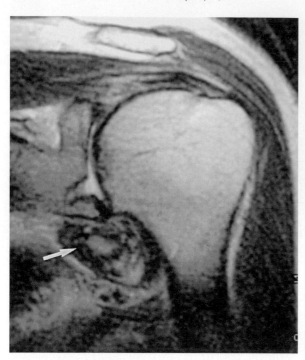

Figure 12–88
Pigmented villonodular synovitis: MR imaging. A coronal oblique fast spin echo (TR/TE, 2616/96) MR image shows fluid of high signal intensity and hemosiderin (arrow) of low signal intensity in the glenohumeral joint. Cartilage and bone destruction are evident. (Courtesy of S. Eilenberg, M.D., San Diego, California.)

ies of the glenohumeral joint,[294] significant osteoarthritis of this joint generally has been regarded as unusual in the absence of local trauma. In fact, the detection of considerable degenerative or destructive alterations during radiographic examination of the glenohumeral joint, particularly in patients without known accidental or occupational trauma, is believed to require a search for other disorders, such as alkaptonuria, acromegaly, epiphyseal dysplasia, calcium pyrophosphate dihydrate or hydroxyapatite crystal deposition disease, neuropathic osteoarthropathy (Fig. 12–92), and hemophilia. Osteoarthritis may affect the glenohumeral joint, however, even in patients without prior physical injury (see Fig. 12–92).[295–297]

The most frequent abnormality accompanying osteoarthritis in this site is the formation of osteophytes along the articular margin of the humeral head and the line of attachment of the labrum to the glenoid fossa. These osteophytes, which may result from functional stress provided by capsular traction, predominate in the anterior and inferior aspects of the joint margin. A second abnormality accompanying osteoarthritis of the glenohumeral joint is focal or global eburnation of the articular surface of the humeral head. As thinning of the articular cartilage predominates in that portion of the humeral head that is in contact with the glenoid fossa when the arm is abducted between 60 and 100 degrees (on a frontal radiograph in neutral position, this part of the humerus lies superomedially),[297] eburnation of subchondral bone occurs in the superior and middle regions of the head of the humerus. Similar eburnation as well as erosion of bone is most evident in the central portion of the glenoid fossa. Osseous excrescences with occasional areas of pitting or cystic change are observed in the anatomic neck of the humerus, greater and lesser tuberosities, and bicipital groove. Those abnormalities in the tuberosities are indicative, in part, of pathologic

alterations in the musculotendinous rotator cuff. Beginning in the third decade of life and increasing in each successive decade, the rotator cuff with its synovial lining gradually is pulled away from the margin of the articular cartilage in the humerus. This movement creates an interval of exposed bone in the anatomic neck, between the periphery of the articular surface and the inner aspect of the rotator cuff. The extent of bone proliferation, pitting, or cystic change that occurs in this region is in direct proportion to the severity of cuff degeneration.

A significant association appears to exist between osteoarthritis of the glenohumeral joint and rotator cuff degeneration. Autopsy studies have indicated that approximately 75 per cent of shoulders with cartilage degeneration also have evidence of attrition or rupture of the cuff. It is not clear, however, if osteoarthritis of the glenohumeral joint and deterioration of the rotator cuff represent independent and somewhat frequent phenomena of aging or if a common pathogenetic mechanism connects them. Two such mechanisms are possible. A penetrating or full-thickness injury of the rotator cuff may lead to leakage of synovial fluid, reduction in intracapsular pressure, and decreased perfusion of nutrients to the articular cartilage. Progressive superior migration of the humeral head then produces instability, increasing wear of cartilaginous surfaces, and osteoarthritis (a phenomenon designated *cuff-tear arthropathy*). Alternatively, the relationship of glenohumeral joint and rotator cuff degeneration may lie in the abnormal accumulation of calcium hydroxyapatite crystals. Release of these crystals into the synovial fluid may induce the release of collagenase and neutral protease, resulting in an attack on the periarticular tissues, including the rotator cuff. The eventual arthropathy, which is designated the *Milwaukee shoulder*, resembles rheumatoid arthritis or neuropathic osteoarthropathy.

Degenerative changes in the acromioclavicular joint

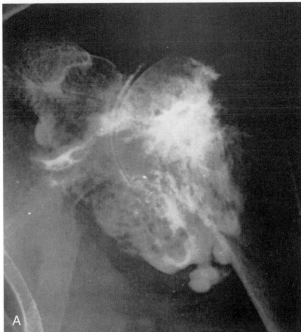

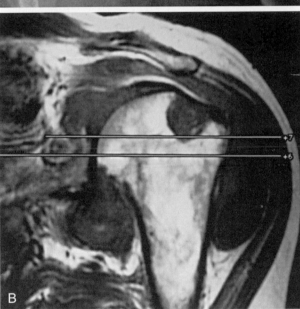

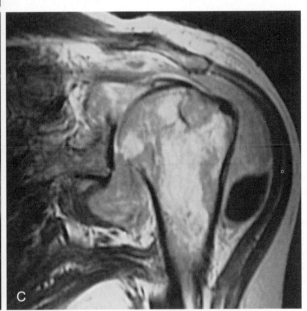

Figure 12–89

Pigmented villonodular synovitis: Glenohumeral joint arthrography and MR imaging.

A The arthrogram reveals gross irregularity of the synovial membrane, sacculations and diverticula, and multiple filling defects.

B On a coronal oblique T1-weighted (TR/TE, 749/16) spin echo MR image, observe distention of the joint and subdeltoid bursa and erosion of the humeral head.

C After intravenous administration of a gadolinium compound, irregular enhancement of signal intensity in the synovium of the joint and bursa and in the humeral erosion is seen on a T1-weighted (TR/TE, 749/16) spin echo MR image.

(Courtesy of B. Y. Yang, M.D., Taipei, Taiwan.)

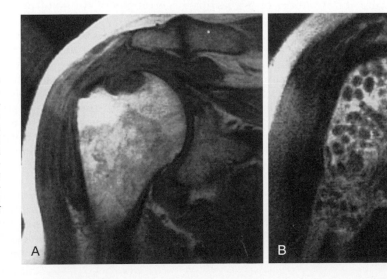

Figure 12–90

Idiopathic synovial (osteo)chondromatosis: MR imaging. Involvement of both the joint and subacromial-subdeltoid bursa with humeral erosion is evident on a coronal oblique T1-weighted (TR/TE, 500/19) spin echo MR image **(A)**, but the multiple synovial bodies in the bursa are better seen on a coronal oblique T2-weighted (TR/TE, 1500/90) spin echo MR image **(B).** (Courtesy of J. Kramer, M.D., Vienna, Austria.)

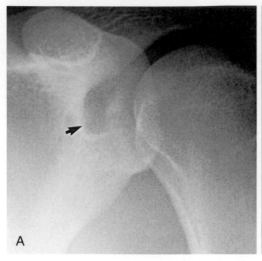

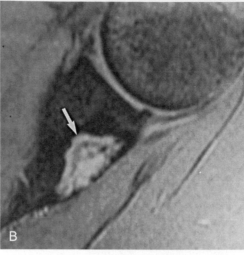

Figure 12–91
Ganglion cysts: MR imaging. Ganglion cysts about the shoulder often are found on the posterior aspect of the scapula where they rarely may lead to bone erosion (arrow, **A**) and, more commonly, to nerve entrapment. MR imaging, in this case a transaxial MPGR (TR/TE, 350/15; flip angle, 25 degrees) MR image **(B)**, is useful in detection of such cysts (arrow).

are almost universal in elderly persons. Diffuse discomfort in the shoulder region, radiating to the upper arm and aggravated by motion, is suggestive of osteoarthritis in the acromioclavicular joint.[298, 299] Such pain is most intense when the arm is elevated between 120 and 180 degrees above the head. Pathologic examination of aging acromioclavicular joints indicates rapid deterioration of the articular disc, beginning as early as the second decade of life and becoming severe by the fifth decade.[300, 301] Changes in this fibrocartilaginous structure are accompanied by rapid loss of articular cartilage, eburnation of subchondral bone, and the formation of osteophytes on both the clavicular and the acromial surfaces.

Osteoarthritis of the sternoclavicular joint also is not uncommon. Its clinical manifestations include pain, tenderness, and palpable enlargement of the articulating bone. Symptoms are aggravated by abduction and elevation of the arm. Pathologic examination of this joint in elderly patients and cadavers indicates degenerative changes, which are not so marked as those in the acromioclavicular joint.[300, 301] The fibrocartilaginous intra-articular disc and the clavicle (Fig. 12–93) are affected more severely than the sternum.[302, 303]

Although routine radiography is effective in demonstrating moderate to severe abnormalities of osteoarthritis in the glenohumeral and acromioclavicular joints, this method is ineffective in documenting early degenerative changes in these locations and any findings of osteoarthritis in the sternoclavicular joint. Specialized radiographic projections (see earlier discussion), CT scanning, and CT arthrography may improve diagnostic sensitivity in some cases. The role of MR imaging in this regard is not clear. Although a number of MR imaging sequences have shown promise in the assessment of articular cartilage in the knee (Chapter 16), these sequences as well as MR arthrography have been less effective in the analysis of the articular cartilage of the glenohumeral joint (Fig. 12–94).[304] Insufficient contrast between cartilage and surrounding structures may lead to errors in the assessment of cartilage thickness, resulting in either underestimation (Fig. 12–95) or overestimation (Fig. 12–96) of this thickness.[304]

The detection of osteocartilaginous bodies in the glenohumeral joint in osteoarthritis or other articular disorders is better accomplished with CT arthrography or MR arthrography than by standard MR imaging.

Glenohumeral Joint Instability

Classification

Glenohumeral joint instability generally is considered a symptomatic clinical situation characterized by altered movement of the humeral head with respect to the glenoid cavity. Such instability, in its classic forms, differs from glenohumeral joint laxity in which asymptomatic passive translation of the humeral head on the glenoid fossa is observed.[305] Glenohumeral joint instability and laxity may coexist. Furthermore, the extent of humeral head translation in patients with glenohumeral joint laxity often is substantial and nearly on a par with that observed in patients with glenohumeral joint instability.[305] Methods of classification of glenohumeral joint instability are based on the degree and direction of instability, its chronology, and its pathogenesis. With regard to the degree of instability, dislocations or subluxations of the joint may be encountered. In the former category, no contact remains between the apposing surfaces of the glenoid cavity and the humeral head. With subluxation, abnormal translation of the humeral head in relation to the glenoid cavity is evident, it is not accompanied by complete separation of the apposing articular surfaces, and it usually is greater than the small amount of translation of the humeral head occurring in the normal range of motion.[306] Subluxation of the glenohumeral joint is transient and often momentary; the humeral head spontaneously returns to its normal position in the glenoid fossa, and the event may be unrecognized by the patient.[307] In one series of patients with anterior subluxation of the glenohumeral joint, a traumatic cause was identified in approximately 90 per cent of cases, and 50 per cent of affected patients were not aware of the problem.[308] Dislocation and subluxation of the glenohumeral joint may occur in several

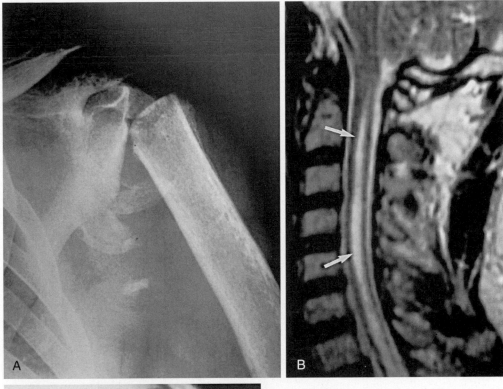

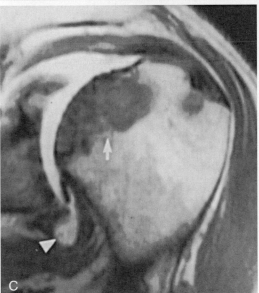

Figure 12–92
Cartilage abnormalities: MR imaging.

A, B Neuropathic osteoarthropathy: Syringomyelia. The detection of destructive abnormalities **(A)** should stimulate a search for a syrinx, well displayed (arrows) on a sagittal fast spin echo (TR/TE, 3600/96) MR image **(B).** (Courtesy of R. Kerr, M.D., Los Angeles, California.)

C Osteoarthritis: Subchondral bone eburnation. A coronal oblique T1-weighted (TR/TE, 650/20) spin echo MR image after the intra-articular injection of gadolinium compound reveals sclerosis, with low signal intensity, in the humeral head (arrow). The rotator cuff is intact, there is sclerosis in the glenoid, and debris (arrowhead) is present in the axillary pouch. The articular cartilage is absent, and portions of the glenoid labrum are disrupted.

different directions: anterior, posterior, superior, and inferior. With anterior or posterior dislocations, the displaced humeral head may become located in a subcoracoid, subglenoid, subclavicular, or intrathoracic location (anterior dislocations) or in a subacromial, subglenoid, or subspinous location (posterior dislocations) (see later discussion). Subluxations and dislocations of the glenohumeral joint may occur at different times in a single patient, and multidirectional instability may lead to different patterns of displacement of the humeral head in a single shoulder.

With regard to chronology, acute dislocations are defined as those seen within the first 24 or 48 hours, and chronic dislocations are defined as those evaluated after this time.[307] In common with subluxations of the glenohumeral joint, dislocations of this joint may be transient, with spontaneous reduction of the humeral head. With dislocations of the glenohumeral joint, the humeral head also may be fixed, or locked, in the abnormal position. If the glenohumeral joint has been unstable on multiple occasions, the instability is classified as recurrent.

Dislocations and subluxations of the glenohumeral joint also may be categorized according to their pathogenesis. They may be traumatic or atraumatic, congenital or acquired, and voluntary or involuntary. The acronym TUBS describes patients with *t*raumatic instability who usually have *u*nilateral involvement, typically have

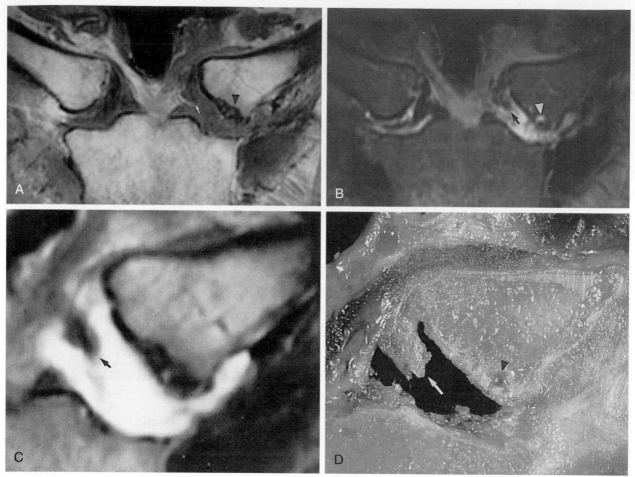

Figure 12–93

Osteoarthritis of the sternoclavicular joint: MR imaging. Cadaveric specimen.

A, B Coronal T1-weighted **(A)** and T2-weighted **(B)** spin echo MR images reveal effusions in both sternoclavicular joints. Note the torn intra-articular disc (arrows) on the left side, associated with a subchondral cyst (arrowheads) in the left clavicle. The articular cartilage of the sternum and clavicle is eroded, particularly in the left joint.

C A T1-weighted coronal spin echo MR image obtained after intra-articular injection of a gadolinium compound confirms the presence of a disrupted disc (arrow) in the left sternoclavicular joint.

D A photograph of a coronal section of the left joint shows the torn disc (arrow), articular cartilage degeneration, and subchondral clavicular cyst (arrowhead).

a *B*ankart lesion, and often require *s*urgery; AMBRI refers to patients with *a*traumatic instability who may have *m*ultidirectional instability, often with *b*ilateral involvement, and may respond to a *r*ehabilitation program or require an *i*nferior capsular shift.[307]

Prevalence and Direction

For a number of reasons, including its propensity for injury and its inherent instability, the glenohumeral joint is the most common site of dislocation and subluxation in the human body. In one study, approximately 45 per cent of more than 8000 dislocations involved the glenohumeral joint.[303] Approximately 85 per cent of all dislocations about the shoulder affect the glenohumeral joint (as opposed to the acromioclavicular or sternoclavicular joint). Glenohumeral joint dislocations can be classified into anterior, posterior, superior, and inferior types.

Figure 12–94

Assessment of articular cartilage of glenohumeral joint: MR imaging. Cadaveric specimen.

A Fat-suppressed T1-weighted (TR/TE, 600/20) spin echo image. Signal intensity of articular cartilage is similar to that of adjacent infraspinatus muscle (arrow).

B Fat-suppressed T1-weighted (TR/TE, 600/20) spin echo image with intra-articular gadolinium contrast agent. Articular cartilage is less intense than the contrast agent. The thickness of humeral head articular cartilage is underestimated dorsally (arrows).

C Fat-suppressed spoiled GRASS image (TR/TE, 60/10; flip angle, 60 degrees). Signal intensity of articular cartilage differs from that of surrounding structures. Three layers of cartilage can be recognized in the anterior portion of the humeral head (arrow).

D Fat-suppressed spoiled GRASS image (TR/TE, 60/10; flip angle, 60 degrees) with intra-articular administration of a gadolinium compound. Articular cartilage is less intense than intra-articular contrast agent. Cartilage thickness is underestimated dorsally (arrows).

E Corresponding anatomic section.

(Reproduced from Hodler, J, et al: AJR *165*:615, 1995. Copyright 1995, American Roentgen Ray Society.)

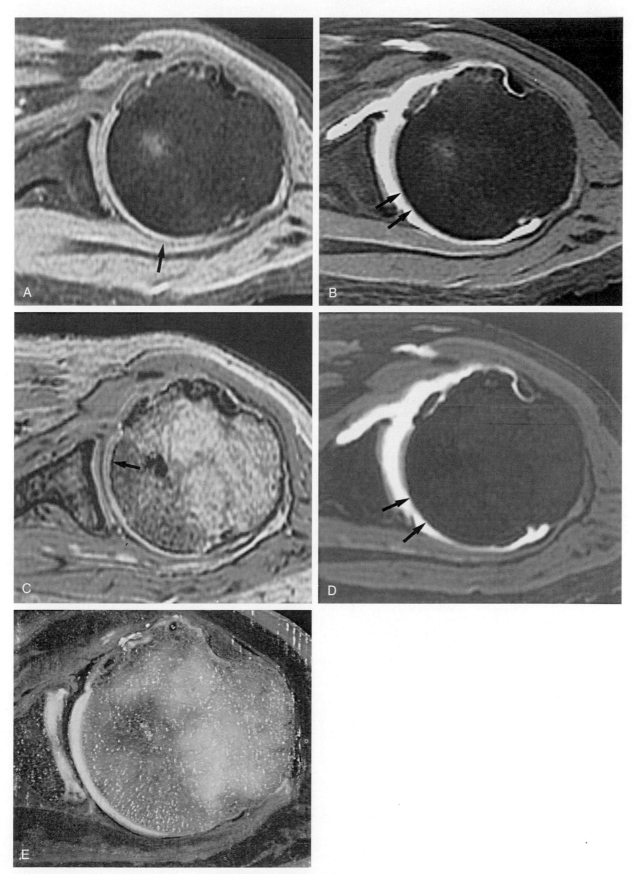

Figure 12–94 *See legend on opposite page*

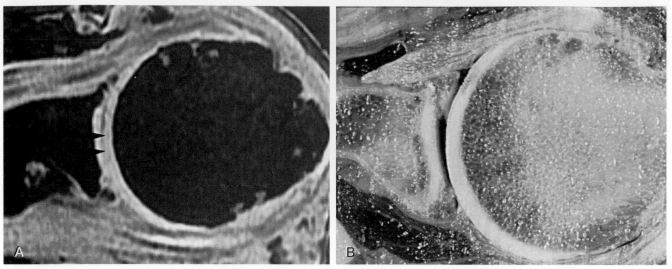

Figure 12–95

Assessment of articular cartilage of glenohumeral joint: MR imaging—cadaveric specimen, underestimation of cartilage thickness.

A Fat-suppressed spoiled GRASS image (TR/TE, 60/10; flip angle, 60 degrees). The superficial hyperintense layer of articular cartilage simulates intra-articular contrast medium (arrows).

B Corresponding anatomic section.

(From Hodler, J, et al: AJR *165*:615, 1995. Copyright 1995, American Roentgen Ray Society.)

Anterior dislocation is by far the most frequent, representing over 95 per cent of such injuries (Fig. 12–97). Anterior dislocations are further classified as subcoracoid (the most common type) (Fig. 12–98A), subglenoid (second in frequency) (Fig. 12–98B), and subclavicular and intrathoracic (rare types) (Figs. 12–99). The usual mechanism causing subcoracoid dislocation is a combination of shoulder abduction, extension, and external rotation.[307] The other types of anterior dislocation usually involve severe trauma. Anterior dislocations (as well as posterior dislocations of the glenohumeral joint) are best evaluated radiographically by the inclusion of a

lateral scapular projection or an axillary projection, or both, in addition to the standard frontal views of the shoulder.

Anterior dislocations are associated with a compression fracture on the posterolateral aspect of the humeral head that is produced by impaction of the humerus against the anterior rim of the glenoid fossa. This osseous defect of the humerus has been recognized for a century,[309] although the report of Hill and Sachs in 1940[310] of the humeral lesion was the first review of the subject in the English language. Because of this, the osseous defect frequently is termed the Hill-Sachs lesion.

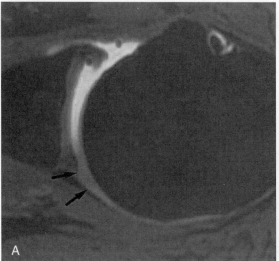
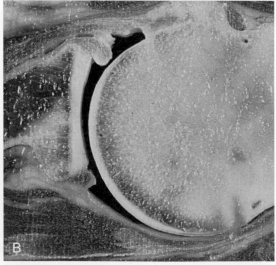

Figure 12–96

Assessment of articular cartilage of glenohumeral joint: MR imaging—cadaveric specimen, overestimation of cartilage thickness.

A Fat-suppressed spoiled GRASS image (TR/TE, 60/10; flip angle, 60 degrees) with intra-articular administration of gadolinium contrast agent. Inadequate mixing of contrast material and joint fluid has led to reduced contrast between fluid and articular cartilage (arrows).

B Corresponding anatomic section.

(From Hodler, J, et al: AJR *165*:615, 1995. Copyright 1995, American Roentgen Ray Society.)

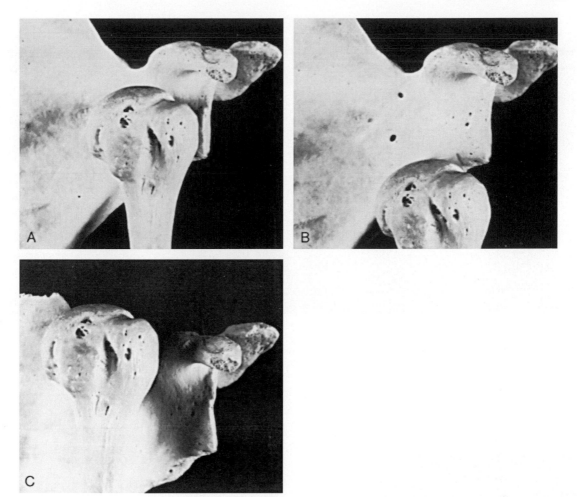

Figure 12–97
Glenohumeral joint: Types of anterior dislocation.

A Subcoracoid type. This is the most common variety of anterior dislocation, resulting from a combination of indirect abduction, extension, and external rotation forces. The head of the humerus is displaced anteriorly and is situated inferior to the coracoid process.

B Subglenoid type. This is the second most common type of anterior dislocation of the glenohumeral joint. The head of the humerus is displaced in an anterior and inferior direction owing to an abduction force that is stronger than the external rotation force. Fracture of the greater tuberosity of the humerus and tearing of the rotator cuff are well-recognized complications of this pattern of dislocation.

C Subclavicular type. This rare type of anterior glenohumeral joint dislocation is characterized by the addition of a lateral force that drives the humeral head medial to the coracoid process and below the midportion of the clavicle.

(From Greenway GD, et al: Med Radiogr Photogr *58*:22, 1982. Reprinted courtesy of Eastman Kodak Company.)

Figure 12–98
Glenohumeral joint: Anterior dislocation—subcoracoid and subglenoid types.

A Subcoracoid type. Note the anterior and medial displacement of the humeral head and fracture of the greater tuberosity.

B Subglenoid type. The humeral head is displaced anteriorly and inferiorly, and the greater tuberosity is fractured.

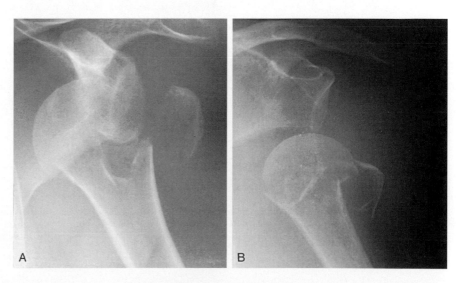

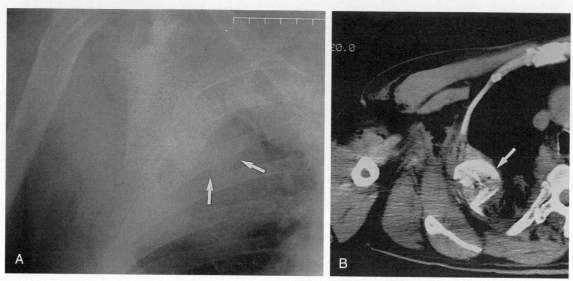

Figure 12–99

Glenohumeral joint: Anterior dislocation—intrathoracic type.

A Routine radiograph reveals a fracture of the proximal portion of the humerus with dislocation of the humeral head (arrows), which now is located in the right hemithorax.

B A transaxial CT scan confirms the presence of the humeral head (arrow) in the right hemithorax.

(Courtesy of P. Kindynis, M.D., Geneva, Switzerland.)

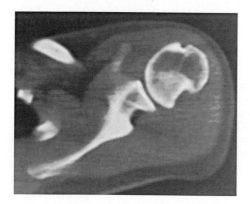

Figure 12–100

Glenohumeral joint: Anterior dislocation—Hill-Sachs lesion. In a transaxial CT image, the Hill-Sachs deformity is readily apparent in the posterolateral aspect of the left humerus. (Courtesy of H. Pavlov, M.D. New York, New York.)

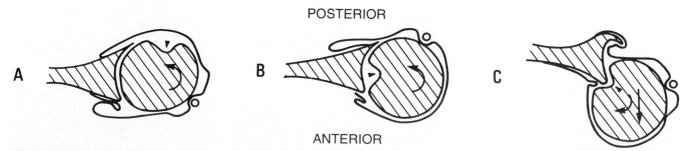

Figure 12–101

Hill-Sachs lesion: Propensity for recurrent dislocation. In a patient with a Hill-Sachs lesion (arrowheads), external rotation **(B)** may allow the lesion to engage the glenoid process so that during subsequent internal rotation **(C),** the humeral head is levered out of the glenoid fossa, producing an anterior dislocation. (**A,** Neutral position.) (Courtesy of G. Greenway, M.D., Dallas, Texas.)

This lesion is observed in many cases of anterior dislocation of the glenohumeral joint. It frequently is larger in those cases that are dislocated for a considerable period of time, those that are recurrent, and those in which the direction of dislocation is anteroinferior rather than purely anterior.[311] The reported frequency of the lesion has varied considerably. Hill and Sachs detected it in 27 per cent of 119 cases of acute anterior dislocation and in 74 per cent of 15 cases of recurrent anterior dislocation.[310] Other investigators have noted the Hill-Sachs defect in 50 to 100 per cent of cases of recurrent dislocations.[312-317] Much of this variation is related to the difference in the radiographic technique used to investigate patients with glenohumeral joint dislocation.[311, 318, 319] In fact, many different radiographic projections have been described in this clinical setting.[677] Films obtained in various degrees of internal rotation are mandatory, as such rotation of the humerus will produce a tangential view of the osseous lesion. Fluoroscopy also can be helpful in equivocal cases. The role of CT in allowing identification of the Hill-Sachs lesion has not been defined precisely (Fig. 12–100). Although ultrasonography also has been used to detect the Hill-Sachs lesion,[678] its role in this regard is also not clear. The radiographic detection of a Hill-Sachs lesion is important, as it delineates the nature of a shoulder injury that may be obscure clinically, implies a propensity for recurrent dislocation, and influences the necessity for and choice of a surgical procedure (Fig. 12–101).

A second type of fracture accompanying anterior dislocation of the humeral head involves the glenoid fossa and is called the Bankart lesion (Fig. 12–102).[320] When osseous fragmentation of the anterior glenoid rim occurs, the abnormality may be apparent on plain film radiographs in frontal or axillary projections, or both.[321]

Specialized radiographic projections such as the Didiee and the West Point views are of further diagnostic help.[319] Although large osseous fractures of the glenoid are apparent occasionally,[322] the fracture may include only the cartilaginous surface of the bone.

A number of other osseous and nonosseous injuries accompany anterior dislocations of the glenohumeral joint. An avulsion fracture of the greater tuberosity of the humerus occurs in 10 to 15 per cent of cases. It is variable in size, and the resulting abnormal contour of the humeral head may simulate that seen with a Hill-Sachs lesion (Fig. 12–103). Disruption of the rotator cuff may complicate anterior dislocation of the glenohumeral joint, particularly in patients who are older than 40 years of age.[323, 324] Various portions of the cuff, including the supraspinatus, infraspinatus, and subscapularis tendons, may be affected, and resulting clinical manifestations (i.e., inability to abduct the arm after reduction of the dislocation) may be falsely attributed to an injury of the axillary nerve. Indeed, injuries to the brachial plexus occur in 7 to 45 per cent of anterior glenohumeral joint dislocations, and such injuries may occur with or without rotator cuff disruption.[325, 694]

Approximately 40 per cent of anterior glenohumeral joint dislocations are recurrent. Recurrent dislocations are more likely in cases of subcoracoid and subglenoid dislocations and in younger persons. Chronic unreduced anterior dislocations with massive Hill-Sachs and Bankart-like lesions also are encountered.[326]

Posterior dislocation of the glenohumeral joint is rare, constituting approximately 2 to 4 per cent of all shoulder dislocations. Specific types of posterior dislocation include the subacromial (the most common type) and the subglenoid and subspinous (rare injuries) varieties (Fig. 12–104). Over 50 per cent of these cases are unrec-

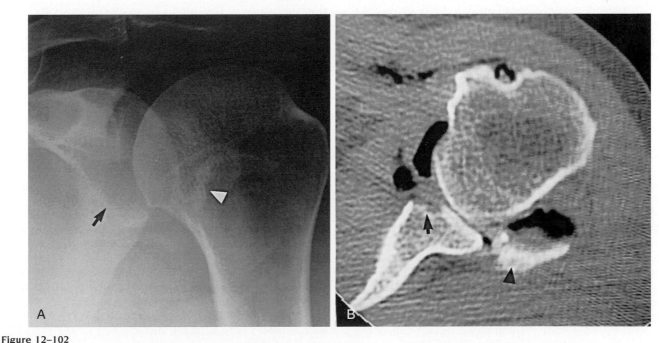

Figure 12–102
Glenohumeral joint: Anterior dislocation—Bankart lesion.
  A Routine radiograph shows disruption of the anterior margin of the glenoid fossa (arrow) and bone fragments (arrowhead).
  B CT arthrography (with air alone) shows the glenoid fracture (arrow) and intra-articular bone fragments (arrowhead).

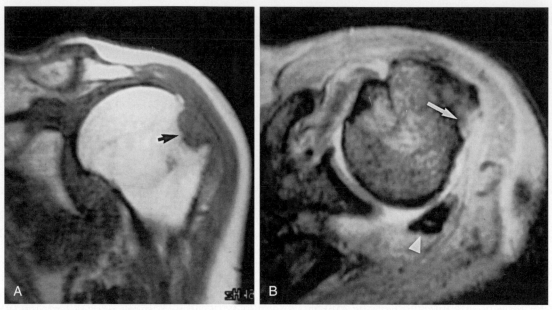

Figure 12–103

Glenohumeral joint: Anterior dislocation—avulsion fracture of humeral head. In a 90 year old woman, a massive tear of the rotator cuff occurred as a result of an anterior glenohumeral joint dislocation. On a coronal oblique T1-weighted (TR/TE, 666/20) spin echo MR image **(A)**, findings include disruption of the rotator cuff with elevation of the humeral head, a joint effusion, and a fracture (arrow) of the humeral head that simulates a Hill-Sachs lesion. A transaxial MPGR (TR/TE, 700/20; flip angle, 45 degrees) MR image **(B)** reveals the avulsed and medially displaced bone fragment (arrowhead) that arose from the greater tuberosity (arrow) owing to the pull of the infraspinatus and, possibly, teres minor tendons. (Courtesy of D. Witte, M.D., Memphis, Tennessee.)

ognized on initial evaluation, despite the presence of a history of trauma, pain, swelling, and limitation of motion. The diagnosis of adhesive capsulitis (frozen shoulder) often is suggested in such cases.[327, 328] Many cases of posterior dislocation result from convulsions, and in these instances, bilateral dislocations may be evident (Fig. 12–105).[329–331] Physical examination reveals a posteriorly displaced humeral head that is held in internal rotation.[332] Absence of external rotation and limitation of abduction are present in virtually all cases of posterior dislocation. Associated injuries include stretching of the posterior capsule, fracture of the posterior aspect of the glenoid rim, an avulsion fracture of the lesser tuberosity of the humerus, and a stretched or detached subscapularis tendon.

Radiographs are diagnostic; the routine examination must include a lateral view of the scapula or an axillary view of the shoulder, or both, and additional projections also may be helpful.[333] On an anteroposterior radiograph, posterior dislocation of the humeral head distorts the normal elliptical radiodense area created by the overlapping of the head and the glenoid fossa (Fig. 12–106). An empty or vacant glenoid cavity is a second radiographic sign of dislocation in this projection; the posterior displacement of the humeral head may create a space between the anterior rim of the glenoid and the humeral head that frequently is greater than 6 mm.[334] In addition, the normal parallel pattern of the articular surfaces of the glenoid concavity and the humeral head convexity is lost. Other radiographic signs of posterior dislocation on frontal radiographs include a fixed position of internal rotation of the humerus and a second cortical line, the trough line, parallel and lateral to the

subchondral articular surface of the humeral head.[335] This line represents the margin of a troughlike impaction fracture of the humeral head created when this structure contacts the posterior glenoid rim during the dislocation.[336] As such, it is analogous to the Hill-Sachs lesion that is seen in association with anterior glenohumeral joint dislocation and is quite diagnostic of a posterior dislocation. The medially located lesser tuberosity that appears during marked internal rotation in the normal shoulder should not be misinterpreted as a trough or as a site of impaction fracture, however.

A tangential view of the glenoid normally demonstrates no overlapping of the humeral head and glenoid rim.[337] In patients with posterior glenohumeral joint dislocation, the humeral head is displaced medially, and abnormal overlapping may be seen. An axillary or lateral scapular projection allows direct delineation of the posterior position of the humeral head with respect to the glenoid. The degree of displacement of the humeral head as evident on these two projections in patients with posterior dislocations of the glenohumeral joint, particularly when associated with large trough fractures of the humeral head, may be less than in those patients with anterior dislocations of the glenohumeral joint, producing some diagnostic difficulty.

CT represents an additional imaging technique that can be used to evaluate patients with acute (or chronic) dislocations of the glenohumeral joint (Fig. 12–107.)[326] This method also is useful in the evaluation of posterior subluxation (without frank dislocation) of the glenohumeral joint.[338]

Owing to a delay in accurate diagnosis of posterior dislocations of the glenohumeral joint,[339] secondary os-

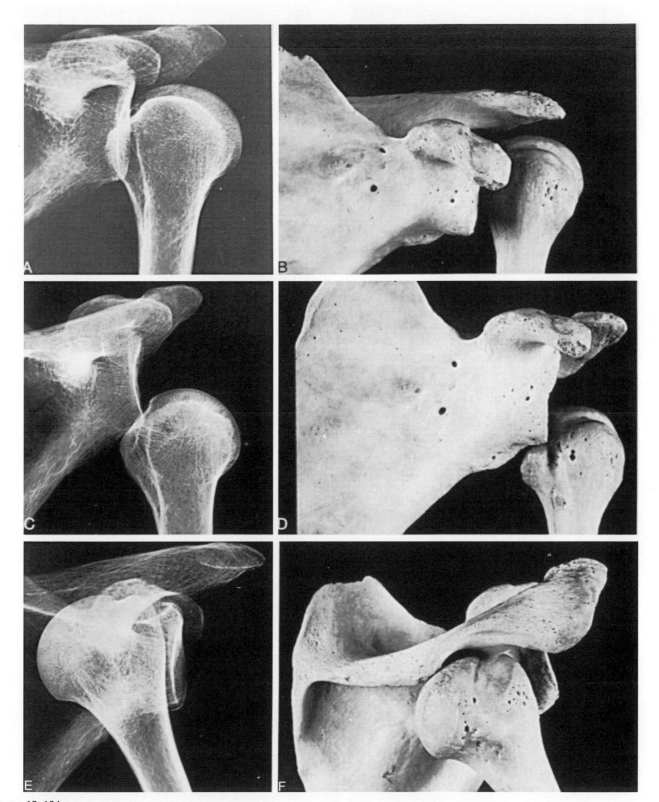

Figure 12–104

Glenohumeral joint: Types of posterior dislocation.

    A, B Subacromial type. This is the most common pattern of posterior dislocation of a glenohumeral joint. The articular surface of the humeral head is directed posteriorly and is behind the glenoid fossa and beneath the acromion process. Note the internal rotation of the humerus.

    C, D Subglenoid type. This is a less common pattern of injury in which the humeral head is displaced posteriorly and inferiorly with respect to the glenoid fossa.

    E, F Subspinous type. In this rare injury, the humeral head becomes situated medial to the acromion process, inferior to the scapular spine, and posterior to the glenoid process. (From Greenway GD, et al: Med Radiogr Photogr *58*:22, 1982. Reprinted courtesy of Eastman Kodak Company.)

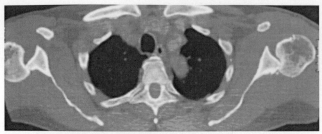

Figure 12–105
Glenohumeral joint: Posterior dislocation—bilateral recurrent dislocations. Transaxial CT shows posterior displacement of both humeral heads and trough fractures of the medial surface of the humeral heads. (Courtesy of M. Schweitzer, M.D., Philadelphia, Pennsylvania.)

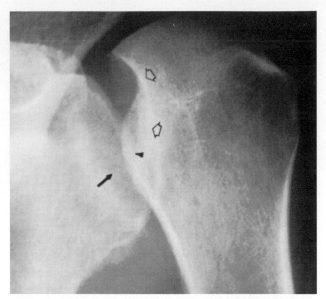

Figure 12–106
Glenohumeral joint: Posterior dislocation. An anteroposterior radiograph in a patient with a posterior glenohumeral joint dislocation. Findings include distortion of the normal elliptical radiodense region created by overlying of the humeral head and glenoid fossa (arrowhead), a "vacant" glenoid cavity (solid arrow), loss of parallelism between the articular surfaces of the glenoid cavity and humeral head, internal rotation of the humerus, and an impaction fracture (open arrows).

teoarthritis in this location is not infrequent.[340] Radiographic findings, including joint space narrowing, osteophytosis, and deformity of the humeral head, simulate those of calcium pyrophosphate dihydrate crystal deposition disease, hydroxyapatite crystal deposition disease, ischemic necrosis of bone, and ochronosis. In untreated chronic dislocations, deformity of the posterior portion of the scapula is seen.

Superior dislocation of the glenohumeral joint is rare (Fig. 12–108).[341] An extreme forward and upward force on the adducted arm can produce extensive damage to the rotator cuff, capsule, biceps tendon, and surrounding musculature and neurovascular structures and fracture of the acromion, clavicle, coracoid process, or humeral tuberosities. Without such fractures, the radiographic appearance of a superior dislocation of the humeral head is identical to that of a primary, massive rotator cuff tear. *Inferior dislocation* of the glenohumeral joint (luxatio erecta) also is rare (Fig. 12–109).[342–348] A direct axial force on a fully abducted arm or a hyperabduction force leading to leverage of the humeral head across the acromion is responsible for this type of dislo-

cation.[348] After this injury, the superior aspect of the articular surface of the humeral head is directed inferiorly and does not contact the inferior glenoid rim. As a result, the arm is held over the patient's head, the inferior aspect of the capsule is torn, and associated injuries, including a fracture of the greater tuberosity of the humerus, of the acromion process, of the coracoid process, of the clavicle, or of the inferior glenoid mar-

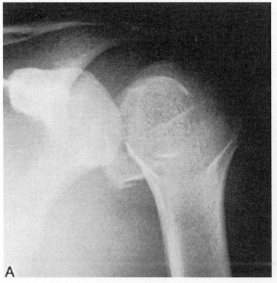
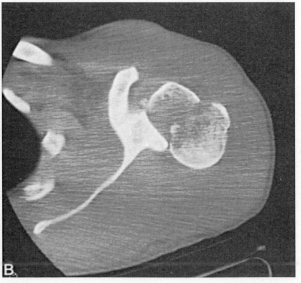

Figure 12–107
Glenohumeral joint: Posterior dislocation—CT scanning in acute injuries. In a 23 year old man, the frontal radiograph (**A**) demonstrates an abnormal relationship of the humeral head and glenoid fossa, an empty glenoid cavity, and avulsion and fragmentation of the lesser tuberosity of the humerus. A transaxial CT scan (**B**) shows a posterior dislocation of the glenohumeral joint and the avulsed tuberosity.

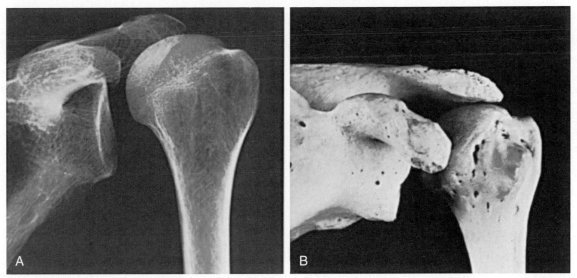

Figure 12–108
Glenohumeral joint: Superior dislocation. In this unusual pattern of dislocation, the humeral head is displaced in a superior direction. Damage to the soft tissues, including the joint capsule, the rotator cuff, the biceps tendon, and the surrounding muscles, is seen. Fractures associated with this dislocation also may be apparent. (From Greenway GD, et al: Med Radiogr Photogr *58*:22,1982. Reprinted courtesy of Eastman Kodak Company.)

gin, may be seen. A lesion of the humeral head, simulating a Hill-Sachs lesion, may accompany luxatio erecta, although it is located more superiorly and laterally.[348] Complications of inferior dislocation of the glenohumeral joint include injuries of the axillary artery and brachial plexus and, later, recurrent subluxation or dislocation and adhesive capsulitis.

In addition to traumatic glenohumeral joint dislocation, *voluntary subluxation or dislocation* may be encountered, especially in adolescents.[349, 350] In these cases, spontaneous displacements of the humeral head on one or both sides occur anteriorly or, more frequently, posteriorly. Although it has been proposed that develop-

mental anomalies of the glenoid cavity or generalized ligamentous laxity may be responsible for this phenomenon[351, 352] and that some patients also may reveal genu valgum and weak arches, widespread abnormalities generally are not evident in patients with voluntary dislocation of the glenohumeral joint.[350] This condition has a favorable prognosis.[353]

A special type of inferior displacement of the humeral head is termed the *drooping shoulder* (Fig. 12–110).[354–357] It can be associated with uncomplicated fractures of the surgical neck of the humerus. The pathogenesis of the displacement is not clear, although relaxation or stretching of the supporting musculature, detachment of the

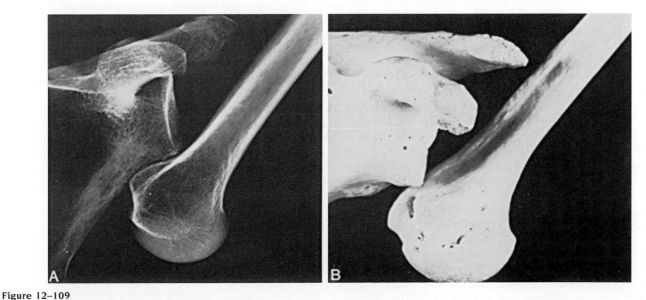

Figure 12–109
Glenohumeral joint: Inferior dislocation.
  A, B In this uncommon pattern of dislocation, the humeral head is driven downward and is inverted. The superior aspect of the articular surface of the humeral head does not contact the inferior aspect of the glenoid rim. (From Greenway GD, et al: Med Radiogr Photogr *58*:22, 1982. Reprinted courtesy of Eastman Kodak Company.)

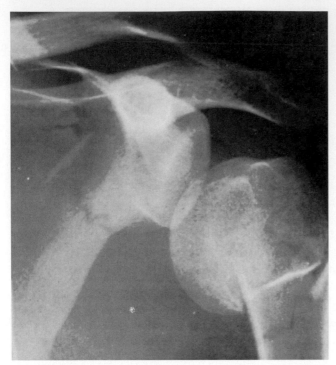

Figure 12–110
Glenohumeral joint: Drooping shoulder. A fracture of the surgical neck of the humerus is associated with inferior subluxation of the head with respect to the glenoid cavity. Observe an associated scapular fracture.

capsule, and hemarthrosis have each been proposed as possible mechanisms. The appearance of a similar displacement in patients with neurologic injuries of the brachial plexus, especially those involving the axillary nerve, supports the view that muscular alterations produce the subluxation, whereas the detection of a drooping shoulder in patients with various articular disorders (e.g., hemophilia) may indicate that joint effusion also can lead to inferior displacement of the humeral head. The degree of inferior displacement of the humeral head varies. In some cases, only subtle widening of the superior portion of the joint space is visible, whereas in others gross displacement is seen. Recognition of this condition will eliminate erroneous diagnosis of fracture-dislocation of the proximal end of the humerus, and conservative therapy will lead to disappearance of the drooping shoulder over a period of weeks.

Etiology and Pathogenesis

Although developmental factors may lead to congenital instability of the glenohumeral joint and such factors combined with emotional and psychiatric problems may promote voluntary subluxations and dislocations of this joint, trauma is the leading cause of subluxations and dislocations of the glenohumeral joint. Indirect forces are more common than direct forces as causes of glenohumeral joint instability. The combination of abduction, extension, and external rotation forces applied to the arm may result in an anterior dislocation of the glenohumeral joint; axial loading of an adducted, internally rotated arm may produce a posterior dislocation.[307]

Although many structures, such as the components of the rotator cuff, the glenoid labrum, the glenohumeral ligaments, the joint capsule and supporting musculature, and the coracoacromial arch, contribute to glenohumeral joint stability (Fig. 12–111), the contributions of each are not agreed on. Both static (passive) and dynamic (active) constraints are believed to contribute to shoulder stability.[358] Static constraints include the bone configuration of the glenohumeral joint, and the capsular and ligamentous complex that surrounds the shoulder; dynamic constraints include the muscle and tendon units that surround the glenohumeral joint, particularly the muscles and tendons of the rotator cuff.[359] Matsen and collaborators[307] have provided an excellent summary of the passive and active constraints, and some of their observations are included here.

With regard to passive mechanisms, the stability of the glenohumeral joint is affected by the size, shape, and tilt of the glenoid fossa. Studies have indicated that the glenoid fossa and its contact area may be smaller in shoulders affected by recurrent glenohumeral joint dislocations than in normal shoulders,[360] and that retroversion of the glenoid cavity may be excessive in shoulders demonstrating posterior glenohumeral joint instability.[361] Conversely, decreased retroversion of the humeral head has been associated with recurrent anterior dislocations of the glenohumeral joint.[362] Whether some of the reported changes are the cause or the effect of glenohumeral joint instability is not clear, however.[363] The glenoid labrum serves to deepen the glenoid cavity, perhaps providing some element of increased stability, but its size is highly variable and often small, such that the contribution of the glenoid labrum to glenohumeral joint stability remains speculative.

The capsule of the glenohumeral joint is large, loose, and redundant, allowing for a great range of motion.[307] Reinforcing the capsule of this joint are the coracohumeral ligament and the three glenohumeral ligaments (Fig. 12–112), whose anatomy has been discussed earlier in this chapter. Although the glenohumeral ligaments are inconstant and variable in size, their importance in providing stability to the glenohumeral joint has been emphasized repeatedly. In combination with the anterior and posterior portions of the joint capsule, the glenohumeral ligaments appear to limit the translation and rotation of the humerus and, therefore, may serve as the last guardian of shoulder stability after all other passive and dynamic mechanisms have been overwhelmed.[307] The role of the joint capsule and glenohumeral ligaments in this regard has been confirmed in a number of cadaveric studies, the results of which have been summarized by Matsen and coworkers[307]:

1. The anteroinferior capsule restrains anterior subluxation of the abducted arm.
2. The middle glenohumeral ligament limits external rotation at 45 degrees of abduction of the arm.
3. The inferior glenohumeral ligament limits external rotation at 45 to 90 degrees of abduction of the arm.
4. The posterior portion of the capsule and the teres minor muscle and tendon restrain internal rotation of the arm.

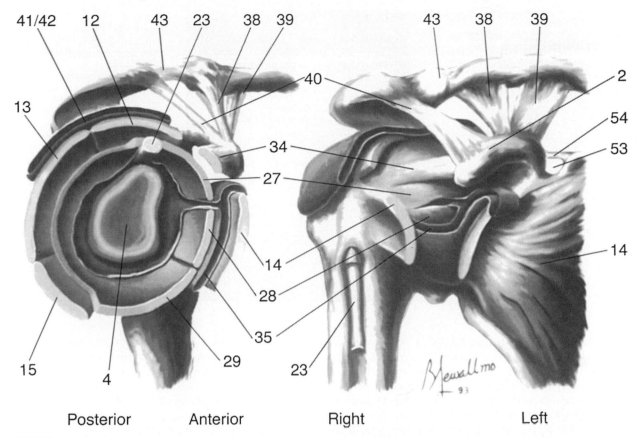

Posterior   Anterior   Right   Left

Figure 12–111
Capsular complex of the glenohumeral joint, rotator cuff, and supraspinatus outlet: Normal anatomy. On the right, a right shoulder is sketched as if all of the muscles have been dissected away to reveal the glenohumeral, coracohumeral, coracoacromial, and coracoclavicular ligaments. The tendons of the long head of the biceps brachii muscle, the subacromial-subdeltoid bursa, and the subscapularis bursa also are depicted. On the left, the relationships of these structures in the sagittal plane are emphasized. In numerical order, the structures that are illustrated are the following:

2. Coracoid process	34. Coracohumeral ligament
4. Glenoid cavity	35. Subscapularis bursa
12. Supraspinatus muscle and tendon	38. Trapezoid ligament
13. Infraspinatus muscle and tendon	39. Conoid ligament
14. Subscapularis muscle and tendon	40. Coracoacromial ligament
15. Teres minor muscle	41. Subacromial bursa
23. Tendon of the long head of the biceps brachii muscle	42. Subdeltoid bursa
27. Superior glenohumeral ligament	43. Acromioclavicular joint and ligaments
28. Middle glenohumeral ligament	53. Suprascapular notch
29. Inferior glenohumeral ligament	54. Superior transverse scapular ligament

(Drawings courtesy of B. O. Sewell, M.D., San Diego, California; from Petersilge CA, et al: MRI Clin North Am *1*:1, 1993.)

5. The lower two thirds of the anterior capsule and the lower portion of the subscapularis muscle and tendon restrain abduction and external rotation of the arm.

Active mechanisms of glenohumeral joint stability include the long head of the biceps brachii muscle and its tendon and the components of the rotator cuff (supraspinatus, infraspinatus, subscapularis, and teres minor muscles and their tendons). The rotator cuff surrounds the humeral head, blending with the capsule of the glenohumeral joint and the capsular ligaments. The components of the rotator cuff can act independently or as a unit, pressing the humeral head into the glenoid fossa and resisting displacing forces resulting from contraction of the major muscles of the shoulder (e.g., deltoid and pectoralis major muscles).[307] This action of the rotator cuff muscles and the stabilizing effect of the biceps brachii muscle form the basis for conservative treatment (e.g., muscle strengthening programs) of shoulder instability.[364] The muscles providing scapular rotation, which include the rhomboids, latissimus dorsi, trapezius, serratus anterior, and levator scapulae, also contribute to glenohumeral joint stability, positioning the scapula to provide a stable platform beneath the humeral head.[365]

The contributions of the anterior glenohumeral ligaments to joint stability have received great emphasis in numerous investigations, the conclusions of which have been summarized by Pagnani and coworkers.[365] The inferior glenohumeral ligament complex has been shown to represent the primary check against anterior instability with the arm abducted 90 degrees. This ligament complex also may serve as the primary static stabilizer against posterior instability when the arm is ab-

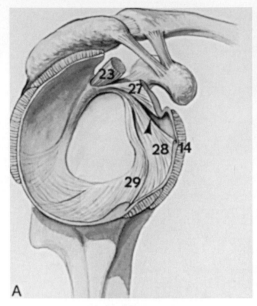
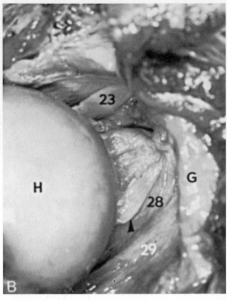

Figure 12–112
Capsular complex of the glenohumeral joint: Normal anatomy. The diagram **(A)** provides a simplified depiction of the anterior capsular complex of the glenohumeral joint; a photograph of a dissected shoulder **(B)** also shows this mechanism. The indicated structures are:

    14. Subscapularis muscle and tendon

    23. Tendon of the long head of the biceps brachii muscle

    27. Superior glenohumeral ligament

    28. Middle glenohumeral ligament

    29. Inferior glenohumeral ligament

    G. Glenoid cavity

    H. Humeral head

    Arrowheads: Opening into the subscapularis bursa.

    (From Zlatkin M, et al: AJR *150*:151, 1988. Copyright 1988, American Roentgen Ray Society.)

ducted 90 degrees. With the shoulder in 90 degrees of abduction and 30 degrees of extension, the anterior band of the inferior glenohumeral ligament complex represents the prime stabilizer against both anterior and posterior translation; with the shoulder in 90 degrees of abduction and 30 degrees of forward flexion, the posterior band of this ligament complex assumes this function. The role of the inferior glenohumeral complex in preventing inferior translation increases with increasing abduction of the arm. The precise contributions of these bands of the inferior glenohumeral ligament complex also are dependent on whether the shoulder is internally or externally rotated. In the adducted arm, the superior glenohumeral ligament limits both inferior and anterior translation, and this ligament also serves to limit posterior translation in the flexed, adducted, and internally rotated arm. The middle glenohumeral ligament limits anterior translation in the midrange of abduction and serves as a secondary restraint in the lower ranges of abduction.

Pagnani and coworkers[365] also have summarized experimental data related to the function of the coracohumeral ligament. These data have not been consistent, with some investigations supporting the view that this ligament has a significant role in controlling inferior translation and others failing to confirm this role. Increasing size of the rotator interval, located between the superior border of the subscapularis tendon and the anterior margin of the supraspinatus tendon and occupied by the coracohumeral and superior glenohumeral ligaments, has been related to anterior and inferior instability in some investigations.

These observations confirm the complexity of the issue of glenohumeral joint stability. Many different structures working independently or in concert provide such stability, and the structures that are operational at any given time depend upon the position of the arm and the type of shoulder movement taking place. Additional factors related to the presence and amount of joint fluid and cohesive and adhesive mechanisms pro-

vided by this fluid also have been identified.[307] Anterior and posterior capsular mechanisms have been defined, underscoring the importance of the coordinated activities of different anatomic structures performing as a functional unit. Instability of the glenohumeral joint occurs when the integrity and coordinated activity of the supporting mechanisms are disrupted (Table 12–3). No single or essential lesion appears to form the basis of anterior or posterior instability of the joint. Identification of a detached portion of the glenoid labrum (Bankart lesion), a compression fracture of the posterolateral surface of the humeral head (Hill-Sachs lesion), a deficiency of one or more of the glenohumeral ligaments, capsular laxity, or detachment or lengthening of the subscapularis muscle as the primary cause of shoulder instability is an oversimplification of a process that is far more complex.

Clinical Abnormalities

The clinical abnormalities related to instability of the glenohumeral joint vary, being influenced by its atraumatic or traumatic pathogenesis and by its acute or chronic nature. Many patients recall an experience in which the humeral head was felt to have been displaced,

Table 12–3. SOME TYPES OF GLENOHUMERAL JOINT INSTABILITY

Type	Abnormal Supporting Structures
Superior	Biceps tendon anchor
	Superior glenohumeral ligament
Anterosuperior	Biceps tendon anchor
	Superior glenohumeral ligament
	Middle glenohumeral ligament
Anterior	Middle glenohumeral ligament
Inferior	Inferior glenohumeral ligament (anterior ± posterior bands)
Posterior	Inferior glenohumeral ligament (posterior band)

whether initiated by trauma or not.[305] Fixed dislocations of the glenohumeral joint usually are identifiable during physical examination of the patient, particularly with anterior dislocation of the glenohumeral joint. Posterior dislocations of this joint are associated with more subtle but definite clinical manifestations, including fixed internal rotation of the affected arm, with limited external rotation and elevation of the arm. The clinical diagnosis of recurrent glenohumeral joint subluxation is more challenging. A history of a minor injury or shoulder discomfort during sporting activities that require movement of the shoulder and physical findings indicative of generalized ligamentous laxity are helpful clues. Manipulative techniques meticulously attempt to document the specific arcs, angles, and directions at which instability is experienced by the patient or the examiner, or by both.[305, 366] Although these provocative tests accomplished during physical examination are used to establish the occurrence of subluxation of the glenohumeral joint, imaging examinations are fundamental to accurate diagnosis.

Routine Radiographic Abnormalities

The routine radiographic abnormalities associated with dislocations of the glenohumeral joint are discussed earlier in this chapter. In addition to confirming an abnormal position of the humeral head with respect to the glenoid cavity, conventional radiographs are useful in the identification of bone injuries that may occur during the dislocation. Foremost among these injuries are the Hill-Sachs lesion of the humerus and a Bankart-type lesion of the anterior portion of the glenoid rim that may occur during anterior dislocation of the glenohumeral joint, and the trough fracture line of the humerus and an impaction fracture of the posterior portion of the glenoid rim (reverse Bankart-type lesion) that may occur during posterior dislocation of the glenohumeral joint. Specialized projections may increase the sensitivity of conventional radiographs to the detection of these associated osseous abnormalities.[319]

The radiographic assessment of recurrent glenohumeral joint instability includes several views obtained during the application of stress to the shoulder.[307] Small amounts of translational movement of the humeral head with respect to the glenoid cavity may be identified, although similar or perhaps superior data are provided by CT.

Arthrographic Abnormalities

Standard arthrography has a limited role in the assessment of glenohumeral joint instability. Anterior dislocations of the glenohumeral joint are associated with soft tissue damage. As the dislocating humeral head moves anteriorly, it tears the articular capsule or it detaches or lifts the articular capsule from the glenoid and neck of the scapula, producing an abnormal recess of variable size between the subscapular and axillary recesses. On arthrography, the abnormal recess fills with contrast material, obscuring the indentation that normally is present between the subscapular and axillary recesses.

This finding is more evident on radiographs taken in internal rotation.

Additional findings related to anterior dislocation are injuries of cartilage and bone. The Bankart deformity involves an avulsion or compression defect of the anteroinferior rim of the glenoid and may be purely cartilaginous. The arthrogram, particularly when performed with double contrast technique, may outline the cartilaginous abnormalities about the glenoid labrum. The second defect associated with previous anterior dislocation is a Hill-Sachs compression deformity on the posterolateral aspect of the humeral head. This finding generally is evident on plain films but may require arthrography for demonstration if the defect is small or involves only cartilage.

Conventional and Computed Arthrotomographic Abnormalities

As the importance of capsular, ligamentous, and labral abnormalities in cases of glenohumeral joint instability became known, tomographic modifications of standard arthrography were applied. Two techniques became popular—conventional arthrotomography and computed arthrotomography.

Conventional arthrotomography was the first of the two techniques to be developed,[367-372] although it rarely is employed today. Thin-section conventional arthrotomography can be accomplished in two ways (prone oblique or supine oblique patient position), each giving a different perspective of the labrum and both requiring considerable experience and expertise on the part of the examiner and meticulous positioning of the patient. Such patients may be positioned in a prone oblique manner, with the affected shoulder facing downward and the neck flexed, with the opposite shoulder moved slightly forward to avoid overlap with the side of interest and the scapula on the involved side directed perpendicular to the table top. Alternatively, a supine oblique position can be used, with the injured shoulder closest to the table. The described techniques of conventional arthrotomography also differ somewhat with regard to the amount of contrast agent that is advocated. In general, 1 or 2 ml of radiopaque contrast material and 10 to 15 ml of air are instilled into the joint.

Computed arthrotomography, the second technique,[373-383] remains popular today. Computed arthrotomography is accomplished after the injection of 10 to 15 ml of air with or without 1 ml of radiopaque contrast material. The patients are examined in the supine position with their arms positioned by their sides and their shoulders in a neutral attitude or in slight internal rotation; to distend the posterior capsule optimally with air, external rotation of the shoulder can be used. Continuous 3 mm sections usually are used, and an average of 15 scans is sufficient. Reformatted coronal or sagittal images rarely are required.

The interpretation of the images obtained with either conventional or computed arthrotomography requires knowledge of the cross-sectional appearance of the normal humeral head and glenoid region of the scapula and of normal soft tissue structures (Figs. 12–113, 12–

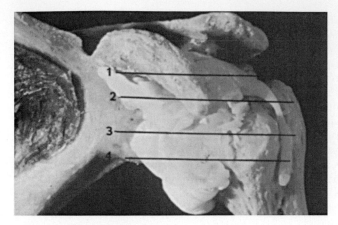

Figure 12–113
Cross-sectional appearance of the glenohumeral joint: Normal anatomy. Four anatomic levels of analysis. As demonstrated in this anatomic specimen, in which the glenohumeral joint has been distended with methylmethacrylate, a simplified approach to the assessment of transaxial images provided by conventional or computed arthrotomography (or MR imaging or MR arthrography) emphasizes findings at four specific levels: the superior aspect of the joint (level 1); the region of the subscapularis recess or bursa (level 2); the midglenoid level (level 3); and the inferior glenoid level (level 4). (From Zlatkin M, et al: AJR *150*:151, 1988. Copyright 1988, American Roentgen Ray Society.)

114, 12–115, 12–116, and 12–117). The head of the humerus is essentially round and smooth on superior sections taken at the level of the coracoid process, which is the appropriate level for evaluation of a Hill-Sachs lesion; the smooth appearance changes to an irregular one at the level of the cartilage-bone junction in the neck of the humerus, where a constant constriction or concavity is evident between the greater tuberosity and the humeral head itself.[384] The bicipital groove, located between the greater and lesser tuberosities of the humerus, varies considerably in both depth and configuration.

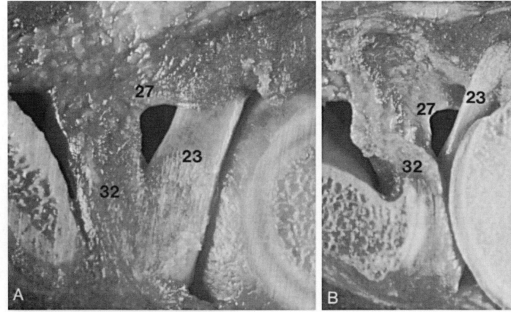

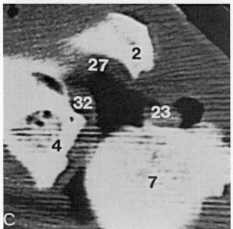

Figure 12–114
Cross-sectional appearance of the glenohumeral joint: Normal anatomy. Level 1—superior aspect of the joint.

  A, B Two sections, **A** slightly above **B**, show the superior portion of the glenoid labrum (32), the capsule and superior glenohumeral ligament (27), and the tendon of the long head of the biceps brachii muscle (23).

  C CT arthrography of the air-distended joint also allows identification of these same structures. The humerus (7), glenoid cavity (4), and coracoid process (2) also are indicated.

  (From Zlatkin M, et al: AJR *150*:151, 1988. Copyright 1988, American Roentgen Ray Society.)

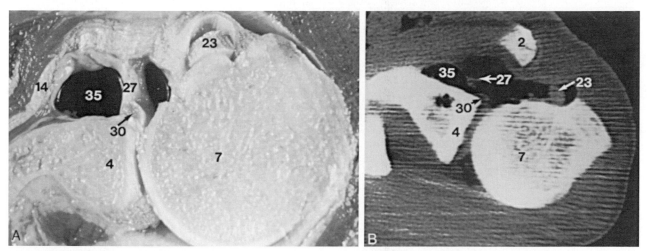

Figure 12–115
Cross-sectional appearance of the glenohumeral joint: Normal anatomy. Level 2—the region of the subscapularis recess or bursa. At this level, the lower portion of the superior glenohumeral ligament (27), opening into the subscapularis bursa (35), anterior portion of the glenoid labrum (30), tendon of the long head of the biceps brachii muscle (23), subscapularis tendon (14), coracoid process (2), glenoid cavity (4), and humerus (7) are identified in the anatomic section (**A**) and CT arthrogram (**B**).

(From Zlatkin M, et al: AJR *150*:151, 1988. Copyright 1988, American Roentgen Ray Society.)

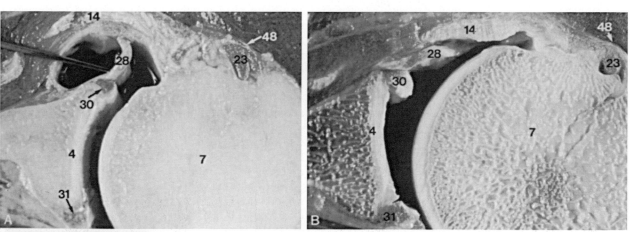

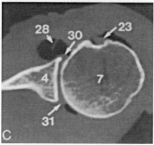

Figure 12–116
Cross-sectional appearance of the glenohumeral joint: Normal anatomy. Level 3—midglenoid level.

A, B Two anatomic sections show variations in the appearance of the middle glenohumeral ligament (28). Also note the subscapularis tendon (14), anterior portion of the glenoid labrum (30), posterior portion of the glenoid labrum (31), tendon of the long head of the biceps brachii muscle (23) within the bicipital groove, transverse humeral ligament (48), glenoid cavity (4), and humeral head (7).

C CT arthrography allows identification of some of these same structures.

(From Zlatkin M, et al: AJR *150*:151, 1988. Copyright 1988, American Roentgen Ray Society.)

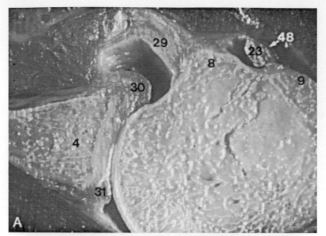

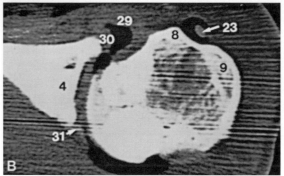

Figure 12–117

Cross-sectional appearance of the glenohumeral joint: Normal anatomy. Level 4—inferior glenoid level.

A An anatomic section shows the prominent inferior glenohumeral ligament (29). Also note the anterior portion of the glenoid labrum (30), posterior portion of the glenoid labrum (31), tendon of the long head of the biceps brachii muscle (23), transverse humeral ligament (48), lesser (8) and greater (9) tuberosities of the humerus, and glenoid cavity (4).

B Some of the same structures can be identified in the CT arthrogram.

(From Zlatkin M, et al: AJR *150*:151, 1988. Copyright 1988, American Roentgen Ray Society.)

The articular surface of the glenoid fossa is gently concave and covered by hyaline cartilage, which is normally thinner at the center than at the periphery. On cross section, the posterior margin of the fossa appears larger and more rounded than the more pointed anterior margin. The inclination of the fossa is characterized by mild retroversion superiorly, changing to slight anteversion on progressively caudal sections. The glenoid labrum is a fibrous structure that is firmly attached to the edge of the fossa. In cross section, the labrum appears essentially triangular (Fig. 12–118). On conventional arthrotomography, the anterior portion often is longer and more pointed than the posterior portion, which frequently appears slightly larger, more rounded, and smoother. On computed arthrotomography, the anterior portion most commonly has a smoothly rounded apex, although on occasion the apex is pointed and closely resembles the appearance on conventional arthrotomography. The base of the labrum abuts on the articular cartilage of the glenoid, somewhat analogous to the meniscus in the knee. Air or contrast material

normally may track between the base of the labrum and the cartilage and should not be mistaken for evidence of partial detachment.

Distention of the glenohumeral joint during conventional or computed arthrotomography (or during MR arthrography) allows identification of the glenohumeral ligaments and sites of capsular insertion. Variability occurs in the size of the glenohumeral ligaments, however, such that it is not possible to visualize all three ligaments in every case. The anterior capsular insertion varies somewhat in appearance; the capsule may insert in or near the labrum (type 1) or more medially along the scapular neck (types 2 and 3) (Fig. 12–119). The importance of a type 3 capsular insertion, representing the most medial type of insertion, as a cause or result of anterior instability of the glenohumeral joint is not clear (Fig. 12–120). The type 1 capsular insertion is the pattern encountered most commonly. The posterior capsule, when normal, invariably inserts in the labrum.

Abnormalities of the glenoid labrum depicted on conventional or computed arthrotomography include foreshortening or thinning or contrast imbibition along its free margin. The labrum also may be completely detached (the true Bankart lesion). An osseous Bankart-type lesion typically is visualized as an elevation of a small sliver of bone and irregularity of the adjacent glenoid rim. A depression along the posterolateral aspect of the humeral head is indicative of a Hill-Sachs lesion.

Both conventional and computed arthrotomographic studies were reported to be highly accurate in the analysis of the glenoid labrum. With regard to the reported series using conventional arthrotomography, Braunstein and O'Connor[368] accurately characterized the anterior labral abnormality seen in all nine of their patients; however, no patients with normal arthrograms were explored, and thus no data on false-negative results are available. Of the 21 patients with surgical confirmation reported by McGlynn and coworkers,[370] the labrum was accurately characterized as normal or abnormal in all cases, and there were no false-positive or false-negative findings. Pappas and collaborators[385] examined 46 patients with prone oblique conventional arthrotomography; 18 patients with positive findings and three normal subjects had operative intervention in which the accuracy of the interpretations was confirmed. In an analysis of 55 patients undergoing conventional arthrotomography, Deutsch and coworkers[375] found that the technique classified the status of the labrum in 13 of the 16 patients who had surgery or arthroscopy (sensitivity, 86 per cent; accuracy, 81 per cent).

Reported studies also have underscored the accuracy of computed arthrotomography in the assessment of the glenoid labrum. In an investigation of 10 patients, Shuman and others[374] observed that, on the basis of surgical confirmation of the findings, computed arthrotomography correctly characterized the labrum as abnormal in five persons and normal in one. Kinnard and collaborators[373] reported that of 10 patients undergoing computed arthrotomography for evaluation of shoulder instability, three had labral abnormalities confirmed at surgery. Deutsch and colleagues,[375] in an investigation

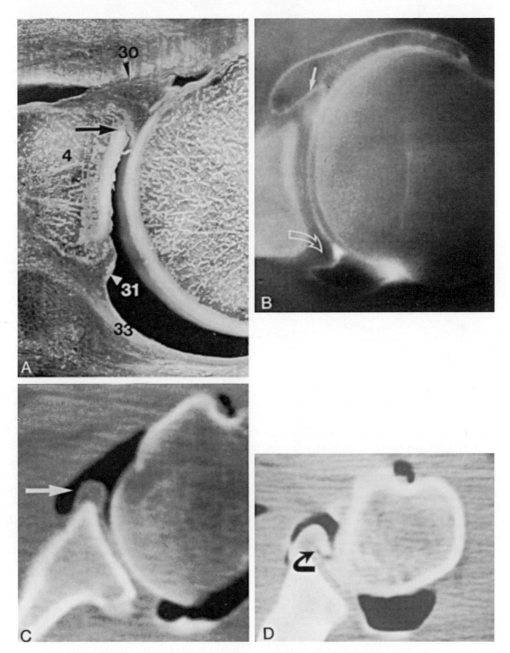

Figure 12–118

Glenoid labrum: Conventional and computed arthrotomography. Normal appearance.

A A transverse anatomic section through the lower third of the glenoid cavity shows the anterior (30) and posterior (31) portions of the labrum. The anterior labrum has a triangular configuration, with a cleft or potential space at its base (arrow) where it abuts the articular cartilage of the glenoid cavity (4). The posterior portion of the glenoid labrum appears smaller and more rounded, and the posterior capsule (33) of the joint attaches directly to it.

B With conventional arthrotomography, the apex of the anterior portion of the labrum (solid arrow) is sharp, in comparison with the rounded appearance of the posterior portion of the labrum (open arrow).

C With CT arthrography, the apex of the anterior portion of the labrum (arrow) commonly appears more rounded than with conventional arthrotomography.

D Air or radiopaque contrast material (curved arrow) normally may be seen between the base of the anterior portion of the labrum and articular cartilage of the glenoid cavity.

(From Deutsch AL, et al: Radiology *153*:603, 1984.)

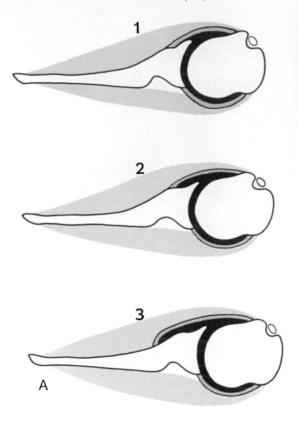

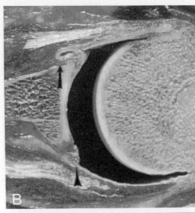

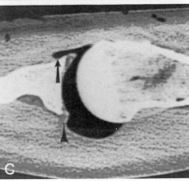

Figure 12–119

Cross-sectional appearance of the glenohumeral joint: Normal anatomy. Types of anterior and posterior capsular insertion.

A The three types of anterior capsular insertion are indicated (see text for details). Note that the posterior portion of the capsule attaches directly to the labrum.

B, C A photograph of a transverse anatomic section (**B**) and CT arthrographic image (**C**), both at the midglenoid level, reveal a type 1 anterior capsular insertion (arrows) and a posterior capsular attachment to the posterior portion of the labrum (arrowheads).

(From Zlatkin M, et al: AJR *150*:151, 1988. Copyright 1988, American Roentgen Ray Society.)

of 81 patients using computed arthrotomography, found that the examination accurately characterized the glenoid labrum as normal, abnormal, or detached in 38 of the 44 patients who had surgery or arthroscopy (sensitivity, 96 per cent; accuracy, 86 per cent). Hill-Sachs defects were seen in 20 of 29 patients with anterior labral abnormalities, and bicipital tendon abnormalities were evident in 6 patients.

The reliability of arthrotomographic methods in defining clinically significant labral abnormalities, however, may be questioned on the basis of an investigation in 1987 by McNiesh and Callaghan.[386] In this investigation, as well as a subsequent one in which MR imaging was assessed,[38] variations in the normal appearance of

the glenoid labrum were described. From material derived from computed arthrotomograms of 72 shoulders in which the labrum had been considered normal at the time of arthroscopy, McNiesh and Callaghan[386] emphasized the occurrence of a notched or cleaved appearance of the anterior labrum, as well as a small labrum, in some cases. Neumann and coworkers,[38] studying the MR images of 50 shoulders in 30 asymptomatic volunteers, expanded on this concept, indicating the presence of many normal variations in labral morphology (see previous discussion). Although these morphologic variations may result from glenohumeral ligamentous attachments to the labrum or from labral degeneration in older persons,[387] ultimately they lead to diagnostic uncertainty with regard to labral integrity in any patient. This diagnostic problem is common to both arthrotomography and MR imaging. Because of this, interpretation of either type of examination commonly relies on the presence or absence of additional abnormalities, such as those of the humeral head (i.e., Hill-Sachs lesion) or glenohumeral capsule or ligaments.

The investigation of Rafii and coworkers[377] in 1986 was the first to provide a detailed analysis of the computed arthrotomographic appearance of the capsular structures of the shoulder. Distention of the glenohumeral joint accomplished during computed arthrotomography (and during MR arthrography) allows visualization of the anterior and posterior capsular insertions of the glenohumeral ligaments, and the coracohumeral ligament. In cases of anterior glenohumeral joint instability, the capsular reflections may appear lax or distorted with either loss or thickening of the anterior subscapular soft tissues (Figs. 12–121, 12–122, 12–123, and 12–124). Although isolated tears of the labrum may

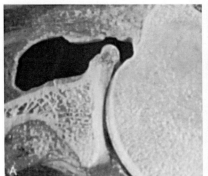

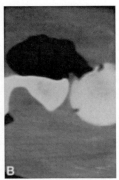

Figure 12–120

Cross-sectional appearance of the glenohumeral joint: Pathologic anatomy. Type 3 insertion of the anterior capsule. An anatomic section (**A**) and a corresponding CT arthrographic image (**B**) reveal a large anterior pouch related to a type 3 capsular insertion. The clinical significance of this finding is not clear. (From Zlatkin M, et al: AJR *150*:151, 1988. Copyright 1988, American Roentgen Ray Society.)

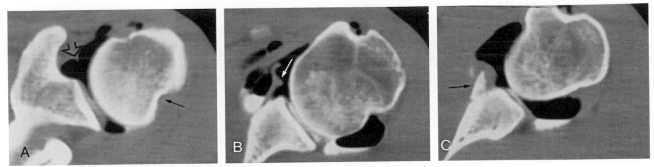

Figure 12–121

Glenohumeral joint instability: Computed arthrotomography. Capsular, ligamentous, and labral abnormalities. Three transaxial CT arthrographic images obtained at the level of the superior aspect of the joint (level 1) **(A),** the midglenoid level (level 3) **(B),** and the inferior glenoid level (level 4) **(C)** show a number of abnormalities indicative of previous anterior glenohumeral joint dislocation. In **A,** observe a Hill-Sachs lesion (arrow), irregularity of the superior glenohumeral ligament (open arrow), and nonvisualization of the superoanterior portion of the labrum. In **B,** findings include avulsion of the anterior portion of the labrum at the site of attachment of the middle glenohumeral ligament (arrow) and a redundant anterior capsule. In **C,** observe a fracture (arrow) of the anterior surface of the glenoid rim.

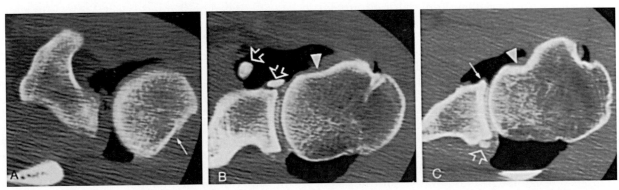

Figure 12–122

Glenohumeral joint instability: Computed arthrotomography. Capsular, ligamentous, and labral abnormalities. Two transaxial CT arthrographic images obtained at the level of the subscapularis bursa (level 2) **(A)** and midglenoid level (level 3) **(B)** show abnormality indicative of anterior instability of the glenohumeral joint. In **A,** note irregularity of the inferior portion of the superior glenohumeral ligament (solid arrow) and absence of the anterior portion of the labrum (open arrow). In **B,** note absence of the anterior portion of the labrum (open arrow) at the site of attachment of the middle glenohumeral ligament (solid arrow).

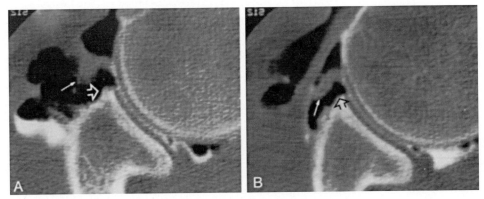

Figure 12–123

Glenohumeral joint instability: Computed arthrotomography. Capsular, ligamentous, and labral abnormalities. Three transaxial CT arthrographic images obtained at the level of the superior aspect of the joint (level 1) **(A),** the midglenoid level (level 3) **(B),** and the inferior glenoid level (level 4) **(C)** show abnormalities indicative of multidirectional instability. In **A,** observe a Hill-Sachs lesion (solid arrow). In **B,** note intra-articular bodies (open arrows) and a trough fracture (arrowhead) in the anterior surface of the humeral head. In **C,** the trough fracture (arrowhead) is more apparent. Additional findings include absence of the anterior portion of the labrum (solid arrow) and a fracture (open arrow) of the posterior glenoid rim.

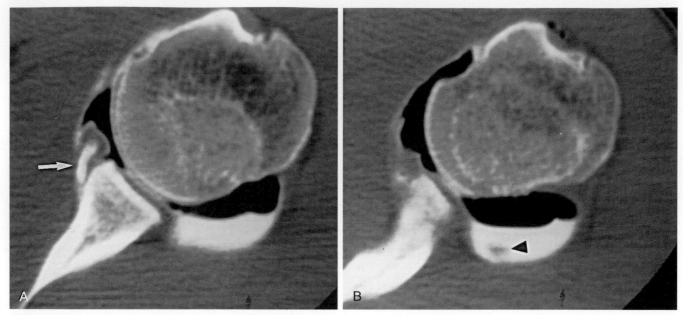

Figure 12–124
Glenohumeral joint instability: Computed arthrotomography. Labral abnormalities and intra-articular bodies. Two transaxial scans, one at the midglenoid level (**A**) and one at the inferior glenoid level (**B**), show labral detachment anteriorly with a bone fragment (arrow) and a posteriorly located body (arrowhead) in the joint in a patient with recurrent anterior glenohumeral joint dislocations. (Courtesy of G. Greenway, M.D., Dallas, Texas.)

be detected, these tears frequently are associated with varying degrees of capsular abnormality and, in some cases, with periostitis involving the anterior portion of the scapula. Detachment of the labrum along with one or more of the glenohumeral ligaments may be apparent. With posterior instability of the glenohumeral joint, the posterior portion of the glenoid labrum may be torn, shredded, or detached, and capsular laxity may be apparent. Both anterior and posterior abnormalities may be seen with computed arthrotomography in patients with multidirectional instability.

Magnetic Resonance Imaging Abnormalities

Numerous publications have examined the value of MR imaging in the analysis of glenohumeral joint instability.[388–400, 679, 680] Most studies have relied upon standard spin echo MR images, although a few have employed gradient echo images,[95, 396, 397, 679] sometimes combined with additional methods such as radial sectioning of the labrum.[390] Few data exist regarding the value of volumetric gradient echo MR imaging in the assessment of the glenoid labrum, although the ability to obtain thin (1 mm or less), contiguous slices with this technique may prove important.[95] MR arthrography, accomplished with the intra-articular injection of gadolinium compounds or saline, also appears to have diagnostic potential,[225, 401–410] although it is invasive and time-consuming, and the added benefits of this technique are not known yet. With standard MR imaging or MR arthrography, the glenoid labrum is best demonstrated in the transaxial plane (Figs. 12–125 and 12–126), although coronal oblique (Fig. 12–127) and sagittal oblique (Fig. 12–128) images provide additional information. Typically, the patient is examined in the supine

position, with the arm at the side in a neutral attitude. External rotation of the arm[397] or abduction and external rotation of the arm (ABER position)[113] also may be used, the latter method being valuable in the assessment of posterosuperior glenoid impingement.

Initial investigations dealing with MR imaging of glenohumeral joint instability described the generally low signal intensity and smooth, wedge-shaped appearance of the normal anterior and posterior portions of the labrum, the irregularity of contour and intermediate or high signal intensity of the torn labrum (Figs. 12–129, 12–130, and 12–131), and slight superiority of this technique when compared with computed arthrotomography in the analysis of labral lesions.[388, 389, 391] In 1991, Legan and associates[392] reported that MR imaging enabled prediction of anterior labral tears with a sensitivity of 95 per cent, a specificity of 86 per cent, and an accuracy of 92 per cent in a series of 88 patients in whom results of arthroscopy were used as the standard. These authors also indicated that MR imaging was less effective in the prediction of tears of the superior portion of the labrum (sensitivity of 75 per cent, specificity of 99 per cent, and accuracy of 95 per cent), and it was unreliable in the prediction of less common, posterior, or inferior labral tears. In this investigation, labral tears were considered to involve the anterior or posterior portion of the labrum if seen on transaxial images and the superior or inferior portion of the labrum if seen on coronal oblique images. The diagnostic criteria for a labral tear included a visibly torn labrum or one that was truncated or absent. A visibly torn labrum was seen as a high signal intensity region traversing the signal void of the normal labrum. The diagnostic value of one additional finding, a glenoid labrum ovoid mass (GLOM), consisting of a rounded, often expanded la-

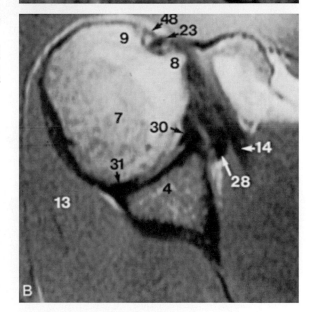

Figure 12–125

Cross-sectional appearance of the glenohumeral joint: Normal anatomy (MR imaging, transaxial T1-weighted [TR/TE, 600/20] spin echo MR images).

A Level 1—superior aspect of the joint. Note the coracoid process (2), glenoid cavity (4), and smooth humeral head (7). The anterior (30) and posterior (31) portions of the glenoid labrum are of low signal intensity. Portions of the superior glenohumeral ligament (27) and coracohumeral (34) ligament and the tendon of the long head of the biceps brachii muscle (23) are seen. Also labeled are the suprascapular neurovascular bundle (55) and infraspinatus muscle (13).

B Level 3—midglenoid level. Note the glenoid cavity (4), humeral head (7), greater (9) and lesser (8) tuberosities of the humerus, tendon of the long head of the biceps brachii muscle (23), transverse humeral ligament (48), anterior (30) and posterior (31) portions of the glenoid labrum, middle glenohumeral ligament (28), subscapular tendon (14), and infraspinatus muscle (13).

bral mass of low signal intensity on proton density and T2-weighted spin echo images as a sign of a torn labrum also was emphasized (see Fig. 12–131). Inherent bias was introduced in this study, however, owing to the high prevalence of labral abnormalities in the predominantly young, athletic patients and to the inclusion of a significant number of patients with recurrent glenohumeral joint subluxations in whom labral abnormalities occur with high frequency. Other investigators[393, 399] were unable to confirm the high sensitivity and specificity of MR imaging in the diagnosis of labral abnormalities that were reported by Legan and collaborators.[392]

The criteria used to diagnose an abnormality of the glenoid labrum with MR imaging include alterations in its morphology and signal intensity. Diagnostic pitfalls exist with regard to the application of either of these criteria, however (Fig. 12–132).

1. *Morphology.* As with computed arthrotomography, MR imaging displays the many variations of labral shape that are evident in asymptomatic persons.[38, 205] A triangular shape of the anterior and posterior portions of the labrum, believed to represent the classic appearance of a normal labrum, has been reported to be evident anteriorly in only 45 per cent of asymptomatic persons and posteriorly in only 73 per cent of asymptomatic persons.[38] Indeed, round, cleaved, notched, triangular, crescent–shaped, or flat labra may be encountered in asymptomatic persons (Fig. 12–133). The presence of a smooth triangular structure generally allows the most confident diagnosis of a normal labrum (Fig. 12–134). The identification of other labral shapes on MR images, however, does not allow a confident diagnosis of a clinically significant abnormality (Fig. 12–135). In elderly patients, such labral variations may be particularly striking, and foci of intralabral calcification may contribute to these modifications in labral shape (Fig. 12–135E, F). The attachment sites of the glenohumeral ligaments and, superiorly, of the tendon of the long head of the biceps brachii muscle also may alter the apparent shape

Text continued on page 260

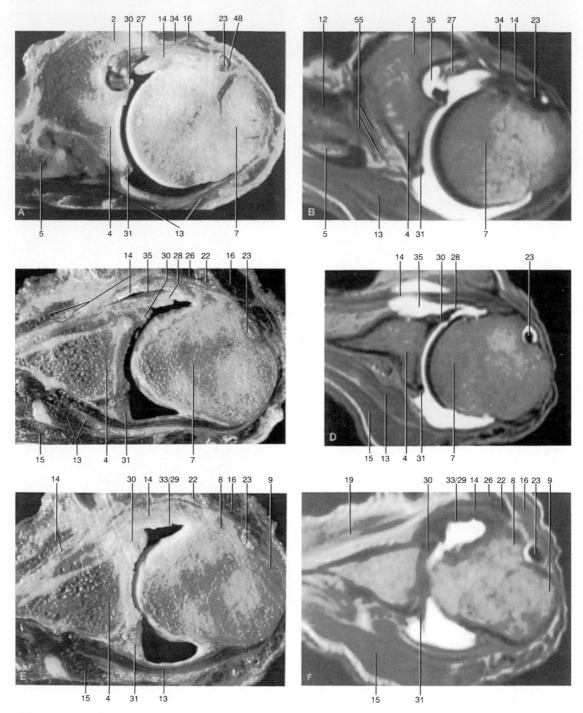

Figure 12–126

Cross-sectional appearance of the glenohumeral joint: Normal anatomy (MR arthrography).

A, B Level 1—superior aspect of the joint. Labeled structures are the coracoid process (2), glenoid cavity (4), scapular spine (5), humeral head (7), supraspinatus muscle (12), infraspinatus muscle (13), subscapularis tendon (14), deltoid muscle (16), tendon of the long head of the biceps brachii muscle (23), superior glenohumeral ligament (27), anterior portion of the glenoid labrum (30), posterior portion of the glenoid labrum (31), coracohumeral ligament (34), subscapularis bursa (35), transverse humeral ligament (48), and suprascapular neurovascular bundle (55).

C, D Level 3—midglenoid level. Labeled structures are the glenoid cavity (4), humeral head (7), infraspinatus muscle and tendon (13), subscapularis tendon (14), teres minor muscle (15), deltoid muscle (16), tendon of the short head of the biceps brachii muscle (22), tendon of the long head of the biceps brachii muscle (23), coracobrachialis muscle (26), middle glenohumeral ligament (28), anterior portion of the glenoid labrum (30), posterior portion of the glenoid labrum (31), and subscapularis bursa (35).

E, F Level 4—inferior glenoid level. Labeled structures are the glenoid cavity (4), lesser tuberosity of the humerus (8), greater tuberosity of the humerus (9), infraspinatus tendon (13), subscapularis tendon (14), teres minor muscle (15), deltoid muscle (16), pectoralis major muscle (19), tendon of the short head of the biceps brachii muscle (22), tendon of the long head of the biceps brachii muscle (23), coracobrachialis muscle (26), inferior glenohumeral ligament (29), anterior portion of the glenoid labrum (30), posterior portion of the glenoid labrum (31), and the joint capsule (33).

(From Petersilge CA, et al: MRI Clin North Am *1*:1, 1993.)

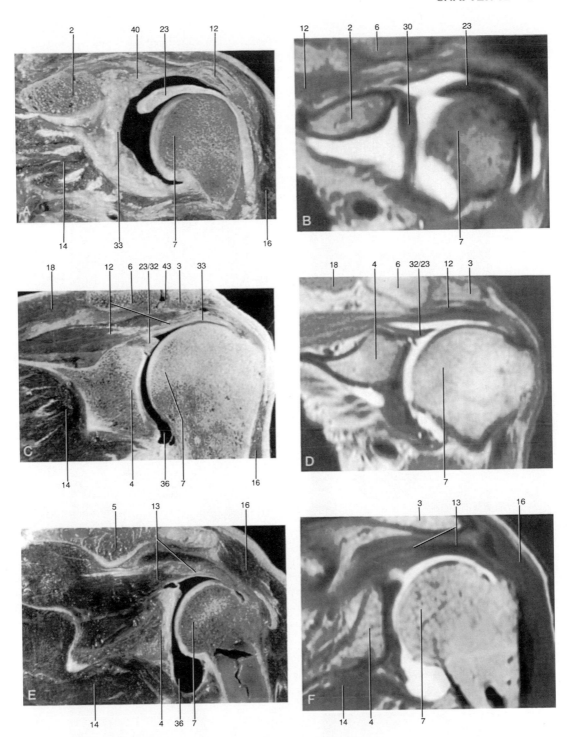

Figure 12–127

Coronal oblique sections of the glenohumeral joint: Normal anatomy (MR arthrography).

A, B Anterior aspect of the joint. Labeled structures are the coracoid process (2), clavicle (6), humeral head (7), supraspinatus tendon (12), subscapularis muscle and tendon (14), deltoid muscle (16), tendon of the long head of the biceps brachii muscle (23), anterior labrum (30), anterior capsule (33), and coracoacromial ligament (40).

C, D Middle aspect of the joint. Labeled structures are the acromion (3), glenoid cavity (4), clavicle (6), humeral head (7), supraspinatus muscle and tendon (12), subscapularis muscle (14), deltoid muscle (16), trapezius muscle (18), tendon of the long head of the biceps brachii muscle (23), superior portion of the glenoid labrum (32), joint capsule (33), axillary recess (36), and acromioclavicular joint and ligaments (43).

E, F Posterior aspect of the joint. Labeled structures are the acromion (3), glenoid cavity (4), scapular spine (5), humeral head (7), infraspinatus muscle and tendon (13), subscapularis muscle (14), deltoid muscle (16), and axillary recess (36).

(From Petersilge CA, et al: MRI Clin North Am *1*:1, 1993.)

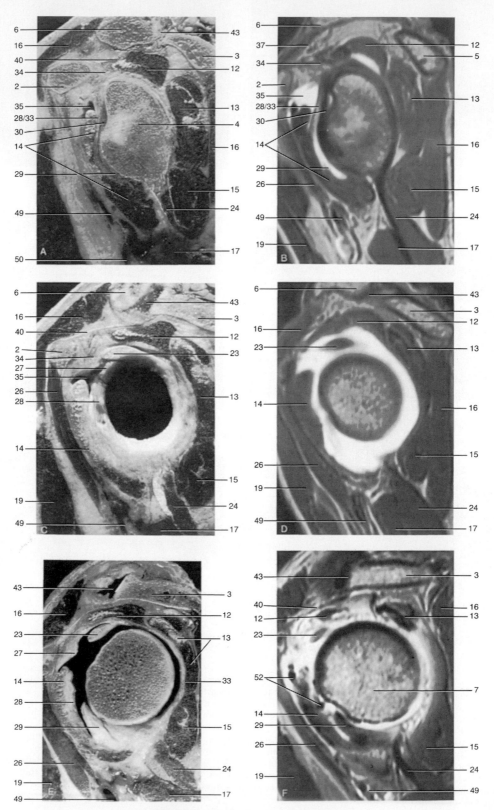

Figure 12–128 *See legend on opposite page*

Figure 12-129
Glenoid labrum: MR arthrography—abnormal appearance. A transaxial T1-weighted (TR/TE, 600/20) spin echo MR image obtained after the intra-articular injection of a gadolinium compound **(A)** reveals a linear region (arrow) of high signal intensity in the anterior portion of the labrum. An anatomic section at the same level **(B)** reveals a subtle, undisplaced tear (arrow) in the anterior portion of the labrum. (From Zlatkin M, et al: AJR *150*:151, 1988.)

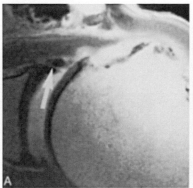

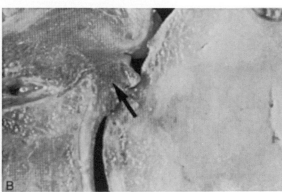

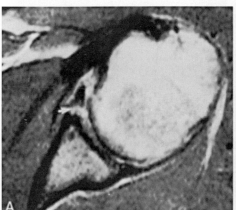

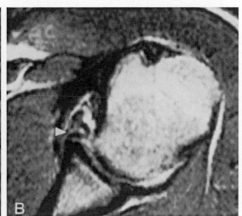

Figure 12-130
Glenoid labrum: MR imaging—abnormal appearance, labral tear and detachment. Two transaxial proton density–weighted (TR/TE, 2116/30) spin echo MR images at the midglenoid **(A)** and lower glenoid **(B)** levels show detachment (arrow) of the anterior portion of the labrum and an intrasubstance labral tear (arrowhead). (Courtesy of M. Rafii, M.D., New York, New York.)

Figure 12-128
Sagittal oblique sections of the glenohumeral joint: Normal anatomy (MR arthrography).

A, B Medial aspect at the level of the glenoid cavity. Labeled structures are the coracoid process (2), acromion (3), glenoid cavity (4), scapular spine (5), clavicle (6), supraspinatus muscle (12), infraspinatus muscle (13), subscapularis muscle and tendon (14), teres minor muscle (15), deltoid muscle (16), teres major muscle (17), pectoralis major muscle (19), tendon of the long head of the triceps muscle (24), coracobrachialis muscle (26), middle glenohumeral ligament (28), inferior glenohumeral ligament (29), anterior portion of the glenoid labrum (30), joint capsule (33), coracohumeral ligament (34), subscapularis bursa (35), coracoclavicular ligaments (37), coracoacromial ligament (40), acromioclavicular joint and ligaments (43), axillary artery and brachial plexus (49), and axillary vein (50).

C, D Middle aspect at the level of the medial aspect of the humeral head. Labeled structures are the coracoid process (2), acromion (3), clavicle (6), supraspinatus tendon (12), infraspinatus muscle and tendon (13), subscapularis tendon (14), teres minor muscle (15), deltoid muscle (16), teres major muscle (17), pectoralis major muscle (19), tendon of the long head of the biceps brachii muscle (23), long head of the triceps muscle and its tendon (24), coracobrachialis muscle (26), superior glenohumeral ligament (27), middle glenohumeral ligament (28), coracohumeral ligament (34), subscapularis bursa (35), coracoacromial ligament (40), acromioclavicular joint and ligaments (43), and axillary artery and brachial plexus (49).

E, F Lateral aspect at the level of the midportion of the humeral head. Labeled structures are the acromion (3), humeral head (7), supraspinatus tendon (12), infraspinatus muscle and tendon (13), subscapularis tendon (14), teres minor muscle (15), deltoid muscle (16), teres major muscle (17), pectoralis major muscle (19), tendon of the long head of the biceps brachii muscle (23), long head of the triceps muscle and its tendon (24), coracobrachialis muscle (26), superior glenohumeral ligament (27), middle glenohumeral ligament (28), inferior glenohumeral ligament (29), joint capsule (33), coracoacromial ligament (40), acromioclavicular joint and ligaments (43), axillary artery and brachial plexus (49), and air bubbles (52).

(From Petersilge CA, et al: MRI Clin North Am *1*:1, 1993.)

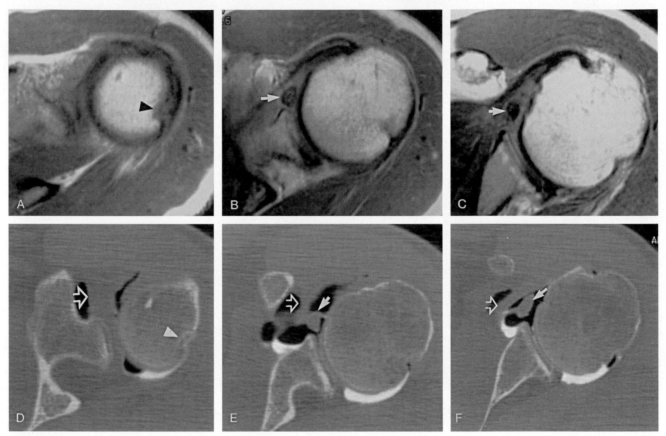

Figure 12–131

Glenoid labrum: MR imaging and CT arthrography—abnormal appearance. Three transaxial proton density–weighted (TR/TE, 2000/19) spin echo MR images **(A–C)** and three transaxial CT arthrographic scans **(D–F)** demonstrate an abnormal anterior portion of the labrum, including a glenoid labrum ovoid mass (GLOM).

A At the level of the base of the coracoid process, note a Hill-Sachs lesion (arrowhead) of the humeral head.

B Slightly below the level of **A,** observe the GLOM (closed arrow) of low signal intensity, diagnostic of a labral tear.

C Slightly below the level of **B,** in the midglenoid region, the GLOM (closed arrow) again is evident.

D At the level of the base of the coracoid process, note the Hill-Sachs lesion (arrowhead) and a thick superior glenohumeral ligament (open arrow).

E Slightly below the level of **D,** note the GLOM (closed arrow) adjacent to the inferior portion of the superior glenohumeral ligament (open arrow).

F Slightly below the level of **E,** in the midglenoid region, the GLOM (closed arrow) is contiguous with the middle glenohumeral ligament (open arrow).

(Courtesy of J. Quale, M.D., Englewood, Colorado.)

Figure 12–132

Glenoid labrum: MR imaging. Tears and pseudotears of the anterior portion of the labrum. Transaxial T1-weighted (TR/TE, 600/20) spin echo MR images **(A, C, E)** and corresponding anatomic sections **(B, D, F).**

A, B Labral tear. Note the region of high signal intensity (solid arrows) representing a true tear (arrowhead), dividing the labrum into two parts (open arrows).

C, D Normal labrum. Note the normal labrum (open arrows) and adjacent joint capsule, synovium, and middle glenohumeral ligament (solid arrows), producing a pseudotear (arrowhead) in the MR image.

E, F Labral degeneration. Irregular signal intensity in the labrum (solid arrow), simulating the appearance of a labral tear, corresponding to sites of mucinous and myxoid degeneration of a labrum that is grossly intact (arrowheads).

(Courtesy of I. Kjellin, M.D., Loma Linda, California.)

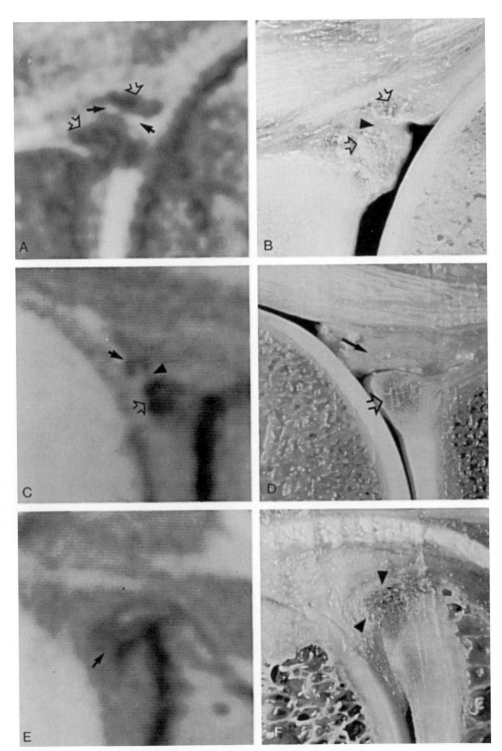

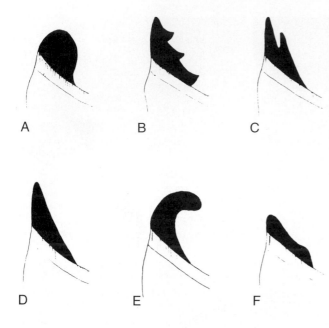

A   B   C

D   E   F

Figure 12–133
Glenoid labrum: MR imaging—variations in labral morphology. **A,** Round; **B,** cleaved; **C,** notched; **D,** triangular; **E,** crescent; **F,** flat.

Figure 12–134
Glenoid labrum: MR imaging—classic normal labral morphology. A photograph of a transverse section of the glenohumeral joint reveals a smooth, triangular anterior portion of the labrum (straight arrow) and a smaller but also smooth and triangular posterior portion of the labrum (curved arrow).

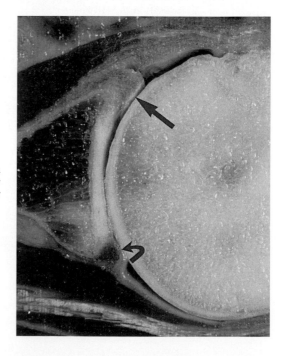

Figure 12–135

Glenoid labrum: MR imaging—variations in labral morphology, midglenoid level.

A, B Crescent-shaped labrum. Transaxial fat-suppressed T1-weighted (TR/TE, 600/20) spin echo MR image with gadolinium compound in joint (**A**) and sectional photograph (**B**) show a crescent-shaped anterior portion of the labrum (arrows). In **B,** note overlying synovial tissue.

C, D Round and flat labrum. Transaxial fat-suppressed T1-weighted (TR/TE, 600/20) spin echo MR image with gadolinium compound in joint (**C**) and sectional photograph (**D**) show a round anterior portion of the labrum (short straight arrows) and flat posterior portion of the labrum (long straight arrows). In **D,** note the middle glenohumeral ligament (curved arrow).

E, F Notch-shaped labrum. Transaxial fat-suppressed T1-weighted (TR/TE, 600/20) spin echo MR image with gadolinium compound in joint (**E**) and sectional photograph (**F**) show a notch-shaped posterior portion of the labrum (arrow, **E**). In **F,** a peripheral thin area of labral tissue (lower arrow) is seen. An adjacent region of calcification (upper arrow) correlates with the more anterior area of hypointense signal intensity in **E,** explaining the notched appearance in the MR image.

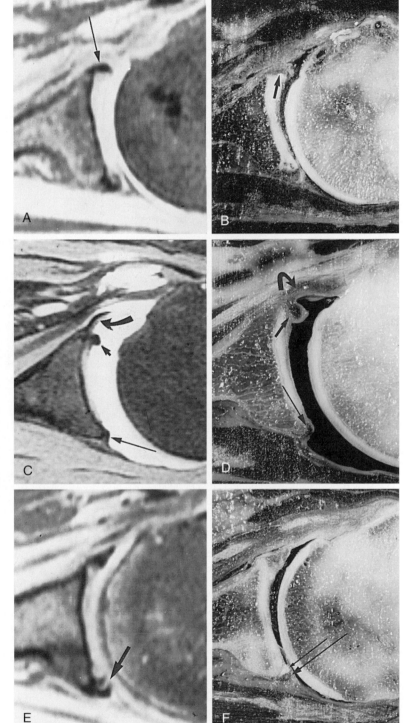

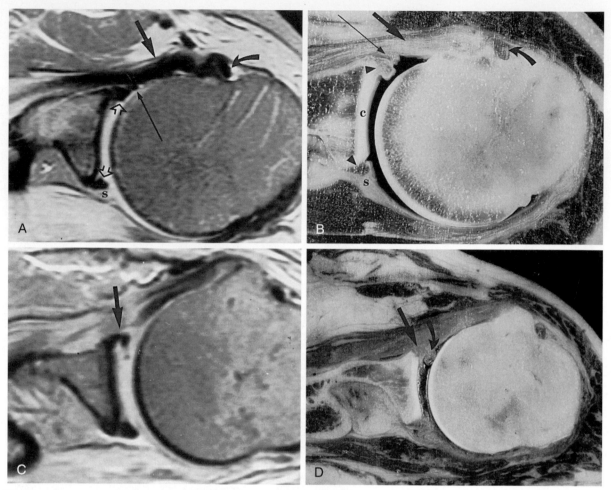

Figure 12–136

Glenoid labrum: MR imaging—variations in labral morphology; capsular and ligamentous contributions to labral appearance, midglenoid level.

A, B A proton density–weighted (TR/TE, 2000/30) spin echo MR image **(A)** shows diffuse hypointense signal intensity in anterior and posterior portions of the labrum (open arrows). Note the subscapularis tendon (upper straight arrow), biceps tendon (curved arrow) in the intertubercular groove, middle glenohumeral ligament (thin straight arrow), and synovial tissue (s). On the sectional photograph **(B)**, the subscapularis tendon (thick straight arrow), biceps tendon (curved arrow), and anterior and posterior portions of the labrum (arrowheads) are identified. The labrum is attached to the scapular periosteum and adjacent cartilaginous (c) tissue.

C, D A proton density–weighted (TR/TE, 2000/30) spin echo MR image **(C)** shows a peculiar composite structure of low signal intensity anteriorly (arrow). The sectional photograph **(D)** reveals a triangular anterior portion of the labrum (straight arrow) and adjacent redundant middle glenohumeral ligament (curved arrow).

of a normal labrum.[128, 681] Although these structures are depicted as being easily separated from the labrum on anatomic or surgical inspection, they often are applied to the surface of the labrum on MR images, particularly when a significant amount of joint fluid is not present (Fig. 12–136). In the presence of a large joint effusion or with MR arthrography, their correct identification is facilitated (Fig. 12–137). Synovial tissue atop the labrum also leads to diagnostic difficulty in interpreting labral morphology on MR images. Further, the pliability of the labrum contributes to its variable shape. For example, with the arm in internal rotation, the labrum may appear more rounded. Detached labral tissue should be regarded as an abnormal finding independent of arm position (Fig. 12–138).

2. *Signal intensity.* The glenoid labrum is composed mainly of dense fibrous connective tissue, and it is continuous with the articular cartilage of the glenoid area

on one side and with the joint capsule on the other side. A sublabral zone or band of tissue reveals transitional histologic characteristics characterized by less organized fibrous tissue than in the labrum and fewer cartilage cell than in the articular cartilage (Fig. 12–139).[398] This sublabral zone of tissue has been designated the transitional zone,[398] and it is uniform in contour, extends a variable distance beneath the labrum, and gradually tapers around the glenoid rim. The transitional zone may be identified both anteriorly and posteriorly or be isolated to either the anterior or posterior portion of the labrum, and its superior-to-inferior extent also varies. This normal transitional zone can lead to regions of intermediate signal intensity beneath the labrum, creating diagnostic difficulty.[398] Furthermore, fibrovascular tissue, mucoid or eosinophilic degeneration, calcification, ossification, synovial tissue, or combinations of these findings can cause alterations in signal intensity

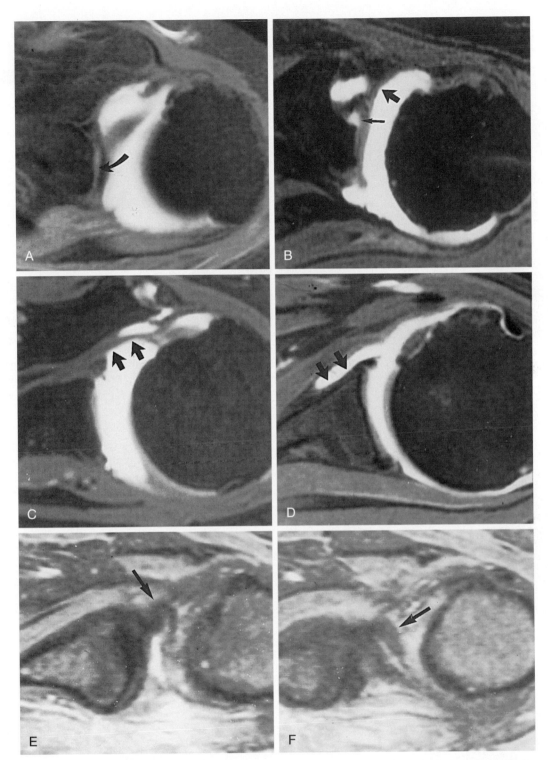

Figure 12–137

Glenoid labrum: MR imaging—variations in labral morphology, capsular and ligamentous contributions to labral appearance (MR arthrography with gadolinium contrast agent).

A Superior glenoid level. The region of intermediate signal intensity (arrow) represents articular cartilage and is not indicative of labral detachment. Transaxial fat-suppressed T1-weighted (TR/TE, 600/20) spin echo MR image.

B Superior glenoid level. Note the superior glenohumeral ligament (thick arrow) and normal sublabral foramen (thin arrow). Transaxial spoiled GRASS (TR/TE, 60/10; flip angle, 60 degrees) MR image.

C Midglenoid level. Note the capsular attachment (arrows) to the anterior portion of the labrum. Transaxial spoiled GRASS (TR/TE, 60/10; flip angle, 60 degrees) MR image.

D Midglenoid level. Note a more medial capsular insertion (arrows). Transaxial T1-weighted (TR/TE, 600/20) fat-suppressed spin echo MR image.

E, F Inferior glenoid level. The anterior (arrow, **E**) and posterior (arrow, **F**) bands of the inferior glenohumeral ligament complex are shown. Transaxial T2-weighted (TR/TE, 2000/80) spin echo MR image.

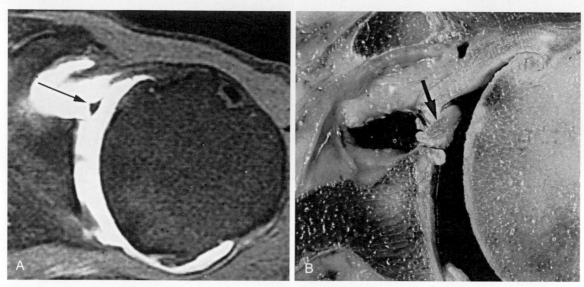

Figure 12–138
Glenoid labrum: MR imaging—labral detachment, superior glenoid level (MR arthrography with gadolinium contrast agent). The labral detachment (arrows) is shown on a fat-suppressed T1-weighted (TR/TE, 600/20) spin echo MR image **(A)** and corresponding sectional photograph **(B)**.

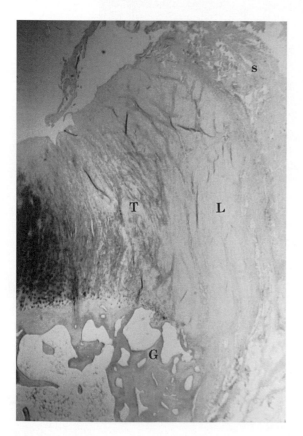

Figure 12–139
Glenoid labrum: Histology. A photomicrograph (safranin O stain, ×16) shows fibrous tissue of normal labrum (L) covered by synovium (s). Note the incomplete zone of transitional fibrocartilage (T) and the glenoid rim (G). (From Loredo R, et al: Radiology *196*:33, 1995.)

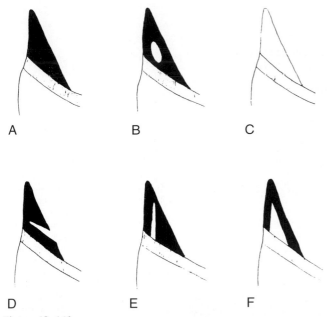

Figure 12–140
Glenoid labrum: MR imaging—variations in labral signal intensity. **A,** Diffuse low signal intensity; **B,** round high signal intensity; **C,** diffuse high signal intensity; **D,** transverse linear high signal intensity; **E,** longitudinal linear high signal intensity; **F,** triangular high signal intensity. (From Loredo R, et al: Radiology *196*:33, 1995.)

on MR images, particularly on gradient echo images and in elderly persons, that simulate those of clinically significant findings.[396, 398]

Loredo and associates[398] identified a number of patterns of increased signal intensity (Fig. 12–140) in the labrum in a cadaveric study that used both spin echo and gradient echo imaging sequences, as well as fat-suppressed sequences and the intra-articular administration of a gadolinium compound. No particular configuration of altered intralabral signal intensity correlated with specific histologic findings (Figs. 12–141, 12–142, and 12–143). Furthermore, there was no prevalence of altered intralabral signal intensity in either the anterior or posterior portions of the labrum or at any particular glenoid level. Although the number of cadavers studied was small and all were of patients who were elderly at the time of death, the results of this study underscore the variation of signal intensity patterns that can be encountered when evaluating the glenoid labrum. The assessment of the glenoid labrum is made even more difficult owing to the occurrence of the magic angle phenomenon, which can cause increased signal intensity in the normal glenoid labrum on short echo time (TE) MR imaging sequences.

Despite the limitations related to normal or clinically insignificant variations in the morphology and signal intensity of the glenoid labrum, MR imaging or MR arthrography allows detection of capsular and ligamentous abnormalities that may be combined with labral alterations in patients with glenohumeral joint instability. The diagnosis of capsular and ligamentous changes is facilitated by the presence of joint fluid, related either to a native effusion or to the intra-articular injection of

a saline solution or gadolinium compound. In MR images, the capsule may appear lax, with an undulating contour, or it may be stripped from the adjacent bone. The labrum may be partially or completely detached and, in some cases, it is displaced into the joint (Fig. 12–144). In elderly persons, disruption of the subscapularis tendon may accompany an anterior glenohumeral joint dislocation. The soft tissue (i.e., ligamentous, capsular, and tendinous) changes may include findings of edema or hemorrhage in the acute stage, appearing as regions of high signal intensity in T2-weighted spin echo and certain gradient echo MR images. Enhancement of signal intensity at the site of acute injury may be evident when intravenous administration of a gadolinium contrast agent is employed (Fig. 12–145). Distribution of the soft tissue abnormalities, including those of the labrum, depends on the direction of glenohumeral joint instability (i.e., anterior, posterior, or multidirectional) (Fig. 12–146).

The major advantage of MR arthrography lies in full distention of the joint, improving dramatically visualization of the glenohumeral ligaments and allowing more accurate categorization of types of anterior capsular insertion (Figs. 12–147, 12–148, 12–149, and 12–150).[409] The method also can provide direct evidence of labral tears when the contrast agent passes into the substance of the labrum.[410] The technique probably is superior to computed arthrotomography, owing to better soft tissue contrast resolution, although it is time-consuming and invasive, and collections of contrast material in normal recesses or about normal structures can simulate the appearance of pathologic labral processes or intra-articular bodies or adhesions.[407, 408] In one study, MR arthrography (using gadolinium agents) was 92 per cent sensitive and 92 per cent specific in showing labral abnormalities and was 76 per cent sensitive and 98 per cent specific in predicting anterior glenohumeral joint instability, when arthroscopic or open surgical findings were used as the gold standard in 121 patients.[406]

A variety of osseous injuries accompanies glenohumeral joint instability and may be detected with MR imaging. These include fractures of the anterior or posterior portion of the glenoid rim, Hill-Sachs and trough lesions, and avulsion fractures of the lesser or greater tuberosity of the humerus (Figs. 12–151, 12–152, and 12–153).

The Hill-Sachs lesion is a specific indicator of a prior anterior glenohumeral joint dislocation (Fig. 12–154*A*). Its radiographic detection is improved when specialized views are used as a supplement to standard methodology. Notch, or Stryker, views, modified Didiee projections, frontal radiographs obtained with varying degrees of internal rotation of the humerus, and fluoroscopy improve the sensitivity of conventional radiography in the identification of this compression fracture.[411] Transaxial images provided by CT and MR imaging (Fig. 12–154*B*) provide further diagnostic sensitivity. In one study, in which agreement of findings in two of three different methods (routine radiography, MR imaging, and arthroscopy) was used as the standard, MR imaging resulted in a sensitivity of 97 per cent, a specificity of 91 per cent, and an accuracy of 94 per cent in the detection

Text continued on page 269

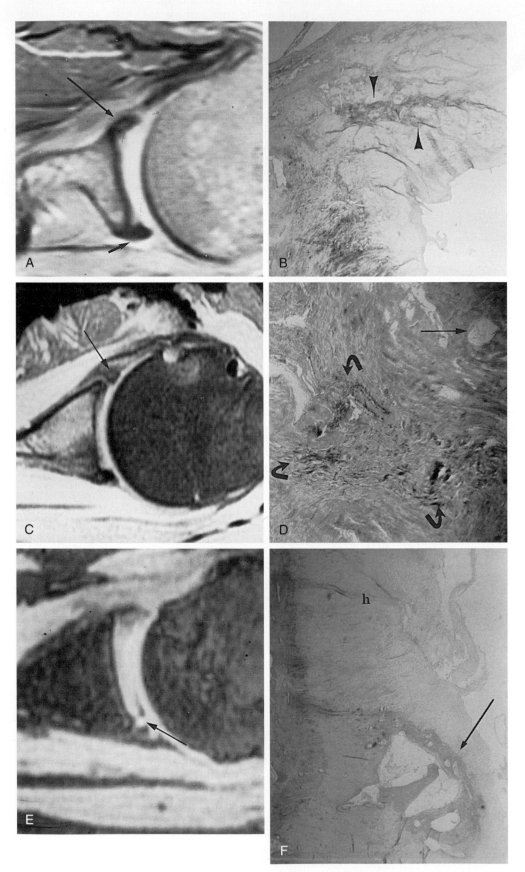

Figure 12–141

Glenoid labrum: MR imaging—variations in labral signal intensity.

A, B Linear pattern of increased intralabral signal intensity correlating with fibrovascular tissue. A transaxial proton density–weighted (TR/TE, 2000/30) spin echo MR image **(A)** demonstrates a linear area of intermediate signal intensity within the anterior portion of the labrum that does not extend to the labral surface (long arrow). Note the normal posterior labrum which maintains low signal intensity and is not blunted or frayed (short arrow). A photomicrograph **(B)** illustrates the correlative linear area of fibrovascular tissue within the fibrous labrum (arrowheads). (Alcian blue stain; original magnification, ×16.)

C, D Triangular pattern of increased intralabral signal intensity correlating with fibrovascular tissue and degeneration. A transaxial proton density–weighted (TR/TE, 2000/30) spin echo MR image **(C)** demonstrates a triangular area of intermediate signal intensity within the anterior portion of the labrum that does not extend to the labral surface (long arrow). A photomicrograph **(D)** illustrates areas of degeneration (straight arrow) and fibrovascular tissue (curved arrows) within the labrum that correlate with the area of altered intralabral signal intensity seen on the MR image. (Alcian blue stain; original magnification, ×100.)

E, F Round pattern of increased intralabral signal intensity correlating with intralabral ossification. A transaxial three-dimensional Fourier transformation gradient echo MR image (TR/TE, 50/10; flip angle, 10 degrees) **(E)** demonstrates a round area of increased signal intensity within the posterior portion of the labrum (arrow). A photomicrograph **(F)** illustrates a small focus of fatty marrow and trabecular bone within the fibrous labrum (arrow). The hyaline cartilage (h) is labeled. (H&E stain; original magnification, ×4.)

(From Loredo R, et al: *Radiology* *196*:33, 1995.)

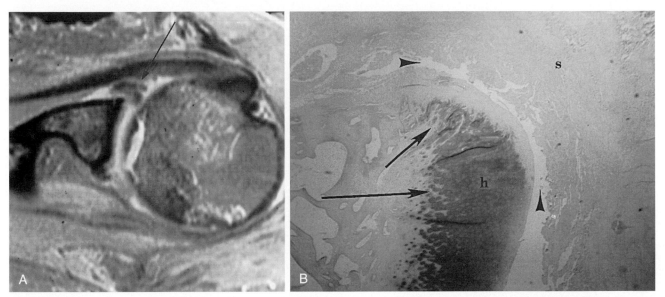

Figure 12–142
Glenoid labrum: MR imaging, variations in labral signal intensity. Diffuse pattern of increased intralabral signal intensity correlating with synovium. A transaxial proton density–weighted (TR/TE, 2000/30) spin echo MR image **(A)** demonstrates altered signal intensity in the anterior portion of the labrum (arrow). Osteonecrosis involving the humeral head is an incidental finding. A photomicrograph **(B)** illustrates a gap (arrowheads) between unattached synovial tissues and the hyaline cartilage (h) of the glenoid bone. Note the absence of labral tissue and the subsynovial extent of the hyaline cartilage (long arrow) and the short zone of transitional fibrocartilage (short arrow). (Alcian blue stain, ×16.) (From Loredo R, et al: Radiology *196*:33, 1995.)

Figure 12–143
Glenoid labrum: MR imaging—variations in signal intensity. A transaxial fat-suppressed T1-weighted (TR/TE, 600/20) spin echo MR image obtained after intra-articular instillation of a gadolinium compound demonstrates complete (straight arrow) and incomplete (curved arrow) sublabral bands of intermediate signal intensity that correlate with transitional zones of fibrocartilage. (From Loredo R, et al: Radiology *196*:33, 1995.)

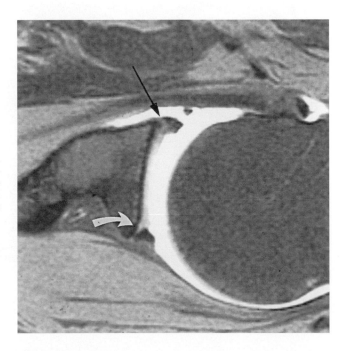

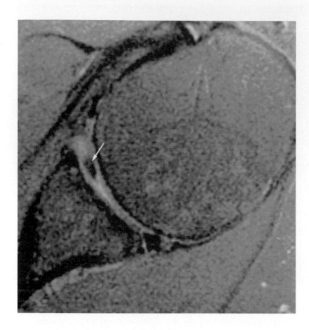

Figure 12–144

Anterior glenohumeral joint instability: MR imaging—labral tear with displacement. A transaxial, fat-suppressed fast spin echo MR image (TR/TE, 2100/21) shows a portion of the anterior aspect of the labrum displaced into the joint (arrow). (Courtesy of S. Eilenberg, M.D., San Diego, California.)

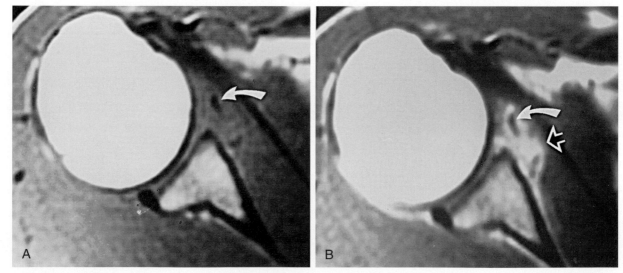

Figure 12–145

Anterior glenohumeral joint instability: MR imaging. Transaxial T1-weighted (TR/TE, 500/20) spin echo MR images obtained before **(A)** and after **(B)** intravenous administration of a gadolinium compound revealed a detached labrum (curved arrows) with perilabral enhancement of signal intensity in **B** (open arrow).

Figure 12–146
Posterior and multidirectional glenohumeral joint instability: MR imaging.

A Posterior glenohumeral joint instability. A transaxial proton density–weighted (TR/TE, 2000/30) spin echo MR image shows a tear of the posterior portion of the labrum (solid arrow), a region of low signal intensity (open arrow) that corresponded to a site of calcification evident in the routine radiographs, capsular stripping, and extra-articular fluid.

B Multidirectional glenohumeral joint instability. A transaxial proton density–weighted (TR/TE, 2116/30) spin echo MR image shows abnormalities of both the anterior (open arrow) and posterior (solid arrow) portions of the labrum.

(Courtesy of M. Rafii, M.D., New York, New York.)

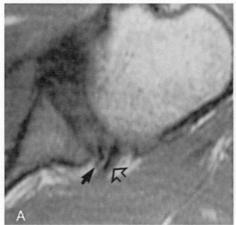
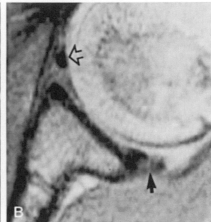

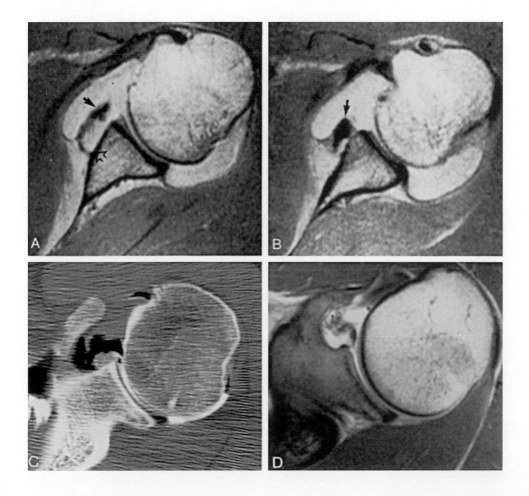

Figure 12–147
Anterior glenohumeral joint instability: MR imaging, MR arthrography, and CT arthrography.

A, B Labral detachment and capsular stripping. Two transaxial proton density–weighted (TR/TE, 1800/30) spin echo MR images, **A** being located at a slightly higher level than **B,** show a large joint effusion, detachment of the anterior portion of the labrum (closed arrows), capsular stripping (open arrow), and extra-articular fluid extravasation. (Courtesy of C. Ho, M.D., Stanford, California.)

C, D Labral tear. A transaxial CT arthrogram (**C**) and a transaxial T1-weighted (TR/TE, 850/16) spin echo MR image obtained after the intra-articular administration of a gadolinium compound (**D**) both reveal irregularity of the anterosuperior portion of the labrum. In **D,** high signal intensity is observed at the base of the labrum.

(Courtesy of V. Chandnani, M.D., Honolulu, Hawaii.)

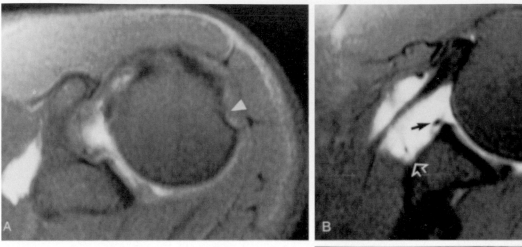

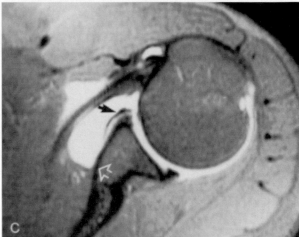

Figure 12–148

Anterior glenohumeral joint instability: MR arthrography—labral tear and detachment, capsular stripping, and Hill-Sachs lesion.

A, B Two transaxial T1-weighed (TR/TE, 600/13) spin echo MR images obtained with chemical presaturation of fat (ChemSat) after the intra-articular injection of a gadolinium compound show, at the higher level **(A),** a Hill-Sachs lesion (arrowhead) and, at the lower level **(B),** labral detachment (solid arrow) and capsular stripping (open arrow).

C In a second patient, a transaxial T1-weighted (TR/TE, 750/20) spin echo MR image obtained with chemical presaturation of fat (ChemSat) after the intra-articular injection of a gadolinium compound shows labral detachment and a tear (solid arrow) and capsular stripping (open arrow).

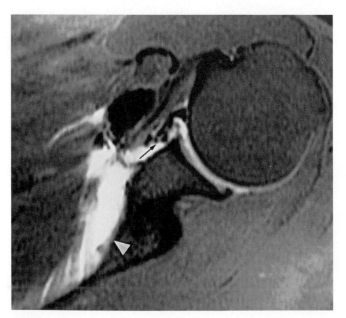

Figure 12–149

Anterior glenohumeral joint instability: MR arthrography—labral detachment and capsular stripping. This fat-suppressed transaxial T1-weighted (TR/TE, 450/12) spin echo MR image obtained after intra-articular administration of a gadolinium compound shows detachment of the anterior portion of the labrum (arrow) at the level of the middle glenohumeral ligament, anterior capsular stripping (arrowhead), and artifacts related to periarticular and intra-articular collections of air.

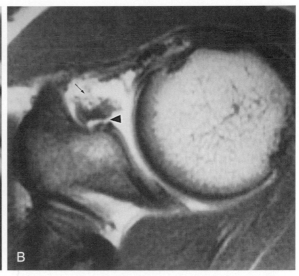

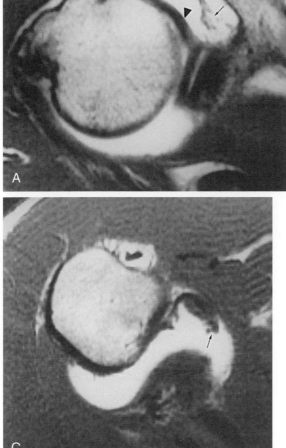

Figure 12–150

Anterior glenohumeral joint instability: MR arthrography—glenohumeral ligament abnormalities, T1-weighted (TR/TE, 600/20) spin echo MR arthrograms (using intra-articular gadolinium contrast agent) with transaxial images.

A Superior glenohumeral ligament tear. Note the torn ligament (arrow) and intact biceps tendon (arrowhead).

B Middle glenohumeral ligament tear. A torn ligament (arrow) and labral tear (arrowhead) are evident.

C Inferior glenohumeral ligament detachment. The detached ligament (arrow) is apparent.

(From Chandnani VP, et al: Radiology *196*:27, 1995.)

of a Hill-Sachs lesion.[412] The presence of a normal groove in the posterolateral aspect of the proximal humeral metaphysis can lead to difficulty in the diagnosis of the Hill-Sachs lesion on transaxial CT and MR images. This groove, however, is located lower than a Hill-Sachs lesion (Fig. 12–155). The latter is apparent almost universally in the first two or three transaxial images through the superior portion of the humeral head (with 3 mm or 5 mm slice thickness). In patients with chronic unreduced glenohumeral joint dislocations, osseous lesions can be far more extensive (Fig. 12–156).

Other Capsulolabral Variations and Abnormalities

A number of normal anatomic variations and specific capsulolabral (and related) abnormalities may be encountered when studying the glenohumeral joint with CT arthrography, MR imaging, and MR arthrography (Table 12–4).

Sublabral Foramen and Buford Complex. Mainly on the basis of observations made during glenohumeral joint arthroscopy, a sublabral foramen has been identi-fied between the anterosuperior portion of the labrum and the articular cartilage of the glenoid cavity.[413] Its frequency, although not certain, appears to be about 10 per cent of normal persons. This foramen has been encountered during CT arthrography owing to the passage of contrast material between the labrum and the glenoid rim,[37] although sometimes a sulcus rather than a true foramen occurs in this region. The sublabral foramen also can be observed during MR arthrography (Fig. 12–157).[682, 695] Generally, it is considered a nonsignificant finding, although its imaging appearance may simulate that of pathologic labral conditions (see Fig. 12–137B) and, rarely, synovial tissue projecting into the sublabral foramen may produce impingement symptoms.[414] A sublabral foramen may increase the severity of glenohumeral joint instability in patients in whom a disrupted middle glenohumeral ligament or a Bankart lesion, or both, are present. Usually, however, a sublabral foramen does not compromise the function of the labrum when the glenohumeral ligaments and muscles of the rotator cuff are intact. A cordlike middle glenohumeral ligament attaching to the anterosuperior portion of the labrum (Fig. 12–158) has been identified in as many as 75 per cent of patients with a sublabral hole.[415]

Text continued on page 275

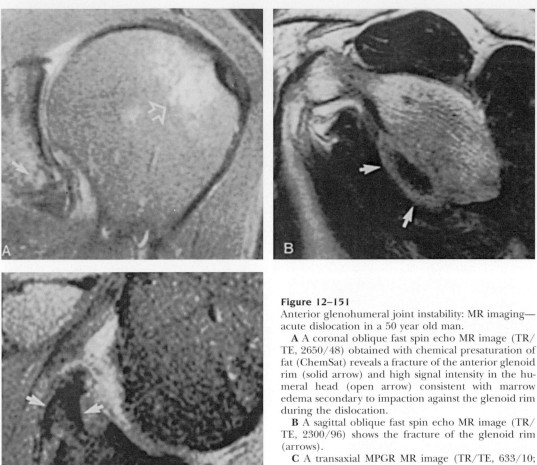

Figure 12–151

Anterior glenohumeral joint instability: MR imaging—acute dislocation in a 50 year old man.

A A coronal oblique fast spin echo MR image (TR/TE, 2650/48) obtained with chemical presaturation of fat (ChemSat) reveals a fracture of the anterior glenoid rim (solid arrow) and high signal intensity in the humeral head (open arrow) consistent with marrow edema secondary to impaction against the glenoid rim during the dislocation.

B A sagittal oblique fast spin echo MR image (TR/TE, 2300/96) shows the fracture of the glenoid rim (arrows).

C A transaxial MPGR MR image (TR/TE, 633/10; flip angle, 35 degrees) reveals the anterior glenoid fracture fragment (arrows).

(Courtesy of S. Eilenberg, M.D., San Diego, California.)

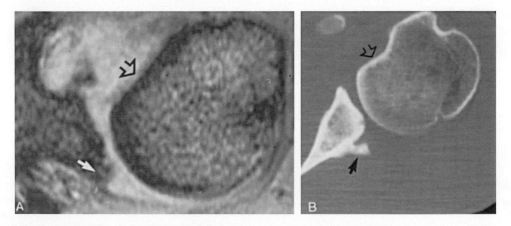

Figure 12–152

Posterior glenohumeral joint instability: MR imaging and CT scanning.

A A transaxial spoiled gradient recalled (SPGR) MR image in the steady state (TR/TE, 45/15; flip angle, 20 degrees) shows posterior subluxation of the humeral head, irregularity of the posterior glenoid rim (solid arrow), and a trough fracture (open arrow) involving the anterior surface of the humeral head.

B A transaxial CT scan at a slightly lower level in the same patient confirms posterior displacement of the humeral head, a fracture of the posterior glenoid region (solid arrow), and a trough fracture (open arrow) of the humeral head.

(Courtesy of M. Schweitzer, M.D., Philadelphia, Pennsylvania.)

Figure 12–153
Posterior glenohumeral joint instability: Routine radiography and MR imaging. Note the fracture (arrows) of the posterior glenoid rim seen on an axillary radiograph **(A)** and sagittal oblique proton density–weighted (TR/TE, 2217/20) spin echo MR image **(B)**.

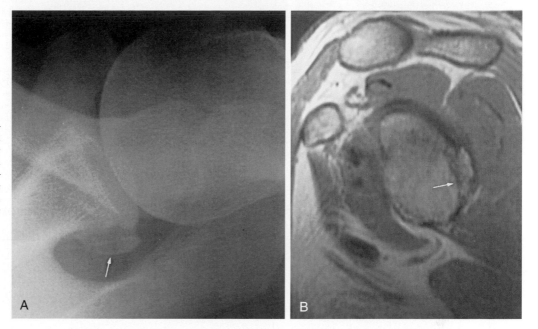

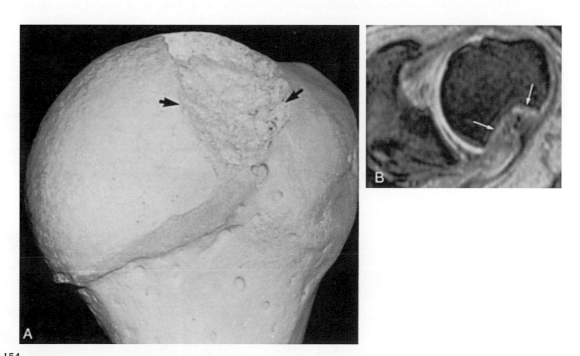

Figure 12–154
Anterior glenohumeral joint instability: Hill-Sachs lesions.
   A A photograph of the posterior surface of the humeral head shows the typical location of the Hill-Sachs lesions (arrows).
   B A transaxial 3DFT spoiled gradient recalled acquisition in the steady state MR image (TR/TE, 63/10; flip angle, 60 degrees) obtained with chemical presaturation of fat (ChemSat) shows a large Hill-Sachs lesions (arrows) appearing as a depression in the posterolateral surface of the humeral head at the level of the coracoid process.

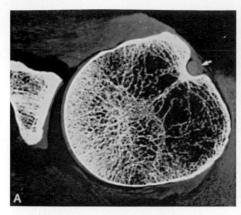 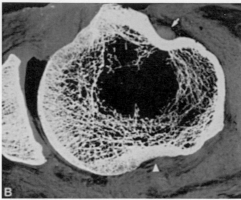

Figure 12–155
Normal groove in the proximal metaphysis of the humerus.

A Humeral head. A radiograph of a transverse section at the level of the humeral head reveals a smooth posterior surface. The intertubercular sulcus is seen anteriorly (arrow).

B Humeral metaphysis. A radiograph of transverse section at the level of the proximal humeral metaphysis shows the normal posterior groove (arrowhead) as well as the intertubercular sulcus anteriorly (arrow).

Table 12–4. SOME TERMS APPLIED TO NORMAL VARIATIONS OR LESIONS OF THE LABROLIGAMENTOUS COMPLEX AND SURROUNDING STRUCTURES OF THE SHOULDER

Term	Description
Hill-Sachs lesion	Fracture of the posterolateral surface of the humeral head indicative of previous anterior glenohumeral joint dislocation
Trough lesion	Fracture of the medial surface of the humeral head indicative of previous posterior glenohumeral joint dislocation
Bankart lesion	Injury of the anteroinferior portion of the glenoid labrum indicative of previous anterior glenohumeral joint dislocation
Sublabral foramen	Normal variation in which a foramen is identified between the anterosuperior portion of the glenoid labrum and the articular cartilage of the glenoid cavity, lying anterior to the biceps anchor
Buford complex	Normal variation in which a cord-like middle glenohumeral ligament is associated with absence of the anterosuperior portion of the glenoid labrum
GLOM sign	Designation for a glenoid labral ovoid mass indicative of an injury with avulsion of a portion of the anterior aspect of the glenoid labrum
ALPSA lesion	Designation for an anterior labroligamentous periosteal sleeve avulsion, which is associated with recurrent anterior glenohumeral joint dislocations owing to incompetence of the anterior portion of the inferior glenohumeral ligament complex
HAGL lesion	Designation for humeral avulsion of the glenohumeral ligament, which is seen usually in older patients and is associated with recurrent anterior glenohumeral joint instability and a tear of the subscapularis tendon
BHAGL lesion	Designation for a humeral avulsion fracture accompanying a HAGL lesion
GLAD lesion	Designation for glenolabral articular disruption, which is associated with a tear of the anteroinferior portion of the labrum and erosion of the articular cartilage of the glenoid fossa and which is not associated with anterior glenohumeral joint instability
SLAP lesion	Designation for superior labral, anterior and posterior tear, often seen in athletes involved in sports requiring repetitive overhead use of the arm and varying in severity but involving the superior portion of the glenoid labrum and, sometimes, the biceps anchor
Bennett lesion	Enthesophyte that arises from the posteroinferior portion of the glenoid rim, often seen in baseball pitchers and probably arising at the site of insertion of the posterior band of the inferior glenohumeral ligament complex
Perilabral ganglion cyst	Ganglion cyst arising adjacent to the glenoid labrum and often associated with a labral tear

Figure 12–156
Chronic unreduced anterior glenohumeral joint dislocation: MR imaging. T1-weighted (TR/TE, 500/12) transaxial **(A)** and sagittal oblique **(B)** spin echo MR images show an anterior dislocated humeral head with a large defect (arrows) in the posterolateral surface of the humeral head.

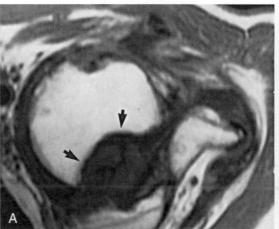 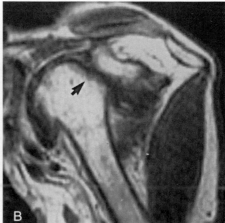

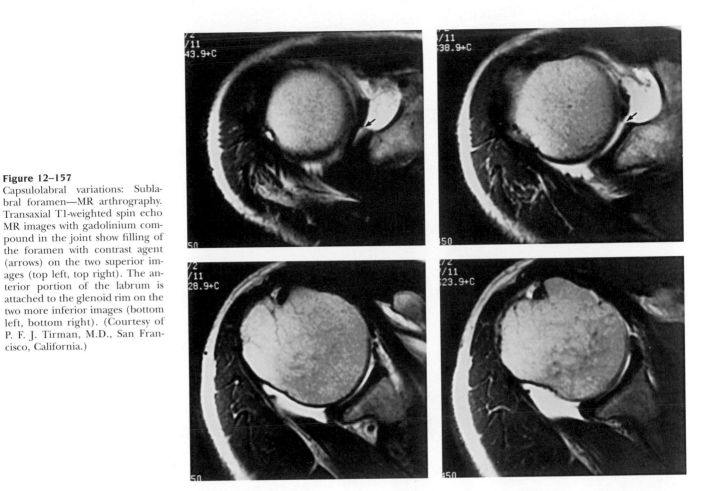

Figure 12–157
Capsulolabral variations: Sublabral foramen—MR arthrography. Transaxial T1-weighted spin echo MR images with gadolinium compound in the joint show filling of the foramen with contrast agent (arrows) on the two superior images (top left, top right). The anterior portion of the labrum is attached to the glenoid rim on the two more inferior images (bottom left, bottom right). (Courtesy of P. F. J. Tirman, M.D., San Francisco, California.)

Figure 12–158
Capsulolabral variations: Sublabral foramen. A schematic illustration shows a sublabral foramen (solid arrow) between the anterosuperior portion of the labrum (open arrow) and glenoid margin and a cord-like middle glenohumeral ligament (arrowhead) attaching to the labrum. (Modified from Williams MM, et al: Arthroscopy 10:241, 1994.)

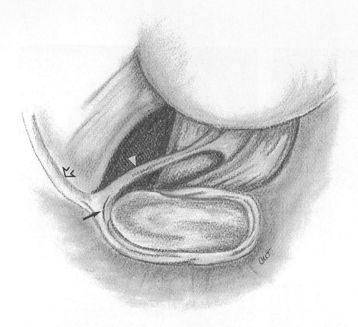

Figure 12–159

Capsulolabral variations: Buford complex. Schematic illustration demonstrates the three essential elements of the Buford complex: a cordlike middle glenohumeral ligament (arrowhead); attachment of this ligament to the superior portion of the labrum (solid arrow) near the base of the biceps tendon (open arrow); and absence of additional labral tissue in the anterosuperior glenoid quadrant. (Modified from Williams MM, et al: Arthroscopy *10*:241, 1994.)

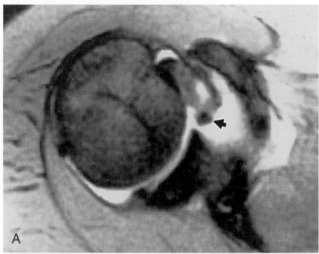

Figure 12–160

Capsulolabral variations: Buford complex—MR arthrography.

A A transaxial gradient echo MR image with gadolinium compound in the joint shows the absence of the anterosuperior portion of the labrum and the presence of a cordlike middle glenohumeral ligament (arrow). (Courtesy of P. F. J. Tirman, M.D., San Francisco, California.)

B, C In a second patient, transaxial (TR/TE, 500/12) (**B**) and sagittal oblique (TR/TE, 800/14) (**C**) fat-suppressed T1-weighted spin echo MR images, obtained after intra-articular administration of a gadolinium compound, show a cordlike middle glenohumeral ligament (arrows) and the absence of the anterosuperior portion of the labrum. At arthroscopy, the thickened ligament appeared bifid and no labral tear was evident.

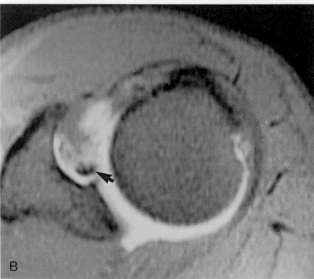

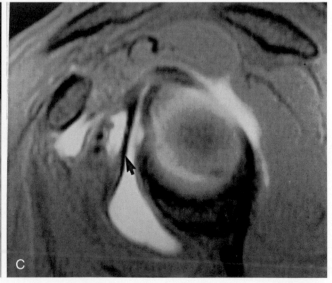

A relatively uncommon variation of caspulolabral anatomy, designated the Buford complex, is characterized by a cordlike middle glenohumeral ligament that originates directly from the superior portion of the labrum at the base of the biceps tendon and crosses the subscapularis tendon to insert on the humerus (Fig. 12–159).[415, 682, 683] No anterosuperior labral tissue is present between this attachment site and the midglenoid notch. The anomaly, which may be present in 2 to 5 per cent of persons, may simulate labral detachment (Fig. 12–160); reattachment of the anomalous ligament may lead to restriction of glenohumeral joint motion.[415]

Anterior Labroligamentous Periosteal Sleeve Avulsion. Recurrent unidirectional anterior instability of the glenohumeral joint may be associated not only with a classic Bankart lesion (an avulsion of the anterior labroligamentous structures from the anterior glenoid rim) but also with an avulsion of the periosteal sleeve of the anterior portion of the scapula (Fig. 12–161).[416] This lesion differs from a Bankart lesion because the anterior scapular periosteum does not rupture, thereby allowing the labroligamentous structures to displace medially and rotate inferiorly on the scapular neck. The anterior labroligamentous periosteal sleeve avulsion (ALPSA lesion) is associated with recurrent anterior dislocation of the glenohumeral joint because of the subsequent incompetence of the anterior portion of the inferior glenohumeral ligament. MR arthrography may allow identification of the ALPSA lesion (Fig. 12–162).

Humeral Avulsion of the Glenohumeral Ligament. The pathologic abnormalities accompanying an initial traumatic anterior dislocation of the glenohumeral joint are influenced by the age of the patient. In patients below the age of 30 years, a Bankart or ALPSA lesion is most typical. In older patients, however, humeral avulsion of the glenohumeral ligament (HAGL) may occur,[129] although such dislocation also may lead to rupture of the rotator cuff or fracture of the greater tuberosity of the humerus. HAGL often is associated with a tear of the subscapularis tendon and recurrent anterior glenohumeral joint instability, and it may be identified with MR arthrography (Fig. 12–163). In one study, the frequency of HAGL in patients with anterior instability of the glenohumeral joint was 9.3 per cent, suggesting it should be suspected when a classic Bankart lesion is not found.[661] Arthroscopic repair of HAGL is feasible with reattachment of the ligament to the humerus through the use of sutures. Rarely, a humeral avulsion fracture (BHAGL lesion) accompanies the HAGL abnormality.[696]

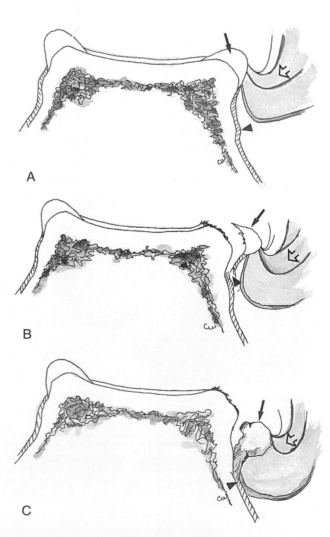

Figure 12–161

Capsulolabral abnormalities: Anterior labroligamentous periosteal sleeve avulsion (ALPSA lesion)—cross-sectional illustrations of the glenoid cavity, with anterior aspect to the right and posterior aspect to the left.

A Normal situation. Note the anteroinferior portion of the labrum (solid arrow), anterior portion of the inferior glenohumeral ligament complex (open arrow), and anterior scapular periosteum (arrowhead).

B Bankart lesion. Note the anteroinferior portion of the labrum (solid arrow), anterior portion of the inferior glenohumeral ligament complex (open arrow), and disruption of the anterior scapular periosteum (arrowhead) with a labral fragment.

C ALPSA lesion. The anteroinferior portion of the labrum (solid arrow) and anterior portion of the inferior glenohumeral ligament complex (open arrow) are displaced and rotated, although the anterior scapular periosteum (arrowhead) is not disrupted.

(Modified from Neviaser TJ: Arthroscopy *9*:17, 1993.)

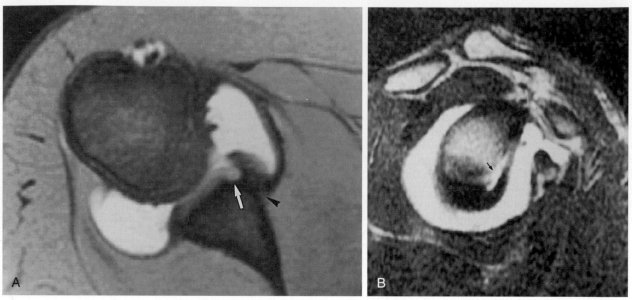

Figure 12–162

Capsulolabral abnormalities: Anterior labroligamentous periosteal sleeve avulsion (ALPSA lesion) (MR arthrography). Transaxial gradient echo (**A**) and sagittal oblique T1-weighted spin echo (**B**) MR images with gadolinium compound in the joint show that the anteroinferior portion of the labrum and adjacent portion of the inferior glenohumeral ligament complex are displaced inferomedially but are still attached to the scapular periosteum (arrowhead, **A**). Contrast material (arrows, **A** and **B**) is seen between the labroligamentous tissue and glenoid bone. (Courtesy of P. F. J. Tirman, M.D., San Francisco, California.)

Glenolabral Articular Disruption. Another specific type of labral lesion has been identified arthroscopically, consisting of a superficial tear of the anteroinferior portion of the labrum.[417] The lesion is always associated with an inferior flap tear with no demonstrable anterior glenohumeral joint instability, and the deep fibers of the inferior glenohumeral ligament remain strongly attached to the labrum and glenoid rim. This lesion has been designated glenolabral articular disruption (GLAD lesion),[417] and it is accompanied by fibrillation and ero-

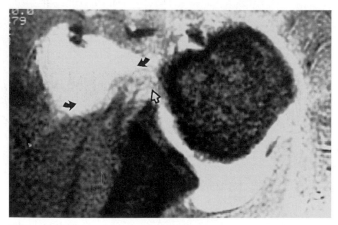

Figure 12–163

Capsulolabral abnormalities: Humeral avulsion of the glenohumeral ligament (HAGL lesion). MR arthrography. Transaxial gradient echo MR image obtained after intra-articular administration of a gadolinium compound demonstrates extravasation of contrast material from the joint through an avulsion of the humeral attachment of the inferior glenohumeral ligament complex (open arrow). The glenoid insertion of this ligament is intact. Note pooling of contrast agent anteriorly (curved arrows). (Courtesy of P. F. J. Tirman, M.D., San Francisco, California.)

sion of the articular cartilage in the anteroinferior quadrant of the glenoid fossa. Arthrography of the glenohumeral joint is normal in these cases, and the MR imaging findings have not been studied.

Superior Labral, Anterior and Posterior Tear. In athletes involved in sports requiring repetitive overhead use of the arm, such as in baseball, volleyball, and tennis, an injury of the superior portion of the glenoid labrum may occur, resulting from sudden forced abduction of the arm.[418–421] This injury, which also occurs occasionally in middle-aged persons, may be related to excessive traction, due to a sudden pull of the tendon of the long head of the biceps brachii muscle, and frequently is referred to as a superior labral, anterior and posterior tear (SLAP lesion). The lesion appears to begin posteriorly and extends anteriorly, terminates prior to or at the midglenoid notch, and includes the anchor of the biceps tendon to the glenoid labrum. A fall on the outstretched arm with the shoulder positioned in abduction and slight forward flexion at the time of impact also is a typical mechanism of injury.

The SLAP lesion initially was divided into four types (Fig. 12–164*A–D*)[421]: type I lesions, representing approximately 10 per cent of all SLAP lesions, are associated with degenerative fraying of the superior portion of the labrum, but the labrum remains firmly attached to the glenoid rim; type II lesions, representing approximately 40 per cent of all SLAP lesions, are characterized by separation of the superior portion of the glenoid labrum and the tendon of the long head of the biceps brachii muscle from the glenoid rim; type III lesions, representing approximately 30 per cent of all SLAP lesions, are bucket-handle tears of the superior portion of the labrum without involvement of the attachment site of the

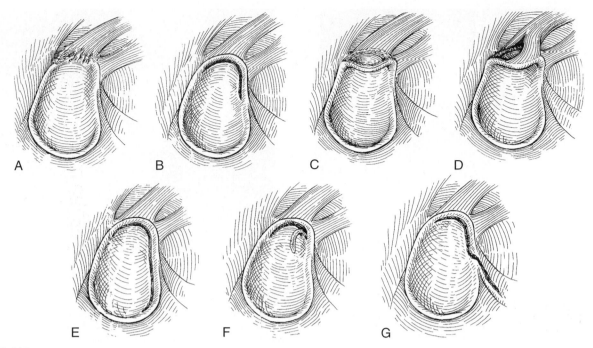

Figure 12–164

Superior labral anterior and posterior tear (SLAP lesion): Classification. (See text for details.)

A Type I lesion.
B Type II lesion.
C Type III lesion.
D Type IV lesion.
E Type V lesion.
F Type VI lesion.
G Type VII lesion.
(From Urban WP Jr, Caborn DNM: Operative Techn Orthop 5:224, 1995.)

tendon of the long head of the biceps brachii muscle; and type IV lesions, representing approximately 15 per cent of all SLAP lesions, are characterized by a bucket-handle tear of the superior portion of the labrum that extends into the biceps tendon. Maffet and collaborators[422] added three further types of SLAP lesions: Type V lesions consist of an anteroinferior Bankart lesion that extends upward to include a separation of the biceps tendon; type VI lesions consist of unstable radial or flap tears that are associated with separation of the biceps anchor; and type VII lesions are characterized by anterior extension of the SLAP lesion beneath the middle glenohumeral ligament. Difficulties in identification and classification of these lesions exist, however, owing to the occurrence of normal foramina (i.e., sublabral foramina) in this region and to labral fraying and irregularity seen in asymptomatic, often elderly persons that simulate types I and II SLAP lesions.[695] Clinical findings of SLAP lesions include painful motion of the shoulder and, at times, audible clicking noises. As a lesion of the superior portion of the labrum that destabilizes the insertion of the biceps tendon results in abnormal glenohumeral translation,[423] stress maneuvers on physical examination may allow diagnosis of some types of SLAP lesions.[424] Lesions of the superior portion of the labrum that do not involve the supraglenoid insertion of the biceps tendon, however, do not result in such abnormal translation, and overt instability (i.e., dislocation or subluxation) of the glenohumeral joint on physical exami-

nation of patients with SLAP lesions need not be present.[423]

The precise pathogenesis of SLAP lesions may vary according to the type of lesion that is present.[425] Athletes using overhead shoulder motion and patients with atraumatic instability often develop type I or type II lesions, whereas patients who develop shoulder instability after an acute traumatic episode may have type V or VII lesions. Acute traction injuries most likely produce type II lesions, whereas a fall on the outstretched hand may produce a type III, IV, or V lesion.

Both computed arthrotomography[426] (Fig. 12–165) and MR imaging[427-430] (Figs. 12–166, 12–167, and 12–168) have been used to detect SLAP lesions of the glenoid labrum-capsular-bicipital tendon complex, with variable success. In a retrospective analysis of computed arthrotomographic images in 17 patients with surgically proved SLAP lesions, Hunter and coworkers[426] indicated that this imaging method showed abnormalities in 16 of the patients and that in 15 the type of labral tear could be determined. Shoulders with type I lesions revealed superior labral irregularities, those with type II lesions showed labral tears with capsular injury or laxity, those with type III lesions showed a rounded core of soft tissue surrounded by a rim of contrast material and air adjacent to the anterior portion of the labrum (a finding that was designated the Cheerio sign), and shoulders with type IV lesions revealed evidence of a rupture of the tendon of the long head of the biceps brachii mus-

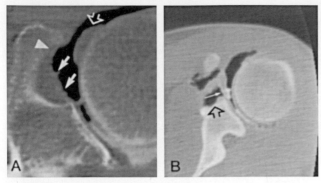

Figure 12–165

Superior labral anterior and posterior tear (SLAP lesion): CT arthrography.

A Type I SLAP lesion. A transaxial CT arthrographic image obtained 4 mm below the scapular insertion of the tendon of the long head of the biceps brachii muscle shows subtle fraying (solid arrows) of the anterosuperior portion of the labrum. The bicipital tendon (open arrow) and superior glenohumeral ligament (arrowhead) are indicated.

B Type II SLAP lesion. A transaxial CT arthrographic image reveals labral-capsular separation (open arrow) and marked irregularity of the free edge of the anterosuperior portion of the labrum (solid arrow).

(Courtesy of J. Quale, M.D., Englewood, Colorado.)

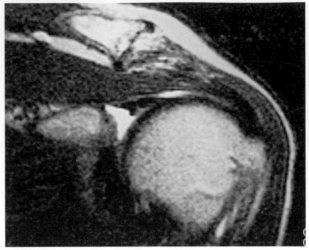

Figure 12–167

Superior labral anterior and posterior tear (SLAP lesion): MR imaging, type IV SLAP lesion. This coronal oblique T2-weighted (TR/TE, 2200/80) spin echo MR image clearly shows detachment of the superior aspect of the labrum along with the biceps tendon from the glenoid rim. At surgery, a partial tear of the biceps tendon also was found. (Courtesy of D. Wilcox, M.D., Kansas City, Missouri.)

cle. Hodler and associates[427] reviewed MR images and arthroscopic reports in nine patients in whom SLAP lesions were present (using arthroscopic findings as the standard). MR imaging did not allow recognition of simple fraying of the superior portion of the labrum, and the differentiation between complete and partial labral detachments of this portion of the labrum was difficult using MR imaging or even MR arthrography (see Fig. 12–168). Detection of abnormalities required analysis of both coronal oblique and transaxial MR images. These authors emphasized the difficulty encountered in the differentiation of significant labral detachment from normal or age-related separation of the labrum.[431, 432] Cartland and colleagues,[428] in a retrospective analysis of MR images in 10 patients with surgically proved SLAP injuries, indicated the usefulness of this imaging method in the detection and classification of these injuries. Type I lesions were characterized by irreg-

ularity of labral contour and a slight increase in its signal intensity, type II lesions were associated with a globular region of high signal intensity interposed between the superior part of the glenoid labrum and the superior portion of the glenoid fossa, type III lesions were accompanied by superior labral tears, and type IV lesions were associated with diffuse high signal intensity in the superior portion of the labrum and in the proximal part of the biceps tendon. Mono and colleagues[430] used standard spin echo MR imaging sequences in all three imaging planes and found the coronal plane to be most sensitive in the diagnosis of SLAP lesions. These authors, too, emphasized the diagnostic value of the Cheerio sign. Analysis of all reported data indicates that careful imaging assessment generally allows the diagnosis of SLAP lesions, that categorizing the lesion more specifically is difficult, that the use of arthrographic technique (i.e., CT arthrography or MR arthrography)

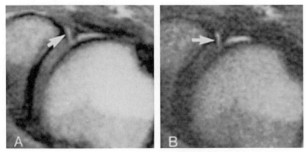

Figure 12–166

Superior labral anterior and posterior tear (SLAP lesion): MR imaging—type II SLAP lesion. Coronal oblique proton density–weighted (TR/TE, 1881/30) **(A)** and T2-weighted (TR/TE, 1881/80) **(B)** spin echo MR images reveal separation (arrows) of the superior portion of the glenoid labrum and the tendon of the long head of the biceps brachii muscle from the superior portion of the glenoid fossa. (Courtesy of P. Fenton, M.D., Toronto, Ontario, Canada.)

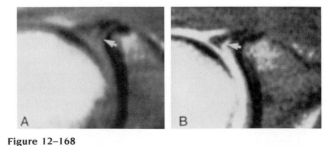

Figure 12–168

Superior labral anterior and posterior tear (SLAP lesion): MR imaging and MR arthrography. Type II SLAP lesion. A coronal oblique proton density–weighted (TR/TE, 2000/20) spin echo MR image **(A)** and a T1-weighted (TR/TE, 600/20) spin echo MR image after the intraarticular administration of a gadolinium compound **(B)** show disruption (arrows) of the superior portion of the glenoid labrum at its site of attachment. The findings are more obvious in **B**. (From Hodler J, et al: AJR *159*:565, 1992. Copyright 1992, American Roentgen Ray Society.)

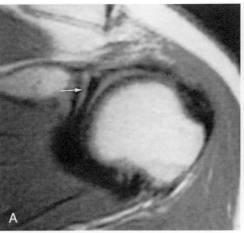
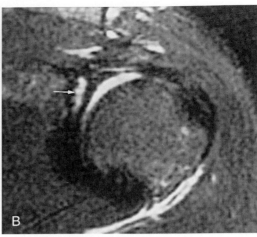

Figure 12–169
Superior labral anterior and posterior tear (SLAP lesion): MR imaging. Coronal oblique proton density–weighted (TR/TE, 1800/23) **(A)** and fat-suppressed T2-weighted (TR/TE, 2300/92) **(B)** fast spin echo MR images show a tear (arrows) of the anterosuperior portion of the labrum with the biceps anchored to a portion of the torn labrum. (Courtesy of D. Salonen, M.D., Toronto, Ontario, Canada.)

improves diagnostic accuracy, that numerous variations exist regarding the extent of the lesion, and that arthroscopy is the most definitive means for defining precisely such variations (Figs. 12–169, 12–170, 12–171, 12–172, and 12–173).

The treatment of SLAP lesions may involve excision of part of the glenoid labrum.[419, 433] Such repairs can be accomplished arthroscopically.[425, 435, 436] The results of such therapy have been inconsistent, however. Indeed, Cooper and coworkers[34] have emphasized the normal

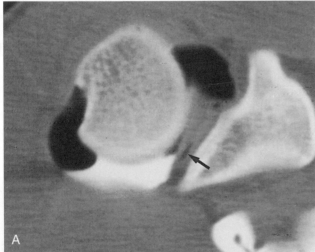

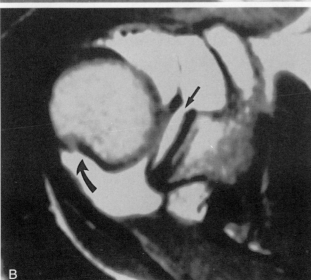
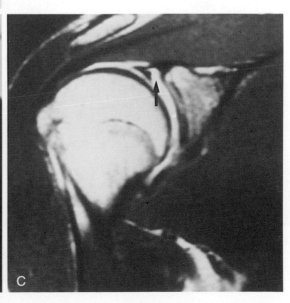

Figure 12–170
Superior labral anterior and posterior tear (SLAP lesion): CT arthrography and MR arthrography.
A A transaxial CT arthrographic image shows a Hill-Sachs lesion and abnormal separation of the superior aspect of the labrum with subjacent air (arrow).
B, C Transaxial **(B)** and coronal oblique **(C)** T1-weighted (TR/TE, 500/23) spin echo MR arthrographic images demonstrate the Hill-Sachs lesion (curved arrow, **B**) and gadolinium contrast agent beneath the separated portion of the labrum (straight arrows, **B** and **C**).

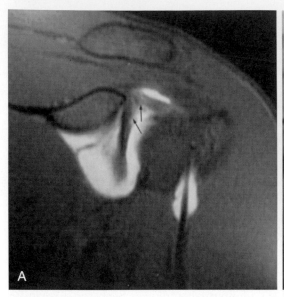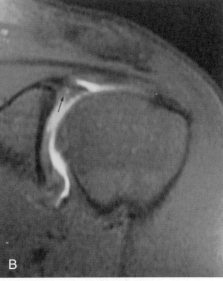

Figure 12–171
Superior labral anterior and posterior tear (SLAP lesion): MR arthrography. Two coronal oblique fat-suppressed T1-weighted (TR/TE, 800/14) spin echo MR arthrographic images, with **A** being more anterior than **B**, show the lesion involving the anterosuperior portion of the labrum with extension into the biceps anchor (arrows, **A**) and involving also labral tissue posterior to this anchor (arrow, **B**). The contrast agent is a gadolinium compound.

laxity of the attachment sites of the superior and anterosuperior portions of the labrum to the glenoid rim that may be difficult to distinguish from a SLAP lesion. This suggests that therapy directed at treating the SLAP lesion in some patients may not be indicated at all.

Perilabral Ganglion Cysts. Certain tears of the anterior, superior, or posterior portion of the labrum are accompanied by the development of perilabral cysts or ganglia (Figs. 12–174 and 12–175).[437] The pathogenesis of the cystic lesions is not certain, although similar lesions have been described in association with meniscal tears of the knee (designated meniscal cysts) and with tears or degeneration of the acetabular labrum (termed

ganglion cysts). In each of these locations, fluid derived from the joint might extend through the tear of the labrum or meniscus into the surrounding soft tissues, leading to cyst formation. In the shoulder, such perilabral cysts or ganglia may extend into the spinoglenoid notch, the suprascapular notch of the scapula, or both notches and produce an entrapment neuropathy (see later discussion).

Bennett Lesion. In 1941, Bennett[438] described a posteroinferior glenoid lesion in throwing athletes (e.g., baseball pitchers) that he believed was caused by traction related to the tendon of the long head of the triceps muscle. Pain was thought to be related to the

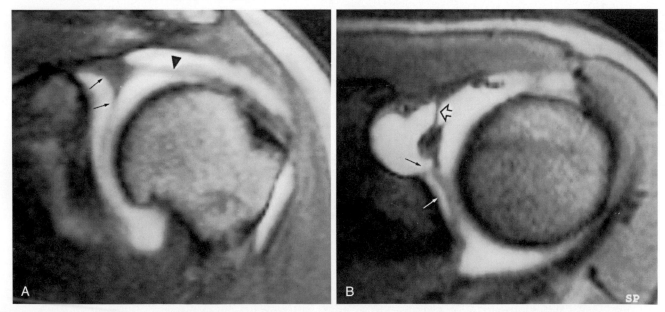

Figure 12–172
Superior labral anterior and posterior tear (SLAP lesion): MR arthrography. Coronal oblique **(A)** and transaxial **(B)** three-dimensional FISP MR images (TR/TE, 32/10; flip angle, 40 degrees) obtained after intra-articular injection of a gadolinium compound show the extent of labral separation (solid arrows) from the glenoid rim. The superior glenohumeral ligament (open arrow) and biceps tendon (arrowhead) are attached to the displaced portion of the labrum. (Courtesy of J. Hodler, M.D., Zurich, Switzerland.)

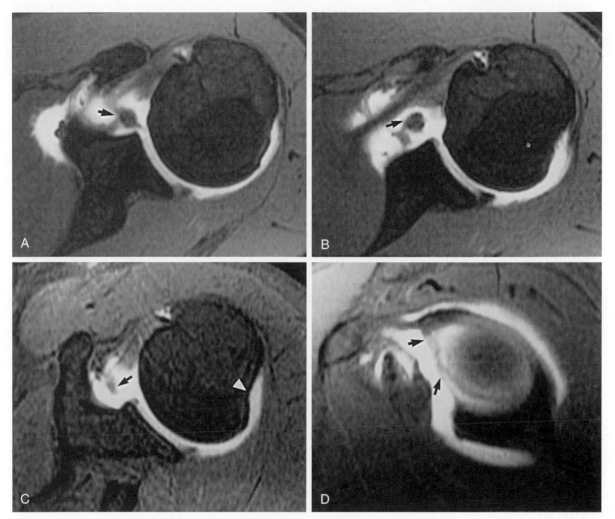

Figure 12–173
Superior labral anterior and posterior tear (SLAP lesion): MR arthrography.

A, B In this patient who had had a repair of a SLAP lesion 2 years previously, transaxial three-dimensional, fat-suppressed SPGR (TR/TE, 58/10; flip angle, 60 degrees) MR images obtained after the intra-articular injection of a gadolinium compound show extension of the lesion (arrows), which now involves the superior **(A)** and middle **(B)** portions of the anterior labrum.

C, D In a second patient, transaxial **(C)** and sagittal oblique **(D)** MR arthrographic images, with identical imaging parameters as in **A** and **B**, show an extensive labral lesion (arrows), which involved the biceps anchor, and a Hill-Sachs deformity (arrowhead).

proximity of the calcified or ossified lesion to the axillary nerve. In 1977, Lombardo and coworkers[439] observed ossification adjacent to the posteroinferior aspect of the glenoid rim in professional baseball players that was found to be in the posterior portion of the joint capsule. The lesion was related to posterior impingement of the humeral head on the glenoid rim during the cocking motion, traction during deceleration of the arm, or a wringing action that occurs during rapid internal rotation of the arm. In 1978, Barnes and Tullos[440] described a posterior capsular syndrome in baseball players that was related to a subperiosteal excrescence at the posteroinferior portion of the glenoid rim, which was associated with posterior labral tears. In 1994, Ferrari and associates,[441] in a study of elite baseball players, used arthroscopy to confirm that ossification posterior to the glenohumeral joint on routine radiographs was associated with posterior labral injury and damage to the posterior inferior surface of the rotator cuff. Furthermore, these investigators suggested that the lesion was unrelated to the attachment of the triceps

tendon but, rather, was related to traction on the posterior band of the inferior glenohumeral complex produced by posterior subluxation of the humeral head during the cocking motion, posterior decelerative forces during the follow-through motion, or a combination of the two. Whatever its precise cause, the Bennett lesion can be studied with routine radiography and MR imaging (Fig. 12–176).

Postsurgical Imaging Abnormalities

Numerous operative techniques are used to correct glenohumeral joint instability (Table 12–5). Recurrent glenohumeral joint instability may occur after any of these techniques, however, related to such factors as persistent abnormalities of the glenoid labrum, joint capsule, or glenohumeral ligaments, compromise of the rotator cuff, or reinjury.[449, 450] In recent years, arthroscopic rather than open stabilization procedures have been used, particularly in patients with anterior glenohumeral joint instability who have a labral detachment with the

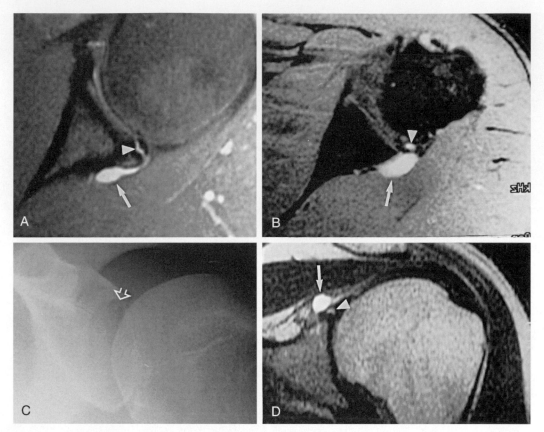

Figure 12–174

Perilabral ganglion cysts: MR imaging. Three examples of ganglion cysts (solid arrows) accompanying labral tears (arrowheads) are shown.

A Posterior portion of the labrum. Transaxial fat-suppressed fast spin echo (TR/TE, 4000/18) MR image.

B Posterior portion of the labrum. Transaxial MPGR (TR/TE, 383/12; flip angle, 15 degrees) MR image.

C, D Superior portion of the labrum. Coronal oblique T2-weighted (TR/TE, 2000/80) spin echo MR image. Note gas within the cyst on the routine radiograph (open arrow, **C**).

(**A,** Courtesy of A.G. Bergman, M.D., Stanford, California; **B,** Courtesy of D. Bates, M.D., San Diego, California.)

inferior glenohumeral ligament attached to the labrum.[684] Open repairs generally are considered more appropriate in patients with anterior glenohumeral joint instability who have a bucket-handle type tear with the labrum detached from the glenoid and the ligamentous structures avulsed from the labrum or in those in whom the quality of the remaining ligamentous tissue is poor. As with open surgical procedures, a variety of arthroscopic techniques have been employed in the treatment of glenohumeral joint instability, including capsulorrhaphy and reattachment of capsulolabral structures, and these techniques use varying arthroscopic approaches and fixation devices. These techniques, when successful, require excellent arthroscopic skills and complete knowledge regarding the type and extent of pathologic abnormalities.[684]

Assessment of the postoperative shoulder with advanced imaging methods such as computed arthrotomography and MR imaging is made difficult owing to surgical distortion of normal soft tissue landmarks, incomplete information regarding the nature of the previous surgery, and unavailability of postoperative baseline studies. In one investigation, computed arthrotomography proved useful in confirming the presence of capsular laxity, subscapularis muscle and tendon abnormalities, and Bankart lesions that were either recurrent or

not identified during previous shoulder operations.[451] The precise role of imaging examinations in the assessment of the postoperative shoulder, however, requires further analysis. MR imaging, for example, of patients who have had arthroscopic or open surgical repairs for glenohumeral joint instability may reveal rounded foci of signal void related to minute metallic shavings that may obscure anatomic detail. These artifacts are more prominent on gradient echo sequences. Furthermore, soft tissue planes and regional anatomy are distorted after surgery, making analysis of MR imaging examinations more difficult.[91] Occasionally, however, a definite role for MR imaging of the postoperative shoulder exists (Fig. 12–177).

Acromioclavicular Joint Dislocation

Subluxation or dislocation of the acromioclavicular joint is a common injury,[452–454] representing approximately 10 per cent of all dislocations involving the shoulder. Acromioclavicular joint injury is observed most commonly in patients between the ages of 16 and 40 years. The abnormality is rare in children,[455] in whom an apparent dislocation of the acromioclavicular joint can

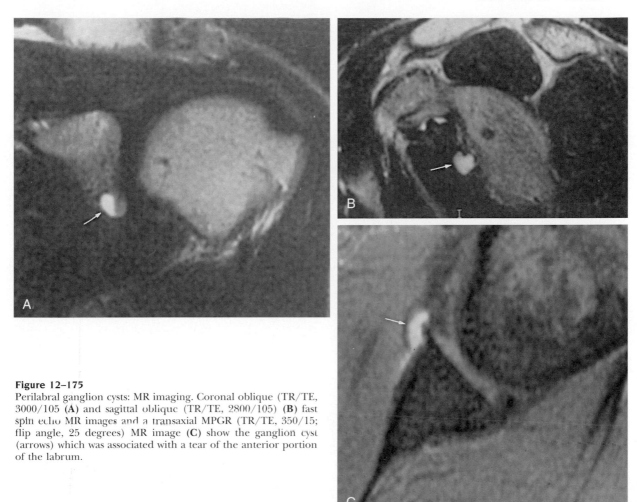

Figure 12–175
Perilabral ganglion cysts: MR imaging. Coronal oblique (TR/TE, 3000/105 (**A**) and sagittal oblique (TR/TE, 2800/105) (**B**) fast spin echo MR images and a transaxial MPGR (TR/TE, 350/15; flip angle, 25 degrees) MR image (**C**) show the ganglion cyst (arrows) which was associated with a tear of the anterior portion of the labrum.

represent, in reality, a displaced fracture of the distal portion of the clavicle. Injury to the acromioclavicular joint can result from indirect or direct forces. An upward indirect force produced by a fall on the outstretched hand can be transmitted from its point of application in the upper extremity along the humerus to the acromioclavicular joint. With the arm in a position of moderate flexion and abduction, the force traverses the glenohumeral joint and is concentrated on the acromion.[456] The scapula is forced in a superior and medial direction. Resulting injuries may include superior dislocation of the glenohumeral joint, acromial fracture, and acromioclavicular capsular stretching and tear. The last-named abnormality, which usually is unassociated with an injury to the coracoclavicular ligament, leads to an acromioclavicular joint sprain or subluxation. A second pattern of indirect injury to the acromioclavicular joint results from a downward force applied by a pull on the upper extremity. A direct injury to the acromioclavicular joint is produced by a fall on the shoulder at a time when the arm is held in adduction, close to the body. In this most common mechanism of injury, the scapula and the clavicle are driven downward. The clavicle may be impacted against the first rib, preventing its further descent. Resulting injuries can include a fracture of the first rib or of the clavicle or, in the absence of such a fracture, injury to the acromioclavicular joint. The degree of disruption of the acromioclavicular and coracoclavicular ligaments varies; the initial injury is to the acromioclavicular ligaments followed by damage to the coracoclavicular ligament.

Injuries of the acromioclavicular joint are classified in several ways, according to the extent of ligamentous damage (Fig. 12–178).[457–459] Although as many as six types of injury are detected (Table 12–6), most investigators refer mainly to the first three of these. A type I injury, indicative of a mild sprain, is associated with stretching or tearing of the fibers of the acromioclavicular ligaments; the acromioclavicular joint remains stable, and the clavicular position is normal. A type II injury, representing a moderate sprain, is associated with disruption of the acromioclavicular ligaments and the aponeurosis of the deltoid and trapezius muscle attachments to the distal portion of the clavicle. The coracoclavicular ligament, the strongest static stabilizer of the acromioclavicular joint, may be strained but otherwise is intact, and the distal aspect of the clavicle may sublux in a posterior or superior direction. With this type of injury, minor elevation of the distal end of the clavicle or widening of the acromioclavicular joint, or both, may be evident on radiographs. A type III injury, represent-

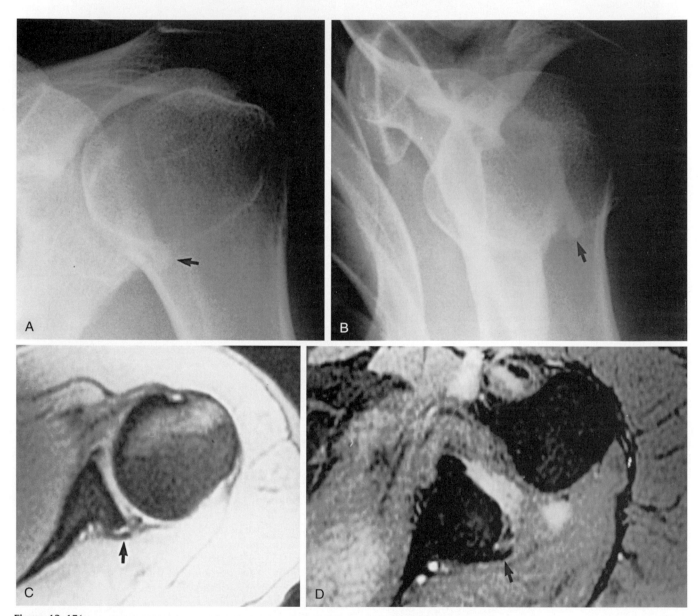

Figure 12–176

Bennett lesion: Routine radiography and MR imaging.

A, B In this 43 year old baseball pitcher, note the osseous excrescence (arrows) arising from the posteroinferior portion of the glenoid cavity.

C In a 17 year old baseball pitcher, a transaxial MPGR (TR/TE, 450/15; flip angle, 10 degrees) MR image shows the area of ossification (arrow), which was visible on routine radiographs (not shown), and an abnormal posterior portion of the labrum.

D In a third patient, a transaxial SPGR (TR/TE, 60/10; flip angle, 60 degrees) fat-suppressed MR image reveals a posterior excrescence (arrow) arising from the scapula.

Table 12–5. SOME TYPES OF SURGICAL PROCEDURES USED FOR RECURRENT ANTERIOR GLENOHUMERAL JOINT DISLOCATIONS

Procedure	Technique
Bankart[320]	Repair of anterior capsular mechanism using drill holes and sutures
Putti-Platt[442]	Shortening of the anterior capsule and subscapularis muscle
Magnuson-Stack[443]	Transfer of the subscapularis tendon from lesser tuberosity to greater tuberosity
Eden-Hybbinette[444, 445]	Bone graft to anterior glenoid region
Oudard[446]	Bone graft to coracoid process
Trillat[447]	Osteotomy with displacement of coracoid process
Bristow-Helfet[448]	Transfer of coracoid process with its attached tendons to neck of the scapula

ing a severe sprain, is characterized by disruption of both the acromioclavicular and coracoclavicular ligaments along with the muscle aponeurosis; on radiographs, elevation of the distal aspect of the clavicle with respect to the acromion is detected. This injury produces an unstable clavicle. Occasionally, the coracoclavicular ligaments remain intact, and an avulsion fracture or epiphyseal separation of the coracoid process is evident.[460–463]

Type I injuries are diagnosed clinically rather than radiographically, although soft tissue swelling and minimal widening of the acromioclavicular joint may be present. The radiographic diagnosis of type II and type III injuries is based on the detection of displacement of the distal portion of the clavicle with relation to the acromion and on the degree of displacement that is evident. Special radiographs may be required, including an angulated frontal projection[464] and films obtained with weight held in the hand (stress radiographs). The stress radiograph should include both shoulders to facilitate comparison between the uninvolved and involved joints (Fig. 12–179). Widening of the acromioclavicular joint without superior displacement of the distal end of the clavicle may be the sole radiographic feature of an injury. Although comparison of the joint width of the injured side with that on the opposite side or of the width of the injured acromioclavicular joint on the routine and stress radiographs may provide diagnostic help, some articular laxity may occur in asymptomatic and noninjured patients. Upward displacement of the distal end of the clavicle provides more definitive evidence of an acromioclavicular joint injury. A difference of 3 to 4 mm in the distance between the superior aspect of the coracoid process and the inferior or superior aspect of the clavicle in the two shoulders indicates an acromioclavicular subluxation or dislocation in which the injured distal clavicle moves superiorly.[465] A complete coracoclavicular ligament disruption is suggested by an increase of the coracoclavicular distance by 40 to 50 per cent.[466] Rarely, inferior dislocation of the clavicle at the acromioclavicular joint occurs in which the bone is forced beneath the acromion or coracoid process.[467] Other, rare patterns of injury include a type III acromioclavicular joint dislocation with superior entrapment of the clavicle above the acromion, preventing reduction,[468] simultaneous dislocations of both the acromioclavicular and sternoclavicular joints (floating clavicle),[469–471] and pseudodislocation of the acromioclavicular articulation owing to a longitudinal rupture in the periosteal envelope of the clavicle.[472] The role of MR imaging in the assessment of these injuries is not known (Fig. 12–180).

Certain complications can be noted after subluxation or dislocation of the acromioclavicular joint. Coracoclavicular ligamentous calcification or ossification can appear after the injury regardless of the type of treatment

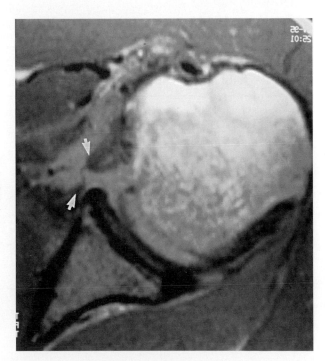

Figure 12–177

Postoperative shoulder: MR imaging. This 21 year old man underwent surgical repair of an anterior labral lesion. Five months later, he developed severe shoulder pain and decreased mobility after a motor vehicle accident. A transaxial proton density (TR/TE, 1813/20) spin echo MR image shows almost complete disruption (arrows) of the subscapularis tendon, as well as a glenohumeral joint effusion. Metal artifact related to the previous surgical procedure is evident.

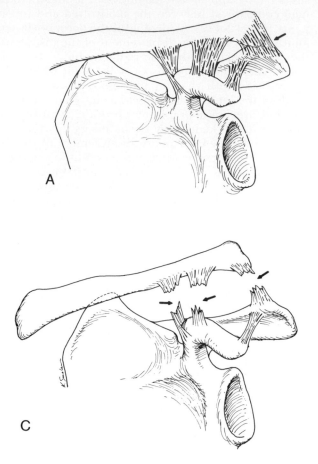

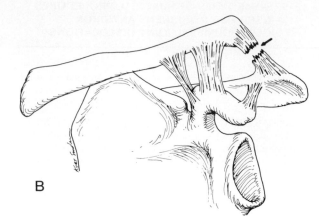

Figure 12–178

Acromioclavicular joint: Classification of injuries.

A Type I injury. Stretching or tearing of the fibers of the acromioclavicular ligaments (arrow) constitutes a mild sprain. The relationship between the distal portion of the clavicle and the acromion remains normal.

B Type II injury. Disruption of the acromioclavicular ligaments (arrow) constitutes a part of this injury, which is classified as a moderate sprain. The coracoclavicular ligament may be strained but otherwise is intact. Minor elevation of the distal portion of the clavicle or widening of the acromioclavicular joint, or both, is the anticipated radiographic abnormality.

C Type III injury. This is a severe sprain and is characterized by disruption of both the acromioclavicular and the coracoclavicular ligaments (arrows) with dislocation of the acromioclavicular joint.

Table 12–6. CLASSIFICATION OF ACROMIOCLAVICULAR JOINT DISLOCATIONS

Type	Injury Pattern	Surgery
I	AC joint capsule partially disrupted	Not indicated
II	AC joint capsule and CC ligaments partially disrupted	Not indicated
III	AC joint capsule and CC ligaments completely disrupted	Optional
IV	Type III + avulsion of CC ligament from clavicle; penetration of clavicle through periosteal sleeve or major soft tissue injury	Indicated
V	Type III + posterior dislocation of clavicle behind acromion	Indicated
VI	Type III + inferolateral dislocation of lateral end of clavicle	Indicated

AC, Acromioclavicular; CC, coracoclavicular.
From Miller ME, Ada JR: Injuries to the shoulder girdle. *In* BD Browner, JB Jupiter, AM Levine, et al [Eds]: Skeletal Trauma: Fractures, Dislocations, Ligamentous Injuries. Philadelphia, WB Saunders Co, 1992, p. 1306.

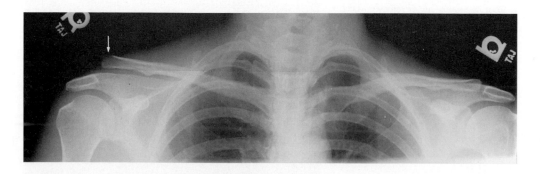

Figure 12–179

Acromioclavicular joint dislocation: Type III injury—stress radiography. Compare the radiographic findings on the normal left side and the abnormal right side. The involved clavicle (arrow) is elevated, with an increased distance between the coracoid process and the inferior surface of the clavicle.

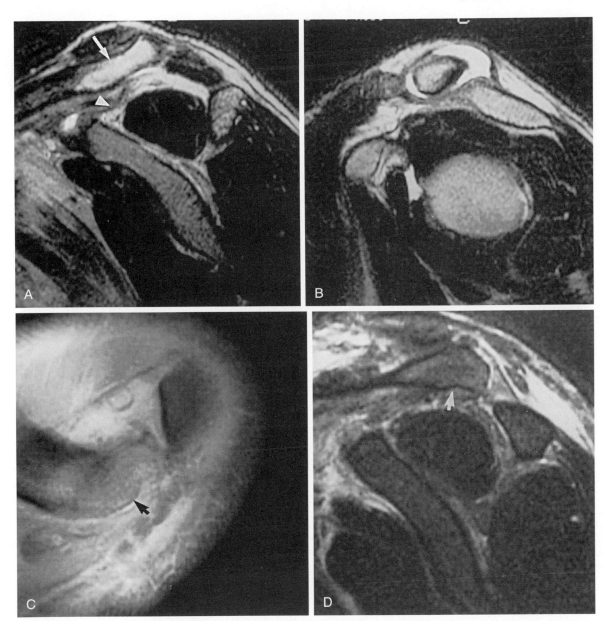

Figure 12–180

Acromioclavicular joint dislocation: MR imaging.

A, B Sagittal oblique fast spin echo (TR/TE, 3883/126) MR images, with **A** more medial to **B,** show the dislocated clavicle with marrow edema (arrow) in **A** and acromioclavicular joint fluid in **B.** Note the disrupted coracoclavicular ligament (arrowhead). The injury had occurred 6 days earlier.

C, D In a second patient, fast spin echo transverse (TR/TE, 3000/14) (**C**) and sagittal oblique (TR/TE, 3000/108) (**D**) fat-suppressed MR images reveal a posteriorly displaced clavicle (arrows) with edema in the adjacent soft tissues.

that is initiated.[473, 474] The radiodense collections may occur within a period of weeks after the traumatic episode, can be prominent in as many as 70 per cent of cases, and do not appear to influence the eventual prognosis of the patient. Additional complications that follow injuries to the acromioclavicular joint include osteoarthritis and posttraumatic osteolysis of the distal end of the clavicle.

Posttraumatic Osteolysis of the Clavicle

Posttraumatic osteolysis can lead to progressive resorption of the outer end of the clavicle.[475–488] The process becomes apparent after single or repeated episodes of local trauma. Frequently the traumatic insult is minor and unassociated with obvious fracture or dislocation; in fact, a similar process has been related to chronic stress (as in weightlifters) without acute injury (see later discussion).[489, 490] The osteolytic process begins as early as 2 to 3 weeks and as late as several years after the injury. When untreated, it leads to lysis of 0.5 to 3 cm of bony substance from the distal end of the clavicle over a period of 12 to 18 months, which may be associated with erosion and cupping of the acromion, soft tissue swelling, and dystrophic calcification (Fig. 12–181).[479] Pain, diminished strength, local crepitation, and restricted mobility may be evident at this stage. After

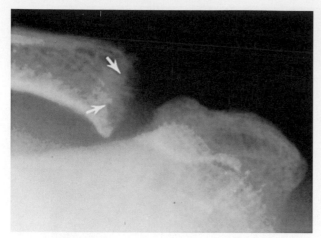

Figure 12–181
Posttraumatic osteolysis of the clavicle: Routine radiography. In a 23 year old weightlifter, irregular erosion of the distal portion of the clavicle (arrows) and, to a lesser extent, the acromion, with widening of the acromioclavicular joint, is seen. (Courtesy of P. Kaplan, M.D., Charlottesville, Virginia.)

the lytic phase stabilizes, reparative changes occur over a period of 4 to 6 months, emphasizing the self-limited nature of the process. Eventually, the subchondral bone becomes reconstituted, although the acromioclavicular joint can remain permanently widened.[479]

Careful analysis of radiographs in the early posttraumatic period may allow identification of prominent soft tissues, osteoporosis, and small gaps in the subchondral bone plate of the clavicle that, when recognized and treated with immobilization, can shorten the course of the process.

The pathogenesis of posttraumatic osteolysis of the clavicle is not certain. Osteoclastic resorption, autonomic nervous system dysfunction, and catabolic hyperemia have been suggested as possible important factors.[491] Levine and coworkers[479] postulated that a slowly progressive, posttraumatic synovial reaction in the acromioclavicular joint could account for the osteolysis, citing such supporting evidence as acromial involvement, the presence of villous hyperplasia and marked vascular proliferation of the synovium after biopsy or resection, and the osseous reconstitution after synovectomy.

Posttraumatic osteolysis of one or both clavicles also is observed in athletes, particularly weightlifters, owing to chronic stress rather than acute injury.[489, 490, 492] A similar process can evolve in persons who lift heavy weights as part of their occupational activities. Clinical and radiologic abnormalities are virtually identical to those that occur after acute injury. Histologic inspection of resected clavicles in athletes has revealed intense osteoblastic activity consistent with a reparative response.[493] Microfractures may be evident in the subchondral bone, and the articular cartilage may contain fissures or other signs of degeneration.[493]

The MR imaging features of posttraumatic osteolysis are not well documented. In a case report of such osteolysis occurring after a significant episode of trauma, Erickson and associates[494] noted high signal intensity in the acromioclavicular joint on T2-weighted spin echo MR images (Fig. 12–182). In a report of seven patients involved in activities leading to repetitive strain of the acromioclavicular joint, Patten[495] emphasized the occurrence of marrow edema in the distal portion of the clavicle (Fig. 12–183), associated in some cases with cortical thinning, small subchondral cysts, and fluid in the acromioclavicular joint. The marrow edema that accompanied this condition was most conspicuous on STIR MR images, and it decreased in extent after conservative treatment.

Sternoclavicular Joint Dislocation

Sternoclavicular joint injuries are rare in comparison to those of the glenohumeral or acromioclavicular joint,

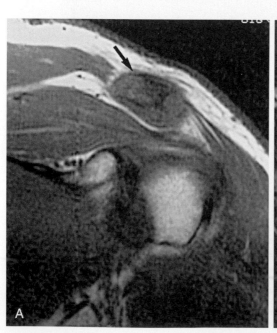
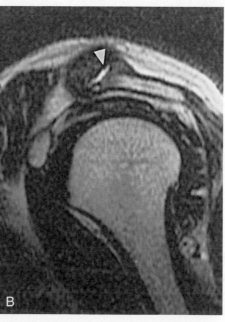

Figure 12–182
Posttraumatic osteolysis of the clavicle: MR imaging. In this 42 year old man, a coronal oblique T1-weighted (TR/TE, 550/15) spin echo MR image **(A)** shows abnormal low signal intensity in the distal portion of the clavicle (arrow) and hypertrophy of capsular tissue about the acromioclavicular joint. A sagittal oblique fast spin echo (TR/TE, 3000/119) MR image **(B)** demonstrates fluid (arrowhead) in the acromioclavicular joint. (Courtesy of R. Kubek, M.D., Atlanta, Georgia.)

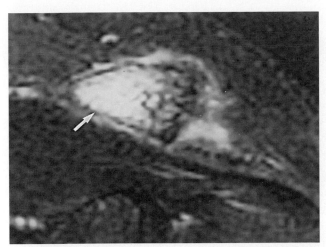

Figure 12–183
Posttraumatic osteolysis of the clavicle: MR imaging. A coronal oblique fat-suppressed fast spin echo (TR/TE, 3000/95) MR image shows marrow edema of high signal intensity in the distal portion of the clavicle (arrow) and a small amount of joint fluid. (Courtesy of P. Kindynis, M.D., Geneva, Switzerland.)

representing only about 2 to 3 per cent of all shoulder dislocations. Anterior dislocations predominate over posterior (retrosternal) dislocations, although the seriousness of posterior dislocations has resulted in many reports of this injury.[496–498] Almost all cases of sternoclavicular subluxation and dislocation are traumatic, although congenital[499] and spontaneous[500] displacements have been recorded. Radiographic analysis is facilitated by a variety of special projections (see previous discussion) and may be supplemented with conventional or computed tomography in some instances.[501, 502] The latter represents the most important technique in the diagnosis of dislocation of the sternoclavicular joint. The role of MR imaging in this regard appears limited, although the technique may allow identification of important ligamentous structures (Fig. 12–184).[503] MR arthrography, however, is superior in this identification (Fig. 12–185).

Traumatic dislocation of the sternoclavicular joint requires a direct or indirect force of great magnitude.[504, 505] Dislocation related to a direct force, the less frequent mechanism of injury, occurs when a force is applied directly to the anteromedial aspect of the clavicle, producing a posterior dislocation of the sternoclavicular joint; anterior sternoclavicular joint dislocation does not occur by direct mechanisms. An indirect force transmitted to the sternoclavicular joint along the longitudinal axis of the clavicle from the shoulder can produce either an anterior or a posterior dislocation. As indicated previously, panclavicular dislocation with displacement of both the sternoclavicular and the acromioclavicular joints is a rare injury.

Prompt recognition of the less common posterior sternoclavicular joint dislocation is required because the displaced clavicle may impinge on the trachea, the esophagus, the great vessels, or the major nerves in the superior mediastinum, leading to vascular compromise, cough, dysphagia, and dyspnea. Death may ensue in unrecognized or severe injuries.[505]

Anterior, or presternal, dislocations are caused by forces that move the shoulder backward and outward or downward. As the distal end of the clavicle is displaced posteriorly, its sternal end, using the first rib and thorax as a fulcrum, springs anteriorly, tearing the sternoclavicular ligaments. An avulsion fracture of the inferior margin of the clavicle may be seen. On physical examination, a prominent anteriorly displaced medial end of the clavicle is visible and palpable and, in the presence of disruption of the costoclavicular ligaments, may be displaced superiorly. Serious complications are rare after this type of dislocation, although a "cosmetic bump" may remain indefinitely.

Posterior, or retrosternal, dislocations of the sternoclavicular joint are an uncommon injury, representing approximately 5 per cent of all of the dislocations at this site (Fig. 12–186). As indicated previously, severe pain may be accompanied by signs related to clavicular impingement on adjacent neurovascular structures and airways. A depression of the skin overlying the displaced medial end of the clavicle may be identified. A pneumothorax or hemothorax may be an associated finding.

An additional injury of the medial end of the clavicle is an epiphyseal fracture or separation. The growth plate at this site is among the last to become obliterated during skeletal maturation, disappearing at approximately 25 years of age. Various types of injuries to the growth plate can occur.[506, 507] Before the medial clavicular epiphysis ossifies at the age of about 18 years, it is extremely difficult to differentiate between a dislocation of the sternoclavicular joint and a fracture through the growth plate. Although MR imaging theoretically could aid in this differentiation, its value in this regard has not been documented.

Fractures of the Proximal Portion of the Humerus

The type of injury that is encountered in the proximal portion of the humerus depends, to a large extent, on the age of the person. In the neonate, physeal separation or, less commonly, fracture of the proximal portion of the humerus may result from birth injury. In the immature skeleton of the child and adolescent, acute or chronic physeal separation or injury with or without associated fractures is encountered (Fig. 12–187), and in the young adult, glenohumeral joint dislocations or subluxations predominate (see previous discussion). It is in middle-aged adults, over the age of 45 years, and in the elderly that fractures of the proximal portion of the humerus typically are seen (Table 12–7). They are more frequent in women than in men, and—in common with fractures of the vertebral bodies, proximal portion of the femur, and distal portion of the radius—their likelihood after injury depends very much on the severity of osteopenia.[508]

The classification of fractures of the proximal region of the humerus on the basis of the level of disruption or the mechanism of injury[509] has been replaced in large part by a scheme proposed by Neer[510] that emphasizes the presence or the absence of significant displacement

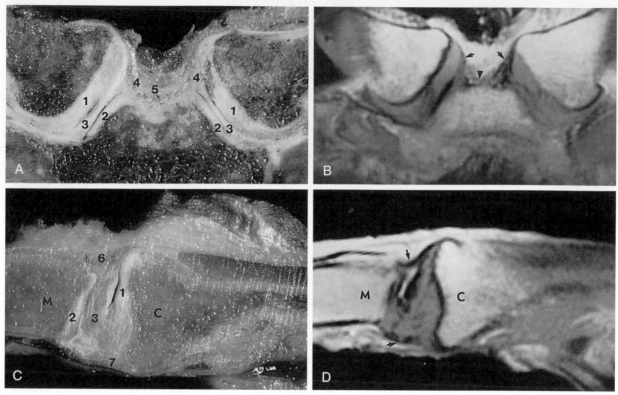

Figure 12–184

Sternoclavicular joint: Normal anatomy (MR imaging, T1-weighted spin echo MR images).

A, B Coronal plane. In the sectional photograph **(A),** identified structures include the articular cartilage of the clavicle (1) and sternum (2), the intra-articular disc (3), the joint capsule (4), and the interclavicular ligament (5). In the MR image **(B),** it is difficult to differentiate between the articular cartilage and articular disc. The joint capsule (arrows) and interclavicular ligament (arrowhead) are seen.

C, D Oblique plane parallel to the long axis of the clavicle. In the sectional photograph **(C),** identified structures are the articular cartilage (1) of the clavicle (C), the articular cartilage (2) of the manubrium sterni (M), the intra-articular disc (3), and the anterior (6) and posterior (7) sternoclavicular ligaments. In the MR image **(D),** the anterior and posterior sternoclavicular ligaments (arrows) coursing between the clavicle (C) and manubrium sterni (M) are seen.

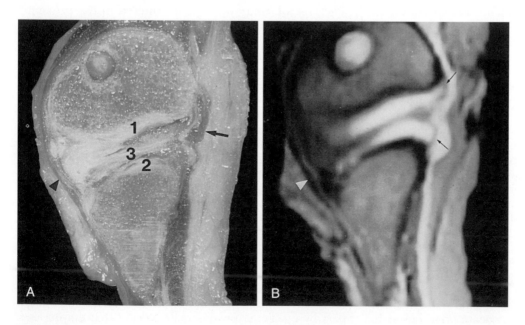

Figure 12–185

Sternoclavicular joint: Normal anatomy (MR arthrography with gadolinium compound). T1-weighted spin echo MR image. In the sectional photograph (sagittal plane with anterior aspect to the right) **(A),** note the articular cartilage of the clavicle (1) and sternum (2), the intra-articular disc (3), and the anterior (arrow) and posterior (arrowhead) capsular and ligamentous (i.e., anterior and posterior sternoclavicular ligaments) structures. A cyst is present in the clavicle. In the MR arthrographic image **(B),** the anterior (arrows) and posterior (arrowhead) capsuloligamentous structures can be identified.

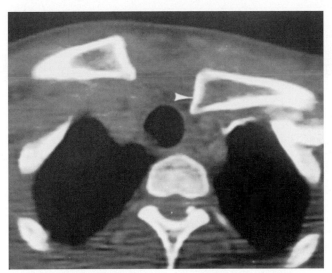

Figure 12–186
Sternoclavicular joint: Posterior dislocation. A transaxial CT scan reveals the posterior position of the injured clavicle (arrowhead) and its relationship to the trachea.

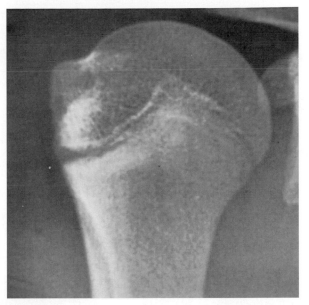

Figure 12–187
Little League shoulder (Salter-Harris type I fracture). A routine radiograph demonstrates mild widening of the lateral aspect of the physis with sclerosis along the metaphyseal aspect. (Courtesy of H. Pavlov, M.D., New York, New York.)

of one or more of the four major osseous segments of this part of the humerus (Fig. 12–188A). These segments are the articular segment containing the anatomic neck, the greater tuberosity, the lesser tuberosity, and the shaft and surgical neck. Approximately 80 per cent of fractures of the proximal portion of the humerus are undisplaced, owing to the protection afforded by the periosteum, joint capsule, and rotator cuff. A displaced fracture exists if any of the four segments is separated by more than 1 cm from its neighbor or is angulated more than 45 degrees. Nondisplaced fractures or fractures with minimal displacement that do not meet these criteria are considered one-part fractures. A two-part fracture is one in which only a single segment is displaced in relation to the other three; two-part fractures represent approximately 15 per cent of all fractures of the proximal portion of the humerus. A three-part fracture, constituting approximately 3 or 4 per cent of humeral fractures, occurs when two segments are displaced in relationship to the other two parts, and a four-part fracture, occurring in approximately 3 or 4 per cent of cases, exists when all the humeral segments are displaced. Neer further uses the term fracture-dislocation to indicate that the articular segment of the humerus is displaced beyond the joint space, and he separates this injury from "impression" or "head-splitting" fractures.

Table 12–7. FRACTURES OF THE HUMERAL METAPHYSES AND SHAFT

Site	Characteristics	Complications
Proximal[508–524]	Middle-aged and elderly adults Classified as one-part to four-part based on the degree and the location of displacement	Lipohemarthrosis Drooping shoulder related to hemarthrosis, capsular tear, muscle or nerve injury Osteonecrosis, especially with displaced fractures of humeral neck and four-part fractures Osteoarthritis Heterotopic ossification Rotator cuff tear Brachial plexus and, less commonly, axillary artery injury Painful arc of motion
Middle[525–533]	Adults > children Most common at junction of distal and middle thirds Associated fractures in 25 per cent of cases (ulna, clavicle, or humerus) Characteristic displacements, related to sites of muscular attachment	Delayed union or nonunion when fracture is transverse or distracted Radial nerve injury in 5 to 15 percent of cases Brachial artery injury
Supracondylar[534–557]	Children >> adults Extension (95 per cent) and flexion (5 per cent) types Paradoxic posterior fat pad sign Supracondylar process may fracture	Brachial artery injury Median, ulnar, or radial nerve injury Heterotopic ossification Volkmann's ischemic contracture

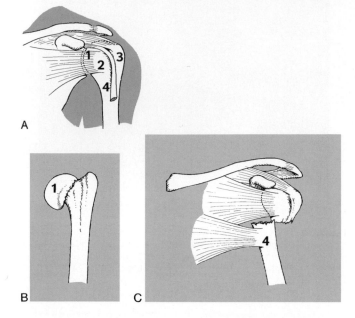

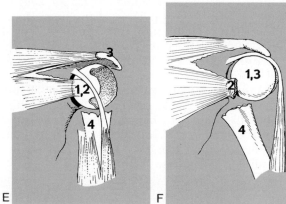

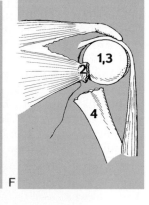

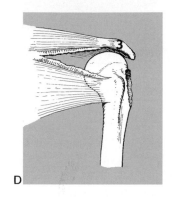

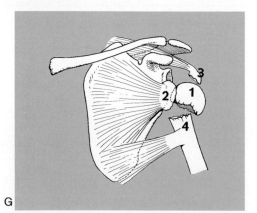

Figure 12–188

Fractures of the proximal end of the humerus: System of classification.

A Normal situation. Four major segments of the proximal portion of the humerus are identified: 1, humeral head; 2, lesser tuberosity; 3, greater tuberosity; 4, humeral shaft.

B Two-part fracture. In this example, a fracture of the anatomic neck has led to displacement of the humeral head (**1**). Ischemic necrosis may complicate this rare injury.

C Two-part fracture. In this example, displacement of the humeral shaft (**4**) relates to the pull of the pectoralis major muscle. The rotator cuff is intact and holds the humeral head in a neutral position. Variations of this fracture pattern relate to the extent of impaction, angulation, and comminution.

D Two-part fracture. In this example, displacement of the greater tuberosity (**3**) occurs owing to the forces generated by a portion of the rotator cuff musculature. Retraction of more than 1.0 cm of the entire greater tuberosity or one of its facets is pathognomonic of a longitudinal tear of the rotator cuff. The fragment tends to be large in younger patients and small in older patients. A complication of this injury is impaired motion of the shoulder.

E Three-part fracture. In this injury, the greater tuberosity (**3**) is displaced and the subscapularis muscle rotates the humeral head (**1,2**) so that its articular surface faces posteriorly. The diaphysis (**4**) is displaced relative to the rotated head owing to the action of the pectoralis major muscle.

F Three-part fracture. In this type of injury, the lesser tuberosity (**2**) is detached and displaced by the action of the subscapularis muscle, and the supraspinatus and external rotators cause the articular surface of the humeral head (**1,3**) to face anteriorly. **4,** Humeral shaft.

G Four-part fracture. The articular segment (**1**) is detached from the tuberosities (**2,3**) and from its circulation and is displaced laterally (as shown), anteriorly, or posteriorly, losing contact with the glenoid cavity. The tuberosities usually are retracted by the attached musculature. **4,** Humeral shaft.

(From Neer CS II: Shoulder Reconstruction. Philadelphia: WB Saunders Co; 1990.)

The Neer classification system underscores the orthopedic surgeon's concern regarding the degree of displacement of fracture fragments of the proximal portion of the humerus, rather than the specific number of such fragments. As such, it has been used widely to aid in determining the choice of appropriate therapy of these fractures. The application of the Neer classification system is not without difficulties, however, as interpretation of the relationship among the fracture fragments on the basis of routine radiography can be a challenge, and wide interobserver variation regarding the specific type of injury present, even among experienced observers, has been documented.[511, 558–560] CT can be employed as an ancillary technique, allowing more accurate determination of the Neer fracture pattern, particularly in cases of complex humeral fractures.[512, 513]

The classic mechanism of injury is a fall on the outstretched arm in which severe abduction of the shoulder produces a fracture of the humeral neck. A second mechanism of injury is a direct blow on the side of the upper arm. In all types of humeral injury, initial symptoms and signs may be obscured by the thickness of the patient's arm so that accurate diagnosis depends on adequate radiographic examination. In some cases, damage to the axillary vessels or brachial plexus provides additional clues regarding the severity of the injury.

The *one-part (nondisplaced) fracture* is the most frequent pattern of injury. The fracture fragments are closely apposed and are not angulated (Fig. 12–189). Rotation of the humerus usually is followed by movement of all of the fragments as a group.

The *two-part fractures* include isolated displacement of the head with fracture of the anatomic neck, displacement of the shaft with a fracture of the surgical neck, displacement of the greater tuberosity, or displacement

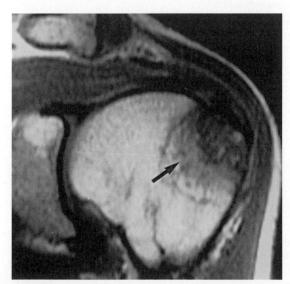

Figure 12–189
Fractures of the proximal end of the humerus: One-part (nondisplaced) fracture. A coronal oblique T1-weighted (TR/TE, 900/12) spin echo MR image shows a subacute (3 weeks old) fracture of the greater tuberosity of the humerus with adjacent marrow edema (arrow).

of the lesser tuberosity.[510] A two-part fracture with isolated displacement of the humeral head is a rare injury, easily overlooked on initial radiographs, and associated with ischemic necrosis of bone (see Fig. 12–188B). A two-part fracture with isolated displacement of the shaft owing to a fracture of the surgical neck is a frequent injury; impaction and anterior angulation at the fracture site may be observed (see Fig. 12–188C). A two-part fracture of the surgical neck can also be associated with anterior and medial displacement of the humeral shaft owing to the pull of the pectoralis major. A third pattern of a two-part surgical neck fracture relates to comminution at the fracture site.

A two-part humeral fracture with displacement of the greater tuberosity is associated with a longitudinal tear of the rotator cuff; the articular segment of the humeral head remains in normal relationship with the shaft (see Fig. 12–188D). The size of the fracture and the degree of displacement of the greater tuberosity vary. A two-part humeral fracture with displacement of the lesser tuberosity can occur as an isolated phenomenon[514, 515] or in association with a nondisplaced surgical neck fracture. The lesser tuberosity is pulled medially by the subscapularis muscle, but normal alignment between the humeral head and neck is present. Similar fractures of the lesser tuberosity may accompany posterior or anterior dislocations of the glenohumeral joint.

Two typical patterns of *three-part fractures* occur in the proximal portion of the humerus; a fracture of the surgical neck may be combined with displacement of either the greater tuberosity or the lesser tuberosity. If the greater tuberosity is avulsed, the subscapularis muscle rotates the humeral head in a posterior direction (see Fig. 12–188E); if the lesser tuberosity is avulsed, the supraspinatus, infraspinatus, and teres minor muscles rotate the humeral head in an anterior direction (see Fig. 12–188F). The pectoralis major produces anteromedial displacement of the humeral shaft. Open surgical methods are required to reduce these fractures.[516]

The severe *four-part fracture* is characterized by isolation of the humeral articular segment and disruption of its blood supply, rendering it ischemic (see Fig. 12–188G).[517–519] Typically, a fracture of the anatomic neck of the humerus is combined with avulsion of the greater and the lesser tuberosities. Common abnormalities include displacements of the lesser tuberosity medially related to the pull of the subscapularis; of the greater tuberosity superiorly owing to the pull of the supraspinatus, infraspinatus, and teres minor; and of the shaft medially owing to traction by the pectoralis major muscle. A specific type of four-part fracture of the proximal end of the humerus results in valgus impaction of the articular segment; the frequency of subsequent osteonecrosis of the humeral head is less than that of other displaced four-part fractures.[520]

In association with two-part, three-part, or four-part fractures, the articular surface of the humeral head may be displaced beyond the joint in either an anterior direction (displacement of the greater tuberosity) or a posterior direction (displacement of the lesser tuberosity). Pericapsular bone formation is frequent after either type of fracture-dislocation.

Several patterns of intra-articular fracture of the humeral head may be encountered. Impaction of the articular surface against the anterior or posterior rim of the glenoid cavity in cases of anterior or posterior glenohumeral joint dislocation has been considered earlier in this chapter. More severe fragmentation or comminution can accompany central impaction of the humeral head against the glenoid cavity. Complications of fractures of the articular head of the humerus include lipohemarthrosis, production of intra-articular osteocartilaginous fragments, inferior displacement of the humeral head (drooping shoulder), and osteoarthritis.

Lipohemarthrosis, with the release of fat and blood into the articular cavity, can follow intracapsular fractures of the humerus (as well as similar fractures at other sites). The source of the fat within the joint space is assumed to be the bone marrow, so that the detection of radiographic evidence of intra-articular fat should alert the physician that a fracture should be present. This rule is not without exception, as it has been proposed that injury to the synovial membrane and surrounding soft tissues also may release fat into the joint. Radiographic demonstration of lipohemarthrosis is facilitated by the inclusion of radiographs obtained with horizontal beam technique. Upright or decubitus films will demonstrate a fat-fluid level with radiolucent fat above and radiodense blood below. CT and MR imaging also allow detection of lipohemarthrosis.

Inferior displacement of the humerus, producing the drooping shoulder, may accompany intra-articular or extra-articular fractures. The findings should not be misinterpreted as a true dislocation of the glenohumeral joint, as the condition is self-limited, the humeral head returning to its normal position with respect to the glenoid cavity over a period of weeks. Its precise pathogenesis is unclear; factors important in its development may include hemarthrosis, detachment of the joint capsule, stretching of the support musculature, or injury to the brachial plexus.[521]

Delayed union or nonunion can accompany any type of fracture of the proximal portion of the humerus and may be accompanied by significant angulation at the site of fracture.[522] *Osteonecrosis* is associated with fractures of the humeral head and neck that lead to loss of the blood supply from both the muscular insertions and the arcuate branch of the internal humeral circumflex artery (Fig. 12–190). This complication, which is reported in 7 to 50 per cent of cases,[523] is most typical of displaced fractures of the anatomic neck of the humerus and a severe fracture or fracture-dislocation of the bone (four-part fracture).[519] The accompanying radiographic features are similar to those that occur in osteonecrosis of the femoral head, including patchy osteolysis and osteosclerosis. Collapse of the articular surface of the humerus after ischemic necrosis is not so marked as in cases of ischemic necrosis of the femoral head owing to the lack of weight-bearing in the upper extremity.

Fractures involving the articular surface of the humeral head may be complicated by *osteoarthritis* with joint space narrowing, sclerosis, and osteophytosis. Fracture-dislocations of the proximal portion of the humerus also can be associated with *heterotopic bone formation* in pericapsular regions. Humeral fractures associated with considerable retraction of the greater tuberos-

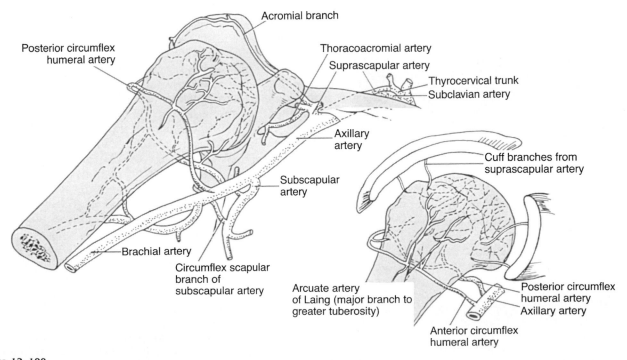

Figure 12–190
Vascular supply to the shoulder region. (From Norris TR: Fractures of the proximal humerus and dislocations of the shoulder. *In* BD Browner, JB Jupiter, AM Levine, PG Traften [Eds]: Skeletal Trauma: Fractures, Dislocations, Ligamentous Injuries. Philadelphia, WB Saunders Co, 1992, p. 1204.)

ity or the lesser tuberosity are characterized by tears in the *rotator cuff*. Abnormal rotation of the humeral head complicating such severe fractures is related to the unopposed action of intact components of the cuff, and these soft tissue attachments provide an important source of blood supply to the humeral head.

Anterior fracture-dislocation of the proximal portion of the humerus can lead to injury of the nearby *brachial plexus* and, less commonly, the *axillary artery*. The axillary artery lies just anterior and medial to the proximal portion of the humerus; injury of this vessel in cases of humeral fracture is rare and relates to its laceration by fracture fragments or stretching or avulsion when one of its branches (humeral circumflex or subscapular arteries) is entrapped at the fracture site.[524] A brachial plexus injury, which results from contusion or mild traction, may be self-limited.

Fractures of the Clavicle

The clavicle is a horizontally oriented and superficial bone that is anchored at both the acromioclavicular and sternoclavicular articulations. It is the subcutaneous location that is responsible, at least in part, for the high frequency of fractures of this bone. Fractures of the clavicle predominate at the junction of its outer and intermediate thirds, where the two osseous curves are continuous. Fracture deformity results from the weight of the arm and the spasm of the musculature crossing from the thorax to the arm. These factors, acting on the coracoclavicular ligament, allow depression of the outer fracture fragment. The proximal fragment is displaced superiorly owing to the action of the sternocleidomastoid muscle. These classic patterns of displacement are modified in the presence of fractures at other clavicular sites.

With regard to the analysis of fractures of the clavicle, it is convenient to divide the bone into three functional segments: a distal or interligamentous segment consisting of the outer 25 to 30 per cent of the bone, the region about and distal to the coracoclavicular ligament; an intermediate segment consisting of the middle 40 to 50 per cent of the bone; and an inner segment consisting of the medial 25 per cent of the bone.[457] Approximately 75 to 80 per cent of clavicular fractures involve the middle segment of the bone, 15 to 20 per cent involve the distal segment, and 5 per cent affect the inner segment. The prognosis of clavicular fractures depends on the precise site of involvement; for example, nonunion is frequent in cases of fracture distal to the coracoclavicular ligament, whereas this complication is rare in cases of fracture of the medial segment of the bone.

The middle segment, located at the junction of the two curvatures of the clavicle, is the most common site of fracture. In adults and children, the mechanism of injury usually is a fall onto the outstretched hand or a fall on the shoulder.[457] Local pain, swelling, and crepitation are evident at the fracture site. In most cases, the radiographic findings permit prompt and accurate

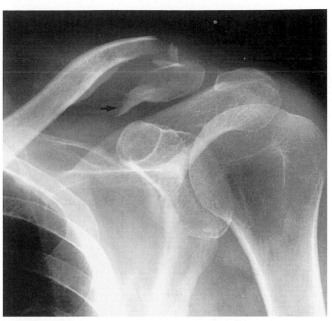

Figure 12–191
Clavicular fracture: Distal segment—type II injury. Disruption of the conoid portion of the coracoclavicular ligament has allowed superior migration of the proximal segment of the clavicle. Note the bone flange (arrow) extending from the distal clavicular segment to which the trapezoid portion of the coracoclavicular ligament inserts.

diagnosis,[561] although specialized oblique and angulated projections may be required.[562]

Fractures of the distal portion of the clavicle, related to a force applied on the shoulder driving the humerus and scapula downward, are divided into two types[563]: type I fractures, in which the coracoclavicular ligaments are intact; and type II fractures, in which a portion (conoid portion) of the coracoclavicular ligaments is severed. A characteristic medial flange of bone extending from the distal clavicular fragment may be evident with type II fractures (Fig. 12–191). Type II fractures have a poorer prognosis related to more significant displacement at the fracture site and to nonunion. The degree of osseous displacement may be obscured on routine radiographic examination, requiring stress views (with a weight tied to the ipsilateral wrist) or oblique projections with the patient erect.[563] Four displacement forces exist with regard to type II fractures: (1) the trapezius, attaching to the entire outer third of the clavicle, draws the larger medial fragment posteriorly within its substance; (2) the weight of the arm pulls the outer fragment downward and forward; (3) the trunk muscles attaching to the humerus and scapula displace the outer fragment in a medial direction toward the apex of the thorax; and (4) the scapular ligaments may rotate the outer fragment as much as 40 per cent.[563] Associated fractures of the coracoid process and ribs may be evident. Rarely, a fracture of the distal aspect of the clavicle is accompanied by a longitudinal rupture in the periosteal envelope and a radiographic appearance simulating that of an acromioclavicular joint dislocation.

Direct trauma accounts for the majority of fractures

of the medial end of the clavicle. They have been divided into two types: transverse fractures, which do not become displaced because of ligamentous and musculature attachments, and intra-articular fractures. When the costoclavicular ligament remains intact and attached to the outer fragment, displacement does not occur.[457] Intra-articular fractures may be overlooked unless conventional tomography is used. They can result in secondary osteoarthritis with persistent pain.

In children, clavicular fractures heal rapidly without significant sequelae. In adults, resultant deformities secondary to extensive callus formation may be observed. Exuberant callus affecting the middle segment of the clavicle can be associated with persistent neurologic defects and circulatory disturbances owing to compression of the subclavian vessels and brachial plexus against the first rib, and surgical removal of the callus may be required.[564–566] Foreshortening of the clavicle in the form of a bayonet deformity at the site of fracture can occur but it usually is unassociated with significant cosmetic problems.

Fracture of the first rib may accompany fracture of the clavicle (or acromioclavicular joint dislocation).[567] In children, an association of clavicular fracture and atlantoaxial rotary fixation has been noted, consistent with a traumatic insult occurring during a fall onto the shoulder and side of the head.[568] Nonunion of a clavicular fracture is uncommon[569] and, when present, is associated with lack of immobilization. Delayed union or nonunion after fractures of the lateral portions of the clavicle usually is related to rupture of the coracoclavicular ligament. In the middle portion of the clavicle, delayed union or nonunion may result from local tissue damage, loss of bone stock, stripping or interposition of soft tissues, inadequate fixation of fracture fragments, or infection.[569–571]

A posttraumatic pseudarthrosis of the clavicle must be differentiated from a congenital pseudarthrosis, a distinction that generally is not difficult. Congenital pseudarthrosis of the clavicle usually is manifested as a painless swelling overlying the middle third of the bone, more frequently on the right side. The patients are infants, commonly within the first few weeks of life. On radiographs, the medial segment of the clavicle is elevated and displaced anteriorly and the lateral segment is depressed and displaced posteriorly. Callus and periosteal bone formation are absent.

Fractures of the Scapula

Scapular fractures are infrequent, constituting approximately 1 per cent of all fractures and 5 to 7 per cent of those about the shoulder. Although they may occur as an isolated phenomenon, more commonly and perhaps in as many as 95 per cent of cases,[572] they are associated with additional injuries, including fractures of the ribs, clavicle, and skull. Scapular fractures may involve one or more of the following anatomic regions: glenoid fossa and articular surface, neck, body, spinous process, acromion process, and coracoid process.[573, 574] They are

found most frequently in the scapular body, followed by the neck and the other regions of the bone.[572, 574]

A fracture of the rim of the glenoid cavity occurs in approximately 20 per cent of traumatic glenohumeral joint dislocations. The fracture fragment may be cartilaginous or osteocartilaginous, requiring for diagnosis careful plain film radiography as well as arthrography or arthrotomography in some cases. Either the anterior glenoid rim (in anterior dislocations) or the posterior glenoid rim (in posterior dislocations) may be affected. Larger portions of the glenoid fossa may be fractured when the humeral head is driven against the glenoid cavity by a direct force.[575, 576] Comminution of the articular surface may require operative intervention.[577] Violent contraction of the triceps muscle, a situation that might occur in an athlete engaged in a throwing sport such as baseball, can lead to avulsion of a portion of the inferior lip of the glenoid cavity.[578]

A fracture in the neck of the scapula typically occurs after a direct blow on the shoulder. When the fracture is complete, the outer fragment is displaced in an inferior direction owing to the effect of gravity on the patient's arm. The fracture line, which may be impacted, extends from the supraclavicular notch above to the coracoid process below. The prognosis is improved if the glenoid cavity is not affected and the coracoclavicular and acromioclavicular ligaments are intact. Combined fractures of the scapular neck and ipsilateral clavicle disrupt the stability of the suspensory structures of the shoulder (i.e., floating shoulder), and muscle forces and the weight of the arm pull the glenoid fragment distally and anteromedially.[579]

Approximately 50 to 70 per cent of scapular fractures involve the body of the bone. The typical mechanism of injury is a direct force of considerable magnitude, which also may result in fractures of neighboring ribs and pneumothorax.[580] Fractures of the body of the scapula due to indirect forces or to muscular avulsion are less frequent.[581] Radiographs will reveal the vertical or horizontal nature of the fracture line or its comminution. Displacement of the osseous fragment is unusual, although a peculiar avulsion fracture of the superior margin of the scapula, probably related to the insertion site of the omohyoid muscle, can be associated with significant upward displacement (Fig. 12–192).[582]

Isolated fractures of the spinous process of the scapula are infrequent and, when present, are the result of direct trauma. Fractures of the acromion process generally follow direct trauma, although muscular traction can rarely produce a similar lesion.[583] On radiographs, a fracture line is evident, usually adjacent to the acromioclavicular joint although occasionally at the base of the acromion process. Significant neurologic injury, although rare in most cases of scapular fracture, is a recognized complication of acromion fractures[574]; depression of the shoulder and contralateral flexion of the neck after these fractures predispose to injuries of the brachial plexus. Of diagnostic importance, the os acromiale, a normal variant of the shoulder, can simulate an acromial fracture. The small osseous density inferior to the acromion that characterizes this extra ossification center is bilateral in approximately 60 per cent of cases.

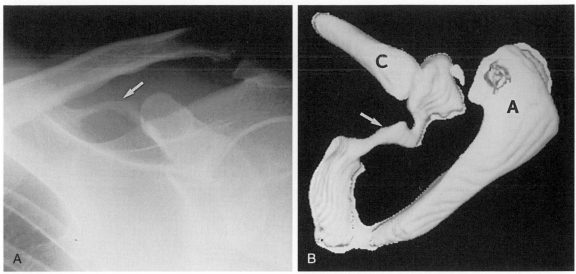

Figure 12–192

Scapular fracture: Avulsion fracture of superior margin of the scapular body. The deformity of the upper margin of the bone (arrows), as shown with routine radiography **(A)** and a three-dimensional CT image of the top of the scapula **(B)** is the result of a recent fracture. It simulates the appearance of a developmental scapular foramen (see Edelson JG: J Bone Joint Surg [Br] 77:505, 1995). A, Acromion; C, clavicle. (Courtesy of G. Bock, M.D., Winnipeg, Manitoba, Canada.)

Fractures of the coracoid process relate to a direct injury from a dislocating humeral head, a direct force on the tip of the coracoid itself, or an avulsion owing to traction on the coracoclavicular ligament (in association with acromioclavicular joint dislocation), the short head of the biceps muscle, or the coracobrachialis muscle.[584, 585] Isolated fractures of the coracoid process are observed in athletes as a result of an avulsion injury or in trapshooters related to repetitive stress from the impact of the recoiling rifle. Anteroposterior radiographs may not demonstrate the coracoid process adequately and must be supplemented with a lateral scapular view or axillary projection, or both. The tip of this process may be displaced in an inferior and medial direction, resembling the appearance of a normal accessory ossification center (infracoracoid bone).

As noted previously, neurologic injury may be a sequela of a scapular fracture, particularly one that involves the acromion process or leads to avulsion of the coracoid process. Vascular compromise is rare after scapular injuries.[586] Fractures of neighboring bones, including the ribs and clavicle, acromioclavicular joint dislocation, pulmonary involvement, skull fractures, and cerebral contusion may accompany scapular injuries. Considering the great degree of force required to fracture this bone, the high frequency of associated injuries is not unexpected.

An intrathoracic dislocation of the scapula producing a "locked scapula" is a rare injury.[587] After a direct blow to the scapula or an outward traction force on the arm, the lower margin of the bone becomes locked between adjacent ribs. Fractures of the scapula or ribs may complicate this injury.

Traumatic lateral displacement of the scapula, scapulothoracic dissociation, also is rare and is accompanied by partial or complete amputation through the soft tissue and injuries to the brachial plexus and the subclavian artery and vein.[588, 589] In addition to the displacement of the scapula, radiographic findings may include disruption of the acromioclavicular joint and fracture of the clavicle (Fig. 12–193).[590]

Fractures of the First and Second Ribs

Fractures of the first or second rib indicate major trauma to the thorax or shoulder.[591–592] Associated ab-

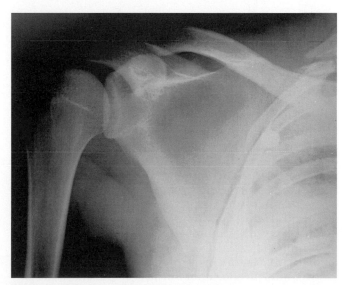

Figure 12–193

Scapulothoracic dissociation. A 2000 kg gate fell on the shoulder of a 20 year old man. Note lateral displacement of the scapula, widening of the acromioclavicular joint, subcutaneous edema, rib fractures, and pulmonary bleeding. (Courtesy of G. Bock, M.D., Winnipeg, Manitoba, Canada.)

normalities are frequent and potentially serious; these include rupture of the apex of the lung or of the subclavian artery, aneurysm of the aortic arch, tracheoesophageal fistula, pleurisy, hemothorax, cardiac alterations, neurologic injury, and additional fractures. Because of the serious implications of these accompanying abnormalities, the detection of a fracture of the first rib requires a careful evaluation of intrathoracic structures to exclude the presence of additional alterations, although there is no uniform agreement regarding the precise indications for aortography.[593–595]

The first rib is not a superficial structure, being protected by the clavicle; fractures of the first rib related to direct trauma may be combined with disruption of the clavicle. Indirect force owing to a sudden strong contracture of the scalenus anterior muscle combined with traction on the arm and on the serratus anterior muscle can produce a fracture about the subclavian sulcus of the rib.[592] Sudden hyperextension of the neck can produce a similar abnormality. Upper rib fractures are observed after median sternotomy, presumably related to surgical trauma.[596] Stress fractures of these ribs are associated with the lifting of heavy weights or the excessive overhead use of the arms and have been described in hikers carrying heavy backpacks.

Fracture and displacement about the first costovertebral articulations are easily overlooked unless the radiographs are interpreted carefully. Direct or indirect force is implicated. Avulsed fragments at the site of osseous attachment of the adjacent ligaments, such as the radiate or costotransverse ligament, probably indicate severe force and may be combined with pulmonary, pleural, or mediastinal abnormality.

Fractures of the Humeral Diaphysis

The diaphyseal portion, or shaft, of the humerus extends from the upper border of the insertion site of the pectoralis major tendon, close to the surgical neck, in a distal direction to the level of the supracondylar ridge. The diaphysis is cylindrical or tubular in its proximal portion and more triangular, with a flattened anterior surface, in its distal portion. Three surfaces can be identified in the humeral shaft: the anterior border, extending from the greater tuberosity proximally to the coronoid fossa distally; the medial border, extending from the lesser tuberosity proximally to the medial supracondylar ridge distally; and the lateral border, extending from the posterior aspect of the greater tuberosity proximally to the lateral supracondylar ridge distally.[597] The deltoid tuberosity and the sulcus for the radial nerve and profunda brachii artery are located on the anterolateral surface of the humerus; the anteromedial surface forms the floor of the intertubercular groove; and the posterior surface of the humerus contains the spiral groove for the radial nerve.[597]

Fractures of the humeral diaphysis account for about 3 to 5 per cent of all fractures (see Table 12–7). These humeral fractures may occur as a response to direct trauma (e.g., motor vehicle accidents, blows received during a physical assault, gunshot wounds) or to indirect forces, including torsional ones that occur in athletic endeavors, such as throwing a ball, shot putting, or arm wrestling.[598–600] Although diaphyseal fractures of the humerus generally heal in a satisfactory fashion, delayed union, nonunion, or malunion of these fractures is well known.[601, 602] An analysis of fractures of the humeral diaphysis reveals the effects of the muscular forces acting on the shaft at varying levels.[597] In fractures occurring above the insertion of the tendon of the pectoralis major muscle, the proximal fragment is displaced into abduction and external rotation, owing to the action of the rotator cuff musculature; fractures occurring in the interval between the insertion of the pectoralis major tendon proximally and the deltoid insertion distally result in adduction of the proximal fragment and lateral displacement of the distal fragment; and fractures occurring distal to the insertion of the deltoid muscle result in abduction of the proximal fragment and proximal displacement of the distal fragment.[597]

The precise fracture configuration depends on the type of injury and its force. Transverse fractures of the humeral shaft are most frequent, representing 50 to 70 per cent of all diaphyseal fractures of the humerus; oblique or spiral fractures, each representing about 20 per cent of all humeral diaphyseal fractures, result from torsional forces; and segmental and comminuted fractures constitute the other patterns of humeral shaft fractures.[603] Approximately three fourths of all such fractures involve the middle third of the bone. Routine radiography generally is sufficient for the diagnosis of fractures of the humeral shaft, although two views acquired at approximately 90 degrees to each other are necessary to allow delineation of the patterns of fracture angulation and displacement. Furthermore, views of the adjacent joints (i.e., shoulder and elbow) are necessary in many cases to exclude associated injuries. Ipsilateral fractures of the radius and ulna, resulting in a "floating elbow," are encountered.[604]

Among the complications of fractures of the humeral diaphysis, neurologic injury is most common. Radial nerve palsy occurs in as many as 18 per cent of closed fractures of the humeral shaft.[597] It is associated most often with transverse fractures of the diaphysis, particularly those occurring in the junction of the middle and distal thirds of the bone. In most cases of radial nerve palsy after such fractures, clinical manifestations, which include wrist drop, are transient and complete recovery is expected. In other cases, transection of the radial nerve or its entrapment between the fracture fragments occurs. Routine radiography in cases of radial nerve entrapment may reveal a sharply marginated notch at the periphery of the fracture or a space, or foramen, within the fracture. MR imaging, however, represents a more appropriate technique for the early diagnosis of entrapment of the radial nerve. Injury to the median or ulnar nerve in cases of humeral diaphyseal fracture is rare. The anterior interosseous nerve also may be affected.

Vascular compromise occurring in patients with fracture of the humeral shaft occurs in less than 5 per cent of cases, and such compromise usually is associated with open fractures or those associated with penetrating injury. Transection or an intimal tear of the brachial artery may occur. As routine radiography provides no evidence of vascular injury, arteriography is indicated when diminution or absence of peripheral pulses is detected.

Delayed union or nonunion of humeral shaft fractures is encountered. In general, transverse, segmental, or open fractures unite more slowly than spiral or oblique fractures or comminuted fractures.[597] Separation of fracture fragments related to excessive traction or interposition of soft tissue contributes to improper fracture healing. Malunion accompanied by shortening, angulation, or rotation also is evident in some cases.

Biceps Tendon Abnormalities

Anatomic Considerations

The tendon of the long head of the biceps brachii muscle arises from the supraglenoid tubercle or the superior portion of the glenoid labrum, or both structures, and it extends obliquely across the top of the humeral head into the intertubercular sulcus or groove (Figs. 12–194 and 12–195). This groove is bounded by the tuberosities of the humerus. The tendon emerges from the joint at the lower portion of the groove, surrounded by a sheath that communicates directly with the joint. The main arterial supply to the intertubercular portion of the biceps tendon is the anterior circumflex humeral artery.

The tendon of the long head of the biceps brachii muscle is restrained at several levels along its course.[605] The intra-articular portion of this tendon lies beneath the coracohumeral ligament in the rotator interval. The primary restraint of the tendon in this area is the thickened joint capsule about the coracohumeral ligament and edges of the subscapularis and supraspinatus tendons. This restraint is believed to be the major obstacle to medial dislocation of the tendon.[606, 607] Within the intertubercular groove, the biceps tendon is held in place by the tendinous expansion from the insertion of the sternocostal portion of the pectoralis major muscle, the falciform ligament.[608] The relative lack of importance of the transverse humeral ligament in keeping the biceps tendon aligned in the groove has been stressed constantly since an early study by Meyer in 1926.[606] Another key structure in this region is the subscapularis muscle and tendon. The subscapularis tendon inserts into the lesser tuberosity of the humerus. Disruption of the subscapularis tendon leaves the biceps tendon unhindered and able to slip medially over the lesser tuberosity into the glenohumeral joint. Similar intra-articular displacement of the biceps tendon may occur if the subscapularis tendon is detached from the lesser tuberosity; in this case, although the subscapularis mechanism may remain intact owing to continuity of its fibers with those of the transverse humeral ligament, the biceps tendon may slip medially, by passing over the lesser tuberosity and underneath the subscapularis tendon.

The osseous anatomy of the bicipital groove has been outlined by Cone and coworkers.[609] In their investiga-tion, the average value for the medial wall angle was 56 degrees and the average depth of the groove was 4.3 mm. Although no correlation between the prevalence of subluxation and low medial wall angle was found in this study, such a correlation has been noted in other investigations.[610, 611]

Tendinitis

Burkhead[605] has divided tendinitis of the long head of the biceps brachii muscle into two categories: impingement tendinitis and attrition tendinitis. The first and more common of these two types of tendinitis occurs in association with the shoulder impingement syndrome and disruption of the rotator cuff. In this situation, the biceps tendon is trapped between the humeral head, the acromion, and the coracoacromial ligament during elevation and rotation of the arm. Synovial inflammation is not present.[605] Attrition tendinitis is accompanied by peritendinous synovitis and affects the intertubercular portion of the tendon. Stenosis of the bicipital groove related to periostitis leads to tendon attrition and, in some cases, tendon rupture.

The frequency of bicipital tendinitis and tenosynovitis (with or without tendon subluxation) is not clear. Its association with anterior shoulder pain in athletes involved in sports requiring throwing of a ball or in golf or swimming has been noted.[612] The pain may extend down the arm or radiate to the humeral insertion site of the deltoid muscle.[605] The findings usually are unilateral but may be bilateral and are most frequent in the fifth or sixth decade of life. Tenderness with palpation of the bicipital groove may be apparent.

Routine radiography generally is nondiagnostic in cases of bicipital tendinitis and tenosynovitis. A specialized view of the bicipital groove may reveal degenerative changes, including bone outgrowths.[609] A bone enthesophyte arising from the medial wall of the groove apparently is produced by tension in the transverse humeral ligament, whereas a similar outgrowth occurring in the floor of the groove may relate to chronic bicipital tendinitis (Fig. 12–196); the detection of both types of enthesophytes requires tangential radiographic projections of the bicipital groove or CT. More extensive bone proliferation in this region narrows the groove and even may create a bicipital tunnel; in either case, interference with the normal excursion of the humeral head on the biceps tendon becomes apparent, leading to attrition of the tendon and, perhaps, its rupture (Fig. 12–197).

Glenohumeral joint arthrography may reveal a corrugated pattern of the contrast material that surrounds the tendon, although the finding is infrequent and of questionable significance. The extent of filling of the sheath about the tendon of the long head of the biceps brachii muscle generally is not useful in the diagnosis of bicipital tendinitis or tenosynovitis. Ultrasonography may be valuable in the assessment of the bicipital tendon; in cases of tenosynovitis, fluid in the tendon sheath or an enlarged tendon may be evident.[613] Absence of the normal fibrillar pattern of the tendon and the presence of enthesophytes about or in the bicipital groove are additional ultrasonographic findings.[614] The value of

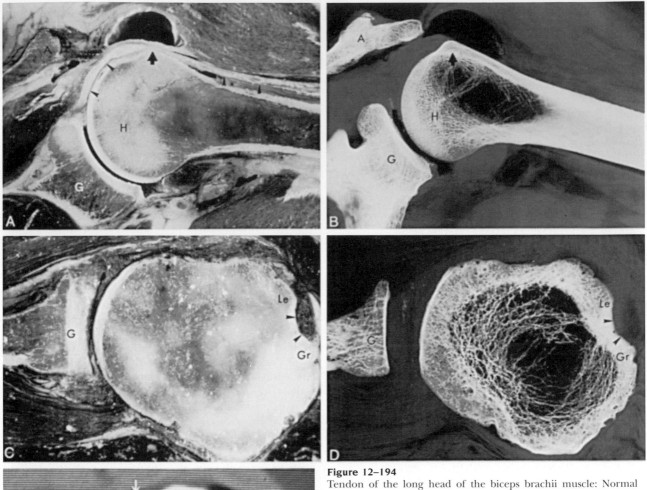

Figure 12–194

Tendon of the long head of the biceps brachii muscle: Normal anatomy.

A, B A photograph and radiograph of a coronal section of a cadaveric shoulder reveal the tendon of the long head of the biceps (arrowheads). It originates at the superior aspect of the glenoid cavity and courses intra-articularly over the humeral head. At the level of the intertubercular sulcus (arrows), the tendon and its synovial sheath leave the joint space. G, Glenoid; A, acromion; H, humeral head.

C, D A photograph and radiograph of a transverse section of a cadaveric shoulder at the level of the intertubercular sulcus (arrowheads) reveal that the latter is bordered by the greater tuberosity (Gr) posteriorly, the lesser tuberosity (Le) anteriorly, and the transverse humeral ligament laterally. G, Glenoid.

E A transaxial CT scan at the level of the intertubercular sulcus after the administration of intra-articular air shows the bicipital tendon (arrow) in its normal position within the sulcus. Gr, Greater tuberosity; Le, lesser tuberosity.

(**A–D,** From Cone RO, et al: AJR *141*:781, 1983. Copyright 1983, American Roentgen Ray Society.)

ultrasonography in the assessment of such enthesophytes has been questioned, however.[685]

The diagnostic role of MR imaging in cases of bicipital tendinitis and tenosynovitis is not clear. Evidence of fluid in the sheath of the tendon of the long head of the biceps brachii muscle has been regarded either as a normal finding[200] or as indicative of inflammation, particularly if there is no associated effusion in the glenohumeral joint.[200, 207] Kaplan and coworkers,[128] in an MR imaging study of 30 shoulders in asymptomatic volunteers, concluded that fluid in the tendon sheath

of the long head of the biceps tendon should be considered abnormal only if it completely surrounds the tendon and a sizable joint effusion is not present. These investigators also indicated that slow blood flow in the anterior circumflex humeral vein may lead to an area of increased signal intensity within the bicipital groove that can be misinterpreted as evidence of tenosynovitis. Tuckman[615] described a number of MR imaging abnormalities indicative of bicipital tendinitis: fluid in the tendon sheath that is out of proportion of that in the glenohumeral joint; a thickened tendon with increased

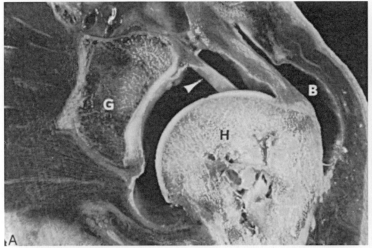

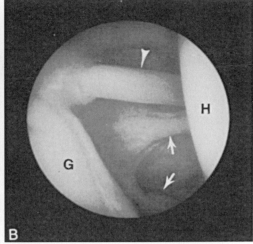

Figure 12–195

Tendon of the long head of the biceps brachii muscle: Normal anatomy.

A A coronal section of a cadaveric shoulder after the introduction of air into the glenohumeral joint shows the articular cartilage of the glenoid cavity (G) and humeral head (H). Note the long head of the bicipital tendon (arrowhead) arising from the supraglenoid tubercle. The subacromial (subdeltoid) bursa is identified (B).

B Arthroscopy reveals the long head of the bicipital tendon (arrowhead) attaching to the supraglenoid tubercle. The superior and middle glenohumeral ligaments are indicated (arrows). G, Glenoid cavity; H, humeral head.

C Transverse section at the midglenoid level reveals the following structures: glenoid cavity (4), humeral head (7), lesser (8) and greater (9) tuberosities of the humerus, infraspinatus muscle (13), subscapularis tendon (14), deltoid muscle (16), tendon of the long head of the biceps brachii muscle (23), anterior (30) and posterior (31) portions of the glenoid labrum, and transverse humeral ligament (48).

signal intensity, particularly on T2-weighted spin echo images; and a diffuse or segmental pattern of disease (Fig. 12–198).

Tendon Subluxation and Dislocation

Medial subluxation or dislocation of the tendon of the long head of the biceps brachii muscle may occur as an isolated lesion but generally is observed in association with massive tears of the rotator cuff. Medial displacement of the biceps tendon also may accompany isolated tears or avulsion of the subscapularis muscle or tendon.[616] Once dislocated, the tendon may relocate spontaneously, but more commonly, owing to the development of scar tissue within the sulcus, the tendon remains in a medially displaced position.[605] Factors predisposing to dislocation of the biceps tendon include anomalies and dysplastic changes of the intertubercular groove,[617] degenerative and attritional changes in the tendon itself, and capsular and ligamentous (i.e., coracohumeral ligament) abnormalities.[618, 619] Even in normal persons, the biceps tendon is pressed against the medial wall of the intertubercular sulcus; hypoplasia of the medial wall of this groove may allow medial subluxation or dislocation of the tendon. Rupture of the coracohumeral ligament may further promote such displacement. Lateral displacement of the tendon of the long head of the biceps brachii muscle does not occur. Posterior dislocation of the tendon may result from a fracture of the greater tuberosity that allows the tendon to slip behind the humerus. It also may occur in association with glenohumeral joint dislocation (Fig. 12–199).

Clinically, none of the findings of a medially dislocated biceps tendon are pathognomonic.[618] The patient may experience a snapping sensation as the tendon moves in and out of the bicipital groove. Abbott and Saunders[608] described a provocative diagnostic test that is performed during the physical examination: with the arm fully abducted, externally rotated and elevated, it is slowly lowered to the side of the patient during which a palpable or audible click is demonstrated as the tendon slips from its groove. A number of other provocative tests also have been described and are summarized by Burkhead.[605]

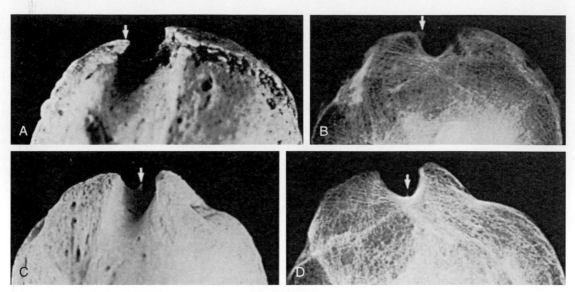

Figure 12–196
Tendon of the long head of the biceps brachii muscle: Bicipital groove enthesophytes.
   A, B Medial wall enthesophyte. Photograph and radiograph reveal large bone enthesophyte (arrows) arising from the medial wall of the intertubercular sulcus at the level of attachment of the transverse humeral ligament.
   C, D Enthesophyte in bicipital floor. In a different specimen, observe a small bone enthesophyte (arrows) arising from the floor of the intertubercular sulcus.
   (From Cone RO, et al: AJR *141*:781, 1983. Copyright 1983, American Roentgen Ray Society.)

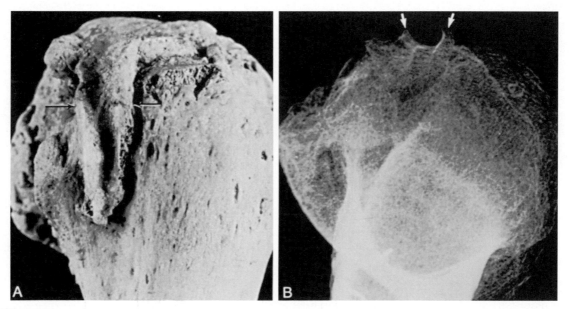

Figure 12–197
Tendon of the long head of the biceps brachii muscle: Bone proliferation about the bicipital groove. Photograph **(A)** and radiograph **(B)** show marked osseous proliferation along the course of the bicipital groove (arrows). It is not clear if this represents enthesophytic response or ossification of the bicipital sleeve. (From Cone RO, et al: AJR *141*:781, 1983. Copyright 1983, American Roentgen Ray Society.)

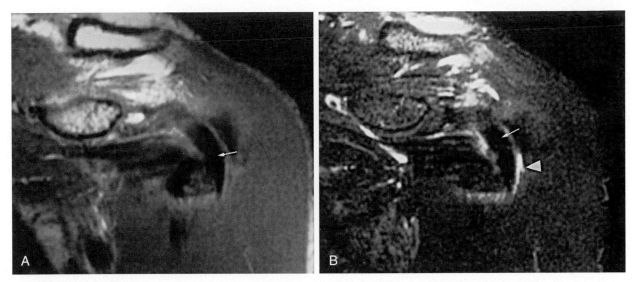

Figure 12–198
Tendon of the long head of the biceps brachii muscle: Tendinitis and tenosynovitis (MR imaging). In a 52 year old man with a clinical diagnosis of bicipital tendinitis, coronal oblique fast spin echo (TR/TE, 2200/21) **(A)** and fat-suppressed fast spin echo (TR/TE, 3000/84) **(B)** MR images show a nondisplaced thickened bicipital tendon (arrows) with tenosynovial fluid, of high signal intensity in **B** (arrowhead).
(Courtesy of S. K. Brahme, M.D., La Jolla, California.)

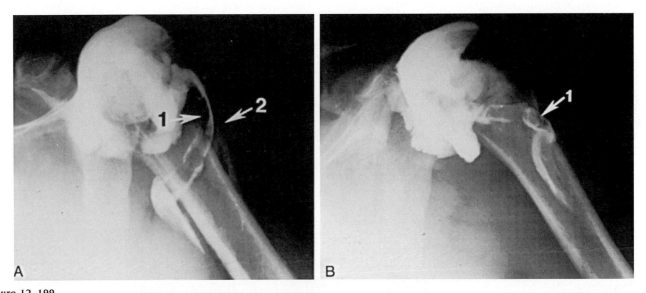

Figure 12–199
Tendon of the long head of the biceps brachii muscle: Posterior dislocation—glenohumeral joint arthrography. This 41 year old man sustained an anterior dislocation of the glenohumeral joint that was manipulated and "reduced." Three months later, he had marked restriction of both active and passive motion of the shoulder. An arthrogram of the glenohumeral joint was performed.
A In internal rotation of the humerus, the dislocated long head of the bicipital tendon is seen in an unusual position (1). A bone fragment is also evident (2).
B In external rotation of the humerus, motion is restricted by the posteriorly displaced long head of the bicipital tendon (1). At surgery, the latter was released from its origin and tenodesis in the bicipital groove was performed, reestablishing full shoulder motion.
(From Freeland AE, Higgins RW: Orthopedics *8:*468, 1985.)

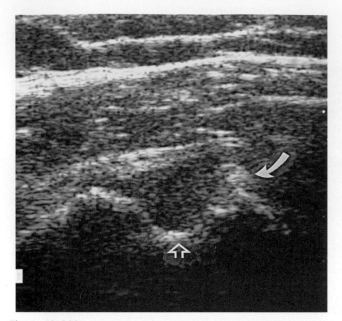

Figure 12–200

Tendon of the long head of the biceps brachii muscle: Medial dislocation (ultrasonography). A transverse sonogram of the upper portion of the humerus shows an empty bicipital groove (open arrow) and a medially displaced hyperechoic biceps tendon (curved arrow), seated atop the lesser tuberosity. (Courtesy of M. van Holsbeeck, M.D., Detroit, Michigan, and J. Jacobson, M.D., San Diego, California.)

Ultrasonography, arthrography, and MR imaging may be used in the assessment of medial dislocation of the biceps tendon. With ultrasonography, the displaced tendon can be identified (Fig. 12–200), and the diagnosis may be facilitated when dynamic scanning is employed with the shoulder in maximal external rotation (Fig. 12–201).[620] Tears of the falciform ligament of the greater pectoral muscle, which may promote dislocation of the biceps tendon, also can be detected with ultrasonography.[614] The arthrographic diagnosis of bicipital tendon displacement is established by direct visualization of a bicipital tendon within its opacified sheath that is not situated in the intertubercular groove and typically is located medial to the lesser tuberosity. A bicipital groove projection accomplished during arthrography

or CT arthrography (Fig. 12–202) may improve the visualization of the tendon and aid in establishing the diagnosis of tendon dislocation. MR imaging also allows this diagnosis.[91, 615, 621–623] The dislocated tendon is seen medial to the bicipital groove, particularly on transaxial (Fig. 12–203) and coronal oblique (Fig. 12–204) MR images. The tendon may appear thickened and may contain abnormal increased signal intensity, and fluid may be seen in the surrounding tendon sheath.[621] Disruption of one or more components of the rotator cuff and the coracohumeral ligament also may be evident. Intra-articular entrapment of the tendon of the long head of the biceps brachii muscle may be documented; access to the joint is provided by disruption of the subscapularis tendon or by detachment of this tendon from the lesser tuberosity of the humerus (Fig. 12–205).[622]

Tendon Rupture

Complete rupture of the tendon of the long head of the biceps brachii muscle may occur proximally, related to impingement or tendon degeneration, or rarely distally, usually resulting from injury (see Chapter 13). The weakest portion of the tendon is the segment just distal to its exit from the joint cavity (extracapsular portion), although intracapsular tears of the bicipital tendon also are encountered.[623] Complete disruption of the bicipital tendon may be accompanied by an audible pop and, later, by ecchymoses and a change in contour of the soft tissues of the arm. The diagnosis usually is obvious on clinical examination and requires no further diagnostic tests. Partial tears of the biceps tendon, however, may be more subtle and, in these cases, ultrasonography, arthrography, and MR imaging again may be useful. The value of MR imaging relates to direct visualization of the entire length of the tendon of the long head of the biceps brachii muscle when images at appropriate levels of the arm are available. The value of arthrography in this clinical setting, however, is less clear. In the normal glenohumeral joint arthrogram, visualization of the tendon sheath and tendon of the long head of the biceps is not constant. Therefore, although the absence of visualization may indeed represent a tear of the biceps, it is not a reliable sign. Occasionally, after exercise,

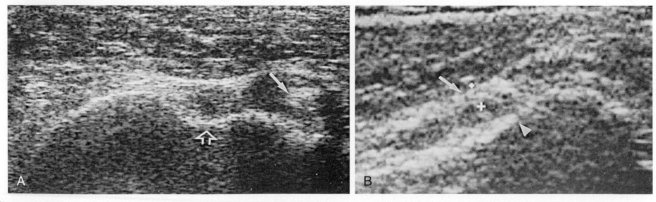

Figure 12–201

Tendon of the long head of the biceps brachii muscle: Medial dislocation (ultrasonography). With the shoulder in maximum external rotation, transverse (**A**) and longitudinal (**B**) sonograms show displacement of the biceps tendon (solid arrows) medially, away from the bicipital groove (open arrow) and surface of the humerus (arrowhead). (From Farin PU, et al: *Radiology 195*:845, 1995.)

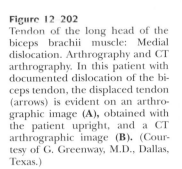

Figure 12 202
Tendon of the long head of the biceps brachii muscle: Medial dislocation. Arthrography and CT arthrography. In this patient with documented dislocation of the biceps tendon, the displaced tendon (arrows) is evident on an arthrographic image **(A),** obtained with the patient upright, and a CT arthrographic image **(B).** (Courtesy of G. Greenway, M.D., Dallas, Texas.)

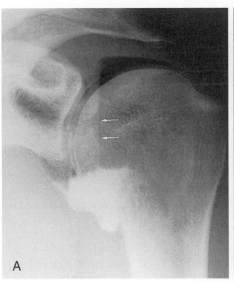

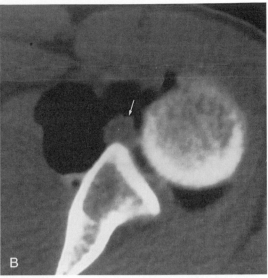

the tendon sheath will be seen when it was not apparent on pre-exercise films. Furthermore, leakage of contrast material from the biceps sleeve can be seen in normal persons, although some investigators regard it as a sign of disruption of the transverse bicipital ligament,[74, 78] rupture of the bicipital tendon itself,[75] or overdistention of the articular cavity.

Considering the wide variation in the arthrographic appearance of the bicipital tendon and sheath in normal persons, the radiologist must not rely too heavily on the arthrogram in establishing the existence of a significant abnormality. Still, when a complete bicipital tendon rupture is apparent clinically, arthrography may

confirm the diagnosis, demonstrating distortion of the synovial sheath and failing to identify the tendon within the opacified sheath (Fig. 12–206). The arthrographic diagnosis of complete rupture is more accurate in cases of acute tears; with less acute ruptures, shrinkage of adjacent tissues may obscure the abnormal findings. Incomplete tears of the bicipital tendon produce increased width of the tendon and distortion of the synovial sheath.

Rupture of the tendon of the short head of the biceps brachii muscle is extremely rare. The mechanism of injury appears to relate to rapid flexion and adduction of the arm with the elbow extended.[623]

Snapping Scapula Syndrome

The snapping, or grating, scapula syndrome refers to an audible and tactile phenomenon originating from the

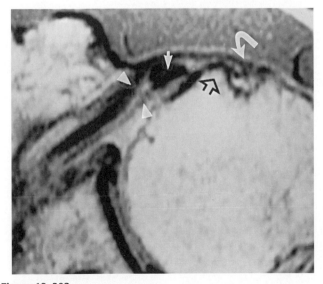

Figure 12–203
Tendon of the long head of the biceps brachii muscle: Medial dislocation (MR imaging). A 54 year old man fell on his shoulder while skiing and subsequently was unable to abduct his arm. A transaxial proton density–weighted (TR/TE, 2000/30) spin echo MR image shows that the biceps tendon (solid straight arrow) has slipped medially over the lesser tuberosity (open arrow) and appears to be lying between the partially displaced fibers (arrowheads) of the subscapularis tendon. The transverse humeral ligament (curved arrow) appears intact.

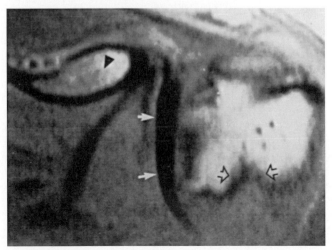

Figure 12–204
Tendon of the long head of the biceps brachii muscle: Medial dislocation (MR imaging). A coronal oblique proton density–weighted (TR/TE, 2500/20) spin echo MR image at the level of the base of the coracoid process (arrowhead) shows a medially located biceps tendon (solid straight arrows) displaced from the bicipital groove (between open arrows).

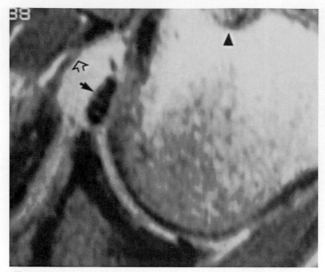

Figure 12–205

Tendon of the long head of the biceps brachii muscle: Medial dislocation with intra-articular entrapment (MR imaging). A transaxial proton density–weighted (TR/TE, 2000/30) spin echo MR image at the midglenoid level reveals an empty intertubercular sulcus (arrowhead) and intra-articular displacement of the biceps tendon (solid arrow). The subscapularis tendon is torn (open arrow).

scapulothoracic articulation during certain movements of the arm.[624, 625] It may or may not be symptomatic, depending on its cause. Although many abnormalities may lead to this syndrome, two basic mechanisms explain its occurrence in most cases[626]: changes in the congruence of the anterior surface of the scapula and the subjacent chest wall; and changes in the interposed soft tissues, muscles, or bursae between the scapula and the chest wall. With regard to the first of these mechanisms, the classic lesion is an osteochondroma (Figs. 12–207 and 12–208) arising from the anterior surface of the scapula, but it is only one of a variety of tumors that can lead to this syndrome. Anomalies of scapular shape (e.g., anterior angulation of the superomedial angle, tubercle of Luschka),[686] scapular sagging (associated with poor posture), subperiosteal excrescences related to injury associated with repetitive and forceful shoulder motion, and deformities of ribs are additional conditions that alter the congruence of the scapula and chest wall. Soft tissue causes of the snapping scapula syndrome include bursitis, interstitial myofibrosis, and muscle atrophy.[627] Routine radiography, including a lateral scapular projection, and CT scanning allow accurate diagnosis in some cases, although the diagnostic value of these methods as well as bone scintigraphy and MR imaging depends on the cause of the syndrome. Similarly, the treatment of the snapping scapula syndrome is influenced by its pathogenesis, with therapeutic options including both conservative and operative measures.[624]

Entrapment Neuropathies

Several entrapment neuropathies occurring about the shoulder are discussed in Chapter 11, and only two of

them are briefly summarized here owing to the importance of MR imaging in their diagnosis.

Suprascapular Nerve Entrapment

The suprascapular nerve is a mixed motor and sensory nerve that carries pain fibers from the glenohumeral and acromioclavicular joints and provides motor supply to the supraspinatus and infraspinatus muscles.[628] It is derived from the upper trunk of the brachial plexus, originating from the fourth, fifth, and sixth cervical nerve roots. The suprascapular nerve passes deep to the trapezius and omohyoid muscles to enter the supraspinatus fossa, passing beneath the superior transverse scapular ligament; it then runs deep to the supraspinatus muscle to enter the infraspinatus fossa through the spinoglenoid notch, passing beneath the inferior transverse scapular ligament at the lateral margin of the spine of the scapula (Fig. 12–209).[628] Two motor branches supplying the supraspinatus muscle are derived from that portion of the suprascapular nerve that is in the supraspinatus fossa and, similarly, two motor branches supplying the infraspinatus muscle are derived from that portion of the suprascapular nerve that is in the infraspinatus fossa. Therefore, depending on the precise site of involvement, entrapment of the suprascapular nerve can lead to weakness and atrophy of both the supraspinatus and infraspinatus muscles or to weakness and atrophy of the infraspinatus muscle alone.

The first pattern, that of proximal involvement, is more frequent in the general population, whereas distal entrapment of the nerve leading to isolated involvement

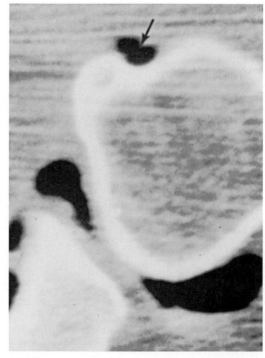

Figure 12–206

Tendon of the long head of the biceps brachii muscle: Rupture (computed arthrotomography). A transaxial CT image after the injection of air into the glenohumeral joint reveals a distended empty bicipital tendon sheath (arrow).

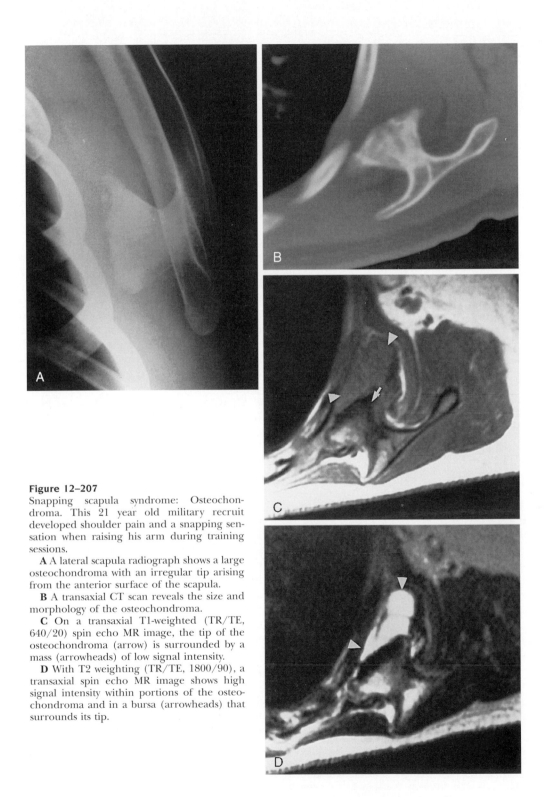

Figure 12–207

Snapping scapula syndrome: Osteochondroma. This 21 year old military recruit developed shoulder pain and a snapping sensation when raising his arm during training sessions.

A A lateral scapula radiograph shows a large osteochondroma with an irregular tip arising from the anterior surface of the scapula.

B A transaxial CT scan reveals the size and morphology of the osteochondroma.

C On a transaxial T1-weighted (TR/TE, 640/20) spin echo MR image, the tip of the osteochondroma (arrow) is surrounded by a mass (arrowheads) of low signal intensity.

D With T2 weighting (TR/TE, 1800/90), a transaxial spin echo MR image shows high signal intensity within portions of the osteochondroma and in a bursa (arrowheads) that surrounds its tip.

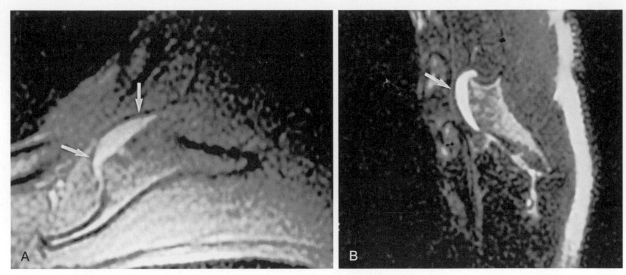

Figure 12–208

Snapping scapula syndrome: Osteochondroma (MR imaging). Transverse STIR (TR/TE, 2800/16; inversion time, 110 msec) **(A)** and sagittal fast spin echo (TR/TE, 3000/95) **(B)** MR images show a large, cartilage-capped osteochondroma (arrows) arising from the anterior aspect of the scapula. (Courtesy of R. Kerr, M.D., Los Angeles, California.)

of the infraspinatus muscle often is seen in male athletes, particularly baseball pitchers and weightlifters. Causes of suprascapular nerve entrapment include fractures of the humerus and scapula, anterior dislocations

![Figure 12-209 anatomical illustration with labels STSL, SN, SA, SS, ITSL, IS, QS, TMi, TMa, TR]

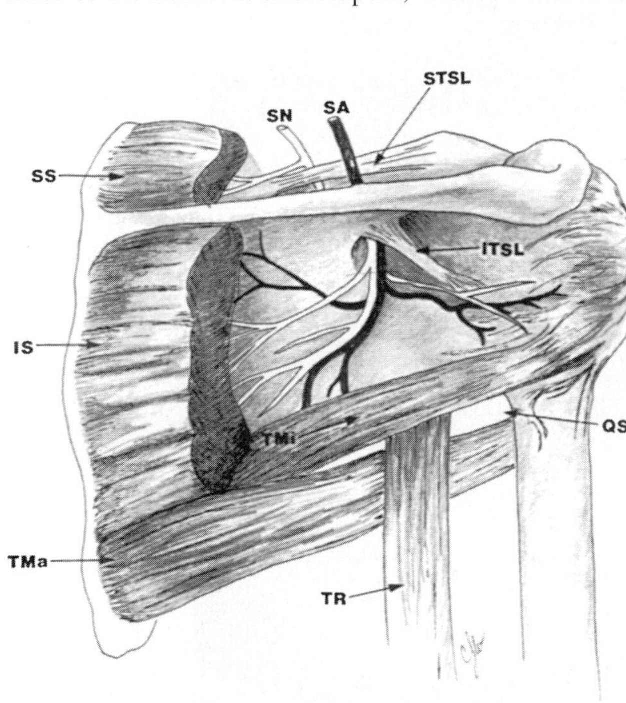

Figure 12–209

Suprascapular nerve: Normal anatomy. The suprascapular nerve (SN) adjacent to the suprascapular artery (SA), passes beneath the superior transverse scapular ligament (STSL) in the suprascapular notch, then runs deep to the supraspinatus muscle (SS) and the inferior transverse scapular ligament (ITSL) to pass through the spinoglenoid notch. The infraspinatus muscle (IS), teres minor muscle (TMi), teres major muscle (TMa), and long head of the triceps muscle (TR) also are indicated. The quadrilateral space (QS) is shown. The axillary nerve and the posterior humeral circumflex artery traverse this space. (Modified from Fritz RC, et al: Radiology 182:437, 1992.)

of the glenohumeral joint, penetrating or surgical trauma, anomalies of the transverse scapular ligaments, tumors, and ganglia.[628–633] A delay in diagnosis is frequent, related in part to the patient's not seeking medical treatment until significant shoulder weakness is observed.

MR imaging, as well as ultrasonography and CT, has been used to investigate patients with findings of suprascapular nerve entrapment.[628, 634] Although a variety of benign and malignant soft tissue and bone lesions cause this entrapment, the documentation of periarticular ganglion cysts with MR imaging has been emphasized (Figs. 12–210 and 12–211).[628] These ganglia may lead to proximal or distal entrapment of the suprascapular nerve and are seen as well-defined, smooth masses of low signal intensity on T1-weighted spin echo MR images and of high signal intensity on T2-weighted spin echo MR images. An associated finding is atrophy of the infraspinatus muscle alone or of both the infraspinatus and supraspinatus muscles. Such ganglia also may be accompanied by tears in the adjacent portion of the glenoid labrum, which suggests that their pathogenesis may be similar to that of meniscal cysts in the knee.[437]

Axillary Nerve Entrapment

The quadrilateral space syndrome represents an entrapment neuropathy of the axillary nerve that occurs within the quadrilateral space of the shoulder. This space is located posteriorly, bounded by the teres minor muscle above, the teres major muscle below, the long head of the triceps muscle medially, and the humeral neck laterally (Figs. 12–209 and 12–212). Passing through this space are the axillary nerve and the posterior humeral circumflex artery.

The quadrilateral space syndrome was described in 1983 by Cahill and Palmer.[635] Clinical findings include

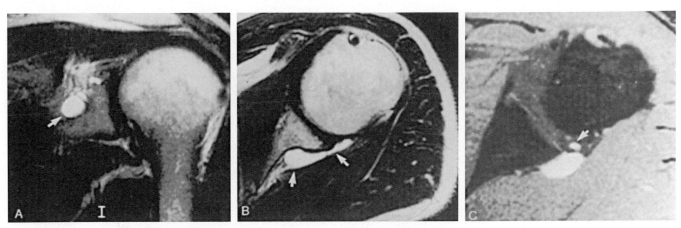

Figure 12–210

Suprascapular nerve: Entrapment related to ganglion cysts.

A, B Coronal oblique (**A**) and transaxial (**B**) T2-weighted (TR/TE, 3200/105) fast spin echo MR images reveal a ganglion cyst (arrows) extending medially from the glenohumeral joint to the region of the spinoglenoid notch of the scapula. Although this patient had clinical evidence of entrapment of the suprascapular nerve, no MR imaging findings of muscle atrophy are evident.

C In a second patient, a transaxial MPGR MR image (TR/TE, 383/12; flip angle, 15 degrees) reveals a ganglion cyst of high signal intensity adjacent to the posterior margin of the glenoid cavity. Observe a tear in the adjacent labrum (arrow).

skin paresthesias in the distribution of the axillary nerve, weakness of the teres minor or deltoid muscle or of both, and tenderness on palpation of the quadrilateral space. Posterior shoulder pain exacerbated by abduction and external rotation of the arm may be evident. A history of trauma may[636] or may not[636] be present. The dominant arm of athletes involved in sports requiring abduction and external rotation of the arm, as in the cocking motion in throwing, may be affected. One documented cause of this syndrome is fibrous bands in the quadrilateral space; treatment may require surgical lysis of these bands and decompression of the quadrilateral space.[637]

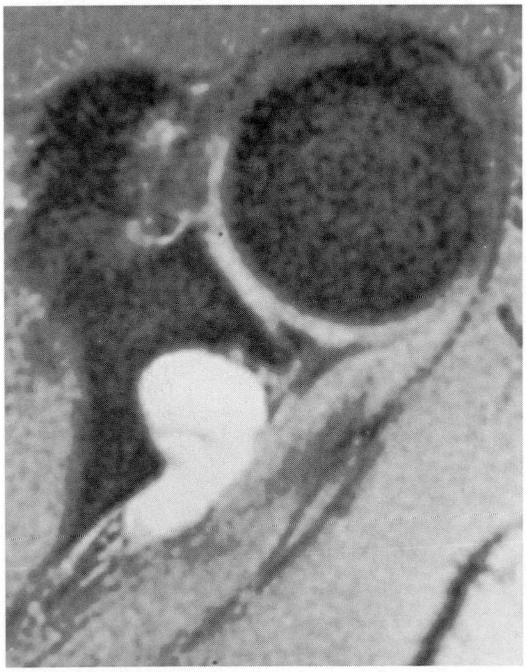

The diagnosis of the quadrilateral space syndrome may be accomplished with arteriography[638] or MR imaging.[639] On subclavian arteriograms, occlusion of the posterior humeral circumflex artery can be documented with the arm in abduction and external rotation, although the artery may be patent when the arm is placed alongside the body. MR imaging reveals atrophy with fatty infiltration of the teres minor muscle or the deltoid muscle, or of both muscles (Fig. 12–213). Of interest, MR angiography has revealed occlusion of the posterior humeral circumflex artery in abducted arms of asymptomatic volunteers as well as in a patient with the quadrilateral space syndrome.[640]

Normal Variations and Developmental Abnormalities

Humeral Pseudocyst

A normal region of rarefaction adjacent to the greater tuberosity of the humerus often is encountered (Fig. 12–214A, B). The finding is designated a humeral pseudocyst,[641, 642] and it may simulate the appearance of a tumor (e.g., chondroblastoma). On MR images, the signal intensity characteristics of the pseudocyst are those of fat (Fig. 12–214C). Lesions containing both fat and fluid also can be seen in this same location (Fig. 12–215).

Os Acromiale

A persistent ossification center at the free end of the acromion occurs in as many as 15 per cent of persons.

Figure 12–211

Suprascapular nerve: Entrapment related to ganglion cysts. A large cystic collection in the posterior aspect of the scapular spinoglenoid fossa is identified clearly in a transaxial multiplanar gradient recalled (MPGR) MR image (TR/TE, 350/20; flip angle, 30 degrees). No associated atrophy of the infraspinatus muscle is present. (Courtesy of H. Pavlov, M.D., New York, New York.)

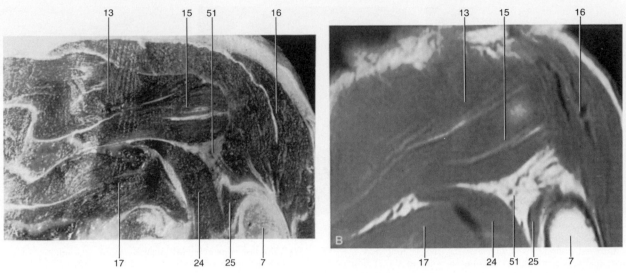

Figure 12–212

Quadrilateral space: Normal anatomy. Coronal oblique section **(A)** and T1-weighted (TR/TE, 600/20) spin echo MR image **(B)**. The posterior humeral circumflex artery and the axillary nerve (51) are located in the quadrilateral space. Other identified structures are the humeral diaphysis (7), infraspinatus muscle (13), teres minor muscle (15), deltoid muscle (16), teres major muscle (17), long head of the triceps muscle (24), and lateral head of the triceps muscle (25). (From Petersilge CA, et al: MRI Clin North Am *1*:1, 1993.)

Typically, this center fuses with the acromion before the person reaches 25 years of age; a separate site of ossification after this age is designated an os acromiale (Figs. 12–216 and 12–217). The os acromiale is variable in size and most commonly is triangular. It usually forms a synchondrosis with the acromion and may articulate also with the clavicle. Pain and a higher prevalence of the shoulder impingement syndrome and tears of the rotator cuff have been associated with an os acromiale. Its appearance simulates that of a fracture of the acromion (Fig. 12–218).

Hypoplasia (Dysplasia) of the Glenoid Neck of the Scapula

This entity also is termed glenoid hypoplasia and dentated glenoid anomaly (Fig. 12–219).[643–652, 687, 688] Men and women are affected with about equal frequency. Although the age at which the diagnosis is established varies, most patients have been evaluated in the third to seventh decades of life. Children and adolescents also may have this abnormality, however.[649] Shoulder pain and limitation of motion frequently are evident[653]; less commonly, the condition may be discovered as an incidental finding. Severe glenohumeral joint instability is infrequent or rare. In one series, however, 25 per cent of affected patients had multidirectional instability of this joint.[653] In another series, 9 of 12 patients with voluntary multidirectional instability of the glenohumeral joint revealed localized posteroinferior glenoid hypoplasia.[687] In a third series, three of nine patients with radiographic evidence of glenoid hypoplasia had findings of glenohumeral joint instability.[688] A family history of similar abnormalities has been apparent in some of the reported patients, suggesting that the changes may represent a hereditary trait, possibly due to a dominant gene with low penetrance.[643]

Radiography reveals abnormalities that usually are confined to the shoulder. Bilateral and relatively symmetric changes predominate, consisting of dysplasia of

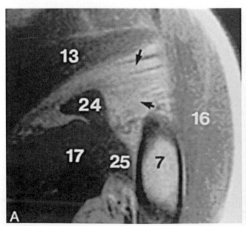
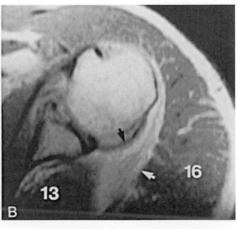

Figure 12–213

Quadrilateral space syndrome: MR imaging. Coronal oblique **(A)** and transaxial **(B)** proton density–weighted (TR/TE, 2000/25) MR images show selective atrophy with fatty replacement of the teres minor muscle (arrows). The infraspinatus muscle (13), deltoid muscle (16), teres major muscle (17), and long (24) and lateral (25) heads of the triceps muscle are identified and are not involved. The humeral diaphysis (7) also is seen. (Courtesy of W. Glenn, M.D., Long Beach, California.)

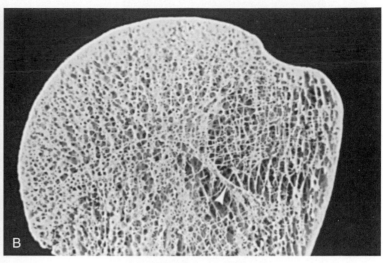

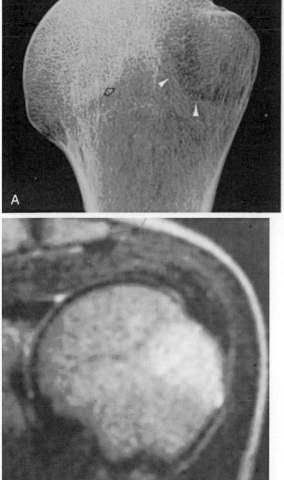

Figure 12–214

Humeral pseudocyst: Routine radiography and MR imaging.

A, B The area of rarefaction adjacent to the greater tuberosity is termed a humeral pseudocyst and is a normal finding. The curvilinear inferior margin (arrowheads) represents a distinct band of trabeculae that separate the relatively porous region laterally and the more compact spongiosa medially. A fusion line, marking the site of closure of a portion of the physis, is faintly visible (arrow).

(From Resnick D, Cone RO III: Radiology *150*:27, 1984.)

C In a patient, a coronal oblique T2-weighted (TR/TE, 2000/80) spin echo MR image reveals that the humeral pseudocyst contains sparse trabeculae and fatty marrow whose signal intensity is greater than that in other portions of the proximal end of the humerus.

(Courtesy of M. Stull, M.D., Washington, D.C.)

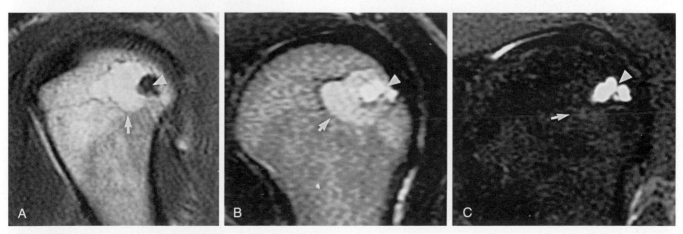

Figure 12–215

Humeral pseudo-pseudocyst: MR imaging. Sagittal oblique T1-weighted (TR/TE, 550/17) spin echo **(A)**, coronal oblique T2-weighted (TR/TE, 2000/80) spin echo **(B)**, and coronal oblique fast spin echo STIR (TR/TE, 4500/42; inversion time, 150 msec) **(C)** MR images show a benign lesion in the proximal portion of the humerus containing both fat (arrows) and fluid (arrowheads). (Courtesy of K. van Lom, M.D., San Diego, California.)

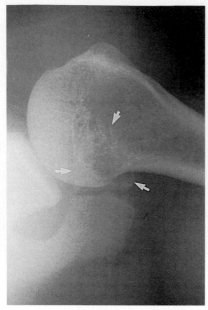

Figure 12–216
Os acromiale: Routine radiography. Note the well-defined triangular piece of bone (arrows) on this axillary radiograph.

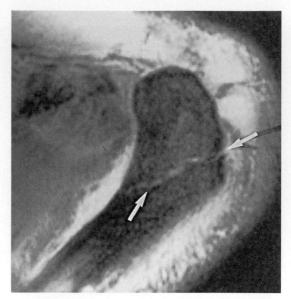

Figure 12–218
Nondisplaced acromial fracture simulating os acromiale: MR imaging. A transaxial fast low angle shot (FLASH) MR image (TR/TE, 500/18; flip angle, 30 degrees) shows the fracture line (arrows).

the scapular neck and irregularity of the glenoid surface. A dentate or notched articular surface becomes apparent (Fig. 12–220*A*).[647] Additional findings may include hypoplasia of the humeral head and neck, varus deformity of the proximal portion of the humerus, and enlargement and bowing of the acromion and the clavicle. The glenohumeral joint appears widened, especially inferiorly. Premature development of osteoarthritis at this site may occur.

Arthrography or computed arthrotomography of the glenohumeral joint reveals smooth, concentric articular surfaces with thick cartilage covering the glenoid cavity, particularly on its inferior aspect.[643, 648, 654, 655] A channel-like collection of contrast material has been observed at the apparent site of the thickened glenoid cartilage (Fig. 12–220*B*).[648] The precise cause of this peculiar arthrographic abnormality is unclear. Such an appearance can result from a developmental splitting or acquired ulceration of the articular cartilage or glenoid labrum. The observation of such channels in symptom-

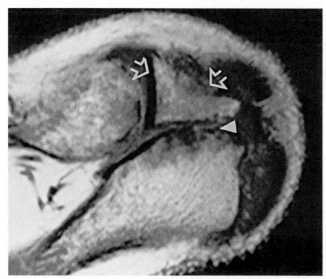

Figure 12–217
Os acromiale: MR imaging. A transaxial proton density–weighted (TR/TE, 1000/20) spin echo MR image shows a triangular os acromiale (arrows) articulating with the clavicle and, in an irregular fashion (arrowhead), with the acromion. (Courtesy of S. Eilenberg, M.D., San Diego, California.)

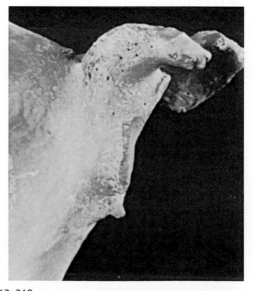

Figure 12–219
Hypoplasia (dysplasia) of the glenoid neck of the scapula. A photograph of the scapula reveals an irregular, dentate, or notched articular surface and hypoplasia of the glenoid neck.

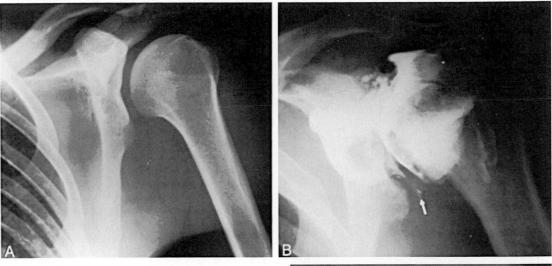

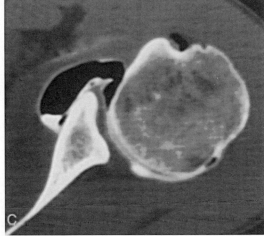

Figure 12–220

Hypoplasia (dysplasia) of the glenoid neck of the scapula.

A Hypoplasia of the scapular neck, an irregular notched glenoid articular surface, and widening of the lower portion of the joint space are evident. The opposite side was affected similarly.

B Arthrography of the glenohumeral joint in a different patient shows a channel-like collection of contrast material inferiorly (arrow).

(**A, B,** From Resnick D, et al: AJR *139*:387, 1982. Copyright 1982, American Roentgen Ray Society.)

C In a third patient, computed arthrotomography shows posterior subluxation of the humeral head and redundancy of the anterior portion of the joint capsule. The findings are compatible with multidirectional instability.

(**C,** Courtesy of G. Greenway, M.D., Dallas, Texas.)

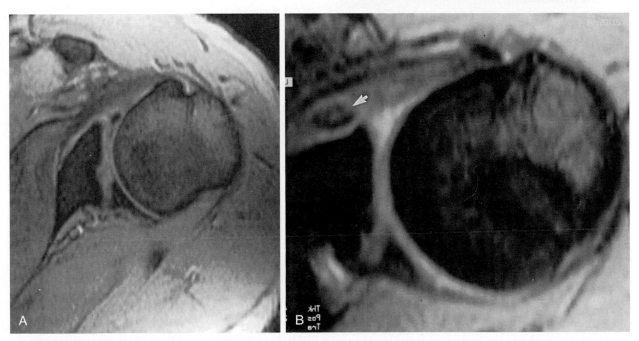

Figure 12–221

Hypoplasia (dysplasia) of the glenoid neck of the scapula: MR imaging.

A In this 24 year old male baseball pitcher with mild shoulder pain, a transaxial FLASH (TR/TE, 550/15; flip angle, 20 degrees) MR image shows the deformed and angular glenoid fossa, thick articular cartilage, large posterior portion of the labrum, and small anterior portion of the labrum.

B In a 17 year old man with anterior instability of the glenohumeral joint, a transaxial FLASH (TR/TE, 550/15; flip angle, 20 degrees) MR image shows similar findings as in **A,** although the anterior portion of the labrum is detached (arrow). The subscapularis tendon also was partially detached.

atic patients suggests also that the cartilaginous abnormalities relate to injury associated with subluxations of the humeral head (Fig. 12–220*C*).[655] Pathologic data, however, are lacking. MR imaging also can be used to assess this anomaly (Fig. 12–221).

The radiographic abnormalities associated with dysplasia of the neck of the scapula are virtually diagnostic. The absence of alterations in other epiphyses eliminates the diagnosis of multiple epiphyseal dysplasia. Similarly, the lack of significant anomalies at other skeletal sites in almost all reported cases of this disorder allows its differentiation from various other skeletal dysplasias. In a few reports of dysplasia of the scapular neck, however, the presence of additional anomalies has been noted, including spina bifida, hemivertebrae, cervical ribs, and webbing of the axillae. Other disorders, such as occupational trauma, ischemic necrosis of bone, osteochondritis dissecans, hemophilia, pigmented villonodular synovitis, ochronosis, and Sprengel's deformity, are not realistic diagnostic choices.

The precise cause and pathogenesis of glenoid hypoplasia are unknown. It is possible that the precartilage destined to ossify and become the inferior segment of the glenoid fails to develop[645, 655]; however, the stimulus for this lack of normal development remains obscure. The radiographic abnormalities resemble those seen in developmental dysplasia of the hip, but a meaningful association of the two conditions has not been established.

Bone Abnormalities

Occult Bone Injuries

A number of radiographically occult bone injuries may lead to significant shoulder disability. These include acute fractures of the tuberosities of the humerus, osteochondritis dissecans of the glenoid cavity or humeral head, stress fractures of the clavicle, scapula, or ribs, and posttraumatic osteolysis of the distal end of the clavicle. When routine radiographs are not rewarding, diagnostic information may be supplied by bone scintigraphy, CT scanning, CT arthrography, or MR imaging (Fig. 12–222).

Condensing Osteitis of the Clavicle

In 1974, Brower and collaborators[662] reported two young women with pain and swelling over the medial end of the clavicle associated with bony eburnation and an intact articular space. Histologic examination delineated thickening of trabeculae within the cancellous bone and periosteal reaction resembling an osteophyte. The pathologic changes were interpreted as a response to mechanical stress, and there was no evidence of inflammation or infection. In 1976, Solovjev[663] further described this entity, and in 1978, Teates and coworkers,[664] examining two other patients with bone-seeking agents, demonstrated that the lesions revealed increased accumulation of radionuclide activity. Additional cases of osteitis condensans of the clavicle have been reported subsequently.[665, 666] Patients are women with an average age of 40 years (range, 20 to 50 years) and with a history of stress to the region of the sternoclavicular joint, usually associated with heavy lifting or sports activity. Pain most commonly is referred to the ipsilateral shoulder and is accentuated with abduction of the arm. No definite association with osteitis pubis or osteitis condensans ilii has been reported.

Radiographs reveal bone sclerosis and mild enlargement of the inferomedial aspect of the clavicle, as well as osteophytes in the inferior margin of the clavicular head (Fig. 12–223*A*). The sternoclavicular joint space is not narrowed, and adjacent soft tissue and osseous structures are not affected. In addition to scintigraphy, which demonstrates increased accumulation of bone-

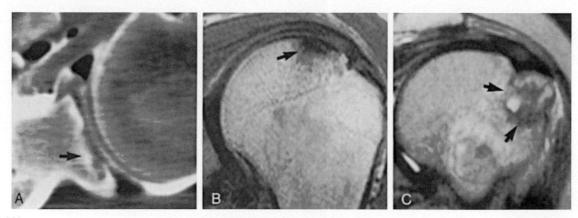

Figure 12–222
Occult bone abnormalities: CT arthrography and MR imaging.
  A Osteochondritis dissecans of the glenoid cavity. A transaxial CT arthrographic image shows a subtle osseous lesion (arrow) in the posterior region of the glenoid cavity in an 18 year old baseball catcher. Although the overlying cartilage appears normal, a detached chondral fragment was evident at arthroscopy. (Courtesy of G. Greenway, M.D., Dallas, Texas.)
  B Osteochondritis dissecans of the humeral head. A coronal oblique T1-weighted (TR/TE, 550/20) spin echo MR image shows a small lesion (arrow) involving the posterior surface of the humeral head. (Courtesy of S. Eilenberg, M.D., San Diego, California.)
  C Fracture of the greater tuberosity. A coronal oblique T2-weighted (TR/TE, 3200/104) fast spin echo MR image shows the fracture site (arrows) with areas of high signal intensity extending into the humeral head.

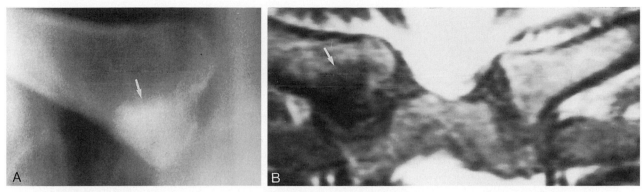

Figure 12–223
Condensing osteitis of the clavicle: MR imaging. A 40 year old woman developed pain and tenderness over the medial end of the right clavicle.
  A Conventional tomography reveals bone sclerosis involving the inferomedial aspect of the bone (arrow).
  B A coronal T1-weighted (TR/TE, 300/11) spin echo MR image shows low signal intensity in this area (arrow). The diminished signal intensity persisted on T2-weighted spin echo and gradient echo images (not shown).
  (Courtesy of G. Greenway, M.D., Dallas, Texas.)

seeking radiopharmaceutical agents, CT scanning and MR imaging can be used to document the extent of bone involvement.[667] Areas of low signal intensity within the clavicle on both T1-weighted and T2-weighted spin echo MR imaging sequences are typical, and these findings are indicative of the presence of sclerotic bone (Fig 12–223B).

Bone Tumors

Virtually any bone tumor can arise about the shoulder (Table 12–8). Of the benign lesions, osteoid osteoma deserves emphasis owing to its characteristic radiographic and dramatic MR imaging abnormalities (Fig. 12–224). When in an intra-articular location, osteoid osteomas can lead to significant synovial inflammation. The nidus of the lesion can be identified with MR imaging, although CT may be a more effective method in this regard.

Both benign (e.g., chondromas) and malignant (e.g., chondrosarcomas) cartilage tumors are not infrequent about the shoulder (Figs. 12–225 and 12–226). Most cartilage neoplasms show high signal intensity on T2-weighted spin echo MR images, and many reveal distinc-

Table 12–8. TUMORS AND TUMOR-LIKE LESIONS OF BONE: FREQUENCY OF INVOLVEMENT OF BONES ABOUT THE SHOULDER

Lesion	Humerus[†]	Scapula	Clavicle	Sternum	Ribs
Enostosis	9	1	<1		12
Osteoid osteoma	7	1			<1
Osteoblastoma	3	3	<1		3
Osteosarcoma	14	2	<1	<1	2
Enchondroma	7	1	<1	1	5
Periosteal chondroma	32				2
Chondroblastoma	22	2	<1	<1	2
Chondromyxoid fibroma	1	1		<1	3
Osteochondroma	19	4	<1	<1	2
Chondrosarcoma	15	4	1	2	9
Nonossifying fibroma	5	<1	<1		1
Desmoplastic fibroma	10	3	2		2
Fibrosarcoma	11	2	1	<1	1
Giant cell tumor	6	<1	<1	<1	1
Malignant fibrous histiocytoma	9	1	1	<1	3
Lipoma	9	<1			8
Hemangioma	3	2	1		9
Hemangiopericytoma	15	2	4	4	8
Hemangioendothelioma	13	3		1	5
Neurofibroma/neurilemoma	3	1			3
Simple bone cyst	56	<1	<1		<1
Aneurysmal bone cyst	9	2	3		3
Adamantinoma	6				1
Ewing's sarcoma	10	5	2	<1	8

*Numbers indicate approximate percentages of the lesions that affect the bones about the shoulder based upon analysis of major reports containing the greatest number of cases.
†Lesions affecting any part of the humerus are included.

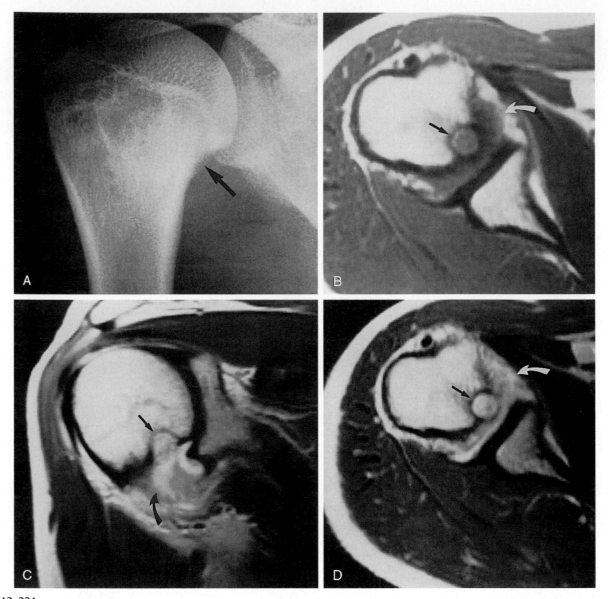

Figure 12–224
Osteoid osteoma: MR imaging.

   A Routine radiograph reveals a small osteolytic lesion (arrow) in the medial cortex of the humeral neck.

   B A transaxial T1-weighted (TR/TE, 500/15) spin echo MR image shows the nidus (straight arrow) and synovial inflammatory tissue and joint fluid (curved arrow).

   C, D After intravenous administration of a gadolinium compound, coronal oblique (C) and transaxial (D) T1-weighted (TR/TE, 550/15) spin echo MR images reveal the nidus (straight arrows) and thickened synovium (curved arrows), both exhibiting enhancement of signal intensity.

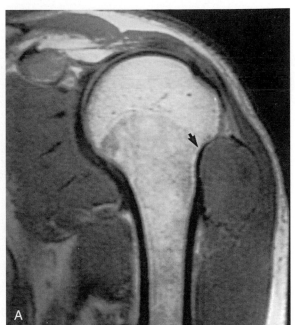

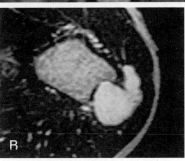

Figure 12–225
Periosteal chondroma: MR imaging. A coronal oblique T1-weighted (TR/TE, 655/22) spin echo MR image (**A**) shows a well-defined periosteal tumor whose signal intensity is identical to that of muscle. It has a rim of very low signal intensity, representing a bone shell, and has eroded the humerus (arrow). The transaxial T2-weighted (TR/TE, 1800/90) spin echo MR image (**B**) reveals high signal intensity in the tumor. (Courtesy of T. Hughes, M.D., Christchurch, New Zealand.)

tive lobulation. They may arise within the bone (e.g., enchondromas and chondrosarcomas) or on the surface of the bone (e.g., periosteal chondromas and juxtacortical chondrosarcomas).

Osteosarcomas also may be encountered about the shoulder. Although their MR imaging appearance usually is not specific, fluid levels occasionally are evident in cases of telangiectatic osteosarcoma (Fig. 12–227). Osteosarcomas, as well as other malignant tumors of bone (Fig. 12–228), may develop after radiation therapy.

Other Bone Lesions

A variety of infectious (Fig. 12–229) and ischemic (Fig. 12–230) disorders may affect the bones of the shoulder girdle. The primary role of MR imaging in these instances is to define the extent of the process.

Soft Tissue Abnormalities

Of the many types of soft tissue tumors that may involve the shoulder, extra-abdominal desmoid tumors and elastofibromas deserve emphasis. Both are not uncommon in the shoulder. Desmoid tumors may lead to infiltration of surrounding structures. Elastofibromas (Fig. 12–231)

may be unilateral or bilateral in distribution, may appear in manual laborers or weightlifters, and commonly are located between the scapula and the chest wall.[434, 689]

Lipomas and liposarcomas also are encountered about the shoulder. Although lipomas often can be diagnosed precisely on the basis of their MR imaging abnormalities, liposarcomas (Fig. 12–232) have nondiagnostic MR imaging features.

Hemangiomas and other vascular tumors and malformations (Fig. 12–233) also are encountered about the shoulder. In some cases, a specific diagnosis of such conditions is provided by MR imaging owing to the identification of serpentine vascular structures and regions of signal void related to rapid blood flow.

SUMMARY

This chapter clearly indicates the diversity of the conditions that may involve the shoulder in a manner in which imaging techniques can be used in their evaluation. With regard to accurate interpretation of the results of these techniques, knowledge of regional anatomy and pathophysiology should be emphasized.

Text continued on page 324

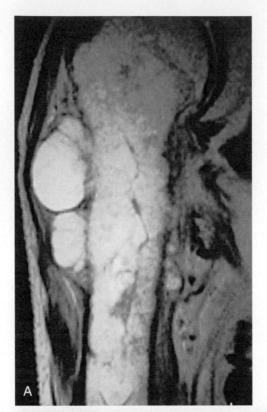

Figure 12–226
Conventional chondrosarcoma, central type: MR imaging.

A This coronal T2-weighted (TR/TE, 2770/100) spin echo MR image reveals the tumor, which is lobulated and of high signal intensity, extending through the lateral and, to a lesser extent, the medial cortex of the humeral shaft.

(Courtesy of T. Claudice-Engle, M.D., Stanford, California.)

B, C In a second patient, coronal oblique T1-weighted (TR/TE, 740/12) (**B**) and sagittal oblique T2-weighted (TR/TE, 3400/119) (**C**) spin echo MR images reveal a low-grade malignant tumor of low signal intensity in **B** and high signal intensity in **C.** It is lobulated and is violating the cortex (arrow).

(Courtesy of S. Siegel, M.D., New York, New York.)

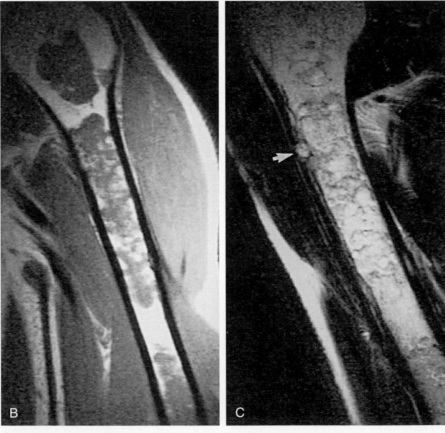

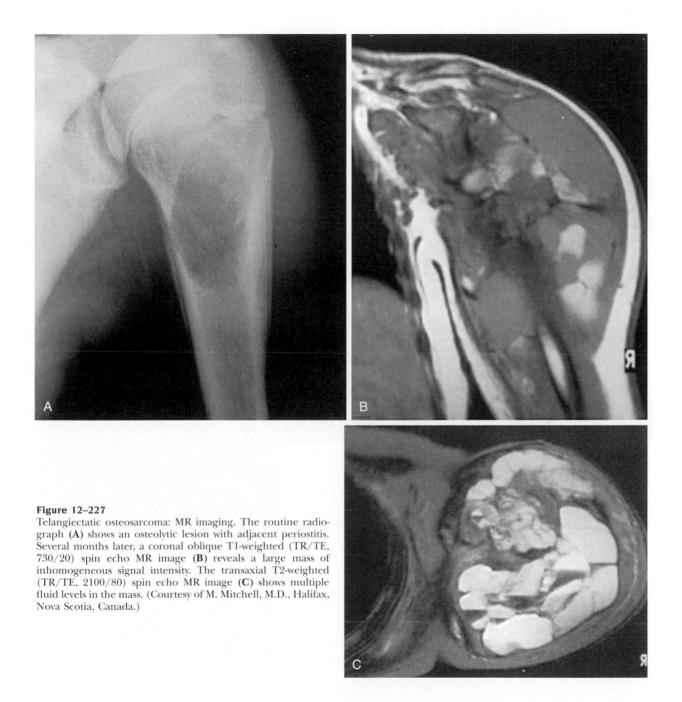

Figure 12–227
Telangiectatic osteosarcoma: MR imaging. The routine radiograph (**A**) shows an osteolytic lesion with adjacent periostitis. Several months later, a coronal oblique T1-weighted (TR/TE, 730/20) spin echo MR image (**B**) reveals a large mass of inhomogeneous signal intensity. The transaxial T2-weighted (TR/TE, 2100/80) spin echo MR image (**C**) shows multiple fluid levels in the mass. (Courtesy of M. Mitchell, M.D., Halifax, Nova Scotia, Canada.)

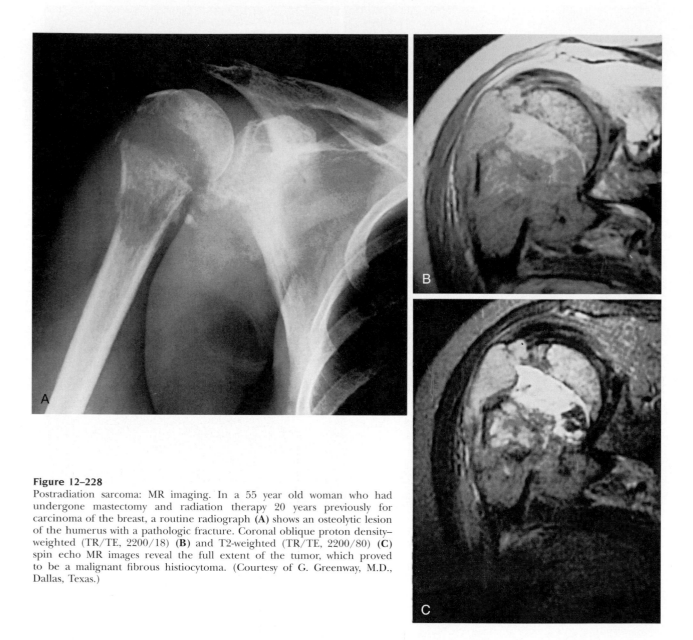

Figure 12–228

Postradiation sarcoma: MR imaging. In a 55 year old woman who had undergone mastectomy and radiation therapy 20 years previously for carcinoma of the breast, a routine radiograph **(A)** shows an osteolytic lesion of the humerus with a pathologic fracture. Coronal oblique proton density–weighted (TR/TE, 2200/18) **(B)** and T2-weighted (TR/TE, 2200/80) **(C)** spin echo MR images reveal the full extent of the tumor, which proved to be a malignant fibrous histiocytoma. (Courtesy of G. Greenway, M.D., Dallas, Texas.)

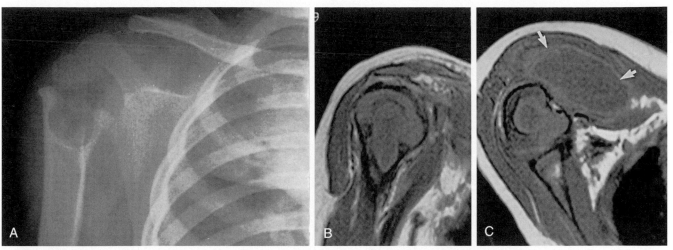

Figure 12–229
Tuberculous osteomyelitis: MR imaging. Routine radiography **(A)** shows metaphyseal destruction of the humerus and pulmonary involvement. Coronal oblique **(B)** and transaxial **(C)** T1-weighted (TR/TE, 500/20) spin echo MR images show osseous and soft tissue (arrows) involvement. (Courtesy of A. Motta, M.D., Cleveland, Ohio.)

Figure 12–230
Osteonecrosis: MR imaging. Coronal oblique fast spin echo (TR/TE, 3300/126) **(A)** and transverse fat-suppressed fast spin echo (TR/TE, 3200/14) **(B)** MR images show classic features of osteonecrosis of the humeral head, including a crescent sign (arrows).

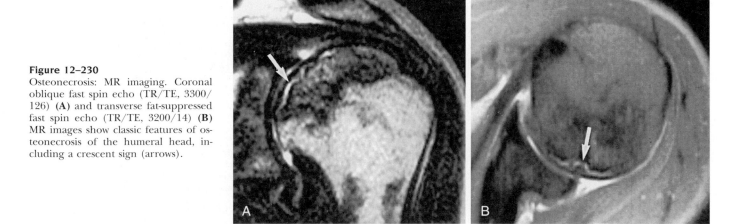

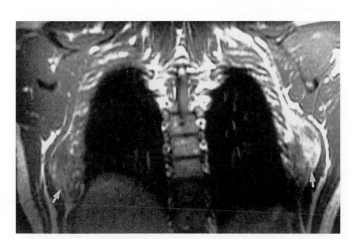

Figure 12–231
Elastofibroma. In a 43 year old woman who was an avid weightlifter, bilateral masses developed between the lower part of the scapula and the chest wall. This coronal T1-weighted (TR/TE, 500/20) spin echo MR image shows the two lesions (arrows), with inhomogeneous but mainly low signal intensity. Note areas of high signal intensity consistent with that of fat, however.

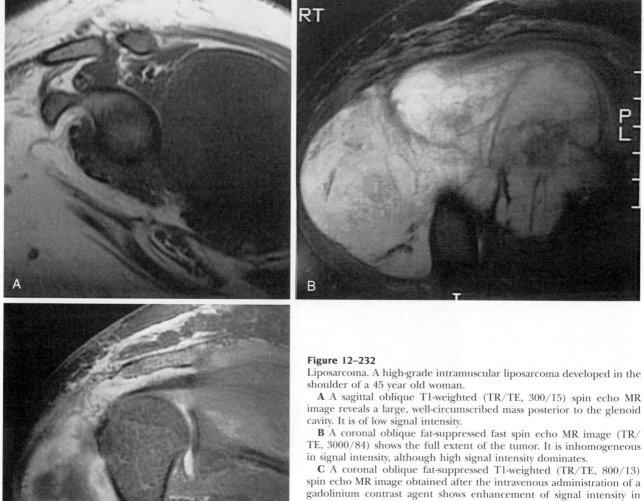

Figure 12–232

Liposarcoma. A high-grade intramuscular liposarcoma developed in the shoulder of a 45 year old woman.

A A sagittal oblique T1-weighted (TR/TE, 300/15) spin echo MR image reveals a large, well-circumscribed mass posterior to the glenoid cavity. It is of low signal intensity.

B A coronal oblique fat-suppressed fast spin echo MR image (TR/TE, 3000/84) shows the full extent of the tumor. It is inhomogeneous in signal intensity, although high signal intensity dominates.

C A coronal oblique fat-suppressed T1-weighted (TR/TE, 800/13) spin echo MR image obtained after the intravenous administration of a gadolinium contrast agent shows enhancement of signal intensity in portions of this tumor, with low signal intensity remaining in its necrotic center.

(Courtesy of S. K. Brahme, M.D., San Diego, California.)

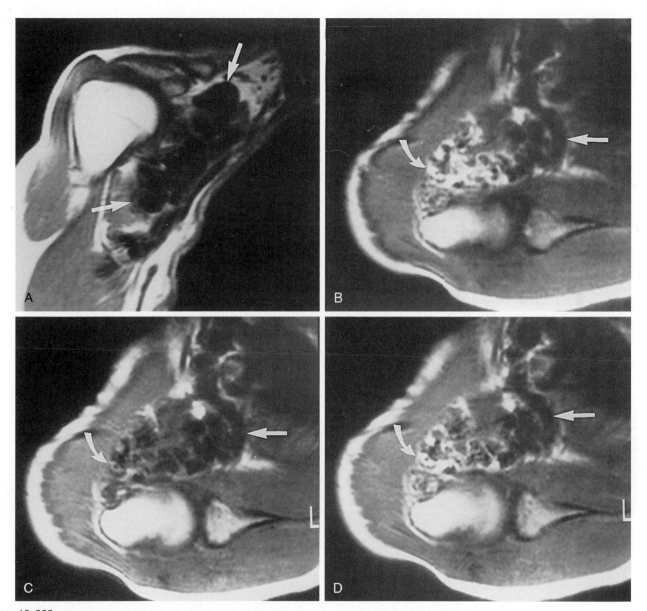

Figure 12–233

Arteriovenous malformation.

   A In a 28 year old woman, a coronal oblique T1-weighted (TR/TE, 500/30) spin echo MR image shows an irregular lesion (arrows) of low signal intensity medial to the humeral head. It has a tubular appearance.

   B On a transaxial T2-weighted (TR/TE, 2000/60) spin echo MR image, note tubular and circular areas of signal void (arrows). Some regions of the malformation show high signal intensity.

   C, D Transaxial T1-weighted (TR/TE, 650/30) spin echo MR images obtained before (**C**) and after (**D**) the intravenous administration of gadolinium contrast agent reveal the malformation (arrows) with some foci of enhancement of signal intensity in **D**.

REFERENCES

1. O'Brien SJ, Arnoczky SP, Warren RF, et al: Developmental anatomy of the shoulder and anatomy of the glenohumeral joint. *In* CA Rockwood Jr, FA Matsen III (Eds): The Shoulder. Philadelphia, WB Saunders Co, 1990, p. 1.
2. Cone RO, Danzig L, Resnick D, et al: The bicipital groove: A radiographic, anatomic, and pathologic study. AJR *141*:781, 1983.
3. Saha AK: Dynamic stability of the glenohumeral joint. Acta Orthop Scand *42*:491, 1971.
4. Sarrafian SK: Gross and functional anatomy of the shoulder. Clin Orthop *173*:11, 1983.
5. Saha AK: Mechanism of shoulder movements and a plea for the recognition of the "zero position" of the glenohumeral joint. Clin Orthop *173*:3, 1983.
6. Friedman RJ, Hawthorne KB, Genez BM: The use of computerized tomography in the measurement of glenoid version. J Bone Joint Surg [Am] *74*:1032, 1992.
7. Petersson CJ, Redlund-Johnell I: Joint space in normal glenohumeral radiographs. Acta Orthop Scand *54*:274, 1983.
8. Petersson CJ, Redlund-Johnell I: The subacromial space in normal shoulder radiographs. Acta Orthop Scand *55*:57, 1984.
9. Gradoyevitch B: Coracoclavicular joint. J Bone Joint Surg *21*:918, 1939.
10. Nutter PD: Coracoclavicular articulations. J Bone Joint Surg *23*:177, 1941.
11. Wertheimer LG: Coracoclavicular joint. J Bone Joint Surg [Am] *30*:570, 1948.
12. Redlund-Johnell I: The costoclavicular joint. Skel Radiol *15*:25, 1986.
13. Cockshott WP: The coracoclavicular joint. Radiology *131*:313, 1979.
14. Uhthoff HK, Piscopo M: Anterior capsular redundancy of the shoulder: Congenital or traumatic? An embryological study. J Bone Joint Surg [Br] *67*:363, 1985.
15. Killoran PJ, Marcove RC, Freiberger RH: Shoulder arthrography. AJR *103*:658, 1968.
16. Weston WJ: Subdeltoid bursa. Australas Radiol *17*:214, 1973.
17. Weston WJ: The enlarged subdeltoid bursa in rheumatoid arthritis. Br J Radiol *42*:481, 1969.
18. Mitchell MJ, Causey G, Berthoty DP, et al: Peribursal fat plane of the shoulder: Anatomic study and clinical experience. Radiology *168*:699, 1988.
19. DePalma AF: Surgical anatomy of the acromioclavicular and sternoclavicular joints. Surg Clin North Am *43*:1541, 1963.
20. Weston WJ: Arthrography of the acromioclavicular joint. Australas Radiol *18*:213, 1974.
21. Ogden JA, Conlogue GJ, Bronson ML: Radiology of postnatal skeletal development. III. The clavicle. Skel Radiol *4*:196, 1979.
22. Bearn JG: Direct observations on the function of the capsule of the sternoclavicular joint in clavicular support. J Anat *101*:159, 1967.
23. Cave AJE: The nature and morphology of the costoclavicular ligament. J Anat *95*:170, 1961.
24. Inman VT, Saunders JB, Abbott LC: Observations on function of the shoulder joint. J Bone Joint Surg *26*:1, 1944.
25. DePalma AF, Callery G, Bennett GA: Shoulder joint: Variational anatomy and degenerative lesions of the shoulder joint. AAOS Instructional Course Lectures *6*:255, 1949.
26. O'Brien SJ, Neves MC, Rozbuck RS, et al: The anatomy and histology of the inferior glenohumeral complex of the shoulder. Paper presented at the Annual Meeting of the Shoulder and Elbow Society, February 1989, Las Vegas, Nevada.
27. Moseley HF, Overgaard B: The anterior capsular mechanism in recurrent anterior dislocation of the shoulder: Morphological and clinical studies with special reference to the glenoid labrum and gleno-humeral ligaments. J Bone Joint Surg [Br] *44*:913, 1962.
28. Turkel SJ, Panio MW, Marshall JL, et al: Stabilizing mechanisms preventing anterior dislocation of the glenohumeral joint. J Bone Joint Surg [Am] *63*:1208, 1981.
29. Schwartz RE, O'Brien SJ, Warren RF, et al: Capsular restraints to anterior-posterior motion of the abducted shoulder: A biomechanical study. Orthop Trans *12*:727, 1988.
30. Edelson JG, Taitz C, Grishkan A: The coracohumeral ligament: Anatomy of a substantial but neglected structure. J Bone Joint Surg [Br] *73*:150, 1991.
31. Neer CS II, Satterlee CC, Dalsey RM, et al: The anatomy and potential effects of contracture of the coracohumeral ligament. Clin Orthop *280*:182, 1992.
32. Basmajian JV, Bazant FJ: Factors preventing downward dislocation of the adducted shoulder joint. J Bone Joint Surg [Am] *41*:1182, 1959.
33. Ovesen J, Nielsen S: Experimental distal subluxation in the glenohumeral joint. Arch Orthop Trauma Surg *104*:78, 1985.
34. Cooper DE, Arnoczky SP, O'Brien SJ, et al: Anatomy, histology, and vascularity of the glenoid labrum: An anatomical study. J Bone Joint Surg [Am] *74*:46, 1992.
35. Prodromos CC, Ferry JA, Schiller AL: Histological studies of the glenoid labrum from fetal life to old age. J Bone Joint Surg [Am] *72*:1344, 1990.
36. Rafii M, Minkoff J, Bonamo J, et al: CT arthrography of shoulder instabilities in athletes. Am J Sports Med *16*:352, 1988.
37. McNeish LM, Callaghan JJ: CT arthrography of the shoulder: Variations of the glenoid labrum. AJR *149*:963, 1987.
38. Neumann CH, Petersen SA, Jahnke AH: MR imaging of the labral-capsular complex: Normal variations. AJR *157*:1015, 1991.
39. Bankart ASB: Recurrent or habitual dislocation of the shoulder joint. Br Med J *2*:132, 1923.
40. Bankart ASB: The pathology and treatment of recurrent dislocation of the shoulder joint. Br J Surg *26*:23, 1938.
41. McLaughlin HL, Cavallaro WU: Primary anterior dislocation of the shoulder. Am J Surg *80*:615, 1950.
42. Jobe CM: Gross anatomy of the shoulder. *In* CA Rockwood Jr, FA Matsen III (Eds): The Shoulder. Philadelphia, WB Saunders Co, 1990, p. 34.
43. Otis JC, Jiang C-C, Wickiewicz TL, et al: Changes in the moment arms of the rotator cuff and deltoid muscles with abduction and rotation. J Bone Joint Surg [Am] *76*:667, 1994.
44. Kronberg M, Németh G, Broström L-A: Muscle activity and coordination in the normal shoulder. Clin Orthop *257*:76, 1990.
45. Keating JF, Waterworth P, Shaw-Dunn J, et al: The relative strengths of the rotator cuff muscles: A cadaver study. J Bone Joint Surg [Br] *75*:137, 1993.
46. Bassett RW, Browne AO, Morrey BF, et al: Glenohumeral muscle force and moment mechanics in a position of shoulder instability. J Biomech *23*:405, 1990.
47. Kannus P, Jozsa L: Histopathological changes preceding spontaneous rupture of a tendon: A controlled study of 891 patients. J Bone Joint Surg [Am] *73*:1507, 1991.
48. Brewer BJ: Aging of the rotator cuff. Am J Sports Med *7*:102, 1979.
49. Clark J, Sidles JA, Matsen FA: The relationship of the glenohumeral joint capsule to the rotator cuff. Clin Orthop *254*:29, 1990.
50. Harryman DT, Sidles JA, Harris SL, et al: The role of the rotator interval capsule in passive motion and stability of the shoulder. J Bone Joint Surg [Am] *74*:53, 1992.
51. Rothman RH, Parke WW: The vascular anatomy of the rotator cuff. Clin Orthop *41*:176, 1965.
52. Brooks CH, Revell WJ, Heatley FW: A quantitative histological study of the vascularity of the rotator cuff tendon. J Bone Joint Surg [Br] *74*:151, 1992.
53. Sarkar K, Taine W, Uhthoff HK: The ultrastructure of the coracoacromial ligament in patients with chronic impingement syndrome. Clin Orthop *254*:49, 1990.
54. Dines DM, Warren RF, Inglis AE, et al: The coracoid impingement syndrome. J Bone Joint Surg [Br] *72*:314, 1990.
55. Edelson JG, Zuckerman J, Hershkovitz I: Os acromiale: Anatomy and surgical implications. J Bone Joint Surg [Br] *74*:551, 1993.
56. Gagey N, Ravaud E, Lassau JP: Anatomy of the acromial arch: Correlation of anatomy and magnetic resonance imaging. Surg Radiol Anat *15*:63, 1993.
57. Edelson JG, Taitz C: Anatomy of the coraco-acromial arch: Relation to degeneration of the acromion. J Bone Joint Surg [Br] *74*:589, 1992.
58. Bigliani LH, Morrison DS, April EW: The morphology of the acromion and its relationship to rotator cuff tears. Orthop Trans *10*:228, 1986.
59. Haygood TM, Langlotz CP, Kneeland JB, et al: Categorization of acromial shape: Interobserver variability with MR imaging and conventional radiography. AJR *162*:1377, 1994.
60. Edelson JG: The "hooked" acromion revisited. J Bone Joint Surg [Br] *77*:284, 1995.
61. Peh WCG, Farmer THR, Totty WG: Acromial arch shape: Assessment with MR imaging. Radiology *195*:501, 1995.
62. Tuite MJ, Toivonen DA, Orwin JF, et al: Acromial angle on the radiographs of the shoulder: Correlation with the impingement syndrome and rotator cuff tears. AJR *165*:609, 1995.
63. Neer CS, Poppen NK: Supraspinatus outlet. Orthop Trans *11*:234, 1987.
64. Kitchel SH, Butters KA, Rockwood CA: The shoulder impingement syndrome. Orthop Trans *8*:510, 1984.
65. Rockwood CA Jr, Lyons FR: Shoulder impingement syndrome: Diagnosis, radiographic evaluation and treatment with a modified Neer acromioplasty. J Bone Joint Surg [Am] *75*:409, 1993.
66. Beaton LE, Anson BJ: Variation of the origin of the m. trapezius. Anat Rec *83*:41, 1942.
67. Vangsness CT Jr, Jorgenson SS, Watson T, et al: The origin of the long head of the biceps from the scapula and glenoid labrum: An anatomical study of 100 shoulders. J Bone Joint Surg [Br] *76*:951, 1994.
68. Warner JJP, McMahon PJ: The role of the long head of the biceps brachii in superior stability of the glenohumeral joint. J Bone Joint Surg [Am] *77*:366, 1995.
69. Norris TR: Fractures of the proximal humerus and dislocations of the shoulder. *In* BD Browner, JB Jupiter, AM Levine, et al (Eds): Skeletal Trauma: Fracture, Dislocations, Ligamentous Injuries. Philadelphia, WB Saunders Co, 1992, p. 1201.
70. Tibone J, Patek R, Jobe FW, et al: Functional anatomy, biomechanics, and kinesiology. *In* JC DeLee, D Drez Jr (Eds): Orthopaedic Sports Medicine: Principles and Practice. Philadelphia, WB Saunders Co, 1994, p. 463.
71. Guanche C, Knatt T, Solomonow M, et al: The synergistic action of the capsule and the shoulder muscles. Am J Sports Med *23*:301, 1995.
72. Perry J: Anatomy and biomechanics of the shoulder in throwing, swimming, gymnastics, and tennis. Clin Sports Med *2*:247, 1983.
73. Killoran PJ, Marcove RC, Freiberger RH: Shoulder arthrography. AJR *103*:658, 1968.
74. Kernwein GA, Roseberg B, Sneed WR Jr: Arthrographic studies of shoulder joint. J Bone Joint Surg [Am] *39*:1267, 1957.

75. Lindblom K: Arthrography and roentgenography in ruptures of the tendons of the shoulder joint. Acta Radiol 20:548, 1939.
76. Nelson DH: Arthrography of the shoulder. Br J Radiol 25:134, 1952.
77. Neviaser JS: Arthrography of shoulder joint: Study of findings in adhesive capsulitis of shoulder. J Bone Joint Surg [Am] 44:1321, 1962.
78. Samilson R, Raphael RL, Post L, et al: Arthrography of shoulder joint. Clin Orthop 20:21, 1961.
79. Reeves B: Arthrography of shoulder. J Bone Joint Surg [Br] 48:424, 1966.
80. Den Herder BA: Clinical significance of arthrography of humeroscapular joint. Radiol Clin Biol 46:185, 1977.
81. Nelson CL: The use of arthrography in athletic injuries of the shoulder. Orthop Clin North Am 4:775, 1973.
82. Nelson CL, Burton RI: Upper extremity arthrography. Clin Orthop 107:62, 1975.
83. Preston BJ, Jackson JP: Investigation of shoulder disability by arthrography. Clin Radiol 28:259, 1977.
84. Schneider R, Ghelman B, Kaye JJ: A simplified injection technique for shoulder arthrography. Radiology 114:738, 1975.
85. Dalinka MK: A simple aid to the performance of shoulder arthrography. AJR 129:942, 1977.
86. Ghelman B, Goldman AB: The double contrast shoulder arthrogram: Evaluation of rotator cuff tears. Radiology 124:251, 1977.
87. Goldman AB, Ghelman B: The double-contrast shoulder arthrogram: A review of 158 studies. Radiology 127:655, 1978.
88. Takagishi K, Makino K, Takahira N, et al: Ultrasonography for diagnosis of rotator cuff tear. Skeletal Radiol 25:221, 1996.
89. Goodwin DW, Pathria MN: Magnetic resonance imaging of the shoulder. Orthopedics 17:1021, 1994.
90. Tirman PFJ, Bost FW, Steinbach LS, et al: MR arthrographic depiction of tears of the rotator cuff: Benefit of abduction and external rotaiton of the arm. Radiology 192:851, 1994.
91. Uri DS, Kneeland JB, Dalinka MK: Update in shoulder magnetic resonance imaging. Magn Reson Q 11:21, 1995.
92. Totterman SM, Miller RJ, Meyers SP: Basic anatomy of the shoulder by magnetic resonance imaging. Topics Magn Reson Imaging 6:86, 1994.
93. Quinn SF, Sheley RC, Demlow TA, et al: Rotator cuff tendon tears: Evaluation with fat-suppressed MR imaging with arthroscopic correlation in 100 patients. Radiology 195:495, 1995.
94. Peterfy CG: Questions and Answers. AJR 165:734, 1995.
95. Loehr SP, Pope TL Jr, Martin DF, et al: Three-dimensional MRI of the glenoid labrum. Skel Radiol 24:117, 1995.
96. Patten RM: Vacuum phenomenon: A potential pitfall in the interpretation of gradient-recalled MR images of the shoulder. AJR 162:1383, 1994.
97. Recht MP, Kramer J, Petersilge CA, et al: Distribution of normal and abnormal fluid collections in the glenohumeral joint: Implications for MR arthrography. J Magn Reson Imaging 4:173, 1994.
98. Kopka L, Funke M, Fischer U, et al: MR arthrography of the shoulder with gadopentetate dimeglumine: Influence of concentration, iodinated contrast material, and time on signal intensity. AJR 163:621, 1994.
99. Neer CS II: Anterior acromioplasty for the chronic impingement syndrome in the shoulder: A preliminary report. J Bone Joint Surg [Am] 54:41, 1972.
100. Neer CS II: Impingement lesions. Clin Orthop 173:70, 1983.
101. Neer CS II, Bigliani LU, Hawkins RJ: Rupture of the long head of the biceps related to subacromial impingement. Orthop Trans 1:111, 1977.
102. Neer CS II, Welsh RP: The shoulder in sports. Orthop Clin North Am 8:583, 1977.
103. Matsen FA III, Arntz CT: Subacromial impingement. In CA Rockwood Jr, FA Matsen III (Eds): The Shoulder. Philadelphia, WB Saunders Co, 1990, p. 623.
104. Rathbun JB, Macnab I: The microvascular pattern of the rotator cuff. J Bone Joint Surg [Br] 52:540, 1970.
105. Sigholm G, Styf J, Körner L, et al: Pressure recording in the subacromial bursa. J Orthop Res 6:123, 1988.
106. Fu FH, Harner CD, Klein AH: Shoulder impingement syndrome: A critical review. Clin Orthop 269:162, 1991.
107. Jobe FW, Kvitne RS: Shoulder pain in the overhand or throwing athlete: The relationship of anterior instability and rotator cuff impingement. Orthop Rev 18:963, 1989.
108. Miniaci A, Fowler PJ: Impingement in the athlete. Clin Sports Med 12:91, 1993.
109. Fowler PJ, Webster MS: Shoulder pain in highly competitive swimmers. Orthop Trans 7:170, 1983.
110. Ticker JB, Fealy S, Fu FH: Instability and impingement in the athlete's shoulder. Sports Med 19:418, 1995.
111. Walch G, Boileau P, Noel E, et al: Impingement of the deep surface of the supraspinatus tendon on the posterior glenoid rim: An arthroscopic study. J Shoulder Elbow Surg 1:238, 1992.
112. Liu SH, Boynton E: Posterior superior impingement of the rotator cuff on the glenoid rim as a cause of shoulder pain in the overhead athlete. Arthroscopy 9:697, 1993.
113. Tirman PFJ, Bost FW, Garvin GJ, et al: Posterosuperior glenoid impingement of the shoulder: Findings at MR imaging and MR arthrography with arthroscopic correlation. Radiology 193:431, 1994.
114. Hawkins RJ, Abrams JS: Impingement syndrome in the absence of rotator cuff tear (Stages 1 and 2). Orthop Clin North Am 18:373, 1987.
115. LeRoux J-L, Thomas E, Bonnel F, et al: Diagnostic value of clinical tests for shoulder impingement syndrome. Rev Rhum Mal Osteoartic [Engl Ed] 62:423, 1995.
116. Flatow EL, Soslowsky LJ, Ticker JB, et al: Excursion of the rotator cuff under the acromion: Patterns of subacromial contact. Am J Sports Med 22:779, 1994.
117. Berens DL, Lockie LM: Ossification of the coraco-acromial ligament. Radiology 74:802, 1959.
118. Cone RO III, Resnick D, Danzig L: Shoulder impingement syndrome: Radiographic evaluation. Radiology 150:29, 1984.
119. Kieft GJ, Bloem JL, Rozing PM, et al: Rotator cuff impingement syndrome: MR imaging. Radiology 166:211, 1988.
120. Seeger LL, Gold RH, Bassett LW, et al: Shoulder impingement syndrome: MR findings in 53 shoulders. AJR 150:343, 1988.
121. Seeger L: Magnetic resonance imaging of the shoulder. Clin Orthop 244:48, 1989.
122. Kanecko K, Demouy EH, Brunet ME: MR evaluation of rotator cuff impingement: Correlation with confirmed full-thickness rotator cuff tears. J Comput Assist Tomogr 18:225, 1994.
123. Farley TE, Neumann CH, Steinbach LS, et al: The coracoacromial arch: MR evaluation and correlation with rotator cuff pathology. Skel Radiol 23:641, 1994.
124. Monu JUV, Pruett S, Vanarthos WJ, et al: Isolated subacromial bursal fluid on MRI of the shoulder in symptomatic patients: Correlation with arthroscopic findings. Skel Radiol 23:529, 1994.
125. Chandnani V, Ho C, Gerharter J, et al: MR findings in asymptomatic shoulders: A blind analysis using symptomatic shoulders as controls. Clin Imaging 16:25, 1992.
126. Epstein RE, Schweitzer ME, Frieman BG, et al: Hooked acromion: Prevalence on MR images of painful shoulders. Radiology 187:479, 1993.
127. Park JG, Lee JK, Phelps CT: Os acromiale associated with rotator cuff impingement: MR imaging of the shoulder. Radiology 193:255, 1994.
128. Kaplan PA, Bryans KC, Davick JP, et al: MR imaging of the normal shoulder: Variants and pitfalls. Radiology 184:519, 1992.
129. Feller JF, Tirman PFJ, Steinbach LS, et al: Magnetic resonance imaging of the shoulder: Review. Semin Roentgenol 30:224, 1995.
130. Gartsman GM: Arthroscopic acromioplasty for lesions of the rotator cuff. J Bone Joint Surg [Am] 72:169, 1990.
131. Hurley J, Bronstein R: Shoulder arthroscopy in the athlete: Practical applications. Sports Med 15:133, 1993.
132. Olsewski JM, Depew AD: Arthroscopic subacromial decompression and rotator cuff debridement for stage II and stage III impingement. J Arthrosc Rel Surg 10:158, 1994.
133. Berg EE, Ciullo JV, Oglesby JW: Failure of arthroscopic decompression by subacromial heterotopic ossification causing recurrent impingement. J Arthrosc Rel Surg 10:158, 1994.
134. Owen RS, Iannotti JP, Kneeland JB, et al: Shoulder after surgery: MR imaging with surgical validation. Radiology 186:443, 1993.
135. Matsen FA III, Arntz CT: Rotator cuff tendon failure. In CA Rockwood Jr, FA Matsen III (Eds): The Shoulder. Philadelphia, WB Saunders Co, 1990, p. 647.
136. Cofield RH: Rotator cuff disease of the shoulder. J Bone Joint Surg [Am] 67:974, 1985.
137. Patte D: Classification of rotator cuff lesions. Clin Orthop 254:81, 1990.
138. Keyes EL: Observations on rupture of the supraspinatus tendon: Based upon a study of 73 cadavers. Ann Surg 97:849, 1933.
139. Wilson CL, Duff GL: Pathologic study of degeneration and rupture of the supraspinatus tendon. Arch Surg 47:121, 1943.
140. Cotton RE, Rideout DF: Tears of the humeral rotator cuff: A radiological and pathological necropsy study. J Bone Joint Surg [Br] 46:314, 1964.
141. Fukuda H, Mikasa M, Ogawa K, et al: The partial thickness tear of the rotator cuff. Orthop Trans 7:137, 1983.
142. Pettersson G: Rupture of the tendon aponeurosis of the shoulder joint in anterior inferior dislocation. Acta Chir Scand (Suppl) 77:1, 1942.
143. Gerber C, Krushell RJ: Isolated rupture of the tendon of the subscapularis muscle: Clinical features in 16 cases. J Bone Joint Surg [Br] 73:389, 1991.
144. Neviaser RJ, Neviaser TJ, Neviaser JS: Concurrent rupture of the rotator cuff and anterior dislocation of the shoulder in the older patient. J Bone Joint Surg [Am] 70:1308, 1988.
145. McAuliffe TB, Dowd GS: Avulsion of the subscapularis tendon: A case report. J Bone Joint Surg [Am] 69:1454, 1987.
146. Kumagai J, Sarkar K, Uhthoff HK: The collagen types in the attachment zone of rotator cuff tendons in the elderly: An immunohistochemical study. J Rheumatol 21:2096, 1994.
147. Riley GP, Harrall RL, Constant CR, et al: Tendon degeneration and chronic shoulder pain: Changes in the collagen composition of the human rotator cuff tendons in rotator cuff tendinitis. Ann Rheum Dis 53:359, 1994.
148. Lohr JF, Uhthoff HK: The microvascular pattern of the supraspinatus tendon. Clin Orthop 254:35, 1990.
149. Meyer AW: The minute anatomy of attrition lesions. J Bone Joint Surg [Am] 13:341, 1931.
150. Brewer BJ: Aging of the rotator cuff. Am J Sports Med 7:102, 1979.
151. Soslowsky LJ, An CH, Johnston SP, et al: Geometric and mechanical properties of the coracoacromial ligament and their relationship to rotator cuff disease. Clin Orthop 304:10, 1994.

152. Ozaki J, Fujimoto S, Nakagawa Y, et al: Tears of the rotator cuff of the shoulder associated with pathological changes in the acromion: A study in cadavera. J Bone Joint Surg [Am] 70:1224, 1988.

153. Hijioka A, Suzuki K, Nakamura T, et al: Degenerative change and rotator cuff tears: An anatomical study in 160 shoulders of 80 cadavers. Arch Orthop Trauma Surg 112:61, 1993.

154. Ogata S, Uhthoff HK: Acromial enthesopathy and rotator cuff tear: A radiologic and histologic postmortem investigation of the coracoacromial arch. Clin Orthop 254:39, 1990.

155. Kjellin I, Ho CP, Cervilla V, et al: Alterations in the supraspinatus tendon at MR imaging: Correlation with histopathologic findings in cadavers. Radiology 181:837, 1991.

156. Itoi E, Berglund LJ, Grabowski JJ, et al: Tensile properties of the supraspinatus tendon. J Orthop Res 13:578, 1995.

157. Jim YF, Hsu HC, Chang CY, et al: Coexistence of calcific tendinitis and rotator cuff tear: An arthrographic study. Skel Radiol 22:183, 1993.

158. Bloom RA: The active abduction view: A new maneuvre in the diagnosis of rotator cuff tears. Skel Radiol 20:255, 1991.

159. Goupille P, Anger C, Cotty P, et al: Diagnostic value of plain radiographs in rotator cuff tear. Rev Rhum Mal Osteoartic [Engl Ed] 60:359, 1993.

160. Kotzen LM: Roentgen diagnosis of rotator cuff tear: Report of 48 surgically proven cases. AJR 112:507, 1971.

161. DeSmet AA, Ting YM: Diagnosis of rotator cuff tear on routine radiographs. Can Assoc Radiol J 28:54, 1977.

162. Kaneko K, DeMouy EH, Brunet ME: Massive rotator cuff tears: Screening by routine radiographs. Clin Imaging 19:8, 1995.

163. Golding C: Radiology and orthopedic surgery. J Bone Joint Surg [Br] 48:320, 1966.

164. Paavolainen P, Ahovuo J: Ultrasonography and arthrography in the diagnosis of tears of the rotator cuff. J Bone Joint Surg [Am] 76:335, 1994.

165. Garcia JF: Arthrographic visualization of rotator cuff tears: Optimal application of stress to the shoulder. Radiology 150:595, 1984.

166. Kilcoyne RF, Matsen FA III: Rotator cuff tear measured by arthropneumotomography. AJR 140:315, 1983.

167. Beltran J, Gray L, Bools JC, et al: Rotator cuff lesions of the shoulder: Evaluation by direct sagittal CT arthrography. Radiology 160:161, 1986.

168. Blum A, Boyer B, Regent D, et al: Direct coronal view of the shoulder with arthrographic CT. Radiology 188:677, 1993.

169. Stiles RG, Resnick D, Sartoris DJ, et al: Rotator cuff disruption: Diagnosis with digital arthrography. Radiology 168:705, 1988.

170. Resnik CS, Fronek J, Frey C, et al: Intra-articular pressure determination during glenohumeral joint arthrography: Preliminary investigation. Invest Radiol 19:45, 1984.

171. Bjorkenheim J-M, Paavolainen P, Ahovuo J, et al: The intraarticular pressure during shoulder arthrography: A diagnostic aid in rotator cuff tear. Acta Orthop Scand 58:128, 1987.

172. Craig EV: The geyser sign and torn rotator cuff: Clinical significance and pathomechanics. Clin Orthop 191:213, 1984.

173. Craig EV: The acromioclavicular joint cyst: An unusual presentation of a rotator cuff tear. Clin Orthop 202:189, 1986.

174. Mink JH, Harris E, Rappaport M: Rotator cuff tears: Evaluation using double-contrast shoulder arthrography. Radiology 157:621, 1985.

175. Fukuda H, Mikasa M, Yamanaka K: Incomplete thickness rotator cuff tears diagnosed by subacromial bursography. Clin Orthop 223:51, 1987.

176. Yamanaka K, Matsumoto T: The joint side tear of the rotator cuff: A followup study by arthrography. Clin Orthop 304:68, 1994.

177. Neviaser TJ, Neviaser RJ, Neviaser JS: Incomplete rotator cuff tears: A technique for diagnosis and treatment. Clin Orthop 306:12, 1994.

178. Goutallier D, Postel J-M, Bernageau J, et al: Fatty muscle degeneration in cuff ruptures: Pre- and postoperative evaluation by CT scan. Clin Orthop 304:78, 1994.

179. Goutallier D, Postel J-M, Bernageau J, et al: Fatty infiltration of disrupted rotator cuff muscles. Rev Rhum Mal Osteoartic [Engl Ed] 62:415, 1995.

180. van Holsbeeck MT, Kolowich PA, Eyler WR, et al: US depiction of partial-thickness tear of the rotator cuff. Radiology 197:443, 1995.

181. Farin PU, Jaroma H: Acute traumatic tears of the rotator cuff: Value of sonography. Radiology 197:269, 1995.

182. Hollister MS, Mack LA, Patten RM, et al: Association of sonographically detected subacromial/subdeltoid bursal effusion and intraarticular fluid with rotator cuff tear. AJR 165:605, 1995.

183. Patten RM, Spear RP, Richardson ML: Diagnostic performance of magnetic resonance imaging for the diagnosis of rotator cuff tears using supplementary images in the oblique sagittal plane. Invest Radiol 29:87, 1994.

184. Recht MP, Resnick D: Magnetic resonance imaging studies of the shoulder: Diagnosis of lesions of the rotator cuff. J Bone Joint Surg [Am] 75:1244, 1993.

185. Burk DL, Karasick D, Kurtz AB, et al: Rotator cuff tears: Prospective comparison of MR imaging with arthrography, sonography, and surgery. AJR 153:87, 1989.

186. Davis SJ, Teresi LM, Bradley WG, et al: Effect of arm rotation on MR imaging of the rotator cuff. Radiology 181:265, 1991.

187. Tuite MJ, Yandow DR, De Smet AA: Effect of field of view on MR diagnosis of rotator cuff tears. Skel Radiol 24:495, 1995.

188. Reinus WR, Shady KL, Mirowitz SA, et al: MR diagnosis of rotator cuff tears of the shoulder: Value of using T2-weighted fat saturated images. AJR 164:1451, 1995.

189. Tuite MJ, Yandow DR, De Smet AA, et al: Diagnosis of partial and complete rotator cuff tears using combined gradient echo and spin echo imaging. Skel Radiol 23:541, 1994.

190. Huber DJ, Sauter R, Mueller E, et al: MR imaging of the normal shoulder. Radiology 158:405, 1986.

191. Kneeland JB, Middleton WD, Carrera WD, et al: MR imaging of the shoulder: Diagnosis of rotator cuff tears. AJR 149:333, 1987.

192. Reeder JD, Andelman S: The rotator cuff tear: MR evaluation. Magn Reson Imaging 5:331, 1987.

193. Evancho AM, Stiles RG, Fajman WA, et al: MR imaging diagnosis of rotator cuff tears. AJR 151:751, 1988.

194. Zlatkin MB, Reicher MA, Kellerhouse LE, et al: The painful shoulder: MR imaging of the glenohumeral joint. J Comput Assist Tomogr 12:995, 1988.

195. Buirski G: Magnetic resonance imaging in acute and chronic rotator cuff tears. Skel Radiol 19:109, 1990.

196. Seeger LL, Ruszkowski JT, Bassett LW, et al: MR imaging of the normal shoulder: Anatomic correlation. AJR 148:83, 1987.

197. Middleton WD, Kneeland JB, Carrera GF, et al: High-resolution MR imaging of the normal rotator cuff. AJR 148:559, 1987.

198. Neumann CH, Holt RG, Steinbach LS, et al: MR imaging of the shoulder: Appearance of the supraspinatus tendon in asymptomatic volunteers. AJR 158:1281, 1992.

199. Miniaci A, Dowdy PA, Willits KR, et al: Magnetic resonance imaging evaluation of the rotator cuff tendons in the asymptomatic shoulder. Am J Sports Med 23:142, 1995.

200. Mirowitz SA: Normal rotator cuff: MR imaging with conventional and fat-suppression techniques. Radiology 180:735, 1991.

201. Fullerton GD, Cameron IL, Ord VA: Orientation of tendons in the magnetic field and its effect on T2 relaxation times. Radiology 155:433, 1985.

202. Erickson SJ, Cox IH, Hyde JS, et al: Effect of tendon orientation on MR imaging signal intensity: A manifestation of the "magic angle" phenomenon. Radiology 181:389, 1991.

203. Vahlensieck M, Pollack M, Lang P, et al: Two segments of the supraspinous muscle: Cause of high signal intensity at MR imaging? Radiology 186:449, 1993.

204. Timins ME, Erickson SJ, Estkowski LD, et al: Increased signal in the normal supraspinatus tendon on MR imaging: Diagnostic pitfall caused by the magic-angle effect. AJR 164:109, 1995.

205. Liou JTS, Wilson AJ, Totty WG, et al: The normal shoulder: Common variations that simulate pathologic conditions at MR imaging. Radiology 186:435, 1993.

206. Zlatkin MB, Iannotti JP, Roberts MC, et al: Rotator cuff tears: Diagnostic performance of MR imaging. Radiology 172:223, 1989.

207. Holt RG, Helms CA, Steinbach L, et al: Magnetic resonance imaging of the shoulder: Rationale and current applications. Skel Radiol 19:5, 1990.

208. Rafii M, Firooznia H, Sherman O, et al: Rotator cuff lesions: Signal patterns at MR imaging. Radiology 177:817, 1990.

209. Meyer SJF, Dalinka MK: Magnetic resonance imaging of the shoulder. Semin Ultrasound CT MR 11:253, 1990.

210. Iannotti JP, Zlatkin MB, Esterhai JL, et al: Magnetic resonance imaging of the shoulder: Sensitivity, specificity, and predictive value. J Bone Joint Surg [Am] 73:17, 1991.

211. Nelson MC, Leather GP, Nirschl RP: Evaluation of the painful shoulder: A prospective comparison of magnetic resonance imaging, computerized tomographic arthrography, ultrasonography, and operative findings. J Bone Joint Surg [Am] 73:707, 1991.

212. Hodler J, Terrier B, von Schulthess GK, et al: MRI and sonography of the shoulder. Clin Radiol 43:323, 1991.

213. Farley TE, Neumann CH, Steinbach LS, et al: Full-thickness tears of the rotator cuff of the shoulder: Diagnosis with MR imaging. AJR 158:347, 1992.

214. Zltakin MB, Falchook FS: Magnetic resonance pathology of the rotator cuff. Topics Magn Reson Imaging 6:94, 1994.

215. Patten RM: Tears of the anterior portion of the rotator cuff (the subscapularis tendon): MR imaging findings. AJR 162:351, 1994.

216. Robertson PL, Schweitzer ME, Mitchell DG, et al: Rotator cuff disorders: Interobserver and intraobserver variations in diagnosis with MR imaging. Radiology 194:831, 1995.

217. Sher JS, Uribe JW, Posada A, et al: Abnormal findings on magnetic resonance images of asymptomatic shoulders. J Bone Joint Surg [Am] 77:10, 1995.

218. Hodler J, Kursunoglu-Brahme S, Snyder SJ, et al: Rotator cuff disease: Assessment with MR arthrography versus standard MR imaging in 36 patients with arthroscopic confirmation. Radiology 182:431, 1992.

219. Karzel RP, Snyder SJ: Magnetic resonance arthrography of the shoulder: A new technique of shoulder imaging. Clin Sports Med 12:123, 1993.

220. Fritz RC, Stoller DW: Fat-suppression MR arthrography of the shoulder. Radiology 185:614, 1992.

221. Palmer WE, Brown JH, Rosenthal DI: Rotator cuff: Evaluation with fat-suppressed MR arthrography. Radiology 188:683, 1993.

222. Andrews JR, Broussard TS, Carson WG: Arthroscopy of the shoulder in the management of partial tears of the rotator cuff: A preliminary report. Arthroscopy 1:117, 1985.

223. Itoi E, Tabata S: Incomplete rotator cuff tears: Results of operative treatment. Clin Orthop 284:128, 1992.

224. Traughber PD, Goodwin TE: Shoulder MRI: Arthroscopic correlation with emphasis on partial tears. J Comput Assist Tomogr 16:129, 1992.
225. Flannigan B, Kursunoglu-Brahme S, Snyder S, et al: MR arthrography of the shoulder: Comparison with conventional MR imaging. AJR 155:829, 1990.
226. Samilson RL, Binder WF: Symptomatic full thickness tears of the rotator cuff: An analysis of 292 shoulders in 276 patients. Orthop Clin North Am 6:449, 1975.
227. Neer CS, Marberry TA: On the disadvantages of radical acromionectomy. J Bone Joint Surg [Am] 63:416, 1981.
228. Ellman H, Hanker G, Bayer M: Repair of the rotator cuff: End-result study of factors influencing reconstruction. J Bone Joint Surg [Am] 68:1136, 1986.
229. Ellman H: Diagnosis and treatment of incomplete rotator cuff tears. Clin Orthop 254:64, 1990.
230. Prietto C: Arthroscopic shoulder treatment—what can and cannot be done. West J Med 159:484, 1993.
231. Liu SH: Arthroscopically-assisted rotator-cuff repair. J Bone Joint Surg [Br] 76:592, 1994.
232. Gerber C, Schneeberger AG, Beck M, et al: Mechanical stregth of repairs of the rotator cuff. J Bone Joint Surg [Br] 76:371, 1994.
233. Gazielly DF, Bleyze P, Montagnon C: Functional and anatomical results after rotator cuff repair. Clin Orthop 304:43, 1994.
234. Calvert PT, Packer NP, Stoker DJ, et al: Arthrography of the shoulder after operative repair of the torn rotator cuff. J Bone Joint Surg [Br] 68:147, 1986.
235. Mack LA, Nyberg DA, Matsen FA III, et al: Sonography of the postoperative shoulder. AJR 150:1089, 1988.
236. Luck JV Jr, Andersson GBJ: Occupational shoulder disorders. In CA Rockwood Jr, FA Matsen III (Eds): The Shoulder. Philadelphia, WB Saunders Co, 1990, p. 1088.
237. Nirschl RP, Pettrone F: Tennis elbow: The surgical treatment of lateral epicondylitis. J Bone Joint Surg [Am] 61:832, 1979.
238. McKendry RJR, Uhthoff HK, Sarkar K, et al: Calcifying tendinitis of the shoulder: Prognostic value of clinical, histologic, and radiologic features in 57 surgically treated cases. J Rheumatol 9:75, 1982.
239. Resnick D: Shoulder pain. Orthop Clin North Am 14:81, 1983.
240. Hayes CW, Conway WF: Calcium hydroxapatite deposition disease. RadioGraphics 10:1031, 1990.
241. Holt PD, Keats TE: Calcific tendinitis: A review of the usual and unusual. Skel Radiol 22:1, 1993.
242. Bosworth BM: Calcium deposits in the shoulder and subacromial bursitis: A survey of 12,122 shoulders. JAMA 116:2477, 1941.
243. Caldwell GA, Unkauf BM: Results of treatment of subacromial bursitis in 340 cases. Ann Surg 132:432, 1950.
244. Young BR: Roentgen treatment of bursitis of the shoulder. AJR 56:626, 1946.
245. Arner O, Lindvall N, Rieger A: Calcific tendinitis (tendinitis calcarea) of shoulder joint. Acta Chir Scand 114:319, 1958.
246. Sandstrom C: Peritendinitis calcarea: A common disease of middle life: Its diagnosis, pathology and treatment. AJR 40:1, 1938.
247. Moseley HF: Shoulder Lesions. Edinburgh, E & S Livingstone, 1969, p. 99.
248. ViGario DG, Keats TE: Localization of calcific deposits in the shoulder. AJR 108:806, 1970.
249. Boulis ZF, Dick R: The greater tuberosity of the humerus: An area for misdiagnosis. Australas Radiol 26:267, 1982.
250. Nidecker A, Hartweg H: Seltene Lokalisationen verkalkender Tendopathien. ROFO 139:658, 1983.
251. Goldman AB: Calcific tendinitis of the long head of the biceps brachii distal to the glenohumeral joint: Plain film radiographic findings. AJR 153:1011, 1989.
252. Chadwick CJ: Tendinitis of the pectoralis major insertion with humeral lesions: A report of two cases. J Bone Joint Surg [Br] 71:816, 1989.
253. Hayes CW, Rosenthal DI, Plata MJ, et al: Calcific tendinitis in unusual locations associated with cortical bone erosion. AJR 149:967, 1987.
254. Winn RS, Melhorn JM, DeSmet AA: Layering of calcifications in synovial effusions. Can Assoc Radiol J 31:66, 1981.
255. Mens J, Van der Korst JK: Calcifying supracoracoid bursitis as a cause of chronic shoulder pain. Ann Rheum Dis 43:758, 1984.
256. Baird LW: Roentgen irradiation of calcareous deposits about the shoulder. Radiology 37:316, 1941.
257. Jones GB: Painful shoulder. J Bone Joint Surg [Br] 31:433, 1949.
258. Plenk HP: Calcifying tendinitis of the shoulder: Critical study of the value of x-ray therapy. Radiology 59:384, 1952.
259. Simon WH: Soft tissue disorders of the shoulder: Frozen shoulder, calcific tendinitis and bicipital tendinitis. Orthop Clin North Am 6:521, 1975.
260. Farin PU, Jaroma H: Sonographic findings of rotator cuff calcifications. J Ultrasound Med 14:7, 1995.
261. Farin PU, Jaroma H, Soimakllio S: Rotator cuff calcifications: Treatment with US-guided technique. Radiology 195:841, 1995.
262. Gärtner J, Heyer A: Tendinosis calcarea der Shulter. Orthopäde 24:284, 1995.
263. Burk DL Jr, Karasick D, Mitchell DG, et al: MR imaging of the shoulder: Correlation with plain radiography. AJR 154:549, 1990.
264. Murnaghan JP: Frozen shoulder. In CA Rockwood Jr, FA Matsen III (Eds): The Shoulder. Philadelphia, WB Saunders Co, 1990, p. 837.

265. Lundberg BJ: The frozen shoulder. Acta Orthop Scand (Suppl) 119:1, 1969.
266. Kay N: The clinical diagnosis and management of frozen shoulders. Practitioner 225:164, 1981.
267. Withers RJW: The painful shoulder: Review of one hundred personal cases with remarks on the pathology. J Bone Joint Surg 31:414, 1949.
268. Reeves B: Arthrographic changes in frozen and post-traumatic stiff shoulders. Proc R Soc Med 59:827, 1966.
269. Neviaser JS: Adhesive capsulitis of the shoulder: A study of the pathological findings in periarthritis of the shoulder. J Bone Joint Surg 27:211, 1945.
270. McLaughlin HL: On the frozen shoulder. Bull Hosp Joint Dis 12:383, 1951.
271. Simmonds FA: Shoulder pain with particular reference to the frozen shoulder. J Bone Joint Surg 31:834, 1949.
272. Macnab I: Rotator cuff tendinitis. Ann R Coll Surg Engl 53:271, 1973.
273. Lippman RK: Frozen shoulder; periarthritis; bicipital tenosynovitis. Arch Surg 47:283, 1943.
274. Lidström A: Den "frusna" skuldran. Nord Med 69:125, 1963.
275. Uitvlugt G, Detrisac DA, Johnson LL, et al: Arthroscopic observations before and after manipulation of frozen shoulder. Arthroscopy 9:181, 1993.
276. Bunker TD, Anthony PP: The pathology of frozen shoulder: A Dupuytrenlike disease. J Bone Joint Surg [Br] 77:677, 1995.
277. Weber J, Kecskés S: Arthrografie bei Periarthritis humeroscapularis. ROFO 124:573, 1976.
278. Andrén L, Lundberg BJ: Treatment of rigid shoulders by joint distention during arthrography. Acta Orthop Scand 36:45, 1965.
279. Binder AI, Balgen DY, Hazleman BL, et al: Frozen shoulder: An arthrographic and radionuclear scan assessment. Ann Rheum Dis 43:365, 1984.
280. Resnick D: Frozen shoulder. Ann Rheum Dis 44:805, 1985.
281. Resnik CS, Fronek J, Frey C, et al: Intra-articular pressure determination during glenohumeral joint arthrography. Preliminary investigation. Invest Radiol 19:45, 1984.
282. Gilula LA, Schoenecker PL, Murphy WA: Shoulder arthrography as a treatment modality. AJR 131:1047, 1978.
283. Emig EW, Schweiter ME, Karasick D, et al: Adhesive capsulitis of the shoulder: MR diagnosis. AJR 164:1457, 1995.
284. Ryu KN, Lee SW, Rhee YG, et al: Adhesive capsulitis of the shoulder joint: Usefulness of dynamic sonography. J Ultrasound Med 12:445, 1993.
285. Ryu KN, Lee SW, Rhee YG, et al: Adhesive capsulitis of the shoulder joint: Usefulness of dynamic sonography. J Ultrasound Med 12:445, 1993.
286. Wright MG, Richards AJ, Clarke MB: 99-m pertechnetate scanning in capsulitis. Lancet 2:1265, 1975.
287. Ogilvie-Harris DJ, Wiley AM: Arthroscopic surgery of the shoulder. J Bone Joint Surg [Am] 68:201, 1986.
288. Neviaser TJ: Arthroscopy of the shoulder. Orthop Clin North Am 18:361, 1987.
289. Pollock RG, Durald XA, Flatow EL, et al: The use of arthroscopy in the treatment of resistant frozen shoulder. Clin Orthop 304:30, 1994.
290. Allen AA, Warner JJP: Management of the stiff shoulder. Operat Techniq Orthop 5:238, 1995.
291. Schweitzer ME, Magbalon MJ, Frieman BG, et al: Acromioclavicular joint fluid: Determination of clinical significance with MR imaging. Radiology 192:205, 1994.
292. Schweitzer ME, Magbalon MJ, Fenlin JM, et al: Effusion criteria and clinical importance of glenohumeral joint fluid: MR imaging evaluation. Radiology 194:821, 1995.
293. Ko J-Y, Shih C-H, Chen W-J, et al: Coracoid impingement caused by a ganglion from the subscapularis tendon: A case report. J Bone Joint Surg [Am] 76:1709, 1994.
294. Meachim G, Emery IH: Cartilage fibrillation in shoulder and hip joints in Liverpool necropsies. J Anat 116:161, 1973.
295. Barton NJ: Arthrodesis of the shoulder for degenerative conditions. J Bone Joint Surg [Am] 54:1759, 1972.
296. Neer CS II: Degenerative lesions of the proximal humeral articular surface. Clin Orthop 20:116, 1961.
297. Neer CS II: Replacement arthroplasty for glenohumeral osteoarthritis. J Bone Joint Surg [Am] 56:1, 1974.
298. Oppenheimer A: Arthritis of acromio-clavicular joint. J Bone Joint Surg 25:867, 1943.
299. Zanca P: Shoulder pain: Involvement of the acromioclavicular joint (analysis of 1,000 cases). AJR 171:493, 1971.
300. DePalma AF: Degenerative Changes in Sternoclavicular and Acromioclavicular Joints in Various Decades. Springfield, Ill, Charles C Thomas, 1957.
301. DePalma AF: Surgical anatomy of acromioclavicular and sternoclavicular joints. Surg Clin North Am 43:1541, 1963.
302. Sokoloff L, Gleason IO: The sternoclavicular articulations in rheumatic diseases. Am J Clin Pathol 24:406, 1954.
303. Kopp S, Carlsson GE, Hansson T, et al: Degenerative disease in the temporomandibular, metatarsophalangeal and sternoclavicular joints: An autopsy study. Acta Odontol Scand 34:23, 1976.
304. Hodler J, Loredo RA, Long C, et al: Assessment of articular cartilage thickness of the humeral head: MR-anatomic correlation in cadavers. AJR 165:615, 1995.
305. Minkoff J, Cavaliere G: Glenohumeral instabilities and the role of magnetic resonance imaging techniques: The orthopedic surgeon's perspective. MRI Clin North Am 1:105, 1993.

306. Howell SM, Galinat BJ, Renzi AJ, et al: Normal and abnormal mechanics of the glenohumeral joint in the horizontal plane. J Bone Joint Surg [Am] 70:227, 1988.

307. Matsen FA III, Thomas SC, Rockwood CA Jr: Glenohumeral instability. *In* CA Rockwood Jr, FA Matsen III (Eds): The Shoulder. Philadelphia, WB Saunders Co, 1990, p. 526.

308. Rowe CR, Zarins B: Recurrent transient subluxation of the shoulder. J Bone Joint Surg [Am] 63:863, 1981.

309. Joessel D: Ueber die Recidive der Humerusluxationen. Dtsch Z Chir 13:167, 1880.

310. Hill HA, Sachs MD: The grooved defect of the humeral head: A frequently unrecognized complication of dislocations of the shoulder joint. Radiology 35:690, 1940.

311. Hermodsson I: Röntgenologische Studien über die traumatischen und habituellen Schultergelenkverrenkungen nach Vorn und nach Unten. Acta Radiol (Suppl) 20:1, 1934.

312. Symeonides PP: The significance of the subscapularis muscle in the pathogenesis of recurrent anterior dislocation of the shoulder. J Bone Joint Surg [Br] 54:476, 1972.

313. Eyre-Brook AL: Recurrent dislocation of the shoulder. Physiotherapy 57:7, 1971.

314. Rowe CR: Prognosis in dislocations of the shoulder. J Bone Joint Surg [Am] 38:957, 1956.

315. Brav EA: Recurrent dislocation of the shoulder. Ten years' experience with Putti-Platt reconstruction procedure. Am J Surg 100:423, 1960.

316. Palmar I, Widen A: The bone-block method for recurrent dislocation of the shoulder joint. J Bone Joint Surg [Br] 30:53, 1948.

317. Adams JC: Recurrent dislocations of the shoulder. J Bone Joint Surg [Br] 30:26, 1948.

318. Hall RH, Isaac F, Booth CR: Dislocations of the shoulder with special reference to accompanying small fractures. J Bone Joint Surg [Am] 41:489, 1959.

319. Pavlov H, Warren RF, Weiss CB Jr, et al: The roentgenographic evaluation of anterior shoulder instability. Clin Orthop 194:153, 1985.

320. Bankart ASB: Recurrent or habitual dislocation of the shoulder joint. Br Med J 2:1132, 1923.

321. Pavlov H, Freiberger RH: Fractures and dislocations about the shoulder. Semin Roentgenol 13:85, 1978.

322. Aston JW Jr, Gregory CF: Dislocation of the shoulder with significant fracture of the glenoid. J Bone Joint Surg [Am] 55:1531, 1973.

323. Neviaser RJ, Neviaser TJ, Neviaser JS: Concurrent rupture of the rotator cuff and anterior dislocation of the shoulder in the older patient. J Bone Joint Surg [Am] 70:1308, 1988.

324. Gonzalez D, Lopez RA: Concurrent rotator-cuff tear and brachial plexus palsy associated with anterior dislocation of the shoulder: A report of two cases. J Bone Joint Surg [Am] 73:620, 1991.

325. de Laat EAT, Visser CPJ, Coene LNJEM, et al: Nerve lesions in primary shoulder dislocations and humeral neck fractures. J Bone Joint Surg [Br] 76:381, 1994.

326. Kirtland S, Resnick D, Sartoris DJ, et al: Chronic unreduced dislocations of the glenohumeral joint: Imaging strategy and pathologic correlation. J Trauma 28:1622, 1988.

327. Hill NA, McLaughlin HL: Locked posterior dislocation simulating a "frozen shoulder." J Trauma 3:225, 1963.

328. McLaughlin HL: Posterior dislocation of the shoulder. J Bone Joint Surg [Am] 34:584, 1952.

329. Shaw JL: Bilateral posterior fracture-dislocation of the shoulder and other trauma caused by convulsive seizures. J Bone Joint Surg [Am] 53:1437, 1971.

330. Vastamaki M, Solenen KA: Posterior dislocation and fracture dislocation of the shoulder. Acta Orthop Scand 51:479, 1980.

331. Din KM: Bilateral four-part fractures with posterior dislocation of the shoulder: A case report. J Bone Joint Surg [Br] 65:176, 1983.

332. Dimon JH III: Posterior dislocation and posterior fracture-dislocation of the shoulder: A report of 25 cases. South Med J 60:661, 1967.

333. Bloom MH, Obata WG: Diagnosis of posterior dislocation of the shoulder with use of Velpeau axillary and angle-up roentgenographic views. J Bone Joint Surg [Am] 49:943, 1967.

334. Arndt JH, Sears AD: Posterior dislocation of the shoulder. AJR 94:639, 1965.

335. Cisternino SJ, Rogers LF, Stufflebam BC, et al: The trough line: A radiographic sign of posterior shoulder dislocation. AJR 130:951, 1978.

336. Bernageau J, Patte D: Diagnostic radiologique des luxations postérieures de l'épaule. Rev Chir Orthop 65:101, 1979.

337. Slikva J, Resnick D: An improved radiographic view of the glenohumeral joint. Can Assoc Radiol J 30:83, 1979.

338. Fronek J, Warren RF, Bowen M: Posterior subluxation of the glenohumeral joint. J Bone Joint Surg [Am] 71:205, 1989.

339. Hawkins RJ, Neer CS II, Pianta RM, et al: Locked posterior dislocation of the shoulder. J Bone Joint Surg [Am] 69:9, 1987.

340. Samuson RL, Prieto V: Dislocation arthropathy of the shoulder. J Bone Joint Surg [Am] 65:456, 1983.

341. Downey EF Jr, Curtis DJ, Brower AC: Unusual dislocations of the shoulder. AJR 140:1207, 1983.

342. Lynn FS: Erect dislocation of the shoulder. Surg Gynecol Obstet 39:51, 1921.

343. Laskin RS, Sedlin ED: Luxatio erecta in infancy. Clin Orthop 80:126, 1971.

344. Kothari K, Bernstein RM, Griffiths HJ, et al: Luxatio erecta. Skel Radiol 11:47, 1984.

345. Saxena K, Stavas J: Inferior glenohumeral dislocation. Ann Emerg Med 12:718, 1983.

346. Zimmers T: Luxatio erecta: An uncommon shoulder dislocation. Ann Emerg Med 12:716, 1983.

347. Freundlich BD: Luxatio erecta. J Trauma 23:434, 1983.

348. Davids JR, Talbott RD: Luxatio erecta humeri: A case report. Clin Orthop 252:144, 1990.

349. Rowe CR, Pierce DS, Clark JG: Voluntary dislocation of the shoulder. J Bone Joint Surg [Am] 55:445, 1973.

350. Braunstein EM, Martel W: Voluntary glenohumeral dislocation. AJR 129:911, 1977.

351. Howorth MB: Generalized relaxation of the ligaments. Clin Orthop 30:133, 1963.

352. Brewer BJ, Wubben RC, Carrera GF: Excessive retroversion of the glenoid cavity: A cause of non-traumatic posterior instability of the shoulder. J Bone Joint Surg [Am] 68:724, 1986.

353. Huber H, Gerber C: Voluntary subluxation of the shoulder in children: A long-term follow-up study of 36 shoulders. J Bone Joint Surg [Br] 76:118, 1994.

354. Cotton F: Subluxation of the shoulder downward. Boston Med Surg J 185:405, 1921.

355. Hammond R: Relaxation of the shoulder following bone injury. J Bone Joint Surg 5:712, 1923.

356. Laskin RS, Schreiber S: Inferior subluxation of the humeral head: The drooping shoulder. Radiology 98:585, 1971.

357. Lev-Toaff AS, Karasick D, Rao VM: "Drooping shoulder"—nontraumatic causes of glenohumeral subluxation. Skel Radiol 12:34, 1984.

358. Galinat BJ, Warren RF, Buss DD: Pathophysiology of shoulder instability. *In* JB McGinty (Ed): Operative Arthroscopy. New York, Raven Press, 1991.

359. Stiles RG, Otte MT: Imaging of the shoulder. Radiology 188:603, 1993.

360. Cyprien JM, Vasey HM, Burdet A, et al: Humeral retrotorsion and glenohumeral relationship in the normal shoulder and in recurrent anterior dislocation. Clin Orthop 175:8, 1983.

361. Brewer BJ, Wubben RC, Carrera GF: Excessive retroversion of the glenoid cavity: A cause of non-traumatic posterior instability of the shoulder. J Bone Joint Surg [Am] 68:724, 1986.

362. Symeonides PP, Hatzokos I, Christoforides J, et al: Humeral head torsion in recurrent anterior dislocation of the shoulder. J Bone Joint Surg [Br] 77:687, 1995.

363. Dowdy PA, O'Driscoll SW: Recurrent anterior shoulder instability. Am J Sports Med 22:489, 1994.

364. Itoi E, Newman SR, Kuechle DK, et al: Dynamic anterior stabilizers of the shoulder with the arm in abduction. J Bone Joint Surg [Br] 76:834, 1994.

365. Pagnani MJ, Galinat BJ, Warren RF: Glenohumeral instability. *In* JC DeLee, D Drez Jr (Eds): Orthopaedic Sports Medicine: Principles and Practice. Philadelphia, WB Saunders Co, 1994, p. 580.

366. Allen AA, Warner JJP: Shoulder instability in the athlete. Orthop Clin North Am 26:487, 1995.

367. El-Khoury GY, Albright JP, Abu Yousef MM, et al: Arthrotomography of the glenoid labrum. Radiology 131:333, 1979.

368. Braunstein EM, O'Connor G: Double-contrast arthrotomography of the shoulder. J Bone Joint Surg [Am] 64:192, 1982.

369. Kleinman PK, Kanzaria PK, Goss TP, et al: Axillary arthrotomography of the glenoid labrum. AJR 141:993, 1984.

370. McGlynn FJ, El-Khoury G, Albright JP: Arthrography of the glenoid labrum in shoulder instability. J Bone Joint Surg [Am] 64:506, 1982.

371. El-Khoury GY, Kathol MH, Chandler JB, et al: Shoulder instability: Impact of glenohumeral arthrotomography on treatment. Radiology 160:669, 1986.

372. Kneisl JS, Sweeney HJ, Paige ML: Correlation of pathology observed in double contrast arthrotomography and arthroscopy of the shoulder. Arthroscopy 4:21, 1988.

373. Kinnard P, Tricoire J-L, Levesque R-Y, et al: Assessment of the unstable shoulder by computed arthrography: A preliminary report. Am J Sports Med 11:157, 1983.

374. Shuman WP, Kilcoyne RF, Matsen FA, et al: Double-contrast computed tomography of the glenoid labrum. AJR 141:581, 1983.

375. Deutsch AL, Resnick D, Mink JH, et al: Computed and conventional arthrotomography of the glenohumeral joint: Normal anatomy and clinical experience. Radiology 143:603, 1984.

376. Resnik CS, Deutsch AL, Resnick D, et al: Arthrotomography of the shoulder. Radiographics 4:963, 1984.

377. Rafii M, Firooznia H, Golimbu C, et al: CT arthrography of the capsular structures of the shoulder. AJR 146:361, 1986.

378. Wilson AJ, Totty WG, Murphy WA, et al: Shoulder joint: Arthrographic CT and long-term follow-up, with surgical correlation. Radiology 173:329, 1989.

379. Pennes DR, Jonsson K, Buckwalter K, et al: Computed arthrotomography of the shoulder: Comparison of examinations made with internal and external rotation of the humerus. AJR 153:1017, 1989.

380. Ribbans WJ, Mitchell R, Taylor GJ: Computerised arthrotomography of primary anterior dislocation of the shoulder. J Bone Joint Surg [Br] 72:181, 1990.

381. Wilson AJ: Computed arthrotomography of glenohumeral instability. Topics Magn Reson Imaging 6:139, 1994.
382. DeWatre F, Cotten A, LeBlond D, et al: Aspects normaux et pathologiques du bourrelet glenoidien en arthroscanner opaque. J Radiol 75:413, 1994.
383. Turner PJ, O'Connor PJ, Saifuddin A, et al: Prone oblique positioning for computed tomographic arthrography of the shoulder. Br J Radiol 67:835, 1994.
384. Richards RD, Sartoris DJ, Pathria MN, et al: Hill-Sachs lesion and normal humeral groove: MR imaging features allowing the differentiation. Radiology 190:665, 1994.
385. Pappas AM, Goss TP, Kleinman PK: Symptomatic shoulder instability due to lesions of the glenoid labrum. Am J Sports Med 11:279, 1983.
386. McNiesh LM, Callaghan JJ: CT arthrography of the shoulder: Variations of the glenoid labrum. AJR 149:963, 1987.
387. Rafii M, Firooznia H: Variations of normal glenoid labrum. AJR 152:201, 1989.
388. Seeger LL, Gold RH, Bassett LW: Shoulder instability: Evaluation with MR imaging. Radiology 168:695, 1988.
389. Habibian A, Stauffer A, Resnick D, et al: Comparison of conventional and computed arthrotomography with MR imaging in the evaluation of the shoulder. J Comput Assist Tomogr 13:968, 1989.
390. Munk PL, Holt RG, Helms CA, et al: Glenoid labrum: Preliminary work with use of radial-sequence MR imaging. Radiology 173:751, 1989.
391. Gross ML, Seeger LL, Smith JB, et al: Magnetic resonance imaging of the glenoid labrum. Am J Sports Med 18:229, 1990.
392. Legan JM, Burkhard TK, Goff WB II, et al: Tears of the glenoid labrum: MR imaging of 88 arthroscopically confirmed cases. Radiology 179:241, 1991.
393. Garneau RA, Renfrew DL, Moore TE, et al: Glenoid labrum: Evaluation with MR imaging. Radiology 179:519, 1991.
394. Imhoff A, Perrenoud A, Neidl K: MRI bei Schulterinstabilitat-Korrelation zum Arthro-CT und zur Arthroskopie der Schulter. Arthroskopie 5:122, 1992.
395. Gudinchet F, Naggar L, Ginalski JM, et al: Magnetic resonance imaging of nontraumatic shoulder instability in children. Skel Radiol 21:19, 1992.
396. McCauley TR, Pope CF, Jokl P: Normal and abnormal glenoid labrum: Assessment with multiplanar gradient-echo MR imaging. Radiology 183:35, 1992.
397. Tuite MJ, De Smet AA, Norris MA, et al: MR diagnosis of labral tears of the shoulder: Value of T2-weighted gradient-recalled echo images made in external rotation. AJR 164:941, 1995.
398. Loredo R, Longo C, Salonen D, et al: Glenoid labrum: MR imaging with histologic correlation. Radiology 196:33, 1995.
399. Green MR, Christensen KP: Magnetic resonance imaging of the glenoid labrum in anterior shoulder instability. Am J Sports Med 22:493, 1994.
400. Fischbach TJ, Seeger LL: Magnetic resonance imaging of glenohumeral instability. Topics Magn Reson Imaging 6:121, 1994.
401. Hajec PC, Baker LL, Sartoris DJ, et al: MR arthrography: Pathologic investigation. Radiology 163:141, 1987.
402. Chandnani VP, Yeager TD, DeBeradino T, et al: Glenoid labral tears: Prospective evaluation with MR imaging, MR arthrography, and CT arthrography. AJR 161:1229, 1993.
403. Tirman PFJ, Stauffer AE, Crues JU III, et al: Saline magnetic resonance arthrography in the evaluation of glenohumeral instability. J Arthrosc Rel Surg 9:550, 1993.
404. Palmer WE, Brown JH, Rosenthal DI: Labral-ligamentous complex of the shoulder: Evaluation with MR arthrography. Radiology 190:645, 1994.
405. Schweitzer ME: MR arthrography of the labral-ligamentous complex of the shoulder. Radiology 190:641, 1994.
406. Palmer WE, Caslowitz PL: Anterior shoulder instability: Diagnostic criteria determined from prospective analysis of 121 MR arthrograms. Radiology 197:819, 1995.
407. Palmer WE, Caslowitz PL, Chew FS: MR arthrography of the shoulder: Normal intraarticular structures and common abnormalities. AJR 164:141, 1995.
408. Massengill AD, Seeger LL, Yao L, et al: Labrocapsular ligamentous complex of the shoulder: Normal anatomy, anatomic variation, and pitfalls of MR imaging and MR arthrography. Radiographics 14:1211, 1994.
409. Chandnani VP, Gagliardi JA, Murnane TG, et al: Glenohumeral ligaments and shoulder capsular mechanism: Evaluation with MR arthrography. Radiology 196:27, 1995.
410. Kreitner K-F, Grebe P, Kersjes W, et al: Ensatzmöglichkeiten der MR-Arthrographie bei Erkrankungen des Schultergelenkes. ROFO 160:137, 1994.
411. Danzig LA, Greenway G, Resnick D: The Hill-Sachs lesion: An experimental study. Am J Sports Med 8:328, 1980.
412. Workman TL, Burkhard TK, Resnick D, et al: Hill-Sachs lesion: Comparison of detection with MR imaging, radiography, and arthroscopy. Radiology 185:847, 1992.
413. Johnson LL: Arthroscopic Surgery: Principles and Practice. St. Louis, CV Mosby, 1986.
414. Zellner AA, Dihlmann SW, Lehnert M: Impingement symptoms caused by a synovial fold in the glenoid fossa projecting into the sublabral hole. J Arthrosc Rel Surg 11:112, 1995.
415. Williams MM, Snyder SJ, Buford D Jr: The Buford complex—the "cord-like" middle glenohumeral ligament and absent anterosuperior labrum complex: A normal anatomic capsulolabral variant. J Arthrosc Rel Surg 10:241, 1994.
416. Neviaser TJ: The anterior labroligamentous periosteal sleeve avulsion lesion: A cause of anterior instability of the shoulder. J Arthrosc Rel Surg 9:17, 1993.
417. Neviaser TJ: The GLAD lesion: Another cause of anterior shoulder pain. J Arthrosc Rel Surg 9:22, 1993.
418. Snyder SJ: Superior labrum anterior and posterior lesions of the shoulder. Proceedings of the Annual Meeting on Arthroscopic Surgery on the Shoulder, San Diego, 1989.
419. Andrews JR, Carson WG Jr, McLeod WD: Glenoid labrum tears related to the long head of the biceps. Am J Sports Med 13:337, 1985.
420. Yoneda M, Hirooka A, Saito S, et al: Arthroscopic stapling for detached superior glenoid labrum. J Bone Joint Surg [Br] 73:746, 1991.
421. Snyder S, Karzel RP, Del Pizzo W, et al: SLAP lesions of the shoulder. Arthroscopy 6:274, 1990.
422. Maffet MW, Gartsman GM, Moseley B: Superior labrum-biceps tendon complex lesions of the shoulder. Am J Sports Med 23:93, 1995.
423. Pagnani MJ, Deng X-H, Warren RF, et al: Effect of lesions of the superior portion of the glenoid labrum on glenohumeral translation. J Bone Joint Surg [Am] 77:1003, 1995.
424. Kibler WB: Specificity and sensitivity of the anterior slide test in throwing athletes with superior glenoid labral tears. J Arthrosc Rel Surg 11:296, 1995.
425. Urban WP Jr, Caborn DNM: Management of superior labral anterior to posterior lesions. Oper Techniq Orthop 5:223, 1995.
426. Hunter JC, Blatz DJ, Escobedo EM: SLAP lesions of the glenoid labrum: CT arthrographic and arthroscopic correlation. Radiology 184:513, 1992.
427. Hodler J, Kursunoglu-Brahme S, Flannigan B, et al: Injuries of the superior portion of the glenoid labrum involving the insertion of the biceps tendon: MR imaging findings in nine cases. AJR 159:565, 1992.
428. Cartland JP, Crues JV III, Stauffer A, et al: MR imaging in the evaluation of SLAP injuries of the shoulder: Findings in 10 patients. AJR 159:787, 1992.
429. Smith AM, McCauley TR, Jokl P: SLAP lesions of the glenoid labrum diagnosed with MR imaging. Skel Radiol 22:507, 1993.
430. Mono JUV, Pope TL Jr, Chabon SJ, et al: MR diagnosis of superior labral anterior posterior (SLAP) injuries of the glenoid labrum: Value of routine imaging without intraarticular injection of contrast material. AJR 163:1425, 1994.
431. Detrisac DA, Johnson LL: Arthroscopic Shoulder Anatomy. Thorofare, NJ, Slack Inc, 1986, p. 71.
432. DePalma AF: Surgery of the Shoulder. 3rd ed. Philadelphia, JB Lippincott, 1983, p. 211.
433. Matthews IS, Terry G, Vetter WL: Shoulder anatomy for the arthroscopist. Arthroscopy 1:83, 1985.
434. Naylor MF, Nascimento AG, Sherrick AD, et al: Elastofibroma dorsi: Radiologic findings in 12 patients. AJR 167:683, 1996.
435. Warner JJP, Kann S, Marks P: Arthroscopic repair of combined Bankart and superior labral detachment anterior and posterior lesions: Technique and preliminary results. J Arthrosc Rel Surg 10:383, 1994.
436. Terry GC, Friedman SJ, Uhl TL: Arthroscopically treated tears of the glenoid labrum: Factors influencing outcome. Am J Sports Med 22:504, 1994.
437. Tirman PFJ, Feller JF, Janzen DL, et al: Association of glenoid labral cysts with labral tears and glenohumeral instability: Radiologic findings and clinical significance. Radiology 190:653, 1994.
438. Bennett GE: Shoulder and elbow lesions of the professional baseball pitcher. JAMA 117:510, 1941.
439. Lombardo SJ, Jobe FW, Kerlan RK, et al: Posterior shoulder lesions in throwing athletes. Am J Sports Med 5:106, 1977.
440. Barnes DA, Tullos HS: An analysis of 100 symptomatic baseball players. Am J Sports Med 6:62, 1978.
441. Ferrari JD, Ferrari DA, Coumas J, et al: Posterior ossification of the shoulder: The Bennett lesion. Am J Sports Med 22:171, 1994.
442. Osmond-Clarke H: Recurrent dislocation of the shoulder: The Putti-Platt operation. J Bone Joint Surg [Br] 30:19, 1948.
443. Magnuson PB, Stack JK: Bilateral habitual dislocation of the shoulders in twins, a family tendency. JAMA 144:2103, 1940.
444. Eden R: Zur Operation der habituellen Schulterluxation unter mitteilung eines neuen Verfahrens bei Abris am inneren Plafannenrande. Dtsch Ztschr Chir 144:269, 1918.
445. Hybbinette S: De la transplantation d'un fragment osseux pour remédier aux luxations récidivantes de l'épaule: Constatations et résultats opératoires. Acta Chir Scand 71:411, 1932.
446. Oudard P: La luxation récidivante de l'épaule (variété antero-interne): Procédé opératoire. J Chir 23:13, 1924.
447. Trillat A: Traitement de la luxation récidivante de l'épaule: Considérations techniques. Lyon Chir 49:986, 1954.
448. Helfet AJ: Coracoid transplantation for recurring dislocation of the shoulder. J Bone Joint Surg [Br] 40:198, 1958.
449. Rowe CR, Zarins B, Ciullo JV: Recurrent anterior dislocation of the shoulder after surgical repair: Apparent causes of failure and treatment. J Bone Joint Surg [Am] 66:159, 1984.
450. Hovelius L, Thorling J, Fredin H: Recurrent anterior dislocation of the shoulder: Results after the Bankart and Putti-Platt operations. J Bone Joint Surg [Am] 61:566, 1979.

451. Singson RD, Feldman F, Bighani LU, et al: Recurrent shoulder dislocation after surgical repair: Double-contrast CT arthrography. Work in progress. Radiology 164:425, 1987.

452. Uhrist MR: Complete dislocations of the acromioclavicular joint: The nature of the traumatic lesion and effective methods of treatment with an analysis of 41 cases. J Bone Joint Surg 28:813, 1946.

453. Powers JA, Bach PJ: Acromioclavicular separations: Closed or open treatment? Clin Orthop 104:213, 1974.

454. Weaver JK, Dunn HK: Treatment of acromioclavicular injuries, especially complete acromioclavicular separation. J Bone Joint Surg [Am] 54:1187, 1972.

455. Eidman DK, Siff SJ, Tullos HS: Acromioclavicular lesions in children. Am J Sports Med 9:150, 1981.

456. Cox JS: The fate of the acromioclavicular joint in athletic injuries. Am J Sports Med 9:50, 1981.

457. Allman FL Jr: Fractures and ligamentous injuries of the clavicle and its articulation. J Bone Joint Surg [Am] 49:774, 1967.

458. Zlotsky NA, Ballard A: Acromioclavicular injuries in athletes. J Bone Joint Surg [Am] 48:1224, 1966.

459. Post M: Current concepts in the diagnosis and management of acromioclavicular dislocations. Clin Orthop 200:234, 1985.

460. Montgomery SP, Loyd RD: Avulsion fracture of the coracoid epiphysis with acromioclavicular separation: Report of two cases in adolescents and review of the literature. J Bone Joint Surg [Am] 59:963, 1977.

461. Protass JJ, Stampfli FV, Osmer JC: Coracoid process fracture diagnosis in acromioclavicular separation. Radiology 116:61, 1975.

462. Smith DM: Coracoid fracture associated with acromioclavicular dislocation: A case report. Clin Orthop 108:165, 1975.

463. Taga I, Yoneda M, Ono K: Epiphyseal separation of the coracoid process associated with acromioclavicular sprain: A case report and review of the literature. Clin Orthop 207:138, 1986.

464. Zanca P: Shoulder pain: Involvement of the acromioclavicular joint: Analysis of 1000 cases. AJR 112:493, 1971.

465. Väätäinen U, Pirinen A, Mäkelä A: Radiological evaluation of the acromioclavicular joint. Skel Radiol 20:115, 1991.

466. Bearden JM, Hughston JC, Whatley GS: Acromioclavicular dislocation: Method of treatment. J Sports Med Phys Fitness 1:5, 1973.

467. Sage J: Recurrent inferior dislocation of the clavicle at the acromioclavicular joint: A case report. Am J Sports Med 10:145, 1982.

468. Leonard MH, Capen DA: Superior entrapment of the clavicle. Am J Sports Med 11:96, 1983.

469. Jain AS: Traumatic floating clavicle: A case report. J Bone Joint Surg [Br] 66:560, 1984.

470. Gearen PF, Petty W: Panclavicular dislocation: Report of a case. J Bone Joint Surg [Am] 64:454, 1982.

471. Cook F, Horowitz M: Bipolar clavicular dislocation: Report of a case. J Bone Joint Surg [Am] 69:145, 1987.

472. Falstie-Jensen S, Mikkelsen P: Pseudodislocation of the acromioclavicular joint. J Bone Joint Surg [Br] 64:368, 1982.

473. Millbourn E: On injuries to the acromioclavicular joint: Treatment and results. Acta Orthop Scand 19:349, 1950.

474. Arner O, Sandahl U, Ohrling H: Dislocation of the acromioclavicular joint—review of the literature and report of 56 cases. Acta Chir Scand 113:140, 1957.

475. Madsen B: Osteolysis of the acromial end of the clavicle following trauma. Br J Radiol 36:822, 1963.

476. Smart MJ: Traumatic osteolysis of the distal ends of the clavicles. Can Assoc Radiol J 23:264, 1972.

477. Jacobs P: Post-traumatic osteolysis of the outer end of the clavicle. J Bone Joint Surg [Br] 46:705, 1964.

478. Halaby FA, DiSalvo EI: Osteolysis: A complication of trauma. AJR 94:590, 1965.

479. Levine AH, Pais MJ, Schwartz EE: Posttraumatic osteolysis of the distal clavicle with emphasis on early radiologic changes. AJR 127:781, 1976.

480. Seymour EQ: Osteolysis of the clavicular tip associated with repeated minor trauma to the shoulder. Radiology 123:56, 1977.

481. Zsernaviczky J, Horst M: Kasuistischer Beitrag zur Osteolyse am distalen Klavikulaende. Arch Orthop Unfallchir 89:163, 1977.

482. Alnor P: Die posttraumatische Osteolyse des lateralen Claviculaendes. ROFO 75:364, 1951.

483. Hasselmann W: Die sog, posttraumatische Osteolyse des lateralen Claviculaendes. Monatsschr Unfallheilkd 58:242, 1955.

484. Ehricht HG: Die Osteolyse im lateralen Claviculaende nach Pressluftschaden. Arch Orthop Unfallchir 50:576, 1959.

485. Murphy OB, Bellamy R, Wheeler W, et al: Post-traumatic osteolysis of the distal clavicle. Clin Orthop 109:108, 1975.

486. Quinn SF, Glass TA: Posttraumatic osteolysis of the clavicle. South Med J 76:307, 1983.

487. Jeandel P, Garbe L, Dischino M, et al: Ostéolyse post-traumatique de l'extremité distale de la clavicule: Etude anatomopathologique de deux observations. Rev Rhum Mal Osteoartic 59:207, 1992.

488. Matthews LS, Simonson BG, Wolock BS: Osteolysis of the distal clavicle in a female body builder: A case report. Am J Sports Med 21:150, 1993.

489. Cahill BR: Osteolysis of the distal part of the clavicle in male athletes. J Bone Joint Surg [Am] 64:1053, 1982.

490. Scavenius M, Iversen BF, Stürup J: Resection of the lateral end of the clavicle following osteolysis, with emphasis on non-traumatic osteolysis of the acromial end of the clavicle in athletes. Injury 18:261, 1987.

491. Werder H: Posttraumatische Osteolyse des Schlüsselbeinendes. Schweiz Med Wochenschr 34:912, 1950.

492. Kaplan PA, Resnick D: Stress-induced osteolysis of the clavicle. Radiology 158:139, 1986.

493. Cahill BR: Correspondence. J Bone Joint Surg [Am] 65:421, 1983.

494. Erickson SJ, Kneeland JB, Komorowski RA, et al: Post-traumatic osteolysis of the clavicle: MR features. J Comput Assist Tomogr 14:835, 1990.

495. Patten RM: Atraumatic osteolysis of the distal clavicle: MR findings. J Comput Assist Tomogr 19:92, 1995.

496. Nettles JL, Linscheid R: Sternoclavicular dislocations. J Trauma 8:158, 1968.

497. Tyer HDD, Sturrock WDS, Callow FM: Retrosternal dislocation of the clavicle. J Bone Joint Surg [Br] 45:132, 1963.

498. Selesnick FH, Jablon M, Frank C, Post M: Retrosternal dislocation of the clavicle: Report of four cases. J Bone Joint Surg [Am] 66:287, 1984.

499. Newlin NS: Congenital retrosternal subluxation of the clavicle simulating an intrathoracic mass. AJR 130:1184, 1978.

500. Sadr B, Swann M: Spontaneous dislocation of the sternoclavicular joint. Acta Orthop Scand 50:269, 1979.

501. Levinsohn EM, Bunnell WP, Yuan HA: Computed tomography in the diagnosis of dislocations of the sternoclavicular joint. Clin Orthop 140:12, 1979.

502. Lourie JA: Tomography in the diagnosis of posterior dislocation of the sterno-clavicular joint. Acta Orthop Scand 51:579, 1980.

503. Klein MA, Miro PA, Spreitzer AM, et al: MR imaging of the normal sternoclavicular joint: Spectrum of findings. AJR 165:391, 1995.

504. Lee FA, Gwinn JL: Retrosternal dislocation of the clavicle. Radiology 110:631, 1974.

505. McKenzie JM: Retrosternal dislocation of the clavicle: A report of two cases. J Bone Joint Surg [Br] 45:138, 1963.

506. Brooks AL, Henning GD: Injury to the proximal clavicular epiphysis. J Bone Joint Surg [Am] 54:1347, 1972.

507. Lemire L, Rosman M: Sternoclavicular epiphyseal separation with adjacent clavicular fracture. J Pediatr Orthop 4:118, 1984.

508. Rose SH, Melton J III, Morrey BF, et al: Epidemiologic features of humeral fractures. Clin Orthop 168:24, 1982.

509. Dehne E: Fractures of the upper end of the humerus: A classification based on the etiology of trauma. Surg Clin North Am 25:28, 1945.

510. Neer CS II: Displaced proximal humeral fractures. I. Classification and evaluation. J Bone Joint Surg [Am] 52:1077, 1970.

511. Kristiansen B, Anderson ULS, Olsen CA, et al: The Neer classification of fractures of the proximal humerus: An assessment of interobserver variation. Skel Radiol 17:420, 1988.

512. Kilcoyne RF, Shuman WP, Matsen FA III, et al: The Neer classification of displaced proximal humeral fractures: Spectrum of findings on plain radiographs and CT scans. AJR 154:1029, 1990.

513. Castagno AA, Shuman WP, Kilcoyne RF, et al: Complex fractures of the proximal humerus: Role of CT in treatment. Radiology 165:759, 1987.

514. Earwaker J: Isolated avulsion fracture of the lesser tuberosity of the humerus. Skel Radiol 19:121, 1990.

515. LaBriola JH, Mohaghegh HA: Isolated avulsion fracture of the lesser tuberosity of the humerus: A case report and review of the literature. J Bone Joint Surg [Am] 57:1011, 1975.

516. Hawkins RJ, Bell RH, Gurr K: The three-part fracture of the proximal part of the humerus: Operative treatment. J Bone Joint Surg [Am] 68:1410, 1986.

517. Neer CS II: Displaced proximal humeral fractures. II. Treatment of three-part and four-part displacement. J Bone Joint Surg [Am] 52:1090, 1970.

518. Stableforth PG: Four-part fractures of the neck of the humerus. J Bone Joint Surg [Br] 66:104, 1984.

519. Lee DK, Hansen HR: Post-traumatic avascular necrosis of the humeral head in displaced proximal humeral fractures. J Trauma 21:788, 1984.

520. Jakob RP, Miniaci A, Anson PS, et al: Four-part valgus impacted fractures of the proximal humerus. J Bone Joint Surg [Br] 73:295, 1991.

521. Ovesen J, Nielsen S: Experimental distal subluxation in the glenohumeral joint. Arch Orthop Trauma Surg 104:78, 1985.

522. Rooney PJ, Crockshott WP: Pseudarthrosis following proximal humeral fractures: A possible mechanism. Skel Radiol 15:21, 1986.

523. Kofoed H: Revascularization of the humeral head: A report of two cases of fracture-dislocation of the shoulder. Clin Orthop 179:175, 1983.

524. Zuckerman JD, Flugstad DL, Teitz CC, et al: Axillary artery injury as a complication of proximal humeral fractures: Two case reports and a review of the literature. Clin Orthop 189:234, 1984.

525. Stewart MJ: Fractures of the humeral shaft. Curr Pract Orthop Surg 2:140, 1964.

526. Lemperg R, Liliequist B: Dislocation of the upper proximal epiphysis of the humerus in newborns. Acta Paediatr Scand 59:337, 1970.

527. Epps CH Jr: Fractures of the shaft of the humerus. In CA Rockwood Jr, DP Green (Eds): Fractures in Adults. 2nd Ed. Philadelphia, JB Lippincott Co, 1984, p. 653.

528. Klenerman L: Fractures of the shaft of the humerus. J Bone Joint Surg [Br] 48:105, 1966.

529. Whitson RO: Relation of the radial nerve to the shaft of the humerus. J Bone Joint Surg [Am] *36*:85, 1954.

530. Pollock FH, Drake D, Bovill EG, et al: Treatment of radial neuropathy associated with fractures of the humerus. J Bone Joint Surg [Am] *63*:239, 1981.

531. Shah JJ, Bhatti NA: Radial nerve paralysis associated with fractures of the humerus: A review of 62 cases. Clin Orthop *172*:171, 1983.

532. Kaiser TE, Sim FH, Kelly PJ: Radial nerve palsy associated with humeral fractures. Orthopedics *4*:1245, 1981.

533. Collins DN, Weber ER: Anterior interosseous nerve avulsion. Clin Orthop *181*:175, 1983.

534. Eppright RH, Wilkins KE: Fractures and dislocations of the elbow. *In* CA Rockwood Jr, DP Green (Eds): Fractures in Adults. Philadelphia, JB Lippincott Co, 1975, p. 487.

535. DePalma AF: The Management of Fractures and Dislocations. 2nd Ed. Philadelphia, WB Saunders Co, 1970.

536. Hoyer A: Treatment of supracondylar fractures of the humerus by skeletal traction in an abduction splint. J Bone Joint Surg [Am] *34*:623, 1952.

537. Murphy WA, Siegel MJ: Elbow fat pads with new signs and extended differential diagnoses. Radiology *124*:659, 1977.

538. Kamal AS, Austin RT: Dislocation of the median nerve and brachial artery in supracondylar fractures of the humerus. Injury *12*:161, 1980.

539. Symeonides PP, Paschaloglou C, Pagalides T: Radial nerve enclosed in the callus of a supracondylar fracture. J Bone Joint Surg [Br] *57*:523, 1975.

540. Tachdjian MO: Pediatric Orthopedics. Philadelphia, WB Saunders Co, 1972.

541. Arnold JA, Nascu RJ, Nelson CL: Supracondylar fractures of the humerus: The role of dynamic fractures in prevention of deformity. J Bone Joint Surg [Am] *59*:589, 1977.

542. Norman O: Roentgenological studies on dislocations in supracondylar fractures of the humerus. Ann Radiol *18*:395, 1975.

543. Fowles JV, Kassab MT: Displaced supracondylar fractures of the elbow in children. J Bone Joint Surg [Br] *56*:490, 1974.

544. Kamal AS, Austin RT: Dislocation of the median nerve and brachial artery in supracondylar fractures of the humerus. Injury *12*:161, 1980.

545. Rogers LF: Fractures and dislocations of the elbow. Semin Roentgenol *13*:97, 1978.

546. Smith L: Deformity following supracondylar fractures of the humerus. J Bone Joint Surg [Am] *42*:235, 1960.

547. D'Ambrosia RD: Supracondylar fractures of the humerus—prevention of cubitus varus. J Bone Joint Surg [Am] *54*:60, 1972.

548. Dodge HS: Displaced supracondylar fractures of the humerus in children—treatment by Dunlop's traction. J Bone Joint Surg [Am] *54*:1408, 1972.

549. Aitken AP, Smith L, Blackett CW: Supracondylar fractures in children. Am J Surg *59*:161, 1943.

550. Blount WP, Schulz I, Cassidy RH: Fractures of the elbow in children. JAMA *146*:699, 1951.

551. King D, Secor C: Bow elbow (cubitus varus). J Bone Joint Surg [Am] *33*:572, 1951.

552. Parkinson C: The supracondyloid process. Radiology *62*:556, 1954.

553. Engber WD, McBeath AA, Cowle AE: The supracondylar process. Clin Orthop *104*:228, 1974.

554. Barnard LB, McCoy SM: The supracondyloid processes of the humerus. J Bone Joint Surg *28*:845, 1946.

555. Thomsen PB: Processus supracondyloidea humeri with concomitant compression of the median nerve and the ulnar nerve. Acta Orthop Scand *48*:391, 1977.

556. Kolb LW, Moore RD: Fractures of the supracondylar process of the humerus. J Bone Joint Surg [Am] *49*:532, 1967.

557. Symeonides PP: The humerus supracondylar process syndrome. Clin Orthop *82*:141, 1972.

558. Sidor ML, Zuckerman JD, Lyon T, et al: The Neer classification system for proximal humeral fractures: An assessment of interobserver reliability and intraobserver reproducibility. J Bone Joint Surg [Am] *75*:1745, 1993.

559. Siebenrock KA, Gerber C: The reproducibility of classification of fractures of the proximal end of the humerus. J Bone Joint Surg [Am] *75*:175, 1993.

560. Burstein AH: Fracture classification systems: Do they work and are they useful? J Bone Joint Surg [Am] *75*:1743, 1993.

561. Quesada F: Technique for the roentgen diagnosis of fractures of the clavicle. Surg Gynecol Obstet *42*:424, 1926.

562. Weinberg B, Seife B, Alonso P: The apical oblique view of the clavicle: Its usefulness in neonatal and childhood trauma. Skel Radiol *20*:201, 1991.

563. Neer CS II: Fracture of the distal clavicle with detachment of the coracoclavicular ligaments in adults. J Trauma *3*:99, 1963.

564. Miller DS, Boswick JA Jr: Lesions of the brachial plexus associated with fractures of the clavicle. Clin Orthop *64*:144, 1969.

565. Howard FM, Shafer SJ: Injuries to the clavicle with neurovascular complications: A study of fourteen cases. J Bone Joint Surg [Am] *47*:1335, 1965.

566. Kay SP, Eckardt JJ: Brachial plexus palsy secondary to clavicular nonunion: Case report and literature survey. Clin Orthop *207*:219, 1986.

567. Weiner DS, O'Dell HW: Fractures of the first-rib associated with injuries to the clavicle. J Trauma *9*:412, 1969.

568. Goddard NJ, Stabler J, Albert JS: Atlanto-axial rotary fixation and fracture of the clavicle: An association and a classification. J Bone Joint Surg [Br] *72*:72, 1990.

569. Neer CS II: Nonunion of the clavicle. JAMA *96*:1006, 1960.

570. Sakellarides H: Pseudarthrosis of the clavicle: A report of twenty cases. J Bone Joint Surg [Am] *43*:130, 1961.

571. Manske DJ, Szabo RM: The operative treatment of mid-shaft clavicular non-unions. J Bone Joint Surg [Am] *67*:1367, 1985.

572. Ada JR, Miller ME: Scapular fractures: Analysis of 113 cases. Clin Orthop *269*:174, 1991.

573. Imatani RJ: Fractures of the scapula: A review of 53 fractures. J Trauma *15*:473, 1975.

574. McGahan JP, Rab GT, Dublin A: Fractures of the scapula. J Trauma *20*:880, 1980.

575. Varriale PL, Adler ML: Occult fracture of the glenoid without dislocation: A case report. J Bone Joint Surg [Am] *65*:688, 1983.

576. Goss TP: Fractures of the glenoid cavity. J Bone Joint Surg [Am] *74*:299, 1992.

577. Hardegger FJ, Simpson LA, Weber BG: The operative treatment of scapular fractures. J Bone Joint Surg [Br] *66*:725, 1984.

578. Heyse-Moore GH, Stoker DJ: Avulsion fractures of the scapula. Skel Radiol *9*:27, 1982.

579. Herscovici D Jr, Fiennes AGTW, Allgöwer M, et al: The floating shoulder: Ipsilateral clavicle and scapular neck fractures. J Bone Joint Surg [Br] *74*:362, 1992.

580. McLennan JG, Ungersma J: Pneumothorax complicating fracture of the scapula. J Bone Joint Surg [Am] *64*:598, 1982.

581. Banerjee AK, Field S: An unusual scapular fracture caused by a water skiing accident. Br J Radiol *58*:465, 1985.

582. Ishizuki M, Yamaura I, Isobe Y, et al: Avulsion fracture of the superior border of the scapula: Report of five cases. J Bone Joint Surg [Am] *63*:820, 1981.

583. Rask MR, Steinberg LH: Fracture of the acromion caused by muscle forces: A case report. J Bone Joint Surg [Am] *60*:1146, 1978.

584. Benton J, Nelson C: Avulsion of the coracoid process in an athlete. J Bone Joint Surg [Am] *53*:356, 1971.

585. Froimson AI: Fracture of the coracoid process of the scapula. J Bone Joint Surg [Am] *60*:710, 1978.

586. Stein RE, Bone J, Korn J: Axillary artery injury in closed fracture of the neck of the scapula: A case report. J Trauma *11*:528, 1971.

587. Nettrour LF, Krufky EL, Mueller RE, et al: Locked scapula: Intrathoracic dislocation of the inferior angle: A case report. J Bone Joint Surg [Am] *54*:413, 1972.

588. Oreck SL, Burgess A, Levine AM: Traumatic lateral displacement of the scapula: A radiographic sign of neurovascular disruption. J Bone Joint Surg [Am] *66*:758, 1984.

589. Rubenstein JD, Ebraheim NA, Kellam JF: Traumatic scapulothoracic dissociation. Radiology *157*:297, 1985.

590. Kelbel JM, Jardon OM, Huurman WW: Scapulothoracic dissociation: A case report. Clin Orthop *209*:210, 1986.

591. Richardson JD, McElvein RB, Trinkle JK: First rib fracture: A hallmark of severe trauma. Ann Surg *181*:251, 1975.

592. Lorentzen JE, Movin M: Fracture of the first rib. Acta Orthop Scand *47*:632, 1976.

593. Fisher RG, Ward RE, Ben-Menachem Y, et al: Arteriography and the fractured first rib: Too much for too little? AJR *138*:1059, 1982.

594. Woodring JH, Fried AM, Hatfield DR, et al: Fractures of first and second ribs: Predictive value for arterial and bronchial injury. AJR *138*:211, 1982.

595. Livoni JP, Barcia TC: Fracture of the first and second rib: Incidence of vascular injury relative to type of fracture. Radiology *145*:31, 1982.

596. Woodring JH, Royer JM, Todd EP: Upper rib fractures following median sternotomy. Ann Thorac Surg *39*:355, 1985.

597. Ward EF, Savoie FH, Hughes JL: Fractures of the diaphyseal humerus. *In* BD Browner, JB Jupiter, AM Levine, et al (Eds): Skeletal Trauma: Fractures, Dislocations, Ligamentous Injuries. Philadelphia, WB Saunders Co, 1992, p. 1177.

598. Garth WP Jr, Leberte MA, Cool TA: Recurrent fractures of the humerus in a baseball pitcher. J Bone Joint Surg [Am] *70*:305, 1988.

599. Heilbronner DM, Manoli A II, Morawa LG: Fractures of the humerus in arm wrestlers. Clin Orthop *149*:169, 1980.

600. Hartonas GD, Verettas DJ: Fracture of the humerus in a shotput athlete. Injury *18*:68, 1987.

601. Healy WL, White GM, Mick CA, et al: Nonunion of the humeral shaft. Clin Orthop *219*:206, 1987.

602. Reginato AJ, Feldman E, Rabinowitz JL: Traumatic chylous knee effusion. Ann Rheum Dis *44*:793, 1985.

603. Mast JW, Spiegel PG, Harvey JP Jr, et al: Fractures of the humeral shaft: A retrospective study of 240 adult fractures. Clin Orthop *112*:254, 1975.

604. Pierce RA Jr, Hodurski DF: Fractures of the humerus, radius and ulna in the same extremity. J Trauma *19*:182, 1979.

605. Burkhead WZ Jr: The biceps tendon. *In* CA Rockwood Jr, FA Matsen III (Eds): The Shoulder. Philadelphia, WB Saunders Co, 1990, p. 791.

606. Meyer AW: Spontaneous dislocation of the tendon of the long head of the biceps brachii. Arch Surg *13*:109, 1926.

607. Meyer AW: Spontaneous dislocation and destruction of the tendon of the long head of the biceps brachii. Arch Surg *17*:493, 1928.

608. Abbott LC, Saunders LB: Acute traumatic dislocation of the tendon of the long head of the biceps brachii: Report of 6 cases with operative findings. Surgery *6*:817, 1939.

609. Cone RO, Danzig L, Resnick D, et al: The bicipital groove: Radiographic, anatomic, and pathologic study. AJR *41*:781, 1983.

610. Hitchcock HH, Bechtol CO: Painful shoulder: Observations on the role of the tendon of the long head of the biceps brachii in its causation. J Bone Joint Surg [Am] *30*:263, 1948.

611. Habermeyer P, Kaiser E, Knappe M, et al: Functional anatomy and biomechanics of the long biceps tendon. Unfallchirurg *90*:319, 1987.

612. O'Donohue D: Subluxating biceps tendon in the athlete. Clin Orthop *164*:26, 1982.

613. Middleton WD, Remus WR, Totty WG, et al: Ultrasonographic evaluation of the rotator cuff and biceps tendon. J Bone Joint Surg [Am] *68*:440, 1986.

614. Ptasznik R, Hennessy O: Abnormalities of the biceps tendon of the shoulder: Sonographic findings. AJR *164*:409, 1995.

615. Tuckman GA: Abnormalities of the long head of the biceps tendon of the shoulder: MR imaging findings. AJR *163*:1183, 1994.

616. Collier SG, Wynn-Jones CH: Displacement of the biceps with subscapularis avulsion. J Bone Joint Surg [Br] *72*:145, 1990.

617. Levinsohn EM, Santelli ED IV: Bicipital groove dysplasia and medial dislocation of the biceps brachii tendon. Skel Radiol *20*:419, 1991.

618. Slätis P, Aalto K: Medial dislocation of the tendon of the long head of the biceps brachii. Acta Orthop Scand *50*:73, 1979.

619. Paschal SO, Hutton KS, Weatherall PT: Isolated avulsion fracture of the lesser tuberosity of the humerus in adolescents: A report of two cases. J Bone Joint Surg [Am] *77*:1427, 1995.

620. Farin PU, Jaroma H, Harju A, et al: Medial displacement of the biceps brachii tendon: Evaluation with dynamic sonography during maximal external shoulder rotation. Radiology *195*:845, 1995.

621. Chan TW, Dalinka MK, Kneeland JB, et al: Biceps tendon dislocation: Evaluation with MR imaging. Radiology *179*:649, 1991.

622. Cervilla V, Schweitzer ME, Ho C, et al: Medial dislocation of the biceps brachii tendon: Appearance at MR imaging. Radiology *180*:523, 1991.

623. van Leersum M, Schweitzer ME: Magnetic resonance imaging of the biceps complex. MRI Clin North Am *1*:77, 1993.

624. Lyons FR, Rockwood CA Jr: Snapping scapula. *In* JC DeLee, D Drez Jr (Eds): Orthopedic Sports Medicine: Principles and Practice. Philadelphia, WB Saunders Co, 1994, p. 568.

625. de Haart M, van der Linden ES, de Vet HCW, et al: The value of computed tomography in the diagnosis of grating scapula. Skel Radiol *23*:357, 1994.

626. Milch H: Snapping scapula. Clin Orthop *20*:139, 1961.

627. Sisto DJ, Jobe FW: The operative treatment of scapulothoracic bursitis in professional pitchers. Am J Sports Med *14*:192, 1986.

628. Fritz RC, Helms CA, Steinbach LS, et al: Suprascapular nerve entrapment: Evaluation with MR imaging. Radiology *182*:437, 1992.

629. Callahan JD, Scully TB, Shapiro SA, et al: Suprascapular nerve entrapment: A series of 27 cases. J Neurosurg *74*:893, 1991.

630. Ganzhorn RW, Hocker JT, Horowitz M, et al: Suprascapular-nerve entrapment. J Bone Joint Surg [Am] *63*:492, 1981.

631. Garcia G, McQueen D: Bilateral suprascapular-nerve entrapment syndrome. J Bone Joint Surg [Am] *63*:491, 1981.

632. Thompson RC, Schneider W, Kennedy T: Entrapment neuropathy of the inferior branch of the suprascapular nerve by ganglia. Clin Orthop *166*:185, 1982.

633. Demaio M, Drez D Jr, Mullins RC, et al: The inferior transverse scapular ligament as a possible cause of entrapment neuropathy of the nerve to the infraspinatus: A brief note. J Bone Joint Surg [Am] *73*:1061, 1991.

634. Takagishi K, Maeda K, Ikeda T, et al: Ganglion causing paralysis of the suprascapular nerve: Diagnosis by MRI and ultrasonography. Acta Orthop Scand *62*:391, 1991.

635. Cahill BR, Palmer RE: Quadrilateral space syndrome. J Hand Surg *8*:65, 1983.

636. Francel TJ, Dellon AL, Compbell JN: Quadrilateral space syndrome: Diagnosis and operative decompression technique. Plast Reconstr Surg *87*:911, 1991.

637. Redler MR, Ruland LJ III, McCue FC III: Quadrilateral space syndrome in a throwing athlete. Am J Sports Med *14*:511, 1986.

638. Cormier PJ, Matalon TAS, Wolin PM: Quadrilateral space syndrome: A rare cause of shoulder pain. Radiology *167*:797, 1988.

639. Linker CS, Helms CA, Fritz RC: Quadrilateral space syndrome: Findings at MR imaging. Radiology *188*:675, 1993.

640. Mochizuki T, Isoda H, Masui T, et al: Occulsion of the posterior humeral circumflex artery: Detection with MR angiography in healthy volunteers and in a patient with quadrilateral space syndrome. AJR *163*:625, 1994.

641. Resnick D, Cone RO III: The nature of humeral pseudocysts. Radiology *150*:27, 1984.

642. Helms CA: Pseudocysts of the humerus. AJR *131*:287, 1978.

643. Pettersson H: Bilateral dysplasia of the neck of the scapula and associated anomalies. Acta Radiol *22*:81, 1981.

644. Triquet J, Trellu M, Trellu X, et al: Dysplasie monoepiphysaire de la cavité glenoid de l'omoplate. Arch Fr Pediatr *37*:683, 1980.

645. Owen R: Bilateral glenoid hypoplasia: Report of five cases. J Bone Joint Surg [Br] *35*:262, 1953.

646. McClure JG, Raney RB: Anomalies of the scapula. Clin Orthop *110*:22, 1975.

647. Sutro CJ: Dentated articular surface of the glenoid—an anomaly. Bull Hosp Joint Dis *28*:104, 1967.

648. Resnick D, Walter RD, Crudale AS: Bilateral dysplasia of the scapular neck. AJR *139*:387, 1982.

649. Kozlowski K, Colavita N, Morris L, et al: Bilateral glenoid dysplasia: Report of 8 cases. Australas Radiol *29*:174, 1985.

650. Lintner DM, Sebastianelli WJ, Hanks GA, et al: Glenoid dysplasia: A case report and review of the literature. Clin Orthop *283*:145, 1992.

651. Kozlowski K, Scougall J: Congenital bilateral glenoid hypoplasia: A report of four cases. Br J Radiol *60*:705, 1987.

652. Borenstein ZCF, Mink J, Oppenheim W, et al: Case report 655. Skel Radiol *20*:134, 1991.

653. Wirth MA, Lyons FR, Rockwood CA Jr: Hypoplasia of the glenoid: A review of sixteen patients. J Bone Joint Surg [Am] *75*:1175, 1993.

654. Callaghan JJ, York JJ, McNeish LM, et al: Unusual anomaly of the scapula defined by arthroscopy and computed tomographic arthrography: Report of a case. J Bone Joint Surg [Am] *70*:452, 1988.

655. Manns RA, Davies AM: Glenoid hypoplasia: Assessment by computed tomographic arthrography. Clin Radiol *43*:316, 1991.

656. Hulstyn MJ, Fadale PD: Arthroscopic anatomy of the shoulder. Orthop Clin North Am *26*:597, 1995.

657. Edelson JG, Luchs J: Aspects of coracoacromial ligament anatomy of interest to the arthroscopic surgeon. Arthroscopy *11*:715, 1995.

658. Jobe CM: Posterior superior glenoid impingement: Expanded spectrum. Arthroscopy *11*:530, 1995.

659. Traughber P, Czech M: Accuracy of fat-suppressed MR imaging of the shoulder for detection of partial-thickness rotator cuff tears. Radiology *196*:293, 1996.

660. Cardinal E, Buckwalter KA, Braunstein EM, et al: Amyloidosis of the shoulder in patients on chronic hemodialysis: Sonographic findings. AJR *166*:153, 1996.

661. Wolf EM, Cheng JC, Dickson K: Humeral avulsion of the glenohumeral ligaments as a cause of anterior shoulder instability. Arthroscopy *11*:600, 1995.

662. Brower AC, Sweet DE, Keats TE: Condensing osteitis of the clavicle: A new entity. AJR *121*:17, 1974.

663. Solovjev M: Osteitis condensans claviculae. ROFO *125*:375, 1976.

664. Teates CD, Brower AC, Williamson BRJ, et al: Bone scans in condensing osteitis of the clavicle. South Med J *71*:736, 1978.

665. Greenspan A, Gerscovich E, Szabo RM, et al: Condensing osteitis of the clavicle: A rare but frequently misdiagnosed condition. AJR *156*:1011, 1991.

666. Outwater E, Oates E: Condensing osteitis of the clavicle: Case report and review of the literature. J Nucl Med *29*:1122, 1988.

667. Weiner SN, Levy M, Bernstein R, et al: Condensing osteitis of the clavicle: A case report. J Bone Joint Surg [Am] *66*:1484, 1984.

668. Getz JD, Recht MP, Piraino DW, et al: Acromial morphology: Relation to sex, age, symmetry, and subacromial enthesophytes. Radiology *199*:737, 1996.

669. Palmer WE: MR arthrography: Is it worthwhile? Topics Magn Res Imag *8*:24, 1996.

670. Needell SD, Zlatkin MB, Sher JS, et al: MR imaging of the rotator cuff: Peritendinous and bone abnormalities in an asymptomatic population. AJR *166*:863, 1996.

671. Sonin AH, Peduto AJ, Fitzgerald SW, et al: MR imaging of the rotator cuff mechanism: Comparison of spin-echo and turbo spin-echo sequences. AJR *167*:333, 1996.

672. Singson RD, Hoang T, Dan S, et al: MR evaluation of rotator cuff pathology using T2-weighted fast spin-echo technique with and without fat suppression. AJR *166*:1061, 1996.

673. Mormino MA, Gross RM, McCarthy JA: Captured shoulder: A complication of rotator cuff surgery. Arthroscopy *12*:457, 1996.

674. Anzilotti KF Jr, Schweitzer ME, Oliveri M, et al: Rotator cuff strain: A posttraumatic mimicker of tendonitis on MRI. Skeletal Radiol *25*:555, 1996.

675. Farin PU: Consistency of rotator-cuff calcifications. Observations on plain radiography, sonography, computed tomography, and needle treatment. Invest Radiol *31*:300, 1996.

676. Farin PU, Räsänen H, Jaroma H, et al: Rotator cuff calcifications: Treatment with ultrasound-guided percutaneous needle aspiration and lavage. Skeletal Radiol *25*:551, 1996.

677. Gusmer PB, Potter HG: Imaging of shoulder instability. Clin Sports Med *14*:777, 1995.

678. Farin PU, Kaukanen E, Jaroma H, et al: Hill-Sachs lesion: Sonographic detection. Skeletal Radiol *25*:559, 1996.

679. Gusmer PB, Potter HG, Schatz JA, et al: Labral injuries: Accuracy of detection with unenhanced MR imaging of the shoulder. Radiology *200*:519, 1996.

680. Liu SH, Henry MH, Nuccion S, et al: Diagnosis of glenoid labral tears. A comparison between magnetic resonance imaging and clinical examinations. Am J Sports Med *24*:149, 1996.

681. Longo C, Loredo R, Yu J, et al: MRI of the glenoid labrum with gross anatomic correlation. J Comput Assist Tomogr *20*:487, 1996.

682. Tuite MJ, Orwin JF: Anterosuperior labral variants of the shoulder: Appearance on gradient-recalled echo and fast spin-echo MR images. Radiology *199*:537, 1996.

683. Tirman PFJ, Feller JF, Palmer WE, et al: The Buford complex—a variation of normal shoulder anatomy: MR arthrographic imaging features. AJR *166*:869, 1996.

684. Jahnke AH Jr, Greis PE, Hawkins RJ: Arthroscopic evaluation and treatment of shoulder instability. Orth Clin North Am 26:613, 1995.

685. Farin PU, Jaroma H: The bicipital groove of the humerus: Sonographic and radiographic correlation. Skeletal Radiol 25:215, 1996.

686. Edelson JG: Variations in the anatomy of the scapula with reference to the snapping scapula. Clin Orthop Rel Res 322:111, 1996.

687. Edelson JG: Localized glenoid hypoplasia. An anatomic variation of possible clinical significance. Clin Orthop Rel Res 321:189, 1995.

688. Trout TE, Resnick D: Glenoid hypoplasia and its relationship to instability. Skeletal Radiol 25:37, 1996.

689. Yu JS, Weis LD, Vaughan LM, et al: MRI of elastofibroma dorsi. J Comput Assist Tomogr 19:601, 1995.

690. Thomazeau H, Rolland Y, Lucas C, et al: Atrophy of the supraspinatus belly: Assessment by MRI in 55 patients with rotator cuff pathology. Acta Orthop Scand 67:264, 1996.

691. Gaenslen ES, Satterlee CC, Hinson GW: Magnetic resonance imaging for evaluation of failed repairs of the rotator cuff: Relationship to operative findings. J Bone Joint Surg [AM] 78:1391, 1996.

692. Bureau NJ, Dussault RG, Keats TE: Imaging of bursae around the shoulder joint. Skeletal Radiol 25:513, 1996.

693. Griffith JF, Peh WCG, Evans NS, et al: Multiple rice body formation in chronic subacromial/subdeltoid bursitis: MR appearances. Clin Radiol 51:511, 1996.

694. Tuckman GA, Devlin TC: Axillary nerve injury after anterior glenohumeral dislocation: MR findings in three patients. AJR 167:695, 1996.

695. Smith DK, Chopp TM, Aufdemorte TB, et al: Sublabral recess of the superior glenoid labrum: Study of cadavers with conventional nonenhanced MR imaging, MR arthrography, anatomic dissection, and limited histologic examination. Radiology 201:251, 1996.

696. Oberlander MA, Morgan BE, Visotsky JL: The BHAGL lesion: A new variant of anterior shoulder instability. Arthroscopy 12:627, 1996.

The elbow represents the important functional link between the upper arm and the hand and wrist. Through the elbow's movements, the hand can be brought into the myriad positions required for daily activities. The joint about the elbow has three constituents: (1) humeroradial—the area between the capitulum of the humerus and the facet on the radial head; (2) humeroulnar—the area between the trochlea of the humerus and the trochlear notch of the ulna; and (3) superior (proximal) radioulnar—the area between the head of the radius and radial notch of the ulna and the annular ligament. These constituents act in concert during movements of the joint. The primary motions of the elbow, flexion and extension, account for its designation as a hinge joint, although axial rotation also occurs at this joint.

This chapter addresses the complex anatomy and function of the elbow, with consideration given to bony, ligamentous, tendinous, and soft tissue structures. Important pathologic conditions affecting the joint are described, with emphasis placed on assessment of these conditions with advanced imaging methods.

ANATOMY

Osseous Anatomy

The osseous structures about the elbow include the proximal ends of the ulna and radius and the distal end of the humerus (Figs. 13–1 and 13–2).

The proximal end of the ulna contains two processes, the olecranon and the coronoid. The olecranon process is smooth posteriorly at the site of attachment of the triceps tendon. Its anterior surface provides the site of attachment of the capsule of the elbow joint. The coronoid process contains the radial notch, below which is the ulnar tuberosity.

The proximal end of the radius consists of head, neck, and tuberosity. The radial head is disc-shaped, containing a shallow, cupped articular surface, which is intimate with the capitulum of the humerus. The articular circumference of the head is largest medially, where it articulates with the radial notch of the ulna. The radial neck is the smooth, constricted part of the bone below the radial head. The radial tuberosity is located beneath the medial aspect of the neck.

The distal aspect of the humerus is a wide, flattened structure. The medial third of its articular surface, termed the trochlea, is intimate with the ulna. Lateral to the trochlea is the capitulum, which articulates with the radius. The sulcus is between the trochlea and the capitulum. A hollow area is found on the posterior surface of the humerus above the trochlea, termed the olecranon fossa; the posterior capsular attachment of the humerus is located above this fossa. A smaller fossa, the coronoid fossa, lies above the trochlea on the anterior surface of the humerus, and a radial fossa lies adjacent to it, above the capitulum. The anterior capsular attachment to the humerus is located above these fossae. When the elbow is fully extended, the tip of the olecranon process is located in the olecranon fossa, and when the elbow is flexed, the coronoid process of the ulna is found in the coronoid fossa and the margin of the radial head is located in the radial fossa.

The medial epicondyle is a blunt osseous projection of the distal end of the humerus. The posterior smooth surface of this epicondyle is crossed by the ulnar nerve.

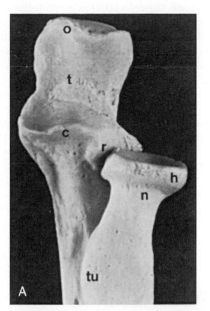

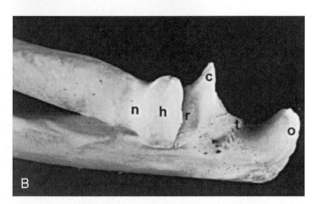

Figure 13–1
Elbow joint: Osseous anatomy. Radius and ulna.
  A Radius and ulna, anterior aspect. Note the olecranon (o), coronoid process (c), trochlear notch (t), radial notch (r), radial head (h), radial neck (n), and radial tuberosity (tu).
  B Radius and ulna, lateral aspect.

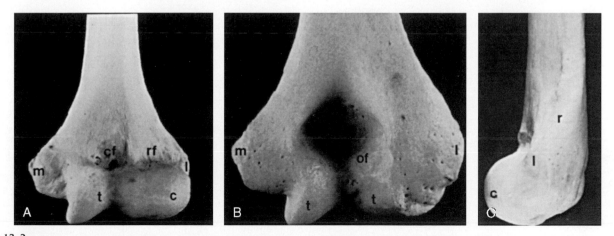

Figure 13–2
Elbow joint: Osseous anatomy. Distal end of the humerus. An anterior view **(A)** reveals the trochlea (t), capitulum (c), medial epicondyle (m), lateral epicondyle (l), coronoid fossa (cf), and radial fossa (rf). A posterior view **(B)**, oriented in the same fashion, outlines some of the same structures and, in addition, the olecranon fossa (of). In a view of the lateral surface of the humerus **(C)**, observe the capitulum (c), lateral epicondyle (l), and lateral supracondylar ridge (r).

The anterior surface of the medial epicondyle is the site of attachment of superficial flexor muscles of the forearm. The lateral epicondyle is located on the lateral surface of the distal end of the humerus. Its lateral and anterior surface represents the site of origin of the superficial group of extensor muscles of the forearm.

The degree of congruity of apposing articulating surfaces of radius, ulna, and humerus varies in different positions of the elbow joint; the greatest congruity exists when the forearm is in a position midway between full supination and full pronation and the elbow is flexed to a right angle. When the elbow is extended, the inferior and posterior aspects of the trochlea contact the ulna; when the elbow is flexed, the trochlear notch slides forward on the anterior aspect of the ulna, exposing the posterior aspect of that bone. The capitulum and the radial head are reciprocally curved; in a midprone position, extensive contact occurs between radius and capitulum.

Articular Anatomy

The articular surface of the humerus consists of a grooved trochlea, the spheroidal capitulum, and a sulcus between them (Fig. 13–3). Almost all of the trochlea is covered with a layer of articular cartilage. The capitulum is also covered with cartilage, which is approximately 2 mm thick. The ulnar articulating surface is the trochlear notch (Fig. 13–4). This notch is covered with cartilage, which is interrupted in a transverse fashion across its deepest aspect. Thus, articular cartilage covering the anterior aspect of the notch (that related to the coronoid process) is separated from articular cartilage located posteriorly in the notch (in the area of the olecranon process) by fatty tissue. A longitudinal ridge in the notch further divides the articular surface into four parts, two anterior and two posterior.[1] The troch-

lear notch of the ulna and the trochlea of the humerus articulate. The radial articulating area is the radial head (see Fig. 13–4), which is covered with articular cartilage except in its anterolateral portion. This portion of the radial head lacks a subchondral bone plate, is relatively weak, and is fractured most often.[1] The cartilage of the radial head is continuous with that along the sides of the radial head, including an area in the superior radioulnar joint. The radial head articulates with the capitulum and the capitulotrochlear groove.

A fibrous capsule completely invests the elbow. The attachments of its broad, thin, and weak anterior part are the anterior humerus along the medial epicondyle and above the coronoid and radial fossae, the anterior surface of the ulnar coronoid process, and the annular ligament. The superior attachments of its thin, weak posterior part are the posterior surface of the humerus behind the capitulum, the olecranon fossa, and the medial epicondyle. Inferomedially the capsule is attached to the upper and lateral margins of the olecranon. Laterally the capsule is continuous with that about the superior radioulnar joint. The fibrous capsule is strengthened by transverse and obliquely directed fibrous bands that originate above the medial aspect of the trochlea and insert into the annular ligament and that originate above the capitulum and insert along the lateral aspect of the coronoid process (Fig. 13–5). The capsule also is strengthened at the sides of the joint by the radial and ulnar collateral ligaments. The anterior aspect of the capsule is lax in flexion and taut in extension of the joint. The normal capacity of the fully distended elbow joint is 25 to 30 ml.

The synovial membrane of the elbow lines the deep surface of the fibrous capsule and annular ligament. It extends from the articular surface of the humerus and contacts the olecranon, radial, and coronoid fossae and the medial surface of the trochlea. A synovial fold projects into the joint between the radius and ulna,

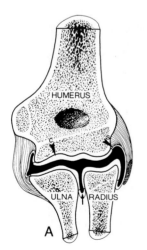
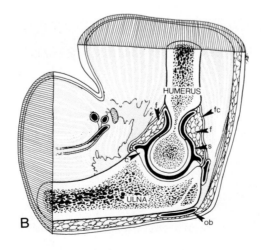
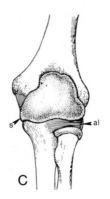
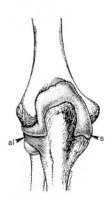

Figure 13–3
Elbow joint: Articular anatomy.
  A, B Drawings of coronal (**A**) and sagittal (**B**) sections. Observe synovium (s), articular cartilage (c), fibrous capsule (fc), anterior and posterior fat pads (f), and olecranon bursa (ob). Note the extension of the elbow joint between radius and ulna as the superior radioulnar joint (arrow).
  C Drawings of the anterior (left) and posterior (right) aspects of the distended elbow joint with the fibrous capsule removed. Observe the synovial membrane (s) and the annular ligament (al) extending around the proximal radius, constricting the joint cavity.
  (From Warwick R, Williams P [Eds]. Gray's Anatomy. 15th British edition. Philadelphia, WB Saunders Co, 1973.)

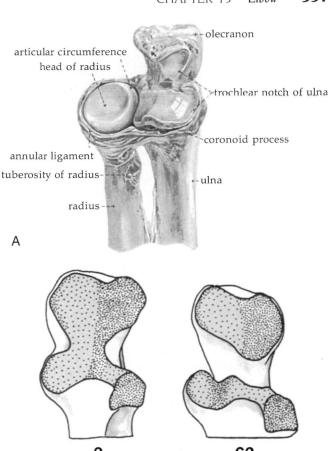

A

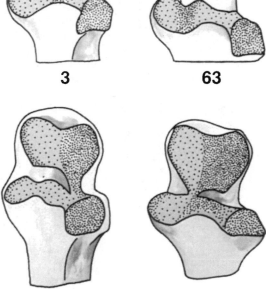

B

3   **63**

32   **2**

Figure 13–4
Elbow joint: Articular anatomy.

A Hyaline cartilage covers approximately 240 degrees of the outside circumference of the radial head, allowing its articulation with the proximal end of the ulna at the radial notch of the ulna. (From Langman J, Woerdeman MW: Atlas of Medical Anatomy. Philadelphia, WB Saunders, 1978.)

B The relative percentage of hyaline cartilage distribution at the end of the ulna is indicated by the number below each drawing. (Redrawn from Tillman B: A Contribution to the Function Morphology of Articular Surfaces. Translated by G Konorza. Stuttgart, George Thieme; Littleton, Mass. P. S. G. Publishing, 1978.)

partially dividing the articulation into humeroulnar and humeroradial portions.

Several fat pads are located between fibrous capsule and synovial membrane (Fig. 13–6). Fat pads are found near the synovial fold between the radius and ulna and over the olecranon, coronoid, and radial fossae. These fat pads are extrasynovial but intracapsular. On lateral radiographs, an anterior radiolucent area represents the summation of radial and coronoid fossae fat pads. These fat pads are pressed into their respective fossae by the brachialis muscle during extension of the elbow. A posterior radiolucent region represents the olecranon fossa fat pad. It is pressed into this fossa by the triceps muscle during flexion of the elbow. The anterior fat pad nor-

mally assumes a teardrop configuration anterior to the distal end of the humerus on lateral radiographs of the elbow exposed in approximately 90 degrees of joint flexion. The posterior fat pad normally is not visible in radiographs of the elbow exposed in flexion. Its occasional appearance on such radiographs may reflect unusually large fat pads or slightly oblique projections. Any intra-articular process that is associated with a mass or fluid may produce a "positive fat-pad sign" characterized by elevation and displacement of anterior and posterior fat pads.

The superior radioulnar joint exists between the radial head and the osseous-fibrous ring formed by the annular ligament and the radial notch of the ulna. This

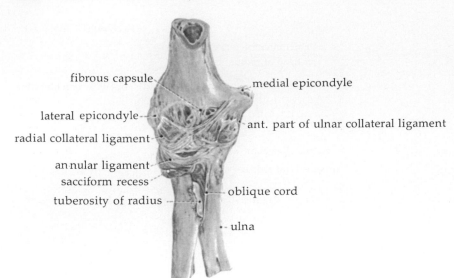

fibrous capsule
medial epicondyle
lateral epicondyle
ant. part of ulnar collateral ligament
radial collateral ligament
annular ligament
sacciform recess
tuberosity of radius
oblique cord
ulna

Figure 13–5
Elbow joint: Articular anatomy. The fibers of the anterior capsule have a cruciate orientation that provides a good deal of its strength. (From Langman J, Woerdeman MW: Atlas of Medical Anatomy. Philadelphia, WB Saunders, 1978.)

notch is lined with articular cartilage that is continuous with that on the lower part of the trochlear notch. The radial head is also covered with cartilage. The annular ligament is attached anteriorly to the anterior margin of the radial notch (Fig. 13–7). It encircles the head of the radius, and posteriorly it contains several bands that attach to the ulna near the posterior margin of the radial notch. The superior portion of the annular ligament is lined with fibrocartilage where it apposes the circumference of the radial head. The inferior portion of the annular ligament is covered with synovial membrane, which extends downward onto the radial neck. The quadrate ligament (ligament of Denucé), a thin, fibrous layer, covers the synovial membrane.

Several bursae may be identified about the elbow. As in other anatomic sites, these bursae often are described as deep or superficial (subcutaneous) in location. Along the posterior aspect of the elbow, a subcutaneous bursa,

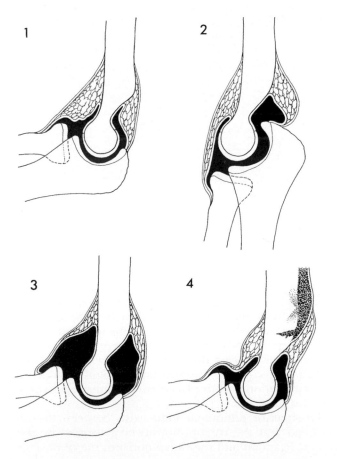

1

2

3

4

Figure 13–6
Elbow joint: Normal and abnormal appearance of intracapsular fat pads. Schematic drawings of anterior and posterior fat pads in normal and abnormal situations. Normally (1), the extrasynovial anterior and posterior fat pads are closely applied to the distal end of the humerus. In extension (2), the anterior fat pad is pressed tightly against the humerus, whereas the posterior fat pad may be elevated by contact between the olecranon and humerus. With a joint effusion (3), both anterior and posterior fat pads may be elevated by intra-articular fluid. With distal humeral fractures (4), a paradoxic elevation of the posterior fat pad may occur. (From Murphy WA, Siegel MJ: Radiology *124*:659, 1977.)

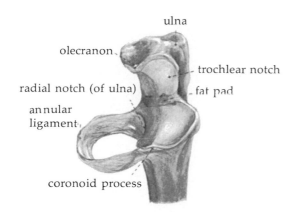

Figure 13–7
Elbow joint: Articular anatomy—annular ligament. The annular ligament constitutes approximately four fifths of a complete circle and stabilizes the radial head in the radial notch of the ulna. (From Langman J, Woerdeman MW: Atlas of Medical Anatomy. Philadelphia, W. B. Saunders, 1976.)

the olecranon bursa, separates the skin from the ulnar olecranon. It is situated like a cap on the olecranon process. Other, less constant bursae are found within or about the triceps tendon, deep to the anconeus muscle, deep to the common extensor tendon, between the biceps tendon and the tuberosity of the radius, between the biceps tendon and the ulna, between the ulnar nerve and the medial epicondyle, and subcutaneously about the medial and lateral epicondyles.[1]

Ligaments

Although classic descriptions of ligamentous anatomy of the elbow emphasize the radial and ulnar collateral ligaments, which reinforce the fibrous capsule of the joint[2] (Figs. 13–8 and 13–9), more recent investigations have indicated some variability in ligamentous anatomy, particularly on the radial aspect of the elbow. According to Morrey,[1] a lateral ligament complex can be identified, consisting of four components (see Fig. 13–8C): radial collateral ligament, annular ligament, lateral ulnar collateral ligament, and accessory lateral collateral ligament. The radial collateral ligament, less distinct and more variable than the ulnar collateral ligament on the medial side of the elbow, is a thick, roughly triangular band of fibrous tissue that attaches superiorly to the lateral epicondyle of the humerus, beneath the common origin of the extensor muscles, and inferiorly to the radial notch of the ulna and annular ligament. The ligament remains taut throughout the normal range of flexion and extension of the elbow. The annular ligament is circular in shape and attaches to the anterior and posterior margins of the radial notch of the ulna. It serves as a restraining ligament, maintaining the radial head in contact with the ulna and preventing withdrawal or inferior displacement of the head of the radius from its socket. The lateral ulnar collateral ligament originates from the lateral epicondyle and blends with the fibers of the annular ligament.[1] It extends distally to insert in the tubercle of the crest of the supinator on the ulna. Morrey[1] believes this ligament provides stability to the ulnohumeral joint, is the main lateral stabilizer of

the elbow, is taut in both flexion and extension of the joint, and is deficient in cases of posterolateral rotary instability of the elbow. An accessory lateral collateral ligament is not present uniformly and represents discrete fibers attaching to the supinator tubercle without a contribution to the posterior portion of the radial collateral ligament. When present, this ligament may serve to stabilize the annular ligament further during varus stress. One additional structure, the oblique cord, is an inconstant bundle of fibrous tissue that extends from the lateral side of the tuberosity of the ulna to the radius just below the radial tuberosity.[1] This structure may have limited functional importance. It is taut with full supination of the forearm, and its contracture may lead to limitation of such supination.

The medial (ulnar) collateral ligament is composed of three distinct bands that are continuous with each other (see Fig. 13–8A). The anterior band extends from the anterior aspect of the medial epicondyle of the humerus to the medial edge of the coronoid process[187]; a posterior band passes from the posterior aspect of the medial epicondyle to the medial edge of the olecranon; a thin intermediate band extends from the medial epicondyle to merge via a transverse or oblique band (the ligament of Cooper) with the anterior and posterior bands on the coronoid process and olecranon. Of these three bands, the anterior band (or bundle) is the most discrete, the posterior band appears as a thickening of the capsule (best defined with the elbow in 90 degrees of flexion), and the intermediate band with its transverse component often cannot be identified. Medial stability is provided mainly by the anterior band of the medial collateral ligament. This band resists valgus stress to the elbow, although additional, or secondary, resistance to valgus stress is provided by the flexor pronator muscle mass, the radiocapitular joint, and the joint capsule of the elbow.[3]

Muscles and Tendons

The many muscles about the elbow can be divided conveniently into four groups: posterior group, anterior group, lateral group, and medial group.[2, 4] The muscles of the posterior group are the triceps and the anconeus (Fig. 13–10). The triceps consists of three muscle bellies: the long head of the triceps muscle arises by a strong tendon from the infraglenoid tubercle of the scapula near the inferior margin of the glenoid cavity, and it descends into the arm between the teres major and teres minor muscles; the lateral head of the triceps muscle originates from the posterior and lateral surfaces of the humerus and from the lateral intermuscular septum; and the medial head of the triceps muscle arises from the posterior surface of the humerus, medial and below the radial groove, and from the medial and lower part of the lateral intermuscular septum. After receiving the muscular fibers, the tendon of the triceps muscle descends to attach to the upper surface of the olecranon process of the ulna and to the antebrachial fascia near the anconeus muscle and tendon. The anconeus muscle is small and triangular, arising from a tendon on the posterior surface of the lateral epicondyle of the hu-

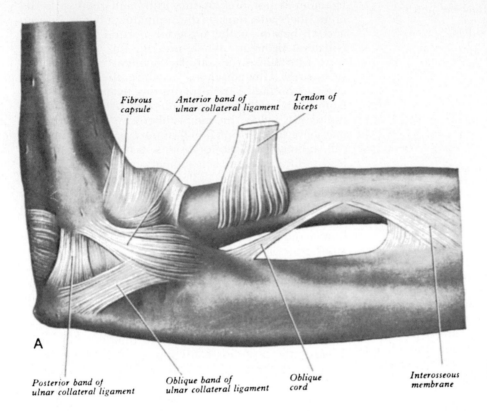

A

Fibrous capsule   *Anterior band of ulnar collateral ligament*   *Tendon of biceps*

Posterior band of ulnar collateral ligament   *Oblique band of ulnar collateral ligament*   *Oblique cord*   *Interosseous membrane*

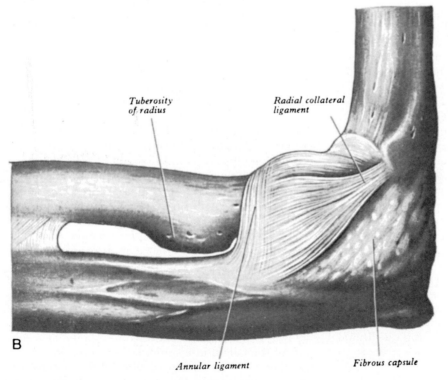

B

Tuberosity of radius   *Radial collateral ligament*

Annular ligament   *Fibrous capsule*

Figure 13–8
Elbow joint: Ligamentous anatomy.
 A Medial aspect of the elbow.
 B Lateral aspect of the elbow.
 (**A, B,** From Williams PL, Warwick R [Eds]: Gray's Anatomy. 36th British edition. Edinburgh, Churchill Livingstone, 1980, p 431.)

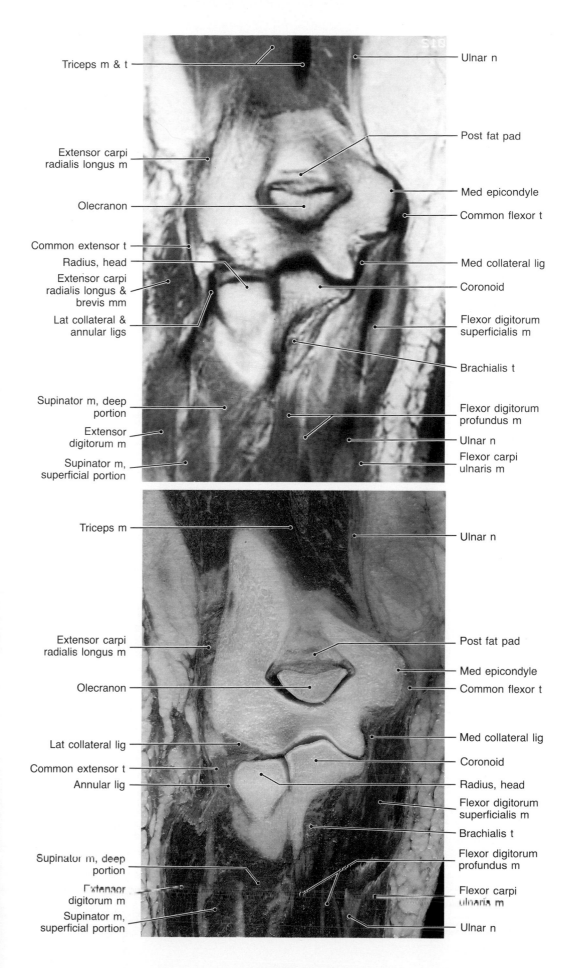

Triceps m & t

Extensor carpi
radialis longus m

Olecranon

Common extensor t

Radius, head

Extensor carpi
radialis longus &
brevis mm

Lat collateral &
annular ligs

Supinator m, deep
portion

Extensor
digitorum m

Supinator m,
superficial portion

Ulnar n

Post fat pad

Med epicondyle

Common flexor t

Med collateral lig

Coronoid

Flexor digitorum
superficialis m

Brachialis t

Flexor digitorum
profundus m

Ulnar n

Flexor carpi
ulnaris m

Triceps m

Extensor carpi
radialis longus m

Olecranon

Lat collateral lig

Common extensor t

Annular lig

Supinator m, deep
portion

Extensor
digitorum m

Supinator m,
superficial portion

Ulnar n

Post fat pad

Med epicondyle

Common flexor t

Med collateral lig

Coronoid

Radius, head

Flexor digitorum
superficialis m

Brachialis t

Flexor digitorum
profundus m

Flexor carpi
ulnaris m

Ulnar n

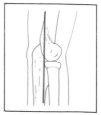

PLATE 13–1

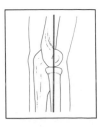

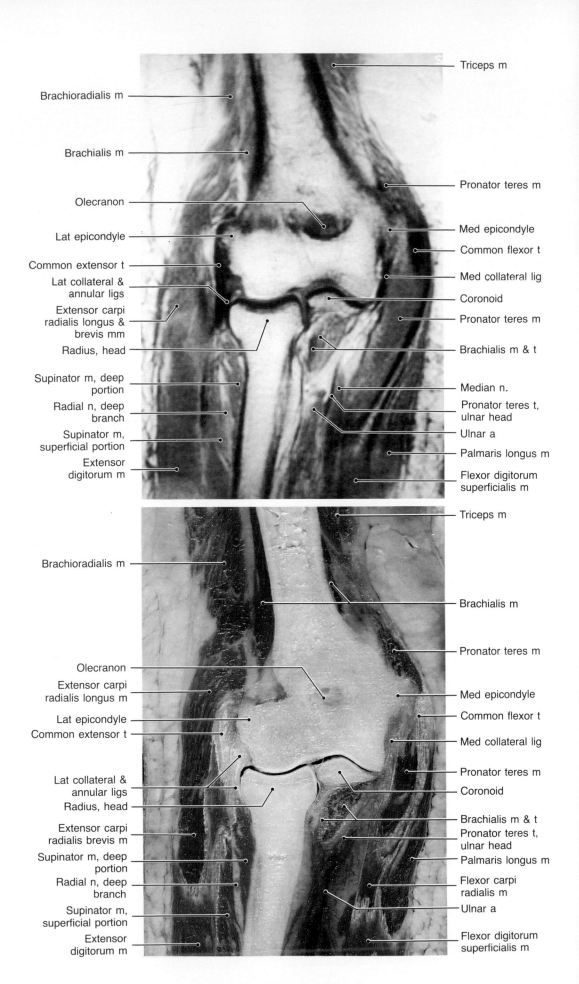

Triceps m

Brachioradialis m

Brachialis m

Olecranon

Lat epicondyle

Common extensor t

Lat collateral &
annular ligs

Extensor carpi
radialis longus &
brevis mm

Radius, head

Supinator m, deep
portion

Radial n, deep
branch

Supinator m,
superficial portion

Extensor
digitorum m

Pronator teres m

Med epicondyle

Common flexor t

Med collateral lig

Coronoid

Pronator teres m

Brachialis m & t

Median n.

Pronator teres t,
ulnar head

Ulnar a

Palmaris longus m

Flexor digitorum
superficialis m

Triceps m

Brachioradialis m

Brachialis m

Pronator teres m

Olecranon

Extensor carpi
radialis longus m

Lat epicondyle

Common extensor t

Med epicondyle

Common flexor t

Med collateral lig

Pronator teres m

Coronoid

Lat collateral &
annular ligs

Radius, head

Extensor carpi
radialis brevis m

Supinator m, deep
portion

Radial n, deep
branch

Supinator m,
superficial portion

Extensor
digitorum m

Brachialis m & t

Pronator teres t,
ulnar head

Palmaris longus m

Flexor carpi
radialis m

Ulnar a

Flexor digitorum
superficialis m

PLATE 13-2

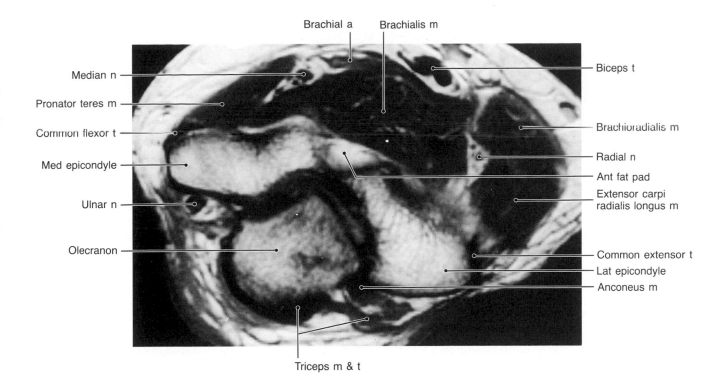

Brachial a — Brachialis m

Median n

Pronator teres m

Common flexor t

Med epicondyle

Ulnar n

Olecranon

Biceps t

Brachioradialis m

Radial n

Ant fat pad

Extensor carpi radialis longus m

Common extensor t

Lat epicondyle

Anconeus m

Triceps m & t

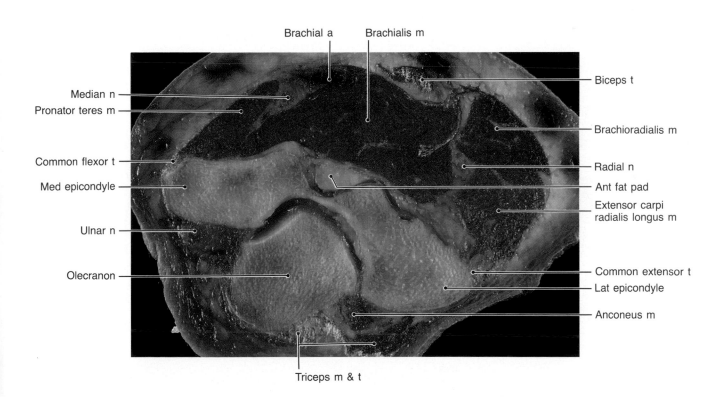

Brachial a — Brachialis m

Median n

Pronator teres m

Common flexor t

Med epicondyle

Ulnar n

Olecranon

Biceps t

Brachioradialis m

Radial n

Ant fat pad

Extensor carpi radialis longus m

Common extensor t

Lat epicondyle

Anconeus m

Triceps m & t

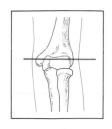

PLATE 13-3

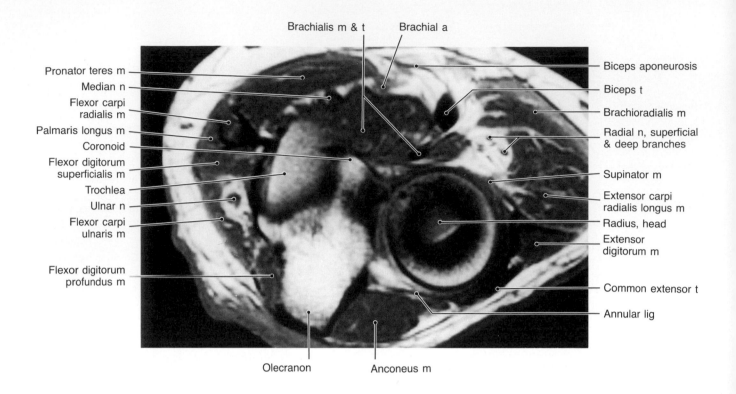

Brachialis m & t — Brachial a

Pronator teres m

Median n

Flexor carpi radialis m

Palmaris longus m

Coronoid

Flexor digitorum superficialis m

Trochlea

Ulnar n

Flexor carpi ulnaris m

Flexor digitorum profundus m

Biceps aponeurosis

Biceps t

Brachioradialis m

Radial n, superficial & deep branches

Supinator m

Extensor carpi radialis longus m

Radius, head

Extensor digitorum m

Common extensor t

Annular lig

Olecranon — Anconeus m

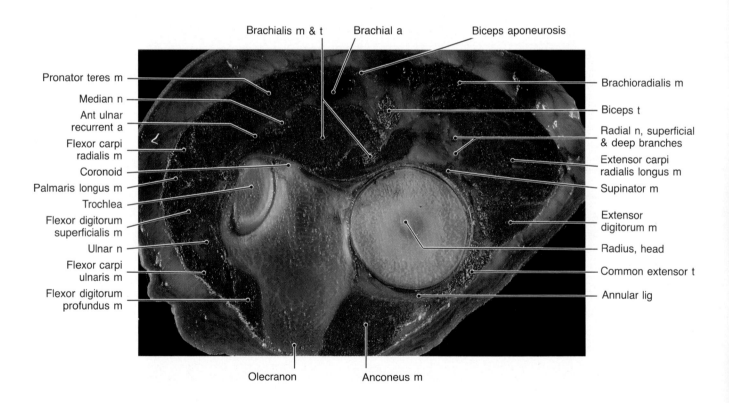

Brachialis m & t — Brachial a — Biceps aponeurosis

Pronator teres m

Median n

Ant ulnar recurrent a

Flexor carpi radialis m

Coronoid

Palmaris longus m

Trochlea

Flexor digitorum superficialis m

Ulnar n

Flexor carpi ulnaris m

Flexor digitorum profundus m

Brachioradialis m

Biceps t

Radial n, superficial & deep branches

Extensor carpi radialis longus m

Supinator m

Extensor digitorum m

Radius, head

Common extensor t

Annular lig

Olecranon — Anconeus m

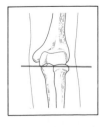

PLATE 13–4

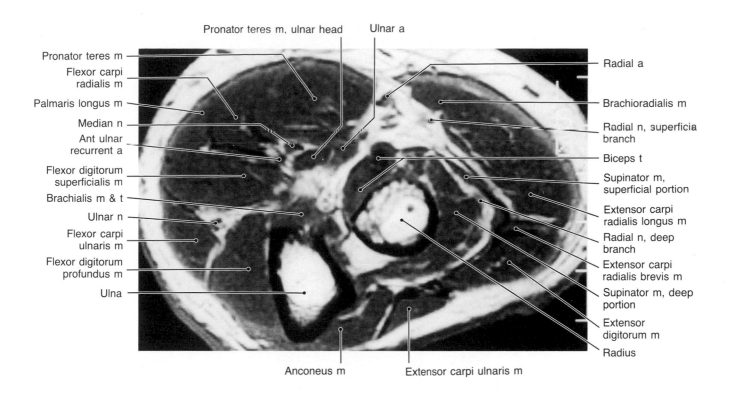

Pronator teres m, ulnar head · Ulnar a

Pronator teres m
Flexor carpi radialis m
Palmaris longus m
Median n
Ant ulnar recurrent a
Flexor digitorum superficialis m
Brachialis m & t
Ulnar n
Flexor carpi ulnaris m
Flexor digitorum profundus m
Ulna

Anconeus m · Extensor carpi ulnaris m

Radial a
Brachioradialis m
Radial n, superficial branch
Biceps t
Supinator m, superficial portion
Extensor carpi radialis longus m
Radial n, deep branch
Extensor carpi radialis brevis m
Supinator m, deep portion
Extensor digitorum m
Radius

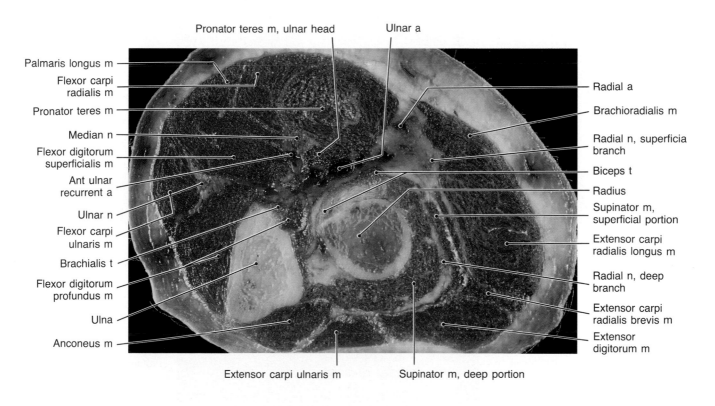

Pronator teres m, ulnar head · Ulnar a

Palmaris longus m
Flexor carpi radialis m
Pronator teres m
Median n
Flexor digitorum superficialis m
Ant ulnar recurrent a
Ulnar n
Flexor carpi ulnaris m
Brachialis t
Flexor digitorum profundus m
Ulna
Anconeus m

Extensor carpi ulnaris m · Supinator m, deep portion

Radial a
Brachioradialis m
Radial n, superficial branch
Biceps t
Radius
Supinator m, superficial portion
Extensor carpi radialis longus m
Radial n, deep branch
Extensor carpi radialis brevis m
Extensor digitorum m

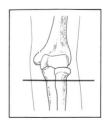

PLATE 13–5

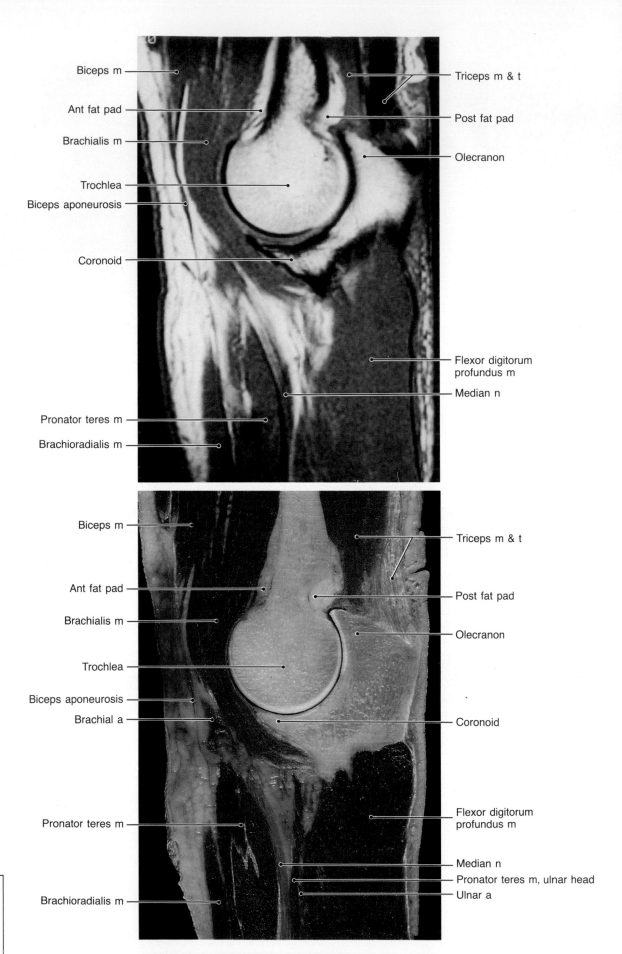

Biceps m

Ant fat pad

Brachialis m

Trochlea

Biceps aponeurosis

Coronoid

Pronator teres m

Brachioradialis m

Triceps m & t

Post fat pad

Olecranon

Flexor digitorum profundus m

Median n

Biceps m

Ant fat pad

Brachialis m

Trochlea

Biceps aponeurosis

Brachial a

Pronator teres m

Brachioradialis m

Triceps m & t

Post fat pad

Olecranon

Coronoid

Flexor digitorum profundus m

Median n

Pronator teres m, ulnar head

Ulnar a

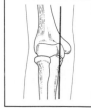

PLATE 13–6

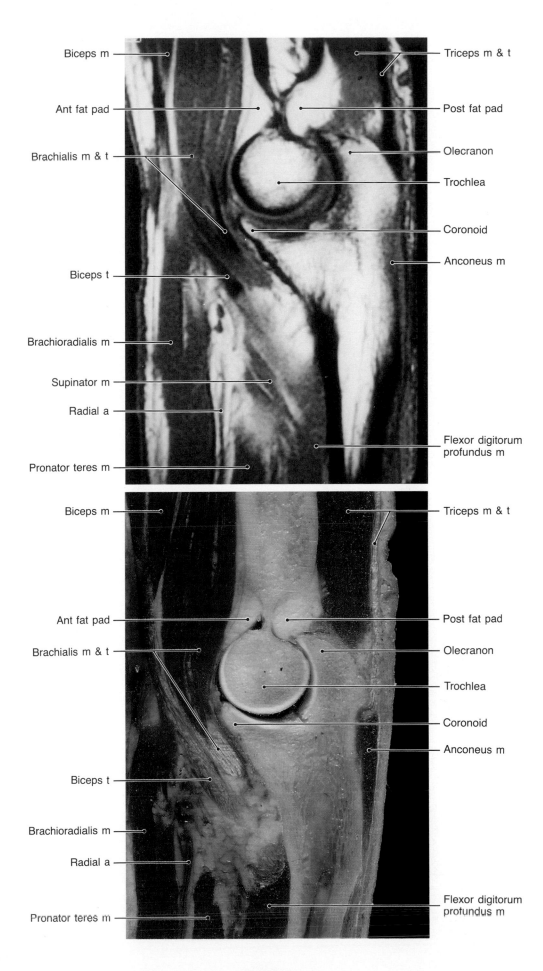

Biceps m	Triceps m & t
Ant fat pad	Post fat pad
Brachialis m & t	Olecranon
	Trochlea
	Coronoid
Biceps t	Anconeus m
Brachioradialis m	
Supinator m	
Radial a	
	Flexor digitorum profundus m
Pronator teres m	

Biceps m	Triceps m & t
Ant fat pad	Post fat pad
Brachialis m & t	Olecranon
	Trochlea
	Coronoid
Biceps t	Anconeus m
Brachioradialis m	
Radial a	
	Flexor digitorum profundus m
Pronator teres m	

PLATE 13–7

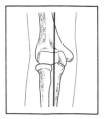

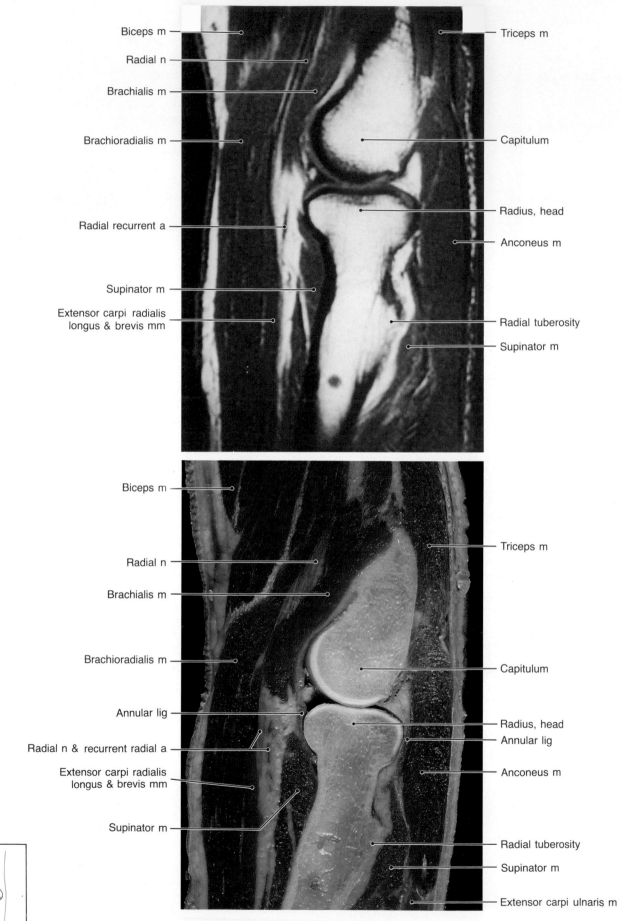

Biceps m — Triceps m

Radial n

Brachialis m

Brachioradialis m — Capitulum

Radial recurrent a — Radius, head

Anconeus m

Supinator m

Extensor carpi radialis longus & brevis mm — Radial tuberosity

Supinator m

Biceps m

Triceps m

Radial n

Brachialis m

Brachioradialis m — Capitulum

Annular lig — Radius, head

Radial n & recurrent radial a — Annular lig

Extensor carpi radialis longus & brevis mm — Anconeus m

Supinator m — Radial tuberosity

Supinator m

Extensor carpi ulnaris m

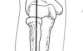

PLATE 13–8

Figure 13–8 (*Continued*)
C Lateral ligament complex. A detailed representation of the radial collateral ligament complex shows a portion termed the radial collateral ligament that extends from the humerus to the annular ligament. This is the portion that is most commonly meant when referring to the radial or lateral collateral ligament. (From Morrey BF [Ed]: The Elbow and Its Disorders. 2nd Ed. Philadelphia, WB Saunders, 1993, p 30.)

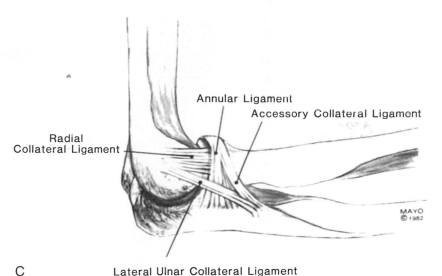

Annular Ligament
Accessory Collateral Ligament
Radial Collateral Ligament
MAYO © 1982
C
Lateral Ulnar Collateral Ligament

merus. It descends toward the ulna, covering the posterior aspect of the annular ligament and attaching to the lateral surface of the olecranon process and upper posterior surface of the shaft of the ulna.

The muscles of the anterior group are the biceps brachii and brachialis. The biceps brachii muscle typically consists of two heads, the short head and the long head, although in approximately 10 per cent of persons an additional head or multiple additional heads also are evident. The short head of the biceps brachii muscle arises from the tip of the coracoid process, in common with the coracobrachialis, and the long head of the biceps brachii muscle arises from the supraglenoid tubercle of the scapula and extends through the glenohumeral joint into the intertubercular groove of the humerus. The two major muscle bellies of the biceps join to form a common tendon approximately 6 or 7 cm above the elbow, which attaches to the posterior aspect of the radial tuberosity. An aponeurosis (i.e., bicipital aponeurosis) arises from the tendon, passes across the brachial artery, and terminates in the fascia that overlies the origin of the flexor muscles of the forearm. The brachialis muscle originates mainly from the anterior aspect of the lower portion of the humerus, descends across the elbow joint, and inserts as a tendon into the tuberosity and anterior surface of the coronoid process of the ulna.[187]

The lateral group of muscles includes the supinator and brachioradialis muscles and the extensor muscles of the wrist and hand (i.e., extensor carpi radialis longus, extensor carpi radialis brevis, extensor digitorum, extensor digiti minimi, and extensor carpi ulnaris muscles). The brachioradialis muscle is located superficially, arising from the lateral supracondylar ridge of the humerus and the anterior surface of the lateral intermuscular septum. After extending below the elbow, this muscle ends as a tendon that is attached to the lateral aspect of the distal portion of the radius, just above the styloid process. The extensor carpi radialis longus muscle is deep to the brachioradialis muscle, also arising from the lateral supracondylar ridge of the humerus and lateral intermuscular septum. Its tendon commences at the

distal one third of the shaft of the radius where it is located laterally, passes beneath the extensor retinaculum, and terminates by attaching to the dorsoradial surface of the base of the second metacarpal bone. At the level of the elbow, the extensor carpi radialis brevis, extensor digitorum, extensor digiti minimi, and extensor carpi ulnaris muscles all appear as a single mass. The supinator is the deepest muscle in the lateral group, originating from the lateral epicondyle of the humerus, from the supinator crest of the ulna, and from the radial collateral and annular ligaments of the elbow and superior radioulnar joint. It courses inferiorly, wrapping about the proximal portion of the radius and inserting on the proximal aspect of the diaphysis of the radius.

The medial group of muscles includes the pronator teres, the palmaris longus, and the flexors of the hand and wrist (flexor carpi radialis, flexor digitorum superficialis, flexor carpi ulnaris, flexor digitorum profundus, and flexor pollicis longus). The most superficial of these muscles is the pronator teres. It has origins from the humerus just above the medial epicondyle (the humeral head) and the medial side of the coronoid process (the ulnar head). The median nerve enters the forearm between these two parts of the muscle and is separated from the ulnar artery by the ulnar head of the muscle. After passing across the forearm, the muscle ends in a tendon that is attached to the lateral aspect of the radial shaft. The other muscles all arise from the common flexor tendon, which also gives rise to a portion of the humeral head of the pronator teres muscle, and these other muscles are arranged from anterior to posterior as the flexor carpi radialis, the palmaris longus, the flexor carpi ulnaris, and the flexor digitorum superficialis. They extend distally, attaching as tendons to various bones in the wrist (e.g., carpus) and hand. The flexor digitorum profundus muscle arises from the upper portion of the anterior and medial surfaces of the ulna, the coronoid process, and the interosseous membrane, and it ends as four tendons that attach to the index, third, fourth, and fifth fingers. The flexor pollicis longus muscle arises from the anterior surface of the radius, near its tuberosity, and the interosseous mem-

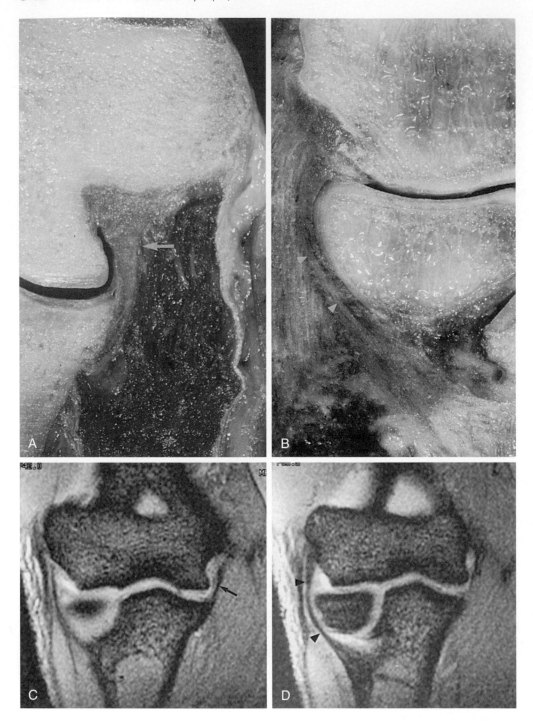

Figure 13–9
Elbow joint: Ligamentous anatomy.

A Medial (ulnar) collateral ligament: Anterior band, coronal oblique section. This part of the ligament (arrow) extends from the anterior aspect of the medial epicondyle of the humerus to the medial edge of the coronoid process.

B Lateral ulnar collateral ligament, coronal oblique section. This ligament originates from the lateral epicondyle and sweeps by the radial head (arrowheads) to insert in the tubercle of the crest of the supinator on the ulna.

C, D Coronal MPGR images (TR/TE, 3000/15; flip angle, 25 degrees) show the anterior band of the medial (ulnar) collateral ligament (arrow, **C**) and the lateral ulnar collateral ligament (arrowheads, **D**).

(**A, B,** Courtesy of A. Cotten, M.D., Lille, France.)

brane and, after passing distally, attaches to the palmar surface of the base of the distal phalanx of the thumb.

Radioulnar Syndesmosis

The diaphyses of the radius and ulna are united by an interosseous membrane whose fibers run in an inferior and medial direction from radius to ulna. This membrane originates approximately 3 cm below the radial tuberosity, extends to the wrist, and contains an aperture for various interosseous vessels. A crest can be noted on both bones at the interosseous border.

Although much of the soft tissue that connects the radial and ulnar shafts is thin, translucent, and mechani-

cally insignificant and properly is referred to as an interosseous membrane, a central portion (i.e., central band) can be identified that grossly and histologically resembles a ligament and is designated the interosseous ligament of the forearm.[5] This ligament is the principal stabilizer of the radius after resection of the radial head.[5]

Vessels and Nerves

The major artery about the elbow is the brachial artery, which extends superficial to the brachialis muscle and medial to the biceps muscle and tendon. Approximately 1 to 2 cm distal to the elbow joint, it divides into the radial and ulnar arteries. The radial artery descends

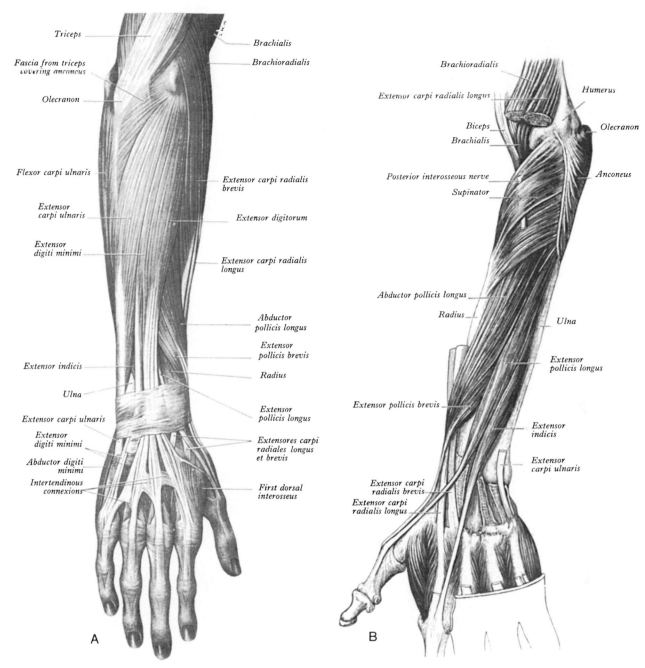

Figure 13–10
Elbow joint and forearm: Muscle and tendon anatomy.
A Superficial muscles of the extensor aspect of the forearm.
B Deep muscles of the extensor aspect of the forearm.
Illustration continued on following page

further between the brachioradialis and pronator teres muscles, and the larger ulnar artery crosses obliquely below the cubital fossa under the pronator teres and flexor muscles. Recurrent branches of the radial and ulnar arteries form a network of vessels about the elbow joint (Fig. 13–11).

Three major nerves exist in the elbow region. The median nerve parallels the course of the brachial artery, courses anterior to it in the cubital area, and descends further between the superficial and deep heads of the pronator teres muscle. The ulnar nerve is present on the posteromedial side of the elbow and passes in a groove between the olecranon process of the ulna and the medial epicondyle of the humerus. The radial nerve descends above the elbow between the brachialis and the brachioradialis muscles and divides near the elbow into deep and superficial branches.

FUNCTION

Although the elbow generally is regarded as a hinge joint, allowing flexion and extension related to the con-

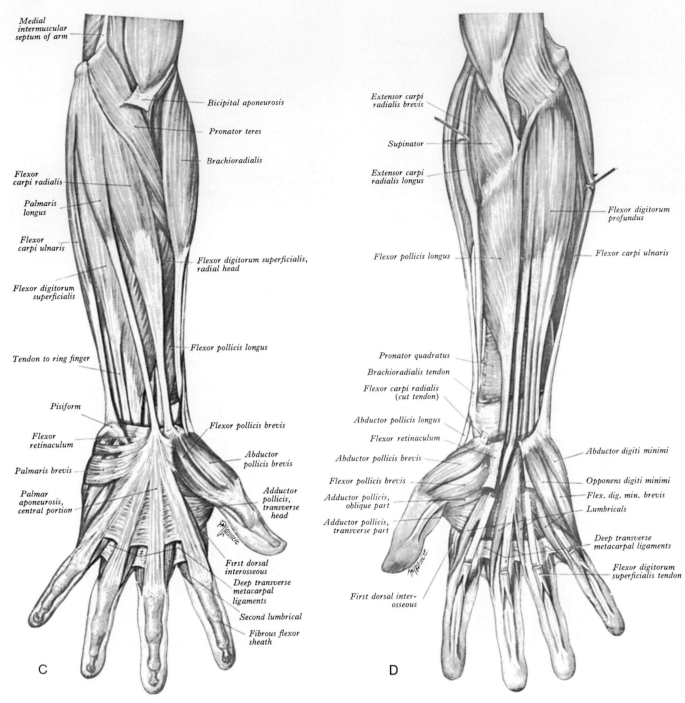

Medial intermuscular septum of arm

Bicipital aponeurosis

Pronator teres

Brachioradialis

Flexor carpi radialis

Palmaris longus

Flexor carpi ulnaris

Flexor digitorum superficialis

Flexor digitorum superficialis, radial head

Flexor pollicis longus

Tendon to ring finger

Pisiform

Flexor retinaculum

Palmaris brevis

Palmar aponeurosis, central portion

Flexor pollicis brevis

Abductor pollicis brevis

Adductor pollicis, transverse head

First dorsal interosseous

Deep transverse metacarpal ligaments

Second lumbrical

Fibrous flexor sheath

C

Extensor carpi radialis brevis

Supinator

Extensor carpi radialis longus

Flexor pollicis longus

Flexor digitorum profundus

Flexor carpi ulnaris

Pronator quadratus

Brachioradialis tendon

Flexor carpi radialis (cut tendon)

Abductor pollicis longus

Flexor retinaculum

Abductor pollicis brevis

Flexor pollicis brevis

Adductor pollicis, oblique part

Adductor pollicis, transverse part

First dorsal inter-osseous

Abductor digiti minimi

Opponens digiti minimi

Flex. dig. min. brevis

Lumbricals

Deep transverse metacarpal ligaments

Flexor digitorum superficialis tendon

D

Figure 13–10 (*Continued*)
  C Superficial muscles of the flexor aspect of the forearm.
  D Deep muscles of the flexor aspect of the forearm.
  (From Williams PL, Warwick R [Eds]: Gray's Anatomy. 36th British edition. Edinburgh, Churchill Livingstone, 1980, pp 574, 576, 580, 581.)

gruity of the ulnohumeral joint, axial rotation of about 5 degrees also is observed.[6, 7] This is seen as internal rotation during early elbow flexion and external rotation during terminal flexion.[7] The axis of rotation for flexion and extension of the elbow passes through the center of the trochlea as well as the humeroradial joint.[8] In addition, the radius rotates around the ulna, allowing for supination and pronation of the forearm. The longitudinal axis of the forearm is considered to pass through the convex head of the radius at the proximal radioul-

nar joint and through the convex articular surface of the ulna at the distal radioulnar joint.[6] With pronation of the forearm, the radius migrates proximally. The carrying angle of the elbow, defined as the angle formed by the long axis of the humerus and the long axis of the ulna, is measured in the frontal plane with the elbow fully extended; this angle is 10 to 15 degrees in men and about 5 degrees greater in women.[6]

Normally, elbow motion ranges from about 0 degrees to about 150 degrees of flexion and from about 75

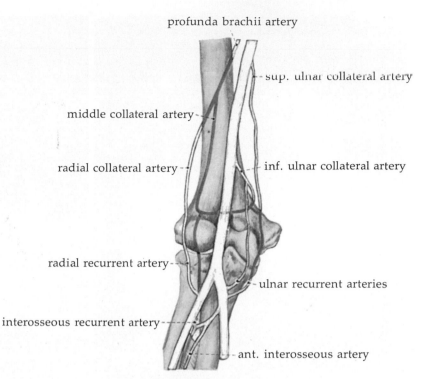

profunda brachii artery

sup. ulnar collateral artery

middle collateral artery

radial collateral artery

inf. ulnar collateral artery

radial recurrent artery

ulnar recurrent arteries

interosseous recurrent artery

ant. interosseous artery

Figure 13–11
Elbow joint: Arterial anatomy. The anterior arterial vascular network about the elbow is shown. (From Langman J, Woerdeman MW: Atlas of Medical Anatomy. Philadelphia, WB Saunders, 1978.)

degrees in pronation to 85 degrees in supination.[8] Factors that limit elbow extension are the impact of the olecranon process in its fossa, the anterior portion of the medial collateral ligament, the joint capsule, and the flexor muscles; flexion of the elbow is limited by the anterior muscle bulk of the arm, tension of the triceps muscle, and the impact of the coronoid process in its fossa.[8] With regard to forearm pronation and supination, restriction of motion relates to passive muscular constraint more than ligamentous structures.[8]

Owing to its congruity, the elbow is one of the most stable joints in the human body. Stabilization of the joint is provided by the articular surfaces and a number of soft tissue structures. Static soft tissue stabilizers include the collateral ligament complexes and the anterior portion of the joint capsule. As summarized by An and Morrey,[6] with elbow extension, the anterior portion of the capsule provides about 70 per cent of the soft tissue restraint to joint distraction, whereas the medial collateral ligament assumes this function at 90 degrees of elbow flexion. Varus stress is checked in extension equally by the articular surfaces and the soft tissues, lateral collateral ligament, and joint capsule; in flexion of the elbow, the articular surfaces contribute about 70 per cent to varus stability.[6] Valgus stress in extension is checked equally by the medial collateral ligament, the capsule, and the articular surfaces; valgus stress in flexion is checked mainly by the anterior portion of the medial collateral ligament.[6] Internal and external rotation of the ulna is limited primarily by the distal portion of the coronoid process.[6]

IMAGING TECHNIQUES

The assessment of disorders of the elbow with imaging methods begins with routine radiography. Standard ra-

diographs can be supplemented with oblique projections, specialized radial head views, and images obtained during the application of varus or valgus stress. Owing to the presence of anterior and posterior fat bodies (or pads) that are intracapsular (although extrasynovial) and applied to the corresponding surfaces of the distal portion of the humerus, any process associated with the accumulation of fluid, blood, synovial inflammatory tissue, or combinations of these, often is accompanied by elevation of the fat pads from the surface of the bone, leading to a positive "fat pad sign."

Arthrography

Arthrography alone or combined with CT scanning represents an effective technique in the evaluation of a number of elbow disorders.[9] In particular, the instillation of air alone or air combined with a small amount of radiopaque contrast material is useful in the detection of intra-articular osteocartilaginous bodies (see later discussion) and of denudation and erosion of the articular cartilage. With regard to arthrographic technique, the injection of iodinated contrast material alone is particularly useful for outlining the presence and extent of synovial disorders, capsular integrity, and synovial cysts, whereas a double contrast study with contrast material and air or a single contrast study with air alone may be superior in demonstrating cartilaginous and osseous defects and free intra-articular bodies.[10, 11] After injection, fluoroscopic spot films and radiographs are obtained, supplemented with conventional tomography or CT scanning when necessary.[12–14]

In the normal situation (Fig. 13–12), on frontal radiographs, a thin layer of contrast material or air is observed between the humerus, radius, and ulna. A peri-

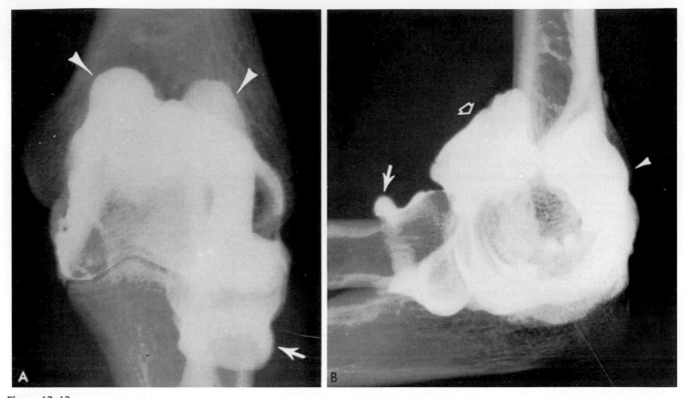

Figure 13–12
Arthrography of the elbow: Normal arthrogram.

A Anteroposterior radiograph. Observe the thin layer of contrast material between humerus and ulna, the proximal extension of material in front of the humerus resembling the ears of a rabbit (arrowheads), and the periradial or annular recess (arrow).

B Lateral radiograph. Note the periradial or annular recess (arrow), the coronoid or anterior recess (open arrow), and the olecranon or posterior recess (arrowhead).

radial prolongation or recess is apparent about the proximal portion of the radius, which is indented where the annular ligament surrounds the bone. Proximal extension of contrast material along the anterior surface of the humerus may resemble the ears of a rabbit, the "Bugs Bunny" sign.[15] On a lateral radiograph, the periradial or annular recess again is apparent. In addition, coronoid (anterior) and olecranon (posterior) recesses are seen. The borders of all recesses and the remainder of the articular cavity appear smooth in configuration with two exceptions: The anterior border of the coronoid recess may be slightly wrinkled in flexion, and the medial border adjacent to the collateral ligament is irregular.[10] Smooth articular cartilage is observed on the humerus, radial head, and ulna; it is of uniform thickness except for a portion of the trochlear notch of the ulna, which lacks cartilage.

Scintigraphy and Ultrasonography

Bone scintigraphy is a sensitive but nonspecific method in the analysis of traumatic, infectious, and neoplastic disorders about the elbow. Ultrasonography is assuming an increasingly important role as a diagnostic technique in the analysis of musculoskeletal disorders.[16] The method, which generally is limited to evaluation of su-

perficial structures, has been used to assess a number of elbow disorders, including effusions, bursitis, tendinitis and tenosynovitis, and soft tissue infections and tumors. In general, however, MR imaging enjoys similar sensitivity and far more specificity in the evaluation of such disorders, although this method is expensive.

MR Imaging

As is addressed in subsequent sections of this chapter, MR imaging has assumed a prominent role in the analysis of osseous, articular, and soft tissue disorders of or about the elbow. The patient usually is placed in a supine position with the arm extended along the side. In this position, an extremity surface coil can be employed. For some patients, a wrist coil, although of small size, can be used; in others, particularly when full extension of the elbow is not possible, a larger coil (e.g., knee or shoulder coil) must be used. Alternatively, the patient can be placed prone in the magnet with the arm extended overhead.[17] If elbow extension is severely limited, the elbow can be examined with 90 degrees of flexion.[18] In this position, a shoulder surface coil or a paired set of coils can be employed. Typical imaging parameters include a field of view of 10 cm to 16 cm (depending on the size of the elbow and degree of elbow extension that is possible) and, for most sequences, images that are 3 to 4 mm thick.

As for other joints, imaging in three planes (transaxial, coronal, and sagittal) usually is necessary for MR examinations of the elbow (Plates 13–1 through 13–8). The axes for the coronal and sagittal images can be derived from a transaxial scout image (e.g., 40 cm field of view). The coronal and sagittal images are obtained parallel and at 90 degrees to the axis of the humeral epicondyles.[19] Standard or fast spin echo MR images are the mainstay of the examination, although these often are supplemented with gradient echo or short tau inversion recovery (STIR) images, or both.[188] Furthermore, fast spin echo MR images coupled with fat suppression are useful in the assessment of marrow edema after injury, and fat-suppressed MR images obtained after the intravenous administration of a gadolinium compound are essential in the analysis of bone and soft tissue infections and tumors. Rarely, as in cases in which intra-articular bodies are suspected, MR arthrography through the use of gadolinium compound or saline solution may be employed (see later discussion).

Evaluation of osseous, articular, and soft tissue structures of the elbow requires attention to MR images in each of the three planes. The transaxial plane generally is the most useful, although the anatomic display is complex in this plane. The ligaments about the elbow are best evaluated in transaxial and coronal planes, and the tendons are well delineated in the transaxial and sagittal planes. Important landmarks in the transaxial MR images include the olecranon, coronoid, and radial fossae, intracapsular fat bodies, ulnar nerve, and triceps and biceps muscles and tendons, although virtually all muscles, tendons, ligaments, and neurovascular structures are seen, as are the bones. In the sagittal MR images, the triceps muscle and tendon, biceps muscle and tendon, brachialis muscle and tendon, and intracapsular fat bodies are important landmarks. In the coronal MR images, the radial head, capitulum, trochlea, common flexor and extensor tendons, and medial and lateral ligamentous complexes are identified.

Several anatomic variations may be seen on MR images that may lead to diagnostic difficulty (Fig. 13–13*A–D*). One, designated the pseudodefect of the capitulum,[20] may simulate the appearance of osteochondritis dissecans. This pseudodefect relates to the presence of a normal groove between the anteriorly located, rounded capitulum and the lateral epicondyle of the humerus. The finding is evident in coronal and sagittal MR images of the elbow. In the coronal images, an apparent interruption of the capitular surface is noted laterally and is highlighted when a joint effusion is present. In the sagittal MR images, a similar notchlike defect is evident posteriorly, which may be deep and angular in appearance.[20]

Another anatomic finding that may produce diagnostic difficulty on MR images is the presence of normal ridges in the trochlea.[19] The trochlear notch, as indicated earlier, is not covered by a continuous surface of hyaline cartilage. Rather, a cartilage-free bone ridge separates the olecranon and coronoid articular surfaces. This transverse trochlear notch is about 2 or 3 mm wide and 2 or 3 mm high.[19] In sagittal MR images, irregular or smooth elevation of the trochlea between the coro-

noid and olecranon articular surfaces is noted, simulating the appearance of an osteophyte.

At the medial and lateral margins of the transverse bone ridge, an indentation of the cortical surface of the trochlea is present normally, leading to a waist-like appearance. These cortical notches also are identified in sagittal MR images as apparent defects in the floor of the trochlear groove.[19] The appearance simulates that of an osteochondral fracture or osteochondritis dissecans. The adjacent marrow, however, is normal with no evidence of edema.

Although the precise role for MR arthrography of the elbow is not defined, this technique does allow full distention of the joint, improving the visualization of synovial recesses, cartilaginous surfaces, and deep portions of the collateral ligaments. Potential diagnostic applications of the technique, therefore, may include the identification of intra-articular osteocartilaginous bodies, chondral defects, and partial deep ligamentous tears. Because of the distention of the joint, five normal synovial recesses can be identified: olecranon recess (located about the olecranon fossa); anterior humeral recess (located against the anterior humeral surface); recess of the ulnar collateral ligament (located under the medial epicondyle of the humerus and applied to the undersurface of portions of the ulnar collateral ligament); recess of the radial collateral ligament (located under the lateral epicondyle of the humerus and applied to the undersurface of portions of the radial collateral ligament); and annular recess (located beneath the annular ligament and around the radial neck). Incomplete filling of these recesses with contrast material may be a normal finding, however, related to the presence of intracapsular fat bodies or synovial folds (see Fig. 13–13*E, F*). Furthermore, as with standard MR imaging of the elbow, MR arthrography may lead to the identification of normal findings simulating pathology, such as the pseudodefect of the capitulum and trochlear notches and ridges.

SPECIFIC ABNORMALITIES

Fractures and Dislocations

Fractures and dislocations about the elbow represent 5 to 8 per cent of all fractures and dislocations. Either direct injury, such as the impact of the radius and ulna against the apposing articular surface of the humerus, or indirect injury, such as that resulting from angular forces transmitted through the bones of the forearm, leads to fractures and dislocations about the elbow.[21] Their detection radiographically is made difficult by the complex anatomy of the elbow and, in the child, by the large number and the irregularity of the adjacent ossification centers. Diagnostic aid is provided by the presence of a traumatic hemarthrosis leading to a positive fat pad sign.[22–25] Although not diagnostic of a fracture, the positive fat pad sign should stimulate a careful search for an adjacent fracture in patients with elbow injuries (Fig. 13–14).

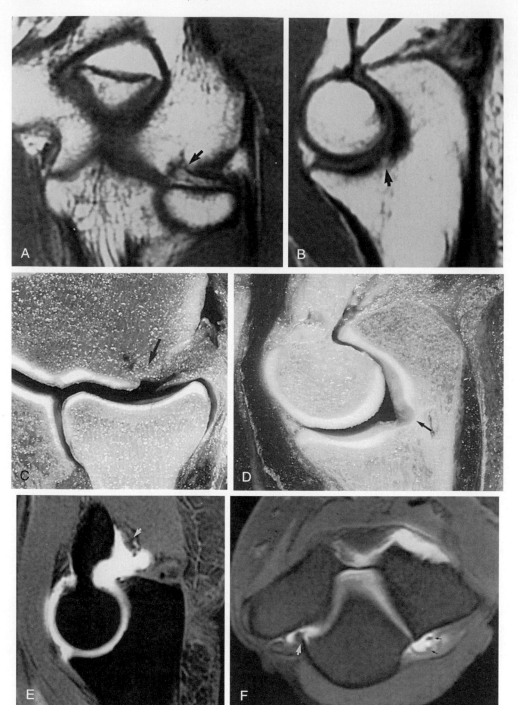

Figure 13–13

MR imaging and MR arthrography of the elbow: Anatomic variations.

A Pseudodefect of the capitulum. On a coronal T1-weighted (TR/TE, 650/19) spin echo MR image, note apparent disruption of the cortex (arrow) at the capitular–distal humeral junction.

B Transverse trochlear ridge. On a sagittal T1-weighted (TR/TE, 500/17) spin echo MR image, note bone irregularity (arrow) produced by this normal anatomic structure.

C, D Normal anatomic variations. The cause of the findings in **A** and **B** is shown in coronal (**C**) and sagittal (**D**) sections of the elbow.

E Olecranon fat. This normal fat pad (arrow) is shown in a sagittal fat-suppressed T1-weighted (TR/TE, 600/20) spin echo MR image obtained after intra-articular gadolinium administration.

F Olecranon fat and synovial folds. A transaxial image with identical parameters as in **E** shows a normal fat pad (white arrow) in the medial olecranon recess and two normal synovial folds (black arrows) in the lateral olecranon recess. (**C–F,** Courtesy of A. Cotten, M.D., Lille, France.)

Elbow Dislocation

Dislocation of the elbow is a relatively frequent injury, especially in the immature skeleton.[26] The elbow joint, accounting for approximately 20 per cent of all dislocations, ranks third (behind the glenohumeral joint and interphalangeal joints of the fingers) as a site of dislocation, and it is the most common site of dislocation in a child.[21] Affected patients usually are between the ages of 5 and 25 years. The usual mechanism of injury is hyperextension (e.g., a fall on the outstretched hand) with the olecranon, driven into the olecranon fossa, serving as a fulcrum to force the elbow apart.[21] The

injury also may relate to axial compression with the elbow slightly flexed. The classification of such injuries is based on the direction of displacement and the presence of radial or ulnar dislocation. In cases of dislocation involving both the radius and the ulna, a posterior (or posterolateral) dislocation (Fig. 13–15) is most frequent (approximately 80 to 90 per cent of all elbow dislocations), as these two bones are displaced in a posterior direction in relation to the distal humerus.[27, 28] In adults, this injury may be complicated by fracture of the coronoid process of the ulna or the radial head, and in children and adolescents, the medial epicondylar ossification center is frequently avulsed and may become

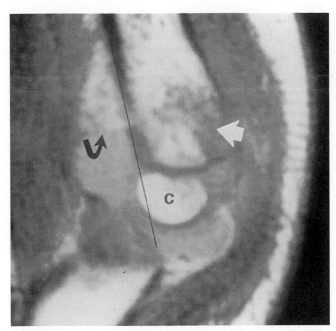

Figure 13–14

MR imaging of the elbow: Supracondylar fracture of the humerus with positive fat pad sign. This sagittal T1-weighted spin echo MR image shows the fracture (straight arrow) and elevation of the anterior intracapsular fat pads (curved arrow). The anterior humeral line passes through the anterior portion of the capitulum (c), an abnormal finding. (Courtesy of L. Steinbach, M.D., San Francisco, California.)

entrapped during reduction.[26] Entrapment of the median nerve in the elbow joint after closed reduction of a posterior dislocation of the elbow with fracture of the medial epicondyle in children can produce a depression in the cortex on the ulnar side of the distal humeral metaphysis.[29-31]

Medial and lateral dislocations of the elbow are not common.[32] Anterior dislocation is also unusual[33] and is associated with severe soft tissue injury. Rarely, elbow dislocations may be recurrent.[34] The cause of the last injury varies, but a residual defect in the articular surface of the trochlea, attenuation of the collateral ligaments, failure of union of the coronoid process, or anterior capsular stripping may be observed.[35] Indeed, instability of the elbow, particularly medial instability with the elbow extended, is common after a dislocation, related to complete rupture of the medial and sometimes the lateral collateral ligaments, as well as to injury of the anterior capsule and the attachment of the brachialis muscle.[36] Also rare is a divergent dislocation of the elbow in which the radius and ulna move in different directions.[37, 38] This divergent dislocation involves all three joints (i.e., radiocapitular, ulnotrochlear, and proximal radioulnar) that constitute the elbow. Extensive ligamentous and soft tissue (i.e., annular ligament, interosseous membrane, capsule of the distal radioulnar joint) disruption accompanies this dislocation, and gross instability of the elbow is present.[21] Translocation of the elbow, in which there is reversal of the normal positions of the proximal radius and ulna with the ulna articulating with the capitulum and the radial head articulating with the trochlea, also has been described.[39]

Isolated dislocation of the ulna at the elbow is unusual. Similarly, isolated radial head dislocation without an associated fracture in the ulna is rare in adults. In the child, subluxation of the radial head, which usually but not invariably is transient,[40] is termed nursemaid's elbow or pulled elbow. It is produced by a sudden pull on the child's arm which, when the forearm is in a pronated position, results in slipping of the radial head beneath the annular ligament as it is torn from its attachment to the radial neck.[21, 41] With supination of the forearm, the ligament is restored to its normal position.[21] Routine radiographs, therefore, are normal. Rarely, the annular ligament becomes entrapped in the joint, requiring surgical reduction.[42] Isolated true dislocations of the radial head, without fracture or plastic bowing of the ulna, occasionally are seen in children.[43] The initial radiographic diagnosis is based on an abnormal position of the radial head, which usually is displaced anteriorly (Fig. 13–16). Within weeks of the injury, curvilinear calcification in the annular ligament may be seen. In the child, traumatic dislocation of the radial head must be differentiated from congenital dislocation of this bone or dislocation associated with osteo-onychodysostosis or hereditary onycho-osteodysplasia (nail-patella syndrome). Because of the rarity of isolated traumatic dislocation of the radial head,[44] all such cases should be investigated extensively for an associated fracture of the ulna.

The combination of an ulnar fracture and radial head dislocation is termed a Monteggia fracture-dislocation.[45-47] Various types of Monteggia fracture-dislocations are recognized: type I—fracture of the middle or upper third of the ulna with anterior dislocation of the radial head and anterior angulation of the ulna; type II—fracture of the middle or upper third of the ulna with posterior dislocation of the radial head and posterior angulation of the ulna; type III—fracture of the

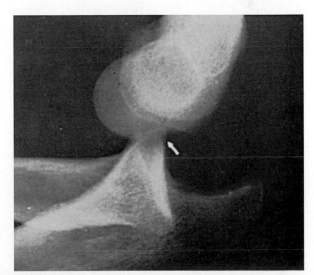

Figure 13–15

Elbow: Posterior dislocation of both the radius and the ulna. Note the posterior displacement of the radius and ulna with respect to the humerus. The trochlea of the humerus and the coronoid process of the ulna contact each other (arrow), resulting in fracture of the articular surfaces.

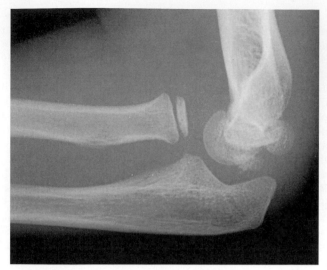

Figure 13–16
Elbow: Dislocation of the radial head. Note the anterior position of the radius with respect to the capitulum and abnormal separation of the radius and ulna.

ulna just distal to the coronoid process with lateral dislocation of the radial head; and type IV—fracture of the upper or middle third of the ulna with anterior dislocation of the radial head and fracture of the upper third of the radius below the bicipital tuberosity.[48] Type I injuries are most frequent (approximately 65 per cent), followed by type II (approximately 18 per cent), type III (approximately 16 per cent), and type IV (approximately 1 per cent).[45] These various patterns emphasize the typical occurrence of injuries to more than one structure in the forearm and the rare occurrence of injury isolated to a single bone in the forearm. Although the classic patterns of the Monteggia fracture-dislocation include an ulnar fracture, ipsilateral radial shaft fracture and dislocation of the radial head without apparent injury to the ulna have been reported.[49] As the Monteggia fracture-dislocation is a common injury in adults (although rare in children[50–54]) and easily overlooked, multiple views of the elbow should be obtained in all patients who demonstrate fractures of the proximal half of the ulna. A line drawn through the radial shaft and radial head should align with the capitulum in any projection.[55]

In infants and young children, separation of the entire distal humeral epiphysis may be confused with elbow dislocation.[56, 57] The correct diagnosis of this injury rests on two observations: a normal relationship between the capitulum and radius; and medial displacement of the radius and ulna with respect to the humerus.

Complications of elbow dislocations include heterotopic calcification and ossification[58–60] and neural and vascular injury.[28, 61] Damaged structures include the brachial artery[62, 63] and the median and ulnar nerves.[64] The brachial artery is injured in association with posterior dislocations of the elbow. Such injury is far more common in open rather than closed dislocations; and when there is disruption of the flexor muscles from the medial epicondyle or from a vertical fracture of the medial epicondyle that allows posterior displacement of or traction on the brachial artery.[65]

Posttraumatic bone formation (Fig. 13–17) occurs as a significant complication in 3 to 5 per cent of elbow injuries, particularly in fracture-dislocations, radial head fractures, and multitrauma patients with head injuries. Calcification or ossification occurs in and around muscles, especially the brachialis muscle, and predominates

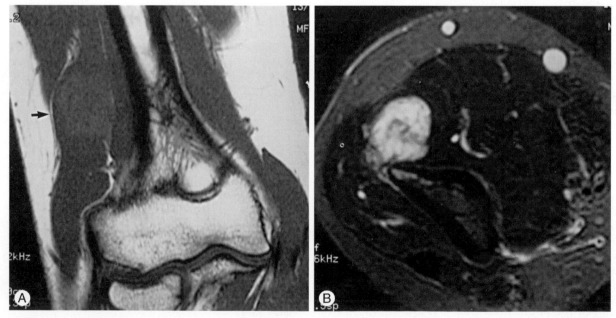

Figure 13–17
Posttraumatic bone formation (myositis ossificans): MR imaging. Three months after an injury, at a time when routine radiographs showed an ossifying soft tissue mass, a coronal T1-weighted (TR/TE, 300/16) spin echo MR image **(A)** reveals a well-defined intramuscular mass (arrow). It is inhomogeneous but mainly of high signal intensity in a transaxial fat-suppressed fast spin echo (TR/TE, 3500/108) MR image **(B)**. (Courtesy of P. Kindynis, M.D., Geneva, Switzerland.)

in the anterior region of the elbow.[21] It usually is visible within 3 to 4 weeks of the injury (see Chapter 10).

Many of the patterns of elbow dislocation are associated with fractures of the radial head or olecranon or coronoid process of the ulna. Such fractures generally indicate a less favorable prognosis owing to increased instability of the joint.

Although routine radiography generally suffices in the assessment of elbow dislocations and their complications, other imaging methods such as CT scanning and MR imaging occasionally are required, particularly in the identification of intra-articular bodies and capsular and ligamentous injury (see later discussion).

Intra-Articular Fractures of the Distal Portion of the Humerus

Intra-articular fractures of the distal portion of the humerus have been classified in several different ways. One traditional method is based on the specific anatomic site of injury (e.g., transcondylar, intercondylar, condylar, epicondylar, transchondral, and miscellaneous)[66] and is considered briefly in the following discussion. A second method is based on a columnar approach to distal humeral anatomy and is summarized later in this discussion.

Transcondylar fractures resemble supracondylar fractures but are intra-articular. The fracture line traverses both condylar surfaces in a horizontal direction. Two types are described: an extension type and a flexion type. The extension variety generally is seen in older patients. Although significant displacement of the fracture fragments generally is not a problem, extensive callus or heterotopic bone formation may be observed and can create mechanical difficulties. The flexion type of transcondylar fracture is associated with significant displacement of the fracture fragments.

Intercondylar fractures of the distal portion of the humerus result in comminuted and complex fracture lines that generally include one component that traverses the supracondylar region of the humerus in a transverse or oblique fashion and a second component, which is vertical or oblique, that enters the articular lumen.[67, 68] These fractures are relatively rare and typically are observed in patients over the age of 50 years.[68, 69] They usually are produced by direct trauma to the elbow in which the ulnar articular surface is driven against the articular surface of the distal portion of the humerus. Indirect forces can produce similar lesions. Complications of intercondylar fractures include soft tissue injury, instability, and loss of elbow function.[70] Other problems, including delay or absence of bone union, injury to nerves (e.g., tardy ulnar palsy) and vessels, and ischemic necrosis of bone, are rare.[71]

The condylar portions of the humerus are separated into medial and lateral structures by the capitulotrochlear sulcus. Each condyle contains an articular and a nonarticular portion. The lateral condyle is composed of the nonarticular lateral epicondyle and the articular capitulum; the medial condyle is composed of the nonarticular medial epicondyle and the trochlea. Condylar fractures imply that the fracture line separates both the articular and the nonarticular portions of one condyle with or without an attached segment of the opposite condyle.[66] These fractures should be distinguished from those involving only an epicondyle (medial or lateral epicondylar fracture) and those affecting the capitulum or the trochlea.

Condylar fractures are relatively uncommon, occurring predominantly in children.[72] The lateral condyle is involved more frequently than the medial condyle. Each of these types can be associated with significant instability and restriction of motion, especially if the fracture fragment is large. In this regard, a classification system has been devised on the basis of the size of the fragment and the presence or absence of disruption of the lateral trochlear ridge.[73] This structure, separating the trochlea and capitulum, is important in providing medial and lateral stability to the elbow. In type I fractures of the condyles, the lateral trochlear ridge is not disrupted, whereas in type II fractures, the larger fracture fragment contains the separated condyle and a portion of this ridge. The latter pattern of injury allows translocation of the radius and the ulna in a mediolateral direction and is termed a fracture-dislocation. Because of this instability, type II fractures require more aggressive orthopedic treatment.

Fractures of the capitulum are rare and involve only the articular surface of the lateral condyle.[74–77] Two types of injury are recognized: type I fractures (Hahn-Steinthal type) are complete and involve a large bony segment of the capitulum; type II fractures (Kocher-Lorenz type) are partial, involving predominantly articular cartilage and producing "uncapping" of the condyle.[75] The mechanism of injury is considered to be a direct force, applied through the radial head.[78, 79] Anteroposterior radiographs may appear surprisingly normal, so that accurate assessment usually depends on the review of optimal lateral radiographs. A semicircular radiopaque shadow representing the displaced capitulum is apparent, usually anterior to the distal portion of the humerus within the radial fossa. An associated injury is fragmentation of the radial head.

The articular surface of the medial condyle, the *trochlea*, rarely is fractured as an isolated event. This structure is well protected owing to its position deep within the elbow.[66]

The *epicondyles*, as well as other osseous structures throughout the elbow, are injured more frequently in the child or adolescent than in the adult. In the mature skeleton, the medial epicondyle is fractured more commonly than the lateral epicondyle, the injury being related in most cases to a direct force applied to the epicondyle. Radiographs reveal a fracture fragment that is displaced in a distal or anterior direction by the action of the forearm flexor muscles.[66] In some cases, it may lodge between the apposing articular surfaces of the humerus and ulna. Injury to the adjacent ulnar nerve also may be apparent.

The *columnar approach* to analysis of distal humeral fractures has been well summarized by Mehne and Jupiter,[80] many of whose observations are repeated here. When viewed from its posterior aspect (and, to a lesser extent, from its anterior aspect), the humeral shaft ex-

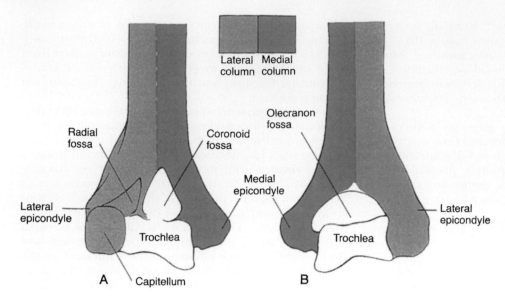

Lateral column Medial column

Radial fossa

Coronoid fossa

Olecranon fossa

Medial epicondyle

Lateral epicondyle

Lateral epicondyle

Trochlea

Trochlea

Capitellum

A

B

Figure 13–18
Humeral fractures: Columnar approach. Anterior (**A**) and posterior (**B**) views of the medial and lateral columns of the distal end of the humerus. (From Jupiter JB: Trauma to the adult elbow and fractures of the distal humerus. In BD Browner, JB Jupiter, AM Levine, et al [Eds]: Skeletal Trauma: Fractures, Dislocations, Ligamentous Injuries. Philadelphia, WB Saunders, 1992, p 1148.)

tends distally in the form of two longitudinal columns, the medial column and the lateral column, that terminate inferiorly in the region of the horizontally oriented trochlea (Fig. 13–18). Fractures involving the distal portion of the humerus can be classified according to their involvement of one or both columns and of the intercalary articular surface (i.e., trochlea). In this fashion, intra-articular fractures may be divided into four categories: single column fractures (medial or lateral), bicolumn fractures (T, Y, H, or lambda patterns), capitulum fractures, and trochlear fractures.[80] Extra-articular fractures can be further classified as intracapsular (or transcolumn) fractures and extracapsular fractures (medial or lateral epicondyle).

Single column fractures represent the condylar fractures in the traditional classification system. According to Mehne and Jupiter,[80] displacement of the fracture fragments relates not to whether the fracture violates the lateral trochlear ridge but to which of the fracture fragments has the greatest capsular attachment and to which of the collateral ligaments is ruptured. Bicolumn fractures correspond to the intercondylar fractures in the traditional classification system. Extra-articular intracapsular fractures, or transcolumn fractures, traverse both columns of the distal portion of the humerus without violating the articular surface. They may be high (supracondylar fractures in the traditional classification system) or low (transcondylar fractures in the traditional classification system) and of the extension or flexion type.

Fractures of the Olecranon and Coronoid Processes of the Ulna

Fractures of the olecranon process, representing approximately 20 per cent of all elbow injuries in adults, result from direct injury, indirect injury, or a combination of the two. A transverse or oblique fracture enters the semiulnar notch, and the pull of the triceps muscle accounts for displacement of the fragment or fragments.[66] Significant posterior displacement of the olec-

ranon fragment combined with anterior movement of the remaining portion of the ulna and the radial head is a serious injury that is termed a fracture-dislocation of the elbow.[81]

No uniformly accepted classification system exists for olecranon fractures of the ulna. Some systems use categories of displaced and nondisplaced fractures, others emphasize the configuration of the fracture line, and still others combine these two features.[66, 82, 83] Prognostic factors include the degree of osseous displacement and the ability of the patient to extend the elbow against gravity; the greater the degree of displacement and the more severe the patient's inability to accomplish elbow extension (indicating disruption of the triceps mechanism), the more likely it is that operative intervention is required.

The complications of olecranon fractures include a decreased range of elbow motion, osteoarthritis, and nonunion (the last occurring in approximately 5 per cent of olecranon fractures).[84, 85] Ulnar nerve damage is evident in approximately 10 per cent of patients.

Isolated fractures of the coronoid process of the ulna are rare.[86] More commonly, coronoid fractures are associated with posterior dislocations of the elbow. Isolated fractures of the coronoid process result from either avulsion of the attached brachialis tendon or impaction against the trochlea.[21, 86] The precise location of the fracture line influences whether or not the injury leads to elbow instability, as it determines the integrity of the soft tissue stabilizers, including the anterior bundle of the medial collateral ligament.[187]

Fractures of the Head and Neck of the Radius

Radial head fractures represent a common injury in adults, resulting principally from indirect trauma. Less frequently, a direct or a violent injury results in a radial head fracture with or without a posterior dislocation of the elbow (in which the head of the radius contacts the capitulum of the humerus).[87] Radial head fractures are

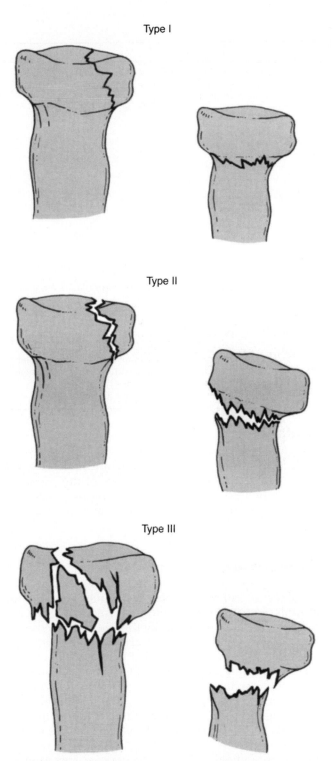

Type I

Type II

Type III

Figure 13–19
Radial head fractures: A modified Mason classification system for radial head fractures is shown. (From Jupiter JB: Trauma to the adult elbow and fractures of the distal humerus. *In* BD Browner, JB Jupiter, AM Levine, et al [Eds]: Skeletal Trauma: Fractures, Dislocations, Ligamentous Injuries. Philadelphia, WB Saunders, 1992, p 1128.)

poorer prognosis, fractures associated with elbow dislocation (Fig. 13–19).[66, 88, 89] In addition, an impaction fracture of the radial neck, without involvement of the radial head, is encountered frequently.

The radiographic abnormalities are important in the accurate diagnosis of these injuries, as the physical findings may be relatively minor or nonspecific. The diagnostic importance of a positive "fat pad sign" as well as that of oblique and specialized radiographic projections is well recognized,[90] and the identification of an associated capitulum fracture or intra-articular osseous fragments has been emphasized.

Complications occurring after radial head fractures are infrequent, consisting of a limited range of motion, osteoarthritis, and, in cases of more severe injuries, heterotopic ossification. Such fractures, however, may be part of a more complex or widespread injury, such as an elbow dislocation, a fracture of the capitulum, subluxation of the distal radioulnar joint (the Essex-Lopresti injury), a Colles' fracture, or a fracture of the scaphoid bone[91] or other carpal bones. The Essex-Lopresti injury consists of a comminuted and displaced radial head fracture and disruption of the distal radioulnar joint. The constant feature of this injury is immediate proximal migration of the radial shaft related to the severity of the radial head fracture.[92] This rare injury results from a longitudinal force applied to the outstretched hand that leads to impaction of the radial head and capitulum. The interosseous membrane is disrupted. Accurate diagnosis requires careful analysis of wrist radiographs. An Essex-Lopresti type injury of the distal radioulnar joint also can result from a fracture-dislocation of the elbow.[93]

Fractures of the Radial and Ulnar Diaphyses
(Table 13–1)

The radius and ulna lie alongside each other, touching at their proximal and distal portions and separated by an interosseous space occupied by the interosseous membrane. This membrane is obliquely oriented, containing fibers that extend from a more proximal position on the radius to a more distal position on the ulna. When a fracture occurs in one or both bones of the forearm, the muscles that join these bones, the pronator quadratus, pronator teres, and supinator muscles, serve to decrease the interosseous space. The final resting position of the radius after fracture depends on the action of these muscles and others, such as the biceps brachii muscle, and is influenced by the level of the fracture itself.[94, 95]

Injuries involving a single anatomic structure in the forearm are rare. In common with the pelvis, mandible, and ankle, the forearm can be considered a ring structure owing to the ligamentous and articular connections of the radius and ulna.[96] Disruption of the ring at one site usually is accompanied by disruption at a second (and even third) site. When both injuries are fractures, accurate diagnosis using routine radiography is not difficult. When a fracture and dislocation represent the components of the two injuries (e.g., Monteggia and Galeazzi fracture-dislocations, Essex-Lopresti injury),

classified as undisplaced fractures (Mason type I), marginal fractures with displacement (e.g., angulation, depression, impaction) (Mason type II), comminuted fractures (Mason type III), and, in recognition of their

Table 13–1. FRACTURES OF THE RADIAL AND ULNAR SHAFTS

Site	Characteristics	Complications
Ulna (alone)	"Nightstick" fracture; direct blow to forearm, distal ulna > middle ulna > proximal ulna	Displacement at fracture site (uncommon)
	Monteggia injury:	Injury to branches of radial nerve (approximately 20 per cent of cases)
	Type I: Fracture of middle or upper third of ulna with anterior dislocation of radial head (65 per cent)	
	Type II: Fracture of middle or upper third of ulna with posterior dislocation of radial head (18 per cent)	
	Type III: Fracture of ulna just distal to coronoid process with lateral dislocation of radial head (16 per cent)	
	Type IV: Fracture of upper or middle third of ulna with anterior dislocation of radial head and fracture of proximal radius (1 per cent)	
Radius (alone)	Proximal and middle segments:	
	Uncommon as usually associated with ulnar fracture	
	Galeazzi's injury: Fracture of the radial shaft with dislocation or subluxation of inferior radiolnar joint, caused by direct blow or fall on the outstretched hand with pronation of forearm, variable degrees of displacement at fracture site	Angulation Entrapment of extensor carpi ulnaris tendon (rare) Delayed union or nonunion
Radius and ulna	Closed or open	Delayed union or nonunion (especially of ulna)
	Nondisplaced or displaced (displacement more common in adults than in children)	Infection, especially in open fractures Nerve and vascular injuries, especially in open fractures and those with severe displacement Compartment syndromes Synostosis between radius and ulna (rare)

routine radiographic diagnosis again is straightforward as long as the entire forearm (i.e., elbow to wrist) is surveyed. When a subluxation represents a component of the injury pattern, however, the initial radiographic examination may be interpreted as showing only a single lesion, particularly if the subluxation is transient or appears only in certain positions of the forearm. Scintigraphy, CT, or MR imaging in such instances may provide diagnostic assistance.

Fractures involving both bones of the forearm are common, resulting usually from direct blows sustained during a motor vehicle accident, fall, or fight. Complications of these fractures include delayed union or nonunion (especially when infection is present), neurologic and vascular injury (representing an uncommon sequela of such fractures), compartment syndrome, and synostoses.[97, 98]

Fractures involving the diaphysis of the ulna may occur as part of a Monteggia fracture-dislocation (see previous discussion) or as an isolated phenomenon. Isolated nondisplaced or minimally displaced fractures of the ulnar shaft are common; typically they result from a direct blow, and are designated nightstick fractures owing to their occurrence during an assault in which the victim raises his or her forearm to protect the head from being struck by a hard object, often a club. Significantly displaced fractures of the ulnar diaphysis rarely occur as an isolated lesion. Rather, they are associated with dislocations of the proximal or distal radioulnar joint, or both joints.[96]

Fractures of the diaphysis of the radius occur most commonly as part of the Galeazzi fracture-dislocation and rarely as an isolated phenomenon. Isolated fractures of the proximal portion of the radial shaft result from a direct blow. A fall on the outstretched hand represents a second cause of a fracture of the proximal radial diaphysis, although associated injuries including dislocation of the radial head and capitular fracture usually are evident.[99]

Ligamentous Abnormalities

The subject of elbow instability is complex. Indeed, no uniformly accepted classification system exists for such instability. Some authors classify the disorder according to five criteria[100]: (1) the specific articular site of involvement (i.e., elbow or isolated radial head instability); (2) the clinical timing of the instability (acute, chronic, or recurrent instability); (3) the direction of displacement (valgus, varus, anterior, posterolateral rotary instability); (4) the degree of displacement (subluxation or dislocation); (5) and the presence or absence of associated fractures.

Elbow instability has been considered a spectrum of injury that can be divided into three stages (Fig. 13–20).[100] In stage 1, posterolateral rotary instability is present in which posterolateral rotational subluxation of the ulna on the humerus is associated with supination or external rotation of the ulna. In this stage, the ulnar part of the lateral ligament complex is disrupted, and other portions of this complex may be disrupted or intact. In stage 2, the elbow dislocates incompletely such that the coronoid process is perched on the trochlea. In this stage, the radial collateral ligament and ulnar part of the lateral ligament complex, as well as the

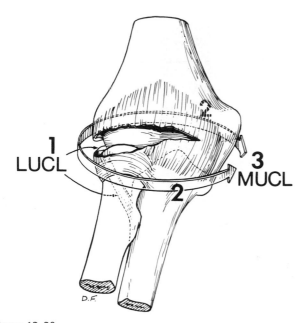

Figure 13–20
Elbow instability. Soft tissue injury progresses in a "circle," from lateral to medial, in three stages. In stage 1, the lateral ulnar collateral ligament (LUCL) is disrupted. In stage 2, the other lateral ligamentous structures and the anterior and posterior capsule are disrupted. In stage 3, disruption of the medial ulnar collateral ligament (MUCL) can be partial with disruption of the posterior MUCL only (3A), or complete (3B). (From O'Driscoll SW, Morrey BF, Korinek S, An KN: Elbow subluxation and dislocation: A spectrum of instability. Clin Orthop *280*:186, 1992.)

anterior and posterior portions of the capsule, are disrupted. In stage 3, the elbow dislocates fully with the coronoid process resting behind the humerus. Stage 3 has been further divided into two separate categories. In stage 3A, in addition to the ligamentous and capsular findings noted in stage 2, the posterior band of the medial collateral ligament is disrupted and the anterior band of the medial collateral ligament is intact. The elbow is stable to valgus stress after reduction of the dislocation. In stage 3B, the anterior band of the medial collateral ligament also is disrupted, and the elbow is unstable in all directions. According to this staging system, dislocation of the elbow represents the final of three sequential stages of instability resulting from posterolateral ulnohumeral rotary subluxation, with soft tissue disruption progressing from a lateral to a medial direction.[100] Clinical manifestations, abnormal movement during stress radiography, and a propensity to develop recurrent dislocations increase as the disorder progresses from stage 1 to stage 3. Although this scheme of elbow instability is but one of many that have been proposed, and elbow dislocations may result from other mechanisms of injury, the importance of the anterior band of the medial collateral ligament and the lateral ulnar collateral ligament in resisting valgus and varus stress applied to the elbow is accepted almost uniformly.[8, 100]

Medial elbow instability may result from a single traumatic event or represent the cumulative effects of repetitive microtrauma.[3] Indeed, the occurrence of medial pain about the elbow in athletes involved in throwing

a ball (e.g., baseball pitcher) or other object is well recognized. Valgus torque applied by the forearm to the elbow during such activities can lead not only to injury of the medial collateral ligament but also to muscle tears, avulsion fractures, and ulnar nerve damage.[101, 102] Flexor tendinitis, repetitive traction, friction, and compression of the ulnar nerve, secondary lateral column compression with valgus elbow laxity, osteochondral injury, and intra-articular osteocartilaginous bodies all can result from medial elbow instability.[3] Physical examination often reveals tenderness to palpation over the medial collateral ligament complex, most often at its distal insertion site.[103] Valgus stability of the elbow is examined with the patient seated and the hand and wrist held securely between the examiner's forearm and trunk.[103] The patient's elbow is flexed beyond 25 degrees to unlock the olecranon process from its fossa, and the medial collateral ligament is palpated while a valgus stress is applied.[103, 104] Additional diagnostic information is provided by radiography obtained during application of stress to the elbow (i.e., increased valgus displacement) (Fig. 13–21),[105] arthrography (i.e., medial extravasation after intra-articular injection of contrast material),[106] and MR imaging (see later discussion).[107, 108]

As indicated earlier, the association of injuries to the medial collateral ligament of the elbow and participation in sports requiring repetitive throwing motions is well established.[101, 103] The main structure involved in the

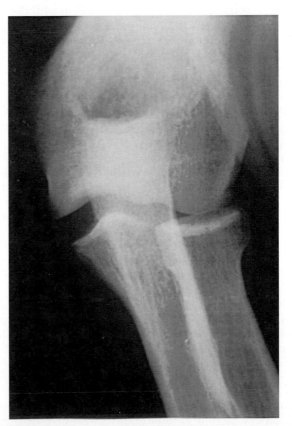

Figure 13–21
Elbow instability: Stress radiography. Radiograph obtained during the application of valgus stress to a partially flexed elbow reveals widening of the medial side of the joint, indicative of injury to the medial collateral ligament.

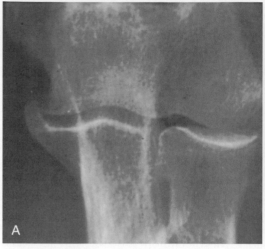

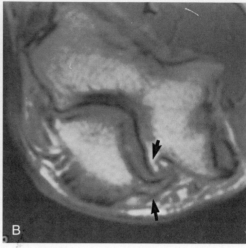

Figure 13–22
Medial elbow instability: Traction enthesophytes and osteophytes.

A Traction enthesophytes. A bone outgrowth in a professional pitcher is seen in the medial aspect of the coronoid tubercle. This relates to traction produced by the medial collateral ligament or the joint capsule. (Courtesy of H. Pavlov, M.D., New York, New York.)

B Osteophytes. In this transaxial T1-weighted (TR/TE, 749/15) spin echo MR image, observe apposing osteophytes (arrows) in the posteromedial corner of the elbow. (Courtesy of L. Steinbach, M.D., San Francisco, California.)

throwing motion is the anterior bundle of the medial collateral ligament. Excessive valgus forces in the medial compartment in the late cocking and acceleration phases of throwing lead to either slow deterioration of portions of this ligament or its acute rupture, either of which is responsible for subsequent elbow instability. Indeed, experimental transection of the medial collateral ligament results in severe instability when valgus stress is applied to the elbow.[109, 110] Associated injuries in these athletes are abnormalities of the annular ligament and triceps tendon which, in combination with the alterations of the medial collateral ligament, are evident only in the dominant extremity. Enthesophytes of the coronoid process commonly are observed in baseball pitchers (Fig. 13–22A). Furthermore, during arm acceleration, excessive valgus stress applied to the elbow causes wedging of the olecranon process into its fossa, resulting in posteromedial impingement.[101, 111] Such impingement is accompanied by osteophyte formation in the posterior and posteromedial aspects of the tip of the olecranon process (Fig. 13–22B), cartilage erosion, and intra-articular bodies.[111] In children and adolescents involved in baseball or other sports requiring overhead throwing motions, acute and chronic injuries involving the ossification center of the medial epicondyle of the humerus are identified (i.e., Little League elbow), including physeal irregularity and fracture and osseous displacement (see later discussion).

Lateral elbow instability related to isolated abnormalities of the lateral collateral ligament complex is not as well described as that on the medial side of the elbow. Although varus stress applied to the elbow may occur as an acute injury, repetitive varus stress (as in athletic endeavors) is not encountered frequently. Indeed, lateral collateral ligament injury rarely occurs after isolated varus stress applied to the elbow; rather, elbow dislocation is the most common cause of deficiency of this ligament.[112] Other causes of lateral collateral ligament deficiency include elbow subluxations and surgical injury (e.g., release of the common extensor tendon or radial head resection). Release or repair of the common extensor tendon for lateral epicondylitis may be complicated by injury to the lateral collateral ligament in as

many as 25 per cent of patients.[113] As in the case of medial elbow instability, careful physical examination supplemented with stress testing (with or without the use of radiography) are fundamental to the diagnosis of lateral instability of the elbow.[112]

MR imaging can be applied to the assessment of acutely or chronically injured ligaments about the elbow.[17, 108, 114–116] Normally, the collateral ligaments, especially the medial collateral ligament, are seen on coronal images of the elbow as thin linear bands of low signal intensity. Coronal oblique MR imaging planes accomplished along the longitudinal axes of the most important components of the collateral ligaments may improve their visualization. With injury to these ligaments, MR imaging findings are laxity, irregularity, poor definition, and increased signal intensity within and around the ligament (Fig. 13–23). The regions of increased signal intensity, which are most prominent on T2-weighted spin echo and gradient echo coronal MR images, reflect the presence of hemorrhage and edema (Fig. 13–24). MR imaging characteristics of the medial collateral ligament in the immature skeleton are more complex and are well described by Sigimoto and Oh-

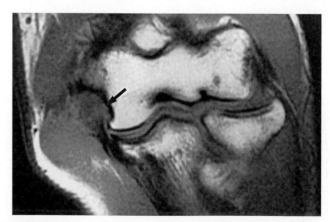

Figure 13–23
Medial collateral ligament injury: MR imaging. In addition to injury of the flexor tendons, a coronal T1-weighted (TR/TE, 700/18) spin echo MR image shows disruption (arrow) of the medial collateral ligament. (Courtesy of D. Wilcox, M.D., Kansas City, Missouri.)

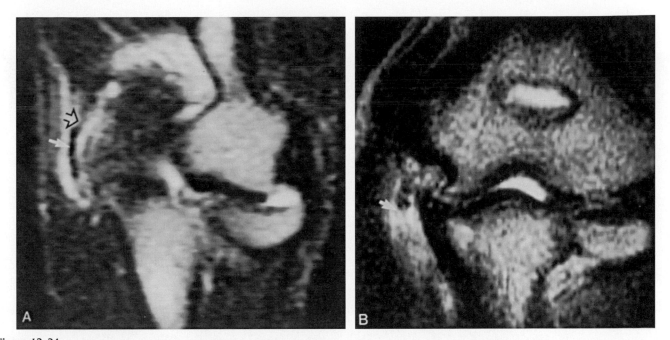

Figure 13–24

Medial collateral ligament injury: MR imaging—tears.

A In a baseball pitcher with a collateral ligament injury, a coronal T2-weighted (TR/TE, 2500/80) spin echo MR image shows an ill-defined medial collateral ligament, with increased signal intensity, indicating fluid surrounding its margins, particularly medially (solid arrow). In addition, a focus of abnormal increased signal intensity is present within the substance of the proximal portion of the ligament (open arrow).

B In a second patient, a complete rupture of the medial collateral ligament is manifest in a coronal T2-weighted (TR/TE, 2250/80) spin echo MR image as thickening and proximal retraction of the ligament (arrow). Increased signal intensity surrounding the medial collateral ligament is indicative of hemorrhage and edema.

Illustration continued on following page

sawa.[116] In the normal elbow, the periosteum of the ulna is an extension of the medial collateral ligament, with signal intensity characteristics that differ from those of the ligament. Prior to fusion of the medial epicondyle with the humerus, valgus stress applied to the elbow produces fragmentation of the epicondylar ossification center as well as subchondral resorption of bone. Subsequent to fusion, more typical findings of ligamentous disruption are seen.[116] In children and adults, the role of MR arthrography in the evaluation of ligamentous injuries about the elbow is not established (Fig. 13–25).[193, 197]

Complications of ligamentous disruptions about the elbow depend on their cause. In cases of elbow dislocation, such complications include chronic instability with recurrent dislocations, associated fractures, intra-articular bodies, stretching of the annular ligament, and entrapment of the brachial artery and median nerve. In children, entrapment of the medial epicondyle of the humerus may result from an elbow dislocation.

Tendinous Abnormalities

Classification and General Abnormalities

The classification of tendon injuries about the elbow can be accomplished in a number of ways. Such injuries can be categorized as medial (common flexor tendon), lateral (common extensor tendon), posterior (tendon of the triceps brachii muscle), or anterolateral (tendon of the distal portion of the biceps brachii muscle). They

can be classified further according to pattern or degree (e.g., partial or complete intratendinous tear, avulsion injury at the site of tendon attachment to bone) or to their acute or chronic (i.e., overuse syndrome) nature. Tendon injury related to a single isolated event is uncommon, although disruption of the bicipital tendon attachment to the radial tuberosity and of the triceps tendon attachment to the ulnar olecranon process is encountered. Tendon disruptions about the elbow also may occur as a complication of systemic diseases such as primary or secondary hyperparathyroidism, systemic lupus erythematosus, rheumatoid arthritis, and osteogenesis imperfecta.[117, 118] More commonly, however, tendinous injuries result from the chronic stress of sports activities that require repetitive elbow motion (e.g., golf and tennis) and often are referred to as epicondylitis (i.e., medial or lateral). A number of excellent reviews of tendon injuries about the elbow,[119–121] as well as more limited descriptions of such injuries,[122–125] are available to the interested reader.

Although the accurate diagnosis of tendinous injury relies foremost on analysis of historical aspects of the injury supplemented by careful physical examination, imaging techniques also can supply important information. Routine radiography may reveal avulsion fractures at sites of tendinous attachment to bone and soft tissue swelling. Although other imaging methods such as CT scanning and ultrasonography may be used to delineate tendinous injuries,[126] MR imaging appears most suitable to this task.[107] Normal tendons about the elbow (and elsewhere) appear as smooth, linear structures of low

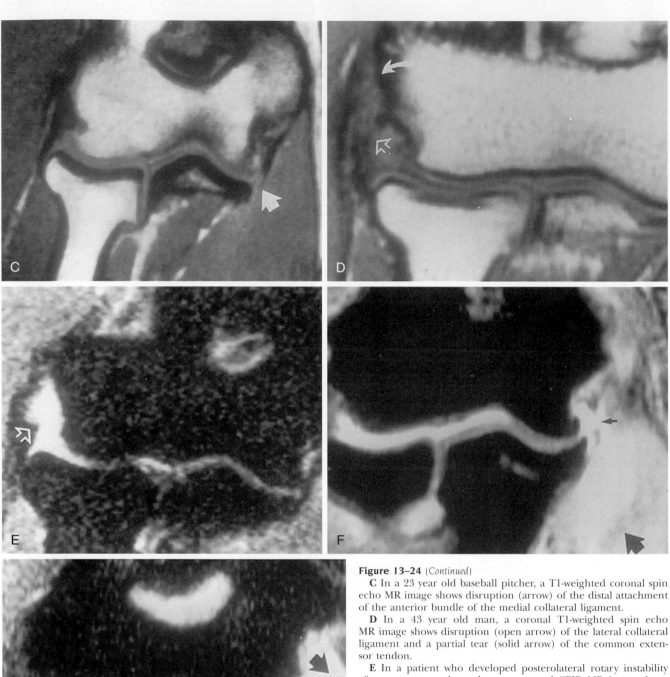

Figure 13–24 (*Continued*)

C In a 23 year old baseball pitcher, a T1-weighted coronal spin echo MR image shows disruption (arrow) of the distal attachment of the anterior bundle of the medial collateral ligament.

D In a 43 year old man, a coronal T1-weighted spin echo MR image shows disruption (open arrow) of the lateral collateral ligament and a partial tear (solid arrow) of the common extensor tendon.

E In a patient who developed posterolateral rotary instability after extensor tendon release, a coronal STIR MR image shows complete disruption (open arrow) of the lateral ulnar collateral ligament.

F In a 30 year old football player, a midsubstance tear (small arrow) of the medial collateral ligament and a strain of the flexor digitorum superficialis muscle (large arrow) are evident on a coronal STIR MR image.

G In a professional baseball player who had had an allograft replacement of the medial collateral ligament, a coronal STIR MR image reveals increased signal intensity (large straight arrow) at the site of the ruptured graft. Increased signal intensity in the lateral portion of the radial head (curved arrow) is the result of impaction forces related to valgus instability. The lateral ulnar collateral ligament (small straight arrows) is intact.

(**A, B**, From Mirowitz SA, et al: Radiology *185*:573, 1992; **C–G**, Courtesy of R. C. Fritz, M.D., San Francisco, California.)

Figure 13–25
Lateral collateral ligament injury: MR arthrography. After the intra-articular injection of saline solution, coronal (TR/TE, 4000/95) **(A)** and transaxial (TR/TE, 5000/105) **(B)** fast spin echo MR images show complete disruption of the lateral collateral ligament complex, with extracapsular extension of the saline solution (of high signal intensity). Distortion of the attachment site of the common extensor tendon is observed. (Courtesy of D. Levey, M.D., Corpus Christi, Texas.)

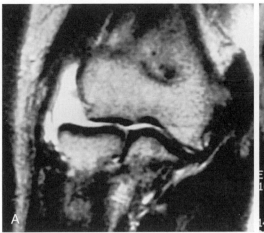
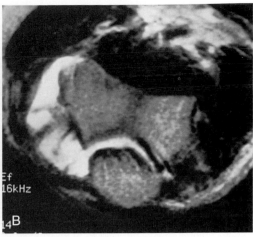

signal intensity on MR imaging sequences. A magic angle phenomenon, however, occasionally leads to regions of intermediate signal intensity within the tendons when MR imaging sequences using short echo times (TE) are employed. Tendinous tears and avulsions are associated with irregular and frayed contours and alterations in signal intensity of the tendons. The extent of abnormality relates to the severity of the injury (i.e., complete or partial tears). Complete tears are accompanied by discontinuity and retraction of the tendon, and partial tears are accompanied by some remaining intact tendinous fibers. Alterations in signal intensity depend on the age of injury, although high signal intensity within the tendon itself and the adjacent soft tissues and bone commonly is present on T2-weighted spin echo MR images. Obliteration of nearby fat planes and local hematomas also are seen. With healing, scar formation develops in the injured tendon that may lead to regions of low to intermediate signal intensity, even on T2-weighted spin echo images.

Injuries of the Biceps Tendon

Rupture of the tendon of the biceps brachii muscle about the elbow is rare, constituting less than 5 per cent of all biceps tendon injuries,[127] although it represents an important injury. Men are affected far more commonly than women, and the elbow in the dominant upper extremity usually is involved. Although the age of the persons with such injuries varies considerably, most are adults in the fourth, fifth, and sixth decades of life. The typical mechanism of injury relates to forceful hyperextension applied to a flexed and supinated forearm, as may occur in competitive weightlifters. Although the injury often occurs acutely after a single traumatic event, its appearance in persons engaged in strenuous and repetitive physical activity, including athletes, underscores the importance of preexisting degenerative changes in the tendon in the pathogenesis of its rupture and supports the general concept that normal tendons rarely rupture. With complete disruption of the distal portion of the biceps tendon, acute and intense pain in the antecubital fossa, a palpable defect about the elbow, and a proximal lump related to the retracted muscle

allow accurate clinical diagnosis. Accurate diagnosis is more difficult in cases of complete tears without such retraction and of partial tears of the tendon. With delayed diagnosis, chronic pain that increases with physical activity and weakness in flexion of the elbow, supination of the forearm, and grip strength occur.[119]

The propensity for rupture of the distal tendinous portion of the biceps brachii muscle to develop at sites of tendon degeneration may explain the occurrence of subtle radiographic abnormalities that may be evident about the radial tuberosity. Irregularity of the osseous surface of the tuberosity, with associated bone proliferation, has been noted,[119] suggesting that irritation of the biceps tendon as it rubs against the irregular surface of the radial tuberosity during pronation and supination of the forearm may eventually lead to its disruption. An accompanying chronic cubital bursitis has been emphasized in some reports.[128] The cubital bursa separates the tendon (and its paratenon) from the radial tuberosity and its inflammation (i.e., bursitis) may be associated with either tendon degeneration or tendon rupture (Fig. 13–26).[129] The clinical differentiation of cubital bursitis, bicipital tendon degeneration, and partial rupture of the bicipital tendon is extremely difficult, and this clinical dilemma is accentuated owing to the simul-

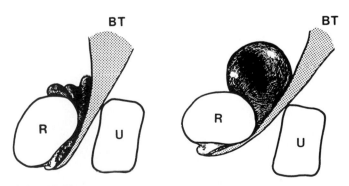

Figure 13–26
Biceps brachii tendon: Degeneration associated with cubital bursitis. Cubital bursitis may occur in association with degeneration of the distal biceps insertion. BT, biceps tendon; R, radius; U, ulna. (With permission from Karanjia ND, Stiles PJ: Cubital bursitis. J Bone Joint Surg [Br] 70:832, 1988.)

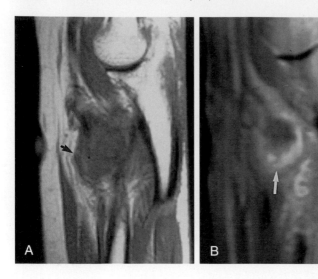

Figure 13–27
Biceps brachii tendon: Degeneration and tear associated with
cubital bursitis. A mass (arrow) is seen surrounding the biceps
tendon in a sagittal T1-weighted (TR/TE, 800/15) spin echo MR
image **(A)**. The periphery of the mass shows enhancement of
signal intensity (arrow) in a sagittal fat-suppressed T1-weighted
(TR/TE, 770/15) spin echo MR image obtained after intravenous administration of a gadolinium compound **(B)**.

taneous occurrence of two or more of these conditions
(Fig. 13–27), as well as irritation of the adjacent median
nerve, which may complicate cubital bursitis or partial
tendon rupture.[129] Ultrasonography, CT scanning, and
MR imaging have all been applied to the assessment of
cubital bursitis.[189, 190]

The identification of partial tears of the biceps tendon
is relatively recent. Indeed, the pathogenesis of such
tears is not agreed on.[119] Some authors regard the initial
pathologic site in cases of incomplete rupture of the
tendon to be the lacertus fibrosus (Fig. 13–28), which
courses from the biceps tendon proximally in a distal
direction to interdigitate with longitudinal fibers of the
antebrachial fascia over the proximal one third of the
flexor-pronator muscle group; primary rupture of the
lacertus fibrosus may lead to secondary elongation of
the biceps tendon, producing an incompetent tendon
whose radial attachment site is intact. Other authors
regard the initial site of injury to be the biceps tendon
itself; partial (and, later, complete) disruption of the
biceps tendon subsequently is accompanied by stretching or tearing of the lacertus fibrosus. Whatever the
precise mechanism, clinical diagnosis is more difficult in
those cases in which the biceps tendon is not disrupted
completely, and a role for imaging assessment, particularly with MR imaging, in such cases appears likely.

The application of MR imaging to evaluation of tears
of the bicipital tendon about the elbow is well described
(Figs. 13–29 to 13–32).[129–131, 194] Transaxial images are
most useful, but these must encompass the entire region
from the musculotendinous junction of the biceps tendon to the insertion of the tendon on the radial tuberosity. The inclusion of comparison images of the opposite
(uninvolved) side is not necessary (except for those who
are not familiar with elbow anatomy) and, indeed, leads
to considerable prolongation of the examination. Sagittal MR images of the involved elbow, however, are useful
in some cases. Classic MR imaging features include absence of the tendon distally, a fluid-filled tendon sheath,
a mass in the antecubital fossa, and muscle edema or
atrophy in cases of complete rupture; in addition, high
signal intensity within the tendon, fluid in the tendon
sheath, and thinning or thickening of the distal tendon
are seen in cases of partial tears.[131] The status of the
lacertus fibrosus can be assessed in the transaxial images, although such assessment may not be critical as
this structure generally is not repaired during surgical
procedures that address the partially or completely ruptured biceps tendon.[129] In cases of complete disruption,
the biceps tendon can be reattached anatomically to the
radial tuberosity (with a potential risk of injury to the
radial nerve) or, alternatively, the biceps tendon can be
inserted into the brachialis muscle. The first of these two

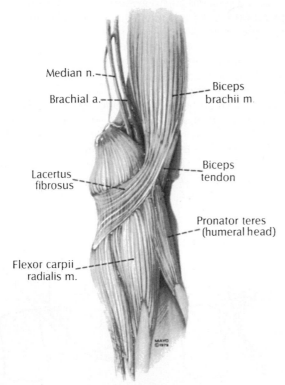

Median n.
Brachial a.
Biceps brachii m.
Lacertus fibrosus
Biceps tendon
Pronator teres (humeral head)
Flexor carpii radialis m.

MAYO ©1975

Figure 13–28
Lacertus fibrosus. Course of the lacertus fibrosus in the antecubital
fossa is shown. The median nerve may be trapped under this structure
as it compresses the origin of the pronator teres. (From Morrey BF
[Ed]: The Elbow and Its Disorders. 2nd Ed. Philadelphia, WB Saunders, 1993, p 827).

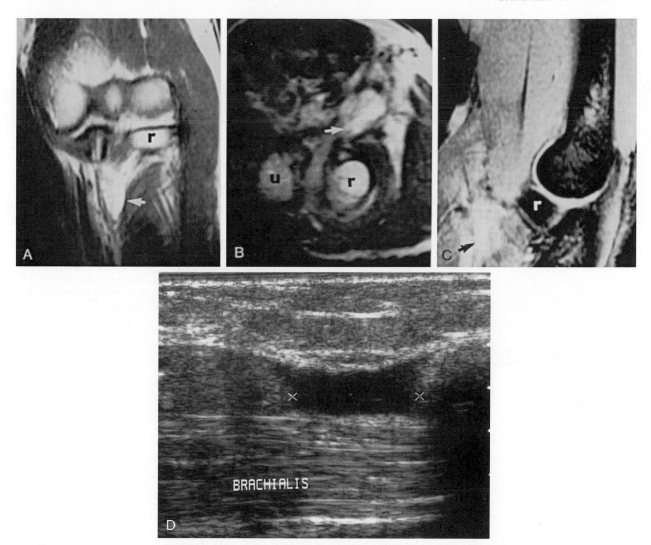

Figure 13–29
Biceps brachii tendon: Tears.

A, B Acute partial avulsive injury in a 78 year old man. Coronal T2-weighted (TR/TE, 2000/70) spin echo MR image **(A)** shows fluid of high signal intensity (arrow) adjacent to the radial tuberosity. The head of the radius (r) is indicated. A transaxial T2-weighted (TR/TE, 2000/80) spin echo MR image **(B)** shows a region of high signal intensity (arrow) anterior to the neck of the radius (r). The ulna (u) also is indicated.

C Acute complete avulsive injury in a 48 year old man. A sagittal MPGR MR image (TR/TE, 500/15; flip angle, 30 degrees) shows regions of high signal intensity (arrow) anterior to the notch of the radius (r). The tendon is retracted, and a prominence of the biceps muscle in the anterior portion of the upper arm is seen. (Courtesy of S.K. Brahme, M.D., La Jolla, California.)

D Ultrasonography can be applied to the assessment of tears of the biceps brachii tendon. In this example, a sonogram of the anterior aspect of the elbow in the sagittal plane demonstrates anechoic fluid between the retracted ends (markers) of the completely torn tendon. (Courtesy of M. van Holsbeeck, M.D., Detroit, Michigan, and J. Jacobson, M.D., San Diego, California.)

techniques is accompanied by more normal function of the forearm, including supination.[119] The treatment of partial tears of the biceps tendon often includes complete removal of the remaining fibers of the tendon, trimming of the torn end of the tendon, and reattachment of this torn end to the radial tuberosity.[119] Heterotopic ossification between the ulna and the radius is a recognized complication of surgical treatment of biceps tendon injury, however.

Injuries of the Triceps Tendon

Disruption of the triceps tendon is not encountered commonly. The extent of injury is variable, although complete tears are more frequent than partial tears.

Both men and women and both adults and children may be affected, with the mean age of involved patients being approximately 30 years. As with other tendons, rupture of the triceps tendon can occur spontaneously (as in primary or secondary hyperparathyroidism and systemic lupus erythematosus) or after injury. Two types of traumatic insult have been noted.[119] Most typically, a deceleration force applied to the extended arm with contraction of the triceps muscle (as in a fall) is responsible for the tendinous injury, although tears or avulsions of the triceps tendon have been noted to result from uncoordinated and excessive contraction of the muscle (as in body builders). A second (and uncommon) mechanism of injury relates to a direct blow to the posterior aspect of the elbow where the triceps

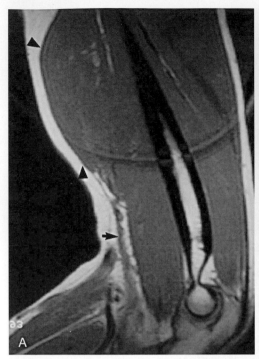
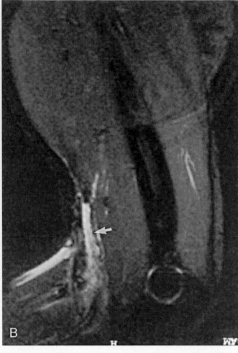

Figure 13–30

Biceps brachii tendon: Tears. Complete rupture in a 41 year old man who noted a popping sensation while lifting a heavy weight.

A A sagittal T1-weighted (TR/TE, 570/15) spin echo MR image shows a corkscrew-like appearance of the biceps brachii tendon (arrow). Note the retracted muscle (arrowheads). A wrap-around artifact relates to patient positioning for the MR imaging examination.

B A sagittal STIR MR image (TR/TE, 6200/22; inversion time, 150 msec) shows the abnormal biceps brachii tendon (arrow).

(Courtesy of C. Wakeley, M.D., Bristol, England.)

tendon attaches to the ulnar olecranon process.[119] Associated findings may include olecranon bursitis and subluxation of the ulnar nerve.[132, 133] Accurate clinical diagnosis of disruption of the triceps tendon relies on the presence of local pain, swelling, and ecchymosis, a palpable defect, and partial or complete loss of the ability to extend the elbow.

Typically, failure of the triceps tendon occurs at its site of insertion in the olecranon process (i.e., avulsion injury), and routine radiographs in such cases often reveal bone fragments of variable size that are diagnostic of the injury. Less commonly, the site of abnormality is the myotendinous junction or the muscle belly itself.[119]

Fractures of the radial head may be an associated injury.[134]

MR imaging has been employed in the evaluation of triceps tendon injuries (Figs. 13–33 and 13–34).[129, 135] Transaxial and sagittal MR images are most useful. In the normal situation, the appearance of the triceps tendon depends on the position of the elbow; the tendon often appears lax and redundant when the elbow is imaged in full extension and taut when the elbow is imaged with mild degrees of flexion.[129] The MR imaging features of a torn triceps tendon are similar to those associated with tears of other tendons. Accompanying findings include olecranon bursitis and edema of the

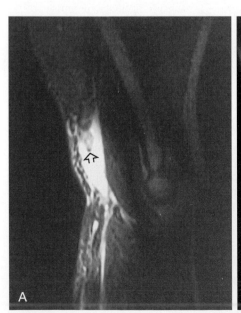
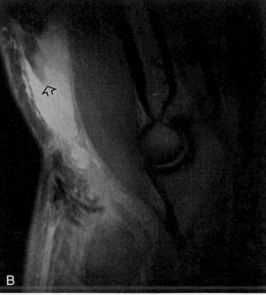

Figure 13–31

Biceps brachii tendon: Tears. Complete rupture at distal insertion site in a 44 year old man. Sagittal STIR (TR/TE, 3000/38; inversion time, 150 msec) **(A)** and fat-suppressed fast spin echo (TR/TE, 3300/17) **(B)** MR images reveal the retracted tendon (arrows) and soft tissue edema and hemorrhage of high signal intensity.

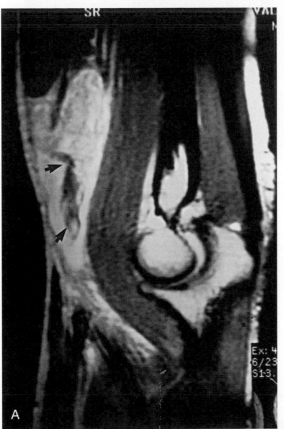

Figure 13–32

Biceps brachii tendon: Tears. Complete rupture at distal insertion site.

A In a sagittal fast spin echo MR image (TR/TE, 4133/19), note the torn and retracted tendon (arrows) with surrounding hematoma.

B A transaxial fast spin echo MR image (TR/TE, 4316/20) at the approximate level of the humeral epicondyle shows the thickened, retracted biceps tendon (arrow) with surrounding hematoma.

C A transaxial fast spin echo MR image (TR/TE, 4316/20) through the distal portion of the humerus and olecranon process demonstrates a hematoma (arrow) with no visualization of the biceps tendon.

(Courtesy of D. Levey, M.D., Corpus Christi, Texas.)

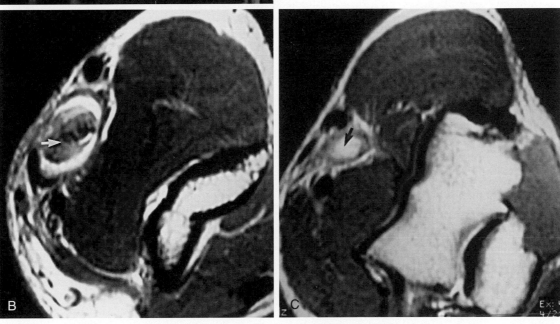

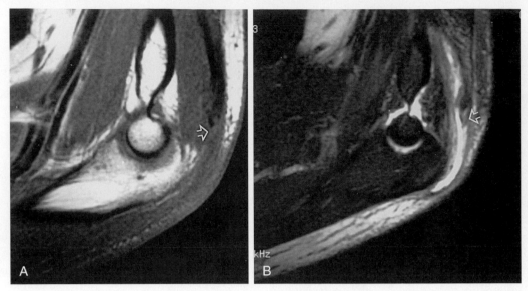

Figure 13–33

Triceps tendon: Tears. Acute complete avulsive injury in a 30 year old man. On a sagittal T1-weighted spin echo (TR/TE, 500/17) **(A)** and a sagittal fast spin echo (TR/TE, 3500/100) **(B)** MR image, the latter obtained with fat suppression, note the torn and retracted tendon (arrows) with surrounding hemorrhage and bursitis. (Courtesy of D. Witte, M.D., Memphis, Tennessee.)

marrow in the olecranon process. The latter finding also may be indicative of a stress fracture of the bone, which may occur in the absence of failure of the tendon.[136]

The treatment of a complete rupture of the triceps tendon is surgical repair with reattachment of the tendon to the olecranon process; partial tears of the triceps tendon may be treated conservatively.

A snapping sensation about the posteromedial aspect of the elbow may have several causes, including subluxation of the ulnar nerve or dislocation of a portion of the triceps mechanism.[119] A snapping triceps tendon syndrome has been described, resulting most often from subluxation of the medial head of the triceps muscle over the medial epicondyle of the humerus.[137] This condition, which also may relate to the presence of an anomalous slip of the triceps tendon, may be associated with irritation of the ulnar nerve.[138]

Overuse Syndromes and Epicondylitis

Chronic stress applied to the elbow is frequent in a number of sporting activities.[120, 121, 136, 139, 191] A spectrum of injuries of varying severity may result. The frequency of involvement of the flexor and extensor tendinous attachments of the medial and lateral epicondyles, respectively, has led to the designation of epicondylitis as a general term applied to these overuse syndromes. Their frequency in tennis players (perhaps affecting as many as 10 to 50 per cent of persons who play tennis regularly) also has led to the designation of tennis elbow. As histologic examination of injured tissue has confirmed the absence of a classic inflammatory reaction, the term epicondylitis (or even tendinitis) is not ideal; since the injury is not confined to tennis players, the term tennis elbow likewise is not suitable. Anatomically, these overuse syndromes can be classified ac-

cording to location: lateral, medial, and posterior. The lateral side of the elbow is involved approximately seven times more frequently than the medial side.[136] Posterior localization, represented by involvement of the triceps tendon at its attachment site to the olecranon process, is uncommon. Reported abnormalities associated with these overuse syndromes have included ulnar nerve neurapraxia, carpal tunnel syndrome, and entrapment of the motor branch of the radial nerve in the radial tunnel.[120]

In general, this tendon injury results from extrinsic tensile overload, which, over a period of time, produces microscopic tears that do not heal properly.[136] The specific location that is affected (i.e., medial or lateral epicondylar region) depends on whether the flexors or extensors of the wrist and digits are the site of stress during any particular sporting activity.[136] Macroscopic inspection of involved tendons reveals a grayish, gelatinous, friable, and edematous tissue that closely resembles scar tissue, and the appearance is similar to that encountered in tendinitis (or tendinosis or tendinopathy) affecting the rotator cuff, patellar tendon, or Achilles tendon or of plantar fasciitis.[120] The reported frequency of macroscopically visible deep or superficial tears of the tendon has varied from about 35 to 70 per cent.[121] Descriptions of microscopic pathologic findings in cases of such tendon injury about the elbow also have not been consistent. In some cases, findings have included infiltration of round cells, tendon necrosis, calcific foci, and scar tissue.[121] In other cases, invasion of the tendon by fibroblasts and vascular granulation tissue has been noted, which has been described as angiofibroblastic hyperplasia.[120] The degree of angiofibroblastic infiltration appears to correlate with the duration of the symptoms, and the involved tendon also may appear hypercellular, degenerative, and fragmented.[120] The absence of a significant inflammatory response has

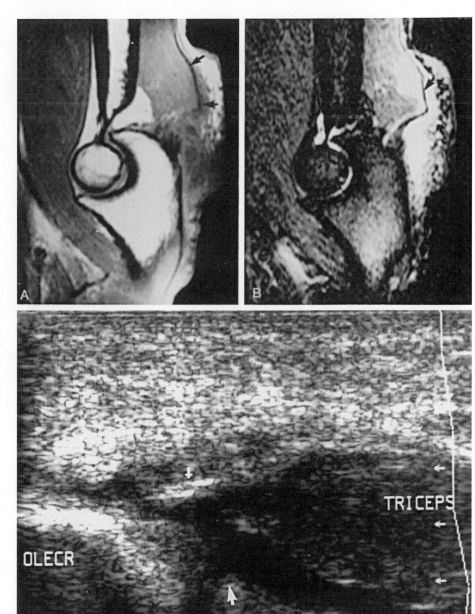

Figure 13–34

Triceps tendon: Tears.

A, B Acute complete avulsive injury in a 51 year old man. Sagittal T1-weighted (TR/TE, 800/20) **(A)** and T2-weighted (TR/TE, 2500/80) **(B)** spin echo MR images show tendon laxity (arrows), disorganization at the ulnar site of attachment, and muscle retraction. Note regions of high signal intensity in **B**.

C In a second patient, ultrasonography in the sagittal plane demonstrates anechoic fluid (arrows) between the olecranon process and retracted triceps tendon. (Courtesy of M. van Holsbeeck, M.D., Detroit, Michigan, and J. Jacobson, M.D., San Diego, California.)

been emphasized repeatedly, however, and may explain the inadequacy of the healing process.

Lateral epicondylitis appears to represent the most common injury of the athlete's elbow. Affected structures include the lateral extensor tendons, particularly the extensor carpi radialis brevis tendon at its site of origin in the lateral epicondyle. It is the backhand stroke in tennis that appears to be most responsible for this lesion; electromyographic studies confirm high activity in this tendon during the backhand stroke, in which the wrist is maintained in extension and radial deviation.[140] Altered mechanics during this stroke when accomplished single-handedly (the lesion is rare in tennis players who use a double-handed backhand tennis stroke) subjects the wrist extensors to greater force. Clinical findings include the insidious onset of lateral elbow pain, with tenderness to palpation of the origin of the extensor carpi radialis brevis tendon or the extensor longus or common digital extensor tendons. Routine radiographs generally are normal, although calcification about the lateral epicondyle has been noted in 20 to 30 per cent of cases.[136] Conservative treatment generally is adequate, although surgical procedures may be employed in recalcitrant cases.[136]

Medial epicondylitis, which also has been designated medial tennis elbow or golfer's or pitcher's elbow, is far less common than lateral epicondylitis. This condition also has been observed in javelin throwers, racquetball and squash players, swimmers, and bowlers. The pronator teres and flexor carpi radialis tendons are involved most frequently resulting in pain and tenderness to palpation over the anterior aspect of the medial epicondyle of the humerus and the origin of the flexor-pronator tendons. Pain results from resisting pronation of the

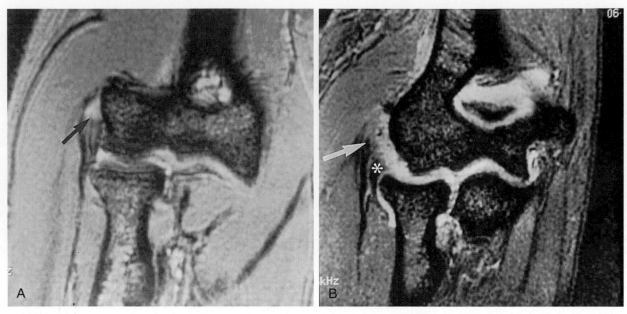

Figure 13–35

Lateral epicondylitis: Degeneration and tears of the extensor carpi radialis brevis tendon.

A Tendon degeneration. A coronal three-dimensional Fourier transform gradient echo MR image (TR/TE, 56/18; flip angle, 10 degrees) in a 40 year old man with a 2 year history of elbow pain shows signal hyperintensity at the origin of the extensor carpi radialis brevis tendon (arrow), with separation between the extensor tendons and the radial collateral ligament. Severe tendon degeneration was noted at the time of surgery.

B Tendon tear. A coronal multiplanar gradient echo recalled (MPGR) MR image (TR/TE, 451/20; flip angle, 45 degrees) in a 51 year old man with a 1 year history of lateral elbow pain (with a recent increase in severity of the pain) shows complete disruption of the extensor origin of the extensor carpi radialis brevis tendon (arrow). The retracted edge of the tendon is focally thickened. A tear of the humeral aspect of the radial collateral ligament (asterisk) also is seen. These findings were confirmed surgically.

(Reproduced with permission from Potter HG, et al: *Radiology 196*:43, 1995.)

forearm or flexion of the wrist.[139] An associated ulnar neuropathy at the elbow has been emphasized in some reports,[139] and the repetitive valgus stress seen in throwing athletes may produce medial collateral ligament injury or laxity.[136] As in the case of lateral epicondylitis, conservative treatment of medial epicondylitis generally is adequate. Surgery may be required in some cases, however, especially in instances of full-thickness tendon tears.

MR imaging has been employed to assess patients with lateral or medial epicondylitis (Figs. 13–35 to 13–38).[17, 114, 115, 129, 141] All three planes (transaxial, coronal, and sagittal) of imaging may be necessary. Spin echo images may require supplementation with STIR images or those obtained after the intravenous administration of a gadolinium compound. The precise appearance of the lesion depends on the severity of the process, which varies from partial or complete tendon tears to tendon degeneration (tendinosis or tendinopathy). Complete tendon tears are associated with gaps between the af-

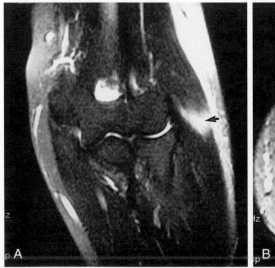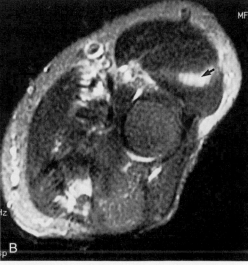

Figure 13–36

Lateral epicondylitis: Tears of the extensor carpi radialis brevis tendon and muscle. These coronal (TR/TE, 3000/100) **(A)** and transaxial (TR/TE, 3000/90) **(B)** fat-suppressed fast spin echo MR images in a patient with tennis elbow show the site of injury (arrows) as a region of high signal intensity.

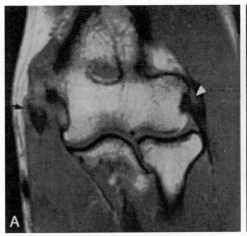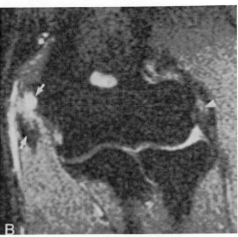

Figure 13–37
Medial epicondylitis: Acute avulsive injury of the common flexor tendon. A coronal T1-weighted (TR/TE, 600/30) spin echo MR image **(A)** shows avulsion of the flexor tendons (arrow) from the medial epicondyle of the humerus. Abnormal signal intensity also is evident in the common extensor tendons (arrowhead). A coronal STIR MR image **(B)** reveals high signal intensity at the site of flexor tendon avulsion (arrows), altered signal intensity in the common extensor tendons (arrowhead), and a joint effusion. (Courtesy of C. Ho, M.D., Palo Alto, California.)

fected tendon and adjacent bone surfaces that may accumulate fluid, leading to high signal intensity on T2-weighted spin echo images. Partial tears are accompanied by thinning of the tendon, with disruption of some of its fibers. Tendinosis or tendinopathy is associated with intermediate signal intensity on T1-weighted spin echo images, with no further increase in signal intensity on T2-weighted spin echo images. STIR and intravenous gadolinium-enhanced MR images generally accentuate the abnormalities of signal intensity in cases of partial or complete tendon tears. As one example, increased signal intensity in the anconeus muscle in STIR images has been observed in some patients with lateral epicondylitis.[142] Volumetric gradient echo MR imaging also may be beneficial owing to the ability to reformat the image data in a nonconventional oblique plane, the appropriate axis depending on the precise tendon that is being studied.[141] The value of MR imaging in the assessment of epicondylitis relates also to the ability to detect any associated abnormalities, including those of the collateral ligaments.

Muscle Abnormalities

Muscle injuries occur about the elbow (Figs. 13–36 and 13–39), especially in professional athletes. These are discussed in Chapter 10.

Nerve Abnormalities

As described in Chapter 11, entrapment and compression neuropathies about the elbow may involve the ulnar, radial, or median nerve.[136, 143, 144] Such neuropathies often result from indirect injuries related to friction, traction, or compression of a nerve, or, far less frequently, these neuropathies may relate to contusion produced by a direct blow.

Nerve injuries about the elbow in athletes involve the ulnar nerve most commonly (Fig. 13–40). The superficial location of this nerve makes it vulnerable to contusion from direct trauma occurring in contact sports. This vulnerability may be increased when the nerve

reveals anterior subluxation, a finding that may be evident in as many as 10 to 20 per cent of the general population.[145] Indirect injury to the ulnar nerve related to compression, traction, or friction also is common in athletes. During the course of elbow motion, the volume of the cubital tunnel (through which the ulnar nerve passes) changes. For each 45 degrees of elbow flexion, the retinaculum of the cubital tunnel stretches nearly 5 mm, and at about 90 degrees of flexion, the proximal edge of this retinaculum becomes taut.[143] This change in configuration of the retinaculum, when combined with relaxation and bulging of the medial collateral ligament that normally occur during elbow flexion, leads to a significant reduction in the volume of the cubital tunnel.[146] Furthermore, during elbow motion, the ulnar nerve normally moves in a mediolateral and longitudinal direction. Narrowing of the cubital tunnel may interfere with this sliding movement, leading to perineurial damage. Resulting ulnar neuritis is especially common in sporting activities that require overhead motion of the arm, such as pitching a baseball. The nerve is stretched as it passes behind the medial epicondyle of the humerus with the elbow flexed in a slight valgus position.[136] The nerve may become tethered by scar formation, traction enthesophytes, calcific deposits in and around the medial collateral ligament, or an irregular osseous surface of the ulna related to osteoarthritis or a remote medial epicondylar separation.[136] One specific type of ulnar nerve entrapment syndrome is termed the Osborne lesion and relates to thickening of the retinaculum of the cubital tunnel with or without hypertrophy of the flexor musculature of the forearm.[136, 147] Other types of entrapment are associated with recurrent anterior dislocation of the ulnar nerve (which may result from developmental laxity of the soft tissue constraints that normally hold the nerve within the epicondylar groove) or hypertrophy of the medial head of the triceps muscles or anconeus epitrochlearis muscle (as in baseball pitchers or weightlifters).[136] Clinical manifestations of ulnar neuritis in athletes are similar to those of the cubital tunnel syndrome related to such diverse causes as osteoarthritis, rheumatoid arthritis, prolonged bed rest, anomalous muscles, masses, and trochlear hypoplasia.[148–150] These manifestations include

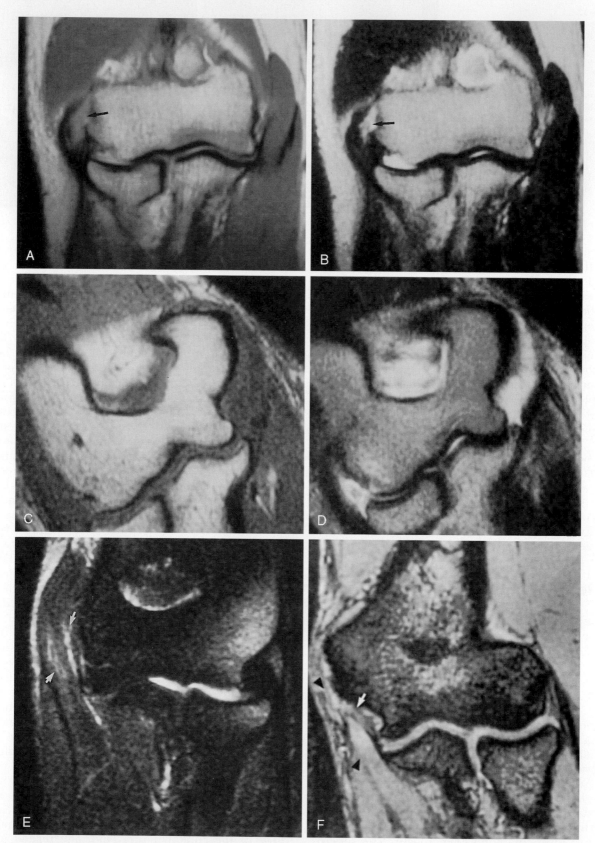

Figure 13–38 *See legend on opposite page*

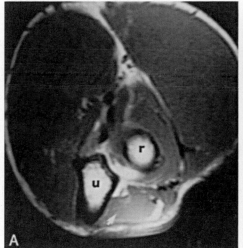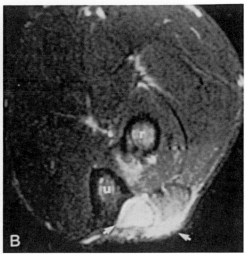

Figure 13–39
Muscle injury: Tear with edema of the anconeus muscle in a 30 year old male body builder who developed acute pain during weightlifting. Transaxial T1-weighted (TR/TE, 500/12) **(A)** and T2-weighted (TR/TE, 4000/68) **(B)** spin echo MR images, the latter obtained with chemical presaturation of fat (ChemSat), show altered morphology, and, in **B**, increased signal intensity in the anconeus muscle and surrounding tissues (arrows). Inflammatory changes in the biceps tendon also are evident. The radius (r) and ulna (u) are indicated. (Courtesy of C. Sebrechts, M.D., San Diego, California.)

weakness of the flexor carpi ulnaris muscle, flexor digitorum profundus muscle of the fourth and fifth fingers, and intrinsic hand muscles. The nerve may be enlarged and tender to palpation.

Although axial radiographs may reveal narrowing of the cubital tunnel related, in part, to osteophytosis,[151] MR imaging represents a far more elegant means to evaluate this syndrome.[115, 129, 152, 153] MR imaging abnormalities include displacement or shift of the ulnar nerve, a soft tissue mass, and enlargement and increased signal intensity in the compressed nerve (Fig. 13–41). Ulnar nerve enlargement may be focal, occurring at the level of the cubital tunnel, with a normal girth noted proximal and distal to the tunnel.[152] Subluxation of the ulnar nerve may be accentuated if MR imaging is performed with the elbow flexed.[153]

A variety of surgical procedures may be employed in the treatment of ulnar nerve entrapment. These include decompression of the nerve, medial epicondylectomy, or subcutaneous, intramuscular, or submuscular transfer (translocation) of the nerve.[195]

Entrapment of a portion of the radial nerve may occur just distal to the elbow where the posterior interosseous, or deep, branch passes into the supinator muscle. The terminology applied to this entrapment syndrome is not constant and has included the posterior interosseous nerve syndrome, the supinator syndrome,

the radial tunnel syndrome, and resistant tennis elbow syndrome. Potential causes of this syndrome include elbow dislocations, fractures, rheumatoid arthritis, soft tissue tumors, and traumatic or developmental fibrous bands.[154, 155] Recurrent radial vessels (the leash of Henry), the arcade of Frohse, and the margin of the extensor carpi radialis brevis muscle also may produce radial nerve entrapment. The affected patient may be unable to extend the fingers partially or completely at the metacarpophalangeal joints. Deep pain in the posterior portion or dorsum of the forearm, gradual fist weakness, and local pain on compression distal to the lateral humeral epicondyle may simulate the clinical manifestations of tennis elbow. Median nerve entrapment near the elbow may result from compression by the ligament of Struthers, extending distally from a supracondylar process; hypertrophy of the pronator teres muscle or fibrous bands leading to compression of the nerve in the antecubital area where the nerve passes between the two heads of the pronator teres muscle and then under the edge of the flexor digitorum sublimis muscle (pronator syndrome); and compression of the anterior interosseous nerve (Kiloh-Nevin syndrome), the motor branch of the ulnar nerve (see Chapter 11). MR imaging in cases of radial or median nerve compression may reveal a mass (e.g., lipoma or ganglion cyst) and displacement and abnormal signal intensity within

Figure 13–38
Medial and lateral epicondylitis: Various lesions.
  A, B A tear (arrows) of the common extensor tendon is evident on coronal proton density–weighted (TR/TE, 3000/21) **(A)** and T2-weighted (TR/TE, 3000/105) **(B)** spin echo MR images.
  C, D In this patient, who sustained an elbow dislocation, coronal T1-weighted (TR/TE, 700/18) **(C)** and proton density–weighted (TR/TE, 3000/15) **(D)** spin echo MR images show disruption of the common flexor tendon and medial collateral ligament.
  E A coronal fat-suppressed T2 weighted fast spin echo MR image reveals abnormal high signal intensity (arrows) indicative of a sprain of the medial collateral ligament and a flexor muscle strain.
  F Coronal gradient echo sequence (TR/TE, 50/15; flip angle, 10 degrees) demonstrates increased signal intensity within the proximal aspect of the common flexor tendon (arrowheads) and in the tissues surrounding the medial epicondyle. Mild increased signal intensity also is present in the proximal attachment of the ulnar collateral ligament (arrow), indicating partial injury. The extensor tendon and radial collateral ligament are normal.
  (A–E, Courtesy of P. Tirman, M.D., San Francisco, California; **F,** Courtesy of H. Pavlov, M.D., New York, New York.)

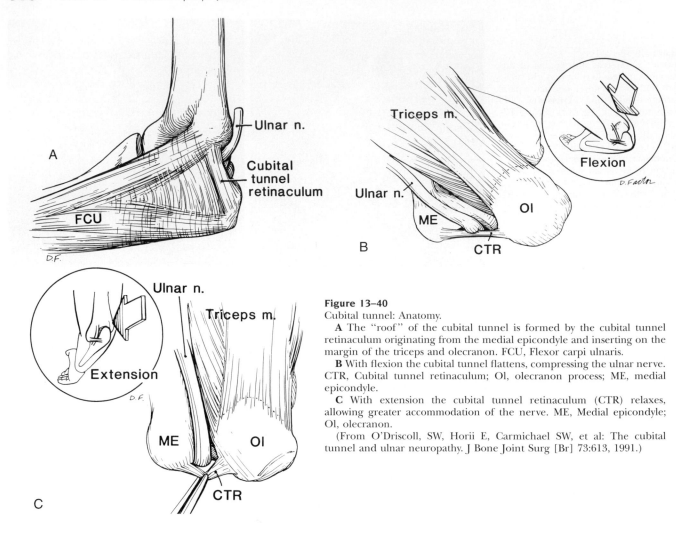

Figure 13–40

Cubital tunnel: Anatomy.

A The "roof" of the cubital tunnel is formed by the cubital tunnel retinaculum originating from the medial epicondyle and inserting on the margin of the triceps and olecranon. FCU, Flexor carpi ulnaris.

B With flexion the cubital tunnel flattens, compressing the ulnar nerve. CTR, Cubital tunnel retinaculum; Ol, olecranon process; ME, medial epicondyle.

C With extension the cubital tunnel retinaculum (CTR) relaxes, allowing greater accommodation of the nerve. ME, Medial epicondyle; Ol, olecranon.

(From O'Driscoll, SW, Horii E, Carmichael SW, et al: The cubital tunnel and ulnar neuropathy. J Bone Joint Surg [Br] 73:613, 1991.)

the affected nerve.[152, 196] Muscles innervated by the affected nerve may reveal abnormal signal intensity related to the presence of extracellular water or fatty infiltration.

Bone Abnormalities

Occult Fractures

As described in Chapter 8, various types of occult fractures of bone are encountered at virtually any anatomic site, including the bones about the elbow. These include acute fractures, trabecular microfractures, and stress fractures.

Most acute fractures about the elbow are readily identifiable on routine radiographs, and no further imaging studies are required. Some acute fractures, such as those of the radial head or neck, may escape radiographic detection unless observation of a positive "fat pad sign" is used as a stimulus to obtain supplementary and specialized radiographic projections. Even when these latter projections are employed, however, some fractures of the radial head or neck remain inapparent. In such cases, options available to the treating physician include prophylactic casting of the elbow with repeat radiographic examinations being performed about 1 week

later or the immediate use of other imaging methods such as bone scintigraphy or MR imaging. Either of these two techniques is highly sensitive in the detection of these fractures and, furthermore, negative results

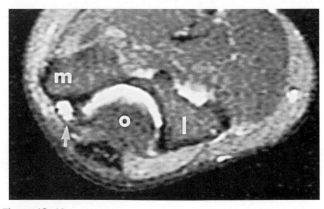

Figure 13–41

Entrapment neuropathy: Cubital tunnel syndrome. A transaxial T2-weighted (TR/TE, 2000/70) spin echo MR image, accomplished with chemical presaturation of fat (ChemSat) shows increased signal intensity in the ulnar nerve (arrow) within the cubital tunnel. The medial (m) and lateral (l) epicondyles of the humerus and the olecranon process (o) of the ulna are indicated. A joint effusion is present. (Courtesy of S.K. Brahme, M.D., La Jolla, California.)

with either of these methods virtually excludes the presence of a fracture. Although the cost effectiveness of acquiring scintigraphic or MR imaging examinations at the time of injury versus casting with delayed routine radiography in instances of such elbow trauma is not established, MR imaging appears to be the better of these two imaging techniques. Its main advantage relates to high specificity. Furthermore, the examination can be shortened significantly through the reliance on T1-weighted spin echo and STIR sequences.

Trabecular microfractures, or bone bruises, about the elbow may result from direct injury or indirect forces occurring in association with ligamentous disruption. As about the knee, these microfractures about the elbow are apparent on MR images owing to the presence of marrow edema and hemorrhage. High signal intensity in the affected marrow is evident on conventional or fast T2-weighted spin echo and STIR MR images (Fig. 13–42A, B). The value of specific patterns of distribution of marrow involvement in predicting sites

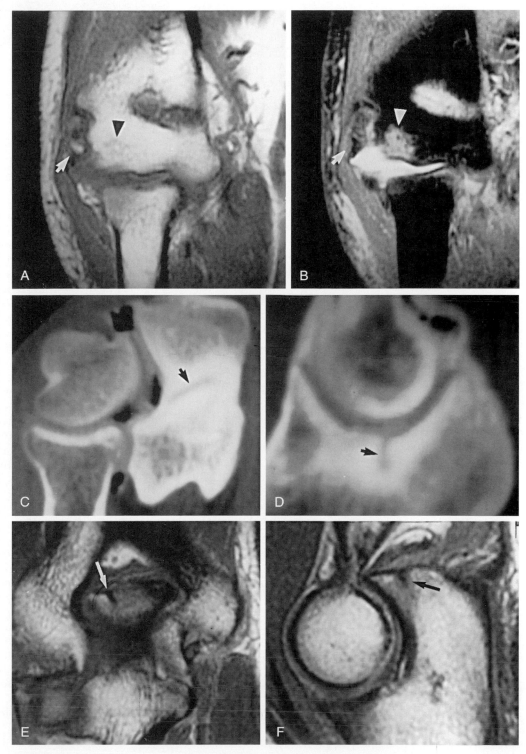

Figure 13–42
Occult fractures: Avulsion fractures, stress fractures, and trabecular microfractures (bone bruises).

A, B In a 25 year old man, oblique coronal T1-weighted (TR/TE, 550/12) spin echo **(A)** and fast spin echo STIR (TR/TE, 4000/17; inversion time, 150 msec) **(B)** MR images of the slightly flexed elbow reveal an avulsion fracture (arrows) of the medial epicondyle (which was evident on routine radiographs) and a bone bruise (arrowheads) of the humerus (which was not apparent on radiographs).

C, D In this basketball player, a stress fracture of the olecranon (arrows) is shown in coronal **(C)** and sagittal **(D)** CT scans during a CT arthrogram. (Courtesy of G. Greenway, M.D., Dallas, Texas.)

E, F In this baseball player, an olecranon stress fracture (arrows) is seen in coronal (TR/TE, 650/17) **(E)** and sagittal (TR/TE, 800/17) **(F)** T1-weighted spin echo MR images. This patient also had evidence of a medial collateral ligament injury.

of ligamentous and capsular injury of the elbow is not clear.

Stress fractures (i.e., fatigue and insufficiency fractures) are far more common in the bones of the lower extremity and pelvis than in those of the upper extremity (see Chapter 8). Stress fractures of the olecranon process, however, have been observed in athletes, particularly javelin throwers and baseball players.[156, 157] These may involve the tip of the olecranon process or its midarticular portion. Clinical and routine radiographic examinations may not allow accurate diagnosis, and bone scintigraphy (or, perhaps, CT scanning or MR imaging) may be required (see Fig. 13–42C–F).[136] Displacement of the fracture fragment or delayed union of the fracture is not uncommon, such that surgery may be used to treat these stress fractures. A similar lesion seen in adolescent baseball pitchers involves the physeal plate of the olecranon process.

Osteochondral Fractures and Osteochondritis Dissecans

As indicated in Chapter 8, the development and refinement of MR imaging have led to the identification of a number of occult injuries of subchondral bone and cartilage that may escape detection on routine radiographic analysis. Such injuries, which have been investigated most completely about the knee, include osteochondral fractures. They result from impaction and shearing forces applied to the articular surfaces, and they are manifested on MR images as irregularity of the chondral coat, fracture lines, and marrow edema. The last of these findings results in increased signal intensity on T2-weighted spin echo, gradient echo, and STIR imaging sequences.

Osteochondritis dissecans about the elbow usually affects the capitulum (see Chapter 8). This disorder differs from a developmental alteration of the capitular ossification center known as Panner's disease (Figs. 13–43 and 13–44). The precise relationship of osteochondritis dissecans of the capitulum and an osteochondral fracture is not clear, but most investigators regard

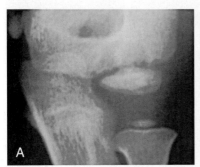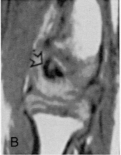

Figure 13–43
Panner's disease: MR imaging abnormalities.
A The frontal radiograph shows slight irregularity and increased density of the capitulum.
B A sagittal T1-weighted (TR/TE, 600/20) spin echo MR image demonstrates the abnormal signal intensity (arrow) in the ossified portion of the capitulum. The cartilage about this portion appears normal.
(Courtesy of A. Stauffer, M.D., Mission Viejo, California.)

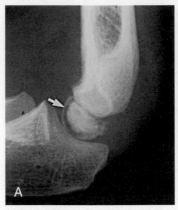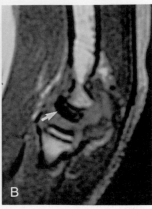

Figure 13–44
Panner's disease: MR imaging abnormalities. A 7 year old boy developed pain and stiffness in the elbow.
A The lateral radiograph demonstrates subtle increased radiodensity of the ossified portion of the capitulum with a peripheral radiolucent band (arrow). A joint effusion is present.
B The sagittal T1-weighted (TR/TE, 600/20) spin echo MR image shows that the capitellar ossification center contains marrow of low signal intensity (arrow).
(Courtesy of E. Bosch, M.D., Santiago, Chile.)

the former condition as a posttraumatic abnormality that may lead to osteonecrosis. In common with osteochondritis dissecans at other sites, such as the femoral condyles, a variety of imaging techniques, including routine radiography, conventional tomography, CT scanning, CT arthrography, and MR imaging, in cases of osteochondritis dissecans about the elbow (Fig. 13–45) may be used to gain information regarding the integrity of the adjacent articular cartilage, the viability of the separated fragment, and the presence or absence of associated intra-articular osseous and cartilaginous bodies.[115, 129, 158, 159] The presence of joint fluid or granulation tissue at the interface between the fragment and the parent bone, manifested as increased signal intensity on T2-weighted spin echo MR images, generally indicates an unstable lesion. A potential role exists for the use of intravenous administration of a gadolinium compound as an adjunct to the MR imaging examination.[159] Enhancement of signal intensity in granulation tissue occurs, which increases the value of the imaging method in allowing assessment of the stability of the lesion. Direct visualization of the articular cartilage with standard MR imaging sequences, however, remains a problem, and MR arthrography employing the intra-articular injection of gadolinium compounds may be advantageous, not only in the delineation of the chondral surface but also in the detection of intra-articular bodies (see later discussion). Injected gadolinium agent is of increased signal intensity on T1-weighted spin echo MR images and may be identified on the surface of the articular cartilage, within defects in the articular cartilage, and in the interface between the osteochondral fragment and subjacent bone. Conventional and computed arthrotomography both provide similar information. With these tomographic techniques, as well as with MR imaging, the extent of bone involvement becomes apparent. Sagittal, coronal, and transaxial images,

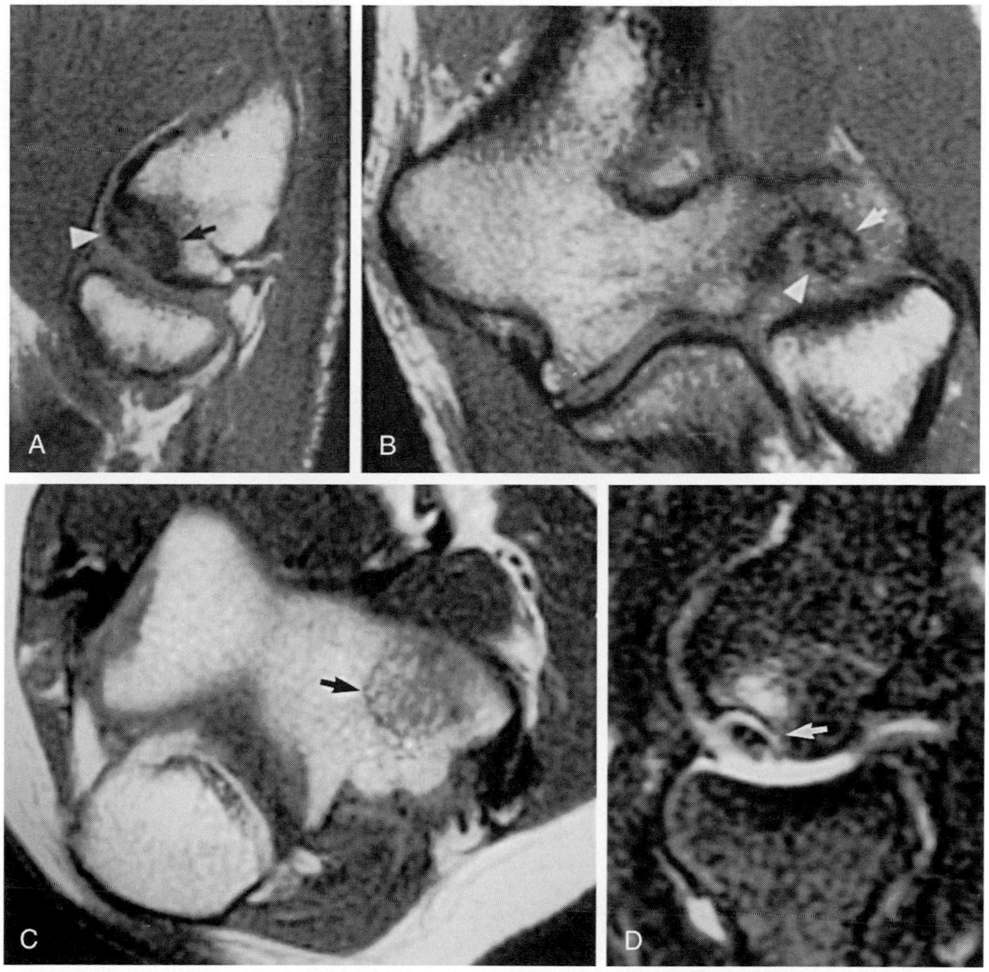

Figure 13–45
Osteochondritis dissecans: Capitulum of the humerus.

A, B In a 16 year old boy, a sagittal T1-weighted (TR/TE, 600/20) spin echo MR image **(A)** shows the concave defect (arrow) of the capitulum containing an ossified body (arrowhead). A coronal proton density–weighted (TR/TE, 2000/20) spin echo MR image **(B)** shows the osseous defect (arrow) containing an ossified body (arrowhead). The integrity of the adjacent articular cartilage cannot be determined. (Courtesy of M. Schweitzer, M.D., Philadelphia, Pennsylvania.)

C, D In a second patient, a similar lesion (arrows) is shown in a transaxial T1-weighted (TR/TE, 500/21) spin echo MR image **(C)** and in a sagittal fat-suppressed fast spin echo (TR/TE, 4000/92) MR image **(D)**. In **D**, note the fluid between a fragment and the parent bone, a joint effusion, and a region of high signal intensity in the capitulum. (Courtesy of D. Goodwin, M.D., Hanover, New Hampshire.)

readily obtained with MR imaging, allow full assessment of the osseous abnormalities.

Ultimately, it is the integrity of the articular cartilage and the stability of the lesion that guide the orthopedic surgeon's choice of therapy. Lesions that have intact cartilage and are not displaced often are treated conservatively; those that have progressed to complete displacement with intra-articular bodies often are treated with arthroscopic or open surgical removal of the bodies; and those lesions that have detached partially may be treated conservatively or surgically, with one option being arthroscopic pinning of the fragment.[136] With this in mind, the accuracy of any imaging method in placing the status of the lesion in the correct category must be compared to that of arthroscopy alone, a comparison that will require further investigation.

Chondroepiphyseal Injuries

Accurate radiographic diagnosis of acute injuries of the elbow in young children is difficult, owing to the large number of developing ossification centers, the normal irregularities of bone in these centers, and the cartilaginous components of these centers that are not visible on routine radiographs. Differentiation among the many types of Salter-Harris lesions of the growth plate (e.g., type II and type IV injuries of the distal portion

of the humerus) may be impossible when standard radiography alone is employed. As such differentiation has prognostic implications and may guide the orthopedic surgeon in his or her choice of therapy (i.e., closed reduction versus open reduction and fixation), a diagnostic role for other imaging methods such as arthrography and MR may exist.[160–162] Arthrography using radiopaque contrast material, perhaps combined with conventional tomography or CT, results in coating of the articular surfaces of the distal portion of the humerus and proximal portions of the radius and ulna. Interruption of the articular surface and opacification of fracture lines in the chondroepiphysis are important arthrographic findings, allowing accurate assessment of the extent of injury. Spin echo or gradient echo MR images provide direct visualization of the cartilaginous and osseous components of the chondroepiphyses about the elbow. Physeal separation and violation, fractures, and edema are readily detectable on such images.[163]

The occurrence of chronic physeal injuries of the elbow in young athletes has received increasing attention in recent years. The association of injuries to the medial epicondyle of the humerus with playing baseball led to the term Little League elbow, although this designation often is used in a global sense to encompass all injuries of the elbow in children and adolescents who are baseball players. In pediatric baseball pitchers, pain and tenderness about the medial epicondyle are very frequent. This epicondyle serves as the attachment site of the medial collateral ligament and flexor (pronator) muscles, and tension on these structures during valgus stress or overhead arm movement may lead to recurrent and progressive injury to the developing epicondylar ossification center. The precise site of injury varies according to the age of the patient, although two basic types of medial epicondylar fracture have been described.[164] In younger children, the entire epicondyle may be displaced and rotated; in adolescents, in whom muscle mass and strength have increased rapidly, avulsion of small fragments of the medial epicondyle may be observed. In the former situation, intra-articular entrapment of the epicondyle may occur; in the latter situation, the fragments may not unite with the parent bone but, rather, may become painful fragments located in the common flexor muscle mass.[165]

Chronic injuries of the medial epicondyle are not confined to baseball players and, furthermore, other physes about the elbow may reveal similar abnormalities. As an example, chronic stress injuries of the apophysis

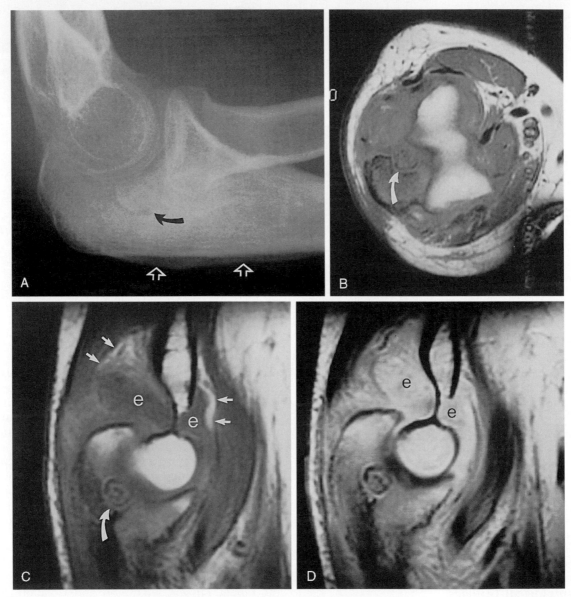

Figure 13–46
Osteoid osteoma: MR imaging.
   A A lateral radiograph reveals the heavily calcified nidus (solid arrow) of an osteoid osteoma of the ulna. Periostitis is seen (open arrows).
   B A transaxial T1-weighted (TR/TE, 500/17) spin echo MR image demonstrates the calcified nidus (arrow).
   C On a sagittal T1-weighted (TR/TE, 500/16) spin echo MR image, note the lesion (curved arrow) and elevation of perihumeral fat pads (straight arrows) owing to the presence of a large joint effusion (e).
   D After intravenous administration of a gadolinium contrast agent, a sagittal T1-weighted (TR/TE, 500/16) spin echo MR image shows the osteoid osteoma, the joint effusion (e), and periarticular enhancement of signal intensity.
   (**A–D,** Courtesy of J.M. Ahn, M.D., Seoul, Korea.)

or physeal plate of the developing olecranon process may be observed in gymnasts, divers, hockey players, tennis players, and javelin throwers.[136]

Developmental Abnormalities

Radioulnar Synostosis

A common site of osseous fusion in the tubular bones of the extremities is between the proximal portions of the radius and ulna.[166] Two distinct types have been recognized: proximal or true radioulnar synostosis, in which the radius and ulna are fused smoothly at their proximal borders for a distance of about 2 to 6 cm; and a second variety, in which fusion just distal to the proximal radial epiphysis is associated with congenital dislocation of the radial head.[167] In both types, interference with normal forearm supination is seen. Other descriptions of radioulnar synostosis indicate additional radiographic types of this anomaly[168] or a spectrum of involvement that can range from fibrous to complete bone fusion. The condition is bilateral in approximately 60 per cent of patients, affecting men and women equally or showing a slight male predominance.[168] Sporadically occurring examples appear more often than familial cases. Radioulnar synostosis is regarded as an anomaly of longitudinal segmentation in which, instead of the formation of the superior radioulnar joint space, the interzonal mesenchyme persists and undergoes chondrification and ossification. Indeed, additional anomalies may accompany radioulnar synostosis.[167, 169, 170]

Congenital Dislocation of the Radial Head

Although it is a rare condition, congenital dislocation of the radial head represents the most common anomaly of the elbow region. It may occur as an isolated phenomenon or in association with other congenital abnormalities, particularly those of the hand.[171-173] In some instances, a familial history of the anomaly, suggesting an autosomal recessive inheritance pattern, is evident.[174] Clinical findings usually appear in infancy or childhood and include a decrease in elbow motion.[172] Radiographic abnormalities include a relatively short ulna or long radius, hypoplasia or aplasia of the capitulum, a partially defective trochlea, prominence of the ulnar epicondyle, a dome-shaped radial head with an elongated radial neck, and grooving of the distal portion of the humerus.[172] Unilateral or bilateral involvement is seen,[175] and progressive subluxation or dislocation of the radial head usually proceeds in a posterior direction.

Synovial Abnormalities

Synovial Proliferation

Synovial proliferation in the elbow may accompany a variety of disease processes, including rheumatoid arthritis, septic arthritis, neuropathic osteoarthropathy, crystal deposition disorders, pigmented villonodular synovitis, idiopathic synovial osteochondromatosis, and osteoid osteoma (Fig. 13–46). The accumulation of joint fluid leads to characteristic displacements of the anterior and posterior intracapsular, extrasynovial fat pads of the elbow, which can be recognized with routine radiography, CT, and MR imaging (Fig. 13–47). The finding lacks specificity, indicating only the presence of an effusion, synovial inflammation, intra-articular mass, or a combination of these findings. With MR imaging, a joint effusion, best seen in the sagittal plane, is of high signal intensity on T2-weighted spin echo and certain gradient echo MR images.

Rheumatoid arthritis and other synovial inflammatory disorders affecting the elbow lead to proliferation of the synovial membrane and accumulation of joint fluid. With conventional arthrography, synovial inflammation with hypertrophy and villous transformation accounts for an irregular outline of contrast material. Lymphatic visualization is common and capsular distention, sacculation, and cystic swelling may be observed. Capsular

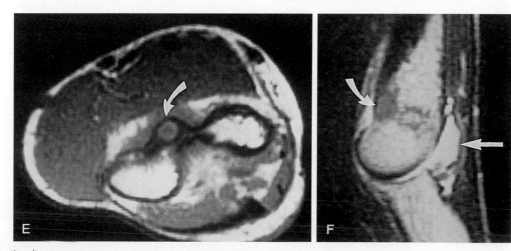

Figure 13–46 (Continued)
   E, F In a 16 year old male patient, the partially calcified nidus (curved arrows) of an osteoid osteoma of the humerus and an accompanying joint effusion (straight arrow) are seen on transaxial T1-weighted (TR/TE, 600/20) (**A**) and sagittal T2-weighted (TR/TE, 200/80) (**B**) spin echo MR images.

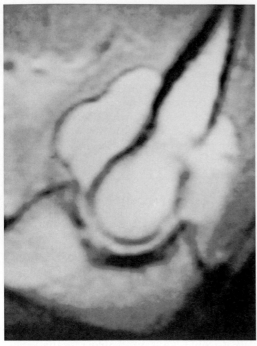

Figure 13–47
Joint effusion: MR imaging. A sagittal T2-weighted (TR/TE, 2000/80) spin echo MR image shows fluid in the anterior and posterior portions of the joint. (Courtesy of S. Fernandez, M.D., Mexico City, Mexico.)

rupture and synovial cyst formation also are seen. Cysts, which may become large, occur anteriorly, medially, laterally, or even posteriorly over the olecranon and are more frequent in patients with elbow flexion contractures. These cysts most frequently occur when the joint itself is involved extensively in the rheumatoid process, but on occasion they may represent a relatively early sign of the disease. Altered dynamics at the proximal radioulnar joint and elbow may be contributing factors in the production of these cysts, and the caput ulnae syndrome frequently is apparent in the ipsilateral wrist. Cysts in the antecubital fossa may produce swelling of the forearm and compression of the interosseous nerve.

The signal intensity characteristics of the abnormal synovium and fluid are similar on standard MR imaging sequences. Intravenous administration of gadolinium compounds leads to enhancement of the signal intensity of the inflammatory tissue, and it does not affect the signal intensity of fluid on MR images obtained immediately after the injection (Fig. 13–48).

Pigmented villonodular synovitis may involve the elbow, leading initially to an effusion and subsequently to osteoporosis and even joint space loss and bone erosions. Although the diagnosis may be suggested on the basis of appropriate clinical history and typical radiographic abnormalities, the deposition of hemosiderin in the affected synovial tissue produces regions of persistent low signal intensity on spin echo and, especially, gradient echo MR images (Fig. 13–49). This finding also may be observed in cases of chronic hemarthrosis, hemophilia, synovial hemangioma, and other conditions.

Idiopathic synovial osteochondromatosis, related to metaplasia of the synovial lining, is accompanied by synovial proliferation and the formation of intrasynovial nodules of cartilage. The fate of these nodules is variable; they may calcify or ossify, or they may become free within the joint cavity and later become embedded in a distant synovial site. Routine radiography is sensitive in the detection of calcified and ossified intra-articular bodies but insensitive in the detection of nonossified bodies. Arthrography, in which the bodies appear as multiple filling defects within the opacified joint, and MR imaging can be helpful diagnostically. The appearance of idiopathic synovial osteochondromatosis on MR images depends on the composition of the cartilage nodules and, specifically, the degree of calcification and ossification. In the absence of such calcification or ossification, the nodules have signal intensity similar to that of fluid; when calcified or ossified, the nodules reveal regions of low signal intensity.

Bursitis

Synovial inflammation and fluid accumulation in the olecranon bursa are seen in rheumatoid arthritis, in septic bursitis, in gout and other crystal deposition diseases, and after injury. With regard to traumatic olecranon bursitis, the subcutaneous location of the bursa makes it vulnerable to contusion in such contact sports as ice hockey, wrestling, and football (particularly when played on artificial turf).[136] The diagnosis of olecranon bursitis generally is apparent on physical examination. Imaging methods such as ultrasonography (Fig. 13–50A), bursography, and MR imaging can be employed in patients with olecranon bursitis but rarely are necessary. A sympathetic effusion in the elbow joint may accompany this condition. In rheumatoid arthritis, subcutaneous nodules may simulate the appearance of olecranon bursitis (Fig. 13–51).

The MR imaging features of olecranon bursitis depend on its cause and chronicity. Blood, synovial fluid, or pus may be present within the bursa, and, in certain conditions, the synovial lining of the bursa may be inflamed or contain fibrous nodules, or rice bodies. Intravenous administration of a gadolinium contrast agent can be employed to study the inflammatory nature of the process (see Fig. 13–50B, C).

Synovial Cysts

Para-articular synovial cysts that communicate with the elbow joint are a recognized manifestation of rheumatoid arthritis,[176–181] but theoretically they could occur with any process leading to elevation of intra-articular pressure in the elbow. As in the knee, a valvelike mechanism may exist between the synovial cyst and the elbow joint. Such cysts predominate in the antecubital region,[177] although synovial cysts posterior to the joint also may be evident.[179] Arthrography, cystography, ultrasonography, CT, and MR imaging are all effective in establishing the diagnosis and determining if there is rupture of the contents of the cyst (Fig. 13–52).

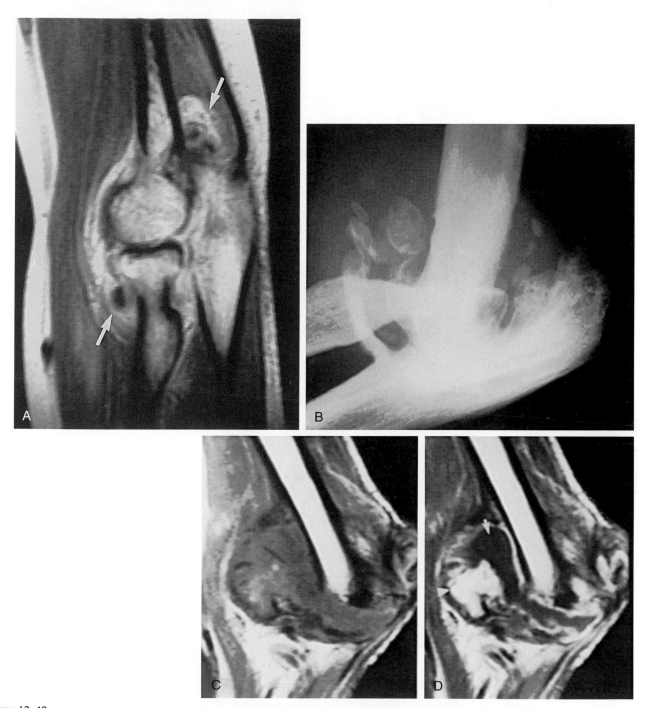

Figure 13–48

Synovitis: MR imaging.

A Rheumatoid arthritis. Immediately after the intravenous injection of a gadolinium compound, a sagittal T1-weighted (TR/TE, 600/15) spin echo MR image shows inflamed synovium of high signal intensity (arrows) and intra-articular fluid of low signal intensity.

B–D Neuropathic osteoarthropathy. A disorganized elbow joint with bone resorption, fragmentation and sclerosis, and multiple intra-articular osseous bodies is evident (**B**). Coronal oblique T1-weighted (TR/TE, 500/30) spin echo MR images are shown. In **C,** prior to the intravenous injection of gadolinium contrast agent, a distorted elbow joint contains material of low signal intensity, presumably representing a combination of fluid and pannus. In **D,** after administration of gadolinium agent, the fluid remains of low signal intensity (arrow), and the pannus exhibits high signal intensity (arrowhead). This patient had syringomyelia.

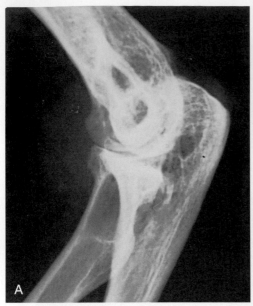

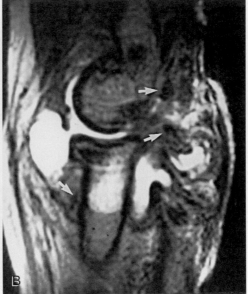

Figure 13–49
Pigmented villonodular synovitis: MR imaging. On a lateral radiograph **(A)**, multiple cystic lesions of variable size are noted in all three bones. A sagittal fat-suppressed fast spin echo (TR/TE, 3600/100) MR image **(B)** shows a joint effusion, thickening of the synovial membrane, and hemosiderin deposition of low signal intensity (arrows) in the synovial membrane. (Courtesy of B.Y. Yang, M.D., Taipei, Taiwan.)

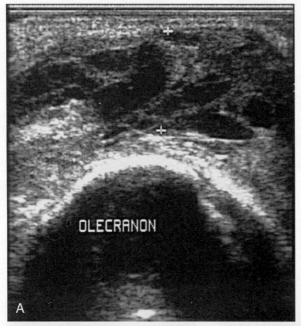

Figure 13–50
Olecranon bursitis.

A Ultrasonography—infection. Sonography of the posterior portion of the elbow in the transverse plane demonstrates a septated fluid-filled olecranon bursa (markers) superficial to the olecranon process. (Courtesy of M. van Holsbeeck, M.D., Detroit, Michigan, and J. Jacobson, M.D., San Diego, California.)

B, C MR imaging. A sagittal T1-weighted (TR/TE, 600/20) spin echo MR image shows enlargement of the olecranon bursa **(B)**. A fat-suppressed, sagittal T1-weighted (TR/TE, 600/20) spin echo MR image obtained immediately after the intravenous administration of gadolinium contrast agent shows enhancement of signal intensity in the inflamed synovial tissue of the bursa and low signal intensity of the bursal fluid **(C)**.

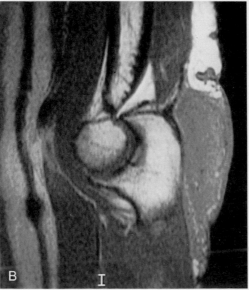

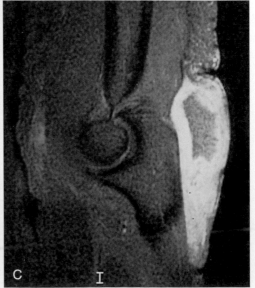

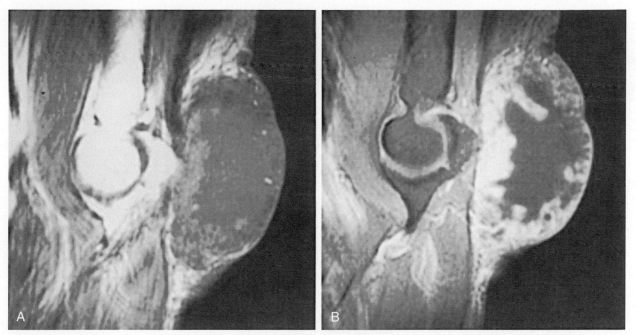

Figure 13–51
Olecranon nodule in rheumatoid arthritis. This 76 year old man had multiple subcutaneous nodules. A sagittal T1-weighted (TR/TE, 700/14) spin echo MR image (**A**) shows a large soft tissue nodule posterior to the olecranon process. It is inhomogeneous but mainly of low signal intensity. Following the intravenous injection of a gadolinium compound, a sagittal T1-weighted (TR/TE, 600/14) fat-suppressed spin echo MR image (**B**) shows enhancement of the wall of this necrotic nodule. Additional diagnostic considerations include an infected subcutaneous nodule and septic olecranon bursitis.

Intra-Articular Osteocartilaginous Bodies

Any process leading to disintegration of the articular surface of the elbow joint may be responsible for intra-articular osteocartilaginous bodies, although trauma remains the most important cause. In common with intra-articular bodies in other locations, bodies originating from the joint surface may be composed of cartilage alone, cartilage and bone together, or rarely bone alone, and they may remain at their site of origin, become partially detached or completely free and, if free, migrate about the joint to become embedded in a distant synovial site. Free bodies in the elbow joint commonly migrate to dependent portions of the joint and to sites of normal depressions in bone, particularly the olecranon fossa. In this last location, intra-articular bodies may prevent full extension of the joint. Once detected, they may be removed arthroscopically.[182–185]

Calcified bodies in the elbow joint can be detected by routine radiography; however, those that lodge in the olecranon fossa may be overlooked unless conventional tomography or CT is employed. Noncalcified bodies are more difficult to detect. Such detection requires arthrography, conventional arthrotomography, computed arthrotomography, or MR imaging (Fig. 13–53). Of these techniques, computed arthrotomography often is preferred; with this method, purely cartilaginous bodies are manifested as radiodense regions that simulate hypertrophied synovial tissue, creating some diagnostic difficulty. MR imaging is relatively insensitive in the diagnosis of small calcified bodies, as the signal void of these bodies is overlooked easily. Furthermore, small noncalcified cartilaginous bodies are characterized by high signal intensity on T2-weighted spin echo images similar to the signal intensity of joint fluid. MR arthrography (Fig. 13–54) may be useful in the detection of small calcified or noncalcified bodies. Large calcified bodies, owing to the presence of prominent foci of low signal intensity, and large ossified bodies, owing to the presence of bone marrow within them, are detected more easily with MR imaging.[186] Whatever technique is employed, careful inspection of the coronoid, radial, and olecranon fossae of the distal portion of the humerus often is fruitful in the search for intra-articular bodies. In such cases, an inspection of other joint surfaces occasionally will uncover a likely site of origin of these bodies.

Soft Tissue Abnormalities

As in other regions of the body, a large number of diverse processes lead to soft tissue masses about the elbow. These include tumors and tumor-like lesions of bone or soft tissue (Figs. 13–55 and 13–56), bursitis, tenosynovitis (Fig. 13–57), ganglia (Fig. 13–58), abscesses, lymph node enlargement (Fig. 13–59), hematomas, and heterotopic ossification. The frequency of heterotopic ossification about the elbow is well established, not only in patients after physical injury but also in patients with burns or neurologic injury.

Cat-scratch disease is an infectious disorder occurring after exposure to a scratch by an animal, usually a cat, and often appearing in a child or adolescent. The elbow region is involved frequently, and resulting lymphadenitis and lymphadenopathy can be confirmed with MR

Text continued on page 384

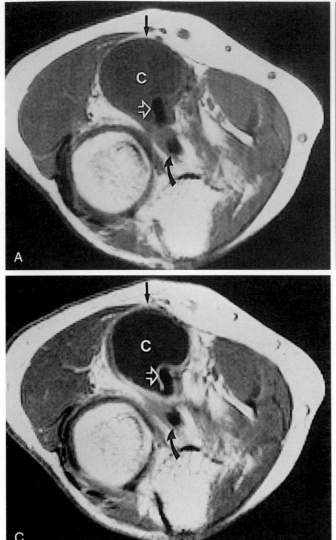

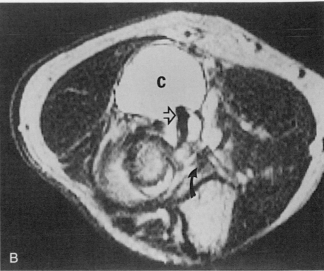

Figure 13–52

Synovial (ganglion) cyst: MR imaging.

A In a 54 year old woman with an enlarging mass about the elbow, a transaxial T1-weighted (TR/TE, 500/15) spin echo MR image shows a cyst (C) (straight solid arrow) intimately related to the biceps tendon (open arrow) and near the brachialis muscle and tendon (curved arrow).

B With T2 weighting (TR/TE, 2500/90), the cyst (C) is of high signal intensity. The biceps tendon (open arrow) and brachialis muscle and tendon (curved arrow) are again seen.

C A transaxial T1-weighted (TR/TE, 500/15) spin echo MR image, obtained with intravenous gadolinium enhancement, shows increased signal intensity in the thin wall (straight solid arrow) of the cyst (C). Open arrow, biceps tendon; curved arrow, brachialis muscle and tendon.

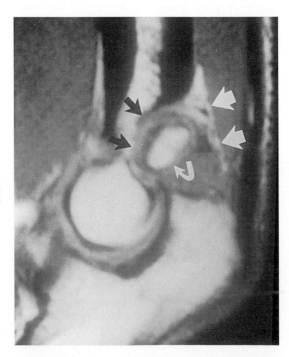

Figure 13–53

Intra-articular osteocartilaginous bodies: MR imaging. A sagittal T1-weighted spin echo MR image shows a large osseous body (curved arrow) lodged in the olecranon fossa (black arrows) with elevation of the posterior (olecranon) fat body (straight white arrows). (Courtesy of L. Steinbach, M.D., San Francisco, California.)

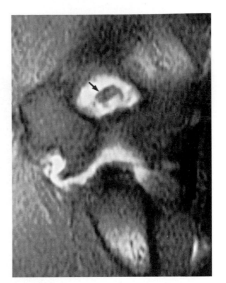

Figure 13–54
Intra-articular osteocartilaginous bodies: MR arthrography. A coronal T1-weighted (TR/TE, 950/13) spin echo MR image, obtained after the intra-articular injection of a gadolinium compound and with chemical presaturation of fat (ChemSat), shows a body (arrow) in the olecranon fossa.

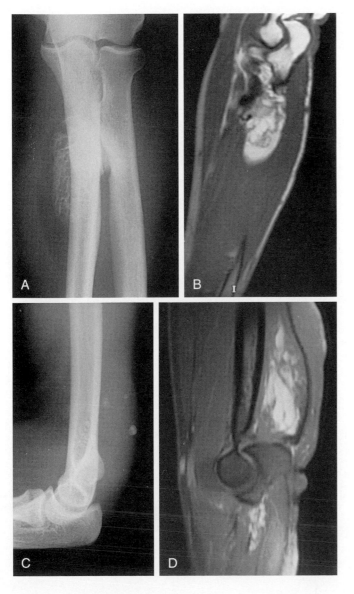

Figure 13–55
Soft tissue tumors.

  A, B Ossifying lipoma. Routine radiography (**A**) and sagittal T1-weighted (TR/TE, 600/20) spin echo MR imaging (**B**) reveal classic features of an ossifying lipoma. Note a radiolucent mass adjacent to the ossification in **A** and typical signal intensity characteristics of fat in **B**. (Courtesy of L. White, M.D., Toronto, Ontario, Canada.)

  C, D Hemangioma. The routine radiograph (**C**) reveals phleboliths typical of this lesion. A sagittal fat-suppressed T1-weighted (TR/TE, 700/12) spin echo MR image obtained after the intravenous administration of a gadolinium contrast agent (**D**) shows channel-like regions of high signal intensity, diagnostic of a soft tissue hemangioma.

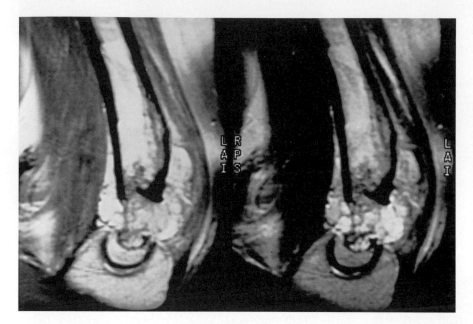

Figure 13–56
Aggressive fibromatosis. In a 15 year old girl who was unable to extend the elbow fully, sagittal proton density–weighted (TR/TE, 3000/20) (image on left) and T2-weighted (TR/TE, 3000/100) (image on right) spin echo MR images show a mass of inhomogeneous signal intensity located posterior to the elbow and extending into the joint. Bone erosion and periostitis are evident. (Courtesy of V. Gylys-Morin, M.D., Cincinnati, Ohio.)

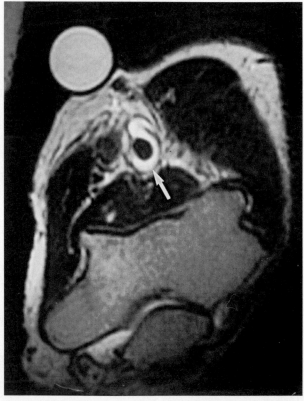

Figure 13–57
Tenosynovitis. Bicipital tenosynovitis is manifested as a fluid-filled collection of high signal intensity about the tendon (arrow) on a transaxial fast spin echo MR image (TR/TE, 4800/112). It had led to a clinically palpable mass (marker on skin) in a 98 year old man.

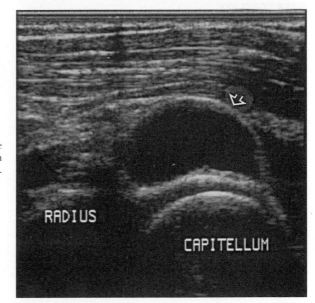

Figure 13–58
Ganglion cyst. Sonogram of the anterior aspect of the elbow in the sagittal plane demonstrates an anechoic fluid collection (arrow) superficial to the capitulum (capitellum). (Courtesy of M. van Holsbeeck, M.D., Detroit, Michigan, and J. Jacobson, M.D., San Diego, California.)

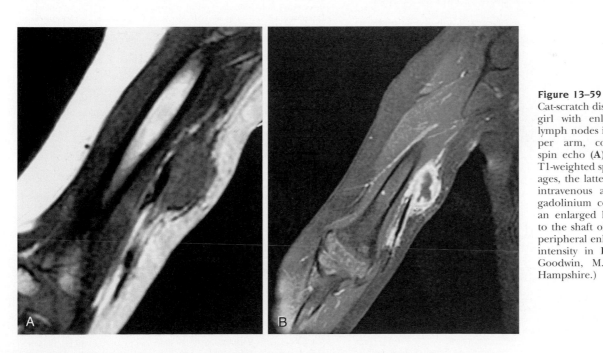

Figure 13–59
Cat-scratch disease. In a 4 year old girl with enlarging and tender lymph nodes in the axilla and upper arm, coronal T1-weighted spin echo (**A**) and fat-suppressed T1-weighted spin echo (**B**) MR images, the latter obtained after the intravenous administration of a gadolinium contrast agent, show an enlarged lymph node medial to the shaft of the humerus, with peripheral enhancement of signal intensity in **B**. (Courtesy of D. Goodwin, M.D., Hanover, New Hampshire.)

imaging.[192] The detection of enlarged lymph nodes with adjacent stranding of soft tissues and with little soft tissue edema, as seen with this imaging method, may have diagnostic significance (see Fig. 13–59).

SUMMARY

This chapter summarizes a variety of processes that affect elbow function. Emphasis is given to anatomic considerations that are fundamental to an understanding of many of these processes. In particular, abnormalities of tendons and ligaments and traumatic disorders of bone are discussed, and their assessment with advanced imaging methods, especially MR imaging, is addressed.

REFERENCES

1. Morrey BF: Anatomy of the elbow joint. *In* BF Morrey (Ed): The Elbow and Its Disorders. 2nd Ed. Philadelphia, WB Saunders, 1993, p 16.
2. Bunnell DH, Fisher DA, Bassett LW, et al: Elbow joint: Normal anatomy on MR images. Radiology 165:527, 1987.
3. Davidson PA, Pink M, Perry J, et al: Functional anatomy of the flexor pronator muscle group in relation to the medial collateral ligament of the elbow. Am J Sports Med 23:245, 1995.
4. Middleton WD, Macrander S, Kneeland JB, et al: MR imaging of the normal elbow: Anatomic considerations. AJR 149:543, 1987.
5. Hotchkiss RN: Injuries to the interosseous ligament of the forearm. Hand Clin 10:391, 1994.
6. An K-N, Morrey BF: Biomechanics of the elbow. *In* BF Morrey (Ed): The Elbow and Its Disorders. 2nd Ed. Philadelphia, WB Saunders, 1993, p 53.
7. Werner FW, An KN: Biomechanics of the elbow and forearm. Hand Clin 10:357, 1994.
8. Pincivero DM, Heinrichs K, Perrin D: Medial elbow stability: Clinical implications. Sports Med 18:141, 1994.
9. Holland P, Davies AM, Cassar-Pullicino VN: Computed tomographic arthrography in the assessment of osteochondritis dissecans of the elbow. Clin Radiol 49:231, 1994.
10. Eto RT, Anderson PW, Harley JD: Elbow arthrography with the application of tomography. Radiology 115:283, 1975.
11. Pavlov H, Ghelman B, Warren RF: Double-contrast arthrography of the elbow. Radiology 130:87, 1979.
12. Roback DL: Elbow arthrography: Brief technical considerations. Clin Radiol 30:311, 1979.
13. Teng MM, Murphy WA, Gilula LA, et al: Elbow arthrography: A reassessment of the technique. Radiology 153:611, 1984.
14. Singson RD, Feldman F, Rosenberg ZS: Elbow joint: Assessment with double-contrast CT arthrography. Radiology 160:167, 1986.
15. Weston WJ, Palmer DG: Soft Tissues of the Extremities: A Radiologic Study of Rheumatic Disease. New York, Springer-Verlag, 1977.
16. Chhem RK, Kaplan PA, Dussault RG: Ultrasonography of the musculoskeletal system. Radiol Clin N Amer 32:275, 1994.
17. Fritz RC, Brody GA: MR imaging of the wrist and elbow. Clin Sports Med 14:315, 1995.
18. Huynh PT, Kaplan PA, Dussault RG: Magnetic resonance imaging of the elbow. Orthopedics 17:1029, 1994.
19. Rosenberg ZS, Beltran J, Cheung Y, et al: MR imaging of the elbow: Normal variant and potential diagnostic pitfalls of the trochlear grove and cubital tunnel. AJR 164:415, 1995.
20. Rosenberg ZS, Beltran J, Cheung Y, et al: Pseudodefect of the capitellum: Potential MR imaging pitfall. Radiology 191:821, 1994.
21. Rogers LF: Radiology of Skeletal Trauma. 2nd Ed. New York, Churchill Livingstone, 1992.
22. Norrell HG: Roentgenologic visualization of extracapsular fat: Its importance in diagnosis of traumatic injuries to the elbow. Acta Radiol Diagn 42:205, 1954.
23. Murphy WA, Siegel MJ: Elbow fat pads with new signs and extended differential diagnosis. Radiology 124:659, 1977.
24. Kohn AM: Soft tissue alterations in elbow trauma. AJR 82:867, 1959.
25. Quinton DN, Finlay D, Butterworth R: The elbow fat pad sign: Brief report. J Bone Joint Surg [Br] 69:844, 1987.
26. Rogers LF: Fractures and dislocations of the elbow. Semin Roentgenol 13:97, 1978.
27. Kini MG: Dislocation of the elbow and its complications. J Bone Joint Surg 22:107, 1940.
28. Linscheid RL, Wheeler DK: Elbow dislocations. JAMA 194:1171, 1965.
29. Matev I: A radiological sign of entrapment of the median nerve in the elbow joint after posterior dislocation: A report of two cases. J Bone Joint Surg [Br] 58:353, 1976.
30. Green NE: Entrapment of the median nerve following elbow dislocation. J Pediatr Orthop 3:384, 1983.
31. Floyd WE III, Gebhardt MC, Emans JB: Intra-articular entrapment of the median nerve after elbow dislocation in children. J Hand Surg [Am] 12:704, 1987.
32. Exarchou EJ: Lateral dislocation of the elbow. Acta Orthop Scand 48:161, 1977.
33. Cohn I: Fractures of the elbow. Am J Surg 55:210, 1942.
34. Symeonides PP, Paschaloglou C, Stavrou Z, et al: Recurrent dislocation of the elbow: Report of three cases. J Bone Joint Surg [Am] 57:1084, 1975.
35. Josefsson PO, Gentz CF, Johnell O, et al: Dislocations of the elbow and intraarticular fractures. Clin Orthop 246:126, 1989.
36. Josefsson PO, Johnell O, Wendeberg B: Ligamentous injuries in dislocations of the elbow joint. Clin Orthop 221:221, 1987.
37. Andersen K, Mortensen AC, Gron P: Transverse divergent dislocation of the elbow: A report of two cases. Acta Orthop Scand 56:442, 1985.
38. Holbrook JL, Green NE: Divergent pediatric elbow dislocation: A case report. Clin Orthop 234:72, 1988.
39. Eklöf O, Nybonde T, Karlsson G: Luxation of the elbow complicated by proximal radio-ulnar translocation. Acta Radiol 31:145, 1990.
40. Frumken K: Nursemaid's elbow: A radiographic demonstration. Ann Emerg Med 14:690, 1985.
41. Salter RB, Zaltz C: Anatomic investigations of the mechanism of injury and pathologic anatomy of "pulled elbow" in young children. Clin Orthop 77:134, 1971.
42. Triantafyllou SJ, Wilson SC, Rychak JS: Irreducible "pulled elbow" in a child: A case report. Clin Orthop 284:153, 1992.
43. Earwaker J: Posttraumatic calcification of the annular ligament of the radius. Skel Radiol 21:149, 1992.
44. Wiley JJ, Pegington J, Horwich JP: Traumatic dislocation of the radius at the elbow. J Bone Joint Surg [Br] 56:501, 1974.
45. Bruce HE, Harvey JP Jr, Wilson JC Jr: Monteggia fractures. J Bone Joint Surg [Am] 56:1563, 1974.
46. Peiro A, Andres F, Fernandez-Esteve F: Acute Monteggia lesions in children. J Bone Joint Surg [Am] 59:92, 1977.
47. Giustra PE, Killoran PJ, Furman RS, Root JA: The missed Monteggia fracture. Radiology 110:45, 1974.
48. Bado JL: The Monteggia Lesion. Springfield, Ill, Charles C Thomas, 1962.
49. Simpson JM, Andreshak TG, Patel A, et al: Ipsilateral radial head dislocation and radial shaft fracture: A case report. Clin Orthop 266:205, 1991.
50. Wiley JJ, Galey JP: Monteggia injuries in children. J Bone Joint Surg [Br] 67:728, 1985.
51. Letts M, Locht R, Wiens J: Monteggia fracture-dislocation in children. J Bone Joint Surg [Br] 67:724, 1985.
52. Kalamchi A: Monteggia fracture-dislocation in children: Late treatment in two cases. J Bone Joint Surg [Am] 68:615, 1986.
53. Papavasiliou VA, Nenopoulos SP: Monteggia-type elbow fractures in childhood. Clin Orthop 233:230, 1988.
54. Olney BW, Menelaus MB: Monteggia and equivalent lesions in childhood. J Pediatr Orthop 9:219, 1989.
55. Storen G: Traumatic dislocation of the radial head as an isolated lesion in children: Report of one case with special regard to roentgen diagnosis. Acta Chir Scand 116:144, 1959
56. Rogers LF, Rockwood CA Jr: Separation of the entire distal humeral epiphysis. Radiology 106:393, 1973.
57. Mizuno K, Hirohata K, Kashiwagi D: Fracture-separation of the distal humeral epiphysis in young children. J Bone Joint Surg [Am] 61:570, 1979.
58. Loomis LK: Reduction and after-treatment of posterior dislocation of the elbow. Am J Surg 63:56, 1944.
59. Thompson HC III, Garcia A: Myositis ossificans (aftermath of elbow injuries). Clin Orthop 50:129, 1967.
60. Josefsson PO, Johnell O, Gentz CF: Long-term sequelae of simple dislocation of the elbow. J Bone Joint Surg [Am] 66:927, 1984.
61. Kerin R: Elbow dislocation and its association with vascular disruption. J Bone Joint Surg [Am] 51:756, 1969.
62. Hofammann KE III, Moneim MS, Omer GE, Ball WS: Brachial artery disruption following closed posterior elbow dislocation in a child—assessment with intravenous digital angiography: A case report with review of the literature. Clin Orthop 184:145, 1984.
63. Grimer RJ, Brooks S: Brachial artery damage accompanying closed posterior dislocation of the elbow. J Bone Joint Surg [Br] 67:378, 1985.
64. Malkawi H: Recurrent dislocation of the elbow accompanied by ulnar neuropathy: A case report and review of the literature. Clin Orthop 161:270, 1981.
65. Goldman MH, Kent S, Schaumburg E: Brachial artery injuries associated with posterior elbow dislocation. Surg Gynecol Obstet 164:95, 1987.
66. DeLee JC, Green DP, Wilkins KE: Fracture and dislocations of the elbow. *In* CA Rockwood Jr, DP Green (Eds): Fractures in Adults. 2nd Ed. Philadelphia, JB Lippincott Co, 1984, p 559.
67. Riseborough EJ, Radin EL: Intercondylar T-fractures of the humerus in the adult (a comparison of operative and non-operative treatment in twenty-nine cases). J Bone Joint Surg [Am] 51:130, 1969.
68. Miller WA: Comminuted fractures of the distal end of the humerus in the adult. J Bone Joint Surg [Am] 46:644, 1964.
69. Bickel WH, Perry RE: Comminuted fractures of the distal humerus. JAMA 184:553, 1963.

70. Gabel GT, Hanson G, Bennett JB, et al: Intraarticular fractures of the distal humerus in the adult. Clin Orthop 216:99, 1987.

71. Mitsunaga MM, Bryan RS, Linscheid RL: Condylar nonunions of the elbow. J Trauma 22:787, 1982.

72. Knight RA: Fractures of the humeral condyles in adults. South Med J 48:1165, 1955.

73. Milch H: Fractures and fracture dislocations of the humeral condyles. J Trauma 4:592, 1964.

74. Kleiger B, Joseph H: Fractures of the capitellum humeri. Bull Hosp J Dis 25:64, 1964.

75. Alvarez E, Patel MR, Nimberg G, Pearlman HS: Fracture of the capitellum humeri. J Bone Joint Surg [Am] 57:1093, 1975.

76. Grantham SA, Norris TR, Bush DC: Isolated fracture of the humeral capitellum. Clin Orthop 161:262, 1981.

77. Schild H, Muller HA, Klose K: The halfmoon sign. Australas Radiol 26:273, 1982.

78. Keon-Cohen BT: Fractures of the elbow. J Bone Joint Surg [Am] 48:1623, 1966.

79. Milch H: Unusual fractures of the capitellum humeri and the capitellum radii. J Bone Joint Surg 13:882, 1931.

80. Mehne DK, Jupiter JB: Fractures of the distal humerus. In BD Browner, JB Jupiter, AM Levine, et al (Eds): Skeletal Trauma: Fractures, Dislocations, Ligamentous Injuries. Philadelphia, WB Saunders Company, 1992, p 1146.

81. Stug LH: Anterior dislocation of the elbow with fracture of the olecranon. Am J Surg 75:700, 1948.

82. Horne JG, Tanzer TL: Olecranon fractures: A review of 100 cases. J Trauma 21:469, 1981.

83. Colton CL: Fractures of the olecranon in adults: classification and management. Injury 5:121, 1973–1974.

84. Eriksson E, Sahlen O, Sandahl U: Late results of conservative and surgical treatment of fracture of the olecranon. Acta Chir Scand 113:153, 1957.

85. Kiviluoto O, Santavirta S: Fractures of the olecranon. Acta Orthop Scand 49:28, 1978.

86. Regan W, Morrey B: Fractures of the coronoid process of the ulna. J Bone Joint Surg [Am] 71:1348, 1989.

87. Gaston SR, Smith FM, Baab OD: Adult injuries of the radial head and neck. Importance of time element in treatment. Am J Surg 78:631, 1949.

88. Mason JA, Shutkin NM: Immediate active motion treatment of fractures of the head and neck of the radius. Surg Gynecol Obstet 76:731, 1943.

89. Swanson AB, Jaeger SH, La Rochelle D: Comminuted fractures of the radial head. The role of silicone-implant replacement arthroplasty. J Bone Joint Surg [Am] 63:1039, 1981.

90. Greenspan A, Norman A: Radial head—capitellum view: An expanded imaging approach to elbow injury. Radiology 164:272, 1987.

91. Funk DA, Wood MB: Concurrent fractures of the ipsilateral scaphoid and radial head. Report of four cases. J Bone Joint Surg [Am] 70:134, 1988.

92. Edwards GS Jr, Jupiter JB: Radial head fractures with acute distal radioulnar dislocation: Essex-Lopresti revisited. Clin Orthop 234:61, 1988.

93. Bock GW, Cohen MS, Resnick D: Fracture-dislocation of the elbow with inferior radioulnar dissociation: a variant of the Essex-Lopresti injury. Skel Radiol 21:315, 1992.

94. Evans EM: Rotational deformity in the treatment of fractures of both bones of the forearm. J Bone Joint Surg [Am] 27:373, 1945.

95. Creasman C, Zaleske D, Ehrlich MG: Analyzing forearm fractures in children: The more subtle signs of impending problems. Clin Orthop 188:40, 1984.

96. Goldberg HD, Young JWR, Reiner BI, et al: Double injuries of the forearm: A common occurrence. Radiology 185:223, 1992.

97. Vince KG, Miller JE: Cross-union complicating fracture of the forearm. I. Adults. J Bone Joint Surg [Am] 69:640, 1987.

98. Vince KG, Miller JE: Cross-union complicating fracture of the forearm. II. Children. J Bone Joint Surg [Am] 69:654, 1987.

99. Billett DM: An uncommon fracture dislocation of the radius. J Trauma 17:243, 1977.

100. O'Driscoll SW: Classification and spectrum of elbow instability: Recurrent instability. In BF Morrey (Ed): The Elbow and Its Disorders. 2nd Ed. Philadelphia, WB Saunders, 1993, p 453.

101. Fleisig GS, Andrews JR, Dillman CJ, et al: Kinetics of baseball pitching with implications about injury mechanisms. Am J Sports Med 23:233, 1995.

102. Schwab GH, Bennett JB, Woods GW, et al: Biomechanics of elbow instability: The role of the medial collateral ligament. Clin Orthop 146:42, 1980.

103. Jobe FW, Elattrache NS: Diagnosis and treatment of ulnar collateral ligament injuries in athletes. In BF Morrey (Ed): The Elbow and Its Disorders. 2nd Ed. Philadelphia, WB Saunders, 1993, p 566.

104. Morrey BF, Tanaka S, An KNA: Valgus stability of the elbow: A definition of primary and secondary constraints. Clin Orthop 201:84, 1991.

105. Rijke AM, Goitz HT, McCue FC, et al: Stress radiography of the medial elbow ligaments. Radiology 191:213, 1994.

106. Kuroda S, Sakamaki K: Ulnar collateral ligament tears of the elbow joint. Clin Orthop 208:266, 1986.

107. Murphy BJ: MR imaging of the elbow. Radiology 184:525, 1992.

108. Mirowitz SA, London SL: Ulnar collateral ligament injury in baseball pitchers: MR imaging evaluation. Radiology 185:573, 1992.

109. Sojbjerg JO, Ovesen J, Nielsen S: Experimental elbow instability after transection of the medial collateral ligament. Clin Orthop 218:186, 1987.

110. Hotchkiss RN, Weiland AJ: Valgus stability of the elbow. J Orthop Res 5:372, 1987.

111. Wilson FD, Andrews JR, Blackburn TA, et al: Valgus extension overload in the pitching elbow. Am J Sports Med 11:83, 1983.

112. Morrey BF, O'Driscoll SW: Lateral collateral ligament injury. p 573.

113. Morrey BF: Reoperation for failed tennis elbow surgery. J Shoulder Elbow Surg 1:47, 1992.

114. Patten RM: Overuse syndromes and injuries involving the elbow: MR imaging findings. AJR 165:1205, 1995.

115. Ho CP: Sports and occupational injuries of the elbow: MR imaging findings. AJR 164:1465, 1995.

116. Sugimoto H, Ohsawa T: Ulnar collateral ligament in the growing elbow: MR imaging of normal development and throwing injuries. Radiology 192:417, 1994.

117. Cirincione RJ, Baker BE: Tendon ruptures with secondary hyperparathyroidism: A case report. J Bone Joint Surg [Am] 57:852, 1975.

118. Match RM, Corrylos EV: Bilateral avulsion fracture of the triceps tendon insertion from skiing with osteogenesis imperfecta tarda. Am J Sports Med 11:99, 1983.

119. Morrey BF: Tendon injuries about the elbow. In BF Morrey (Ed): The Elbow and Its Disorders. 2nd Ed. Philadelphia, WB Saunders, 1993, p 492.

120. Nirschl RP: Muscle and tendon trauma: Tennis elbow. In BF Morrey (Ed): The Elbow and Its Disorders. 2nd Ed. Philadelphia, WB Saunders, 1993, p 537.

121. Morrey BF, Regan WD: Tendinopathies about the elbow. In BF Morrey (Ed): The Elbow and Its Disorders. 2nd Ed. Philadelphia, WB Saunders, 1993, p 860.

122. Jorgensen U, Hinge K, Rye B: Rupture of the distal biceps brachii tendon. J Trauma 26:1061, 1986.

123. Levy M, Fischel RE, Stern GM: Triceps tendon avulsion with or without fracture of the radial head—a rare injury? J Trauma 18:677, 1978.

124. Davis WM, Jassine Z: An etiologic factor in the tear of the distal tendon of the biceps brachii. J Bone Joint Surg [Am] 38:1365, 1956.

125. Farrar EL III, Lippert FG: Avulsion of the triceps tendon. Clin Orthop 161:242, 1981.

126. Barr LL, Babcock DS: Sonography of the normal elbow. AJR 157:793, 1991.

127. Gilcreest EL: Rupture of muscles and tendons. JAMA 84:1819, 1925.

128. Karanjia ND, Stiles PJ: Cubital bursitis. J Bone Joint Surg [Br] 70:832, 1988.

129. Fritz RC: Magnetic resonance imaging of the elbow. Semin Roentgenol 30:241, 1995.

130. Fitzgerald SW, Curry DR, Erickson SJ, et al: Distal biceps tendon injury: MR imaging diagnosis. Radiology 191: 203, 1994.

131. Falchook FS, Zlatkin MB, Erbacher GE, et al: Rupture of the distal biceps tendon: Evaluation with MR imaging. Radiology 190:659, 1994.

132. Clayton ML, Thirupathi RG: Rupture of the triceps tendon with olecranon bursitis: A case report with a new method of repair. Clin Orthop 184:183, 1984.

133. Herrick RT, Herrick S: Ruptured triceps in a powerlifter presenting as cubital tunnel syndrome: A case report. Am J Sports Med 15:514, 1987.

134. Levy M, Fishel RE, Stern GM: Triceps tendon avulsion with or without fracture of the radial head: A rare injury? J Trauma 18:677, 1978.

135. Tiger E, Mayer DP, Glazer R: Complete avulsion of the triceps tendon: MRI diagnosis. Comput Med Imaging Graph 17:51, 1993.

136. Caldwell GL Jr, Safran MR: Elbow problems in the athlete. Orthop Clin North Am 26:465, 1995.

137. Dreyfuss U: Snapping elbow due to dislocation of the medial head of the triceps. J Bone Joint Surg [Br] 60:57, 1978.

138. Rolfsen L: Snapping triceps tendon with ulnar neuritis. Acta Orthop Scand 41:74, 1970.

139. Gabel GT, Morrey BF: Operative treatment of medial epicondylitis: Influence of concomitant ulnar neuropathy at the elbow. J Bone Joint Surg [Am] 77:1065, 1995.

140. Morris M, Jobe FW, Perry J, et al: Electromyographic analysis of elbow function in tennis players. Am J Sports Med 17:241, 1989.

141. Potter HG, Hannafin JA, Morwessel RM, et al: Lateral epicondylitis: Correlation of MR imaging, surgical, and histopathologic findings. Radiology 196:43, 1995.

142. Coel M, Yamada CY, Ko J: MR imaging of patients with lateral epicondylitis of the elbow (tennis elbow): Importance of increased signal of the anconeus muscle. AJR 161:1019, 1993.

143. Jobe FW, Fanton GS, Elattrache NS: Ulnar nerve injury. In BF Morrey (Ed.): The Elbow and Its Disorders. 2nd Ed. Philadelphia, WB Saunders, 1993, p 560.

144. Regan WD, Morrey BF: Entrapment neuropathies about the elbow. In BF Morrey (Ed.): The Elbow and Its Disorders. 2nd Ed. Philadelphia, WB Saunders, 1993, p 844.

145. Childress HM: Recurrent ulnar nerve dislocation at the elbow. Clin Orthop 180:168, 1975.

146. O'Driscoll SW, Horii E, Carmichael SW, et al: The cubital tunnel and ulnar neuropathy. J Bone Joint Surg [Br] 75:613, 1991.

147. Osborne GV: The surgical treatment of tardy ulnar neuritis. J Bone Joint Surg [Br] 39:782, 1957.

148. Bora FW, Osterman AL: Compression neuropathy. Clin Orthop 163:20, 1982.

149. Vanderpool DW, Chalmers J, Lamb DW, et al: Peripheral compression lesions of the ulnar nerve. J Bone Joint Surg [Br] 50:792, 1968.

150. Feindel W, Stratford J: Cubital tunnel compression. Can Med Assoc J *78*:351, 1958.

151. St John JN, Palmaz JC: The cubital tunnel in ulnar entrapment neuropathy. Radiology *158*:119, 1986.

152. Rosenberg ZS, Beltran J, Cheung YY, et al: The elbow: MR features of nerve disorders. Radiology *188*:235, 1993.

153. Beltran J, Rosenberg ZS: Diagnosis of compressive and entrapment neuropathies of the upper extremity: Value of MR imaging. AJR *163*:525, 1994.

154. Lichter R, Jacobson T: Tardy palsy of the posterior interosseous nerve with Monteggia fracture. J Bone Joint Surg [Am] *57*:124, 1975.

155. Millender LH, Nalebuff EA, Holdsworth DE: Posterior interosseous nerve syndrome secondary to rheumatoid synovitis. J Bone Joint Surg [Am] *55*:753, 1973.

156. Nuber GW, Diment MT: Olecranon stress fractures in throwers. Clin Orthop *278*:58, 1992.

157. Hulko A, Orava S, Nikula P: Stress fractures of the olecranon in javelin throwers. Int J Sports Med *7*:210, 1986.

158. Holland P, Davies AM, Cassar-Pullisino VN: Computed tomographic arthrography in the assessment of osteochondritis dissecans of the elbow. Clin Radiol *49*:231, 1994.

159. Peiss J, Adam G, Casser R, et al: Gadopentetate dimeglumine–enhanced MR imaging of osteonecrosis and osteochondritis dissecans of the elbow: Initial experience. Skel Radiol *24*:17, 1995.

160. Yates C, Sullivan JA: Arthrographic diagnosis of elbow injuries in children. J Pediatr Orthop *7*:54, 1987.

161. Jaramillo D, Laor T, Zaleske DJ: Indirect trauma to the growth plate: Results of MR imaging after epiphyseal and metaphyseal injury in rabbits. Radiology *187*:171, 1993.

162. Jaramillo D, Hoffer FA: Cartilaginous epiphysis and growth plate: Normal and abnormal MR imaging findings. AJR *158*:1105, 1992.

163. Beltran J, Rosenberg ZS, Kawelblum M, et al: Pediatric elbow fractures: MRI evaluation. Skel Radiol *23*:277, 1994.

164. Woods GW, Tullos HS: Elbow instability and medial epicondylar fractures. Am J Sports Med *5*:23, 1977.

165. Pappas AM: Elbow problems associated with baseball during childhood and adolescence. Clin Orthop *163*:30, 1982.

166. Green WT, Mital MA: Congenital radio-ulnar synostosis: Surgical treatment. J Bone Joint Surg [Am] *61*:738, 1979.

167. Mital MA: Congenital radioulnar synostosis and congenital dislocation of the radial head. Orthop Clin North Am *7*:375, 1976.

168. Cleary JE, Omer GE Jr: Congenital proximal radio-ulnar synostosis: Natural history and functional assessment. J Bone Joint Surg [Am] *67*:539, 1985.

169. Davenport CB, Taylor HL, Nelson LA: Radio-ulnar synostosis. Arch Surg *8*:705, 1924.

170. Kusswetter W, Heisel A: Die radio-ulnare Synostose als Merkmal von Chromossomen-aberrationen. Z Orthop *119*:10, 1981.

171. Kelly DW: Congenital dislocation of the radial head: Spectrum and natural history. J Pediatr Orthop *1*:295, 1981.

172. Mardam-Bey T, Ger E: Congenital radial head dislocation. J Hand Surg *4*:316, 1979.

173. Campbell CC, Waters PM, Emans JB: Excision of the radial head for congenital dislocation. J Bone Joint Surg [Am] *74*:726, 1992.

174. Cockshott WP, Omololu A: Familial posterior dislocation of both radial heads. J Bone Joint Surg [Br] *40*:484, 1958.

175. McFarland B: Congenital dislocation of the head of the radius. Br J Surg *24*:41, 1936.

176. Leffert RD, Dorfman HD: Antecubital cyst in rheumatoid arthritis—surgical findings. J Bone Joint Surg [Am] *54*:1555, 1972.

177. Ehrlich GE, Guttmann GG: Valvular mechanisms in antecubital cysts of rheumatoid arthritis. Arthritis Rheum *16*:259, 1973.

178. Ehrlich GE: Antecubital cysts in rheumatoid arthritis—a corollary to popliteal (Baker's) cysts. J Bone Joint Surg [Am] *54*:165, 1972.

179. Pirani M, Lange-Mechlen I, Cockshott WP: Rupture of a posterior synovial cyst of the elbow. J Rheumatol *9*:94, 1982.

180. Allan RA, Keen RW, Hine AL: Case report 855. Skel Radiol *23*:462, 1994.

181. Treadwell EL: Synovial cysts and ganglia: The value of magnetic resonance imaging. Semin Arthritis Rheum *24*:61, 1994.

182. Ogilvie-Harris DJ, Schemitsch E: Arthroscopy of the elbow for removal of loose bodies. J Arthrosc Rel Surg *9*:5, 1993.

183. O'Driscoll SW, Morrey BF: Arthroscopy of the elbow: Diagnostic and therapeutic benefits and hazards. J Bone Joint Surg [Am] *74*:84, 1992.

184. Poehling CG, Ekman EF: Arthroscopy of the elbow. J Bone Joint Surg [Am] *76*:1265, 1994.

185. Ekman EF, Poehling GG: Arthroscopy of the elbow. Hand Clin *10*:453, 1994.

186. Quinn SF, Haberman JJ, Fitzgerald SW, et al: Evaluation of loose bodies in the elbow with MR imaging. J Magn Res Imaging *4*:169, 1994.

187. Cage DJN, Abrams RA, Callahan JJ, Botte MJ: Soft tissue attachments of the ulnar coronoid process: An anatomic study with radiographic correlation. Clin Orthop Rel Res *320*:154, 1995.

188. Sonin AH, Fitzgerald SW: MR imaging of sports injuries in the adult elbow: A tailored approach. AJR *167*:325, 1996.

189. Liessi G, Cesari S, Spaliviero B, et al: The US, CT and MR findings of cubital bursitis: A report of five cases. Skeletal Radiol *25*:471, 1996.

190. Matsumoto K, Hukuda S, Fujita M, et al: Cubital bursitis caused by localized synovial chondromatosis of the elbow. A case report. J Bone Joint Surg [Am] *78*:275, 1996.

191. Plancher KD, Halbrecht J, Lourie GM: Medial and lateral epicondylitis in the athlete. Clin Sports Med *15*:283, 1996.

192. Holt PD, de Lange EE: Cat scratch disease: Magnetic resonance imaging findings. Skeletal Radiol *24*:437, 1995.

193. Schwartz ML, Al-Zahrani S, Morwessel RM, et al: Ulnar collateral ligament injury in the throwing athlete: Evaluation with saline-enhanced MR arthrography. Radiology *197*:297, 1995.

194. Le Huec JC, Moinard M, Liquois F, et al: Distal rupture of the biceps brachii. Evaluation by MRI and the results of repair. J Bone Joint Surg [Br] *78*:767, 1996.

195. Geutjiens GG, Langstaff RJ, Smith NJ, et al: Medial epicondylectomy or ulnar-nerve transposition for ulnar neuropathy at the elbow? J Bone Joint Surg [Br] *78*:777, 1996.

196. Hashizume H, Nishida K, Nanba Y, et al: Non-traumatic paralysis of the posterior interosseous nerve. J Bone Joint Surg [Br] *78*:771, 1996.

197. Nakanishi K, Masatomi T, Ochi T, et al: MR arthrography of elbow: Evaluation of the ulnar collateral ligament of the elbow. Skeletal Radiol *25*:629, 1996.

The wrist and, to a lesser extent, the hand are regions of complex anatomy whose proper function, essential to everyday activities, depends on the integrity of a number of joints, bones, and supporting soft tissues. Internal derangements, which are numerous and diverse, compromise such function. The diagnosis of these derangements often is made on the basis of a careful physical examination, supplemented by data derived from questioning the patient regarding the nature of the affliction and, in some instances, by analysis of results of laboratory and imaging examinations. In this chapter, diagnostic imaging of internal derangements of the wrist and hand is reviewed.

ANATOMY

Osseous Anatomy

The distal aspects of the radius and ulna articulate with the proximal row of carpal bones (Fig. 14–1). On the lateral surface of the radius is the radial styloid process, which extends more distally than the remainder of the bone, and from which arises the radial collateral ligament of the wrist joint. The articular surface of the radius is divided into an ulnar and a radial portion by a faint central ridge of bone. The ulnar portion articulates with the lunate and the radial portion articulates with the scaphoid. The articular surface is continuous medially with that of the triangular fibrocartilage. The medial surface of the distal end of the radius contains the concave ulnar notch, which articulates with the distal end of the ulna. The posterior surface of the distal portion of the radius is convex and grooved or irregular in outline to allow passage of tendons and tendon sheaths. A prominent ridge in the middle of this surface is the dorsal tubercle of the radius. The anterior surface of the distal radial end allows attachment of the palmar radiocarpal ligaments.

The distal end of the ulna contains a small round head and a styloid process. The lateral aspect contains an articular surface for contact with the ulnar notch of the radius. The ulna also has a distal articular surface, which is intimate with the triangular fibrocartilage. The ulnar styloid process, which extends distally from the posteromedial aspect of the bone, gives rise to the ulnar collateral ligament. Between the styloid process and inferior articular surface, the ulna has an area for attachment of the triangular fibrocartilage and a dorsal groove for the extensor carpi ulnaris tendon and sheath.

The proximal row of carpal bones consists of the scaphoid, lunate, and triquetrum, as well as the pisiform

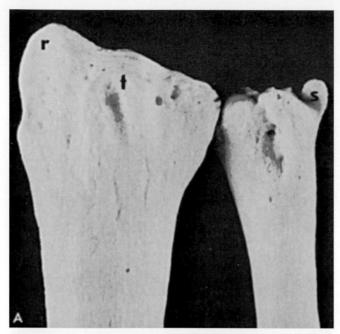

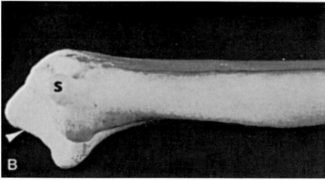

Figure 14–1

Distal portions of the radius and ulna: Osseous anatomy.

A Posterior aspect. Note the convex surface of the distal end of the radius with radial styloid process (r), dorsal tubercle (t) with grooves for passage of various tendons and tendon sheaths, and the surface of the distal end of the ulna with styloid process (s) and groove for the extensor carpi ulnaris tendon and tendon sheath.

B Ulnar aspect. Observe the ulnar styloid (s) and the articular surface of distal end of the radius (arrowhead).

bone within the tendon of the flexor carpi ulnaris. The distal row of carpal bones contains the trapezium, trapezoid, capitate, and hamate bones. The dorsal surface of the carpus is convex from side to side, and the palmar surface presents a deep concavity, termed the carpal groove or canal. The medial border of this palmar carpal groove contains the pisiform and hook of the hamate. The lateral border of the carpal groove contains the tubercles of the scaphoid and the trapezium. A strong fibrous retinaculum attaches to the palmar surface of the carpus, converting the groove into a carpal tunnel, through which pass the median nerve and flexor tendons.

The distal row of carpal bones articulates with the bases of the metacarpals. The trapezium has a saddle-shaped articular surface for the first metacarpal. The trapezoid fits into a deep notch in the second metacar-

pal. The capitate articulates mainly with the third metacarpal, but also with the second and fourth metacarpals. The hamate articulates with the fourth and fifth metacarpals. The bases of the metacarpals articulate not only with the distal row of carpal bones but also with each other.

At the metacarpophalangeal joints, the metacarpal heads articulate with the proximal phalanges. The medial four metacarpal bones lie side by side; the first metacarpal lies in a more anterior plane and is rotated medially along its long axis through an angle of 90 degrees. In this fashion, the dorsal surface of the thumb is aligned in a radial direction, whereas its ulnar surface is oriented superiorly. This position allows the thumb to appose the other four metacarpals during flexion and rotation.

The metacarpal heads are smooth and round, extending farther on the palmar than on the dorsal aspect of the bone. On the palmar aspect, the articular surface of the metacarpal head is divided in such a fashion that it resembles condyles. The head of the first metacarpal is less convex than those of the other metacarpals and has two palmar articular eminences, which relate to sesamoid bones. Tubercles are found on the heads of all metacarpals; these tubercles occur at the sides of the metacarpal heads where the dorsal surface of the body of the bone extends onto the head. Collateral ligaments attach to the metacarpal tubercles. The bases of the phalanges contain concave oval surfaces that articulate with the metacarpal heads.

The interphalangeal joints of the hand consist of four distal interphalangeal joints, four proximal interphalangeal joints, and one interphalangeal joint of the first digit.

At the proximal interphalangeal joints, the head of the proximal phalanx articulates with the base of the adjacent middle phalanx. The articular surface of the phalangeal head is wide (from side to side), with a central groove and ridges on either side for attachment of the collateral ligaments. The base of the middle phalanx contains a ridge that fits into the groove on the head of the proximal phalanx.

At the distal interphalangeal joints, the head of the middle phalanx articulates with the base of the distal phalanx. This phalangeal head, like that of the proximal phalanx, is pulley-like in configuration and conforms to the base of the adjacent phalanx. This latter structure is relatively large.

The interphalangeal joint of the thumb separates the proximal and distal phalanges of that digit. These phalanges are similar in structure to those of the other digits but in general are shorter and broader.

Articular Anatomy

The wrist consists of a series of joints or compartments (Fig. 14–2):

1. Radiocarpal compartment.
2. Distal (inferior) radioulnar compartment.
3. Midcarpal compartment.

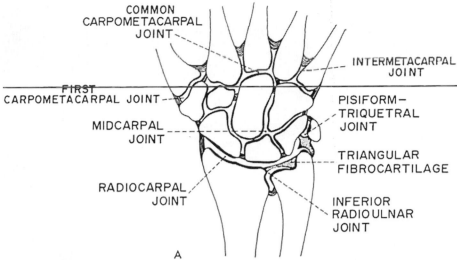

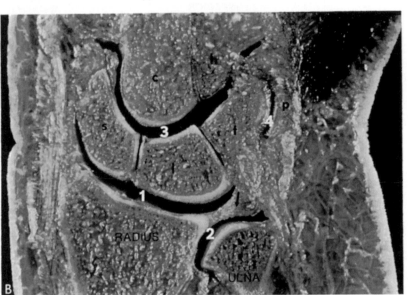

Figure 14–2
Articulations of the wrist: General anatomy. Observe the various wrist compartments on a schematic drawing (**A**) and photograph (**B**) of a coronal section. These include the radiocarpal (1), inferior radioulnar (2), midcarpal (3), and pisiform-triquetral (4) compartments. Note the triangular fibrocartilage (arrow). s, Scaphoid; l, lunate; t, triquetrum; p, pisiform; h, hamate; c, capitate.

4. Pisiform-triquetral compartment.
5. Common carpometacarpal compartment.
6. First carpometacarpal compartment.
7. Intermetacarpal compartments.

Radiocarpal Compartment

The radiocarpal compartment (Figs. 14–3 and 14–4) is formed proximally by the distal surface of the radius and the triangular fibrocartilage and distally by the proximal row of carpal bones exclusive of the pisiform. In the coronal plane, the radiocarpal compartment is a C-shaped cavity with a smooth, shallow curve, which is concave distally. In the sagittal plane, this compartment also is C-shaped, but the curve is more acute. Interosseous ligaments extend between the carpal bones of the proximal row and prevent communication of this compartment with the midcarpal compartment (see later discussion). A triangular fibrocartilage prevents communication of the radiocarpal and inferior radioulnar compartments, whereas a meniscus may attach to the trique-

trum, preventing communication of the radiocarpal and pisiform-triquetral compartments.

The radial collateral ligament is located at the radial limit of the radiocarpal compartment, whereas the ulnar limit of this compartment is the point at which the meniscus is firmly attached to the triquetrum. This ulnar area is Y-shaped; a proximal limb or diverticulum, termed the prestyloid recess, approaches the ulnar styloid and a distal limb is intimate with two thirds of the proximal aspect of the triquetrum.

Palmar radial recesses extend proximally from the radiocarpal compartment beneath the distal articulating surface of the radius. These recesses vary in number and size.

Distal (Inferior) Radioulnar Compartment

The inferior radioulnar compartment (see Figs. 14–2 to 14–4) is an L-shaped joint whose proximal border is the cartilage-covered head of the ulna and ulnar notch of the radius. Its limit is the triangular fibrocartilage. This latter ligament is a band of tough fibrous tissue that

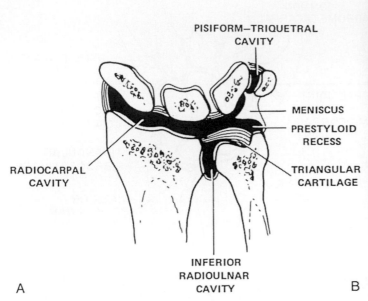

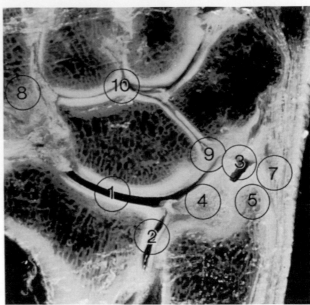

Figure 14–3

Radiocarpal compartment.

 A Detailed drawing of the radiocarpal compartment. Note its C shape, with a Y-shaped ulnar limit produced by the meniscus. The proximal limb or diverticulum at the ulnar limit of the radiocarpal compartment is the prestyloid recess, which is intimate with the ulnar styloid. The distal limb extends along the triquetrum and may, in some instances, communicate with the pisiform-triquetral compartment.

 B Coronal section of cadaveric wrist. Identified structures are the radiocarpal compartment (1), inferior radioulnar compartment (2), prestyloid recess (3), triangular fibrocartilage (4), ulnar styloid (5), ulnar collateral ligament (7), scaphoid (8), interosseous ligament between lunate and triquetrum (9), and midcarpal compartment (10).

 (From Resnick D: Radiology *113*:331, 1974.)

extends from the ulnar aspect of the distal end of the radius to the base of the ulnar styloid (see later discussion).

Midcarpal Compartment

The midcarpal compartment (see Figs. 14–2 and 14–5) extends between the proximal and distal carpal rows. On the ulnar aspect of this compartment, the head of the capitate and the hamate articulate with a concavity produced by the scaphoid, lunate, and triquetrum. This ulnar side widens between the triquetrum and hamate. On the radial aspect of the midcarpal compartment, the trapezium and trapezoid articulate with the distal aspect of the scaphoid. The radial side of this compartment is termed the trapezioscaphoid space.

Pisiform-Triquetral Compartment

The pisiform-triquetral compartment (see Figs. 14–2 and 14–5) exists between the palmar surface of the triquetrum and the dorsal surface of the pisiform. A large proximal synovial recess can be noted. The pisiform-triquetral compartment is surrounded by a loose fibrous articular capsule.

Common Carpometacarpal Compartment

The common carpometacarpal compartment exists between the base of each of the four medial metacarpals and the distal row of carpal bones. This synovial cavity extends proximally between the distal portion of the

carpal bones and distally between the bases of the metacarpals to form three small intermetacarpal joints. Occasionally, the joint between the hamate and the fourth and fifth metacarpals is a separate synovial cavity, produced by a ligamentous attachment between the hamate and fourth metacarpal (see Fig. 14–2).

First Carpometacarpal Compartment

The carpometacarpal compartment of the thumb is a separate saddle-shaped cavity between the trapezium and base of the first metacarpal (see Fig. 14–2). It possesses a loose, fibrous capsule, which is thickest laterally and dorsally.

Intermetacarpal Compartments

Three intermetacarpal compartments extend between the bases of the second and third, the third and fourth, and the fourth and fifth metacarpals (see Fig. 14–2). These compartments usually communicate with each other and with the common carpometacarpal compartment.

Metacarpophalangeal and Interphalangeal Joints

At the metacarpophalangeal joints, articular cartilage covers the osseous surfaces of metacarpals and phalanges, and the synovial membrane is attached to the articular margin of the metacarpal head (Fig. 14–6). This membrane is particularly prominent on the volar aspect

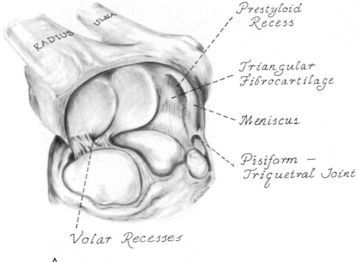

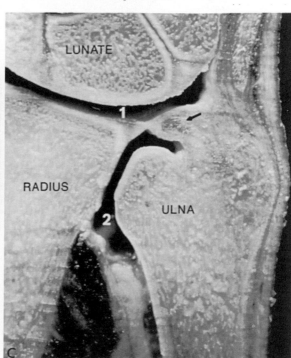

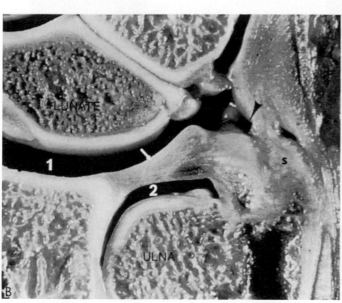

Figure 14–4
Radiocarpal and inferior radioulnar compartments.

A Radiocarpal compartment, open and flexed. The prestyloid recess approaches the ulnar styloid process. Observe the palmar (volar) radial recesses and the pisiform-triquetral joint, which communicates with the radiocarpal compartment in this drawing. (From Lewis OJ, et al: The anatomy of the wrist joint. J Anat *106*:539, 1979. Courtesy of Cambridge University Press.)

B Ulnar limit of radiocarpal compartment (coronal section). Note the extent of this compartment (1), its relationship to the inferior radioulnar compartment (2), the intervening triangular fibrocartilage (arrow), and the prestyloid recess (arrowhead), which is intimate with the ulnar styloid (s).

C Inferior radioulnar compartment (coronal section). This L-shaped compartment (2) extends between the distal radius and ulna and is separated from the radiocarpal compartment (1) by the triangular fibrocartilage (arrow). Note the saclike proximal contour of the inferior radioulnar compartment.

of the metacarpal head and neck. The capsule about the metacarpophalangeal joint is somewhat loose, allowing motion of the proximal phalanx. It attaches to the elevated bony crest surrounding the smooth articular surface of the metacarpal head to the bony ridge about the articular surface of the base of the phalanx. On the dorsal surface of the metacarpophalangeal joints, the fibrous capsule is thin; in this location, a bursa separates the capsule from the extensor tendon.

Each metacarpophalangeal joint has a palmar ligament and two collateral ligaments. The palmar ligament is located on the volar aspect of the joint and is firmly attached to the base of the proximal phalanx and loosely united to the metacarpal neck. Laterally, the palmar ligament blends with the collateral ligaments, and, volarly, the palmar ligament blends with the deep transverse metacarpal ligaments, which connect the pal-

mar ligaments of the second through fifth metacarpophalangeal joints. The palmar ligament also is grooved for the passage of the flexor tendons, whose fibrous sheaths are attached to the sides of the groove. The collateral ligaments reinforce the fibrous capsule laterally. These ligaments pass obliquely from the posterior tubercles and depressions on the radial and ulnar aspects of the metacarpal to attach to the base of the proximal phalanx.

Active movements of the metacarpophalangeal joints include flexion, extension, adduction, abduction, circumduction, and limited rotation. Accessory movements include rotation, gliding, and distraction. The metacarpophalangeal joint of the thumb, in general, has less extensive movement than the others; movement of the thumb occurs in two planes, that parallel to the remainder of the hand and that at right angles to this first plane.

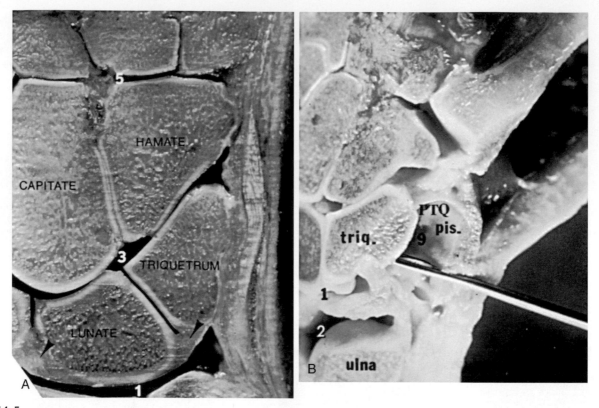

Figure 14–5
Midcarpal and pisiform-triquetral compartments.

A Midcarpal compartment (coronal section). The ulnar side of the midcarpal compartment (3) is well shown. This compartment is separated from the radiocarpal compartment (1) by interosseous ligaments (arrowheads) extending between bones of the proximal carpal row. Observe the common carpometacarpal compartment (5) between the distal carpal row and the bases of the four ulnar metacarpals.

B Pisiform-triquetral compartment (coronal section). This compartment (PTQ 9) exists between the triquetrum (triq.) and pisiform (pis.). The radiocarpal (1) and inferior radioulnar (2) compartments also are indicated.

At the proximal and distal interphalangeal joints, apposing surfaces of bone are covered by articular cartilage. A fibrous capsule surrounds each joint, and on its inner aspect the capsule is covered by synovial membrane, which extends over intracapsular bone not covered by articular cartilage. At the interphalangeal joints, synovial pouches exist proximally on both dorsal and palmar aspects of the articulation. The interphalangeal joints have a palmar and two collateral ligaments whose anatomy is similar to those about the metacarpophalangeal joints. Active movements at these joints include flexion and extension, both of which may be accompa-

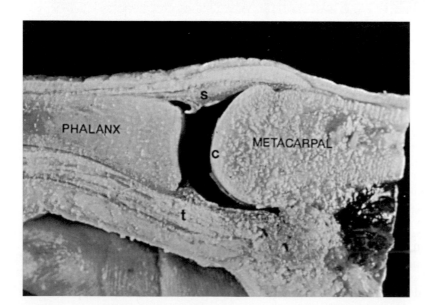

Figure 14–6
Metacarpophalangeal joints: General anatomy. Sagittal section. Observe the articular cavity, cartilage (c), synovial membrane (s), and flexor tendon (t).

nied by a small amount of rotation; accessory movements are rotation, abduction, adduction, and gliding.

Anatomy of the Triangular Fibrocartilage Complex

The distal radioulnar joint is stabilized primarily by the triangular fibrocartilage complex (TFCC) of the wrist.[1–6] In addition, the TFCC serves as a cushion between the carpus and distal portion of the ulna and as an extension of the articular surface of the radius and provides a site of anchorage for the ulnar-sided carpal bones. The components of the TFCC are not agreed on but include the triangular fibrocartilage (TFC) itself, the dorsal and volar radioulnar ligaments, the ulnomeniscal homologue, the ulnar collateral ligament, and the sheath of the extensor carpi ulnaris tendon. The TFC is thicker peripherally than centrally and may be fenestrated centrally, especially in middle-aged and elderly persons (Fig. 14–7A). The central portion of the TFC is avascular and consists of obliquely oriented sheets of collagen fibers.[3] The thick and strong marginal portions of the TFC, composed of lamellar collagen, often are referred to as the dorsal and volar radioulnar ligaments. The TFCC arises from the ulnar aspect of the lunate fossa of the radius, courses toward the ulna, and inserts into the fovea at the base of the ulnar styloid process.[7] As it extends distally, it is joined by fibers of the ulnar collateral ligament, becomes thickened in the form of the meniscus homologue, and inserts distally into the lunate, triquetrum, hamate, and base of the fifth metacarpal bone.[7] On its volar aspect, the TFCC is attached strongly to the triquetrum (the ulnotriquetral ligament)

and to the lunotriquetral interosseous ligament and less strongly to the lunate bone (the ulnolunate ligament); on its dorso-ulnar aspect, the TFCC is incorporated into the floor of the sheath of the extensor carpi ulnaris tendon.[7]

When the radius and ulna are of equal length, a situation designated neutral ulnar variance, the distal portion of the radius transmits approximately 80 per cent of the axial load across the wrist, and the distal portion of the ulna transmits approximately 20 per cent.[8, 9] Surgical removal of the TFCC decreases the load borne by the distal portion of the ulna by approximately 12 per cent, and removal of the distal portion of the ulna eliminates the load borne across the ulnar aspect of the wrist. When the ulna is short relative to the radius, a situation designated minus ulnar variance and occurring in association with Kienböck's disease, a diminution in the force borne by the distal portion of the ulna is evident. When the ulna is long relative to the radius, a situation designated positive ulnar variance and occurring in association with disruption of the TFCC, lunotriquetral interosseous ligament tears, and the ulnar impaction syndrome, an increase in the force borne by the distal portion of the ulna is apparent.[7]

The blood supply of the TFCC (Fig. 14–8) originates from the ulnar artery through its radiocarpal branches and the dorsal and palmar branches of the anterior interosseous artery.[3] These vessels supply the TFCC in a radial fashion; they penetrate only the peripheral 10 to 40 per cent of the TFCC.[3] The central section is avascular. The radial insertion of the TFCC, until now, also has been considered to be avascular,[3] although new evidence suggests otherwise.[5] This vascularity may be significant with regard to tissue healing after surgical reconstructive procedures.[5]

Figure 14–7
Age-related fenestrations of the triangular fibrocartilage and interosseous ligaments.

A In elderly persons, fenestrations (arrow) may develop in the triangular fibrocartilage, allowing communication of the radiocarpal (1) and inferior radioulnar (2) compartments.

B In elderly persons, progressive deterioration of the scapholunate interosseous ligament (arrow) eventually may allow communication of the radiocarpal (1) and midcarpal (3) compartments.

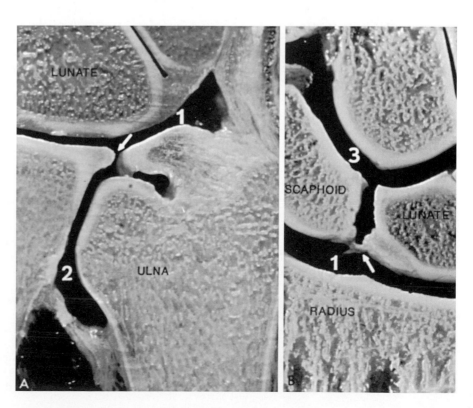

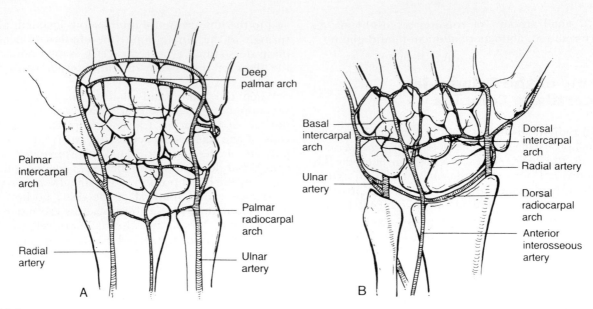

Figure 14–8

Arterial supply of the wrist. Anastomoses from the radial, ulnar, and anterior interosseous arteries form three transverse arches.

   A Arterial supply of palmar aspect of the wrist.

   B Arterial supply of the dorsal aspect of the wrist.

   (Reproduced with permission from McCue FC, Bruce JF Jr. The wrist. *In* JC DeLee, D. Drez Jr [eds]: Orthopaedic Sports Medicine. Philadelphia, WB Saunders Co, 1994, p 915.)

Ligamentous Anatomy

A number of ligaments about the distal ends of the radius and ulna and the carpal bones have been described. Some of these are considered intrinsic ligaments, arising and inserting on carpal bones, and others are considered extrinsic ligaments, joining the distal portion of the radius and the carpal bones (Fig. 14–9).

Interosseous Ligaments

The bones of the proximal carpal row are joined by two interosseous (or intrinsic) ligaments, the scapholunate interosseous ligament (joining the proximal surfaces of the scaphoid and lunate) and the lunotriquetral interosseous ligament (joining the proximal surfaces of the lunate and triquetrum). These ligaments connect the corresponding bones from their palmar to dorsal surfaces. They are C-shaped and thickened both dorsally and volarly, with a relatively thin and structurally weaker central membranous portion.[10] They may have a triangular configuration when sectioned in the coronal plane, are reinforced by fibers derived from the extrinsic radiocarpal ligaments (see later discussion) and, when intact, separate the radiocarpal and midcarpal compartments of the wrist. Disruption of these proximal intercarpal ligaments allows communication of the radiocarpal and midcarpal compartments of the wrist (see Fig. 14–7B). Failure of the scapholunate interosseous ligament requires less force than that needed to produce failure of the lunotriquetral interosseous ligament, and both ligaments elongate by as much as 50 to 100 per cent of their original length prior to failure.[10] Disruption of the scapholunate interosseous ligament, when combined with disruption of one or more of the volar extrinsic

radiocarpal ligaments, allows separation of the scaphoid and lunate bones, designated scapholunate dissociation.[11]

Three additional interosseous ligaments are found in the distal carpal row. These ligaments, which seldom fail clinically, unite the trapezium and the trapezoid bones, the trapezoid and the capitate bones, and the capitate and the hamate bones. These distal interosseous ligaments do not extend from the volar to the dorsal portions of the wrist capsule, explaining the communication of the midcarpal and common carpometacarpal compartments of the wrist.[2]

Palmar Radiocarpal Ligaments

Radiocarpal (extrinsic) ligaments of the wrist commonly are considered in two groups: palmar radiocarpal ligaments and dorsal radiocarpal ligaments. The former are more important to wrist function than the latter, representing significant stabilizers of wrist motion.[10, 12–15] The terminology applied to these ligaments is not constant, and only one system of nomenclature is emphasized here (see Fig. 14–9).

There are three volar (or palmar) radiocarpal ligaments: the radioscaphocapitate (radiocapitate) ligament, the radiolunotriquetral (radiotriquetral) ligament, and the radioscapholunate (radioscaphoid and radiolunate) ligament. The strong radioscaphocapitate ligament arises from the volar and radial aspects of the radial styloid process and extends in a distal and ulnar direction. It traverses a groove in the waist of the scaphoid bone, to which it attaches, and terminates in the center of the volar aspect of the capitate.[2] The insertion of this ligament into the scaphoid bone has been reported to be stronger than the capitate insertion site.[15] Some fibers of the radioscaphocapitate ligament may extend

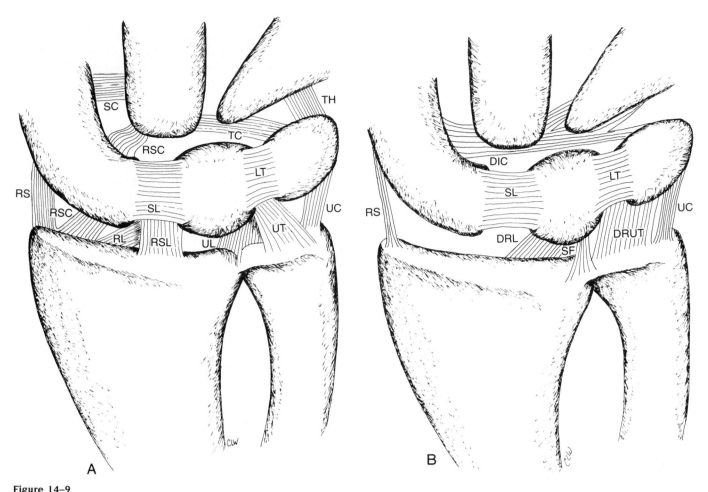

Figure 14–9
Ligamentous anatomy: Extrinsic and intrinsic ligaments.

A Palmar aspect of the wrist. Illustrated structures include the radioscaphoid (RS) portion of the radial collateral ligament, radioscaphocapitate ligament (RSC), radiolunotriquetral ligament (RL), radioscapholunate ligament (RSL), scaphocapitate ligament (SC), triquetrocapitate ligament (TC), triquetrohamate ligament (TH), ulnar collateral ligament (UC), ulnolunate ligament (UL), ulnotriquetral ligament (UT), and scapholunate (SL) and lunotriquetral (LT) interosseous ligaments.

B Dorsal aspect of the wrist. Illustrated structures include the radioscaphoid (RS) portion of the radial collateral ligament, scapholunate (SL) and lunotriquetral (LT) interosseous ligaments, dorsal intercarpal ligament (DIC), dorsal radiolunate ligament (DRL), dorsal radioulnotriquetral ligament (DRUT), ulnar collateral ligament (UC), and a prominent synovial fold (SF).

(From North ER, Thomas S: J Hand Surg [Am] *13*:815, 1988. © 1988, Churchill Livingstone, on behalf of the Journal of Hand Surgery, New York.)

to the triquetrum, although other fibers connecting the scaphoid to the triquetrum sometimes are referred to as the palmar scaphotriquetral ligament.[16] The large radiolunotriquetral ligament arises from the volar lip and styloid process of the radius adjacent to the radioscaphocapitate ligament, and it is directed distally in an ulnarward direction across the volar aspect of the lunate bone to attach to the palmar aspect of the triquetrum.[2] This ligament serves as volar sling for the lunate. The radioscapholunate ligament is located more medially and deeper than the other two volar ligaments. It arises from the volar aspect of the distal portion of the radius and inserts into the proximal and volar surface of the scapholunate space. This ligament reinforces the scapholunate interosseous ligament, and its disruption, along with that of the scapholunate interosseous ligament, leads to scapholunate dissociation.[2] Separate bundles of fibers in the region of the scapholunate interosseous ligament sometimes are referred to as radiolunate

and radioscaphoid ligaments.[17] Failure of any of the volar radiocarpal ligaments appears to require less force than that necessary to disrupt the interosseous ligaments of the proximal carpal row.[10]

Volar Ulnocarpal Ligaments

Two bands of ligamentous tissue arise from the anterior margin of the TFC and the base of the ulnar styloid process and extend distally, downward, and laterally to the lunate and triquetral bones, respectively.[2] The band inserting on the lunate is designated the ulnolunate ligament, and that inserting on the triquetrum is designated the ulnotriquetral ligament (Fig. 14–10); a distal portion of the ulnotriquetral ligament extends onto the volar aspect of the capitate and hamate.[2]

Other Volar Carpal Ligaments

Ligamentous tissue connects the volar aspects of the capitate and triquetral bones. This tissue sometimes is

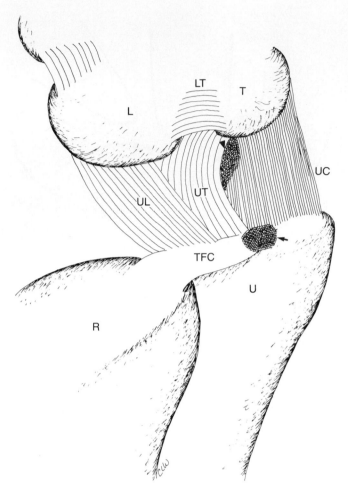

Figure 14–10
Ligamentous anatomy: Volar ulnocarpal ligaments. The lunate (L), triquetrum (T), radius (R), and ulna (U) are indicated. Illustrated structures include the ulnolunate (UL) and ulnotriquetral (UT) ligaments, triangular fibrocartilage (TFC), and lunotriquetral interosseous (LT) and ulnar collateral (UC) ligaments. The two shaded areas represent the prestyloid recess (arrow) and entrance site to the pisiform-triquetral joint (arrowhead). (From North ER, Thomas S: J Hand Surg [Am] *13*:815, 1988. © 1988, Churchill Livingstone, on behalf of the Journal of Hand Surgery, New York.)

designated the capitotriquetral (intrinsic) ligament. In other instances, ligamentous tissue arising from the volar aspect of the capitate is described as having a V-shape, representing a deltoid or arcuate ligament, whose ulnar arm extends to the triquetrum (triquetrocapitate ligament) and whose radial arm extends to the scaphoid bone (radioscaphocapitate ligament). Disruption of the ulnar arm of the arcuate ligament may be responsible for volar intercalated carpal instability, or VISI (see later discussion). Furthermore, the space of Poirier, representing an area of normal weakness in the volar aspect of the capsule just proximal to the deltoid ligament, is the site through which volar dislocation of the lunate occurs.

Dorsal Radiocarpal Ligaments

The dorsal capsule of the wrist contains an area of thickening that extends from the articular surface of the radius toward the lunate and triquetral bones. This area sometimes is viewed as a single structure or as several separate structures, leading to such designations as the radioscapholunotriquetral ligament, the radioscaphoid ligament, the radiolunate ligament, and the radiotriquetral ligament (see Fig. 14–9). The radiotriquetral component of these ligaments appears to be the most consistent of the structures, although its site of origin may be Lister's tubercle of the radius, the radial styloid process, or both structures.[18, 19] Although variation in the terminology applied to the dorsal radiocarpal ligaments exists, they are thin and few in number and generally are regarded as functionally less important than the volar radiocarpal ligaments. They are reinforced by the floor and septa of the fibrous tunnels through which the extensor tendons pass.[20]

Other Dorsal Carpal Ligaments

Several intrinsic dorsal ligaments bind together the carpal bones. Among these, the dorsal intercarpal ligament, consisting of the triquetroscaphoid and triquetrotrapezial fascicles, appears most prominent.[19]

Collateral Ligaments

The collateral ligaments of the wrist, the radial collateral ligament and the ulnar collateral ligament (see Fig. 14–9), represent thickenings of the fibrous capsule and functionally are less important than the collateral ligaments in other joints such as the knee and elbow. The radial collateral ligament extends from the tip of the styloid process of the radius to attach to the waist of the scaphoid bone, with fibers continuing to the trapezium and blending with the transverse carpal ligament and the dorsal capsular ligament. The ulnar collateral ligament is attached proximally to the base and body of the styloid process of the ulna with an extension into the TFC; distally, it attaches to the triquetrum, pisiform, hamate, and fifth metacarpal bone and the transverse carpal ligament.[2]

Soft Tissue Anatomy

Tendons

Those musculotendinous units that move the hand or wrist originate at the elbow and insert on the metacarpal bones; no muscles attach to the bones in the proximal carpal row.[10] The primary flexors are the flexor carpi radialis and flexor carpi ulnaris muscles; the primary extensors are the extensor carpi radialis longus and extensor carpi radialis brevis muscles; the primary radial deviator is the abductor pollicis longus muscle; and the primary ulnar deviator is the extensor carpi ulnaris muscle.[10]

Flexor Retinaculum

On the volar aspect of the wrist, a strong broad ligament, the flexor retinaculum or transverse carpal ligament, extends from its lateral attachment to the tuberos-

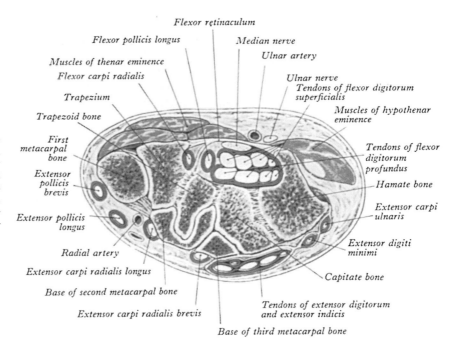

Figure 14–11
Flexor retinaculum and carpal tunnel. A transverse section through the wrist shows the tendons and their synovial sheaths passing beneath the flexor retinaculum. The section is slightly oblique and divides the distal row of the carpus and the bases of the first, second, and third metacarpal bones. (From Williams PL, Warwick R [Eds]: Gray's Anatomy. 36th British edition. Edinburgh, Churchill Livingstone, 1980, p. 583.)

ities of the trapezium and scaphoid to its medial attachment to the pisiform bone and hook of the hammate bone (Fig. 14–11). Its functions may include maintenance of the contour of the carpus and fixation of the flexor tendons during flexion of the wrist, preventing the loss of power that would occur with bowstringing of the tendons.[2]

Carpal Tunnel

Beneath the carpus on the palmar aspect of the wrist, the carpal tunnel is a confined soft tissue compartment that is bounded volarly by the flexor retinaculum and dorsally, medially, and laterally by the carpal bones (see Fig. 14–11). Coursing through the carpal tunnel are a number of structures that include the median nerve, the eight deep and superficial flexor tendons and tenosynovial sheaths, the tendon and synovial sheath of the flexor pollicis longus muscle, the radial and ulnar bursae, and fat. The precise relationship among the structures varies according to the specific level within the canal (i.e., proximal, intermediate, and distal portions) and the position of the wrist (i.e., neutral, flexion, and extension).[21, 22] At the level of the proximal portion of the carpal tunnel, its walls include the trapezium and scaphoid bones laterally, the capitate, hamate, and triquetrum bones dorsally, the pisiform bone medially, and the flexor retinaculum superficially.[21] At this proximal level, the median nerve is just deep to the flexor retinaculum and palmaris longus tendon and is located between the flexor pollicis longus deeply and laterally and the flexor digitorum superficialis tendons deeply and medially. The median nerve is slightly flattened by the adjacent tendons. At the level of the intermediate portion, or midportion, of the carpal tunnel, the relationships of the median nerve are similar to those evident in the proximal portion, although the nerve may be located more deeply.[21] At this level, the hook of the hamate bone forms the ulnar wall of the carpal tunnel. At the distal portion of the carpal tunnel, the flexor retinaculum attaches to the hook of the hamate, and the median nerve still maintains a flattened appearance.[21] With the wrist in neutral position, the median nerve within the carpal tunnel is found either anterior to the superficial flexor tendon of the index finger or interposed more posterolaterally between this tendon and the flexor pollicis longus tendon.[22] With wrist extension, the median nerve assumes (or maintains) an anterior position between the superficial index finger flexor tendon and the flexor retinaculum, while the flexor tendons move posteriorly; with wrist flexion, the flexor tendons shift anteriorly toward the retinaculum and the position of the median nerve is more variable.[22]

Ulnar Tunnel (Guyon's Canal)

The ulnar nerve passes through a fibro-osseous tunnel known as Guyon's canal, in the anteromedial portion of the wrist (see Chapter 11). The tunnel is approximately 4 cm in length, extending from the proximal edge of the pisiform bone to the origin of the hypothenar muscles at the level of the hamulus.[23, 24] The volar margin of the tunnel is the pisohamate interosseous ligament. The ulnar artery and, occasionally, communicating veins accompany the ulnar nerve through the canal.[23]

Digital Flexor Tendon Sheaths and Synovial Sacs of the Palm

The flexor tendons of the fingers, the sublimis digitorum and profundus digitorum, are enveloped by digital sheaths from a line of insertion of the flexor profundus to a line 1 cm proximal to the proximal border of the deep transverse ligament (Fig. 14–12).[25] This arrangement, which is not constant, is most frequent in the index, middle, and ring fingers.[26] Any of these three

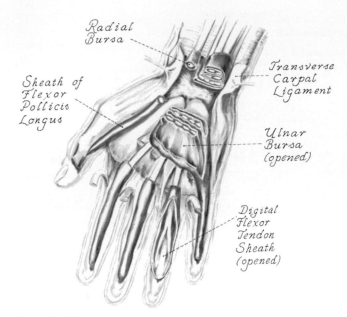

Figure 14–12

Digital flexor tendon sheaths and synovial sacs of the palm. The digital flexor tendon sheaths of the second through fourth fingers terminate proximal to the metacarpophalangeal joint. That of the fifth finger communicates with the ulnar bursa. The sheath of the flexor pollicis longus is continuous with the radial bursa. Note the three invaginations of the ulnar bursa and, in this drawing, absence of communication between radial and ulnar bursae.

sheaths may extend to the wrist.[27] The flexor sheath of the thumb extends from the terminal phalanx to a point 2 to 3 cm proximal to the proximal volar crease of the wrist, although on occasion a septum separates proximal and distal halves of the sheath.[26] The synovial sheath of the little finger also commences at its terminal phalanx. It may end near the deep transverse ligament or continue into the palm, expanding to envelop the adjacent tendons of the second, third, and fourth fingers.[25, 26] The digital sheath of the thumb lies distally near the proximal phalanx, but as it ascends toward the palm it separates from the metacarpal head.

Communication between the individual digital tendon sheaths and synovial sacs or bursae in the palm is not constant[27]; most frequently, such continuation is noted involving the first digit (Fig. 14–13). Not uncommonly the digital sheath of the fifth finger also continues into the palm.[26] Such communication is uncommon in the second, third, and fourth fingers.

The ulnar bursa on the medial aspect of the palm comprises three communicating invaginations[25, 26]; a superficial extension lies in front of the flexor sublimis, a middle one lies between the tendons of the sublimis and the profundus, and a deep extension is found behind the flexor profundus. The bursa, beginning at the proximal end of the digital sheaths, spreads out proximally, overlying the third, fourth, and fifth metacarpals. A statistical analysis of the tendon sheath patterns in the hand using air insufflation techniques in 367 cases demonstrated that the ulnar bursa communicated with the sheaths of the little finger in 81 per cent, of the index finger in 5.1 per cent, of the middle finger

in 4.0 per cent, and of the ring finger in 3.5 per cent of cases.[27]

The radial bursa is the expanded proximal continuation of the digital sheath of the flexor pollicis longus muscle. It is found on the radial aspect of the palm overlying the second metacarpal. It continues proximally along the volar radial aspect of the wrist, terminating about 2 cm above the transverse carpal ligament.[25]

Intercommunications between the ulnar and radial bursae may be noted in 50 per cent of cases (see Fig. 14–13). Such connection is made via intermediate bursae. These accessory synovial sacs may be located posteriorly, between the carpal canal and flexor profundus digitorum of the index finger, or, less commonly, anteriorly, between the superficial and deep tendons of the index finger. A separate carpal sheath that does not communicate with either radial or ulnar bursa may be found enveloping the index flexor tendons.[25] Additionally, a small synovial sac may enclose the tendon of the flexor carpi radialis as it passes under the crest of the trapezium.[25]

Extensor Tendon Sheaths

Several synovial sheaths are located in the dorsum of the wrist beneath the dorsal carpal ligament; they extend for a short distance proximal and distal to that ligament (Fig. 14–14). By insular attachments of the dorsal carpal ligament on the posterior and lateral surfaces of the radius and ulna, six distinct avenues are created for transport of ligamentous structures. The most medial compartment (sixth compartment) contains the extensor carpi ulnaris tendon and sheath (4 to 5 cm in length), lying at the dorsomedial aspect of the distal

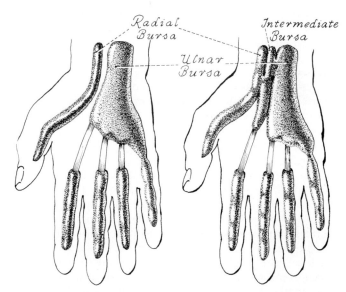

Figure 14–13

Digital flexor tendon sheaths and synovial sacs of the palm. The radial and ulnar bursae may be separate, distinct cavities or may communicate via an intermediate bursa. Note the flexor tendon sheaths which, in the second, third, and fourth fingers, usually terminate just proximal to the metacarpophalangeal joints. The tendon sheaths in the first and fifth fingers usually communicate with the bursae in the wrist. (From Resnick D: AJR *124:*44, 1975. Copyright 1975 American Roentgen Ray Society.)

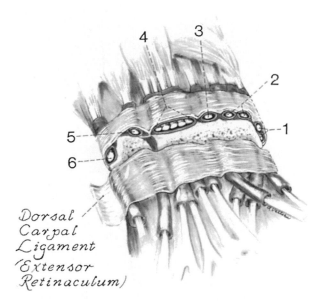

Figure 14–14
Extensor tendons and tendon sheaths. Drawing shows dorsal carpal ligament and extensor tendons surrounded by synovial sheaths traversing dorsum of wrist within six separate compartments. These compartments are created by the insular attachment of the dorsal carpal ligament on the posterior and lateral surfaces of the radius and ulna. The extensor carpi ulnaris tendon and its sheath are in the medial compartment (6) and are closely applied to the posterior surface of the ulna. (From Resnick D: Med Radiogr Photogr 52:50, 1976.)

ulna. In the fifth compartment, a long sheath (6 to 7 cm in length) covers the extensor digiti quinti proprius, which lies in close proximity to and may communicate with the inferior radioulnar joint. The fourth compartment on the posteromedial aspect of the radius contains a large sheath (5 to 6 cm in length) enclosing the tendons of the extensor digitorum communis and the extensor indicis proprius. In the third compartment are the sheath (6 to 7 cm in length) and tendon of the extensor pollicis longus. The sheath may extend as far distally as the trapezium or first metacarpal bone. Lateral to this in the second compartment are sheaths (5 to 6 cm in length) covering the extensor carpi radialis longus and extensor carpi radialis brevis, which may communicate with the sheath of the extensor pollicis longus. Finally, a compartment along the lateral aspect of the radius (first compartment) contains a common synovial sheath (5 to 6 cm in length) enclosing the abductor pollicis longus and extensor pollicis brevis.

FUNCTION

Normal function of the wrist requires coordinated motion among the bones that compose it. The distal ends of the radius and ulna, although moving between positions of supination and pronation of the forearm, generally are considered to be stable.[28] Similarly, little motion occurs between the bones of the distal carpal row and the bases of the metacarpal bones. Rather, it is the varying relationships of the eight carpal bones during movement of the wrist that have received a great deal

of attention.[10, 28, 29] Normally, as the wrist moves from a neutral position to one of full flexion (80 degrees) and full extension (70 degrees), it describes an arc of about 150 degrees. Approximately 50 per cent of this motion occurs at the radiocarpal joint and 50 per cent occurs at the midcarpal joint.[10] Similarly, under normal circumstances, as the wrist moves from a neutral position to one of full radial deviation (20 degrees) and full ulnar deviation (30 degrees), it describes an arc of about 50 degrees. Sixty per cent of this motion occurs at the midcarpal joint and 40 per cent occurs at the radiocarpal joint.[10] These movements of the wrist are accompanied by a change of relationship between the bones of the proximal carpal row and those of the distal carpal row. To understand the complex biomechanical principles that govern carpal motion, investigators have described functional anatomy in a variety of ways.

The link key mechanism governing wrist motion (Fig. 14–15) was defined by Gilford and associates[30] in 1943. This theory proposed that the distal portion of the radius, the proximal carpal row, and the distal carpal row functioned as links in a chain that was stable in tension but inherently unstable in compression.[29] The scaphoid bone, by bridging the two carpal rows, provided stability and helped to control motion. In 1978, Taleisnik[31] described a columnar approach to wrist anatomy (Fig. 14–16) in which the scaphoid bone represented a mobile lateral column, the triquetrum represented a rotary medial column, and lunate and bones of the distal carpal row functioned as a flexion-extension column.[29] In 1980, Weber[32] divided the carpus into two longitudinal columns (Fig. 14–17): The radial side of the carpus functioned as a force-bearing column and the ulnar side of the carpus served to control the position of the lunate bone relative to the capitate bone.[29] In 1981, Lichtman and associates[33] proposed the con-

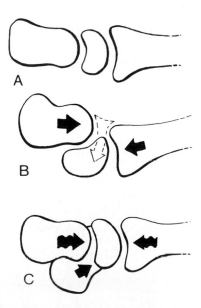

Figure 14–15
Link key mechanism of wrist motion. The scaphoid bridges the proximal and distal carpal rows, providing stability in compression. (Redrawn from Gilford WW, Bolton RH, Lambrinudi C: Guy's Hosp Rep 92:52, 1943.)

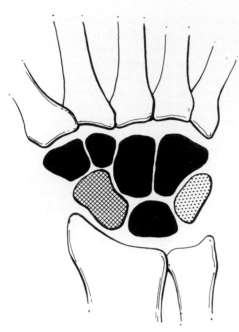

Figure 14–16
Columnar approach to wrist anatomy. (Redrawn from Lichtman DM, Schneider JR, Swafford AR, et al: J Hand Surg *6*:522, 1981.)

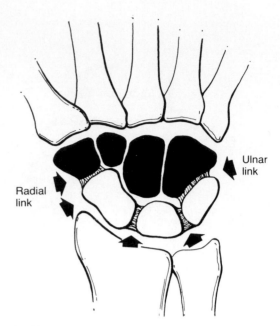

Figure 14–18
Oval ring concept of wrist anatomy. (Redrawn from Lichtman DM, Schneider JR, Swafford AR, et al: J Hand Surg *6*:522, 1981.)

cept of an oval ring (Fig. 14–18) consisting of two mobile links (i.e., radial and ulnar links) that allowed reciprocal motion between the proximal and distal carpal rows.[29] The movement between the links occurred at the trapezioscaphoid and triquetrohamate joints. Whatever the precise mechanism, proper function of the wrist requires smooth and synchronous motion between and within the two carpal rows.[10]

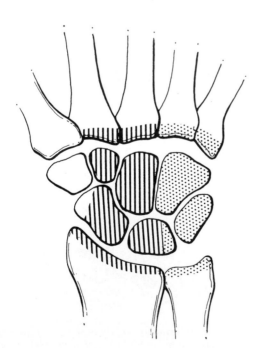

Figure 14–17
Longitudinal column approach to wrist anatomy. (Redrawn from Weber ER: Orthop Clin North Am *15*:196, 1984.)

IMAGING TECHNIQUES

Any number of imaging methods, either alone or in combination, can be used to evaluate the hand and wrist. These techniques include routine radiography, scintigraphy, diagnostic ultrasonography, CT scanning, arthrography, and MR imaging. In this chapter, the diagnostic role assumed by many of these methods is addressed in discussions of individual abnormalities of the wrist and hand. Some additional information regarding two advanced techniques—arthrography and MR imaging—that are fundamental to accurate diagnosis of many of these abnormalities is provided here.

Arthrography

Arthrography of the wrist is a safe procedure, which sometimes is useful in the diagnosis of traumatic and other articular disorders.[34-41]

With standard arthrography technique, under fluoroscopic control, a 22 gauge, 1.5 inch long needle is introduced into the wrist from a dorsal approach. Most often, the radiocarpal compartment is the site of injection, although other compartments of the wrist may be studied (see later discussion). A total of 1.5 to 2.5 ml of iodinated contrast material is administered. Posteroanterior, lateral, and oblique radiographs are obtained before and after mild exercise.

In recent years, several modifications in this technique have been emphasized. Fluoroscopic monitoring combined with sequential spot filming or videotaping during the injection of contrast material allows more precise delineation of sites of abnormal compartmental communication.[42-44, 409] Magnification radiography, analysis of joint motion, and application of stress are additional techniques that have been advocated for more definitive diagnosis.[43, 45] Conventional tomography or CT scanning after the introduction of the contrast agent has allowed the identification of exact sites of perforation of the triangular fibrocartilage[16, 17] as well as ligamentous disruption and cartilage loss,[48] although the time required for the examination is significantly prolonged. Selective injection of the midcarpal compartment, rather than the radiocarpal compartment, has been introduced as a superior method for analysis of the scapholunate and lunotriquetral ligaments,[49] owing to less obscuration by the contrast material although, by itself, it will not allow identification of a tear of the triangular fibrocartilage in the presence of intact intercarpal ligaments (see later discussion).

Digital arthrography can be used successfully in the examination of the wrist. The technique combines the advantages of fluoroscopic monitoring and videotaping and provides the examiner with the opportunity to view the dynamics of the injection process in both the positive and negative mode.[51–55] The technique used involves an initial test exposure and subsequent multiple exposures obtained at the rate of approximately one exposure each second for 20 to 30 sec during the administration of the contrast agent (Fig. 14–19). An image acquired before the appearance of the contrast medium is used as a mask that is subtracted from the remaining frames in the run. The digital technique has many other advantages, including the ability to subtract the carpal bones from the sequential images, providing a clear view of the distribution of the contrast material during the injection process. Furthermore, if more than one wrist compartment is injected (see later discussion), digital technique with subtracted images can eliminate any contrast that had resulted from previous opacification of other compartments.[54, 55]

In recent years, great interest has developed regarding the technique of three-compartment wrist arthrography, in which separate injections into the radiocarpal, midcarpal, and inferior radioulnar compartments are employed. This method was popularized by Levinsohn and colleagues.[55–58] The rationale for this technique was based on the existence of abnormalities involving only the proximal surface of the triangular fibrocartilage or of disruptions of this fibrocartilage or the interosseous ligaments of the wrist that allowed passage of contrast material in only one direction and not the other; such abnormalities might not be detected with radiocarpal arthrography alone. Other investigators have questioned the need for multicompartmental arthrography of the wrist and have emphasized the importance of full distention of the radiocarpal compartment (or other compartments) to ensure visualization of all sites of compartmental communication.[59, 60]

Based on an analysis of reported data, three-compartment wrist arthrography represents the most reliable arthrographic method in the detection of communications among the various compartments of the wrist. The procedure, however, is more time consuming than single compartment arthrography. Furthermore, it is not clear if those tears of the triangular fibrocartilage or interosseous ligaments in the proximal carpal row that allow contrast material to pass in only one direction are of clinical significance. Indeed, communications

among the compartments of the wrist have been documented in asymptomatic persons, and identical arthrographic abnormalities may be encountered when bilateral wrist examinations are performed and comparison is made between symptomatic and asymptomatic sides.[61–64, 410] Some reports have indicated that arthrographic results correlate better with ulnar-sided rather than with radial-sided pain.[65] The advantages of wrist arthrography when compared with wrist arthroscopy continue to be debated, however.[411, 412]

Normally, contrast opacification of the radiocarpal compartment reveals a concave sac with smooth synovial surfaces extending between the distal end of the radius and proximal carpal row (Fig. 14–20A and B). The prestyloid recess appears as a finger-like projection that approaches the ulnar styloid process from the ulnar limit of the radiocarpal joint. One or more volar radial recesses are located beneath the distal end of the radius. If the midcarpal joint is injected, contrast material normally will extend proximally between the scaphoid and lunate and between the lunate and triquetrum to the level of the scapholunate and lunotriquetral interosseous ligaments. It will extend distally into the common carpometacarpal and intermetacarpal compartments. If the distal radioulnar joint is injected, contrast material sits like a cap on the articular surface of the ulna.[66] A small diverticulum extending into the proximal surface of the triangular fibrocartilage has been reported as a normal variation.[67]

Communication between the radiocarpal compartment and other compartments in the wrist during arthrography may be observed in "normal" persons or cadavers. The radiocarpal compartment may communicate with the midcarpal compartment (see Fig. 14–20C and D) in 13 to 47 per cent of the population and with the inferior radioulnar compartment in 7 to 35 per cent.[35, 36, 68] The prevalence of these findings increases in older persons.[69] Arthrographic communication between the radiocarpal and pisiform-triquetral compartments is frequent, particularly with forceful injection of contrast material into either compartment.[38, 70] It is observed in more than 50 per cent of cases.[69] Arthrographic communication between the pisiform-triquetral and midcarpal compartments, however, is considered abnormal.[52]

Opacification of tendon sheaths and lymphatics generally is not observed in "normal" wrist arthrograms,[35] although Trentham and associates[68] indicated that tendon sheath visualization may be apparent in 6 per cent of such normal examinations.

Magnetic Resonance Imaging

The evaluation of the wrist (and hand) with MR imaging is best accomplished with high-field (>1.0 T) MR imaging systems. Surface coils are fundamental to achieving high-resolution images with thin slices and a small field of view (8 to 12 cm). Commercially available wrist imaging coils, paired, phased-array temporomandibular joint receiver coils, transmit-receive quadrature coils, and research prototype coils are among the types of surface coils that have been used by previous investigators to image the wrist.[71–74] In certain clinical situations,

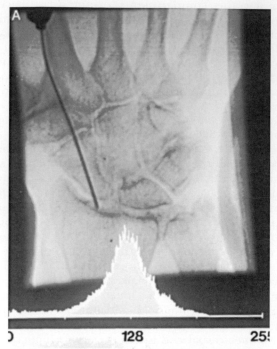

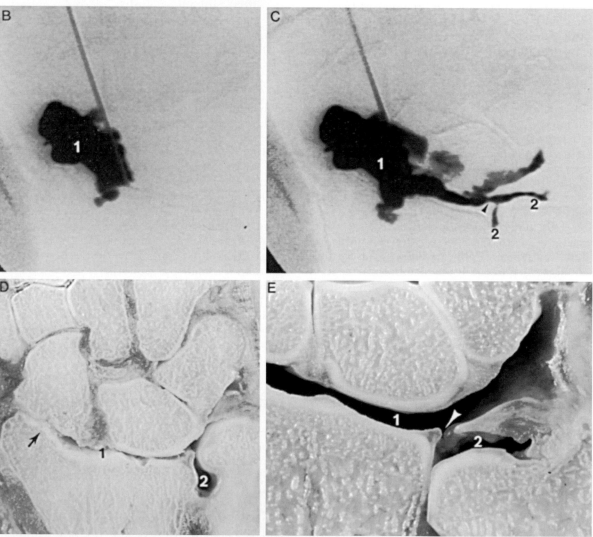

Figure 14–19

Wrist arthrography: Digital technique—radiocarpal joint injection.

A A test exposure is obtained prior to the introduction of the contrast material and is evaluated by computer algorithm to ensure adequate radiographic technique.

B, C Subtraction images are shown after the injection of 0.5 ml (**B**) and 1.0 ml (**C**) of the contrast agent into the radiocarpal joint. In **B**, there is slight irregularity of the contrast agent in the radial aspect of the radiocarpal joint (1). In **C**, most of the radiocarpal compartment (1) has been opacified and filling of the inferior radioulnar joint (2) is occurring through a small defect in the triangular fibrocartilage (arrowhead).

D, E Coronal sections of the wrist confirm minimal irregularity of the articular cartilage of the radius and scaphoid (arrow) and a perforation in the triangular fibrocartilage (arrowhead).

(**B–E** From Resnick D, et al: AJR *142*:1187, 1984. Copyright 1984, American Roentgen Ray Society.)

imaging of both wrists simultaneously may be required, for which a head coil may be used. Depending on the size of the patient, the type of surface coil employed, and the specific clinical information required, the patient may be placed in the magnet either in the supine position with the arm at the side or in the prone position with the arm or arms extended above the head. In general, the prone position with the arm extended is less well tolerated and results in a greater number of motion-degraded studies,[74] but it may be required in the assessment of conditions such as distal radioulnar joint subluxation, when examination of both wrists is necessary. Basically, the more comfortable the patient is at the time of the study, the more likely it is that a diagnostically effective examination will be obtained.

In the examination of masses about the wrist or of patients with point tenderness, taping a vitamin E capsule or other marker to the skin at the site of suspected abnormality is helpful.[74] Also, as is discussed later in this chapter, provocative exercise of the wrist prior to MR imaging, kinematic studies of the wrist in different positions of flexion or extension and radial or ulnar deviation, and application of stress to the joint at the time of imaging may provide additional information.

MR images of the wrist (or hand) usually are accomplished in one or more of three basic planes—coronal, sagittal, and transaxial—although oblique planes programmed according to the anatomy of a specific structure occasionally are used to study certain of the ligaments and tendons (Plates 14–1 through 14–9). The coronal plane is particularly important in the analysis of the TFCC and interosseous ligaments of the wrist, the sagittal plane is fundamental to analysis of wrist instability, the transaxial plane is important in the assessment of the carpal tunnel syndrome and instability of the distal radioulnar joint, and all of these planes may be required in detection and delineation of tumorous and infective processes.

Conventional or fast spin echo techniques are employed most commonly in the analysis of disorders of the wrist and hand. As is indicated in subsequent sections of this chapter, application of additional imaging sequences and methods, including standard or volume gradient echo imaging, the intravenous or intra-articular administration of a gadolinium compound, and fat suppression and short tau inversion recovery (STIR) MR imaging, may be required in the analysis of certain disorders. The highest quality MR images of the wrist, to date, have been provided by Totterman and Miller,[71] who have used a 1.5 T MR imaging unit, a custom-designed wrist coil, and a three-dimensional gradient echo imaging protocol. Although such high-quality images appear to be important in the analysis of some of the wrist ligaments and portions of the TFCC, they may not be essential in other clinical situations.

SPECIFIC ABNORMALITIES
Fractures of the Distal Ends of the Radius and Ulna

The most common mechanism of injury to the wrist is a fall on the outstretched hand causing axial compression combined with a bending moment, which leads to dorsiflexion of the joint. Far less frequently, the wrist is in palmar flexion at the time of injury. It is the precise position of the wrist, which also may include varying degrees of radial or ulnar deviation and supination or pronation, combined with other factors, including the age of the patient and the severity of the forces involved, that dictates the type of injury that will occur. With regard to the influence of age alone, metaphyseal fractures of the radius and ulna in young children, physeal separations of the radius in adolescents, scaphoid fractures in young adults, and fractures of the distal portion of the radius or of both radius and ulna in middle-aged and elderly patients typically follow a fall on the outstretched hand.[75] Fractures of the distal ends of the radius and ulna are approximately 10 times more frequent than those of the carpal bones, and the latter are especially infrequent in children.[76] It generally is believed that the distal portion of the radius yields to a lower level of force and lower angle of dorsiflexion than the carpus.[77]

Many eponyms are used to describe the fractures of the distal ends of the radius and ulna (Table 14–1). Examples include Colles' fracture (fracture of the distal portion of the radius with dorsal displacement), Smith's fracture (fracture of the distal portion of the radius with palmar displacement), Barton's fracture (fracture of the dorsal rim of the radius), and Hutchinson's fracture (fracture of the radial styloid process). It should be understood, however, that fractures about the wrist often do not fall precisely into these specific categories. Rather, with regard to treatment recommendations and prognostic implications, characteristics of the fracture pattern that are most important include articular involvement (i.e., radiocarpal and inferior radioulnar joints) and degree of displacement, angulation, depression, and comminution of the fracture fragments. Two-part (e.g., Barton's fracture, Hutchinson's fracture, die-punch fracture), three-part (e.g., some types of Colles' fractures), four-part (e.g., some types of Colles' fractures), and five-part (or more) (i.e., severely comminuted fracture) fractures are encountered, with each part representing a fragment of bone of sufficient size to be functionally significant and capable of being manipulated or internally fixed, or both (Figs. 14–21 to 14–23).[78]

The classic Colles' fracture is a transverse fracture, with or without comminution, that extends from the volar to the dorsal surface of the distal end of the radius and is accompanied by impaction and displacement of the dorsal surface of the radius. A number of classification systems exist for Colles' fractures; many are complex, and some are based upon the number of joints (i.e., radiocarpal, inferior radioulnar) that are violated and the presence or absence of a fracture of the ulnar styloid process. A fracture of the ulnar styloid process occurs in approximately 50 to 60 per cent of cases, and violation of one or both of these joints occurs in the majority of cases. Radial shortening and dorsal inclination of the articular surface of the radius (which normally has a 5 to 15 degree volar inclination) are emphasized sequelae of Colles' fractures that, if not corrected,

Table 14–1. FRACTURES OF THE DISTAL PORTIONS OF THE RADIUS AND ULNA

Fracture	Mechanism	Characteristics	Complications
Colles' (Pouteau's)	Dorsiflexion	Fracture of distal portion with dorsal displacement	Deformity related to radial shortening and angulation
		Classification system based on extra-articular versus intra-articular location, presence or absence of ulnar fracture	Subluxation or dislocation of inferior radioulnar joint
		Varying amounts of radial displacement, angulation, and shortening	Reflex sympathetic dystrophy syndrome
		Ulnar styloid fracture in about 50 to 60 per cent of cases	Injury to median or, less commonly, radial or ulnar nerve
		Associated injuries to carpus, elbow, humerus, and femur (in osteoporotic patients), inferior radioulnar joint	Osteoarthritis
			Tendon rupture
			Ulnar impaction syndrome
Barton's	Dorsiflexion and pronation	Fracture of dorsal rim of radius with intra-articular extension	Similar to those of Colles' fracture
Radiocarpal fracture-dislocation	Dorsiflexion	Uncommon and severe injury	Entrapment of ulnar nerve and artery, tendons
		Associated fractures of dorsal rim and styloid process of radius, ulnar styloid process	
		May be irreducible	
Hutchinson's (chauffeur's)	Avulsion by radial collateral ligament	Fracture of styloid process of radius	Scapholunate dissociation
		Usually nondisplaced	Osteoarthritis
			Ligament damage
Smith's (reverse Colles')	Variable	Fracture of distal portion of radius with palmar displacement	Similar to those of Colles' fracture
		Less common than Colles' fracture	
		Varying amounts of radial comminution, articular involvement	
		Associated fracture of ulnar styloid process	
Ulnar styloid process	Dorsiflexion or avulsion by ulnar collateral or triangular fibrocartilage complex	Usually associated with radial fractures, rarely isolated	Nonunion
		Usually nondisplaced	

may influence subsequent wrist function.[78, 79] Therefore, precise measurement of such parameters as radial tilt, radial inclination, and ulnar variance on routine radiographs assumes some importance[80] and requires meticulous and sometimes modified radiographic technique.[80, 81] Complications of Colles' fractures include unstable reduction, articular incongruity, subluxation or dislocation of the distal radioulnar joint, median nerve compression resulting in the carpal tunnel syndrome, ulnar nerve injury, entrapment of flexor tendons, reflex sympathetic dystrophy, carpal malalignment or fracture, posttraumatic osteolysis of the ulna, and malunion, delayed union, or nonunion.[82–85]

A distal radial fracture similar in position to that of the Colles' fracture but associated with volar (or palmar) angulation or displacement of the distal fragment is known as Smith's fracture. In contrast to Colles' fractures, the distal radial fragment is displaced anteriorly with palmar angulation of the radial articular surface in a Smith's fracture.[75] Complications of Smith's fractures are similar to those of Colles' fractures and may include injury to the extensor tendons.[86, 87]

A Barton's fracture involves an injury to the dorsal rim of the distal portion of the radius, generally related to dorsiflexion and pronation of the forearm on the fixed wrist and occurring frequently in young patients involved in motorcycle accidents. Classically it does not violate the volar surface of the radius and is accompanied by dorsal displacement of the carpus. A variant of Barton's fracture affects the volar rim of the distal radial end and sometimes is referred to as a reverse Barton's fracture or a type of Smith's fracture. Complications of fractures of the dorsal or volar rim of the distal end of the radius are similar to those of Colles' fracture.

Figure 14–20

Wrist arthrography: Normal and abnormal arthrograms—radiocarpal joint injection.

A, B Frontal and lateral views. Observe the contrast-filled radiocarpal compartment (1), which is communicating with the pisiform-triquetral compartment (9). Also note the prestyloid recess (3) and volar radial recesses (8).

C, D Radiocarpal-midcarpal compartment communication. A frontal radiograph after opacification of the radiocarpal compartment (1) reveals its communication with the midcarpal (6) and common carpometacarpal (7) compartments. This communication is possible when a defect exists in the interosseous ligaments extending between bones of the proximal carpal row. On a photograph of a coronal section of the cadaveric wrist, observe disruption of the scapholunate ligament (arrowhead). The inferior radioulnar compartment (2) and volar radial recesses (8) also are indicated.

E, F Radiocarpal-inferior radioulnar compartment communication. A frontal radiograph after opacification of the radiocarpal compartment (1) reveals its communication with the inferior radioulnar compartment (2). This communication is possible when a defect exists in the triangular fibrocartilage. Such a defect (arrowhead) is illustrated in a photograph of a coronal section of the wrist. Other indicated structures are the midcarpal compartment (6), volar radial recesses (8), and prestyloid recess (3).

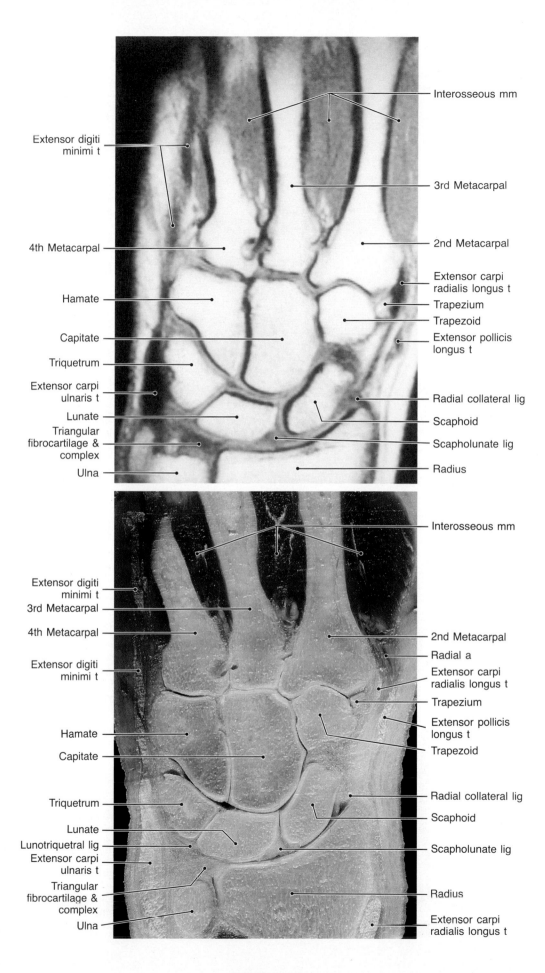

Interosseous mm

Extensor digiti minimi t

3rd Metacarpal

2nd Metacarpal

4th Metacarpal

Extensor carpi radialis longus t

Hamate

Trapezium

Trapezoid

Capitate

Extensor pollicis longus t

Triquetrum

Extensor carpi ulnaris t

Lunate

Radial collateral lig

Triangular fibrocartilage & complex

Scaphoid

Scapholunate lig

Ulna

Radius

Interosseous mm

Extensor digiti minimi t

3rd Metacarpal

4th Metacarpal

2nd Metacarpal

Radial a

Extensor digiti minimi t

Extensor carpi radialis longus t

Trapezium

Hamate

Extensor pollicis longus t

Capitate

Trapezoid

Triquetrum

Radial collateral lig

Lunate

Scaphoid

Lunotriquetral lig

Extensor carpi ulnaris t

Scapholunate lig

Triangular fibrocartilage & complex

Ulna

Radius

Extensor carpi radialis longus t

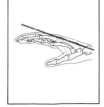

PLATE 14–1

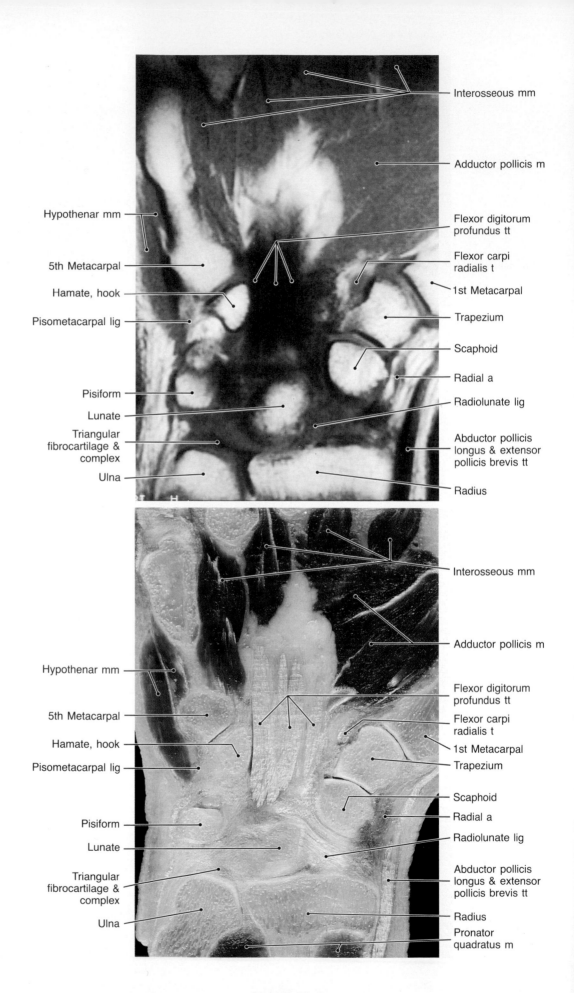

Interosseous mm

Adductor pollicis m

Hypothenar mm

Flexor digitorum profundus tt

Flexor carpi radialis t

5th Metacarpal

1st Metacarpal

Hamate, hook

Trapezium

Pisometacarpal lig

Scaphoid

Radial a

Pisiform

Radiolunate lig

Lunate

Triangular fibrocartilage & complex

Abductor pollicis longus & extensor pollicis brevis tt

Ulna

Radius

Interosseous mm

Adductor pollicis m

Hypothenar mm

Flexor digitorum profundus tt

Flexor carpi radialis t

5th Metacarpal

1st Metacarpal

Hamate, hook

Trapezium

Pisometacarpal lig

Scaphoid

Radial a

Pisiform

Radiolunate lig

Lunate

Triangular fibrocartilage & complex

Abductor pollicis longus & extensor pollicis brevis tt

Ulna

Radius

Pronator quadratus m

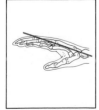

PLATE 14–2

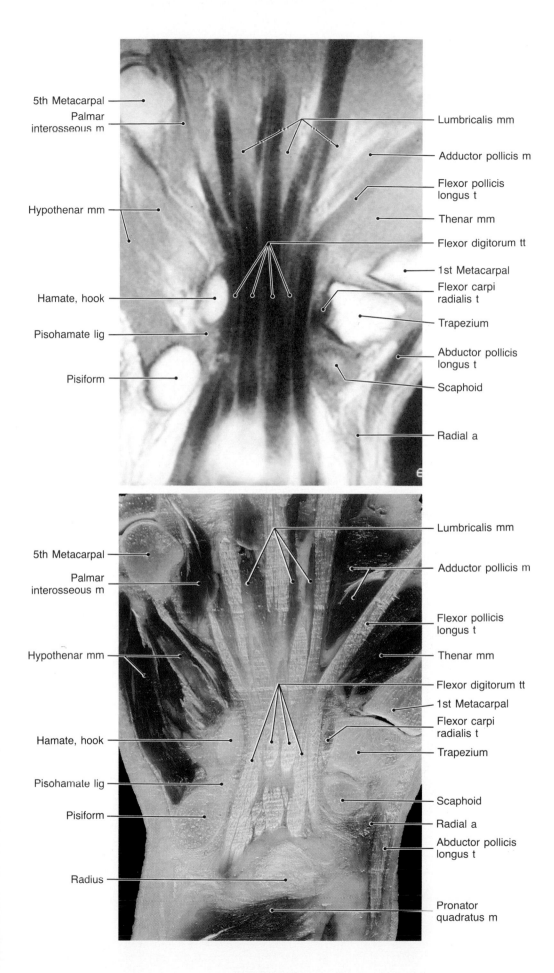

5th Metacarpal

Palmar
interosseous m

Hypothenar mm

Hamate, hook

Pisohamate lig

Pisiform

Lumbricalis mm

Adductor pollicis m

Flexor pollicis
longus t

Thenar mm

Flexor digitorum tt

1st Metacarpal

Flexor carpi
radialis t

Trapezium

Abductor pollicis
longus t

Scaphoid

Radial a

5th Metacarpal

Palmar
interosseous m

Hypothenar mm

Hamate, hook

Pisohamate lig

Pisiform

Radius

Lumbricalis mm

Adductor pollicis m

Flexor pollicis
longus t

Thenar mm

Flexor digitorum tt

1st Metacarpal

Flexor carpi
radialis t

Trapezium

Scaphoid

Radial a

Abductor pollicis
longus t

Pronator
quadratus m

PLATE 14–3

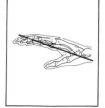

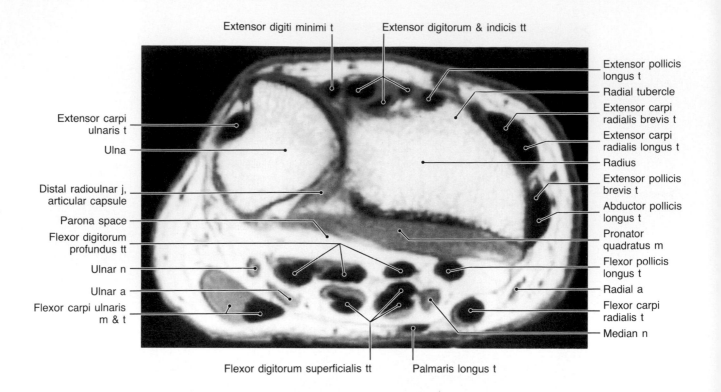

Extensor digiti minimi t

Extensor digitorum & indicis tt

Extensor pollicis longus t

Radial tubercle

Extensor carpi radialis brevis t

Extensor carpi radialis longus t

Radius

Extensor pollicis brevis t

Abductor pollicis longus t

Pronator quadratus m

Flexor pollicis longus t

Radial a

Flexor carpi radialis t

Median n

Extensor carpi ulnaris t

Ulna

Distal radioulnar j, articular capsule

Parona space

Flexor digitorum profundus tt

Ulnar n

Ulnar a

Flexor carpi ulnaris m & t

Flexor digitorum superficialis tt

Palmaris longus t

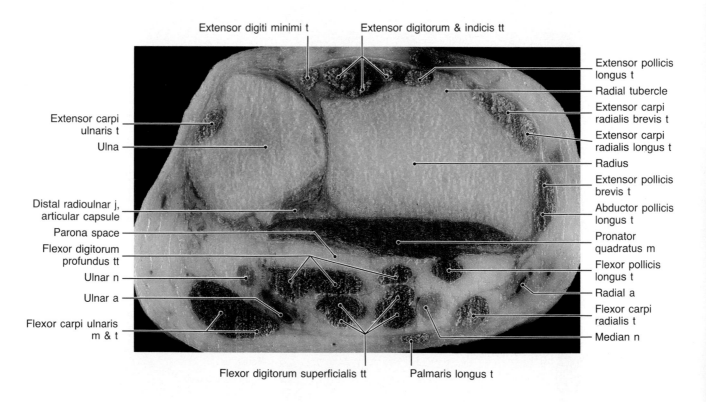

Extensor digiti minimi t

Extensor digitorum & indicis tt

Extensor pollicis longus t

Radial tubercle

Extensor carpi radialis brevis t

Extensor carpi radialis longus t

Radius

Extensor pollicis brevis t

Abductor pollicis longus t

Pronator quadratus m

Flexor pollicis longus t

Radial a

Flexor carpi radialis t

Median n

Extensor carpi ulnaris t

Ulna

Distal radioulnar j, articular capsule

Parona space

Flexor digitorum profundus tt

Ulnar n

Ulnar a

Flexor carpi ulnaris m & t

Flexor digitorum superficialis tt

Palmaris longus t

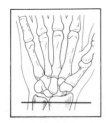

PLATE 14–4

Extensor digitorum & indicis tt

Extensor digiti minimi t

Extensor carpi ulnaris t

Hamate

Triquetrum

Flexor digitorum profundus tt

Pisiform

Hypothenar mm

Ulnar n

Flexor carpi ulnaris t

Ulnar a

Flexor retinaculum

Dorsal intercarpal lig

Extensor carpi radialis brevis t

Extensor pollicis longus t

Extensor carpi radialis longus t

Capitate

Deltoid (V) lig

Scaphoid

Radial a

Flexor pollicis longus t

Extensor pollicis brevis t

Abductor pollicis longus t

Flexor carpi radialis t

Median n

Flexor digitorum superficialis tt

Palmaris longus t

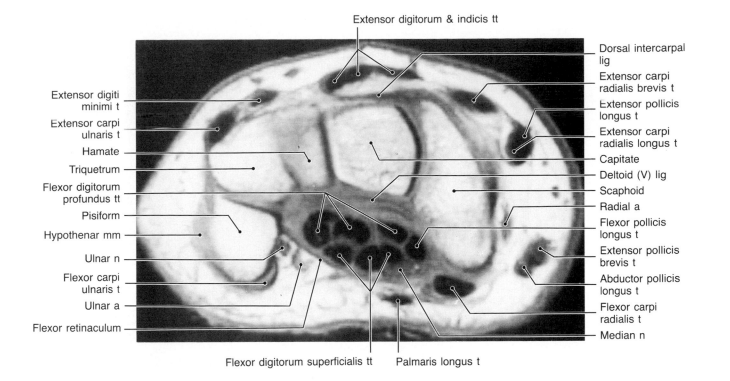

Extensor digiti minimi t

Extensor digitorum & indicis tt

Dorsal intercarpal lig

Extensor carpi radialis brevis t

Capitate

Extensor carpi radialis longus t

Extensor pollicis longus t

Deltoid (V) lig

Scaphoid

Radial a

Flexor pollicis longus t

Extensor pollicis brevis t

Abductor pollicis longus t

Flexor carpi radialis t

Median n

Extensor carpi ulnaris t

Hamate

Triquetrum

Flexor digitorum profundus tt

Pisiform

Hypothenar mm

Ulnar n

Flexor carpi ulnaris t

Ulnar a

Flexor retinaculum

Flexor digitorum superficialis tt

Palmaris longus t

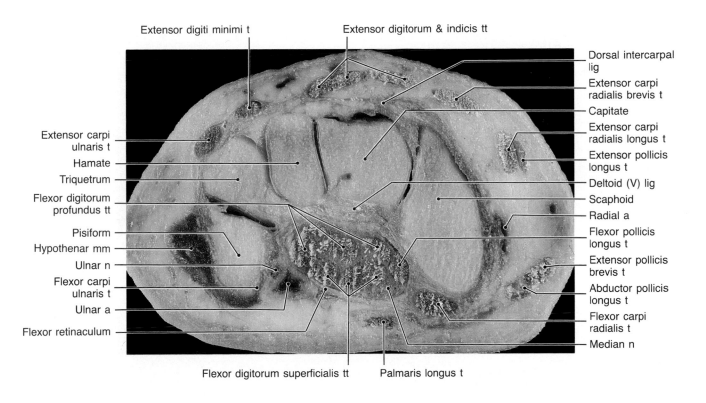

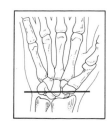

PLATE 14–5

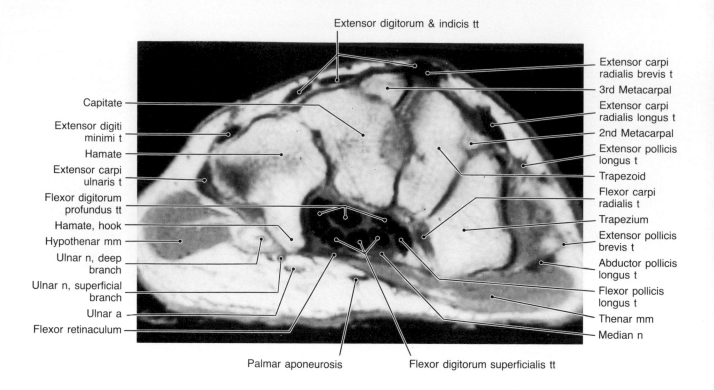

Extensor digitorum & indicis tt

Capitate

Extensor digiti minimi t

Hamate

Extensor carpi ulnaris t

Flexor digitorum profundus tt

Hamate, hook

Hypothenar mm

Ulnar n, deep branch

Ulnar n, superficial branch

Ulnar a

Flexor retinaculum

Extensor carpi radialis brevis t

3rd Metacarpal

Extensor carpi radialis longus t

2nd Metacarpal

Extensor pollicis longus t

Trapezoid

Flexor carpi radialis t

Trapezium

Extensor pollicis brevis t

Abductor pollicis longus t

Flexor pollicis longus t

Thenar mm

Median n

Palmar aponeurosis

Flexor digitorum superficialis tt

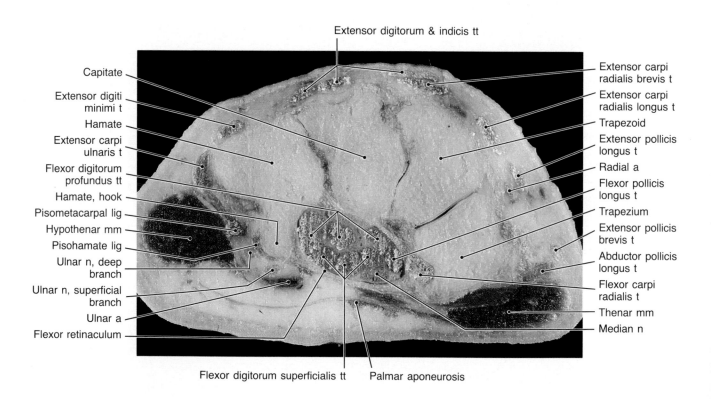

Extensor digitorum & indicis tt

Capitate

Extensor digiti minimi t

Hamate

Extensor carpi ulnaris t

Flexor digitorum profundus tt

Hamate, hook

Pisometacarpal lig

Hypothenar mm

Pisohamate lig

Ulnar n, deep branch

Ulnar n, superficial branch

Ulnar a

Flexor retinaculum

Extensor carpi radialis brevis t

Extensor carpi radialis longus t

Trapezoid

Extensor pollicis longus t

Radial a

Flexor pollicis longus t

Trapezium

Extensor pollicis brevis t

Abductor pollicis longus t

Flexor carpi radialis t

Thenar mm

Median n

Flexor digitorum superficialis tt

Palmar aponeurosis

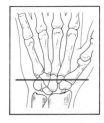

PLATE 14-6

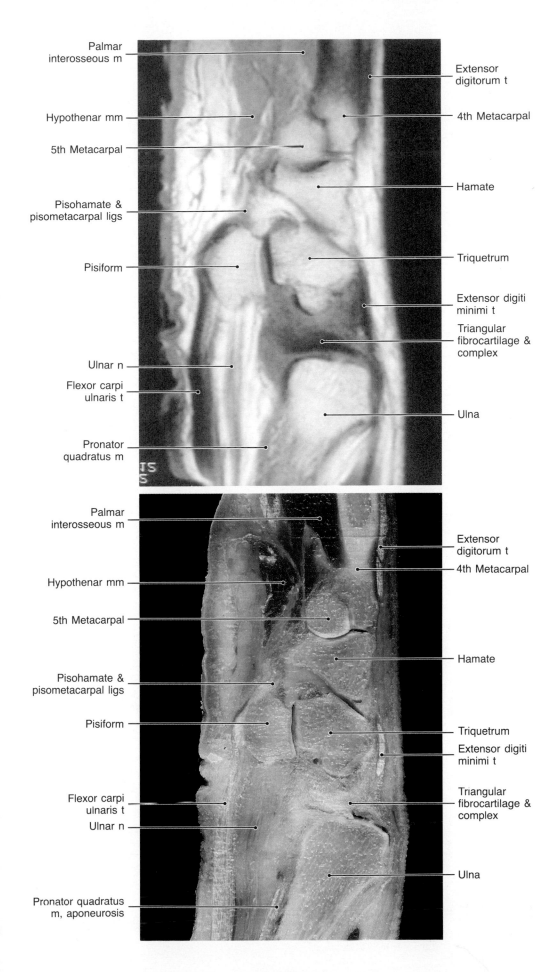

Palmar interosseous m

Hypothenar mm

5th Metacarpal

Pisohamate & pisometacarpal ligs

Pisiform

Ulnar n

Flexor carpi ulnaris t

Pronator quadratus m

Extensor digitorum t

4th Metacarpal

Hamate

Triquetrum

Extensor digiti minimi t

Triangular fibrocartilage & complex

Ulna

Palmar interosseous m

Hypothenar mm

5th Metacarpal

Pisohamate & pisometacarpal ligs

Pisiform

Flexor carpi ulnaris t

Ulnar n

Pronator quadratus m, aponeurosis

Extensor digitorum t

4th Metacarpal

Hamate

Triquetrum

Extensor digiti minimi t

Triangular fibrocartilage & complex

Ulna

PLATE 14-7

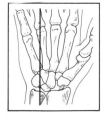

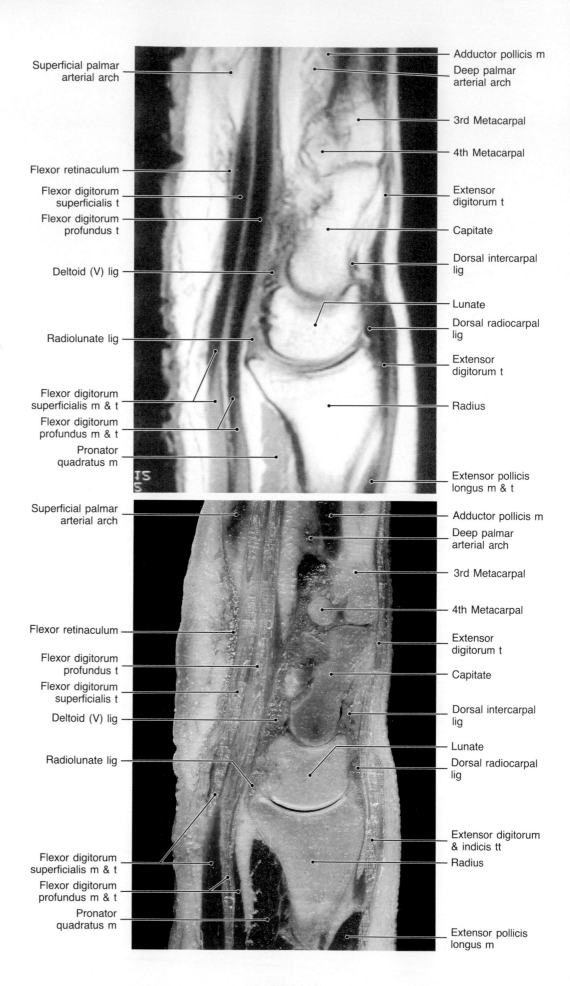

Superficial palmar arterial arch

Flexor retinaculum

Flexor digitorum superficialis t

Flexor digitorum profundus t

Deltoid (V) lig

Radiolunate lig

Flexor digitorum superficialis m & t

Flexor digitorum profundus m & t

Pronator quadratus m

Adductor pollicis m

Deep palmar arterial arch

3rd Metacarpal

4th Metacarpal

Extensor digitorum t

Capitate

Dorsal intercarpal lig

Lunate

Dorsal radiocarpal lig

Extensor digitorum t

Radius

Extensor pollicis longus m & t

Superficial palmar arterial arch

Flexor retinaculum

Flexor digitorum profundus t

Flexor digitorum superficialis t

Deltoid (V) lig

Radiolunate lig

Flexor digitorum superficialis m & t

Flexor digitorum profundus m & t

Pronator quadratus m

Adductor pollicis m

Deep palmar arterial arch

3rd Metacarpal

4th Metacarpal

Extensor digitorum t

Capitate

Dorsal intercarpal lig

Lunate

Dorsal radiocarpal lig

Extensor digitorum & indicis tt

Radius

Extensor pollicis longus m

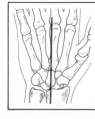

PLATE 14–8

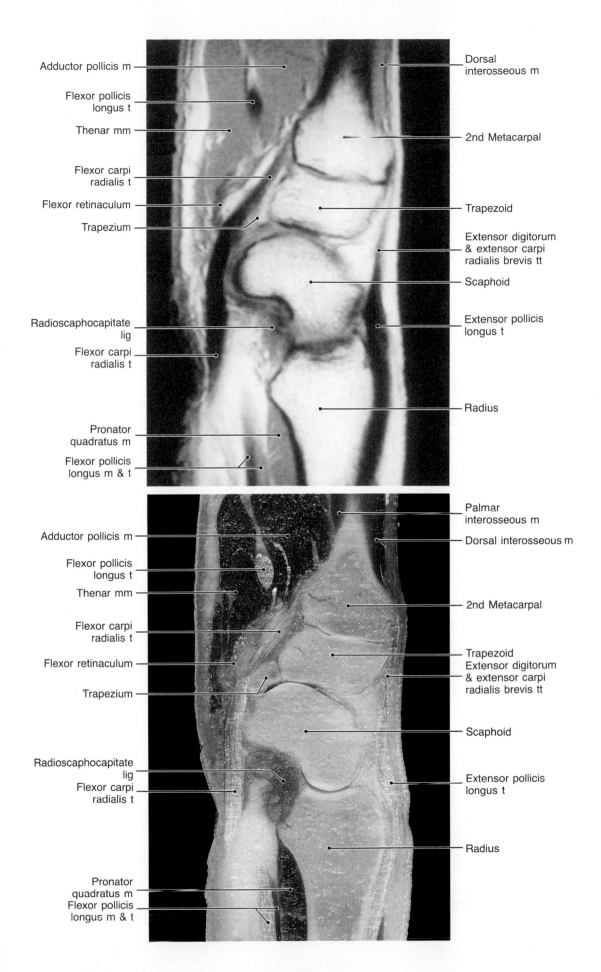

Adductor pollicis m

Flexor pollicis longus t

Thenar mm

Flexor carpi radialis t

Flexor retinaculum

Trapezium

Radioscaphocapitate lig

Flexor carpi radialis t

Pronator quadratus m

Flexor pollicis longus m & t

Dorsal interosseous m

2nd Metacarpal

Trapezoid

Extensor digitorum & extensor carpi radialis brevis tt

Scaphoid

Extensor pollicis longus t

Radius

Palmar interosseous m

Dorsal interosseous m

Adductor pollicis m

Flexor pollicis longus t

Thenar mm

Flexor carpi radialis t

Flexor retinaculum

Trapezium

Radioscaphocapitate lig

Flexor carpi radialis t

Pronator quadratus m

Flexor pollicis longus m & t

2nd Metacarpal

Trapezoid

Extensor digitorum & extensor carpi radialis brevis tt

Scaphoid

Extensor pollicis longus t

Radius

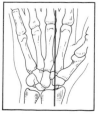

PLATE 14–9

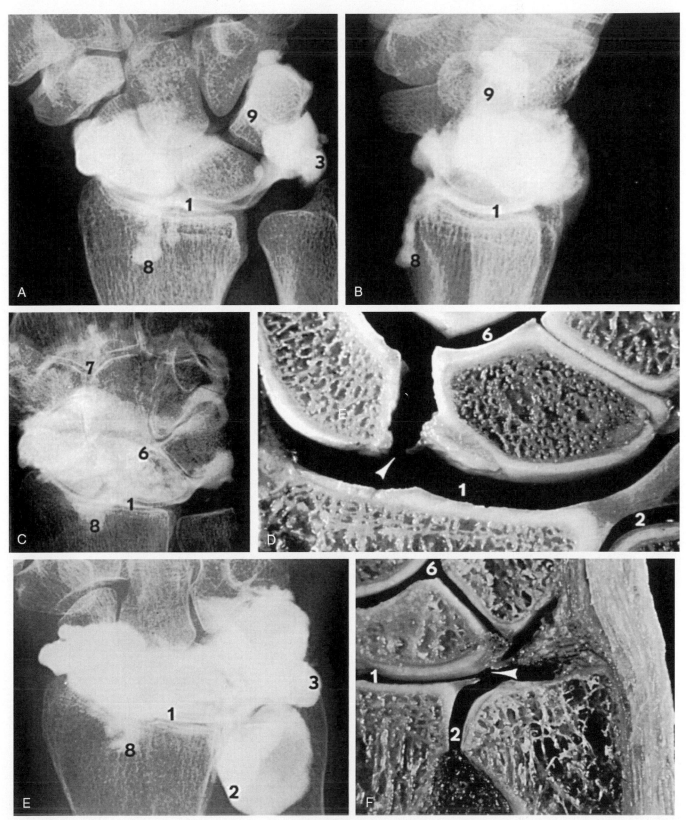

Figure 14–20
See legend on opposite page

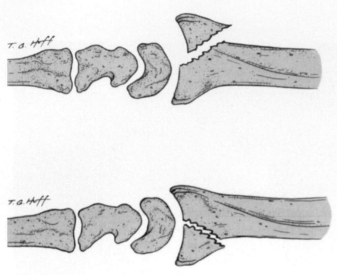

Figure 14–21
Wrist fractures: Two-part fractures of the distal portion of the radius. (From McMurtry RY, Jupiter JB: Fractures of the distal radius. *In* BD Browner, JB Jupiter, AM Levine, et al [Eds]: Skeletal Trauma: Fractures, Dislocations, Ligamentous Injuries. Philadelphia, WB Saunders, 1992, p. 1066.)

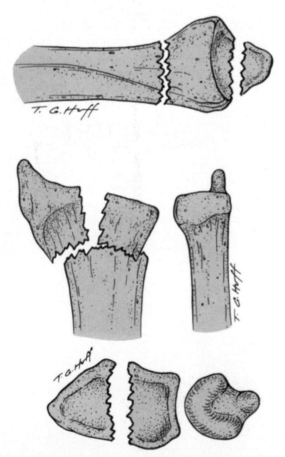

Figure 14–22
Wrist fractures: Three-part fractures of the distal portion of the radius. (From McMurtry RY, Jupiter JB: Fractures of the distal radius. *In* BD Browner, JB Jupiter, AM Levine, et al [Eds]: Skeletal Trauma: Fractures, Dislocations, Ligamentous Injuries. Philadelphia, WB Saunders, 1992, p. 1067.)

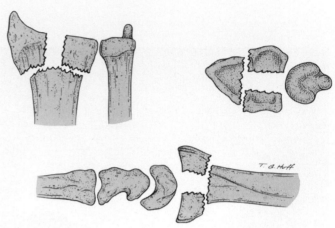

Figure 14–23
Wrist fractures: Four-part fractures of the distal portion of the radius. (From McMurtry RY, Jupiter JB: Fractures of the distal radius. *In* BD Browner, JB Jupiter, AM Levine, et al [Eds]: Skeletal Trauma: Fractures, Dislocations, Ligamentous Injuries. Philadelphia, WB Saunders, 1992, p 1070.)

Radiocarpal joint dislocations are rare; they may occur in a dorsal, volar, or radial direction, may appear as an isolated finding or in association with fractures of the dorsal or volar radial rim or radial or ulnar styloid process, and are accompanied by injuries of the radiocarpal ligaments. Very rarely, they are irreducible owing to entrapment of bone fragments within the joint. Neurovascular and tendinous structures also may be compromised.

A fracture of the styloid process of the radius (Fig. 14–24) often is referred to as a Hutchinson's fracture or a chauffeur's fracture. It appears to represent an avulsion injury related to the sites of attachment of the radiocarpal ligaments or radial collateral ligament, but such fractures also can occur from a direct blow. In some cases, a fracture of the radial styloid process is a component of a more complex injury of the wrist,[88]

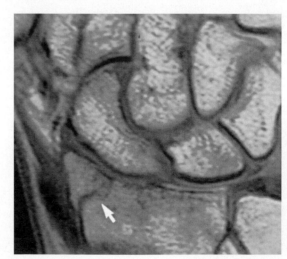

Figure 14–24
Wrist fractures: Hutchinson's fracture. A coronal T1-weighted (TR/TE, 733/20) spin echo MR image reveals a fracture (arrow) of the radial styloid process. (Courtesy of S. Eilenberg, M.D., San Diego, California.)

including radiocarpal joint dislocations. The fracture line may enter the space between the scaphoid and lunate fossae in the articular surface of the radius and, in such cases, it may be associated with scapholunate dissociation and lesser arc injuries of the wrist[89] (see later discussion).

Although fractures of the styloid process of the ulna usually are a component of a more extensive wrist injury, including a Colles' fracture, an injury isolated to the ulnar styloid process occasionally is observed, perhaps related to an avulsion produced by the ulnar collateral ligament or TFCC. Hypertrophy of the fragment with fracture nonunion is encountered infrequently and may be a source of chronic wrist pain.[85]

Significant intra-articular injuries of the wrist may accompany many of these fractures of the distal portions of the radius and ulna. These injuries include disruptions of the TFCC, interosseous ligaments, ulnocarpal ligaments, and extrinsic ligaments, with their frequency increasing in association with displacement of the radial fractures. Accurate diagnosis of the intra-articular injuries requires arthroscopy or advanced imaging methods such as MR imaging or arthrography.

One type of distal radial fracture to which arthroscopy has been applied both as a diagnostic and as a therapeutic method is the die-punch fracture. This fracture resembles a tibial plateau fracture and relates to impaction of the articular surface of the radius by the lunate bone. Complex fracture lines are produced that generally have both coronal and sagittal components, and the degree of compression of the articular surface varies. The ultimate prognosis of this injury is related directly to the degree of articular incongruity. Arthroscopy in combination with manipulation and use of an external fixator can be employed for reduction and stabilization of the fracture fragments. Variations of this fracture pattern, including those with a volarly displaced spike of bone (spike fracture) that may influence structures in the carpal canal, also have been treated using arthroscopic methods, although open reduction and internal fixation of some of these injuries are required.

Distal Radioulnar Joint Abnormalities

Functional Anatomy

The functional anatomy and pathomechanics of the distal radioulnar joint have received a great deal of emphasis.[90–92] Nathan and Schneider[93] have emphasized those features that are fundamental to optimal function of this joint:

1. The articulating surface between the ulnar head and the sigmoid notch of the radius must be intact. The sigmoid notch and two thirds of the ulnar head are covered with articular cartilage. The ulnar head has two surfaces that articulate with the TFC and sigmoid notch of the radius, respectively.[93] The articulation of the ulnar head with the concave sigmoid notch is not congruous; the radius of curvature of the concave surface of the notch is larger than that of the corresponding convex

articular surface of the ulna. This situation implies limited joint congruency, and it enables simultaneous sliding and rotation when the forearm is pronated and supinated. As the forearm moves from supination to pronation, the ulnar head rotates up to 150 degrees and also glides several millimeters in a proximal to distal direction within the sigmoid notch.[93] The radius translates on the seat of the ulnar head; in full supination, the ulnar head rests on the palmar aspect of the notch, and in full pronation it rests against the dorsal lip of the notch.[92]

2. The soft tissue and ligamentous support system of the distal radioulnar joint must be intact. The precise structures providing stability to this joint are not agreed on entirely, although recent evidence has implicated various components of the TFCC (consisting of the TFC or articular disc, the dorsal and volar radioulnar ligaments, the ulnar collateral ligament, the meniscus homologue, and the sheath of the extensor carpi ulnaris tendon) in this regard.[94] Ekenstam and Hagert[95] and Nathan and Schneider[93] considered the TFCC to consist of three parts: a cartilaginous central portion (the disc or TFC) and surrounding thick dorsal and volar radioulnar ligaments. These authors emphasized that the central portion serves as a cushion for the ulnar head and ulnar-sided carpal bones and as the load-bearing component of the TFCC and that the dorsal and volar radioulnar ligaments primarily are responsible for stabilization of the distal radioulnar joint. This hypothesis is consistent with the occurrence of defects of the articular disc itself that may exist without joint instability. In addition to the TFCC, the annular ligament and interosseous membrane of the forearm constrain the radius and the ulna.[91, 413]

3. A proper relationship between the lengths of the radius and ulna must exist (Fig. 14–25). As indicated earlier, changes in the length of the ulna relative to that of the radius, designated positive and negative ulnar variance, alter the distribution of compressive forces across the wrist. The consequences of a short ulna, or minus ulnar variance, include increased force applied to the radial side of the wrist and to the lunate bone, which may explain the association of negative ulnar variance and Kienböck's disease. With such variance, the TFC is thicker, and abnormalities of the TFCC are

ULNAR VARIANCE

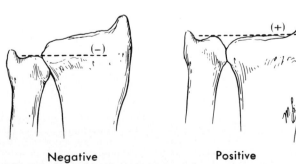

Negative　　　　　Positive

Figure 14–25
Ulnar variance. Diagrams of negative and positive ulnar variance are shown.

uncommon.[94] A consequence of a long ulna, a positive ulnar variance, is the ulnar impaction or ulnar abutment syndrome (see later discussion), with resulting limitation of rotation and subsequent relaxation of the ligamentous fixation of the wrist.[24] The TFC is thinner in instances of positive ulnar variance, and degenerative perforation of this structure (as well as disruption of the lunotriquetral interosseous ligament) may be observed.

Pathologic Anatomy

A variety of systems have been used to classify disorders of the distal radioulnar joint.[93, 94, 96–98] Palmer[94] used two major categories, traumatic lesions and degenerative lesions, to describe such disorders, indicating the relative infrequency of the traumatic lesions (Fig. 14–26). Traumatic abnormalities (Class 1) were subdivided further according to their precise anatomic location. A Class 1A lesion represented a tear or perforation of the horizontal portion of the TFCC, usually occurring as a 1 to 2 mm slit located 2 to 3 mm medial to the radial attachment of the TFCC. A Class 1B lesion represented a traumatic avulsion of the TFCC from its insertion site

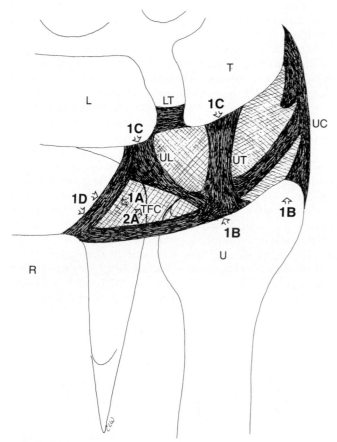

Figure 14–26
Pathologic anatomy of the distal radioulnar joint. Illustrated structures are the radius (R), ulna (U), lunate (L), triquetrum (T), triangular fibrocartilage (TFC), ulnolunate (UL) and ulnotriquetral (UT) ligaments, ulnar collateral ligament (UC), and lunotriquetral interosseous ligament (LT). The sites of the lesions mentioned in the text under the categories of 1A, 1B, 1C, 1D, and 2A are indicated. (Modified from Palmer AK: J Hand Surg [Am] *14*:594, 1989. © 1989, Churchill Livingstone, on behalf of the Journal of Hand Surgery, New York.)

in the distal portion of the ulna that could be associated with a fracture of the base of the styloid process of the ulna. This type of lesion was considered evidence of instability of the distal radioulnar joint. A Class 1C lesion represented a distal avulsion of the TFCC at its site of attachment to the lunate bone (ulnolunate ligament) or triquetrum (ulnotriquetral ligament). Once again, such a lesion implied instability of the distal radioulnar joint. A Class 1D lesion represented an avulsion of the TFCC from its attachment to the radius at the distal aspect of the sigmoid notch that could be associated with an avulsion fracture.

Degenerative abnormalities (Class 2) also were subdivided according to their extent and location. Five types of degenerative lesions were detailed: wear of the central region of the horizontal portion of the TFCC without perforation (Class 2A lesion); similar wear with evidence of chondromalacia of the ulnar aspect of the lunate bone or the radial aspect of the ulnar head, or both areas (Class 2B lesion); perforation of the horizontal portion of the TFCC, occurring in a more ulnar location than a traumatic perforation (Class 2C lesion); such perforation combined with degenerative changes of the articular surfaces of the lunate bone and ulnar head and disruption of the lunotriquetral interosseous ligament (Class 2D lesion); and the ulnar impaction syndrome with complete absence of the horizontal portion of the TFCC, disruption of the lunotriquetral interosseous ligament, osteoarthritis of the distal radioulnar joint, and degenerative changes about the ulnocarpal space (Class 2E lesion).

The anatomic basis of this classification system is valuable, but this system is very extensive and may be difficult to apply clinically. A simpler method has been described by Nathan and Schneider,[93] in which four possible categories of pathologic lesions are considered: (1) instability of the distal radioulnar joint (including traumatic disruption of the TFCC with or without dislocation of the joint or fracture of the radius or ulna, or of both bones; disruption of the TFCC associated with inflammatory diseases such as rheumatoid arthritis; and ulnar head excision); (2) impingement of the ulna on the carpus; (3) incongruity of the distal radioulnar joint (including that related to traumatic or inflammatory disorders); and (4) isolated lesions of the articular disc (which occur without instability of the distal radioulnar joint). This system, with some modifications, is used in the following discussion.

Lesions of the Triangular Fibrocartilage Complex

Lesions of the TFCC are variable in extent; they may be confined to the horizontal or flat portion of the TFCC (referred to as the TFC or articular disc) or involve one or more components of the TFCC with or without instability of the distal radioulnar joint. Those lesions confined to the TFC, a load-bearing structure only, may or may not be symptomatic (manifested as ulnar-sided wrist pain and tenderness and, in some instances, a palpable or audible click during rotation of the forearm) and are not associated with instability of the distal radioulnar joint.[93] Such isolated lesions of the articular disc generally are related to degeneration or trauma, although a congenital basis also has been suggested.[99, 414] An increased frequency of degenerative lesions with advancing age of the patient has been documented arthrographically, and similar data have been derived from cadaveric studies.[100] Such degenerative lesions can lead to full-thickness tears, of which two patterns have been noted[415]: a central oval pattern and a linear defect extending in a dorsal and ulnar direction close to the radial attachment of the TFCC. More extensive lesions of the TFCC, including avulsions from its proximal, distal, or radial sites of attachment, as indicated earlier, usually are regarded as traumatic in pathogenesis.[94]

Degenerative lesions of the TFC are more common than traumatic lesions. Either type may result in full-thickness defects, as can be documented with arthrography and MR imaging. Although such full-thickness defects commonly are referred to as tears, Gilula and Palmer[101] have objected to the use of this word, indicating that it implies that a structure has been torn, as commonly is seen with trauma, and that most of these defects relate to progressive wear. The terms communicating (or full-thickness) and noncommunicating (or partial-thickness) defects are used in the following discussion, although the term defect also is not an ideal designation for a finding that may be a normal variation and clinically insignificant.[102]

The role of arthrography in the diagnosis of defects of the articular disc is well established,[37, 38, 103–106] although disagreement exists regarding the optimal arthrographic technique and, more specifically, the need for injection of contrast material into more than one wrist compartment (i.e., radiocarpal and distal radioulnar joints). The presence of contrast material in the inferior radioulnar compartment after radiocarpal compartmental opacification (see Fig. 14–20E, F) or in the radiocarpal compartment after inferior radioulnar compartmental injection is the sine qua non of a communicating, or complete, defect in the TFC. Partial, or noncommunicating, defects involving the proximal aspect of the TFC can be opacified with injection of contrast material into the inferior radioulnar joint, and those involving the distal aspect of the TFC can be opacified with injection of contrast material into the radiocarpal joint. Intrasubstance degeneration, or tears within the TFC, are invisible to the arthrographer. Other traumatic abnormalities of the TFCC, as described by Palmer,[94] may be associated with distinctive arthrographic findings. Traumatic avulsion of the TFCC from its insertion into the distal ulna (Class 1B lesion) is not visualized during arthrography when the radiocarpal joint is injected but may be seen as extravasation of contrast material when arthrography is performed using an injection into the distal radioulnar joint; traumatic avulsion of the TFCC from its distal attachment to the lunate or the triquetrum (Class 1C lesion) will not lead to a communicating defect of the TFC itself but may be accompanied by capsular leakage of contrast material when either the radiocarpal or the midcarpal compartment is injected; and traumatic avulsion of the TFCC from its attachment to the radius at the distal aspect of the sigmoid notch generally is seen

as a communicating defect at the site of disruption when either the radiocarpal or the distal radioulnar joint is opacified.[94]

The occurrence of communicating defects of the TFC in asymptomatic persons severely limits the clinical usefulness of arthrography (and MR imaging).[62–64, 107] Although this finding increases in frequency with advancing age of the person, it is encountered in young adults as well.[107] The detection of a communicating defect of the TFC assumes greater clinical importance when symptoms and signs correlate with the site of abnormality and, perhaps, when an arthrogram of the contralateral asymptomatic wrist fails to reveal a similar finding.[64] A negative arthrogram is effective in eliminating the diagnosis of a communicating defect of the TFC, with rare exceptions in which fibrosis and scarring may block the flow of contrast material through the defect.[107]

The role of MR imaging in the evaluation of lesions of the TFCC has received increased attention.[71, 108–118, 416, 417] In young persons, the normal TFC is characterized by homogeneously low signal intensity on virtually all MR pulse sequences and in the coronal, sagittal, and transverse planes. In the coronal plane, the normal TFC usually appears as an elongated triangle with its apex attaching to the articular cartilage of the radius (Fig. 14–27). The triangle may be thinner in persons with positive ulnar variance and thicker in those with negative ulnar variance. The ulnar attachment of the TFC may appear bifurcated, with two bands of low signal intensity separated by a region of higher signal intensity. The prestyloid recess of the radiocarpal joint, which extends toward the tip of the styloid process of the ulna, also may reveal higher signal intensity. Adjacent struc-

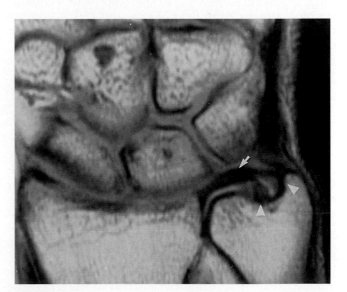

Figure 14–27

Triangular fibrocartilage complex: MR imaging—normal appearance. In a coronal proton density–weighted (TR/TE, 2000/20) spin echo MR image, observe the low signal intensity of the triangular fibrocartilage (arrow), with bifurcated bands of low signal intensity (arrowheads) attaching to the styloid process of the ulna. The scapholunate and lunotriquetral interosseous ligaments are not well seen in this image. Note two bone islands, appearing as foci of low signal intensity, in the lunate and capitate. (Courtesy of A. G. Bergman, M.D., Stanford, California.)

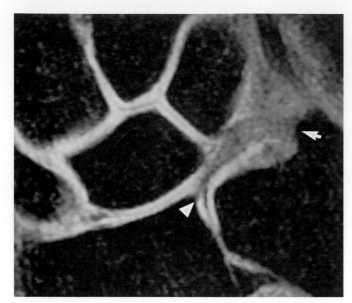

Figure 14–28

Triangular fibrocartilage complex: MR imaging—normal appearance. A three-dimensional coronal SPGR (TR/TE, 69/15; flip angle, 30 degrees) fat-suppressed MR image (approximately 1 mm in thickness) shows the ulnar attachment (arrow) of the triangular fibrocartilage. Note the hyaline cartilage (arrowhead) at the radial site of attachment. The scapholunate and lunotriquetral interosseous ligaments were better seen on other images. (Courtesy of D. Goodwin, M.D., Hanover, New Hampshire.)

tures of the TFCC including the meniscus homologue are identifiable. These structures are better seen when three-dimensional gradient echo sequences are used to obtain contiguous sections of the wrist that are 1 mm thick or less (Fig. 14–28).[71] In one study, this technique coupled with an 8 cm field of view and 256 × 256 matrix provided coronal images that allowed delineation of variations in the pattern of insertion of the TFCC to the distal portion of the ulna and of the ulnolunate and ulnotriquetral ligaments (Fig. 14–29).[71, 119]

Although low signal intensity characterizes the MR imaging appearance of the normal TFC, two regions of higher signal intensity that are encountered normally may simulate the appearance of a lesion (Fig. 14–30)[436]:

1. The articular cartilage of the distal portion of the radius separates the apex of the TFC from the adjacent bone. The linear configuration of this region of articular cartilage is similar to that of a tear, but its signal intensity characteristics are those of cartilage and not those of fluid. A radial avulsion of the TFCC is associated with fluid accumulation in this same region, an appearance not evident in the normal situation.

2. The ulnar limit of the TFC is of higher signal intensity than that of the flat portion of the TFC. The signal intensity characteristics of this area usually are not those of fluid. Differentiation of this normal appearance from an avulsion of the proximal attachment site of the TFCC may prove difficult.

On sagittal images, the normal TFC is of low signal intensity and reveals a discoid shape lying adjacent to the articular cartilage of the distal end of the ulna. Its central portion may appear thinner than its volar and dorsal portions. On transaxial images, a triangular region of low signal intensity characterizes the normal TFC.

Although the previous description of the MR imaging characteristics of the normal TFC has emphasized its low signal intensity, regions of higher signal intensity within the TFC on T1-weighted spin echo MR images are encountered regularly (Fig. 14–31).[114, 117] The basis for this hyperintensity is the presence of histologic changes (including mucinous and myxoid alterations) related to the age of the person and typically considered degenerative.[120–121] In one cadaveric study, no degenerative lesions or communicating defects of the TFC were detected in the first two decades of life, whereas after the fifth decade of life, 100 per cent of wrists had degenerative lesions in the TFC and more than 40 per cent of the wrists had communicating defects of the TFC.[120] Degeneration of the TFC invariably is situated in the thinner central portion; it occurs initially and is much more severe on the ulnar, or proximal, surface of the TFC, owing to more intensive biomechanical forces in this region.[114] The rotational movements that occur during pronation and supination of the hand produce a drilling effect on the ulnar surface of the TFC that is much more stressful than the gliding movements of the carpal condyle on the carpal surface of the TFC. Progression of degeneration on the surface of the TFC leads to erosion, thinning, and finally perforation of this structure. A close correlation exists between the changes in the TFC and those in the articular cartilage of the lunate and distal portion of the ulna.[120]

The increased signal intensity in the degenerative TFC on T1-weighted spin echo MR images can simulate the appearance of traumatic lesions of the TFC, and in extreme cases, the MR imaging findings may be falsely attributed to a traumatically induced communicating defect. The detection of less high signal intensity in the TFC on T2-weighted spin echo MR images is useful in differentiating TFC degeneration from TFC perforation in which high signal intensity on T2-weighted spin echo MR images is evident.[114] These data support the concept that reliance on T1-weighted spin echo MR images alone in the analysis of lesions of the TFC creates diagnostic difficulty, as such images, in instances of severe degeneration of the TFC, often reveal alterations in signal intensity and morphology of the TFC that simulate those of perforation. The situation encountered in the analysis of the TFC with MR imaging is similar to that resulting from mucinous change within the menisci of the knee and the glenoid labrum.

Although it is difficult to differentiate between a traumatically induced communicating defect of the TFC and one related to degeneration using MR imaging (or standard arthrography), characteristic MR imaging features frequently allow an accurate diagnosis of some type of communicating defect or perforation of the structure. Linear regions of altered signal intensity, identical to that of fluid, traversing the entire thickness of the TFC on T1-weighted and T2-weighted spin echo MR images (or gradient echo images) are strong evidence that a communicating defect is present (Figs. 14–32 and 14–33). Although similar regions of high

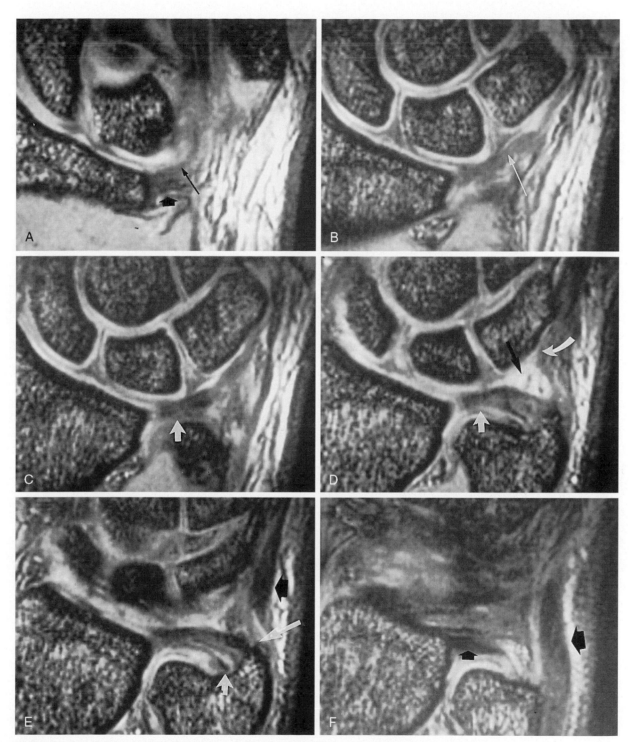

Figure 14–29
Triangular fibrocartilage complex: MR imaging—normal appearance. Coronal three-dimensional gradient echo MR images (TR/TE, 69/17; flip angle, 20 degrees) obtained with an 8 cm field of view, 256 × 256 matrix, and slice thickness of 1 mm show the various components of the triangular fibrocartilage complex. **A** is the most volar section and **F** is the most dorsal section. Identified structures are the following: In **A,** volar radioulnar ligament (black arrow), ulnolunate ligament (long thin black arrow); in **B,** ulnotriquetral ligament (long white arrow); in **C,** volar aspect of disc (short white arrow); in **D,** central disc (short white arrow), prestyloid recess (black arrow), meniscus homologue (curved white arrow); in **E,** extensor carpi ulnaris tendon (short thick black arrow), attachment of TFCC to tip of the styloid (long white arrow), attachment of TFCC to the base of the styloid (short white arrow); in **F,** dorsal radioulnar ligament (short black arrow), extensor carpi ulnaris tendon (short thick black arrow). (Courtesy of S.M.S. Totterman, M.D., Ph.D., Rochester, New York.)

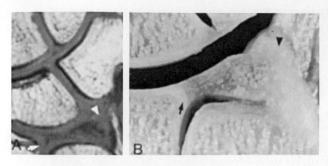

Figure 14–30

Triangular fibrocartilage complex: MR imaging—normal appearance.

A Coronal T1-weighted (TR/TE, 800/20) spin echo MR image shows inhomogeneous low signal intensity in the triangular fibrocartilage. Note intermediate signal intensity in the region of the articular cartilage (arrow) of the radius and at the ulnar limit of the triangular fibrocartilage complex (arrowhead).

B In a coronal section of the ulnar side of the wrist, observe the articular cartilage (arrow) of the radius and fibrofatty tissues (arrowhead) in the ulnar aspect of the triangular fibrocartilage complex.

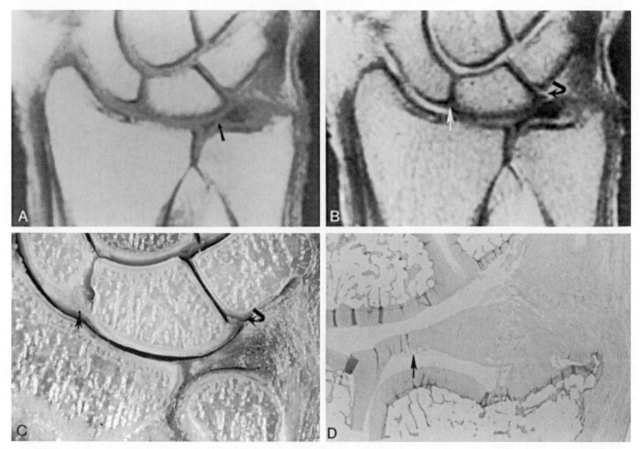

Figure 14–31

Triangular fibrocartilage complex: MR imaging—degenerative changes.

A Coronal T1-weighted (TR/TE, 600/20) spin echo MR image. The triangular fibrocartilage shows bandlike low signal intensity except for its radial and ulnar attachment sites. Apparent discontinuity of the triangular fibrocartilage (arrow) is seen near its radial attachment. The scapholunate and lunotriquetral ligaments are not well shown.

B Coronal T2-weighted (TR/TE, 2000/60) spin echo MR image at the same level as **A.** The triangular fibrocartilage is of low signal intensity and appears to be intact. Perforated lunotriquetral (curved arrow) and intact scapholunate (straight arrow) interosseous ligaments are depicted clearly.

C Coronal section of the specimen. The triangular fibrocartilage and scapholunate interosseous ligament (arrow) are not perforated. The lunotriquetral interosseous ligament (curved arrow) is perforated.

D Histologic preparation of a coronal section of the specimen. The portion of the triangular fibrocartilage that showed discontinuity on the T1-weighted spin echo MR image is not perforated, but it is degenerated (arrow). Mucoid degeneration and surface fibrillation are more severe on the ulnar surface of the triangular fibrocartilage. The articular cartilage is seen at the radial attachment of the triangular fibrocartilage.

(From Kang HS, et al: *Radiology 181*:401, 1991.)

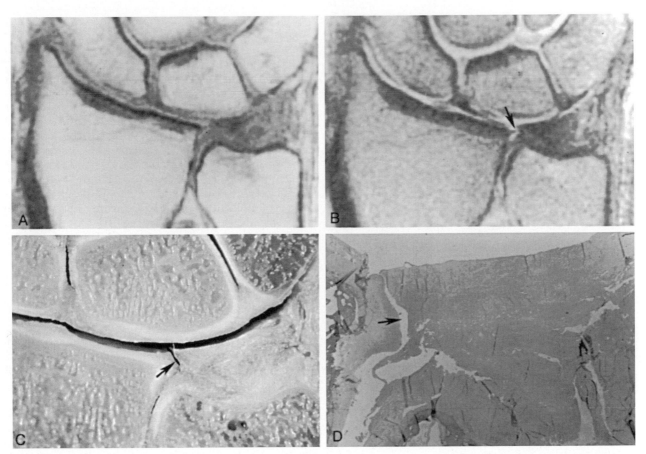

Figure 14–32

Triangular fibrocartilage complex: MR imaging—communicating defect.

A Coronal T1-weighted (TR/TE, 600/20) spin echo MR image. The signal intensity of the triangular fibrocartilage and scapholunate and lunotriquetral interosseous ligaments is diffusely increased.

B T2-weighted (TR/TE, 2000/60) spin echo MR image. The signal intensity of the triangular fibrocartilage and the scapholunate and lunotriquetral interosseous ligaments is lower than in the T1-weighted spin echo MR image. Focal high signal intensity (arrow) near the radial attachment of the triangular fibrocartilage is consistent with the presence of a communicating defect.

C Coronal section of the specimen. The triangular fibrocartilage is perforated (arrow) near its radial attachment. The scapholunate and lunotriquetral interosseous ligaments are not perforated.

D Histologic section. The triangular fibrocartilage is perforated near its radial attachment (arrow). Degeneration of the triangular fibrocartilage is more severe on its ulnar surface and adjacent to the edge of the perforation.

(From Kang HS, et al: Radiology *181*:401, 1991.)

Figure 14–33

Triangular fibrocartilage complex: MR imaging—communicating defect.

A Coronal proton density (TR/TE, 2500/20) spin echo MR image. Note the linear region of increased signal intensity (arrow) in the triangular fibrocartilage.

B T2-weighted (TR/TE, 2500/80) spin echo MR image. Fluid of high signal intensity is present in the defect (arrow) within the triangular fibrocartilage and in the distal radioulnar joint. Fluid also is present in the midcarpal joint.

(Courtesy of M. Zlatkin, M.D., Hollywood, Florida.)

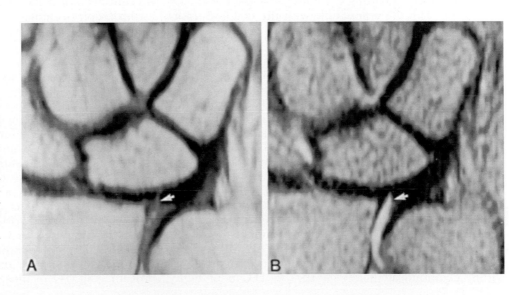

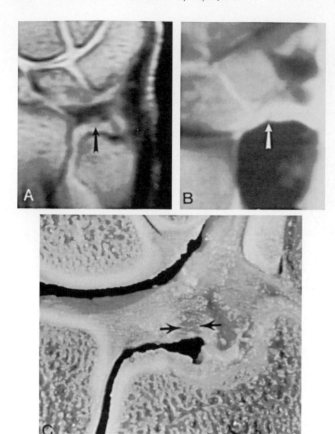

Figure 14–34

Triangular fibrocartilage complex: MR imaging—noncommunicating defect.

A Coronal T2-weighted (TR/TE, 2000/80) spin echo MR image. Note a region of abnormal signal intensity (arrow) in the proximal surface of the triangular fibrocartilage.

B Digital arthrogram with injection of the distal radioulnar joint. This is the third part of a three-part wrist arthrogram in which the inferior radioulnar joint was opacified. Observe a linear collection of contrast material (arrow) consistent with a partial tear of the proximal surface of the triangular fibrocartilage.

C Coronal section of the wrist. The region of the noncommunicating defect of the triangular fibrocartilage (arrows) is evident.

signal intensity extending partially through the thickness of the TFC are compatible with the diagnosis of a noncommunicating defect (Fig. 14–34), the accuracy of this finding is not established. The presence of fluid in the distal radioulnar joint represents a secondary MR imaging finding of perforation of the TFCC,[116] but, as an isolated abnormality, this finding is not diagnostic of such a perforation. Separation of the TFCC from the distal portion of the ulna with high signal intensity proximal to the TFCC may be seen in association with disruptions of the ulnolunate and ulnotriquetral ligaments (a type 1B lesion by the Palmer classification system[94]) (Fig. 14–35).

Most previous investigations of the value of MR imaging in the assessment of the TFC have relied on findings derived from spin echo sequences. Gradient echo imaging sequences also may be valuable, however. On multiplanar gradient recalled (MPGR) MR images in which a low flip angle is used, fluid accumulating within communicating defects in the TFC is of high signal intensity (Fig. 14–36). When gradient recalled imaging is combined with volumetric acquisition, thin sections of the TFC may be obtained, which may accentuate the abnormalities associated with such defects.[71, 416] With volumetric acquisition of image data, radial reconstructions of the TFC also are possible.[102] In one study, STIR MR imaging was found to be more useful than spin echo sequences in the assessment of the TFCC (Fig. 14–37).[116] The role of MR arthrography in this assessment is not clear; however, this procedure requires at least one injection into the radiocarpal or distal radioulnar joint and perhaps two separate injections into the radiocarpal and distal radioulnar joints; therefore, it is more complicated and time-consuming than standard MR imaging (Figs. 14–38 to 14–40).

The relative diagnostic value of MR imaging and standard arthrography in the detection of defects of the TFC has been studied.[112, 116] The lack of a standard of reference in the diagnosis of TFC defects makes such comparisons difficult, however, as even arthroscopy performed by expert orthopedic surgeons is not without diagnostic error. For example, surface irregularities of the TFC may be interpreted as communicating defects by some arthroscopists. Close agreement appears to exist in the results of MR imaging and arthrography in the assessment of defects of the TFC.[116] At this time, state-of-the-art MR imaging and arthrography can be considered equally accurate in this assessment. With either technique, however, the presence of degenerative communicating or noncommunicating defects of the TFC in middle-aged and elderly persons who are asymptomatic, and of degenerative or traumatically induced communicating or noncommunicating defects of the TFC in patients without ulnar-sided wrist pain, makes assessment of the clinical relevance of the findings more difficult.[122, 123]

Despite the widespread availability of wrist arthrography and the increasing availability of MR imaging as a means to study the TFCC, there are those who maintain steadfastly that the advantages of wrist arthroscopy outweigh those of either imaging method, and that arthroscopy, even when used alone (without other diagnostic methods), is effective in the assessment of the TFCC.[124] Recent technical advances have led to more reliable arthroscopic examinations of the wrist, in which the TFCC (as well as other intra-articular structures) can be inspected directly.[125] When compared with conventional open procedures of the wrist, arthroscopy is associated with reduced morbidity; when compared with arthrography and MR imaging, arthroscopy provides a truer three-dimensional display of the TFCC.[124] Instruments introduced through one or more portals can be used to allow arthroscopic treatment of lesions of the TFCC, particularly Class 1A and 2C lesions.[3, 5, 126–128] Reports have indicated therapeutic success after excision of unstable tissue fragments in the central portion of the TFCC and after repair (with sutures) of peripheral separations, or detachments, of the TFCC.[124] Complications of such arthroscopy include infection, painful incisions, injury to cutaneous nerves, and reflex sympathy dystrophy, but they are infrequent. Further investigation is required to determine the benefits of arthrography or MR imaging vis-à-vis those of arthroscopy in the analysis

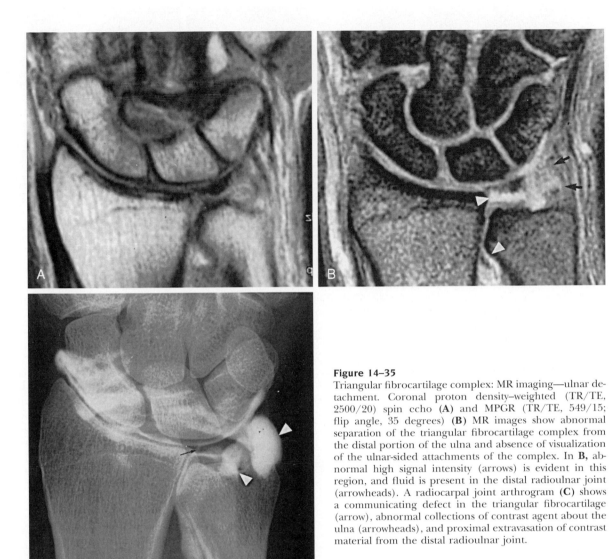

Figure 14–35
Triangular fibrocartilage complex: MR imaging—ulnar detachment. Coronal proton density–weighted (TR/TE, 2500/20) spin echo **(A)** and MPGR (TR/TE, 549/15; flip angle, 35 degrees) **(B)** MR images show abnormal separation of the triangular fibrocartilage complex from the distal portion of the ulna and absence of visualization of the ulnar-sided attachments of the complex. In **B**, abnormal high signal intensity (arrows) is evident in this region, and fluid is present in the distal radioulnar joint (arrowheads). A radiocarpal joint arthrogram **(C)** shows a communicating defect in the triangular fibrocartilage (arrow), abnormal collections of contrast agent about the ulna (arrowheads), and proximal extravasation of contrast material from the distal radioulnar joint.

Figure 14–36
Triangular fibrocartilage complex: MR imaging—communicating defect. Spin echo versus multiplanar gradient recalled (MPGR) MR imaging.

A Coronal T1-weighted (TR/TE, 600/20) spin echo MR image. Discontinuity (arrow) in the low signal intensity of the triangular fibrocartilage is seen. Note fluid of intermediate signal intensity about the distal portion of the ulna.

B Coronal MPGR (TR/TE, 500/15; flip angle, 20 degrees) MR image. Fluid of high signal intensity is seen in the defect (arrow) in the triangular fibrocartilage and about the distal portion of the ulna.

(Courtesy of C. Sebrechts, M.D., San Diego, California.)

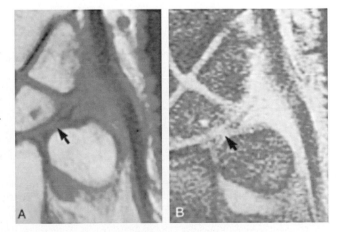

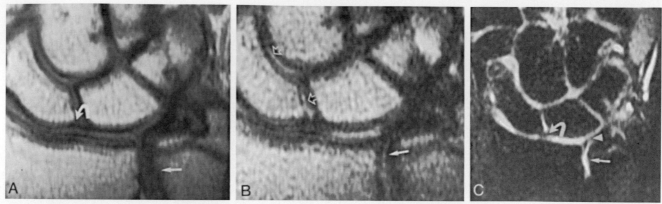

Figure 14–37

Triangular fibrocartilage complex: MR imaging—communicating defect (spin echo versus short tau inversion recovery [STIR] MR images).

A Coronal proton density–weighted (TR/TE, 1700/20) spin echo MR image. The triangular fibrocartilage is of low signal intensity and appears normal. Fluid is seen in the distal radioulnar joint (straight arrow), and the scapholunate interosseous ligament (curved arrow) is normal.

B Coronal T2-weighted (TR/TE, 1700/70) spin echo MR image. Fluid in the distal radioulnar joint (straight arrow) is of high signal intensity. There is questionable extension of this fluid into the substance of the triangular fibrocartilage. Note the fluid in the midcarpal joint, including the space between the scaphoid and the lunate (open arrows).

C STIR (TR/TE, 1650/25; inversion time, 160 msec) MR image. Fluid of high signal intensity in the distal radioulnar joint (straight arrow) extends into a defect (arrowhead) in the triangular fibrocartilage. The scapholunate ligament (curved arrow) appears normal.

(From Schweitzer ME, et al: *Radiology 182*:205, 1992.)

of various abnormalities of the TFCC. Ultimately, as immobilization often is used to treat patients with suspected acute injuries of the TFCC, the role of either of these imaging methods or of arthroscopy may be limited to assessment of such injuries that do not respond to conservative treatment or that are accompanied by evidence of instability of the distal radioulnar or radiocarpal joint.

Ulnar Impaction Syndrome

The ulnar impaction syndrome, also termed ulnocarpal abutment, ulnolunate impaction syndrome, and ulnar abutment syndrome, is defined as a degenerative condition characterized by ulnar-sided wrist pain, swelling, and limitation of motion related to excessive load bearing across the ulnar aspect of the wrist.[80, 129] Additional clinical findings include decreased grip strength and a painful click; instability of the wrist is not evident.[130, 131] Chronic impaction of the ulnar head against the TFCC and ulnar-sided carpal bones results in progressive deterioration of the TFCC, chondromalacia of the lunate and head of the ulna, synovitis, and attrition of the lunotriquetral interosseous ligament.[129] The ulnar impaction syndrome is almost always associated with a positive ulnar variance severe enough to allow transfer of excessive compressive forces from the ulna to the triquetrum and the lunate via the TFCC.[80] This syndrome is distinguished from a second condition, the ulnar impingement syndrome, which, as classically described, consists of a short ulna impinging on the distal portion of the radius, causing a painful, disabling pseud-

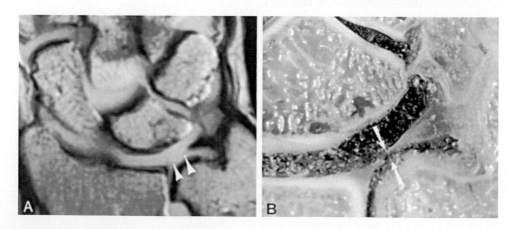

Figure 14–38

Triangular fibrocartilage complex: MR imaging—communicating defect (MR arthrography).

A Coronal T1-weighted (TR/TE, 800/20) spin echo MR image following intra-articular injection of a copper sulfate solution into the radiocarpal compartment of a cadaveric wrist. Note the communicating defect (arrowheads) in the triangular fibrocartilage. The lunotriquetral interosseous ligament also is disrupted, allowing filling of the midcarpal joint.

B Coronal section of the wrist. The defect (arrows) in the triangular fibrocartilage is evident. The abnormality of the lunotriquetral interosseous ligament is not seen well in this section.

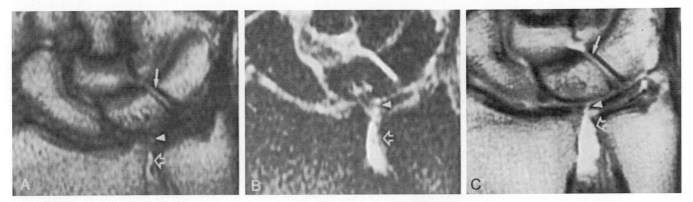

Figure 14–39

Triangular fibrocartilage complex: MR imaging—communicating defect (spin echo and STIR MR images and MR arthrography).

A Coronal T2-weighted (TR/TE, 1700/70) spin echo MR image. Note fluid of high signal intensity (open arrow) in the distal radioulnar joint and the increased signal intensity (arrowhead) in the triangular fibrocartilage, consistent with a defect. Fluid also is present in the midcarpal joint between the lunate and the triquetrum (solid arrow), although the lunotriquetral and scapholunate interosseous ligaments appear intact.

B Coronal STIR (TR/TE, 1650/25; inversion time, 160 msec) MR image. Fluid of high signal intensity is seen in the distal radioulnar joint (open arrow) and in the defect (arrowhead) in the triangular fibrocartilage. The lunotriquetral and scapholunate interosseous ligaments appear intact.

C MR arthrography with radiocarpal compartment injection of gadolinium compound. A coronal T1-weighted (TR/TE, 200/20) spin echo MR image shows that the injected material extends through a defect (arrowhead) in the triangular fibrocartilage into the distal radioulnar joint (open arrow), and through a defect in the lunotriquetral interosseous ligament into the space between the lunate and the triquetrum (solid arrow) and other portions of the midcarpal joint.

(From Schweitzer ME, et al: Radiology *182*:205, 1992.)

arthrosis.[132] Although the ulnar impaction syndrome has been identified in patients with a neutral or a positive ulnar variance, it is not associated with a negative ulnar variance.[129] Causes of this syndrome include developmental alterations in ulnar length, malunion of a fracture of the distal portion of the radius, premature growth arrest of the distal radial physis, an Essex-Lopresti fracture-dislocation, and radial head resection.

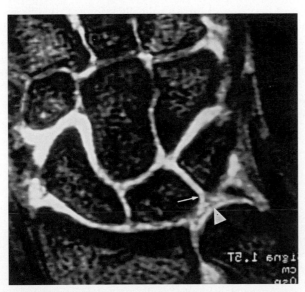

Figure 14–40

Triangular fibrocartilage complex: MR imaging—communicating defect (MR arthrography). After the introduction of a gadolinium compound into the radiocarpal joint, a coronal three-dimensional gradient echo MR image (TR/TE, 60/10; flip angle, 15 degrees) reveals a communicating defect (arrowhead) in the triangular fibrocartilage and disruption of the lunotriquetral interosseous ligament (arrow), the lesions allowing contrast material to reach the inferior radioulnar and midcarpal compartments. (Courtesy of S.K. Brahme, M.D., San Diego, California.)

Routine radiographs in patients with the ulnar impaction syndrome may reveal alterations in the ulnar side of the proximal portion of the lunate, the radial side of the proximal portion of the triquetrum, and the ulnar head or, rarely, the ulnar styloid process (Fig. 14–41). Findings include bone sclerosis, cysts, and osteophytes.[80] Arthrography often demonstrates communicating defects of the TFC and disruption of the lunotriquetral interosseous ligament. MR imaging also documents these abnormalities of the TFC and lunotriquetral interosseous ligament, and chondromalacia and alterations in the subchondral bone of the proximal surfaces of the lunate and triquetrum may be evident (Figs. 14–42 to 14–44).[133]

Partial excision of the TFC accomplished arthroscopically commonly is not successful in patients with a positive ulnar variance and the ulnar impaction syndrome. More extensive procedures, such as shortening of the ulna or resection of the ulnar head, in these patients appear to be more beneficial. A more limited resection of the subchondral bone of the distal portion of the ulna (i.e., wafer procedure) has been emphasized as a therapeutic alternative in some patients.[130, 131]

Ulnar Impingement Syndrome

The ulnar impingement syndrome is associated with clinical manifestations that are similar to but often more disabling than those accompanying the ulnar impaction syndrome. Pain may be aggravated during pronation and supination of the forearm.[129] Three radiographic features are characteristic of the ulnar impingement syndrome: an ulnar minus variance such that the ulna does not articulate with the sigmoid notch of the radius; a scalloped concavity of the distal portion of the radius; and convergence of the ulna to the distal portion of the radius (Fig. 14–45).[132] Causes of this syndrome include

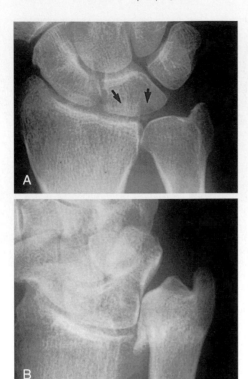

Figure 14–41
Ulnar impaction syndrome: Routine radiography.

A Note cysts and sclerosis (arrows) in the lunate bone. (Courtesy of D. Goodwin, M.D., Hanover, New Hampshire.)

B In this dramatic example, note the positive ulnar variance with flattening and sclerosis of the distal portion of the ulna and triquetrum.

resection of the distal portion of the ulna (Darrach procedure) and growth arrest of the ulna. The latter condition may occur secondary to trauma or a developmental abnormality (e.g., multiple hereditary exostoses).

Instability of the Distal Radioulnar Joint

The distal radioulnar joint is involved in pronation and supination of the forearm, during which the radius moves with respect to a relatively fixed ulna. Although, by convention, subluxation or dislocation of the distal radioulnar joint is described as that of the ulna subluxing or dislocating relative to the radius, in actuality, it is the radiocarpal mass that subluxes or dislocates in relation to the relatively stationary ulnar head.[134] Conventional terminology, however, is used in the following discussion.

Although there is general agreement that the stability of the distal radioulnar joint depends on a number of structures, including the dorsal and volar radioulnar ligaments, (volar) ulnocarpal ligaments, ulnar collateral ligament, extensor carpi ulnaris tendon, and the pronator quadratus and flexor carpi ulnaris muscles, the contributions of each to such stability in attitudes of pronation and supination of the forearm are controversial.[90–93, 95, 135] The importance of the dorsal and volar radioulnar ligaments as a stabilizing factor, preventing subluxations and dislocations of the distal radioulnar joint, appears certain, but their precise role in this respect is not clear. Linscheid,[92] in a discussion of stability of the distal radioulnar joint, indicated that the dorsal radioulnar ligament is under tension, or is taut, in pronation, and the volar radioulnar ligament is under tension in supination; Ekenstam[90] reported the opposite. Nathan and Schneider[93] emphasized the popularly held opinion that distal radioulnar joint instability is caused by a deficiency or disruption of various components of the TFCC. All of these views have emphasized the importance of alterations about the wrist in causing distal radioulnar joint instability, but additional considerations are necessary owing to the functional link between the wrist and elbow. Indeed, the TFCC is but one of three major soft tissue structures that connect the radius to the ulna, the other two being the interosseous ligament (membrane) of the forearm and the annular ligament of the elbow.[136] The encirclement of the distal radioulnar joint by the TFCC stabilizes the coronal relationship of the radius and ulna and, to some extent, resists longitudinal displacement of one bone with respect to the other (as

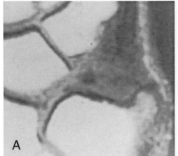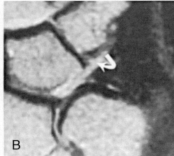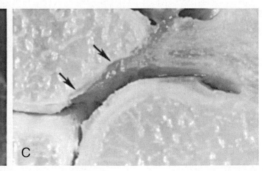

Figure 14–42
Ulnar impaction syndrome: MR imaging.

A Coronal T1-weighted (TR/TE, 600/20) spin echo MR image. There is a large communicating defect of the triangular fibrocartilage and a mild positive ulnar variance. The lunotriquetral interosseous ligament is not well seen. Note the irregularity of the ulnar aspect of the proximal portion of the lunate.

B Coronal T2-weighted (TR/TE, 2000/60) spin echo MR image. Fluid of high signal intensity in the radiocarpal and distal radioulnar joints outlines the large communicating defect in the triangular fibrocartilage. Note a defect (curved arrow) of the lunotriquetral interosseous ligament and irregularity of the proximal articular surface of the lunate.

C Coronal section of the wrist. Defects are seen in the triangular fibrocartilage and lunotriquetral interosseous ligament. The articular cartilage and subchondral bone of the lunate are eroded (straight arrows).

(From Kang HS, et al: Radiology *181*:401, 1991.)

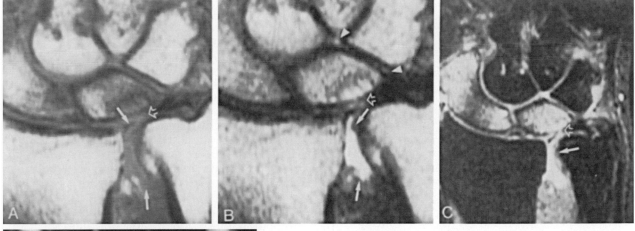

Figure 14-43

Ulnar impaction syndrome: MR imaging.

A Coronal proton density–weighted (TR/TE, 1700/20) spin echo MR image. A large communicating defect (open arrow) in the triangular fibrocartilage is evident. Fluid (solid arrows) is apparent in the distal radioulnar joint. The lunotriquetral interosseous ligament is not well seen. Note abnormal regions of low signal intensity in the lunate and scaphoid, consistent with marrow edema. The lunate changes have occurred as a consequence of the ulnar impaction syndrome.

B Coronal T2-weighted (TR/TE, 1700/70) spin echo MR image. The communicating defect (open arrow) of the triangular fibrocartilage again is evident. Fluid fills the distal radioulnar joint (solid arrows). Fluid (arrowheads) is seen in the midcarpal joint, including the space between the lunate and triquetrum. High signal intensity in the proximal portion of the lunate is indicative of marrow edema.

C Coronal STIR MR image (TR/TE, 1650/25; inversion time, 160 msec). Defects are seen in the triangular fibrocartilage (open arrow) and lunotriquetral interosseous ligament. Fluid fills the distal radioulnar joint (solid arrow) and portions of the radiocarpal and midcarpal joints. Marrow edema in the scaphoid and lunate is manifest as regions of increased signal intensity.

D A coronal short tau inversion recovery (STIR) MR image (TR/TE, 1200/25; inversion time, 120 ms) in a second patient shows a long ulna (open arrow), disruption of the triangular fibrocartilage, fluid in the inferior radioulnar (solid arrow), radiocarpal and midcarpal compartments, and a cyst (arrowhead) in the lunate.

(**A–C,** From Schweitzer ME, et al: Radiology *182*:205, 1992.)

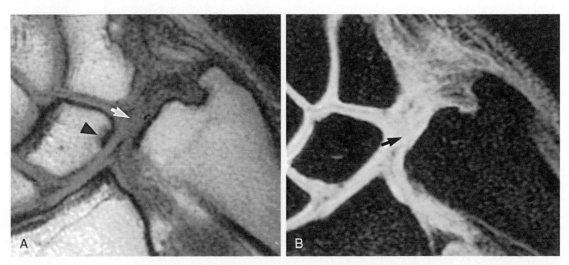

Figure 14-44

Ulnar impaction syndrome: MR imaging. Coronal T1-weighted (TR/TE, 450/19) spin echo (**A**) and three-dimensional fat-suppressed SPGR (TR/TE, 69/15; flip angle, 30 degrees) (**B**) MR images show a full-thickness defect (arrows) in the triangular fibrocartilage and a region of low signal intensity in the lunate (arrowhead) in **A.** (Courtesy of D. Goodwin, M.D., Hanover, New Hampshire.)

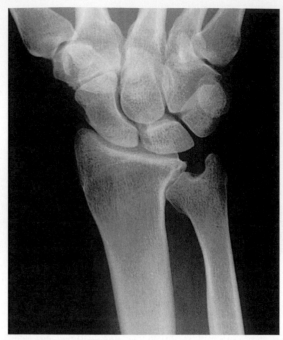

Figure 14–45

Ulnar impingement syndrome: Routine radiography. In this patient with wrist pain during pronation and supination of the forearm, a routine radiograph shows a minus ulnar variance and irregularity of the joint between the distal portions of radius and ulna.

occurs in the Essex-Lopresti injury).[136] The annular ligament, by encircling the proximal portion of the radius, also is better suited to maintain coronal stability than longitudinal stability. The interosseous ligament of the forearm is essential to longitudinal stability.[136]

Distal radioulnar joint instability may occur in association with complex soft tissue and bone injuries of the forearm and elbow, or it may appear as an isolated phenomenon related to injury, as a finding accompanied by a fracture (e.g., Colles' fracture, fracture of the styloid process of the ulna), or as a consequence of inflammatory diseases such as rheumatoid arthritis. Clinical manifestations include pain, weakness, loss of forearm rotation, and snapping. Dorsal instability predominates, and physical examination confirms a dorsal prominence of the ulnar head, especially in a position of forearm pronation.

The detection of subluxation of the distal portion of the ulna by routine radiography may be quite difficult, as slight variations in wrist position alter the relationship of the radius and ulna. Although a number of radiographic measurements can be employed to assess the positions of the distal portions of the radius and ulna more accurately,[137, 138] they are time-consuming and difficult to apply clinically. Tomographic techniques, such as CT scanning and MR imaging, which provide transverse or cross-sectional data, may be advantageous in the diagnosis of distal radioulnar joint instability[139–142]; evaluation of the wrist in the neutral position and with pronation and supination of the forearm and comparison of the injured and opposite wrists commonly are required. Even with these techniques, accurate appraisal of the relative position of the ulna with respect to the radius requires construction of a number of lines, typi-

cally drawn (1) along the dorsal surface of the radius from Lister's tubercle to the dorsal ulnar border of the bone, (2) as a perpendicular to this line through the dorsal ulnar border of the radius, and (3) as a perpendicular to the second line through the palmar border of the ulnar head (Fig. 14–46).[143, 439] In the normal situation, the bulk of the ulnar head is located between lines 1 and 3, slight changes in its position are detected when volar or dorsal stress is applied to the wrist, and little difference in the position of the ulnar heads (with respect to the distal portion of the radii) in the two extremities is evident. Furthermore, the anatomic landmarks required for construction of these lines are constant and usually identified easily. As subtle displacements may characterize minor degrees of distal radioulnar joint instability, however, a comparison of findings in the injured and noninjured wrist is essential. Although both CT and MR imaging allow such comparison, the advantages of MR imaging include direct multiplanar analysis of the distal radioulnar joint, visualization of the dorsal and volar radioulnar ligaments, and assessment of nearby structures such as the extensor carpi ulnaris tendon and other components of the TFCC that also may be affected.[142]

Although isolated dislocations of the inferior radioulnar joint are seen infrequently, dislocation or subluxation of this joint may occur in association with a fracture of the radius. This combination of findings is termed a Galeazzi fracture-dislocation.[144–148] Classically, the shaft of the radius is fractured in this injury; fractures of the distal end of the radius, which may be associated with dislocation of the ulnar head,[148] and of the radial neck and head, which may be associated with a dislocation of the inferior radioulnar joint, are not regarded as Galeazzi fracture-dislocations unless the radial shaft also is fractured.[149] Comminuted fractures of the radial head combined with dislocations of the distal radioulnar joint are termed Essex-Lopresti injuries. Most commonly, the fracture accompanying the Galeazzi fracture-dislocation occurs at the junction of the middle and distal thirds of the radius and has a short oblique or transverse configuration. The distal radial fragment is displaced in an ulnar direction. Usually, the dislocation of the ulnar head readily is apparent, although, in some cases, ulnar head subluxation may be more apparent on clinical evaluation. In equivocal cases, arthrography of the radiocarpal joint can be helpful in establishing the existence of an injury to the distal portion of the ulna or surrounding structures.[150] Disruption of the inferior radioulnar joint requires injury to the triangular fibrocartilage, the major stabilizing structure of the distal portion of the ulna. Thus, contrast opacification of the radiocarpal joint will be associated with filling of the inferior radioulnar joint due to perforation of the intervening triangular fibrocartilage.[147] Fracture of the ulnar head or styloid process also may be identified. Dislocation of the ulna usually occurs in a distal, dorsal, and medial direction; volar dislocation is less frequent.

Carpal Abnormalities

Carpal Instability

Since the landmark publications by Linscheid and co-workers[151] and Dobyns and collaborators,[152] the subject

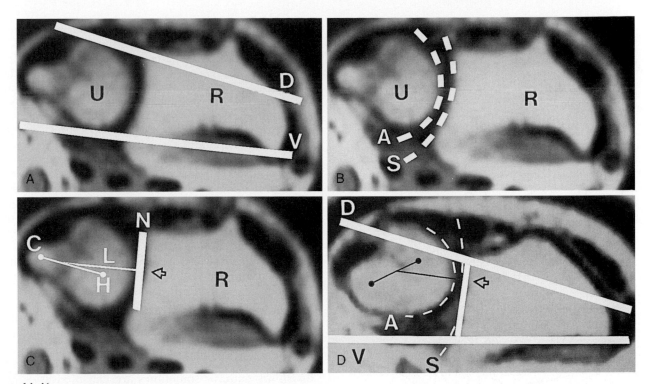

Figure 14–46

Instability of the distal radioulnar joint: MR imaging.

A–C Methods of measurement. Transaxial T1-weighted spin echo MR images are shown. With the radioulnar line method **(A)**, lines are constructed through the dorsal (D) and volar (V) radial (R) borders. The ulnar head (U) normally lies between these lines. With the congruity method **(B)**, arcs outlining the ulnar (U) head (A) and sigmoid notch (S) of the radius (R) are congruent. With the epicenter method **(C)**, a line (L) perpendicular to the chord of the sigmoid notch (N) of the radius (R) extends to a point midway between the centers of the ulnar styloid process (C) and ulnar head (H). The line normally intersects the middle portion (arrow) of the sigmoid notch.

D In this abnormal situation, a T1-weighted spin echo MR image shows ulnodorsal distal radioulnar joint subluxation by all methods. A, Arc of ulnar head; S, arc of sigmoid notch; D, line through the dorsal radial border; V, line through the volar radial border. The arrow marks the intersection of the chord of the sigmoid notch with the line perpendicular to it.

(From Staron RB, et al: Skel Radiol 23:369, 1994.)

of carpal instability has received a great deal of attention. Stability of the wrist depends on the integrity of both the bones and surrounding ligaments. The latter are arranged in three layers: the most superficial layer consists of the antebrachial fascia and the transverse carpal ligament; a second layer contains the extrinsic ligaments generally coursing between the carpal bones and the radius, ulna, or metacarpals, including the radial collateral ligament, volar radiocarpal ligaments, meniscus homologue, triangular fibrocartilage, ulnolunate and ulnotriquetral ligaments, ulnar collateral ligament, and dorsal ligaments; and a third or deep layer consisting of intrinsic ligaments, coursing between individual carpal bones in a circular fashion. Both the extrinsic and the intrinsic ligaments of the wrist contribute to carpal stability, whereas the role of the collateral ligament system in this function is limited. Biomechanically, the extrinsic ligaments are stiffer than the intrinsic ligaments, and the intrinsic ligaments are capable of greater elongation before permanent deformity occurs.[153] The volar radiocarpal and intercarpal ligaments generally are regarded as the most important structures stabilizing the carpus.

Two important concepts regarding the radiographic anatomy of the wrist should be emphasized. On the posteroanterior view, three smooth carpal arcs define the normal intercarpal relationships.[154, 155] Arc 1 follows the proximal surfaces of the scaphoid, lunate, and triquetrum; arc 2 is located along the distal surfaces of these same carpal bones; and arc 3 defines the curvature of the proximal surfaces of the capitate and hamate. In the normal situation, these curvilinear arcs are roughly parallel, without disruption, and the interosseous spaces are approximately equal in size. Second, the lateral radiograph of the normal wrist (in neutral position) is characterized by a specific relationship of the longitudinal axes of the radius, scaphoid, lunate, capitate, and third metacarpal (Fig. 14–47). A continuous line can be drawn through these axes of the radius, lunate and capitate, and this line will intersect a second line through the longitudinal axis of the scaphoid, creating an angle of 30 to 60 degrees. Alterations in these relationships (as well as others) indicate carpal instability, which, in most instances, is related to trauma.

As indicated earlier in this chapter, smooth and synchronous motion between and within the two carpal rows is essential for proper function of the wrist.[10] As summarized by Stanley and Trail,[28] flexion and extension of the wrist result from movements between the radius and the lunate, between the lunate and the capitate, between and among the trapezium, trapezoid, and scaphoid, and between the triquetrum and the hamate.

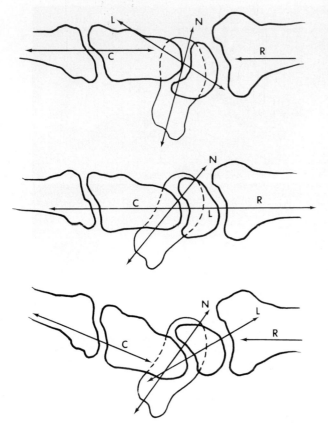

Figure 14–47

Dorsal and volar intercalated segmental instability. Lateral projection. Line drawings of longitudinal axes of third metacarpal, navicular (N) or scaphoid, lunate (L), capitate (C), and radius (R) in dorsal intercalated segmental instability (DISI) (upper drawing), in normal situation (middle drawing), and in volar intercalated segmental instability (VISI) (lower drawing). When the wrist is normal, a continuous line can be drawn through the longitudinal axes of the capitate, the lunate, and the radius, and this line will intersect a second line through the longitudinal axis of the scaphoid, creating an angle of 30 to 60 degrees. In DISI, the lunate is flexed toward the back of the hand and the scaphoid is displaced vertically. The angle of intersection between the two longitudinal axes is greater than 60 degrees. In VISI, the lunate is flexed toward the palm and the angle between the two longitudinal axes is less than 30 degrees. (From Linscheid RL, et al: J Bone Joint Surg [Am] *54*:1612, 1972.)

Approximately half the range of flexion and extension occurs at the radiocarpal joint and half at the midcarpal joint. In radial deviation, the distance between the trapezium and styloid process of the radius shortens, and in ulnar deviation it lengthens.[28] In radial deviation, the scaphoid slides into the lunate fossa of the radius; in ulnar deviation, the lunate slides into the scaphoid fossa of the radius. Furthermore, in radial deviation, the scaphoid flexes; in ulnar deviation the scaphoid undergoes passive extension.[28] The triquetrum moves in these positions of radial and ulnar deviation in a pattern that follows those of the scaphoid and lunate bones, although flexion of the triquetrum is less than that of the scaphoid. Therefore, the lunate bone becomes an intercalated torque converter between the scaphoid and triquetral bones during radial and ulnar deviation of the wrist, and the lunate bone functions as an intercalated segment between the radius and the capitate bones.[28]

The patterns of carpal instability commonly are divided into dissociated and nondissociated types. The dissociated instability patterns, which usually indicate more extensive ligamentous damage than the nondissociated, may be recognized on routine radiographic analysis owing to disruptions in the normal relationships among the carpal bones.[80] Dissociative instability patterns include transscaphoid fractures and complete tears of the scapholunate or lunotriquetral interosseous ligament (or both ligaments), which may occur in association with attenuation or disruption of the palmar or the dorsal extrinsic ligaments, or of both. Nondissociative instability patterns represent abnormalities of alignment or relationship of the carpal bones with intact interosseous ligaments.[80] Nondissociative instability patterns are less common than dissociative instability patterns and may result from attenuation of the palmar or dorsal radiocarpal or ulnocarpal ligaments in the presence of intact scapholunate and lunotriquetral interosseous ligaments. Such intact interosseous ligaments are suggested by routine posteroanterior radiographs of the wrist in which carpal alignment appears normal.[80] Therefore, a normal radiographic appearance does not exclude the presence of carpal instability. Indeed, carpal instability patterns sometimes are classified as static or dynamic, on the basis of the presence (i.e., static instability) or absence (i.e., dynamic instability) of radiographically detectable carpal abnormalities.[156] Patients with dynamic instability of the carpal bones may be able to change the carpal alignment voluntarily from normal to abnormal during certain movements of the wrist, or such abnormal carpal alignment may be elicited during manipulation of the wrist during physical examination.

Anatomically, three types of carpal instability may occur: lateral instability, which usually takes place between the scaphoid and the lunate; medial instability, which occurs between the triquetrum and the lunate or between the triquetrum and the hamate; and proximal instability, which occurs when the abnormal carpal alignment is secondary to an injury of the radius or to massive radiocarpal disruption.[156] The patterns of instability that result from ligamentous disruption in the proximal carpal row (i.e., between the scaphoid and lunate or between the lunate and triquetrum) include scapholunate dissociation, which produces dorsal intercalated segmental instability, and lunotriquetral dissociation, which leads to volar intercalated segmental instability (see Fig. 14–47). *Dorsal intercalary segment carpal instability* (also termed DICI, DISI, dorsiflexion carpal instability) (Fig. 14–48), in which the lunate is tilted dorsally, the scaphoid is flexed, and the scapholunate angle is greater than 70 degrees, is the more common of the two; *volar intercalary segment carpal instability* (VICI, VISI, palmar flexion carpal instability), occurs when the lunate is tilted in a palmar direction and the scapholunate angle is decreased below the normal value of approximately 47 degrees.[157] Although precise analysis of the amount of dorsal or volar lunate tilting requires careful measurements on well-positioned lateral radiographs or tomographic studies, survey of the frontal radiograph alone may allow determination of whether the lunate is tilted in a volar or dorsal direction; with

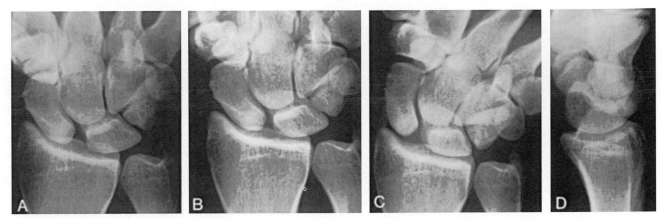

Figure 14–48

Scapholunate dissociation and dorsal intercalated segmental instability (DISI): Routine radiography with specialized projections. Routine posteroanterior (PA) radiograph **(A)**, PA radiograph with the patient clenching his fist **(B)**, and PA radiograph with ulnar deviation of the wrist **(C)** show widening of the scapholunate interosseous space and a rounded distal border of the lunate, indicative of dorsal tilting of the lunate with visualization of its volar surface. The lateral radiograph **(D)** confirms the presence of DISI. (Courtesy of G. Greenway, M.D., Dallas, Texas.)

dorsal tilting the distal contour of the lunate (representing its volar margin) usually is round, and with volar tilting the distal contour of the lunate (representing its dorsal margin) may be angular.[158] Dorsiflexion instability commonly occurs after scaphoid fractures with scapholunate separation, or dissociation, as well as after fractures of the proximal portion of the radius; palmar flexion instability may be seen after disruption of the lunotriquetral interosseous ligament, excision of the triquetrum, and sprains of the midcarpal joint that attenuate the extrinsic ligaments,[159] as well as in patients using wheelchairs.[160] Similar patterns of instability are seen as a normal variant in persons with ligamentous laxity and in those with various articular disorders, including rheumatoid arthritis and calcium pyrophosphate dihydrate crystal deposition disease.[161]

Stanley and Trail[28] have summarized the precise steps that lead to DISI and VISI, and their observations are included here. When ligaments supporting the scaphoid are disrupted, longitudinal compression forces the scaphoid into a flexed position. As the lunate is narrower anteriorly than dorsally, it tends to extend under such compression. Because the scaphoid and lunate are moving in different directions, the ligamentous connections between them are disrupted, and DISI occurs. This instability pattern classically arises from a fall on the outstretched, extended wrist. Conversely, when the hypothenar eminence strikes the ground, pronation results in disruption of the dorsal ulnotriquetral ligament complex, the lunotriquetral interosseous ligament, and the anterior midcarpal capsule. These injuries allow the capitate to hyperextend with respect to the lunate, which compensates by flexing into the palm. Such injuries produce VISI.[28]

The terminology applied to other patterns of carpal instability is not consistent. With regard to medial instability, previous reports have emphasized one type that occurs at the joint between the triquetrum and the hamate and has been termed *triquetrohamate dissociation* (or *instability*).[162–164] It leads to painful clicking on the ulnar aspect of the wrist and is related to traumatically

induced pronation and radial flexion.[162] Abnormal motion between the triquetrum and the hamate is observed during fluoroscopy. Another type of medial carpal instability is termed *triquetrolunate dissociation,* indicating abnormal motion at the intervening articulation.[163]

Proximal carpal instability results from disruption of the radiocarpal ligaments or distal radioulnar joint surfaces. Several types exist.[163] *Ulnar translocation* occurs when the carpus shifts in an ulnar direction, which may follow severe capsular injury or articular disorders such as rheumatoid arthritis. An increased space between the scaphoid and the radial styloid process is an important, although not invariable, diagnostic feature. *Dorsal carpal translocation* usually is associated with malunited fractures involving the dorsal rim of the radius and the radial styloid process. *Palmar carpal translocation* accompanies Barton's fractures or disruptions of the volar rim of the radius. *Proximal midcarpal instability,* which may result from malunited fractures of the distal portion of the radius that do not extend into the radiocarpal joint, leads to disabling pain, tenderness, and occasionally, a loud snapping sound when the hand is brought voluntarily into ulnar deviation.

The diagnosis of all of these abnormalities requires routine radiography supplemented with special views, including posteroanterior projections in neutral and in ulnar and radial deviation, an anteroposterior projection with tightly clenched fist, and oblique and lateral projections.[154, 165] Fluoroscopic monitoring also can be useful in detecting transient subluxations in the wrist,[166–169] and may be combined with the application of stress.[169, 170] Such extensive radiographic protocols for wrist instability usually are not required, however, as radiographic views tailored to the analysis of specific types of instability generally suffice.[171]

Dissociated scapholunate movements may accompany tears of the ventral radiocarpal ligaments and scapholunate interosseous ligament complex. This may occur as a complication of lunate or perilunate dislocation, rheumatoid arthritis, and other articular diseases or as an isolated injury. *Scapholunate dissociation* (rotary sub-

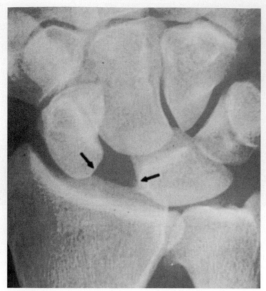

Figure 14–49
Scapholunate dissociation (rotatory subluxation of the scaphoid). Findings include widening of the scapholunate distance (arrows) and a foreshortened scaphoid.

luxation of the scaphoid)[172] is suggested when the distance between the scaphoid and lunate is 2 mm or wider and can be diagnosed almost unequivocally when this distance is 4 mm or wider (Fig. 14–49).[154] Some variability in this width, however, with measurements as great as 5 mm, has been noted in normal persons[173] as well as in those with lunotriquetral coalitions. The finding of a widened scapholunate space implies that an abnormality

exists in the scapholunate interosseous ligament,[174] and, perhaps, in the volar or dorsal radiocarpal ligaments as well.[175] When the scaphoid is tilted in a palmar direction, a ventral radiocarpal ligament tear also is present. Rotary subluxation of the scaphoid is associated with radiographic findings in addition to widening of the scapholunate space (Terry-Thomas sign) and palmar tilting of the scaphoid.[176–180] These findings include, on the posteroanterior view, a ring produced by the cortex of the distal pole of the scaphoid and a foreshortened scaphoid. Radiographs exposed during radial or ulnar deviation of the wrist or in a posteroanterior position with 10 degrees of tube angulation from the ulna toward the radius may accentuate the gap or space between the scaphoid and the lunate,[176, 181] although a false-positive ring sign also may be seen with wrist deviation in the coronal plane.

Arthrography can be used for the diagnosis of communicating defects of the scapholunate and lunotriquetral interosseous ligaments (see Fig. 14–20C, D). Such defects, however, may relate not to injury but to progressive deterioration, a process that increases in frequency with advancing age. Indeed, as noted earlier in this chapter, when bilateral arthrography is employed, patterns of communication between the radiocarpal and midcarpal joints in the injured and symptomatic side also may be observed in the uninjured and asymptomatic side.[62, 64] Furthermore, the identification of all full-thickness defects of the scapholunate and lunotriquetral ligaments, in the opinion of some experts, requires sequential opacification of the radiocarpal and midcarpal compartments, owing to the presence of some defects that allow flow of contrast material in only one

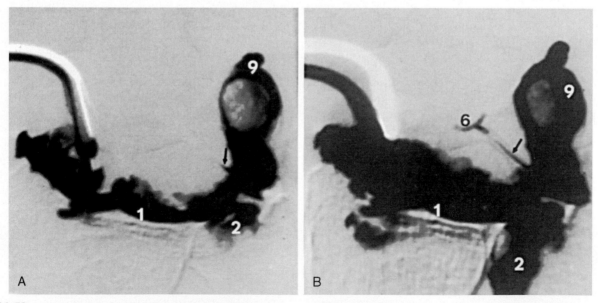

A   B

Figure 14–50
Intercarpal ligaments: Digital arthrography—communicating defect of lunotriquetral interosseous ligament (and triangular fibrocartilage). In a cadaver, subtraction images are provided after the injection of 1.0 ml **(A)** and 2.0 ml **(B)** of contrast material into the radiocarpal compartment (1). In **A,** opacification of this compartment, the inferior radioulnar compartment (2) (indicating a tear of the triangular fibrocartilage), and the pisiform-triquetral compartment (9) is seen. A small amount of contrast agent is present in the space between the lunate and triquetrum (arrow). In **B,** opacification of the midcarpal compartment (6) has begun through a tear in the lunotriquetral interosseous ligament (arrow). (From Resnick D, et al: AJR *142*:1187, 1984. Copyright 1984, American Roentgen Ray Society.)

direction. The demonstration of communications between the radiocarpal and midcarpal compartments may depend not only on which compartment is injected but also on which joint is injected first, the amount of contrast material introduced, and the delay between injections.[60] Accurate analysis of arthrographic findings also requires careful monitoring during the injection process; such monitoring can be accomplished with fluoroscopy, videorecording, or digital technique (Fig. 14–50).

Although MR imaging does not resolve the question of the clinical significance of the ligamentous abnormalities, the technique has been found useful for the identification of defects of the scapholunate and lunotriquetral interosseous ligaments[108, 111, 113, 115, 116, 437] and, in a preliminary fashion, for the assessment of the dorsal and volar radiocarpal and carpal ligaments.[17, 19, 182–184] The coronal plane is most useful for delineation of the interosseous ligaments, although the transaxial plane also demonstrates these ligaments, and the sagittal plane provides additional information regarding the relationship among the carpal bones and, hence, may be valuable in the identification of dorsal or palmar tilting of the lunate (Fig. 14–51). Of the two interosseous ligaments, the scapholunate interosseous ligament is visualized more consistently, although some investigators have indicated that the lunotriquetral ligament also can be identified regularly.[185] On coronal spin echo or gradient echo images, the normal scapholunate interosseous ligament typically is seen as a thin or triangular (delta-shaped) structure of low signal intensity traversing the space between the scaphoid and the lunate (Fig. 14–52). Variations in this normal appearance include a linear shape and circular or linear regions of intermediate signal intensity within the ligament.[72] Indeed, when three-dimensional gradient echo sequences are employed, the dorsal, middle, and volar portions of the scapholunate ligament have been found to have slightly different appearances.[418] When visualized, the normal lunotriquetral interosseous ligament has a similar appearance, extending between the lunate and the trique-

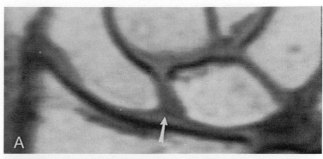
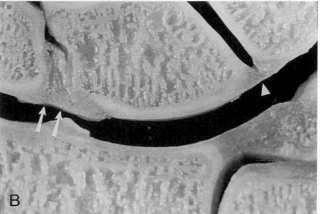

Figure 14–52

Intercarpal ligaments: MR imaging—Normal scapholunate interosseous ligament.

A Coronal T1-weighted (TR/TE, 800/20) spin echo MR image. Note the linear region of low signal intensity (arrow) representing the normal scapholunate interosseous ligament. The lunotriquetral interosseous ligament is not well seen.

B Coronal section of the wrist. The normal scapholunate interosseous ligament (arrows) is evident. The lunotriquetral interosseous ligament (arrowhead) also is normal.

trum. An abnormality of the scapholunate interosseous ligament is suggested when it is elongated, incomplete, courses other than in a horizontal direction, or is not seen at all (Figs. 14–53 and 14–54). An abnormality of the lunotriquetral interosseous ligament is suggested when it is elongated, incomplete, or extends in a direction other than horizontal. Although the successful visualization of a lunotriquetral interosseous ligament depends on the specific imaging parameters employed, its nonvisualization on MR images often has not been a reliable indicator of abnormality.[114, 116, 185] A secondary (although nonspecific) finding associated with a defect of the scapholunate or lunotriquetral interosseous ligament is the presence of fluid in the adjacent portions of the midcarpal joint and in the scapholunate or lunotriquetral interosseous space, respectively. The application of stress to the wrist during the MR imaging examination may improve accuracy in the diagnosis of these ligamentous abnormalities.[186]

Volumetric gradient echo imaging provides thin contiguous sections of the wrist (Fig. 14–55). With this method, the scapholunate and lunotriquetral interosseous ligaments generally are delineated well. Nonvisualization of either ligament, but particularly the scapholunate interosseous ligament, with volumetric imaging is strong evidence that an abnormality exists.

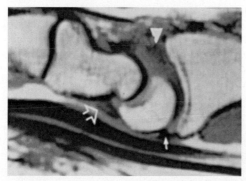

Figure 14–51

Dorsal intercalated segmental instability (DISI): MR imaging. Sagittal MPGR MR image (TR/TE, 533/15; flip angle, 35 degrees). Note dorsal tilting of the lunate with respect to the radius and capitate. Parts of the dorsal radiocarpal ligament (arrowhead), volar radioscaphocapitate ligament (open arrow), and volar radioscapholunate ligament (solid arrow) are seen. (Courtesy of S. Eilenberg, M.D., San Diego, California.)

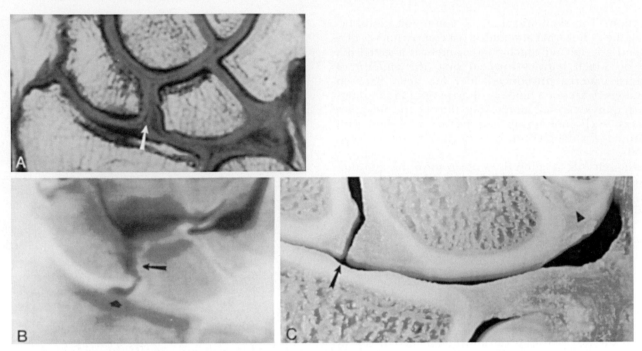

Figure 14–53
Intercarpal ligaments: MR imaging and digital arthrography—communicating defect of the scapholunate interosseous ligament.
   A Coronal T1-weighted (TR/TE, 800/20) spin echo MR image shows discontinuity of the scapholunate interosseous ligament (arrow). The lunotriquetral interosseous ligament is not seen.
   B Digital arthrographic image obtained after a midcarpal injection shows leakage of contrast material through the scapholunate interosseous space (upper arrow) with opacification of the radiocarpal compartment (lower arrow).
   C Coronal section reveals the defect (arrow) in the scapholunate interosseous ligament. The lunotriquetral interosseous ligament (arrowhead) and triangular fibrocartilage are intact.

Schweitzer and coworkers,[116] in a study of the value of MR imaging of patients with chronic wrist pain, employed routine spin echo images, STIR images, and MR arthrography (with injection of gadolinium compound into the radiocarpal joint) (Fig. 14–56). The results of the MR imaging examinations were tabulated using conventional arthrography and arthroscopy as two standards of reference. These investigators found that failure to visualize the scapholunate interosseous ligament on technically optimal MR images can be moderately helpful as a sign of a defect. Abnormal morphology of this ligament resulted in decreased sensitivity but markedly increased specificity in cases of ligamentous disruption. The standard T1-weighted spin echo MR sequence proved to be the most accurate, and this accuracy was better than that of conventional arthrography. When conventional arthrography was the standard, the MR arthrography images were slightly more accurate than the other sequences. The presence of fluid in the midcarpal compartment had a high sensitivity for allowing detection of scapholunate interosseous ligament abnormality. For analysis of the lunotriquetral interosseous ligament, failure of its visualization with MR imaging was not a useful sign of abnormality; however, when the morphology of the lunotriquetral interosseous ligament was assessed, the specificity of the MR imaging observations was high. The presence of fluid in the midcarpal joint also was a helpful indicator of a lunotriquetral interosseous ligament tear and had high sensitivity, similar to that noted for the scapholunate interosse-

ous ligament. With conventional arthrography as the standard, all of the MR imaging sequences showed similar accuracy with regard to assessment of the lunotriquetral interosseous ligament; with arthroscopy as the standard, conventional T1-weighted spin echo MR images and MR arthrography were most accurate. Arthrography alone showed similar accuracy to MR imaging in the evaluation of the lunotriquetral interosseous ligament.

These results suggest that although MR arthrography may improve accuracy in the assessment of the interosseous ligaments (and the TFCC), its invasiveness and time requirements do not appear to justify the procedure; that the presence of fluid in the midcarpal joint is an important secondary indicator of abnormality in the scapholunate or lunotriquetral interosseous ligament and, because of this, T2-weighted spin echo MR images are required; and that conventional arthrography and standard MR imaging generally provide similar information in the assessment of these interosseous ligaments.

Evaluation of the dorsal and volar extrinsic radiocarpal ligaments and many intrinsic carpal ligaments with MR imaging is best accomplished with volumetric gradient echo MR sequences (Fig. 14–57A, B). The oblique orientation of many of these ligaments makes analysis of sequential images mandatory, and reformatted images in these oblique planes may be required (see Fig. 14–57C and D).[17, 19] The clinical usefulness of such MR imaging in the detection of alterations in these ligaments is not established yet,[108] and, ultimately, comparison of findings in the injured and noninjured wrist may

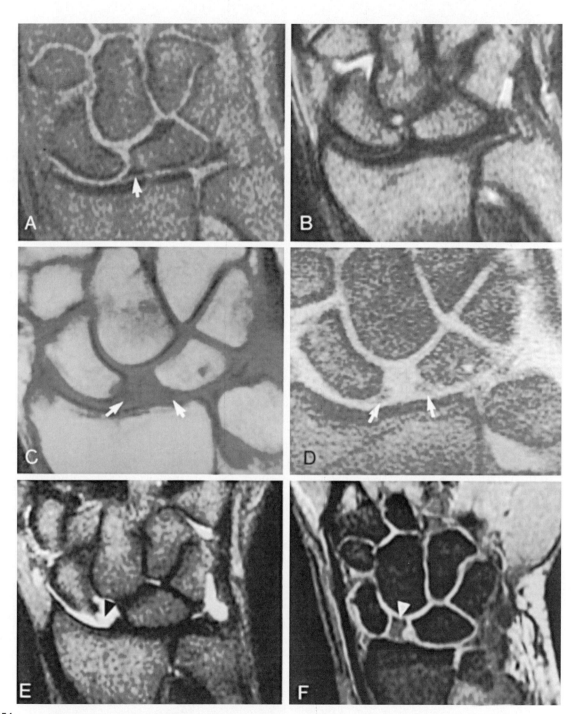

Figure 14–54

Intercarpal ligaments: MR imaging—communicating defect of the scapholunate interosseous ligament.

A, B Coronal T1-weighted (TR/TE, 600/20) spin echo MR image obtained with chemical presaturation of fat (ChemSat) **(A)** and coronal T2-weighted (TR/TE, 2000/80) spin echo MR image **(B).** In **A,** altered morphology of the scapholunate interosseous ligament (arrow) is seen. The triangular fibrocartilage is normal. In **B,** the scapholunate ligament is not well seen. Note fluid of high signal intensity in the midcarpal joint, including the region of the scapholunate interosseous space.

C, D Coronal T1-weighted (TR/TE, 600/20) spin echo MR image **(C)** and MPGR MR image (TR/TE, 500/15; flip angle, 20 degrees) **(D)** in a second patient. Note the altered morphology of the scapholunate interosseous ligament (arrows) with scapholunate widening or dissociation. The triangular fibrocartilage also is disrupted. (Courtesy of C. Sebrechts, M.D., San Diego, CA.)

E, F Coronal T2-weighted (TR/TE, 3600/105) fast spin echo MR image **(E)** and coronal spoiled gradient recalled (SPGR) MR image (TR/TE, 58/10; flip angle, 60 degrees) obtained with three-dimensional Fourier transform (3DFT) and chemical presaturation of fat (ChemSat) **(F)** in a third patient. Fluid (arrowheads) of high signal intensity in **E** and of low signal intensity in **F** in the scapholunate interosseous space is evident.

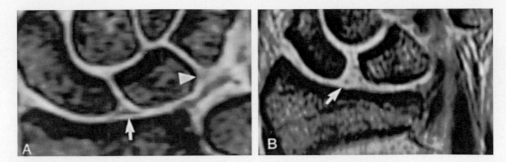

Figure 14–55
Intercarpal ligaments: MR imaging—three-dimensional Fourier transform (3DFT) gradient recalled MR imaging; normal and abnormal scapholunate interosseous ligament.

A Normal scapholunate interosseous ligament. A coronal 3DFT (TR/TE, 60/11; flip angle, 10 degrees) MR image shows the low signal intensity and linear morphology that characterize the normal scapholunate (arrow) and lunotriquetral (arrowhead) interosseous ligaments. The triangular fibrocartilage also is normal. (Courtesy of S. K. Brahme, M.D., La Jolla, California.)

B Communicating defect of the scapholunate interosseous ligament. A coronal oblique 3DFT (TR/TE, 60/10; flip angle, 30 degrees) MR image shows altered morphology (arrow) of the scapholunate interosseous ligament.

be required. The role of MR arthrography in this regard also is not clear (Figs. 14–58 and 14–59).[184]

Arthroscopy of the wrist has been employed as both diagnostic and therapeutic modalities in patients with carpal instability.[187-189, 419] A number of entrance portals may be required for complete assessment during the arthroscopic procedure. Treatment options depend upon the precise site and extent of injury and include simple débridement of abnormal tissue, pinning using one or more Kirschner wires, or a combination of the two.

Dislocations and Fractures

Virtually any of the carpal bones may be dislocated after an injury; reports describe isolated dislocations of the scaphoid,[190-192] capitate,[193] triquetrum,[194] trapezium,[195-197]
trapezoid,[198-200] and pisiform.[201-203] Furthermore, unusual dislocations or displacements of more than a single carpal bone are encountered,[204] including scaphoid dislocation with axial carpal dislocation,[205] dislocation of the scaphoid and lunate,[206] dislocation of the triquetrum with rotatory subluxation of the scaphoid,[207] dislocation of the lunate and triquetrum,[208] and longitudinal disruption of the ulnar aspect of the carpus.[209] Such injuries are rare, however. Because the lunate and the proximal part of the scaphoid are protected to some extent by the distal end of the radius, a common pattern of injury is a perilunate or transscaphoid perilunate dislocation. In a perilunate dislocation, the lunate remains aligned with the distal part of the radius and the other carpal bones dislocate, usually dorsally, although on rare occasions in a volar direction.[210, 211] When the wrist is hyperextended, the dorsal cortex of the distal radial articular

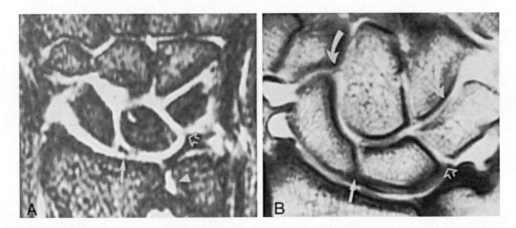

Figure 14–56
Intercarpal ligaments: MR imaging—STIR MR imaging and MR arthrography; communicating defects of the scapholunate and lunotriquetral interosseous ligaments and the triangular fibrocartilage.

A Coronal STIR (TR/TE, 1650/25; inversion time, 160 msec) MR image. Observe fluid in the distal radioulnar joint (arrowhead), altered morphology in the radial aspect of the triangular fibrocartilage and the scapholunate interosseous ligament (solid arrow), and nonvisualization of the lunotriquetral interosseous ligament (open arrow).

B MR arthrography after injection of gadolinium compound into the radiocarpal compartment. A coronal T1-weighted (TR/TE, 500/20) spin echo MR image shows the communicating defect in the lunotriquetral interosseous ligament (open arrow) with opacification of the midcarpal compartment (curved arrows). The scapholunate interosseous ligament (straight arrow) and triangular fibrocartilage appear intact. Standard arthrography and arthroscopy confirmed communicating defects of the triangular fibrocartilage and scapholunate and lunotriquetral interosseous ligaments.

(From Schweitzer ME, et al: Radiology *182*:205, 1992.)

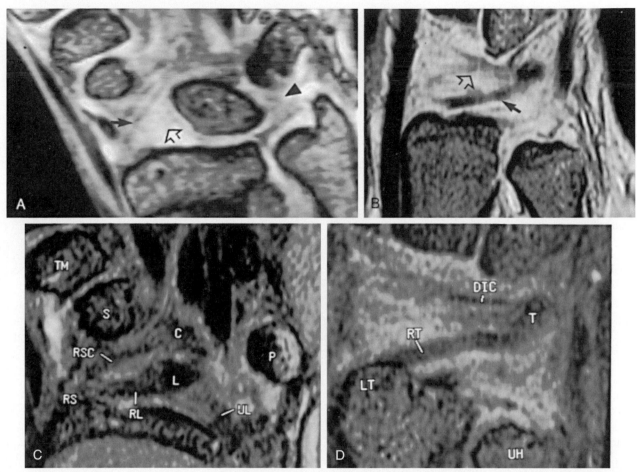

Figure 14–57

Volar and dorsal extrinsic radiocarpal and intrinsic carpal ligaments: MR imaging.

A Normal volar ligaments. Coronal oblique 3DFT gradient recalled MR image (TR/TE, 60/10; flip angle, 30 degrees). Illustrated structures include radioscaphocapitate ligament (solid arrow), radiolunate segment of the radiolunotriquetral ligament (open arrow), and possibly, a portion of the ulnotriquetral ligament (arrowhead).

B Normal dorsal ligaments. Coronal oblique 3DFT gradient recalled MR image (TR/TE, 60/10; flip angle, 30 degrees). Illustrated structures include radiotriquetral ligament (closed arrow) and dorsal intercarpal ligament (open arrow).

C Normal volar ligaments. Paracoronal 3DFT gradient recalled MR image (TR/TE, 37/8; flip angle, 12 degrees). Illustrated structures include radioscaphocapitate ligament (RSC), radiolunate segment (RL) of radiolunotriquetral ligament, and a portion of the ulnolunate ligament (UL). Also identified are the radial styloid process (RS), lunate bone (L), distal pole of scaphoid bone (S), capitate bone (C), trapezium bone (TM), and pisiform bone (P).

D Normal dorsal ligaments. Identical MR imaging sequence as in **E.** Note Lister's tubercle (LT), ulnar head (UH), and dorsal tubercle of triquetral bone (T). Identified structures are the dorsal intercarpal ligament (DIC) and, in this case, a single radiotriquetral ligament (RT).

(**C, D,** Courtesy of D. K. Smith, M.D., San Antonio, Texas; from Smith DK: AJR *161:*119–125, 352–357, 1993.)

surface fixes the lunate in place and apposes the scaphoid waist. A fall on the hyperextended hand, creating an abnormal force through the radius, can produce a fracture of the scaphoid,[212] and, with sufficient stress, a dislocation of the carpus occurs. The distal fragment of the scaphoid may move with the distal carpal row, and the proximal fragment may move with the proximal carpal row. With continued hyperextension force, the capitate may force the lunate ventrally, thus converting the perilunate dislocation into a lunate dislocation (Fig. 14–60), in which the lunate is displaced in a palmar direction and the capitate appears to be aligned with the distal end of the radius.[213, 214] Variations in the classic patterns of dislocation and associated fractures are common, depending on the exact position of the wrist at the time of injury.[215] Transscaphoid, transcapitate, and transtriquetral fracture-dislocations are encountered,

and the radial and ulnar styloid processes also may be affected. Proper radiographic interpretation requires multiple projections, including frontal, lateral, and oblique views. Difficulty in interpretation arises when a fragment is displaced for a considerable distance or when a fracture fragment rotates (e.g., the proximal end of the capitate)[212, 216–218] so that its site of origin is obscure.

Closer inspection of the functional anatomy of the wrist and the patterns of injury has indicated that a predictable sequence of events generally occurs after trauma (Fig. 14–61). The impact and loading conditions in these injuries usually commence about the thenar eminence, initially injuring the radial side of the wrist. Four stages in the resulting abnormalities are defined, with each successive stage indicating increased carpal instability.[219, 220] The stage I injury represents scapholu-

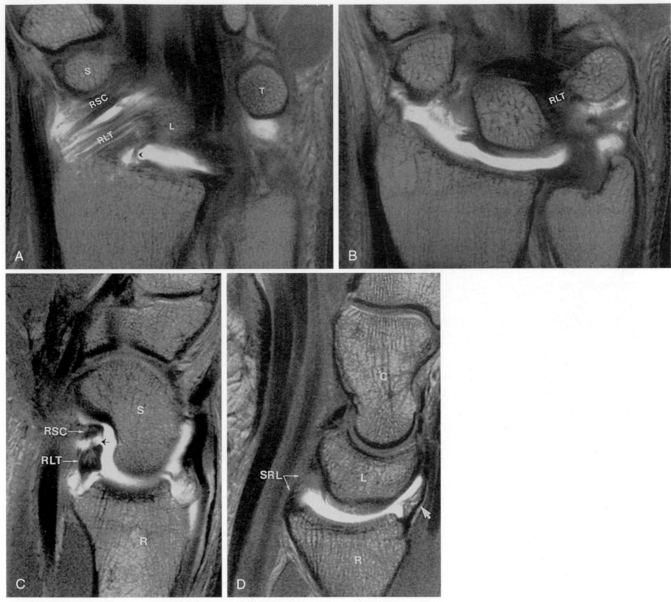

Figure 14–58

Volar and dorsal extrinsic radiocarpal ligaments: MR arthrography.

A, B After injection of a gadolinium compound into the radiocarpal joint, coronal T1-weighted (TR/TE, 500/35) fat-suppressed spin echo MR images, with **A** more volar than **B**, show the radioscaphocapitate (RSC) and radiolunotriquetral (RLT) ligaments. Note the striated appearance of these ligaments. The radioscapholunate ligament also is seen in **A** (arrowhead). L, Lunate bone; R, radius; S, scaphoid bone; T, triquetrum.

C, D Sagittal fat-suppressed T1-weighted (TR/TE, 500/35) spin echo MR images after the introduction of a gadolinium compound into the radiocarpal joint reveal volar and dorsal ligaments to good advantage. In **C**, at the level of the scaphoid (S) and radius (R), note the radioscaphocapitate (RSC) and radiolunotriquetral (RLT) ligaments, with a sulcus (arrow) between them. In **D**, at the level of the lunate (L), radius (R), and capitate (C), observed structures are the short radiolunate ligament (SRL) and a portion of the dorsal radiocarpal ligament (arrow).

(Reproduced with permission from Timins ME, et al: RadioGraphics *15*:575, 1995.)

nate dissociation with rotary subluxation of the scaphoid; the stage II injury is characterized by perilunar instability owing to failure of the radiocapitate ligament or a fracture of the radial styloid process, and leads to a perilunate dislocation; the stage III injury creates ligamentous disruption at the triquetrolunate joint related to partial or complete failure or avulsion of the volar radiotriquetral ligament and dorsal radiocarpal ligaments and may be accompanied by radiographically

evident triquetral malrotation, triquetrolunate diastasis, or triquetral fracture; the final stage IV injury is associated with disruption of the dorsal radiocarpal ligaments, freeing the lunate and allowing it to become volarly displaced (lunate dislocation). This series of events affecting ligaments and joint spaces takes place about the circumference of the lunate and is termed a *lesser arc injury*. *Greater arc injuries* represent fracture-dislocation patterns as this arc passes through the scaphoid, capi-

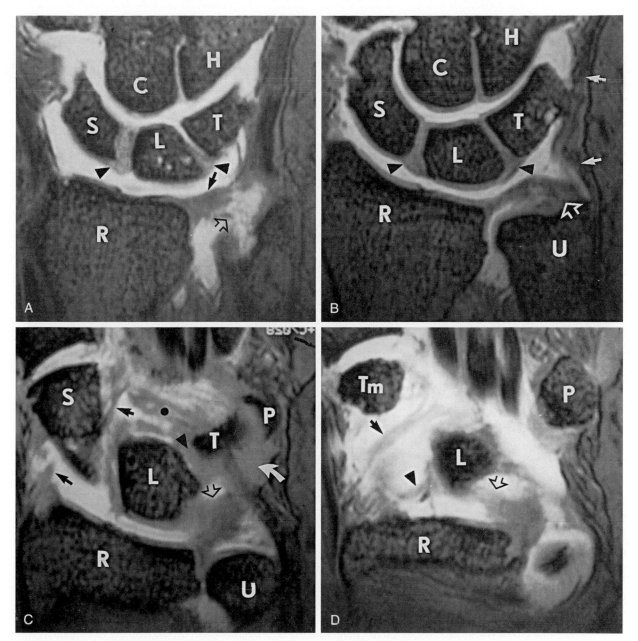

Figure 14–59
Extrinsic and intrinsic ligaments of the wrist: MR arthrography. Three-dimensional, fat-suppressed SPGR (TR/TE, 69/17; flip angle, 20 degrees) MR images with gadolinium compound in radiocarpal, distal radioulnar, and midcarpal compartments.

A–D Coronal plane. In the most dorsal image (**A**), visualized structures include the dorsal portions of the scapholunate and lunotriquetral interosseous ligaments (arrowheads), the dorsal radioulnar ligament (closed arrow), and a part of the most dorsal origin of the TFCC from the ulna (open arrow). In a slightly more volar image (**B**), the interosseous ligaments again are identified (arrowheads), and the ulnar attachment site of the TFCC is evident (open arrow). Note the extensor carpi ulnaris tendon and sheath (closed arrows). In a still more volar image (**C**), note portions of the radioscaphocapitate ligament (closed arrows), radiolunotriquetral ligament (arrowhead), and ulnolunate and ulnotriquetral ligaments (open arrow). The region of the meniscal homologue is also evident (curved arrow). Some fibers of the triquetrocapitate ligament are identified (black dot). In the most volar image (**D**), identified structures are the radioscaphocapitate ligament (closed arrow), radiolunotriquetral ligament (arrowhead), and ulnolunate ligament (open arrow).

Illustration continued on following page

tate, hamate, and triquetrum. Examples include the relatively common transscaphoid perilunate fracture-dislocation; the transscaphoid, transcapitate, perilunate fracture-dislocation (scaphocapitate syndrome); and the severe and infrequent transscaphoid, transcapitate, transhamate, transtriquetral fracture-dislocation.[219] These injuries also may be divided into various stages

based on their severity: stage I, transradial styloid fracture-dislocation; stage II, transscaphoid fracture-dislocation; stage III, transscaphoid, transcapitate fracture-dislocation; stage IV, transscaphoid (or radial styloid), transcapitate, transtriquetral fracture-dislocation; and stage V, complete palmar lunate dislocation associated with carpal fractures.[221]

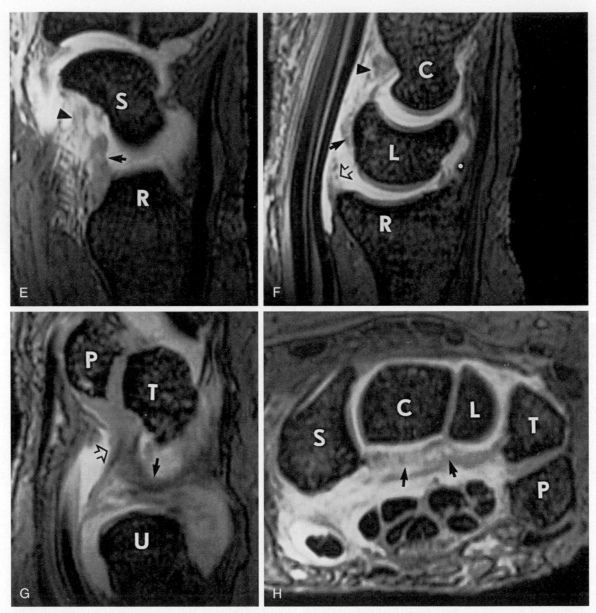

Figure 14–59 *Continued*

E–G Sagittal plane. In the most lateral, or radial, image (**E**), portions of the radioscaphocapitate (arrowhead) and radiolunotriquetral (arrow) ligaments are seen. Slightly more medially (**F**), visualized structures include the radioscaphocapitate ligament (arrowhead), radiolunotriquetral ligament (closed arrow), a portion (radiolunate portion) of the radioscapholunate ligament (open arrow), and a portion (radiolunate portion) of the dorsal radiocarpal ligament (white dot). In the most medial image (**G**), the ulnotriquetral ligament (open arrow) is seen to arise from the volar aspect of the TFC (closed arrow).

H Transaxial plane. At the level of the pisiform, a ligamentous structure is seen volarly, extending from the triquetrum to the scaphoid and probably representing the triquetroscaphoid ligament.

R, radius, S, scaphoid, L, lunate, T, triquetrum, P, pisiform, C, capitate, H, hamate, Tm, trapezium, U, ulna.

The imaging assessment of greater and lesser arc injuries of the wrist begins with routine radiography. Routine radiographic projections, sometimes supplemented with special views, allow assessment of the integrity of the carpal arcs (see previous discussion), the presence or absence of parallelism of the carpal bones, and the presence or absence of carpal fractures. Bone scintigraphy, although sensitive to the presence of an abnormality, lacks specificity and, when employed, serves only as a screening method. Arthrography provides evidence of communicating defects in the interosseous carpal ligaments and TFCC, but the clinical significance of the findings often is unclear. Tomographic sections provided by CT scanning and MR imaging are useful in delineating malalignment among the carpal bones and associated fractures. A potential role exists for MR imaging in defining abnormalities of extrinsic ligaments of the wrist, although this role, to date, is unproved.

Dislocations about the common carpometacarpal joint are rare injuries, most typically involving the ulnar aspect of the wrist. They may be isolated to a single metacarpal[222, 223] or, more commonly, involve two or

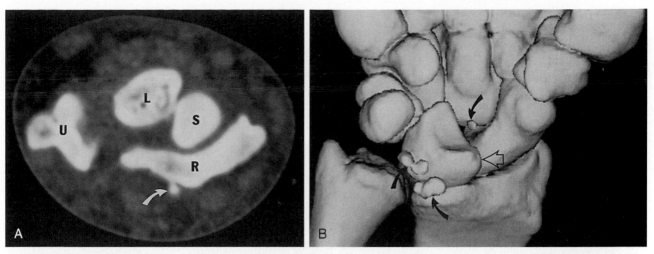

Figure 14–60
Lunate dislocation.

A A transverse CT scan at the level of this distal portion of the radius (R) shows a volarly dislocated lunate bone (L) adjacent to but not aligned with the scaphoid bone (S) and a bone fragment (arrow). U, Ulna.

B A three-dimensional CT display viewed from the volar aspect of the wrist reveals the dislocated and rotated lunate bone (open arrow) and multiple bone fragments (solid arrows).

more of the metacarpal bones.[224–227] Dorsal dislocation predominates. Radiographic abnormalities often are subtle, requiring specialized projections in addition to standard techniques.[228] CT with coronal and sagittal images also is useful. Recognized complications include injuries to the ulnar nerve (in dislocation of the metacarpohamate joint) or median nerve, rupture of extensor tendons, and fractures of one or more metacarpals. Dislocation of the first carpometacarpal joint also is infrequent and, when present, usually is combined with fractures of the base of the first metacarpal bone (Bennett's fracture-subluxation).[229] In cases of such dislocation without fracture, disruption of a volar oblique ligament extending from the trapezium to the volar aspect of the base of the first metacarpal bone sometimes is evident.

With regard to *fractures of the carpal bones,* these are observed most frequently in the scaphoid (Fig. 14–62). Fractures of the scaphoid are classified principally according to their location (proximal pole, waist, distal body, tuberosity, and distal articular), owing to the influence of the site of involvement on the likelihood of ischemic necrosis and the rate of healing.[77] In general, the prognosis of distal fractures is better than that of proximal fractures because of more rapid osseous healing and less extensive vascular interruption. The most frequent scaphoid fracture occurs in the waist (approximately 70 per cent) or proximal pole (approximately 20 per cent) of the bone, although in children, avulsion fractures of the distal portion of the scaphoid are typical and, with reportable exceptions,[230] generally heal well.[231, 232] Unusual patterns of scaphoid injury in-

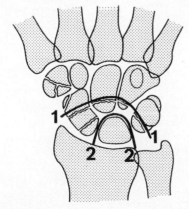

Figure 14–61
Wrist injuries: Greater and lesser arcs. The locations of the greater (1) and lesser (2) arcs are shown, as are the common sites of carpal fractures that can be produced experimentally. A pure greater arc injury consists of a transscaphoid, transcapitate, transhamate, transtriquetral fracture-dislocation; a pure lesser arc injury is a perilunate or lunate dislocation. Various combinations of these injury patterns are seen clinically. (From Johnson RP: Clin Orthop *149*:33, 1980.)

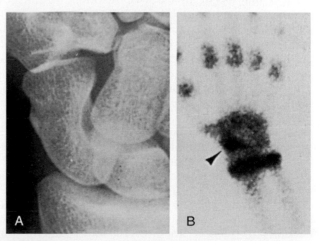

Figure 14–62
Carpal scaphoid fractures: Bone scintigraphy. In this 15 year old boy, the fracture is not evident on initial radiographic examination **(A).** It is apparent as an area of increased accumulation of the radionuclide (arrowhead) on the bone scan **(B).** (Courtesy of G. Greenway, M.D., Dallas, Texas.)

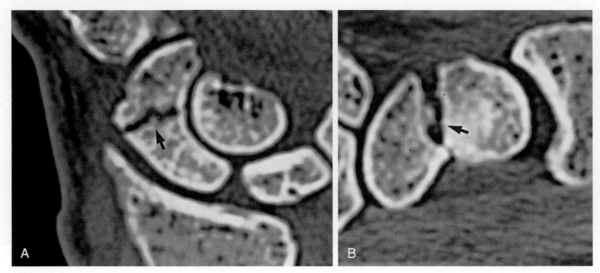

Figure 14–63
Carpal scaphoid fractures: CT scanning. Programming the CT sections along the true coronal **(A)** and longitudinal **(B)** axes of the scaphoid bone is valuable in the detection and characterization of scaphoid fractures (arrows).

clude dorsal avulsion fractures[233] and fractures of the osteochondral interface in young children.[234] In any type of fracture, accurate radiographic diagnosis depends on high quality routine and supplementary radiographs[235, 236] and even fluoroscopy, magnification radiography,[237] scintigraphy,[238–243, 420] or conventional or computed tomography.[244–248] Diagnostic difficulties arise in the detection of associated fractures or ligamentous instability[249] and in the determination of the age of the fracture when historical data are either lacking or inconclusive.[77] Older scaphoid fractures may possess sclerotic margins with adjacent cysts, although these findings are not present uniformly.

With regard to routine radiography, obliteration, distortion, or displacement of the "scaphoid fat stripe" (which is related to the common tendon sheath of the extensor pollicis brevis and the abductor pollicis longus muscles) may occur in cases of scaphoid fracture, although the diagnostic value of these changes is not clear.[250, 251] Scaphoid fractures, particularly those of the waist, generally are transverse or slightly oblique in orientation and rarely are vertical, and such fractures usually are identified most readily on posteroanterior radiographs and "scaphoid views."[252] When initial radiographs are not diagnostic, proper management is determined by the results of a careful clinical examination.[253] Dorsal tilting of the lunate simulating that occurring in dorsal segmental instability accompanies displacement of a scaphoid waist fracture.[254]

Bone scintigraphy, when performed carefully, is effective in confirming the presence or absence of an acute fracture of the scaphoid bone (see Fig. 14–62*B*). With rare exceptions, a negative examination eliminates the possibility of such a fracture. In some patients with pain in the snuff-box of the wrist after an injury, bone scintigraphy documents the presence of a fracture of a carpal bone other than the scaphoid, particularly the trapezoid or trapezium. CT scanning also can be employed in the detection of acute fractures of the scaph-

oid (or subsequent complications of these injuries). Images obtained both parallel and at right angles to the longitudinal axis of the bone are particularly helpful (Fig. 14–63). The clinical importance of MR imaging in the assessment of acute scaphoid fractures is not clear, despite the known sensitivity and specificity of the technique in the analysis of bone injuries at other sites (Figs. 14–64 and 14–65).

The time required for healing of a scaphoid fracture varies according to its location. Those in the tuberosity usually heal in 4 to 6 weeks, whereas fractures of the scaphoid waist may require 6 to 8 weeks or longer to heal.[255] The frequency of delayed union or nonunion is greatest in fractures of the proximal pole of the bone

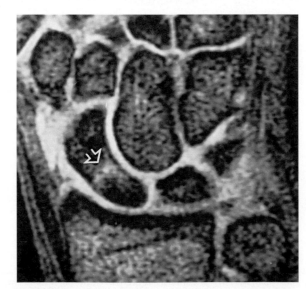

Figure 14–64
Carpal scaphoid fractures: MR imaging. This coronal MPGR MR image (TR/TE, 500/11; flip angle, 15 degrees) reveals an occult scaphoid fracture (arrow). (Courtesy of S.K. Brahme, M.D., San Diego, California.)

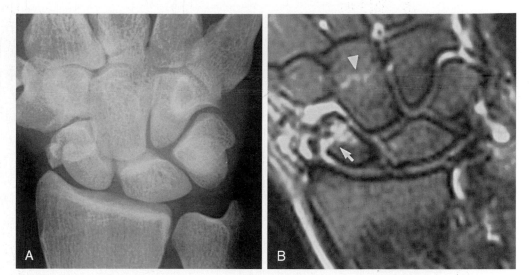

Figure 14–65

Carpal scaphoid fractures: MR imaging—Scaphocapitate syndrome. Although the routine radiograph **(A)** shows the scaphoid fracture, a coronal fat-suppressed fast spin echo MR image (TR/TE, 3500/ 102) **(B)** reveals a fracture not only of the scaphoid bone (arrow) but also of the capitate bone (arrowhead). (Courtesy of P. Kindynis, M.D., Geneva, Switzerland.)

and in those associated with displacement of the fragments.[256] Other factors contributing to delayed union or nonunion of scaphoid fractures include inadequate immobilization, interposition of soft tissue in the fracture gap, and a tenuous blood supply.[256] Routine radiography provides some information regarding the diagnosis of delayed union or nonunion, although interobserver disagreement in the interpretation of the radiographs is encountered.[255] Uncertainty regarding the presence or absence of trabeculae traversing the fracture line is common when conventional radiographs alone are analyzed. Radiographic abnormalities of scaphoid nonunion, which occur in approximately 5 to 15 per cent of cases,[257] include bone sclerosis, cyst formation, widening of the scapholunate space, bone resorption, and, subsequently, osteoarthritis.[258–262] Tendon ruptures may occur as a complication of such nonunion,[263] and CT may reveal hypertrophy of Lister's tubercle on the dorsum of the radius that may predispose to tendon disruption.[264] The frequency of ischemic necrosis after scaphoid fractures is approximately 10 to 15 per cent; this frequency rises to 30 to 40 per cent in

case of nonunion. Owing to the vascular anatomy of the scaphoid, the proximal portion of the bone is the site of osteonecrosis, with reportable exceptions.[265]

MR imaging, as a tomographic technique, shares many of the advantages of CT in the diagnosis of delayed union or nonunion of scaphoid fractures (Figs. 14–66 and 14–67). The fracture site can be identified readily, and the degree of displacement or angulation of the fracture fragments can be determined if coronal, sagittal, and transaxial images are obtained. High signal intensity in the fracture defect on T2-weighted spin echo and certain gradient echo MR images is consistent with the presence of fluid, a certain sign of fracture nonunion. Persistent low signal intensity on T1-weighted and T2-weighted spin echo MR images may indicate the presence of fibrosis at the fracture site. Marrow continuity across the fracture line represents strong evidence that fracture healing has occurred. Furthermore, with MR imaging, additional bone, ligament, and tendon injuries can be detected.

Isolated fractures of the other carpal bones are less frequent than those of the scaphoid. Triquetral fractures

Figure 14–66

Carpal scaphoid fractures: Nonunion and osteonecrosis.

A A direct coronal CT scan shows a large fracture gap with increased density of the proximal portion of the scaphoid bone.

B In a second patient, a nonunion of a scaphoid fracture is shown on a sagittal CT scan. (Courtesy of D. Goodwin, M.D., Hanover, New Hampshire.)

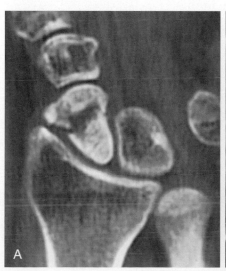
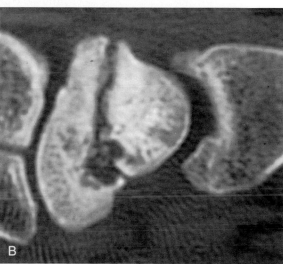

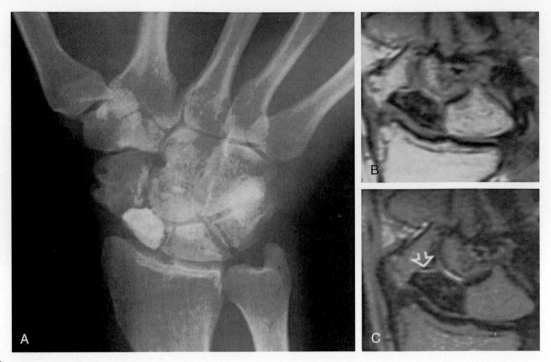

Figure 14–67
Posttraumatic osteonecrosis of the carpal scaphoid: MR imaging.

A Routine radiography reveals typical features of osteonecrosis involving the proximal pole of the bone. No evidence of bone union at the fracture site in the midportion of the scaphoid bone is evident.

B, C Coronal proton density–weighted (TR/TE, 2500/30) **(B)** and T2-weighted (TR/TE, 2500/80) **(C)** spin echo MR images document the abnormally low signal intensity of the marrow in the proximal pole of the bone. In **C**, observe fluid in the midcarpal joint with extension into the fracture gap (arrow).

represent 3 to 4 per cent of all carpal fractures.[266] It is the dorsal surface of the triquetrum that typically is fractured, related either to contact with the hamate or ulnar styloid process or to avulsion by the dorsal radiotriquetral ligaments.[267, 268] Such fractures are seen best on lateral and steep oblique projections. Fractures of the body of the triquetrum, which relate to direct blows in most cases, are rare. Avulsion fractures of the volar aspect of the triquetrum, related to the sites of attachment of the volar capsular ligaments, also are rare and easily overlooked during standard radiographic examination.[421] Isolated fractures of the lunate constitute 2 to 7 per cent of all carpal fractures.[266, 269] They may involve the dorsal or volar surfaces of the bone, representing avulsion injuries, or any portion of its body,[270] including the medial facet.[271] Fractures of the hamate represent 2 to 4 per cent of carpal fractures. Fractures of the hamate may involve any portion of the bone,[272] including the body in which coronal or sagittal fractures occur,[273–276] but those of the hook of the hamate deserve emphasis.[277–279] These latter injuries may result from a fall on the dorsiflexed wrist with a force

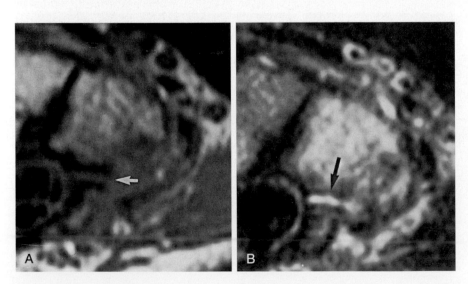

Figure 14–68
Carpal fractures: Hamate. Transverse T1-weighted (TR/TE, 850/14) spin echo **(A)** and fat-suppressed fast spin echo (TR/TE, 4883/115) **(B)** MR images show nonunion of a fracture of the hook of the hamate with fluid in the fracture gap (arrows). (Courtesy of D. Levey, M.D., Corpus Christi, Texas.)

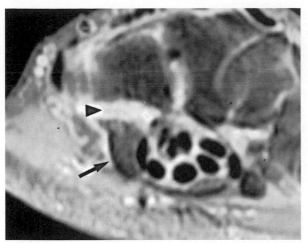

Figure 14–69
Carpal fractures: Hamate. In this patient with an acute injury, a transverse fat-suppressed fast spin echo (TR/TE, 3500/14) MR image shows a displaced fracture (arrow) of the hamate hook, with fluid (arrowhead) in the fracture gap. A rupture of the flexor digitorum profundus tendon in the fifth finger was confirmed in other images.

transmitted through the transverse carpal and pisohamate ligaments or from a direct force, such as occurs in athletes involved in sports that use racquets, bats, or clubs.[280, 281] Accurate clinical and radiographic diagnosis is difficult and specialized techniques, particularly conventional tomography, CT scanning, or MR imaging may be required (Figs. 14–68 and 14–69).[282] Complications of fractures of the hook of the hamate include nonunion,[283] osteonecrosis,[284] injuries to the ulnar or medial nerve,[285] and tendon rupture (Fig. 14–70).[286] Ulnar nerve damage also may follow fractures of the pisi-

form.[287, 288] Isolated fractures of the capitate,[289] trapezium,[290, 291] and trapezoid are infrequent. Those of the capitate (Fig. 14–71) predominate in the neck of the bone, often are combined with metacarpal fractures, and may be associated with scaphoid fractures (scaphocapitate syndrome) (Fig. 14–72). Trapezial fractures involve either the body or the palmar ridge of the bone (Fig. 14–73).[292, 293]

Osteonecrosis

Osteonecrosis of the carpal bones affects three principal sites: the lunate bone (i.e., Kienböck's disease), the scaphoid bone (particularly its proximal portion after a fracture of the waist of the bone), and less commonly, the capitate bone (typically its proximal portion either idiopathically or after an injury). Rarely, other carpal bones such as the hamate are sites of ischemic necrosis. Only the MR imaging aspects of these conditions are emphasized here.

MR imaging currently is regarded as the most sensitive and specific imaging method for the detection of osteonecrosis.[294–296] Although much of the reported data concerning this sensitivity of MR imaging relates to osteonecrosis of the femoral head, similar sensitivity certainly is expected regarding the diagnosis of ischemic necrosis in other bones, including the carpus.[111, 113, 115] Bone scintigraphy, particularly single photon emission computed tomography (SPECT), possesses similar diagnostic sensitivity in cases of osteonecrosis; however, advantages of MR imaging, which include anatomic and diagnostic specificity, tomographic display allowing analysis of the integrity of the articular surfaces, and simultaneous delineation of soft tissues, ensure its general superiority in the evaluation of osteonecrosis. The signal

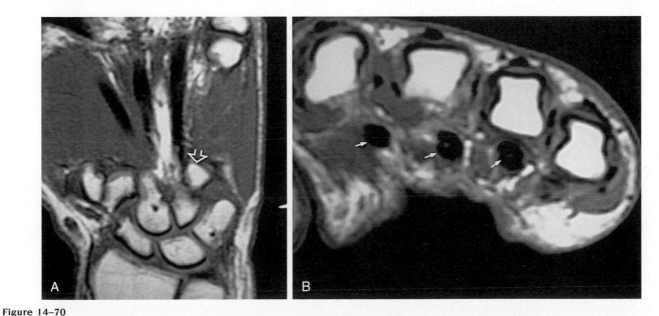

Figure 14–70
Carpal fractures: Hamate. A fracture of the hook of the hamate was associated with rupture of the flexor tendons in the fifth digit.
  A A coronal T1-weighted (TR/TE, 400/15) spin echo MR image shows displacement of the hook of the hamate (arrow), indicative of a fracture. Although the flexor digitorum tendons of the second, third, and fourth fingers are visible, those of the fifth finger are not seen.
  B A transverse T1-weighted (TR/TE, 400/15) spin echo MR image at the level of the second through fifth metacarpal heads shows intact flexor digitorum superficialis and profundus tendons in the second, third, and fourth digits (arrows) and absence of these tendons in the fifth digit.

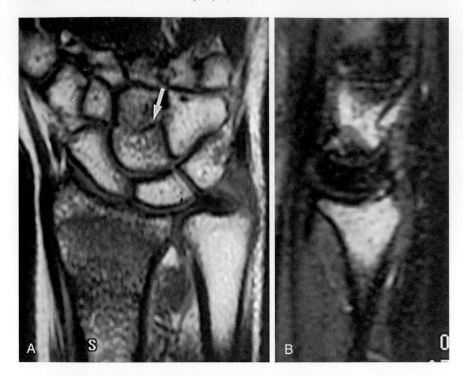

Figure 14–71

Carpal fractures: Capitate. This 18 year old woman developed an acute fracture of the capitate and a bone bruise of the distal portion of the radius after an injury. A coronal T1-weighted (TR/TE, 600/16) spin echo MR image **(A)** shows the fracture (arrow) of the capitate, with surrounding hemorrhage and edema, and a more diffuse abnormality of the radius. A sagittal fat-suppressed fast spin echo (TR/TE, 2300/42) MR image **(B)** reveals high signal intensity in these same regions. (Courtesy of D. Berthoty, M.D., Las Vegas, Nevada.)

intensity characteristics of the infarcted zone that have been used to judge the severity and ultimate prognosis of osteonecrosis of the femoral head have not been tested yet in instances of carpal osteonecrosis.[422]

MR imaging in case of Kienböck's disease (Figs. 14–74 and 14–75) is superior in diagnostic sensitivity when compared with routine radiography and, in some cases, bone scintigraphy.[297–299] The diagnostic specificity of MR imaging in Kienböck's disease is high. In instances in which the entire lunate is affected with or without bone collapse, the imaging pattern is almost specific, particu-larly when adjacent bones, including the distal portion of the radius, are not affected and a negative (minus) ulnar variance also is observed. MR imaging is less specific when only a portion of the lunate is involved, as other conditions such as an intraosseous ganglion may lead to similar alterations. A radiocarpal joint effusion and adjacent synovial inflammation may accompany Kienböck's disease and, in such cases, the improper diagnosis of a systemic articular disease such as rheumatoid arthritis may be offered. On T1-weighted spin echo MR images, the typical appearance of Kienböck's disease is that of diffuse or focal regions of low signal intensity; on T2-weighted spin echo MR images, regions of low or high signal intensity within portions of the lunate are seen. These regions may correspond not only to sites of bone necrosis and reactive granulation tissue but also to areas of surrounding marrow edema. Therefore, an overestimation of the extent of bone necrosis is possible on the basis of the distribution of marrow abnormalities

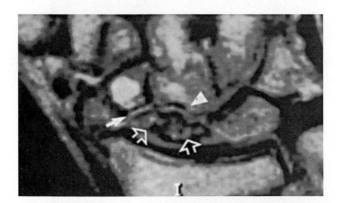

Figure 14–72

Carpal fractures: Scaphocapitate syndrome. This patient had a fracture of the midportion of the scaphoid bone and of the proximal portion of the capitate bone (scaphocapitate syndrome) that was followed by osteonecrosis at both sites. A coronal proton density–weighted (TR/TE, 2000/35) spin echo MR image reveals nonunion of the scaphoid fracture (solid arrow) with osteonecrosis of its proximal pole (open arrows) manifest as decreased size, an irregular contour, and low signal intensity. The proximal pole of the capitate bone (arrowhead) also is irregular, and cystic lesions in the capitate bone and distal portion of the scaphoid are manifested as regions of high signal intensity.

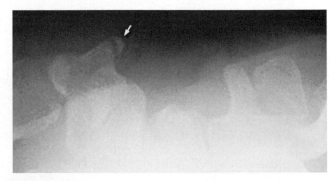

Figure 14–73

Carpal fractures: Trapezium. A fracture of the palmar ridge (arrow) of the trapezium, shown in a carpal tunnel projection, simulated a scaphoid fracture on clinical examination.

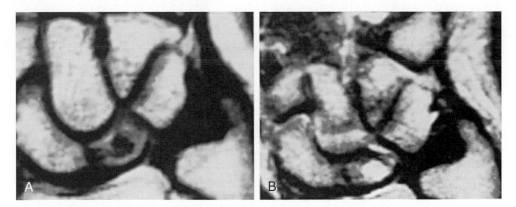

Figure 14–74
Kienböck's disease: MR imaging.

A The coronal T1-weighted (TR/TE, 600/20) spin echo MR image demonstrates a central region of low signal intensity in the lunate, and the remaining marrow in this bone is inhomogeneous in signal intensity.

B With T2 weighting (TR/TE, 1700/80), the central region now demonstrates hyperintensity, and the remaining marrow in the lunate shows regions of high and low signal intensity. The findings are consistent with osteonecrosis, although alternative diagnoses, such as an intraosseous ganglion, could be considered.

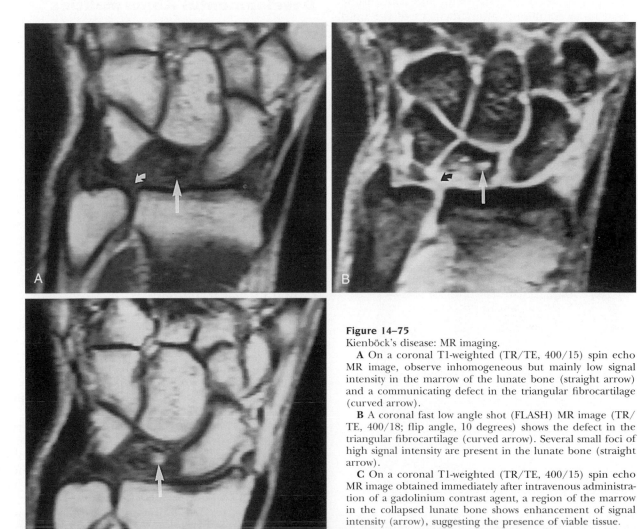

Figure 14–75
Kienböck's disease: MR imaging.

A On a coronal T1-weighted (TR/TE, 400/15) spin echo MR image, observe inhomogeneous but mainly low signal intensity in the marrow of the lunate bone (straight arrow) and a communicating defect in the triangular fibrocartilage (curved arrow).

B A coronal fast low angle shot (FLASH) MR image (TR/TE, 400/18; flip angle, 10 degrees) shows the defect in the triangular fibrocartilage (curved arrow). Several small foci of high signal intensity are present in the lunate bone (straight arrow).

C On a coronal T1-weighted (TR/TE, 400/15) spin echo MR image obtained immediately after intravenous administration of a gadolinium contrast agent, a region of the marrow in the collapsed lunate bone shows enhancement of signal intensity (arrow), suggesting the presence of viable tissue.

delineated with MR imaging. This overestimation of the disease process may be accentuated on STIR MR images. The extent of collapse of the lunate bone in Kienböck's disease varies and can be defined precisely by conventional tomography, CT, or MR imaging. The sagittal plane is especially valuable in delineating the degree of bone collapse and, with MR imaging, sagittal sections also can reveal the relationship of the elongated and fragmented lunate bone to the flexor tendons. The extent of bone collapse, when combined with other factors such as rotation of the scaphoid bone, proximal migration of the capitate bone, and osteoarthritis of the radiocarpal joint, has been used to stage the disease and influences the choice of a therapeutic option. These options include immobilization alone, radial shortening or lunate revascularization procedures, scaphocapitate or triscaphe fusion, wrist arthrodesis, and proximal row carpectomy.

Osteonecrosis of the scaphoid bone is an important complication of its fracture (see previous discussion). Almost universally, posttraumatic osteonecrosis involves the proximal portion of the scaphoid, and this finding is observed most commonly after fractures of the waist or proximal pole of the bone. Routine radiography eventually will reveal regions of increased density and cyst formation within the necrotic zone, but scintigraphic and MR imaging abnormalities will antedate the radiographic findings. Both of these last two imaging methods are sensitive in the diagnosis of scaphoid osteonecrosis, although the specificity of MR imaging is greater (Figs. 14–76 and 14–77). Osteonecrosis of the scaphoid bone also may occur secondary to corticosteroid medication and, rarely, on an idiopathic basis. A type of idiopathic osteonecrosis of the scaphoid bone has been described in which the proximal pole of the bone is affected, a positive ulnar variance is common, and interference of blood supply to the bone through the scapholunate interosseous ligament may be a causative factor.[300]

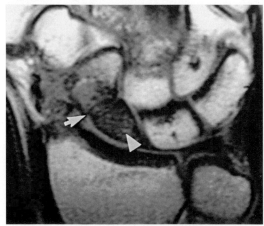

Figure 14–76
Osteonecrosis of the scaphoid bone after a fracture. A coronal T1-weighted (TR/TE, 583/20) spin echo MR image shows the site (arrow) of a previous fracture of the midportion of the scaphoid bone. Note the low signal intensity in the proximal pole of the scaphoid bone (arrowhead). (Courtesy of S. Eilenberg, M.D., San Diego, California.)

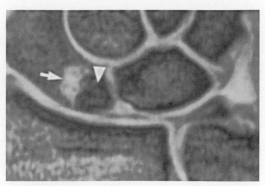

Figure 14–77
Osteonecrosis and cyst formation of the scaphoid bone after fracture. A coronal MPGR MR image (TR/TE, 200/15; flip angle, 25 degrees) shows a cyst (arrow) occurring adjacent to a fracture line in the scaphoid bone, with altered signal intensity in the proximal pole of the scaphoid bone (arrowhead) secondary to osteonecrosis. Note the normal appearance of the triangular fibrocartilage and the scapholunate and lunotriquetral interosseous ligaments.

Developmental Abnormalities

Carpal Boss (Os Styloideum)

A commonly occurring bony protuberance on the dorsum of the wrist at the base of the second and third metacarpal bones adjacent to the capitate and trapezoid is termed a carpal boss or carpe bossu.[301–306] It relates to either an osteophyte or an accessory ossification center, the os styloideum. Although generally asymptomatic or associated only with a lump or bump, the carpal boss occasionally can lead to pain and limitation of hand motion owing to an overlying ganglion, bursitis, osteoarthritis, or slippage of an extensor tendon.[304] Radiographs obtained with 30 degrees of supination and ulnar deviation of the wrist demonstrate the osteophyte or os styloideum to good advantage[304] and may be supplemented with bone scintigraphy, conventional tomography, ultrasonography, or CT scanning (Fig. 14–78).

Carpal Fusion (Coalition)

Carpal fusion or coalition is a relatively common abnormality that may occur as an isolated phenomenon or as part of a generalized congenital malformation syndrome. As a rule, isolated fusions involve bones in the same carpal row (proximal or distal), whereas syndrome-related fusions may affect bones in different rows (proximal and distal).[307, 308]

The most common site of the isolated fusion is between the triquetrum and the lunate bones; in this location the fusion occurs in 0.1 to 1.6 per cent of the general population, more frequently in men and in blacks,[309] and has little or no clinical significance (Fig. 14–79).[310] The fusion is bilateral in approximately 60 per cent of cases.[311] Widening of the scapholunate interosseous space is a frequent finding in cases of lunotriquetral fusion, although the scapholunate interosseous ligament generally is intact. Less common isolated coalitions that may be encountered include capitate-hamate fusion,[312] trapezium-trapezoid fusion, and pisi-

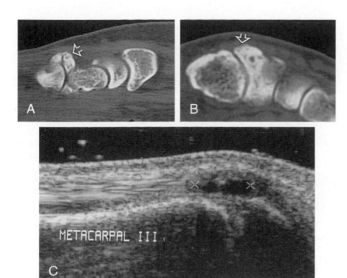

Figure 14–78

Carpal boss (os styloideum).

A, B Sagittal **(A)** and transverse **(B)** CT scans show a typical carpal boss (arrows) partially fused to the capitate and third metacarpal bones. (Courtesy of S.K. Brahme, M.D., San Diego, California.)

C In a second patient, a sonogram of the dorsal aspect of the wrist in the sagittal plane demonstrates anechoic bursal fluid ("X" markers) superficial to the third carpometacarpal joint. The underlying bone abnormality is not well seen in this image. (Courtesy of M. van Holsbeeck, M.D., Detroit, Michigan, and J. Jacobson, M.D., San Diego, California.)

form-hamate fusion.[313, 314] In fact, isolated fusions have been described in almost all possible combinations,[315] including those affecting more than two bones.[316] The presence and exact location of coalition are not always easy to identify on radiographic examination. This difficulty relates to the partial or incomplete nature of the ankylosis in some cases, the need for multiple projections because of the obliquity of the osseous surfaces of the normal carpal bones, and the requirement that congenital and acquired coalition must be dif-

ferentiated. In most cases, symptoms and signs are entirely lacking, although pain has been noted in some cases,[317] especially in association with partial or nonosseous fusions and cystic changes in the adjacent bones (Fig. 14–80),[318–320] and a definite risk of fracture exists in the presence of a fused carpus.[321, 322]

The anomaly develops from a failure of segmentation of the primitive cartilaginous canals and absence of joint formation.[312, 323] The osseous centers of the involved carpus coalesce at variable ages, usually between 6 and 15 years of age. On radiographs, continuous trabeculae can be traced from one bone to the next, although a small notch or cleft may remain at the site of fusion. Discrete intraosseous cysts adjacent to the area of coalition sometimes are seen. The changes usually can be differentiated from acquired ankylosis that may accompany infection, certain arthritides (such as juvenile chronic arthritis and rheumatoid arthritis), trauma, and surgery.

Madelung's Deformity

This painful wrist deformity is characterized by bowing of the distal end of the radius.[324–330] Typically, the radial bowing occurs in a volar direction while the ulna continues to grow in a straight fashion. The curvature and growth disturbance of the radius result in its being shorter than the ulna. The carpal angle, which normally is 130 to 137 degrees, is decreased.[331, 332]

Madelung's deformity has been classified into several types, including posttraumatic (due to extension injuries to the radial epiphysis), dysplastic (due to dyschondrosteosis and multiple hereditary exostoses), genetic (in association with Turner's syndrome), and idiopathic.[330] This classification system is complicated by the fact that the wrist abnormality in some of these conditions is not a typical Madelung's deformity but rather is a "reverse" deformity in which the distal end of the radius is tilted dorsally, the carpus is shifted dorsally, and the distal end of the ulna appears to be dislocated anteriorly.[333]

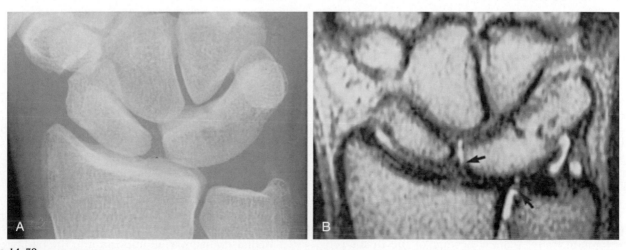

Figure 14–79

Carpal fusion (coalition): MR imaging. On a routine radiograph **(A),** note a solid bony lunotriquetral coalition and a widened scapholunate interosseous space. A coronal T2-weighted (TR/TE, 1000/80) spin echo MR image **(B)** shows fluid of high signal intensity (arrows) that outlines defects in the scapholunate interosseous ligament and triangular fibrocartilage. Usually, in such cases, the scapholunate interosseous ligament is intact.

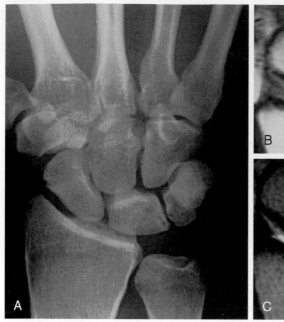

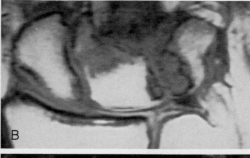

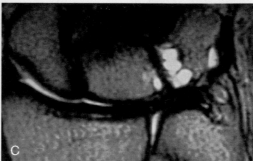

Figure 14–80

Carpal fusion (coalition): MR imaging. In this 46 year old man with ulnar-sided wrist pain, a routine radiograph (**A**) reveals narrowing and irregularity of the lunotriquetral interosseous space, indicative of a nonosseous coalition. On coronal T1-weighted (TR/TE, 500/15) (**B**) and T2-weighted (TR/TE, 3200/120) (**C**) spin echo MR images, abnormalities of signal intensity (low signal intensity in **B** and high signal intensity in **C**) in the marrow of the lunate and triquetrum about the fusion are evident. Fluid is evident in the radiocarpal and inferior radioulnar joints.

The isolated variety of Madelung's deformity is more commonly bilateral than unilateral, is asymmetric, and, if not restricted to women, is at least three to five times more common in female patients. Clinical manifestations usually become evident in the adolescent or young adult, in whom visible deformity, pain, fatigue, and limited range of motion, especially dorsal extension, ulnar deviation, and supination, are noted. The carpal tunnel syndrome may be evident.[334] Rarely, spontaneous rupture of extensor tendons may occur.[335]

Carpal and Ulnar Tunnel Abnormalities

Carpal Tunnel Syndrome

As indicated in Chapter 11, the carpal tunnel syndrome is a relatively common entrapment neuropathy affecting the median nerve within the carpal tunnel in the palmar aspect of the wrist (Fig. 14–81). In most cases, accurate diagnosis based on clinical history and the results of physical examination and electromyographic studies is straightforward. Diagnostic imaging plays a minor role in the assessment of the carpal tunnel syndrome. Ultrasonography, CT, and MR imaging have been used for this purpose.[111, 113, 115, 336–339] The MR imaging findings of the carpal tunnel syndrome have been delineated in detail by Mesgarzadeh and coworkers,[340] who emphasize four consistent findings: swelling of the median nerve, best evaluated at the level of the pisiform bone; flattening of the median nerve, best evaluated at the level of the hamate bone; palmar bowing of the flexor retinaculum, best evaluated at the level of the hamate bone; and increased signal intensity of the median nerve on T2-weighted spin echo images (Figs. 14–82 and 14–83). The pattern of enlargement of the median nerve varies, however; the nerve may be diffusely or focally enlarged,

especially at the level of the pisiform bone.[339] Focal enlargement of the median nerve at this latter level may result in a nerve that is two to three times larger than at the level of the distal portion of the radius. Thus, careful assessment of the size of the median nerve on transaxial images, extending from the region of the distal end of the radius to that of the pisiform bone, is required for accurate diagnosis and, indeed, the use of ratios of nerve size at various levels of the wrist may aid in this diagnosis.[21, 340] The ratio of the cross-sectional area of the median nerve at the pisiform level divided by that at the level of the distal end of the radius is approximately 1 in normal persons, whereas in those with the carpal tunnel syndrome it may be greater than 2. As the median nerve may appear flattened at the level of the hamate bone in patients with the carpal tunnel syndrome, using this region as a site for measuring the cross-sectional area of the median nerve in ratio calculations may be misleading diagnostically. Although quantitative analysis of the size of the median nerve on MR images at various levels of the wrist is a complicated process and one not commonly employed in clinical practice, swelling of the median nerve at the level of the pisiform bone and compression of the median nerve at the level of the hamate bone can be judged qualitatively, and these remain important observations in diagnosis of the carpal tunnel syndrome. Similarly, increased signal intensity in the medial nerve on T2-weighted spin echo and gradient echo MR images is a valuable diagnostic sign that may be apparent at multiple levels of the wrist. Although such increased signal intensity may extend as far distally as the base of the metacarpal bones, it rarely extends proximal to the distal radioulnar joint.

Vascular events may be important in the pathogenesis of the carpal tunnel syndrome, suggesting a potential role for gadolinium-enhanced MR imaging in its diagnosis in some patients. In one study, intravenous administration of a gadolinium compound and positioning the wrist in neutral, flexed, and extended positions were

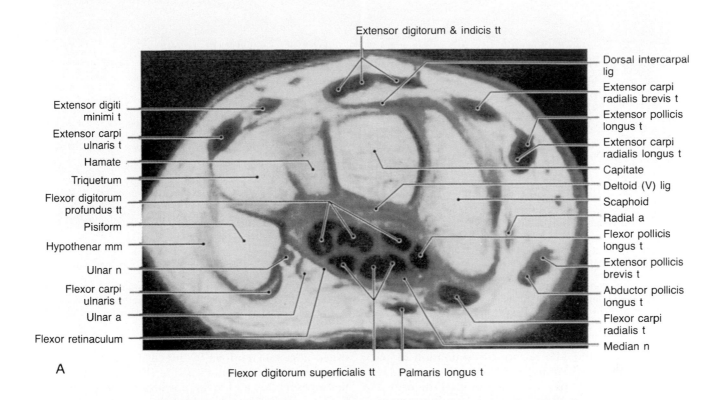

Extensor digitorum & indicis tt

Extensor digiti minimi t

Extensor carpi ulnaris t

Hamate

Triquetrum

Flexor digitorum profundus tt

Pisiform

Hypothenar mm

Ulnar n

Flexor carpi ulnaris t

Ulnar a

Flexor retinaculum

Dorsal intercarpal lig

Extensor carpi radialis brevis t

Extensor pollicis longus t

Extensor carpi radialis longus t

Capitate

Deltoid (V) lig

Scaphoid

Radial a

Flexor pollicis longus t

Extensor pollicis brevis t

Abductor pollicis longus t

Flexor carpi radialis t

Median n

A

Flexor digitorum superficialis tt   Palmaris longus t

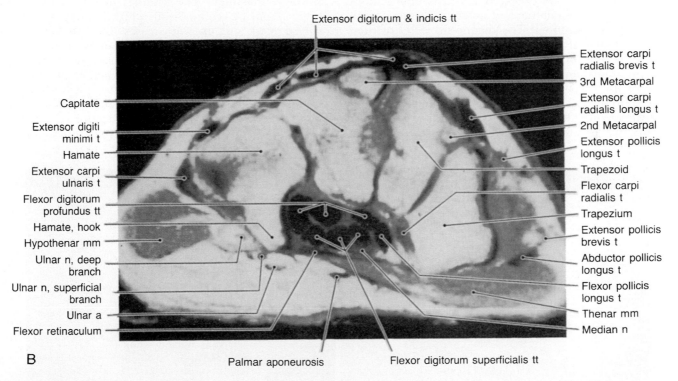

Extensor digitorum & indicis tt

Capitate

Extensor digiti minimi t

Hamate

Extensor carpi ulnaris t

Flexor digitorum profundus tt

Hamate, hook

Hypothenar mm

Ulnar n, deep branch

Ulnar n, superficial branch

Ulnar a

Flexor retinaculum

Extensor carpi radialis brevis t

3rd Metacarpal

Extensor carpi radialis longus t

2nd Metacarpal

Extensor pollicis longus t

Trapezoid

Flexor carpi radialis t

Trapezium

Extensor pollicis brevis t

Abductor pollicis longus t

Flexor pollicis longus t

Thenar mm

Median n

B

Palmar aponeurosis   Flexor digitorum superficialis tt

Figure 14–81

Normal carpal tunnel: MR imaging.

A Transaxial T1-weighted (TR/TE, 600/20) spin echo MR image of the wrist at the level of the pisiform bone.

B Transaxial T1-weighted (TR/TE, 600/20) spin echo MR image of the wrist at the level of the hook of the hamate bone.

(From Kang HS, Resnick D: MRI of the Extremities: An Anatomic Atlas. Philadelphia, WB Saunders Co, 1991.)

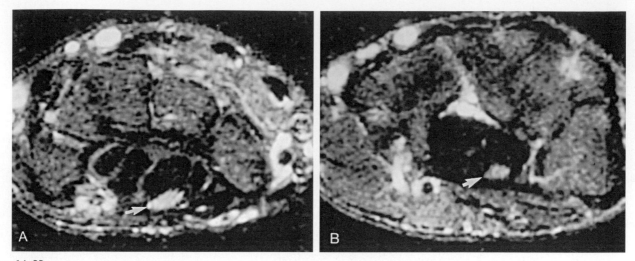

Figure 14–82
Carpal tunnel syndrome: MR imaging.

A Transaxial T2-weighted (TR/TE, 3000/66) fat-suppressed fast spin echo MR image of the wrist at the level of the pisiform bone. Note the diffuse enlargement of and increased signal intensity in the median nerve (arrow).

B Transaxial T2-weighted (TR/TE, 3000/66) fat-suppressed fast spin echo MR image of the wrist at the level of the hook of the hamate bone. Although the signal intensity in the median nerve (arrow) is increased, the nerve is smaller at this level than at the level of the pisiform bone.

(Courtesy of M. Schweitzer, M.D., Philadelphia, Pennsylvania.)

employed during the MR imaging examination of patients with the carpal tunnel syndrome. Two distinctly abnormal patterns of enhancement of signal intensity in the median nerve were observed: marked enhancement, attributed to nerve edema; and no enhancement, attributed to nerve ischemia. The diagnostic value of these supplementary MR techniques requires further analysis.

Inflammation of the flexor tendon sheaths is considered an important and, perhaps, the most common cause of the carpal tunnel syndrome, based mainly on surgical findings. The MR imaging abnormalities of such tenosynovitis include enlargement of individual tendon sheaths due to effusions and increased separation be-

tween adjacent tendons in the carpal tunnel, increased signal intensity resulting from fluid in the enlarged tendon sheaths, and volar bowing, or convexity, of the flexor retinaculum. The findings may be subtle, however, requiring comparison with the opposite uninvolved wrist and, in some cases, the intravenous administration of gadolinium compounds. Tenosynovitis resulting from rheumatoid arthritis, gout, calcium pyrophosphate dihydrate crystal deposition disease, and other systemic articular disorders generally leads to similar MR imaging findings, although additional bone and joint alterations may be evident. Regions of persistent low signal intensity within the carpal tunnel on T2-

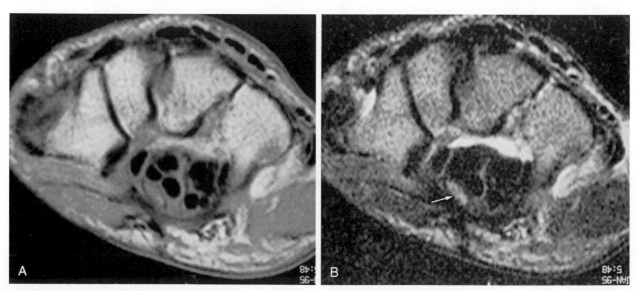

Figure 14–83
Carpal tunnel syndrome: MR imaging. Transverse proton density–weighted (TR/TE, 1800/20) **(A)** and T2-weighted (TR/TE, 1800/80) **(B)** spin echo MR images in a patient with clinical evidence of severe carpal tunnel syndrome show bowing of the flexor retinaculum, fluid dorsal to the flexor tendons and sheaths, and increased signal intensity of the median nerve (arrow) in **B.**

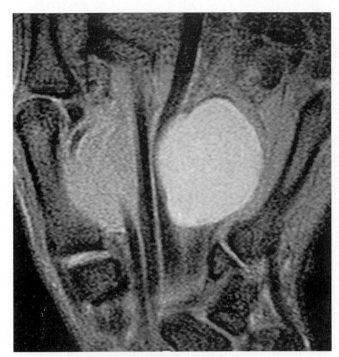

Figure 14–84
Carpal tunnel syndrome: MR imaging. A large neurofibroma involving the carpal tunnel and displacing the flexor tendons is shown in a coronal MPGR (TR/TE, 800/13; flip angle, 20 degrees) MR image. (Courtesy of A.O. Motta, M.D., Cleveland, Ohio.)

weighted spin echo and gradient echo MR images may be encountered in patients with gout or amyloidosis (primary or secondary to long-term hemodialysis). MR imaging findings accompanying some tumors in the carpal tunnel (Fig. 14–84) are diagnostic. One such lesion is fibrolipomatous hamartoma,[341–342, 423] in which gross enlargement of the median nerve (or other nerves) is caused by fatty and fibrous infiltration. Macrodactyly may be an associated finding. On MR images, the documentation of fat in and around the involved nerve permits accurate diagnosis, allowing differentiation from other lesions, including neurofibromatosis (Fig. 14–85).

The role of MR imaging in the evaluation of persistent or recurrent carpal tunnel syndrome after carpal tunnel release is not clear yet. Typically, such release, which may be done operatively or endoscopically, is accomplished by dividing the transverse carpal ligament (flexor retinaculum) near its ulnar insertion on the hook of the hamate. After such surgery, incomplete visualization or palmar displacement of the transverse carpal ligament is evident, and the contents of the carpal tunnel also are displaced volarly.[340] Potential MR imaging findings associated with persistent or recurrent carpal tunnel syndrome after such surgery are incomplete resection of the transverse carpal ligament, scar formation associated with low signal intensity about the incised flexor retinaculum, and persistent or recurrent flexor tenosynovitis (Fig. 14–86).

As in other regions of the body, the differentiation of fluid, which may indicate significant inflammatory disease, and fat within the carpal tunnel on the basis of

findings on standard MR imaging sequences may be difficult. Chemical presaturation of fat with or without prior intravenous injection of gadolinium compounds or STIR MR imaging sequences may be useful in this differentiation.

Ulnar Tunnel Syndrome

Compression of the ulnar nerve as it courses through the ulnar tunnel, or Guyon's canal, in the volar aspect of the wrist is well recognized (see Chapter 11). Causes of such entrapment include masses (e.g., tumors and ganglion cysts), vascular injury (e.g., aneurysms or thrombosis of the ulnar artery) (Fig. 14–87), anatomic variations (e.g., presence of abductor digiti minimi muscles within the canal), muscle hypertrophy (e.g., enlargement of the palmaris brevis muscle), fractures (e.g., fractures of the hook of the hamate bone or the pisiform bone), and hypertrophy of the transverse carpal ligament.[23] Although the MR imaging abnormalities associated with the ulnar tunnel syndrome are not well documented, findings similar to those of the carpal tunnel syndrome are likely.

Abnormalities of the Extensor and Flexor Tendons and Tendon Sheaths

Tendinitis and Tenosynovitis

Inflammation may affect either the extensor tendons and sheaths (Fig. 14–88) or the flexor tendons and sheaths, or both. De Quervain's syndrome (Fig. 14–89) relates to tendinitis and tenosynovitis affecting the abductor pollicis longus and extensor brevis tendons and sheaths in the first extensor compartment. Persons involved in sporting activities that require repetitive ulnar deviation of the wrist are susceptible to development of this syndrome. Involvement occurs at the level of or just proximal to the styloid process of the radius. On physical examination, ulnar deviation of the wrist with the thumb fully adducted, the Finkelstein test, produces pain.[343] MR imaging findings include increased thickness of the involved tendons, tenosynovial fluid, and surrounding soft tissue edema.[424] If conservative treatment of this syndrome is not effective, surgical release with decompression of the slips of the involved tendons may be required.

Inflammation of the flexor carpi ulnaris and flexor carpi radialis tendons (Fig. 14–90) is common, leading to local pain and swelling. The flexor carpi radialis tendon occupies a narrow fibro-osseous tunnel at the level of the crest of the trapezium.[344] At this level, tendinitis may develop as a primary process or secondary to fractures of the scaphoid bone, to osteoarthritis of the first carpometacarpal joint or trapezioscaphoid joint, or to both. In some cases, surgical decompression of the tendon in this tunnel may be required, with operative findings including adhesions, tendon attrition or rupture, an anomalous tendon, osteophytes, or a ganglion cyst.[345] Similarly, involvement of the extensor carpi ul-

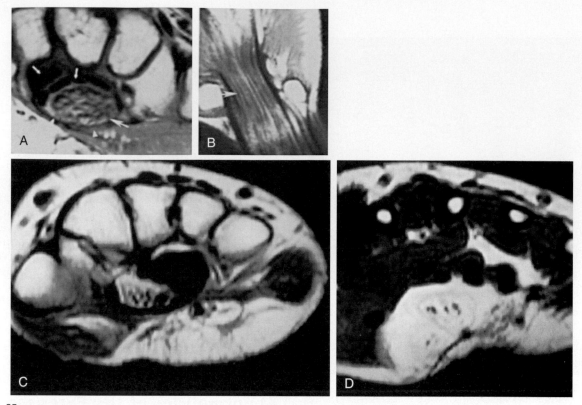

Figure 14–85

Carpal tunnel syndrome related to fibrolipomatous hamartoma of the median nerve: MR imaging.

A Transaxial T1-weighted (TR/TE, 500/15) spin echo MR image of the wrist at the level of the base of the first metacarpal bone shows a large mass (large arrow) of the median nerve that has led to dorsal displacement of the flexor tendons (small arrows) and volar bowing of the flexor retinaculum (arrowheads). Note the inhomogeneous signal intensity of the tumor, resulting from its fibrous and fatty components.

B Coronal T1-weighted (TR/TE, 500/15) spin echo MR image of the volar aspect of the wrist in the same patient shows a mass (arrow) composed of longitudinally oriented cylindrical regions of low and high signal intensity.

C, D In a young woman with a volar mass and findings of a carpal tunnel syndrome, transverse T1-weighted (TR/TE, 600/15) spin echo MR images at the levels of the proximal (**C**) and distal (**D**) portions of the metacarpal bones show enlargement of the median nerve in **C** with signal intensity characteristics compatible with fibrofatty tissue. In **D**, the abnormal tissue extends into the palm. (Courtesy of G. Bock, M.D., Winnipeg, Manitoba, Canada.)

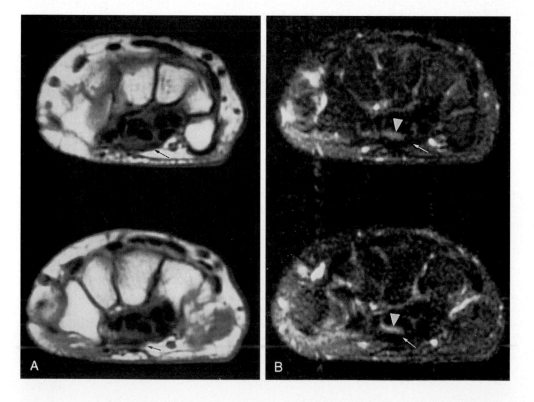

Figure 14–86

Recurrent carpal tunnel syndrome: MR imaging. Transaxial T1-weighted (TR/TE, 600/14) (**A**) and fat-suppressed T2-weighted (TR/TE, 1800/82) (**B**) spin echo MR images are shown. The upper images in **A** and **B** are located at the level of the pisiform bone, and the lower images are close to the level of the hook of the hamate bone. A curvilinear region of low signal intensity (arrows) represents either an inadequately resected transverse ligament or scar tissue. In **B**, the median nerve is flattened and is of high signal intensity (arrowheads). Tenosynovitis also is present. (Courtesy of S.K. Brahme, M.D., San Diego, California.)

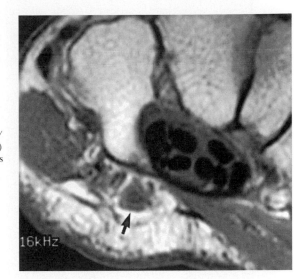

Figure 14–87
Ulnar tunnel syndrome: MR imaging. This transaxial T1-weighted (TR/TE, 600/18) spin echo MR image reveals an enlarged and irregular ulnar artery (arrow) adjacent to the hook of the hamate bone, findings that related to a thrombus within the artery.

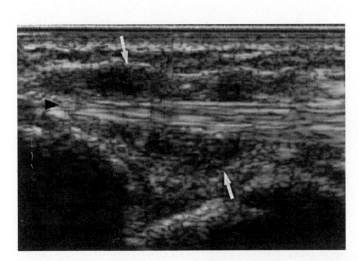

Figure 14–88
Tenosynovitis of the extensor tendon sheaths: Ultrasonography. Tenosynovitis on the dorsal surface of the wrist related to sarcoidosis is seen on a sagittal sonogram as a collection of anechoic fluid (arrows) surrounding the hyperechoic tendon (arrowhead). (Courtesy of M. van Holsbeeck, M.D., Detroit, Michigan, and J. Jacobson, M.D., San Diego, California.)

Figure 14–89
De Quervain's tenosynovitis: MR imaging. On a T1-weighted spin echo MR image **(A)**, a soft tissue mass of low signal intensity is seen adjacent to the radial styloid process. After intravenous administration of a gadolinium compound, a fat-suppressed T1-weighted spin echo MR image **(B)** shows high signal intensity indicative of tenosynovitis. (Courtesy of S.K. Brahme, M.D., San Diego, California.)

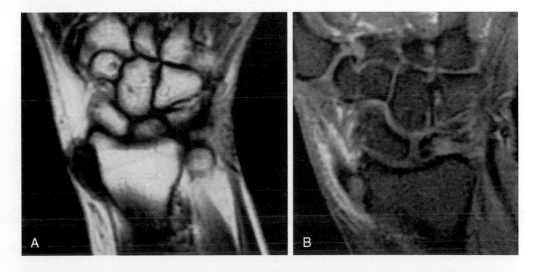

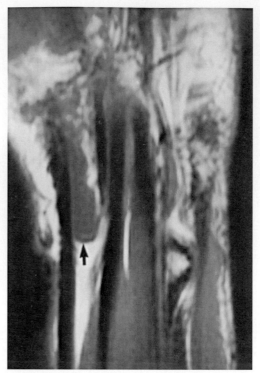

Figure 14–90
Tenosynovitis of the flexor carpi radialis tendon sheath: MR imaging. A coronal T1-weighted (TR/TE, 600/14) spin echo MR image of the volar aspect of the wrist shows the enlarged tendon sheath (arrow) containing fluid or inflammatory tissue.

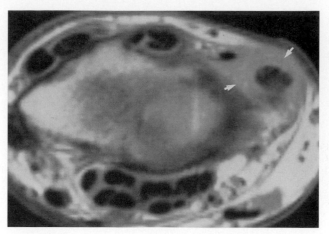

Figure 14–91
Tenosynovitis of the extensor carpi ulnaris tendon sheath: MR imaging. Transaxial T1-weighted (TR/TE, 600/20) spin echo MR image of the wrist at the level of the radiocarpal joint shows fluid of intermediate signal intensity (arrows) about the extensor carpi ulnaris tendon in the sixth extensor compartment. (Courtesy of S.K. Brahme, M.D., San Diego, California.)

naris tendon and sheath in the sixth extensor compartment at the level of the distal portion and styloid process of the ulna may be evident (Fig. 14–91). Furthermore, subluxation of the extensor carpi ulnaris tendon may occur, leading to pain and a snap during pronation and supination of the forearm.[346] Pain developing where the abductor pollicis longus and extensor pollicis brevis tendons pass over the extensor tendons, seen in canoeists and weightlifters, is termed the intersection syndrome.[29]

The MR imaging abnormalities of tendinitis and tenosynovitis include enlargement of its sheath owing to the accumulation of fluid (Fig. 14–92). Although the findings usually are quite apparent, misdiagnosis is possible owing to the magic angle phenomenon.[347, 348] This phenomenon results from variations in the T2 times of poorly hydrated tissues, such as tendons, related to their orientation with the magnetic field. T2 augmentation of tendons (and other structures) is maximum at the magic angle, in which the tendon orientation is 55 degrees with respect to the orientation of the main magnetic field, and such augmentation decreases proportionately with orientation angles greater or less than 55 degrees. The resulting increase signal intensity within the tendon is evident only when short (e.g., 10 to 25 msec) echo times (TE) are employed, and it is not apparent when the tendon is parallel to the main magnetic field. Portions of the extensor tendons of the wrist (as well as the tendons about the shoulder and ankle) are oriented at or close to the magic angle.[348] Thus, increased signal intensity within such tendons on short TE MR imaging sequences (i.e., routine T1-weighted

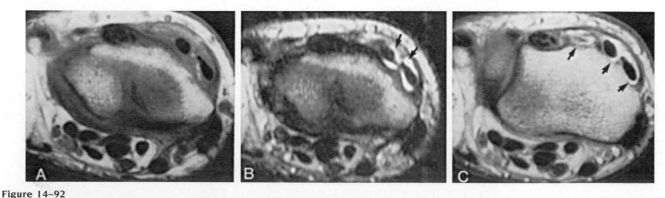

Figure 14–92
Tenosynovitis of the tendon sheaths of the extensor pollicis longus and the extensor carpi radialis brevis and longus tendons: MR imaging. Transaxial T1-weighted (TR/TE, 700/17) **(A)** and T2-weighted (TR/TE, 2000/80) **(B)** spin echo MR images and a transaxial T1-weighted (TR/TE, 650/20) spin echo MR image after the intravenous administration of gadolinium compound **(C)** show the enlarged tendon sheaths. The high signal intensity (arrows) in **B** and **C** is consistent with the presence of synovial inflammatory tissue.

and proton density–weighted spin echo sequences) should not be misinterpreted as evidence of tendinitis or tendon degeneration. The magic angle effect disappears on long TE MR imaging sequences (i.e., T2-weighted spin echo sequences).

In common with MR imaging of tendons at other anatomic sites, ME imaging of those in the wrist and hand is associated with other diagnostic difficulties. For example, few data exist regarding the amount of fluid in the tendon sheaths that would indicate a clinically significant abnormality.[436] The detection of small collections of tenosynovial fluid is not diagnostic of inflammation. Furthermore, differentiation of tenosynovial fluid and an enlarged tendon is difficult on the basis of findings on T1-weighted spin echo MR images. The benefits of MR imaging relative to ultrasonography in the evaluation of tendinitis and tenosynovitis also are not clear.

Infective tenosynovitis and bursitis of the hand and wrist deserve special emphasis. A variety of microorganisms, including bacterial, mycobacterial, and fungal species, may cause infection of flexor and extensor tendons and tendon sheaths as well as of the radial and ulnar bursae in the volar aspect of the wrist. Indeed, tuberculosis represents an important cause of such infection.[425] Either ultrasonography or MR imaging can be used as an effective means of delineating the extent of soft tissue involvement (Figs. 14–93 to 14–95), although the clinical necessity of these techniques is not certain.

Tendon Injury

Any of the extensor or flexor tendons of the wrist or fingers can rupture as a response to an acute injury or

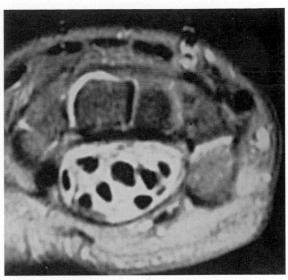

Figure 14–94

Infective tenosynovitis: Flexor tendons of wrist. A transverse fat-suppressed fast spin echo (TR/TE, 4000/19) MR image shows tenosynovial fluid of high signal intensity in the carpal tunnel (at the level of the pisiform bone). Bowing of the flexor retinaculum is evident. Tuberculosis was the cause of this infection. (Courtesy of K. Hoffman, M.D., Stanford, California.)

chronic inflammation as in rheumatoid arthritis. Interruption of the tendon and surrounding fluid or inflammatory tissue are the findings noted on MR images (Fig. 14–96).[349] The degree of tendon retraction and the distance between the torn ends of the tendon can be determined.[73] Classic examples of tendon ruptures in the hand include the mallet finger, in which a flexion deformity of the distal interphalangeal joint results from loss of continuity of the extensor tendon; avulsion of the flexor digitorum profundus tendon at its insertion into the base of the distal phalanx; and the boutonnière deformity, caused by disruption of the central slip of the extensor tendon combined with tearing of the triangular ligament on the dorsum of the middle phalanx.

Injuries involving the flexor tendons of the fingers are varied and complex. Because their precise location (as well as extent) has important therapeutic and prognostic implications, an anatomic system based on five flexor zones has been developed. These zones are as follows: zone I—area distal to the insertion sites of the flexor digitorum superficialis (FDS) tendons in the middle phalanges; zone II—area from the palmar plates of the metacarpophalangeal joints to the FDS tendon insertions (including the region of the fibroosseous tunnels); and zones III, IV, and V—other areas of the hand and wrist that are distal to (zone III), at (zone IV), and proximal to (zone V) the carpal tunnel.[426] Clinical diagnosis of injuries in any of these zones generally is easy, although diagnostic difficulty arises in cases of partial tendon tears and in patients with peritendinous adhesions or joint contractures. In such instances, MR imaging may provide useful information,[426–428] and the technique also can be employed in patients with complications (e.g., adhesions or tendon rupture) after repair of previous flexor tendon injuries.[429, 430] Postoperative

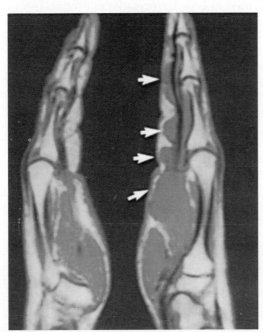

Figure 14–93

Infective tenosynovitis: Flexor tendons of finger. Atypical mycobacterial infection in a farmer. A sagittal T1-weighted (TR/TE, 600/20) spin echo MR image shows lobulated fluid collections (arrows) of low signal intensity extending along the course of the flexor digitorum superficialis and flexor digitorum profundus tendons of the index finger of one hand. Compare with the opposite (normal) hand.

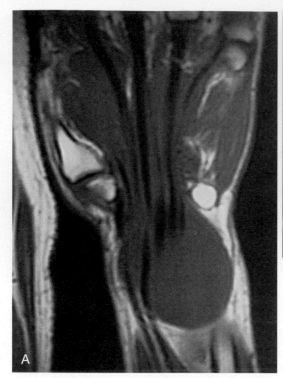

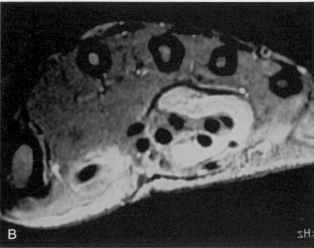

Figure 14–95

Tuberculous bursitis: Radial and ulnar bursae of the wrist.

A A coronal T1-weighted (TR/TE, 300/11) spin echo MR image reveals fluid-filled tendon sheaths and bursae in the volar aspect of the wrist.

B A transverse fat-suppressed fast spin echo MR image (TR/TE, 4000/19) shows high signal intensity in the involved structures.

(Courtesy of K. Hoffman, M.D., Stanford, California.)

adhesions and disruption of the suture can prevent active flexion of the finger in patients who have had repair of an injured flexor tendon, making clinical assessment more difficult. Because treatment of these two complications differ (i.e., tenolysis of adhesions and tendon suturing or grafting at sites of tendon rupture), an imaging technique (such as MR imaging) in this situation may have practical importance.[430]

Traumatic dislocations of the common extensor tendons of the fingers occur in patients with rheumatoid arthritis or other articular disorders and after trauma. Such dislocations result from tearing of the sagittal bands of the extensor hood, which wraps around the metacarpal head and, when intact, serves as a stabilizer of the common extensor tendon. One recent investiga-

tion indicated that MR imaging is effective in delineating these sagittal bands and their disruption after acute trauma.[350]

Giant Cell Tumor of Tendon Sheath

As indicated in Chapter 6, giant cell tumors of soft tissue may arise from tendon sheaths (as well as from joint capsules and ligamentous tissue). Although they may be observed about the wrist, they are far more frequent in the fingers. Soft tissue swelling or a mass with or without erosion of the subjacent bone and without calcification is evident. The relationship of giant cell tumors of the tendon sheath to diffuse or localized (pigmented) villonodular or nodular synovitis is not clear (see Chapter 6),

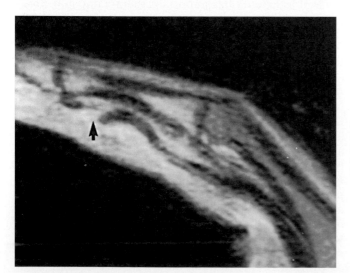

Figure 14–96

Flexor tendon injury: MR imaging. A sagittal fast spin echo (TR/TE, 3700/23) MR image shows the site (arrow) of tendon rupture that resulted from an American football injury. (Courtesy of D. Witte, M.D., Memphis, Tennessee.)

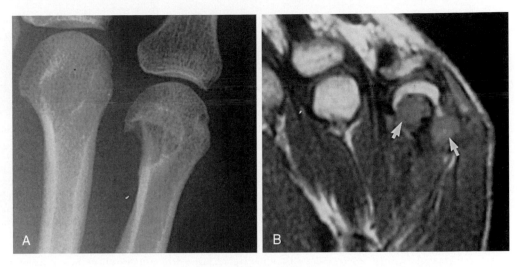

Figure 14–97
Giant cell tumor of tendon sheath: MR imaging.

A The routine radiograph demonstrates well-delineated erosions on the radial and ulnar aspects of the fifth metacarpal head.

B A coronal T1-weighted (TR/TE, 749/29) spin echo MR image shows a lobulated mass (arrows) of intermediate signal intensity with subjacent erosion of bone.

(Courtesy of M. Tartar, M.D., San Diego, California.)

although the tumors may contain hemosiderin deposits. Owing to the presence of hemosiderin deposition or dense acellular fibrous tissue, the lesions may be of low signal intensity on both T1- and T2-weighted spin echo MR images (Fig. 14–97). This pattern, however, is not invariable, and regions of high signal intensity on T2-weighted spin echo MR images or after the intravenous administration of gadolinium contrast agent are encountered (Fig. 14–98).[351]

Abnormalities of the Joint Synovium and Capsule

Ganglion Cysts

Ganglion cysts about the wrist are common, although their precise cause is debated. Ganglion cysts represent as many as 70 per cent of soft tissue masses of the hand and occur most frequently in the second, third, and fourth decades of life. In about 70 per cent of cases, ganglion cysts appear on the dorsum of the wrist, al-

though they also occur volarly and in other locations. The site of origin may be the joint capsule, tendon, or tendon sheath. Ganglion cysts contain fluid that may be slightly more viscous than joint fluid. Such cysts are surrounded by fibrous tissue without a synovial lining. They rarely calcify. A soft tissue mass is evident on radiographic examination. Anechoic oval, round, or lobulated cystic masses are seen with ultrasonography (Fig. 14–99).[352, 353] Arthrography occasionally reveals communication between the opacified joint and the cyst. Indeed, in the evaluation of wrist ganglia, contrast material injected directly into the swelling may fail to opacify the wrist. This phenomenon of a "one-way valve" between the ganglion and articular cavity is similar to that noted with synovial cysts about any joint. It therefore is logical to first inject the joint itself. This usually will demonstrate the site of communication with filling of the soft tissue mass, although, in some cases, it is necessary to decompress the cyst initially. If, in fact, an arthrogram does not opacify the cystic mass, a second injection directly into the mass can be attempted. Tenography also may reveal communication between the opacified

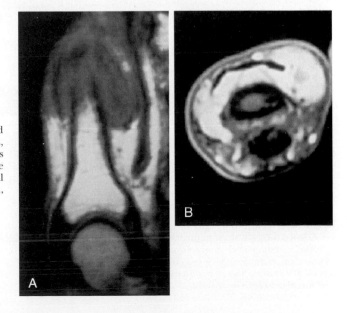

Figure 14–98
Giant cell tumor of a tendon sheath: MR imaging. Coronal T1-weighted (TR/TE, 500/20) **(A)** and transverse fat-suppressed T1-weighted (TR/TE, 700/19) **(B)** spin echo MR images, the latter obtained after intravenous administration of gadolinium contrast agent, reveal the lesion about the proximal phalanx of the second finger. Diffuse enhancement of signal intensity in the giant cell tumor is evident in **B.** (Courtesy of C. Neumann, M.D., Palm Springs, California.)

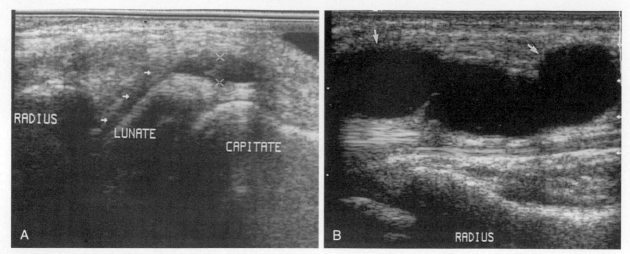

Figure 14–99

Ganglion cysts: Ultrasonography.

A A sonogram of the volar aspect of the wrist in the sagittal plane demonstrates an anechoic ganglion ("X" markers) superficial to the lunate and capitate bones with communication via a channel (arrows) with the radiocarpal joint.

B In a second patient, a sagittal sonogram of the volar aspect of the wrist shows a much larger lobulated anechoic ganglion (arrows) superficial to the radius.

(Courtesy of M. van Holsbeeck, M.D., Detroit, Michigan, and J. Jacobson, M.D., San Diego, California.)

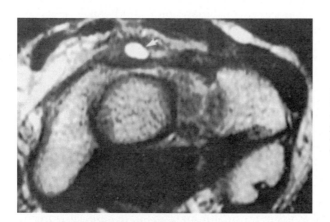

Figure 14–100

Ganglion cysts: MR imaging. A transaxial T2-weighted (TR/TE, 2000/80) spin echo MR image of the wrist at the level of the midcarpal joint shows a small ganglion cyst (arrow) just superficial to the dorsal intercarpal ligament and deep to the extensor tendons. (Courtesy of A. G. Bergman, M.D., Stanford, California.)

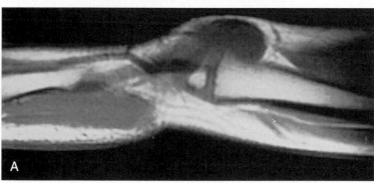

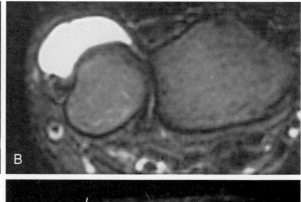

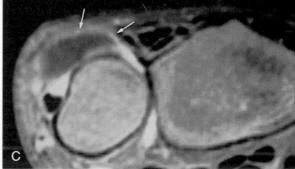

Figure 14–101

Ganglion cysts: MR imaging. This 10 year old boy developed a mass in the dorsum of the wrist.

A A sagittal T1-weighted (TR/TE, 550/14) spin echo MR image shows a mass with slightly inhomogeneous but mainly low signal intensity dorsal to the distal portion of the ulna.

B A transaxial fat-suppressed fast spin echo MR image (TR/TE, 3600/95) demonstrates high signal intensity in the mass, which is intimate with the extensor carpi ulnaris tendon sheath.

C With intravenous administration of a gadolinium compound, the wall of the ganglion cyst shows enhancement of signal intensity (arrows), as shown on a transaxial fat-suppressed T1-weighted (TR/TE, 800/14) spin echo MR image. Also note enhancement of signal intensity in the synovium of the distal radioulnar joint.

(Courtesy of S.K. Brahme, M.D., San Diego, California.)

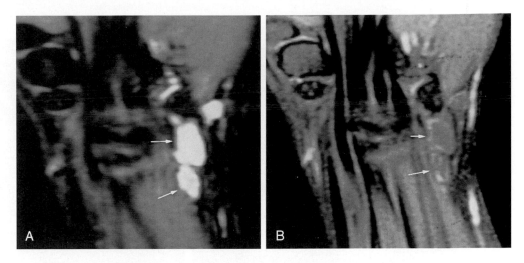

Figure 14–102
Ganglion cysts: MR imaging. A coronal STIR (TR/TE, 3215/19; inversion time, 140 msec) MR image **(A)** and a coronal fat-suppressed T1-weighted (TR/TE, 770/15) spin echo MR image **(B)** obtained after intravenous administration of a gadolinium contrast agent show the ganglion cyst (arrows) communicating with the pisiform-triquetral joint. It is of high signal intensity in **A.** In **B,** enhancement of signal intensity in the wall of the cyst is evident.

tendon sheath and the ganglion cyst. Low to intermediate signal intensity on T1-weighted spin echo MR images and high signal intensity on T2-weighted spin echo MR images within the ganglion cyst are typical (Figs. 14–100 to 14–102).[431] In one study, MR imaging and ultrasonography were found to be equally effective in the detection of occult dorsal wrist ganglia, leading to the conclusion that ultrasonography, because of its dynamic capabilities and lower cost, should be the initial imaging procedure for assessment of these lesions.[353]

Adhesive Capsulitis

Adhesive capsulitis is encountered most frequently in the shoulder, although involvement of the ankle, hip, and wrist also is seen. Physical and neurologic injury are two potential causes of this condition. In two articles, Maloney, Hanson, and their coworkers[354, 355] described 10 patients in whom persistent pain and limited range of motion in the wrist developed after trauma. Radiocarpal joint arthrography showed decreased capacity, small volar and prestyloid recesses, and adhesions preventing complete opacification of the joint (Fig. 14–103). Extravasation of contrast material along the needle track also was evident. Other authors have reported similar observations.[356] Closed manipulation of the wrist under general anesthesia may lead to clinical improvement. MR imaging of adhesive capsulitis is not rewarding unless intra-articular administration of gadolinium contrast agent (MR arthrography) is employed.

Articular Diseases

MR imaging has been used to assess the extent of rheumatoid arthritis and other synovial inflammatory diseases in the wrist (and in other locations) (see Chapter 4). Its advantages when compared with routine radiography include more accurate assessment of cartilage and bone destruction, the extent of synovial inflammation, and the activity of the disease process (Figs. 14–104 and 14–105). Marginal and central bone erosions and subchondral cystic lesions can be identified owing to the tomographic nature of the study and to the high signal intensity of synovial fluid and inflammatory tissue

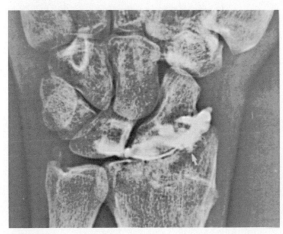

Figure 14–103
Adhesive capsulitis: Arthrography. In this 20 year old man, only 0.5 ml of contrast material could be introduced into the radiocarpal joint. Observe incomplete filling of this compartment and small volar recesses (arrow). Note evidence of remote fractures of the radius and ulnar styloid. (From Maloney MD, et al: Radiology *167*:187, 1988.)

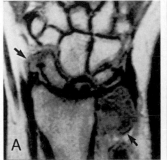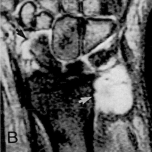

Figure 14–104
Rheumatoid arthritis: MR imaging.
A A coronal T1-weighted (TR/TE, 600/25) spin echo MR image shows abnormal synovial tissue and fluid in the distal radioulnar joint and radial aspect of the radiocarpal joint (arrows). Note erosions of the scaphoid, lunate, and triquetral bones.
B A coronal MPGR MR image (TR/TE, 500/15; flip angle, 30 degrees) shows regions (arrows) of high signal intensity, corresponding to sites of abnormal synovial tissue and fluid, and changes in signal intensity in the lunate and triquetrum.
(Courtesy of W. Glenn, M.D., Long Beach, California.)

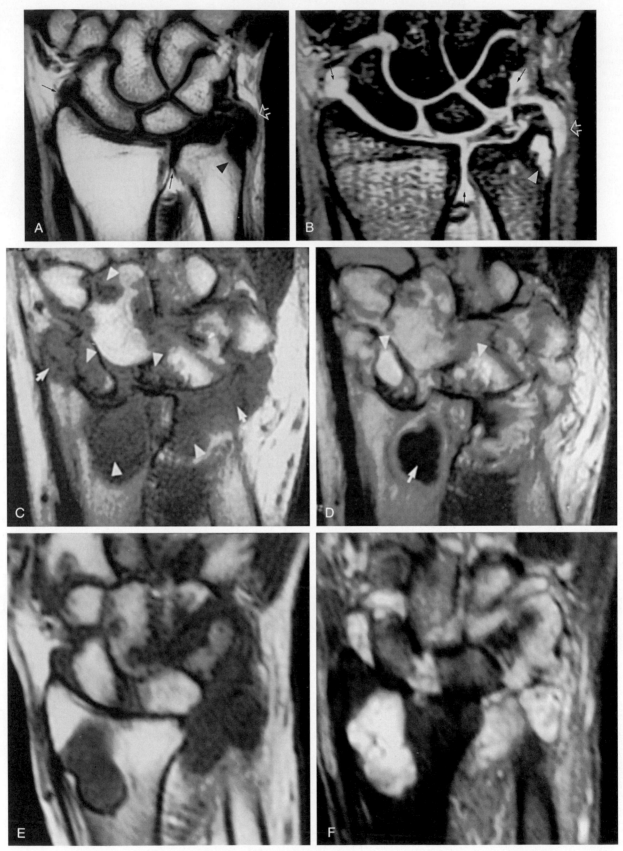

Figure 14–105
See legend on opposite page

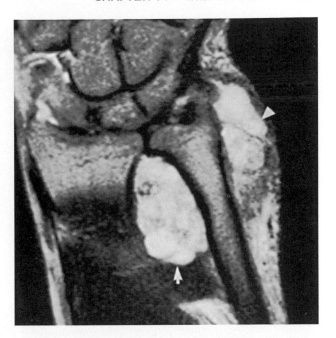

Figure 14–106

Idiopathic synovial (osteo)chondromatosis: MR imaging. A coronal T2-weighted (TR/TE, 1800/80) spin echo MR image reveals cartilage nodules of high signal intensity in the distal radioulnar joint (arrow) and about the outer surface of the ulna (arrowhead). Regions of low signal intensity represent foci of calcification or ossification.

on the T2-weighted spin echo and gradient echo MR images. Differentiation between such fluid and synovial pannus is difficult on the basis of findings derived from standard MR imaging sequences. The use of intravenous injected gadolinium compounds has been emphasized; enhancement of signal intensity within inflamed synovial tissue allows its differentiation from joint fluid (which does not show such enhancement) on T1-weighted spin echo MR images obtained immediately after the injection of gadolinium contrast agent (see Chapter 4).[440] Owing to leakage of the gadolinium agent into the joint fluid, delayed MR images after intravenous administration of gadolinium contrast material are not useful in this differentiation. In a similar fashion, routine or gadolinium-enhanced MR imaging can be used to evaluate the extent of tendon sheath involvement in rheumatoid arthritis and other synovial inflammatory diseases. As enhancement of signal intensity in synovial tissue after the intravenous administration of a gadolinium contrast agent generally implies active inflammation, this technique may be beneficial in monitoring

the therapeutic response of the disease. In one report, gadolinium-enhanced MR imaging and positron emission tomography (PET) both allowed quantification of volumetric and metabolic changes in joint inflammation of the wrist and assessment of efficacies of anti-inflammatory drugs.[357]

The diagnosis of pigmented villonodular synovitis and idiopathic synovial (osteo)chondromatosis (Fig. 14–106) can be established effectively with MR imaging (see Chapter 6). Similarly, MR imaging (or CT scanning) can be used to investigate patients with other articular disorders of the wrist (Fig. 14–107). Although additional imaging methods, such as scintigraphy and arthrography, can be used for this same purpose, the findings often are less specific.

Soft Tissue Masses

Although the most commonly encountered soft tissue masses about the hand and wrist are ganglia, lipomas,

---

Figure 14–105

Synovitis: MR imaging.

A, B Seronegative rheumatoid-like arthritis. This 47 year old man developed pain and swelling on the ulnar aspect of the wrist. Coronal T1-weighted (TR/TE, 400/16) spin echo (**A**) and MPGR (**B**) MR images reveal the extent of disease. Note fluid or synovial inflammatory tissue, or both, in the radiocarpal and inferior radioulnar joints (closed arrows), enlargement and distortion of the prestyloid recess of the radiocarpal joint (open arrows), erosion of the ulnar styloid process (arrowheads), and apparent disruption of the ulnar aspect of the TFCC. (Courtesy of J. Depper, M.D., Bend, Oregon.)

C, D Calcium pyrophosphate dihydrate crystal deposition disease. On a coronal T1-weighted (TR/TE, 700/16) spin echo MR image (**C**), regions of low signal intensity are observed (arrows), consistent with synovial fluid and inflammatory tissue. These regions extend into the scaphoid, lunate, capitate, radius, and ulna (arrowheads). Note scapholunate diastasis and excavation of the distal portion of the radius. After the intravenous injection of gadolinium contrast agent, a similar image (TR/TE, 750/16) (**D**) shows a persistent region of low signal intensity in the radius (arrow), representing fluid, which is surrounded by a rim of higher intensity, consistent with inflammatory or edematous tissue. Regions of high signal intensity are present in the scaphoid and lunate (arrowheads) and in the radiocarpal, inferior radioulnar, and midcarpal joints, presumably indicative of synovial inflammatory tissue. (Courtesy of M. Zlatkin, M.D., Hollywood, Florida.)

E, F Rheumatoid arthritis. Coronal T1-weighted (TR/TE, 450/16) spin echo (**E**) and fat-suppressed fast spin echo (TR/TE, 4000/60) (**F**) MR images show diffuse involvement of the wrist. Note the large cystic lesion of the radius, multiple carpal erosions, and extensive synovial inflammatory tissue, particularly about the distal portion of the ulna.

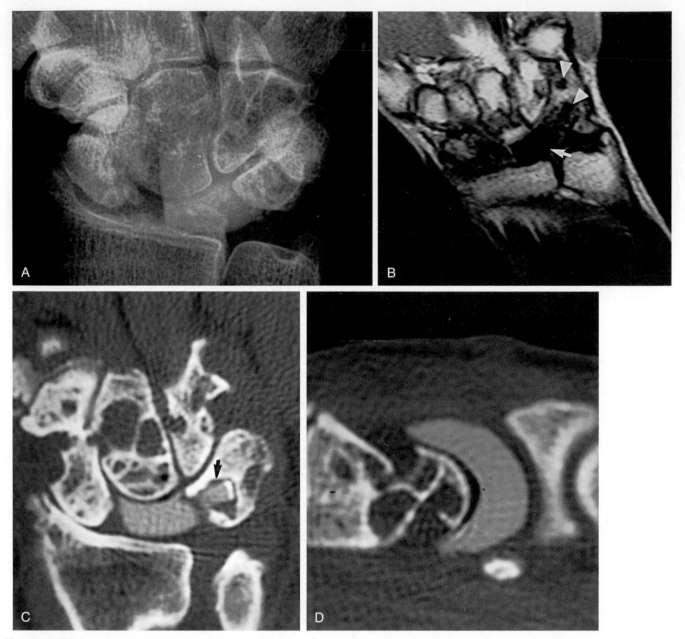

Figure 14–107
Silastic synovitis: MR imaging.

A Routine radiography reveals a Silastic lunate prosthesis (which is displaced and tilted) and cystic changes in many of the carpal bones.

B A coronal proton density–weighted (TR/TE, 2500/20) spin echo MR image shows the very low signal intensity of the prosthesis (arrow) and Silastic particles (arrowheads) in the wrist.

C, D In a second patient, coronal (**C**) and sagittal (**D**) CT scans show a Silastic lunate prosthesis with Silastic fragments (arrow) and carpal cysts.

and giant cell tumors of the tendon sheath,[358] a variety of other tumors and tumor-like lesions occur in this region. These include both benign (Figs. 14–108 to 14–110) and malignant neoplasms, synovial cysts, hematomas and other posttraumatic abnormalities (Figs. 14–111 and 14–112), gouty tophi, rheumatoid nodules, mucous cysts,[432] and even sarcoidosis.

Accessory or anomalous muscles of the hand and wrist are relatively frequent.[359–364, 438] These accessory muscles, which commonly are related to variations of the palmaris longus muscle, may be asymptomatic but also may lead to a soft tissue mass with or without findings of

nerve entrapment. In particular, involvement of the median nerve in the carpal tunnel or of the ulnar nerve in Guyon's canal may be enountered. Examples of specific anomalous muscles include the extensor digitorum brevis manus muscle along the ulnar side of the extensor tendon of the index finger, an accessory flexor digitorum superficialis muscle in the palm, and accessory muscles related to the abductor digiti minimi manus muscle in Guyon's canal. Diagnosis is best accomplished with electromyography and MR imaging, the latter technique revealing a mass with signal intensity characteristics of muscle (Fig. 14–113). Scanning of both hands

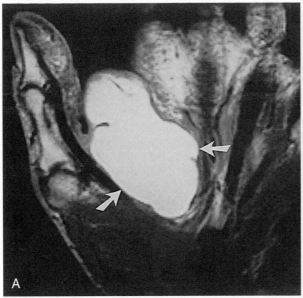
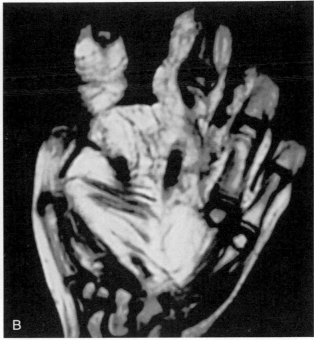

Figure 14–108
Lipomatous lesions: MR imaging.
 A Lipoma. A coronal T1-weighted (TR/TE, 550/15) spin echo MR image shows a typical lipoma (arrows) in the thenar space.
 B Macrodystrophia lipomatosa. A T1-weighted (TR/TE, 600/20) spin echo MR image shows fatty infiltration involving mainly the palm and second and third digits.
 (Courtesy of S. Wootton, M.D., Denver, Colorado.)

may be helpful, although anomalous or accessory muscles may have a bilateral distribution.

Hand Injuries

Metacarpophalangeal and Interphalangeal Joint Dislocations

Dislocation of a metacarpophalangeal joint (excluding the thumb) is considerably less frequent than that of a proximal interphalangeal joint of a finger and results from a fall on the outstretched hand that forces the joint into hyperextension. The index finger is involved most commonly, dislocations of multiple metacarpophalangeal joints are uncommon, and open dislocations of these joints are rare.[365] Dorsal dislocations predominate. The volar plate is disrupted, allowing dorsal displacement of the base of the proximal phalanx.[366] Such dislocations are classified as simple (reducible) and complex (potentially irreducible) injuries.[75] An adjacent sesamoid or volar plate can become displaced into the joint space.[367]

 Volar dislocation of the metacarpophalangeal joint is

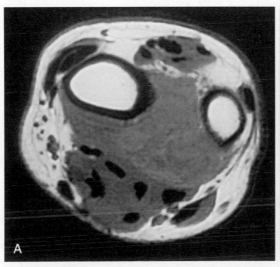
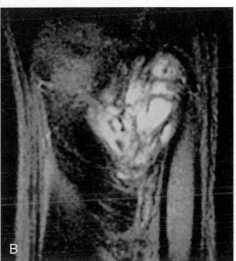

Figure 14–109
Hemangioma: Intramuscular type. Transaxial T1-weighted (TR/TE, 800/20) **(A)** and coronal T2-weighted (TR/TE, 2000/80) **(B)** spin echo MR images show an intramuscular hemangioma with intermediate and low signal intensity in **A** and inhomogeneous but mainly high signal intensity in **B.** The flexor muscles and tendons are displaced in a volar direction.

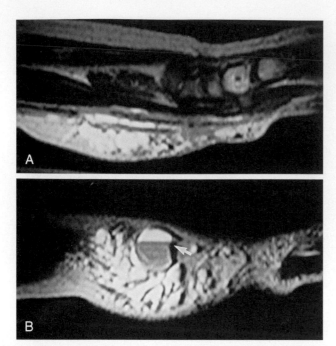

Figure 14–110

Hemangioma: Superficial type. Sagittal T2-weighted (TR/TE, 1800/80) spin echo MR images of the wrist, with **B** located more ulnarly than **A,** show the lesion of high signal intensity. A prominent fluid level (arrow) is seen in **B.** (Courtesy of G. S. Huang, M.D., Taipei, Taiwan.)

rare,[368] but it too may be complex and irreducible.[365] Inability to reduce the dislocation is indicative of injury to the volar plate, the dorsal capsule, the collateral ligaments, or combinations of these structures. Lateral

subluxations, often with spontaneous reduction, are common, are designated sprains, are accompanied by injury of the collateral ligament (usually the radial collateral ligament), and generally are characterized by an intact volar plate.

Dislocations of the proximal interphalangeal joints are very common, usually involve only one joint, and may occur with or without a major adjacent phalangeal fracture.[369, 370] These dislocations can occur in a posterior or, more rarely, anterior direction. Posterior dislocation results from a hyperextension injury. Ligamentous and volar plate disruption is a frequent associated finding.[371, 372] Posterior dislocation of a distal interphalangeal joint or the interphalangeal joint of the thumb also can be encountered. Such dislocations may be irreducible owing to interposition of the volar plate or flexor tendon.[373, 374]

A Bennett's fracture-dislocation is a relatively common intra-articular injury that occurs at the base of the first metacarpal (Fig. 14–114).[375–378] After an axial blow to a partially flexed first metacarpal bone, an oblique fracture line separates the major portion of the bone from a small (or sometimes large) fragment of the volar lip. The base of the metacarpal is pulled dorsally and radially. The Bennett's fracture represents only one of several different fracture patterns that occur at the base of the thumb and should not be confused with a second type of intra-articular fracture, the Rolando fracture, in which a Y- or T-shaped comminuted fracture line is evident. Transverse or oblique extra-articular fractures of the base of the first metacarpal bone also are encountered, as are pure dislocations of the first carpometacarpal joint.

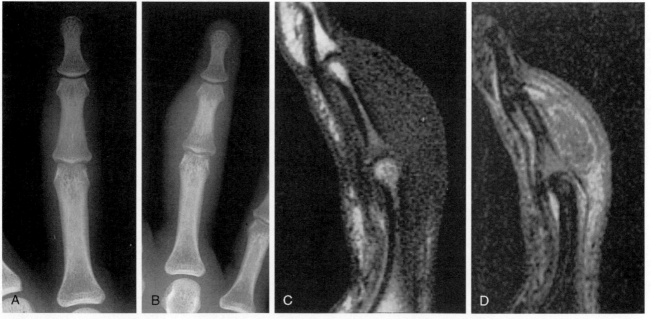

Figure 14–111

Florid reactive periostitis: MR imaging. This 20 year old woman developed progressive swelling of the ring finger.

A, B Radiographs obtained 2 weeks apart show increasing soft tissue swelling and periostitis of the middle phalanx in **B.**

C, D Two weeks after **B,** sagittal T1-weighted (TR/TE, 200/17) spin echo **(C)** and STIR (TR/TE, 2000/40; inversion time, 165 msec) **(D)** MR images document a mass dorsal to the middle phalanx of the ring finger, with low signal intensity in **C** and inhomogeneous but higher signal intensity in **D.** A joint effusion is present in the proximal interphalangeal joint, and subcutaneous edema also is evident.

(Courtesy of R. Kerr, M.D., Los Angeles, California.)

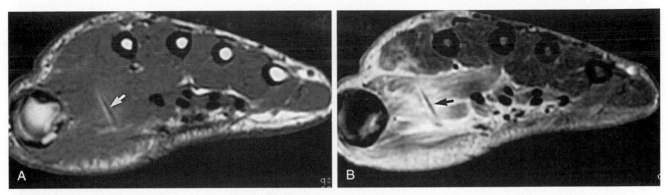

Figure 14–112
Wood splinter: MR imaging. The splinter (arrows) within the musculature between the thumb and index finger is well shown on transaxial T1-weighted (TR/TE, 400/16) spin echo MR images obtained before **(A)** and after **(B)** the intravenous injection of a gadolinium compound. The inflammatory reaction is better shown in **B,** a fat-suppressed image. (Courtesy of D. Goodwin, M.D., Hanover, New Hampshire.)

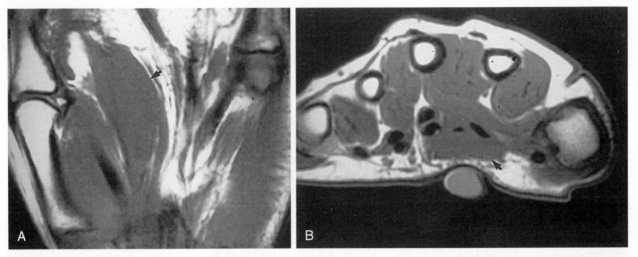

Figure 14–113
Accessory muscle: MR imaging. T1-weighted coronal (TR/TE, 700/15) **(A)** and sagittal (TR/TE, 500/15) **(B)** spin echo MR images show an accessory muscle (arrows) with signal intensity characteristics identical to those of normal muscle. (Courtesy of S. Eilenberg, M.D., San Diego, California.)

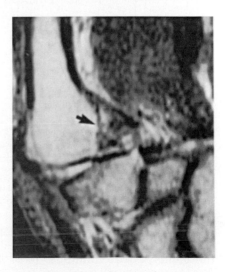

Figure 14–114
Bennett's fracture of the first metacarpal bone: MR imaging. A coronal T2-weighted (TR/TE, 2000/80) spin echo MR image shows a fracture (arrow) in the ulnar portion of the base of the first metacarpal bone, associated with radial displacement of the remaining portion of the bone and an effusion in the first carpometacarpal joint.

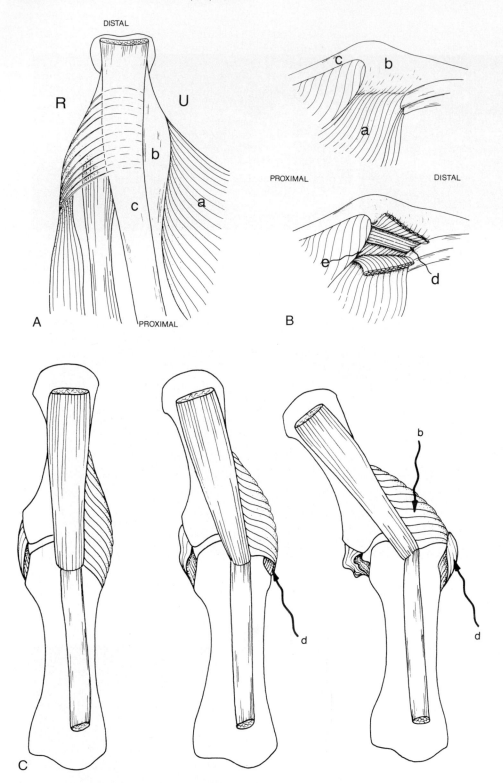

Figure 14–115

Gamekeeper's thumb: Mechanism of injury, anatomy of ligaments of metacarpophalangeal joint of thumb.

A Dorsal aspect showing radial (R) and ulnar (U) sides of metacarpophalangeal joint. Tendon of extensor pollicis longus (c) passes over the metacarpophalangeal joint, running from the proximal to the distal aspect of the digit. The adductor pollicis (a) inserts in part on the proximal phalanx, some of its fibers fusing with a portion of the dorsal aponeurosis, termed the adductor aponeurosis (b).

B Ulnar aspect showing adductor pollicis (a), adductor aponeurosis (b), and tendon of the extensor pollicis longus (c). In lower drawing, the adductor pollicis has been incised and opened, exposing the ulnar collateral (d) and accessory collateral (e) ligaments.

C Dorsal aspect of first metacarpophalangeal joint following rupture of the ulnar collateral ligament. With time, the torn ligament (d) can protrude from the proximal edge of the adductor aponeurosis (b), the latter preventing its return.

(From Resnick D, Danzig LA: AJR *126:*1046, 1976. Copyright 1976, American Roentgen Ray Society.)

Dislocations and collateral ligament injuries of the first metacarpophalangeal joint are important complications of trauma.[379] Although several types of injuries can be identified, that related to a sudden valgus stress applied to the metacarpophalangeal joint of the thumb, the gamekeeper's thumb, is most important (see later discussion). Dorsal subluxation or dislocation of the metacarpophalangeal joint of the thumb results from forcible hyperextension. Locking of the joint after this injury may indicate interposition of a sesamoid bone or ligamentous abnormality.[379, 380]

Fractures of the Metacarpal Bones and Phalanges

Fractures of the metacarpal bones, which predominate in the first and fifth digits, generally are classified ac-

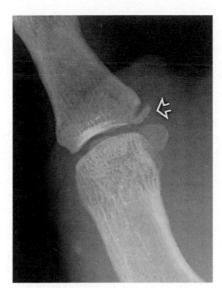

Figure 14–116
Gamekeeper's thumb: Routine radiography. Note slight displacement of a small fragment (open arrow) arising from the ulnar aspect of the proximal phalanx of the thumb.

cording to anatomic location: metacarpal head, metacarpal neck, metacarpal shaft, and metacarpal base. Typical locations of fractures include the shaft and neck of the fifth metacarpal (boxer's fracture), the shaft of the third or fourth metacarpal, or both, and the articular surface of the second metacarpal.[381, 382] Displacement, angulation, or rotation commonly is encountered, and the rotation, if not corrected, may lead to serious disability.[383]

Phalangeal fractures are more frequent than those of the metacarpal bones and most typically involve the distal phalanges,[384] followed in order of frequency by the proximal phalanges and the middle phalanges. Important varieties include the mallet fracture (in which an avulsion injury at the base of the dorsal surface of the terminal phalanx is produced by damage to the extensor mechanism),[385, 386] the volar plate fracture (in which a dorsal dislocation of a proximal interphalangeal joint may be associated with an avulsion fracture in the middle phalanx at the site of attachment of the volar plate), any fracture with intra-articular extension or significant rotational deformity, a fracture of the shaft of the proximal or middle phalanx (whose volar surface forms the floor of the flexor tendon sheath so that accurate reduction is desirable), a fracture of the base of the proximal phalanx (in which angulation is easily overlooked owing to superimposition of other bones on the lateral radiograph), and, in the immature skeleton, a physeal separation at the base of the distal phalanx (the nailbed injury, in which an open skin surface leads to secondary infection).[383] The diagnostic value of multiple radiographic projections, including an internally rotated oblique projection,[387] in the analysis of phalangeal fractures should be recognized.

Gamekeeper's Thumb

Initially described as an occupational hazard in English gamewardens, who, in killing rabbits by twisting their

necks, sustained repeated stresses about the first metacarpophalangeal joint, gamekeeper's thumb now is recognized to occur in various settings,[388–392] including skiing[393–395] and breakdancing.[396] Attenuation or disruption of the ligamentous apparatus along the ulnar aspect of the thumb is seen (Fig. 14–115), which may be associated with pain, swelling, tenderness, edema, and pinch instability. The findings may occur acutely after a single injury or, as classically described, as a result of chronic stretching with failure of the ulnar collateral ligament. Initial radiographs can be negative, although small avulsed fragments from the base of the proximal phalanx can be delineated in some instances (Fig. 14–116). These fragments may be displaced proximally and rotated from 45 to 90 degrees. Radiographs obtained with radial stress applied to the first metacarpophalangeal joint can reveal subluxation,[397, 398] and arthrography may outline leakage of contrast material from the ulnar aspect of the joint and an abnormal folded position of the ulnar collateral ligament (Fig. 14–117).[399, 400] Neither test is ideal, however. If stress radiographs are employed, some type of local or regional anesthesia is required and the examination should be performed with the first metacarpophalangeal joint placed in positions of flexion and extension. The criteria regarding a positive examination are not agreed on, although most authorities regard measurements of the extent of abduction of the thumb derived from the radiographs to be more accurate than those based on clinical examination. A measurement of more than 35 or 45 degrees of abduction or of more than 10 degrees of abduction greater than the opposite (uninjured) side generally is regarded as positive. Routine radiographs should be obtained prior to stress testing as an avulsion fracture may become more displaced with the application of stress.

When disrupted, the torn end of the ulnar collateral ligament can become displaced superficial to the adductor pollicis aponeurosis, a finding known as the Stener lesion.[391] The interposed aponeurosis interferes with

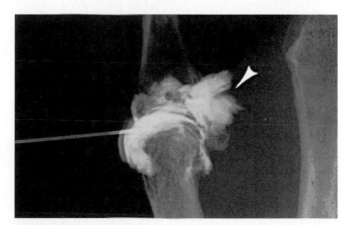

Figure 14–117
Gamekeeper's thumb: Arthrography. After injury to the ulnar aspect of the first metacarpophalangeal joint, arthrography may reveal extravasation of contrast material. Note the contrast extravasation (arrowhead) along the ulnar side of the metacarpal head and proximal phalanx.

(From Resnick D, Danzig L: AJR *126*:1046, 1976. Copyright 1976, American Roentgen Ray Society.)

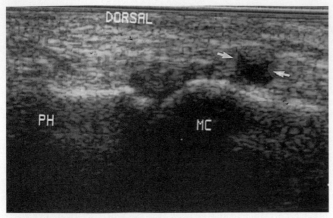

Figure 14–118
Gamekeeper's thumb: Ultrasonography. In this patient with a documented Stener lesion, a sonogram of the first metacarpophalangeal joint in the coronal plane demonstrates the displaced proximal stump (arrows) of the torn ulnar collateral ligament. PH, proximal phalanx; MC, first metacarpal head. (Courtesy of M. van Holsbeeck, M.D., Detroit, Michigan, and J. Jacobson, M.D., San Diego, California.)

healing, and surgery has been advocated for the treatment of displaced tears of the ulnar collateral ligament. Occasionally, displacement of this ligament can be inferred from the presence of an avulsed bone fragment. The absence of bone avulsion, however, does not eliminate the possibility of a Stener lesion. Interposition of the adductor aponeurosis can occur whether the site of rupture is the distal attachment of the ulnar collateral ligament to the proximal phalanx (the most common site of disruption) or the midsubstance of the ligament. Arthrography of the first metacarpophalangeal joint in case of gamekeeper's thumb may reveal a filling defect representing the Stener lesion, although the sensitivity of this arthrographic finding is not clear.

Ultrasonography has been used to assess gamekeeper's thumb.[401–405] The technique appears to be reliable in the identification of a torn ulnar collateral ligament, but the delineation of a Stener lesion with this technique is more difficult. A hypoechogenic structure, usually round, located on the ulnar aspect of the first metacarpal head generally is indicative of a torn and retracted ulnar collateral ligament (Fig. 14–118).

MR imaging can be employed successfully for the identification of the Stener lesion,[405–408] although reported results have not been consistent.[433] In one study, the technique was judged superior to ultrasonography in the evaluation of the torn ulnar collateral ligament.[405] On coronal MR images of the first metacarpophalangeal joint, the normal ulnar collateral ligament appears as a band of low signal intensity medial to the joint (Fig. 14–119A). The adductor aponeurosis often is visible as a paper-thin band of low signal intensity superficial to the ulnar collateral ligament and extending from the distal half of the ulnar collateral ligament over the base of the proximal phalanx. A nondisplaced tear of the ulnar collateral ligament appears as discontinuity of the ligament distally, without ligamentous retraction and with the adductor aponeurosis covering the distal end of the ulnar collateral ligament (see Fig. 14–119B). Displacement of the ulnar collateral ligament, or the Stener lesion, is associated with proximal retraction or folding of the ligament. The proximal margin of the adductor aponeurosis may be seen to abut on the folded ulnar collateral ligament, creating a rounded region of low signal intensity designated a "yo-yo on a string" appearance (see Figs. 14–119C and 14–120).[408] Rarely, other patterns of injury are identified (Figs. 14–121 and 14–122).

In general, conservative therapy is employed in cases of partial tears, or sprains, of the ulnar collateral liga-

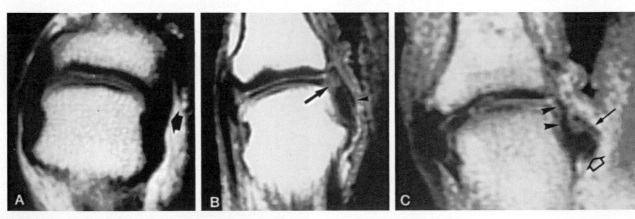

Figure 14–119
Gamekeeper's thumb: MR imaging.

A Normal appearance of the ulnar collateral ligament. A coronal T1-weighted (TR/TE, 500/20) spin echo MR image of the first metacarpophalangeal joint shows the normal ulnar collateral ligament (arrow) as a band of low signal intensity. The adductor aponeurosis is not visible.

B Nondisplaced tear of the ulnar collateral ligament. A coronal T1-weighted (TR/TE, 500/20) spin echo MR image of the first metacarpophalangeal joint shows disruption of the ulnar collateral ligament (arrow) and a superficial curvilinear structure of low signal intensity (arrowhead), representing the adductor aponeurosis.

C Displaced tear of the ulnar collateral ligament (Stener lesion). A coronal T1-weighted (TR/TE, 500/20) spin echo MR image of the first metacarpophalangeal joint reveals a yo-yo appearance. The adductor pollicis aponeurosis (arrowheads) looks like a string holding a yo-yo, the balled-up, displaced ulnar collateral ligament (open arrow). The thin region of low signal intensity (solid arrow) represents an avulsed bone fragment.

(From Spaeth HJ, et al: Radiology *188*:553, 1993.)

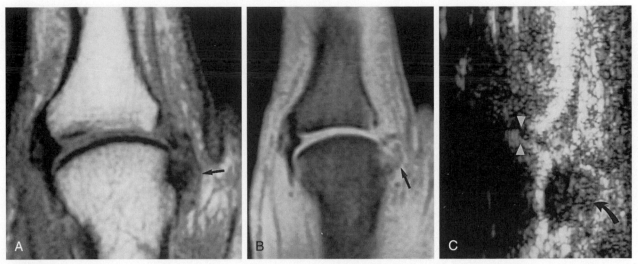

Figure 14–120
Gamekeeper's thumb: MR imaging and ultrasonography. In this 70 year old male skier, coronal T1-weighted (TR/TE, 600/27) spin echo **(A)** and fat-suppressed fast spin echo (TR/TE, 1100/19) **(B)** MR images show the torn and retracted ulnar collateral ligament (arrows). The course of the adductor pollicis aponeurosis cannot be traced completely. An ultrasonographic image **(C)** in the coronal plane and oriented precisely the same as **A** and **B** demonstrates a round hypoechoic structure (arrow) representing the displaced proximal portion of the ulnar collateral ligament. The first metacarpophalangeal joint is indicated with arrowheads. (Courtesy of D. Goodwin, M.D., Hanover, New Hampshire.)

ment. Complete tears, especially those with a Stener lesion, usually are treated surgically. Operative treatment also is employed frequently when large fractures involving a significant portion of the articular surface or fractures displaced by more than 5 mm are identified. Arthroscopic reduction of Stener lesions also has been used.[434]

Other Abnormalities

Occult Bone Injuries

The use of MR imaging to evaluate occult bone injuries is discussed in Chapter 8. Such injuries include acute infractions and chronic stress fractures. Although most reported data related to this use of MR imaging are based on studies of occult bone injuries about the knee and hip, a similar role exists for MR imaging in cases of wrist and hand fractures (Figs. 14–123 and 14–124). Occult fractures of the distal portion of the radius in elderly persons and of scaphoid fractures in young adults are two examples of injuries that can be detected with MR imaging. The sensitivity of the MR imaging examination in this regard is at least equal and probably superior to that of bone scintigraphy, and a negative MR imaging examination virtually excludes the presence of a fracture. Bone scintigraphy, however, still represents an effective, sensitive method for the diagnosis of occult

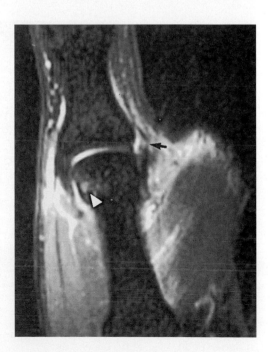

Figure 14–121
Gamekeeper's thumb: MR imaging. In this example, a fast spin echo STIR (TR/TE, 4400/23; inversion time, 160 msec) MR image in the coronal plane shows a disrupted, nonretracted ulnar collateral ligament (arrow), a bone contusion (arrowhead), joint effusion, and periarticular soft tissue edema. The proximal aspect of the radial collateral ligament also looks abnormal. (Courtesy of S. Kingston, M.D., Los Angeles, California.)

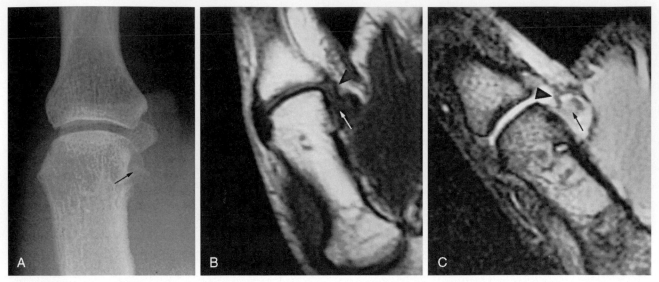

Figure 14–122
Gamekeeper's thumb: MR imaging.

   A In this patient, routine radiography reveals an avulsion fracture (arrow) arising at the proximal site of attachment of the ulnar collateral ligament to the first metacarpal bone.

   B A coronal T1-weighted (TR/TE, 500/25) spin echo MR image shows redundancy of the adductor pollicis aponeurosis (arrowhead) and a balled-up ulnar collateral ligament (arrow).

   C These findings (arrowhead, arrow) are better seen on a coronal multiplanar gradient recalled (MPGR) MR image (TR/TE, 500/20; flip angle, 20 degrees).

   (Courtesy of D. Artenian, M.D., Fresno, California.)

bone injuries, and CT is both sensitive and specific (Fig. 14–125).

Bone Tumors and Tumor-Like Lesions

Although virtually any tumor or tumor-like lesion may involve the bones of the hand and wrist, benign lesions are encountered far more frequently than malignant lesions (Table 14–2). Commonly observed benign processes include enchondromas (typically occurring in the

proximal and middle phalanges of the hand and often containing calcification), intraosseous ganglion cysts (usually occurring in the carpal bones, especially the lunate) (Fig. 14–126),[435] inclusion, or epidermoid, cysts

Table 14–2. TUMORS AND TUMOR-LIKE LESIONS OF BONE: FREQUENCY OF INVOLVEMENT OF BONES IN THE HAND AND WRIST

Lesion	Frequency, %*
Osteoid osteoma	9
Osteoblastoma	3
Osteosarcoma	<1
Enchondroma	57
Periosteal chondroma	22
Chondroblastoma	2
Chondromyxoid fibroma	2
Osteochondroma	5
Chondrosarcoma	3
Nonossifying fibroma	1
Desmoplastic fibroma	1
Fibrosarcoma	<1
Giant cell tumor	8†
Malignant fibrous histiocytoma	<1
Lipoma	<1
Hemangioma	2
Glomus tumor‡	75
Hemangiopericytoma	2
Hemangioendothelioma	2
Neurofibroma/neurilemoma	8
Simple bone cyst	1
Aneurysmal bone cyst	5
Epidermoid cyst	70
Adamantinoma	1
Ewing's sarcoma	1

Figure 14–123
Occult fractures of the hand and wrist: MR imaging. A coronal MPGR (TR/TE, 533/10; flip angle, 30 degrees) MR image shows a fracture of high signal intensity in the midportion of the scaphoid bone. (Courtesy of B.Y. Yang, M.D., Taipei, Taiwan.)

*Approximate figures based upon analysis of major reports containing the greatest number of cases.
†Includes lesions of the distal portions of the radius and ulna.
‡Often involves the fingertips without involvement of adjacent bone.

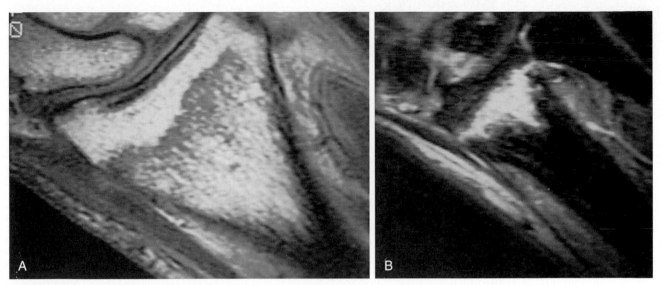

Figure 14–124
Occult fractures of the hand and wrist: MR imaging. An occult fracture of the distal portion of the radius is shown on coronal T1-weighted (TR/TE, 667/17) spin echo **(A)** and fast spin echo STIR (TR/TE, 3400/28; inversion time, 150 msec) **(B)** MR images.

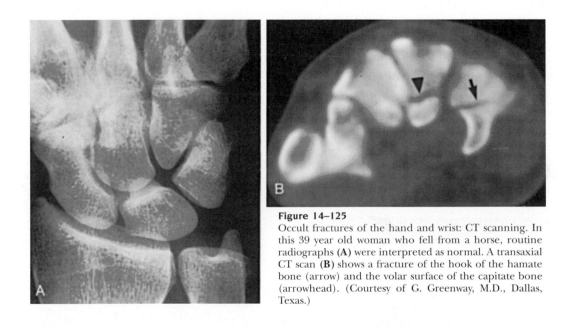

Figure 14–125
Occult fractures of the hand and wrist: CT scanning. In this 39 year old woman who fell from a horse, routine radiographs **(A)** were interpreted as normal. A transaxial CT scan **(B)** shows a fracture of the hook of the hamate bone (arrow) and the volar surface of the capitate bone (arrowhead). (Courtesy of G. Greenway, M.D., Dallas, Texas.)

Figure 14–126
Intraosseous ganglion cysts: MR imaging—lunate. Coronal T1-weighted (TR/TE, 600/20) **(A)** and T2-weighted (TR/TE, 2000/80) **(B)** spin echo MR images reveal a well-marginated lesion involving the radial aspect of the lunate bone. The lesion is of low signal intensity in **A** and of high signal intensity in **B.** Surrounding edema of the bone marrow is evident.

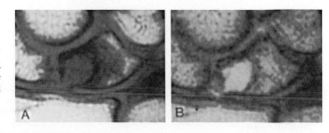

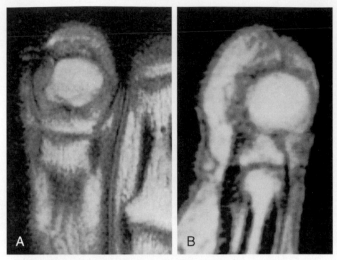

Figure 14–127
Epidermoid cyst: MR imaging. T1-weighted coronal (TR/TE, 616/25) **(A)** and sagittal (TR/TE, 800/25) **(B)** spin echo MR images reveal a cyst of high signal intensity. Note the erosion of the dorsal aspect of the terminal phalanx of the finger. (Courtesy of J. Kirkham, M.D., Minneapolis, Minnesota.)

(predominating in the terminal phalanges) (Fig. 14–127), giant cell tumors (classically seen in the distal portion of the radius and about the metacarpophalangeal joints), giant cell reparative granulomas (inconsistently associated with previous injury and simulating the imaging appearance of giant cell tumors), aneurysmal bone cysts (leading to osseous expansion), glomus tumors (soft tissue lesions often seen at the base of the nail and that may involve the terminal phalanx) (Fig. 14–128), and sarcoidosis (producing a coarsened trabecular pattern and cystic or erosive changes of bone). Although MR imaging allows assessment of the extent of these lesions, specific diagnosis is better accomplished with routine radiography.

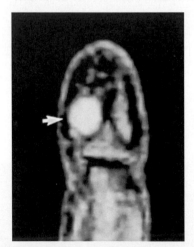

Figure 14–128
Glomus tumor: MR imaging. In a 67 year old woman, a coronal multiplanar gradient recalled (MPGR) MR image (TR/TE, 500/15; flip angle, 30 degrees) shows a lesion (arrow) of high signal intensity applied to the radial aspect of the terminal phalanx of the fifth finger. (Courtesy of W. Glenn, M.D., Long Beach, California.)

SUMMARY

This chapter provides a summary of imaging techniques that can be applied to the assessment of internal derangements (and associated lesions) of the wrist and hand. Two techniques, MR imaging and arthrography, are emphasized, as they both represent excellent methods in this assessment. Others, such as scintigraphy, ultrasonography, and CT scanning, also are useful, and each of these advanced methods should be regarded as supplementary to more standard analysis based on clinical examination and routine radiography. Accurate analysis of imaging data requires, foremost, knowledge of regional anatomy, which in the wrist is complicated by inconsistent terminology that has been used in the literature.

REFERENCES

1. Mikic ZD: Detailed anatomy of the articular disc of the distal radioulnar joint. Clin Orthop *245*:123, 1989.
2. Bogumill GP: Anatomy of the wrist. *In* DM Lichtman (Ed): The Wrist and Its Disorders. Philadelphia, WB Saunders Co, 1988, p. 14.
3. Bednar JM, Osterman AL: The role of arthroscopy in the treatment of traumatic triangular fibrocartilage injuries. Hand Clin *10*:605, 1994.
4. Uchiyama S, Nakatsuchi Y: Anatomical and radiological evaluation of the triangular fibrocartilage complex of the wrist. J Hand Surg [Br] *19*:319, 1994.
5. Jantea CL, Baltzer A, Ruther W: Arthroscopic repair of radial-sided lesions of the fibrocartilage complex. Hand Clin *11*:31, 1995.
6. Sennwald GR, Lauterburg M, Zdravkovic V: A new technique of reattachment after traumatic avulsion of the TFCC at its ulnar insertion. J Hand Surg [Br] *20*:178, 1995.
7. Palmer AK: The distal radioulnar joint. *In* DM Lichtman (Ed): The Wrist and Its Disorders. Philadelphia, WB Saunders Co, 1988, p. 220.
8. Palmer AK, Werner FW: The triangular fibrocartilage complex of the wrist—anatomy and function. J Hand Surg *6*:153, 1981.
9. Palmer AK, Werner FW: Biomechanics of the distal radioulnar joint. Clin Orthop *187*:26, 1984.
10. Ruby LK: Carpal instability. J Bone Joint Surg [Am] *77*:476, 1995.
11. Mayfield JK: Pathogenesis of wrist ligament instability. *In* DM Lichtman (Ed): The Wrist and Its Disorders. Philadelphia, WB Saunders Co, 1988, p. 53.
12. Taleisnik J: The ligaments of the wrist. J Hand Surg *1*:110, 1976.
13. Mayfield JK, Johnson RP, Kilcoyne RF: The ligaments of the human wrist and their functional significance. Anat Rec *186*:417, 1976.
14. Kauer JMG: Functional anatomy of the wrist. Clin Orthop *149*:9, 1980.
15. Berger RA, Landsmeer JMF: The palmar radiocarpal ligaments: A study of adult and fetal human wrist joints. J Hand Surg [Am] *15*:847, 1990.
16. Sennwald GR, Zdravkovic V, Oberlin C: The anatomy of the palmar scapho-triquetral ligament. J Bone Joint Surg [Br] *76*:147, 1993.
17. Smith DK: Volar carpal ligaments of the wrist: Normal appearance on multiplanar reconstructions of three-dimensional Fourier transform MR imaging. AJR *161*:353, 1993.
18. Mizuseki T, Ikuta Y: The dorsal carpal ligaments: Their anatomy and function. J Hand Surg [Br] *14*:91, 1989.
19. Smith DK: Dorsal carpal ligaments of the wrist: Normal appearance on multiplanar reconstructions of three-dimensional Fourier transform MR imaging. AJR *161*:119, 1993.
20. Steinberg BD, Plancher KD: Clinical anatomy of the wrist and elbow. Clin Sports Med *14*:299, 1995.
21. Mesgarzadeh M, Schneck CD, Bonakdarpour A: Carpal tunnel: MR imaging. I. Normal anatomy. Radiology *171*:743, 1989.
22. Zeiss J, Skie M, Ebraheim N, et al: Anatomic relations between the median nerve and flexor tendons in the carpal tunnel: MR evaluation in normal volunteers. AJR *153*:533, 1989.
23. Zeiss J, Jakab E, Khimji T, et al: The ulnar tunnel at the wrist (Guyon's canal): Normal MR anatomy and variants. AJR *158*:1081, 1992.
24. Gross MS, Gelberman RH: The anatomy of the distal ulnar tunnel. Clin Orthop *196*:238, 1985.
25. Kaplan E: Functional and Surgical Anatomy of the Hand. 2nd Ed. Philadelphia, JB Lippincott, 1965.
26. Lampe E: Surgical anatomy of the hand with special reference to infections and trauma. Clin Symp *21*:66, 1969.
27. Scheldrup E: Tendon sheath patterns in hand. Surg Gynecol Obstet *93*:161, 1951.
28. Stanley JK, Trail IA: Carpal instability. J Bone Joint Surg [Br] *76*:691, 1994.
29. McCue FC III, Bruce JF Jr: The wrist. *In* JC DeLee, D Drez Jr (Eds):

Orthopedic Sports Medicine: Principles and Practice. Philadelphia, WB Saunders Co., 1994, p. 913.

30. Gilford W, Baltar R, Lambrinudi C: The mechanics of the wrist joint. Guy's Hosp Rep *92*:52, 1943.

31. Taleisnik J: Wrist: Anatomy, function, and injury. Instr Course Lect *27*:61, 1978.

32. Weber ER: Biomechanical implications of scaphoid wrist fractures. Clin Orthop Rel Res *149*:83, 1980.

33. Lichtman DM, Schneider JR, Mack GR, et al: Ulnar midcarpal instability. J Hand Surg *6*:515, 1981.

34. Ranawat CS, Freiberger RH, Jordan LR, et al: Arthrography in the rheumatoid wrist joint: A preliminary report. J Bone Joint Surg [Am] *51*:1269, 1969.

35. Harrison MO, Freiberger RH, Ranawat CS: Arthrography of the rheumatoid wrist joint. AJR *112*:480, 1971.

36. Kessler I, Silberman Z: Experimental study of the radiocarpal joint by arthrography. Surg Gynecol Obstet *112*:33, 1961.

37. Ranawat CS, Harrison MO, Jordan LR: Arthrography of the wrist joint. Clin Orthop *83*:6, 1972.

38. Resnick D: Arthrography in the evaluation of arthritic disorders of the wrist. Radiology *113*:331, 1974.

39. Dalinka MK, Osterman AL, Albert AS, et al: Arthrography of the wrist and shoulder. Orthop Clin North Am *14*:193, 1983.

40. Kricun ME: Wrist arthrography. Clin Orthop *187*:65, 1984.

41. Mrose HE, Rosenthal DI: Arthrography of the hand and wrist. Hand Clin *7*:201, 1991.

42. Gilula LA, Totty WG, Weeks PM: Wrist arthrography: The value of fluoroscopic spot viewing. Radiology *146*:555, 1983.

43. Schwartz AM, Ruby LK: Wrist arthrography revisited. Orthopedics *5*:883, 1982.

44. Gilula LA, Hardy DC, Totty WG, et al: Fluoroscopic identification of torn intercarpal ligaments after injection of contrast material. AJR *149*:761, 1987.

45. Braunstein EM, Louis DS, Green TL, et al: Fluoroscopic and arthrographic evaluation of carpal instability. AJR *144*:1259, 1985.

46. Berger RA, Blair WF, El-Khoury GY: Arthrotomography of the wrist: The triangular fibrocartilage complex. Clin Orthop *172*:257, 1983.

47. Quinn SF, Belsole RS, Greene TL, et al: Work in progress: Postarthrography computed tomography of the wrist: Evaluation of the triangular fibrocartilage complex. Skel Radiol *17*:565, 1989.

48. Blair WF, Berger RA, El-Khoury GY: Arthrotomography of the wrist: An experimental and preliminary clinical study. J Hand Surg [Am] *10*:350, 1985.

49. Tirman RM, Weber ER, Snyder LL, et al: Midcarpal wrist arthrography for detection of tears of the scapholunate and lunotriquetral ligaments. AJR *144*:107, 1985.

50. Gilula LA, Reinus WR, Totty WG: Midcarpal wrist arthrography. AJR *146*:645, 1986.

51. Resnick D, André M, Kerr R, et al: Digital arthrography of the wrist: A radiographic and pathologic investigation. AJR *142*:1187, 1984.

52. Manaster BJ: Digital wrist arthrography: Precision in determining the site of radiocarpal-midcarpal communication. AJR *147*:563, 1986.

53. Pittman CC, Quinn SF, Belsole R, et al: Digital subtraction wrist arthrography: Use of double contrast technique as a supplement to single contrast arthrography. Skel Radiol *17*:119, 1988.

54. Quinn SF, Pittman CC, Belsole R, et al: Digital subtraction wrist arthrography: Evaluation of the multiple-compartment technique. AJR *151*:1173, 1988.

55. Belsole RJ, Quinn SF, Greene TL, et al: Digital subtraction arthrography of the wrist. J Bone Joint Surg [Am] *72*:846, 1990.

56. Levinsohn EM, Palmer AK, Coren AB, et al: Wrist arthrography: The value of the three compartment injection technique. Skel Radiol *16*:539, 1987.

57. Zinberg EM, Palmer AK, Coren AB, et al: The triple-injection wrist arthrogram. J Hand Surg [Am] *13*:803, 1988.

58. Levinsohn EM, Rosen ID, Palmer AK: Wrist arthrography: Value of the three-compartment injection method. Radiology *179*:231, 1991.

59. Manaster BJ: The clinical efficacy of triple-injection wrist arthrography. Radiology *178*:267, 1991.

60. Wilson AJ, Gilula LA, Mann FA: Unidirectional joint communications in wrist arthrography: An evaluation of 250 cases. AJR *157*:105, 1991.

61. Herbert TJ, Faithfull RG, McCann DJ, et al: Bilateral arthrography of the wrist. J Hand Surg [Br] *15*:233, 1990.

62. Cantor RM, Stern PJ, Wyrick JD, et al: The relevance of ligament tears or perforations in the diagnosis of wrist pain: An arthrographic study. J Hand Surg [Am] *19*:945, 1994.

63. Brown JA, Janzen DL, Adler BD, et al: Arthrography of the contralateral, asymptomatic wrist in patients with unilateral wrist pain. Can Assoc Radiol J *45*:292, 1994.

64. Romaniuk CS, Butt WP, Coral A: Bilateral three-compartment wrist arthrography in patients with unilateral wrist pain: Findings and implications for management. Skel Radiol *24*:95, 1995.

65. Manaster BJ, Mann RJ, Rubenstein S: Wrist pain: Correlation of clinical and plain film findings with arthrographic results. J Hand Surg [Am] *14*:466, 1989.

66. Gilula LA, Hardy DC, Totty WG: Distal radioulnar joint arthrography. AJR *150*:864, 1988.

67. Hardy DC, Totty WG, Carnes KM, et al: Arthrographic surface anatomy of the carpal triangular fibrocartilage complex. J Hand Surg [Am] *13*:823, 1988.

68. Trentham CE, Hamm RL, Masi AT: Wrist arthrography: Review and comparison of normal, rheumatoid arthritis and gout patients. Semin Arthritis Rheum *5*:105, 1975.

69. Mikic ZDJ: Arthrography of the wrist joint: An experimental study. J Bone Joint Surg [Am] *66*:371, 1984.

70. Resnick D: Early abnormalities of the pisiform and triquetrum in rheumatoid arthritis. Ann Rheum Dis *35*:46, 1976.

71. Totterman SMS, Miller RJ: Triangular fibrocartilage complex: Normal appearance on coronal three-dimensional gradient-recalled-echo MR images. Radiology *195*:521, 1995.

72. Smith DK: Scapholunate interosseous ligament of the wrist: MR appearances in asymptomatic volunteers and arthrographically normal wrists. Radiology *192*:217, 1994.

73. Dalinka MK: MR imaging of the wrist. AJR *164*:1, 1995.

74. Fritz RC, Brody GA: MR imaging of the wrist and elbow. Clin Sports Med *14*:315, 1995.

75. Rogers LF: Radiology of Skeletal Trauma. 2nd Ed. New York, Churchill Livingstone, 1992.

76. Tachdjian MO: Pediatric Orthopedics. Philadelphia, WB Saunders Co, 1972.

77. Dobyns JH, Linscheid RL: Fractures and dislocations of the wrist. *In* CA Rockwood Jr, DP Green (Eds): Fractures in Adults. 2nd Ed. Philadelphia, JB Lippincott Co, 1984, p. 411.

78. McMurtry RY, Jupiter JB: Fractures of the distal radius. *In* BD Browner, JB Jupiter, AM Levine, et al (Eds): Skeletal Trauma. Philadelphia, WB Saunders Co, 1992, p. 1063.

79. Porter M, Stockley I: Fractures of the distal radius: Intermediate and end results in relation to radiologic parameters. Clin Orthop *220*:241, 1987.

80. Mann FA, Wilson AJ, Gilula LA: Radiographic evaluation of the wrist: What does the hand surgeon want to know? Radiology *184*:15, 1992.

81. Johnson PG, Szabo RM: Angle measurements of the distal radius: A cadaver study. Skel Radiol *22*:243, 1993.

82. Atkins RM, Duckworth T, Kanis JA: Features of algodystrophy after Colles' fracture. J Bone Joint Surg [Br] *72*:105, 1990.

83. Bickerstaff DR, Bell MJ: Carpal malalignment in Colles' fractures. J Hand Surg [Br] *14*:155, 1989.

84. Paley D, McMurtry RY: Median nerve compression by volarly displaced fragments of the distal radius. Clin Orthop *215*:139, 1987.

85. Burgess RC, Watson HK: Hypertrophic ulnar styloid nonunions. Clin Orthop *228*:215, 1988.

86. Itoh Y, Horiuchi Y, Takahashi M, et al: Extensor tendon involvement in Smith's and Galeazzi's fractures. J Hand Surg [Am] *12*:535, 1987.

87. Thomas WG, Kershaw CJ: Entrapment of extensor tendons in a Smith's fracture: Brief report. J Bone Joint Surg [Br] *70*:491, 1988.

88. Helm RH, Tonkin MA: The chauffeur's fracture: Simple or complex? J Hand Surg [Br] *17*:156, 1992.

89. Mudgal CS, Jones WA: Scapho-lunate diastasis: A component of fractures of the distal radius. J Hand Surg [Br] *15*:503, 1990.

90. Ekenstam FA: Anatomy of the distal radioulnar joint. Clin Orthop *275*:14, 1992.

91. Kauer JMG: The distal radioulnar joint. Anatomic and functional considerations. Clin Orthop *275*:37, 1992.

92. Linscheid RL: Biomechanics of the distal radioulnar joint. Clin Orthop *275*:46, 1992.

93. Nathan R, Schneider LH: Classification of distal radioulnar disorders. Hand Clin *7*:239, 1991.

94. Palmer AK: Triangular fibrocartilage complex lesions: A classification. J Hand Surg [Am] *14*:594, 1989.

95. Ekenstam F, Hagert CG: Anatomical studies of the geometry and stability of the distal radioulnar joint. Scand J Plast Reconstr Surg *19*:17, 1985.

96. Vesely DG: The distal radio-ulnar joint. Clin Orthop *51*:75, 1967.

97. Bowers WH: Problems of the distal radioulnar joint. Adv Orthop Surg *7*:289, 1984.

98. Milch H: So-called dislocation of the lower end of the ulna. Ann Surg *116*:282, 1942.

99. Weigl K, Spira E: The triangular fibrocartilage of the wrist joint. Reconstr Surg Traumatol *11*:139, 1969.

100. Fortems Y, De Smet L, Dauwe D, et al: Incidence of cartilaginous and ligamentous lesions of the radio-carpal and distal radio-ulnar joint in an elderly population. J Hand Surg [Br] *19*:572, 1994.

101. Gilula LA, Palmer AK: Is it possible to diagnose a tear at arthrography or MR imaging? Radiology *187*:581, 1993.

102. Sugimoto H, Shinozaki T, Ohsawa T: Triangular fibrocartilage in asymptomatic subjects: Investigations of abnormal signal intensity. Radiology *191*:193, 1994.

103. Rieunau G, Gay R, Martinez C, et al: Lésions de l'articulation radio-cubitale inférieure dans les traumatismes de l'avant-bras et du poignet. Intérêt de l'arthrographie. Rev Chir Orthop *57*(Suppl 1):253, 1971.

104. Ganel A, Engel J, Ditzian R, et al: Arthrography as a method of diagnosing soft-tissue injuries of the wrist. J Trauma *19*:376, 1979.

105. Palmer AK, Levinsohn EM, Kuzma GR: Arthrography of the wrist. J Hand Surg *8*:15, 1983.

106. Levinsohn EM, Palmer AK: Arthrography of the traumatized wrist: Correlation with radiography and the carpal instability series. Radiology *146*:647, 1983.

107. Kirschenbaum D, Sieler S, Solonick D, et al: Arthrography of the wrist: Assessment of the integrity of the ligaments in young asymptomatic adults. J Bone Joint Surg [Am] *77*:1207, 1995.

108. Zlatkin MB, Chao PC, Osterman AL, et al: Chronic wrist pain: Evaluation with high-resolution MR imaging. Radiology *173*:723, 1989.

109. Golimbu CN, Firooznia H, Melone CP Jr, et al: Tears of the triangular fibrocartilage of the wrist: MR imaging. Radiology *173*:731, 1989.

110. Skahen JR III, Palmer AK, Levinsohn EM, et al: Magnetic resonance imaging of the triangular fibrocartilage complex. J Hand Surg [Am] *15*:552, 1990.

111. Greenan T, Zlatkin MB: Magnetic resonance imaging of the wrist. Semin Ultrasound CT MR *11*:267, 1990.

112. Cerofolini E, Luchetti R, Pederzini L, et al: MR evaluation of triangular fibrocartilage complex tears in the wrist: Comparison with arthrography and arthroscopy. J Comput Assist Tomogr *14*:963, 1990.

113. Dalinka MK, Meyer S, Kricun ME, et al: Magnetic resonance imaging of the wrist. Hand Clin *7*:87, 1991.

114. Kang HS, Kindynis P, Brahme SK, et al: Triangular fibrocartilage and intercarpal ligaments of the wrist: MR imaging. Cadaveric study with gross pathologic and histologic correlation. Radiology *181*:401, 1991.

115. Brahme SK, Resnick D: Magnetic resonance imaging of the wrist. Rheum Dis Clin North Am *17*:721, 1991.

116. Schweitzer ME, Brahme SK, Hodler J, et al: Chronic wrist pain: Spin-echo and short tau inversion recovery MR imaging and conventional and MR arthrography. Radiology *182*:205, 1992.

117. Metz VM, Schratter M, Dock WI, et al: Age-associated changes of the triangular fibrocartilage of the wrist: Evaluation of the diagnostic performance of MR imaging. Radiology *184*:217, 1992.

118. Haramati N, Deutsch A: Proximal wrist imaging. Clin Imaging *18*:79, 1994.

119. Miller RJ, Totterman SMS: Triangular fibrocartilage in asymptomatic subjects: Investigation of abnormal MR signal intensity. Radiology *196*:22, 1995.

120. Mikic ZD: Age changes in the triangular fibrocartilage of the wrist joint. J Anat *126*:367, 1978.

121. Mikic Z, Somer L, Somer T: Histologic structure of the articular disk of the human distal radioulnar joint. Clin Orthop *275*:29, 1992.

122. Metz VM, Mann FA, Gilula LA: Three-compartment wrist arthrography: Correlation of pain site with location of uni- or bidirectional communications. AJR *160*:819, 1993.

123. Metz VM, Mann FA, Gilula LA: Lack of correlation between site of wrist pain and location of noncommunicating defects shown by three-compartment wrist arthrography. AJR *160*:1239, 1993.

124. Whipple TL, Geissler WB: Arthroscopic management of wrist triangular fibrocartilage complex injuries in the athlete. Orthopedics *16*:1061, 1993.

125. Whipple TL, Marotta JJ, Powell JH III: Techniques of wrist arthroscopy. Arthroscopy *2*:244, 1986.

126. Buterbaugh GA: Radiocarpal arthroscopy portals and normal anatomy. Hand Clin *10*:567, 1994.

127. Whipple TL: Arthroscopy of the distal radioulnar joint. Indications, portals, and anatomy. Hand Clin *10*:589, 1994.

128. Adolfsson L: Arthroscopic diagnosis of ligament lesions of the wrist. J Hand Surg [Br] *19*:505, 1994.

129. Friedman SL, Palmer AK: The ulnar impaction syndrome. Hand Clin *7*:295, 1991.

130. Schuurman AH, Bos KE: The ulno-carpal abutment syndrome: Follow-up of the wafer procedure. J Hand Surg [Br] *20*:171, 1995.

131. Wnorowski DC, Palmer AK, Werner FW, et al: Anatomic and biomechanical analysis of the arthroscopic wafer procedure. J Arthroscop Rel Surg *8*:204, 1992.

132. Bell MJ, Hill RJ, McMurtry RY: Ulnar impingement syndrome. J Bone Joint Surg [Br] *67*:126, 1985.

133. Escobedo EM, Bergman AG, Hunter JC: MR imaging of ulnar impaction. Skel Radiol *24*:85, 1995.

134. King GJ, McMurtry RY, Rubenstein JD, et al: Kinematics of the distal radioulnar joint. J Hand Surg [Am] *11*:798, 1986.

135. Adams BD: Partial excision of the triangular fibrocartilage complex articular disk: A biomechanical study. J Hand Surg [Am] *18*:334, 1993.

136. Hotchkiss RN: Injuries to the interosseous ligament of the forearm. Hand Clin *10*:391, 1994.

137. Törnvall AH, Ekenstam FA, Hagert CG, et al: Radiologic examination and measurement of the wrist and distal radio-ulnar joint: New aspects. Acta Radiol Diagn *27*:581, 1986.

138. Nakamura R, Horii E, Imaeda T, et al: Distal radioulnar joint subluxation and dislocation diagnosed by standard roentgenography. Skel Radiol *24*:91, 1995.

139. Mino DE, Palmer AK, Levinsohn EM: The role of radiography and computerized tomography in the diagnosis of subluxation and dislocation of the distal radioulnar joint. J Hand Surg *8*:23, 1983.

140. Mino DE, Palmer AK, Levinsohn EM: Radiography and computerized tomography in the diagnosis of incongruity of the distal radio-ulnar joint. J Bone Joint Surg [Am] *67*:247, 1985.

141. Olerud C, Kongsholm J, Thuomas K-A: The congruence of the distal radioulnar joint: A magnetic resonance imaging study. Acta Orthop Scand *59*:183, 1988.

142. Staron RB, Feldman F, Haramati N, et al: Abnormal geometry of the distal radioulnar joint: MR findings. Skel Radiol *23*:369, 1994.

143. Pirela-Cruz MA, Goll SR, Klug M, et al: Stress computed tomography analysis of the distal radioulnar joint: A diagnostic tool for determining translational motion. J Hand Surg [Am] *16*:75, 1991.

144. Hughston JC: Fracture of the distal radial shaft: Mistakes in management. J Bone Joint Surg [Am] *39*:249, 1957.

145. Wong PCN: Galeazzi fracture-dislocations in Singapore 1960–1964: Incidence and results of treatment. Singapore Med J *8*:186, 1967.

146. Reckling FW, Cordell LD: Unstable fracture-dislocations of the forearm: The Monteggia and Galeazzi lesions. Arch Surg *96*:999, 1968.

147. Mikic ZD: Galeazzi fracture-dislocations. J Bone Joint Surg [Am] *57*:1071, 1975.

148. Walsh HPJ, McLaren CAN, Owen R: Galeazzi fractures in children. J Bone Joint Surg [Br] *69*:730, 1987.

149. Khurana JS, Kattapuram SV, Becker S, et al: Galeazzi injury with an associated fracture of the radial head. Clin Orthop *234*:70, 1988.

150. Rienau G, Gay R, Martinez C, Mansat C, Mansat M: Lésions de l'articulation radio-cubitale inférieure dans les traumatismes de l'avantbras et du poignet: Intérêt de l'arthrographie. Rev Chir Orthop *57*(Suppl 1):253, 1971.

151. Linscheid RL, Dobyns JH, Beabout JW, et al: Traumatic instability of the wrist: Diagnosis, classification, and pathomechanics. J Bone Joint Surg [Am] *54*:1612, 1972.

152. Dobyns JH, Linscheid RL, Chao EYS, et al: Traumatic instability of the wrist. *In* Instructional Course Lectures. American Academy of Orthopaedic Surgeons. Vol. 24. St Louis, CV Mosby, 1975, p. 182.

153. Logan SE, Nowak MD, Gould PL, et al: Biomechanical behavior of the scapholunate ligament. Biomed Sci Instrum *22*:81, 1986.

154. Gilula LA, Weeks PM: Post-traumatic ligamentous instabilities of the wrist. Radiology *129*:641, 1978.

155. Gilula LA: Carpal injuries: Analytic approach and case exercises. AJR *133*:503, 1979.

156. Taleisnik J: Carpal instability. J Bone Joint Surg [Am] *70*:1262, 1988.

157. Linscheid RL, Dobyns JH, Beabout JW, Bryan RS: Traumatic instability of the wrist: Diagnosis, classification, and pathomechanics. J Bone Joint Surg [Am] *54*:1612, 1972.

158. Cantor RM, Braunstein EM: Diagnosis of dorsal and palmar rotation of the lunate on a frontal radiograph. J Hand Surg [Am] *13*:187, 1988.

159. Linscheid RL, Dobyns JH, Beckenbaugh RD, et al: Instability patterns of the wrist. J Hand Surg *8*:682, 1983.

160. Pennes DR, Shirazi KK, Martel W: Bilateral palmar flexion instability: A complication of wheelchair use. AJR *141*:1327, 1983.

161. Resnick D, Niwayama G: Carpal instability in rheumatoid arthritis and calcium pyrophosphate deposition disease: Pathogenesis and roentgen appearance. Ann Rheum Dis *36*:311, 1977.

162. Fisk GR: The wrist. J Bone Joint Surg [Br] *66*:396, 1984.

163. Taleisnik J: Classification of carpal instability. Bull Hosp J Dis *44*:511, 1984.

164. Lichtman DM, Schneider JR, Swafford AR, Mack GR: Ulnar midcarpal instability—clinical and laboratory analysis. J Hand Surg *6*:515, 1981.

165. Jones WA: Beware the sprained wrist: The incidence and prognosis of scapholunate instability. J Bone Joint Surg [Br] *70*:293, 1988.

166. Braunstein EM, Louis DS, Greene TL, et al: Fluoroscopic and arthrographic evaluation of carpal instability. AJR *144*:1259, 1985.

167. Protas JM, Jackson WT: Evaluating carpal instabilities with fluoroscopy. AJR *135*:137, 1980.

168. Jackson WT, Protas JM: Snapping scapholunate subluxation. J Hand Surg *6*:590, 1981.

169. White SJ, Louis DS, Braunstein EM, Hankin FM, Greene TL: Capitate-lunate instability: Recognition by manipulation under fluoroscopy. AJR *143*:361, 1984.

170. Fortems Y, Mawhinney I, Lawrence T, et al: Traction radiographs in the diagnosis of chronic wrist pain. J Hand Surg [Br] *19*:334, 1994.

171. Truong NP, Mann FA, Gilula LA, et al: Wrist instability series: Increased yield with clinical-radiologic screening criteria. Radiology *192*:481, 1994.

172. Watson H, Ottoni L, Pitts EC, et al: Rotary subluxation of the scaphoid: A spectrum of instability. J Hand Surg [Br] *18*:62, 1993.

173. Cautilli GP, Wehbé MA: Scapho-lunate distance and cortical ring sign. J Hand Surg [Am] *16*:501, 1991.

174. Ruby LK, An KN, Linscheid RL, et al: The effect of scapholunate ligament section on scapholunate motion. J Hand Surg [Am] *12*:767, 1987.

175. Berger RA, Blair WF, Crowninshield RD, et al: The scapholunate ligament. J Hand Surg [Am] *7*:87, 1982.

176. Hudson TM, Caragol WJ, Kaye JJ: Isolated rotatory subluxation of the carpal navicular. AJR *126*:601, 1976.

177. Boyes JG: Subluxation of the carpal navicular bone. South Med J *69*:141, 1976.

178. Frankel VH: The Terry-Thomas sign. Clin Orthop *129*:321, 1977.

179. Howard FM, Fahey T, Wojcik E: Rotatory subluxation of the navicular. Clin Orthop *104*:134, 1974.

180. Crittenden JJ, Jones DM, Santarelli AG: Bilateral rotational dislocation of the carpal navicular: Case report. Radiology *94*:629, 1970.

181. Kindynis P, Resnick D, Kang HS, et al: Demonstration of the scapholunate space with radiography. Radiology *175*:278, 1990.

182. Smith DK, Snearly WN: Lunotriquetral interosseous ligament of the wrist: MR appearances in asymptomatic volunteers and arthrographically normal wrists. Radiology *191*:199, 1994.
183. Berger RA, Linscheid RL, Berquist TH: Magnetic resonance imaging of the anterior radiocarpal ligaments. J Hand Surg [Am] *19*:295, 1994.
184. Timins ME, Jahnke JP, Krah SF, et al: MR imaging of the major carpal stabilizing ligaments: Normal anatomy and clinical examples. RadioGraphics *15*:575, 1995.
185. Yu JS: Magnetic resonance imaging of the wrist. Orthopedics *17*:1041, 1994.
186. Ton ERTA, Pattynama PMT, Bloem JL, et al: Interosseous ligaments: Device for applying stress in wrist MR imaging. Radiology *196*:863, 1995.
187. Poehling GG, Chabon SJ, Ruch DS: Carpal instabilities. *In* GG Poehling, LA Koman, TL Pope Jr, et al (Eds): Arthroscopy of the Wrist and Elbow. New York, Raven Press, 1993, p. 73.
188. Osterman AL, Seidman GD: The role of arthroscopy in the treatment of lunatotriquetral ligament injuries. Hand Clin *11*:41, 1995.
189. Zachee B, De Smet L, Fabry G: Frayed ulno-triquetral and ulno-lunate ligament rupture. J Hand Surg [Br] *19*:570, 1994.
190. Maki NJ, Chuinard RG, D'Ambrosia R: Isolated, complete radial dislocation of the scaphoid: A case report and review of the literature. J Bone Joint Surg [Am] *64*:615, 1982.
191. Sides D, Laorr A, Greenspan A: Carpal scaphoid: Radiographic pattern of dislocation. Radiology *195*:215, 1995.
192. Szabo R, Newland CC, Johnson PG, et al: Spectrum of injury and treatment options for isolated dislocation of the scaphoid: A report of three cases. J Bone Joint Surg [Am] *77*:608, 1995.
193. Lowrey DG, Moss SH, Wolff TW: Volar dislocation of the capitate: Report of a case. J Bone Joint Surg [Am] *66*:611, 1984.
194. Soucacos PN, Hartofilakidis-Garofalidas GC: Dislocation of the triangular bone: Report of a case. J Bone Joint Surg [Am] *63*:1012, 1981.
195. Boe S: Dislocation of the trapezium (multangulum majus). A case report. Acta Orthop Scand *50*:85, 1979.
196. Holdsworth BJ, Shackleford I: Fracture dislocation of the trapezio-scaphoid joint—the missing link? J Hand Surg [Br] *12*:41, 1987.
197. Stevanovic MV, Stark HH, Filler BC: Scaphotrapezial dislocation: A case report. J Bone Joint Surg [Am] *72*:449, 1990.
198. Ostrowski DM, Miller ME, Gould JS: Dorsal dislocation of the trapezoid. J Hand Surg [Am] *15*:874, 1990.
199. Inoue G, Inagaki Y: Isolated palmar dislocation of the trapezoid associated with attritional rupture of the flexor tendon: A case report. J Bone Joint Surg [Am] *72*:446, 1990.
200. Goodman ML, Shankman GB: Palmar dislocation of the trapezoid—a case report. J Hand Surg *8*:606, 1983.
201. Sundaram M, Shively R, Patel B, Tayob A: Isolated dislocation of the pisiform. Br J Radiol *53*:911, 1980.
202. Minami M, Yamazaki J, Ishii S: Isolated dislocation of the pisiform: A case report and review of the literature. J Hand Surg [Am] *9*:125, 1984.
203. McCarron RF, Coleman W: Dislocation of the pisiform treated by primary resection: A case report. Clin Orthop *241*:231, 1989.
204. Pai C-H, Wei D-C, Hu S-T: Carpal bone dislocations: An analysis of twenty cases with relative emphasis on the role of crushing mechanisms. J Trauma *35*:28, 1993.
205. Richards RS, Bennett JD, Roth JH: Scaphoid dislocation with radial-axial carpal disruption. AJR *160*:1075, 1993.
206. Coll GA: Palmar dislocation of the scaphoid and lunate. J Hand Surg [Am] *12*:476, 1987.
207. Goldberg B, Heller AP: Dorsal dislocation of the triquetrum with rotary subluxation of the scaphoid. J Hand Surg [Am] *12*:119, 1987.
208. Fowler JL: Dislocation of the triquetrum and lunate: Brief report. J Hand Surg [Br] *70*:665, 1988.
209. Norbeck DE Jr, Larson B, Blair SJ, et al: Traumatic longitudinal disruption of the carpus. J Hand Surg [Am] *12*:509, 1987.
210. Pournaras J, Kappas A: Volar perilunar dislocation: A case report. J Bone Joint Surg [Am] *61*:625, 1979.
211. Klein A, Webb LX: The crowded carpal sign in volar perilunar dislocation. J Trauma *27*:82, 1987.
212. Stein F, Siegel MW: Naviculocapitate fracture syndrome: A case report—new thoughts on the mechanism of injury. J Bone Joint Surg [Am] *51*:391, 1969.
213. MacAusland WR: Perilunar dislocation of the carpal bones and dislocation of the lunate bone. Surg Gynecol Obstet *79*:256, 1944.
214. Dunn AW: Fractures and dislocations of the carpus. Surg Clin North Am *52*:1513, 1972.
215. Mayfield JK, Johnson RP, Kilcoyne RK: Carpal dislocations: Pathomechanics and progressive perilunar instability. J Hand Surg *5*:226, 1980.
216. El-Khoury GY, Usta HY, Blair WF: Naviculocapitate fracture-dislocation. AJR *139*:385, 1982.
217. Resnik CS, Gelberman RH, Resnick D: Transscaphoid, transcapitate, perilunate fracture dislocation (scaphocapitate syndrome). Skel Radiol *9*:192, 1983.
218. Brekkan A, Karlsson J, Thorsteinsson T: Case report 252. Skel Radiol *10*:291, 1983.
219. Yeager BA, Dalinka MK: Radiology of trauma to the wrist. Dislocations, fracture dislocations, and instability patterns. Skel Radiol *13*:120, 1985.
220. Mayfield JK: Patterns of injury to carpal ligaments: A spectrum. Clin Orthop *187*:36, 1984.
221. Cooney WP, Bussey R, Dobyns JH, et al: Difficult wrist fractures: Perilunate fracture-dislocations of the wrist. Clin Orthop *214*:136, 1987.
222. Chen VT: Dislocation of carpometacarpal joint of the little finger. J Hand Surg [Br] *12*:260, 1987.
223. Ho PK, Choban SJ, Eshman SJ, et al: Complex dorsal dislocation of the second carpometacarpal joint. J Hand Surg [Am] *12*:1074, 1987.
224. Lawlis JF III, Gunther SF: Carpometacarpal dislocations: Long-term follow-up. J Bone Joint Surg [Am] *73*:52, 1991.
225. Hazlett JW: Carpometacarpal dislocations other than the thumb: A report of 11 cases. Can J Surg *71*:315, 1968.
226. Hsu JD, Curtis RM: Carpometacarpal dislocations on the ulnar side of the hand. J Bone Joint Surg [Am] *52*:927, 1970.
227. Joseph RB, Linscheid RL, Dobyns JH, Bryan RS: Chronic sprains of the carpometacarpal joints. J Hand Surg *6*:172, 1981.
228. Fisher MR, Rogers LF, Hendrix RW: Systematic approach to identifying fourth and fifth carpometacarpal joint dislocations. AJR *140*:319, 1983.
229. Gunther SF: The carpometacarpal joints. Orthop Clin North Am *15*:259, 1984.
230. Mody BS, Belliappa PP, Dias JJ, et al: Nonunion of fractures of the scaphoid tuberosity. J Bone Joint Surg [Br] *75*:423, 1993.
231. Vahvanen V, Westerlund M: Fracture of the carpal scaphoid in children: A clinical and roentgenological study of 108 cases. Acta Orthop Scand *51*:909, 1980.
232. Cockshott WP: Distal avulsion fractures of the scaphoid. Br J Radiol *53*:1037, 1980.
233. Compson JP, Waterman JK, Spencer JD: Dorsal avulsion fractures of the scaphoid: Diagnostic implications and applied anatomy. J Hand Surg [Br] *18*:58, 1993.
234. Larson B, Light TR, Ogden JA: Fracture and ischemic necrosis of the immature scaphoid. J Hand Surg [Am] *12*:122, 1987.
235. Tiel-van Buul MMC, van Beek EJR, Dijkstra PF, et al: Radiography of the carpal scaphoid: Experimental evaluation of "the carpal box" and first clinical results. Invest Radiol *27*:954, 1992.
236. Lindequist S, Larsen CF: Radiography of the carpal scaphoid: An experimental investigation evaluating the use of oblique projections. Acta Radiol (Diagn) *27*:97, 1986.
237. Nicholl JE, Spencer JD, Buckland-Wright C: Pattern of scaphoid fracture union detected by macroradiography. J Hand Surg [Br] *20*:189, 1995.
238. Young MRA, Lowry JH, Laird JD, et al: ⁹⁹Tc-MDP bone scanning of injuries of the carpal scaphoid. Injury *19*:14, 1988.
239. Brismar J: Skeletal scintigraphy of the wrist in suggested scaphoid fracture. Acta Radiol (Diagn) *29*:101, 1988.
240. Tiel-van Buul MMC, van Beek EJR, Broekhuizen AH, et al: Radiography and scintigraphy of suspected scaphoid fracture: A long-term study in 160 patients. J Bone Joint Surg [Br] *75*:61, 1993.
241. Tiel-van Buul MMC, van Beek EJR, Dijkstra PF, et al: Significance of a hotspot on the bone scan after carpal injury—evaluation by computed tomography. Eur J Nucl Med *20*:159, 1993.
242. Holder LE, Mulligan ME, Gillespie TE: Diagnosis of scaphoid fractures: The role of nuclear medicine. J Nucl Med *36*:48, 1995.
243. Waizenegger M, Wastie ML, Barton NJ, et al: Scintigraphy in the evaluation of the "clinical" scaphoid fracture. J Hand Surg [Br] *19*:750, 1995.
244. Smith DK, Linscheid RL, Amadio PC, et al: Scaphoid anatomy: Evaluation with complex motion tomography. Radiology *173*:177, 1989.
245. Tehranzadeh J, Davenport J, Pais MJ: Scaphoid fracture: Evaluation with flexion-extension tomography. Radiology *176*:167, 1990.
246. Pennes DR, Jonsson K, Buckwalter KA: Direct coronal CT of the scaphoid bone. Radiology *171*:870, 1989.
247. Nakamura R, Imaeda T, Horii E, et al: Analysis of scaphoid fracture displacement by three-dimensional computed tomography. J Hand Surg [Am] *16*:485, 1991.
248. Bain GI, Bennett JD, Richards RS, et al: Longitudinal computed tomography of the scaphoid: A new technique. Skel Radiol *24*:271, 1995.
249. Cooney WP III, Dobyns JH, Linscheid RL: Fractures of the scaphoid: A rational approach to management. Clin Orthop *149*:90, 1980.
250. Andersen JL, Grøn P, Langhoff O: The scaphoid fat stripe in the diagnosis of carpal trauma. Acta Radiol (Diagn) *29*:97, 1988.
251. Corfitsen M, Christensen SE, Cetti R: The anatomical fat pad and the radiological "scaphoid fat stripe." J Hand Surg [Br] *14*:326, 1989.
252. Brøndum V, Larsen CF, Skov O: Fracture of the carpal scaphoid: Frequency and distribution in a well-defined population. Eur J Radiol *15*:118, 1992.
253. Dias JJ, Thompson J, Barton NJ, et al: Suspected scaphoid fractures: The value of radiographs. J Bone Joint Surg [Br] *72*:98, 1990.
254. Smith DK, Gilula LA, Amadio PC: Dorsal lunate tilt (DISI configuration): Sign of scaphoid fracture displacement. Radiology *176*:497, 1990.
255. Dias JJ, Taylor M, Thompson J, et al: Radiographic signs of union of scaphoid fractures: An analysis of inter-observer agreement and reproducibility. J Bone Joint Surg [Br] *70*:299, 1988.
256. Szabo RM, Manske D: Displaced fractures of the scaphoid. Clin Orthop *230*:30, 1988.
257. Duppe H, Johnell O, Lundborg G, et al: Long term results of fracture of the scaphoid: A follow-up study of more than thirty years. J Bone Joint Surg [Am] *76*:249, 1994.
258. Dias JJ, Brenkel IJ, Finlay DBL: Patterns of union in fractures of the waist of the scaphoid. J Bone Joint Surg [Br] *71*:307, 1989.

259. Gelberman RH, Wolock BS, Siegel DB: Fractures and non-unions of the carpal scaphoid. J Bone Joint Surg [Am] 71:1560, 1989.
260. Black DM, Watson HK, Vender MI: Scapholunate gap with scaphoid nonunion. Clin Orthop 224:205, 1987.
261. Mack GR, Bosse MJ, Gelberman RH: The natural history of scaphoid nonunion. J Bone Joint Surg [Am] 66:504, 1984.
262. Ruby LK, Stinson J, Belsky MR: The natural history of scaphoid nonunion: A review of fifty-five cases. J Bone Joint Surg [Am] 67:428, 1985.
263. McLain RF, Steyers CM: Tendon ruptures with scaphoid nonunion: A case report. Clin Orthop 255:117, 1990.
264. Quinn SF, Murray W, Watkins T, et al: CT for determining the results of treatment of fractures of the wrist. AJR 149:109, 1987.
265. Sherman SB, Greenspan A, Norman A: Osteonecrosis of the distal pole of the carpal scaphoid following fracture—a rare complication. Skel Radiol 9:189, 1983.
266. Botte MJ, Gelberman RH: Fractures of the carpus, excluding the scaphoid. Hand Clin 3:149, 1987.
267. Levy M, Fischel RE, Stern GM, Goldberg I: Chip fractures of the os triquetrum: The mechanism of injury. J Bone Joint Surg [Br] 61:355, 1979.
268. Hocker K, Menschik A: Chip fractures of the triquetrum: Mechanism, Classification and results. J Hand Surg [Br] 19:584, 1994.
269. Cetti R, Christensen S-E, Reuther K: Fracture of the lunate bone. Hand 14:80, 1982.
270. Teisen H, Hjarbaek J: Classification of fresh fractures of the lunate. J Hand Surg [Br] 13:458, 1988.
271. Viegas SF, Wagner K, Patterson R, et al: Medial (hamate) facet of the lunate. J Hand Surg [Am] 15:564, 1990.
272. Ogunro O: Fracture of the body of the hamate bone. J Hand Surg 8:353, 1983.
273. Takami H, Takahashi S, Hiraki S: Coronal fractures of the body of the hamate: Case reports. J Trauma 32:110, 1992.
274. Loth TS, McMillan MD: Coronal dorsal hamate fractures. J Hand Surg [Am] 13:616, 1988.
275. Gillespy T III, Stork JJ, Dell PC: Dorsal fracture of the hamate: Distinctive radiographic appearance. AJR 151:351, 1988.
276. Ebraheim NA, Skie MC, Savolaine ER, et al: Coronal fracture of the body of the hamate. J Trauma 38:169, 1995.
277. Schlosser H, Murray JF: Fracture of the hook of the hamate. Can J Surg 27:587, 1984.
278. Murray WT, Meuller PR, Rosenthal DI, Jauernek RR: Fracture of the hook of the hamate. AJR 133:899, 1979.
279. Parker RD, Berkowitz MS, Brahms MA, Bohl WR: Hook of the hamate fractures in athletes. Am J Sports Med 14:517, 1986.
280. Stark HH, Chao E-K, Zemel NP, et al: Fracture of the hook of the hamate. J Bone Joint Surg [Am] 71:1202, 1989.
281. Futami T, Aoki H, Tsukamoto Y: Fractures of the hook of the hamate in athletes: Eight cases followed for 6 years. Acta Orthop Scand 64:469, 1993.
282. Papilion JD, DuPuy TE, Aulicino PL, et al: Radiographic evaluation of the hook of the hamate: A new technique. J Hand Surg [Am] 13:437, 1988.
283. Carter PR, Eaton RG, Littler JW: Ununited fracture of the hook of the hamate. J Bone Joint Surg [Am] 59:583, 1977.
284. Failla JM: Osteonecrosis associated with nonunion of the hook of the hamate. Orthopedics 16:217, 1993.
285. Manske PR: Fracture of the hook of the hamate presenting as carpal tunnel syndrome. Hand 10:181, 1978.
286. Minami A, Ogino T, Usui M, Ishii S: Finger tendon rupture secondary to fracture of the hamate: A case report. Acta Orthop Scand 56:96, 1985.
287. Fleege MA, Jebson PJ, Renfrew DL, et al: Pisiform fractures. Skel Radiol 20:169, 1991.
288. Georgoulis A, Hertel P, Lais E: Die Fraktur und die Luxationsfraktur des Os pisiforme. Unfallchirurg 94:182, 1991.
289. Rand JA, Linscheid RL, Dobyns JH: Capitate fractures: A long-term follow-up. Clin Orthop 165:209, 1982.
290. Shirazi KK, Agha FP, Amendola MA: Isolated fracture of greater multangular. Br J Radiol 55:923, 1982.
291. Abbitt PL, Riddervold HO: The carpal tunnel view: Helpful adjuvant for unrecognized fractures of the carpus. Skel Radiol 16:45, 1987.
292. Griffen AC, Gilula LA, Young VL, et al: Fracture of the dorsoulnar tubercle of the trapezium. J Hand Surg [Am] 13:622, 1988.
293. Botte MJ, von Schroeder HP, Gellman H, et al: Fracture of the trapezial ridge. Clin Orthop 276:202, 1992.
294. Mitchell DG, Kressel HY: MR imaging of early avascular necrosis. Radiology 169:281, 1988.
295. Mitchell DG: Using MR imaging to probe the pathophysiology of osteonecrosis. Radiology 171:25, 1989.
296. Mitchell DG, Rao VM, Dalinka MK, et al: Femoral head avascular necrosis: Correlation of MR imaging, radiographic staging, radionuclide imaging and clinical findings. Radiology 162:709, 1987.
297. Koenig H, Lucas D, Meissner R: The wrist: A preliminary report on high-resolution MR imaging. Radiology 160:463, 1986.
298. Reinus WR, Conway WF, Totty WG, et al: Carpal avascular necrosis: MR imaging. Radiology 160:689, 1986.
299. Sowa DT, Holder LE, Patt PG, et al: Application of magnetic resonance imaging to ischemic necrosis of the lunate. J Hand Surg [Am] 14:1008, 1989.
300. Herbert TJ, Lanzetta M: Idiopathic avascular necrosis of the scaphoid. J Hand Surg [Br] 19:174, 1994.
301. Lamphier TA: Carpal bossing. Arch Surg 81:1013, 1960.
302. Bassoe E, Bassoe HH: The styloid bone and carpe bossu disease. AJR 74:886, 1955.
303. Carter RM: Carpal boss: Commonly overlooked deformity of the carpus. J Bone Joint Surg 23:935, 1941.
304. Conway WF, Destouet JM, Gilula LA, et al: The carpal boss: An overview of radiographic evaluation. Radiology 156:29, 1985.
305. Hultgren T, Lugnegoerd H: Carpal boss. Acta Orthop Scand 57:547, 1986.
306. Keats TE: Normal variants of the hand and wrist. Hand Clinics 7:153, 1991.
307. Poznanski AK: The Hand in Radiologic Diagnosis. Philadelphia, WB Saunders Co, 1974.
308. Cope JR: Carpal coalition. Clin Radiol 25:261, 1974.
309. Garn SM, Frisancho AR, Poznanski AK, et al: Analysis of triquetral-lunate fusion. Am J Phys Anthropol 34:431, 1971.
310. Dean RFA, Jones PRM: Fusion of triquetral and lunate bones shown in several radiographs. Am J Phys Anthropol 17:279, 1959.
311. Knezevich S, Gottesman M: Symptomatic scapholunatotriquetral carpal coalition with fusion of the capitatometacarpal joint: Report of a case. Clin Orthop 251:153, 1990.
312. Cockshott WP: Carpal fusions. AJR 89:1260, 1963.
313. Cockshott WP: Pisiform hamate fusion. J Bone Joint Surg [Am] 51:778, 1969.
314. Ganos DL, Imbriglia JE: Symptomatic congenital coalition of the pisiform and hamate. J Hand Surg [Am] 16:646, 1991.
315. O'Rahilly R: A survey of carpal and tarsal anomalies. J Bone Joint Surg [Am] 35:626, 1953.
316. Smith-Hoefer E, Szabo RM: Isolated carpal synchondrosis of the scaphoid and trapezium: A case report. J Bone Joint Surg [Am] 67:318, 1985.
317. Carlson DH: Coalition of the carpal bones. Skel Radiol 7:125, 1981.
318. Resnik CS, Grizzard JD, Simmons BP, et al: Incomplete carpal coalition. AJR 147:301, 1986.
319. Simmons BP, McKenzie WD: Symptomatic carpal coalition. J Hand Surg [Am] 10:190, 1985.
320. Gross SC, Watson K, Strickland JW, et al: Triquetral-lunate arthritis secondary to synostosis. J Hand Surg [Am] 14:95, 1989.
321. McGoey PF: Fracture-dislocation of fused triangular and lunate (congenital). Report of a case. J Bone Joint Surg 25:928, 1943.
322. Smitham JH: Some observations on certain congenital abnormalities of the hand in African natives. Br J Radiol 21:513, 1948.
323. McCredie J: Congenital fusion of bones: Radiology, embryology, and pathogenesis. Clin Radiol 26:47, 1975.
324. Madelung OW: Die spontane Subluxation der Hand nach vorne. Verh Dtsch Ges Chir 7:259, 1878.
325. Anton JI, Reitz GB, Spiegel MB: Madelung's deformity. Ann Surg 108:411, 1938.
326. Felman AH, Kirkpatrick JA Jr: Madelung's deformity: Observations in 17 patients. Radiology 93:1037, 1969.
327. Nielsen JB: Madelung's deformity: A follow-up study of 26 cases and a review of the literature. Acta Orthop Scand 48:379, 1977.
328. Dannenburg M, Anton JI, Spiegel MB: Madelung's deformity: Consideration of its roentgenological diagnostic criteria. AJR 42:671, 1939.
329. Ranawat CS, DeFiore J, Straub LR: Madelung's deformity: An end-result study of surgical treatment. J Bone Joint Surg [Am] 57:772, 1975.
330. Henry A, Thorburn MJ: Madelung's deformity: A clinical and cytogenetic study. J Bone Joint Surg [Br] 49:66, 1967.
331. Kosowicz J: The carpal sign in gonadal dysgenesis. J Clin Endocrinol Metab 22:949, 1962.
332. Kosowicz J: The roentgen appearance of hand and wrist in gonadal dysgenesis. AJR 93:354, 1965.
333. Fagg PS: Reverse Madelung's deformity with nerve compression. J Hand Surg [Br] 13:23, 1988.
334. Luchetti R, Mingione A, Monteleone M, et al: Carpal tunnel syndrome in Madelung's deformity. J Hand Surg [Br] 13:19, 1988.
335. Goodwin DRA, Michels CH, Weissman SL: Spontaneous rupture of extensor tendons in Madelung's deformity. Hand 71:72, 1979.
336. Gooding GAW: Tenosynovitis of the wrist: A sonographic demonstration. J Ultrasound Med 7:225, 1988.
337. John V, Nau HE, Nahsen HC, et al: CT of carpal tunnel syndrome. AJNR 4:770, 1983.
338. Merhar GL, Clark RA, Schneider HJ, et al: High-resolution computed tomography of the wrist in patients with carpal tunnel syndrome. Skel Radiol 15:549, 1986.
339. Zucker-Pinchoff B, Hermann G, Srinivasan R: Computed tomography of the carpal tunnel: A radioanatomical study. J Comput Assist Tomogr 5:525, 1981.
340. Mesgarzadeh M, Schneck CD, Bonakdarpour A, et al: Carpal tunnel: MR imaging. II. Carpal tunnel syndrome. Radiology 171:749, 1989.
341. Boren WL, Henry REC Jr, Wintch K: MR diagnosis of fibrolipomatous hamartoma of nerve: Association with nerve territory-oriented macrodactyly (macrodystrophia lipomatosa). Skel Radiol 24:296, 1995.
342. Warhold LG, Urban MA, Bora W Jr, et al: Fibrofibromatous hamartomas of the median nerve. J Hand Surg [Am] 18:1032, 1993.
343. Finkelstein H: Stenosing tenovaginitis at the radial styloid process. J Bone Joint Surg [Am] 12:509, 1930.

344. Bishop AT, Gabel G, Carmichael SW: Flexor carpi radialis tendinitis. I. Operative anatomy. J Bone Joint Surg [Am] 76:1009, 1994.

345. Gabel G, Bishop AT, Wood MB: Flexor carpi radialis tendinitis. II. Results of operative treatment. J Bone Joint Surg [Am] 76:1015, 1994.

346. Burkhart SS, Wood MB, Linscheid RL: Post traumatic recurrent subluxation of the extensor carpi ulnaris tendon. J Hand Surg 7:1, 1982.

347. Fullerton GD, Cameron IL, Ord VA: Orientation of tendons in the magnetic field and its effect on T2 relaxation times. Radiology 155:433, 1985.

348. Erickson SJ, Cox IH, Hyde JS, et al: Effect of tendon orientation on MR imaging signal intensity: A manifestation of the "magic angle" phenomenon. Radiology 181:389, 1991.

349. Scott JR, Cobby M, Taggart I: Magnetic resonance imaging of acute tendon injury in the finger. J Hand Surg [Br] 20:286, 1995.

350. Drape J-L, Dubert T, Silbermann O, et al: Acute trauma of the extensor hood of the metacarpophalangeal joint: MR imaging evaluation. Radiology 192:469, 1994.

351. Jelinek JS, Kransdorf MJ, Shmookler BM, et al: Giant cell tumor of the tendon sheath: MR findings in nine cases. AJR 162:919, 1994.

352. Bianchi S, Abdelwahab IF, Zwass A, et al: Ultrasonographic evaluation of wrist ganglia. Skel Radiol 23:201, 1994.

353. Cardinal E, Buckwalter KA, Braunstein EM, et al: Occult dorsal carpal ganglion: Comparison of US and MR imaging. Radiology 193:259, 1994.

354. Maloney MD, Sauser DD, Hanson EC, et al: Adhesive capsulitis of the wrist: Arthrographic diagnosis. Radiology 167:187, 1988.

355. Hanson EC, Wood VE, Thiel AE, et al: Adhesive capsulitis of the wrist. Diagnosis and treatment. Clin Orthop 234:51, 1988.

356. Brandser EA, Renfrew DL, Schenck RR: Adhesive capsulitis of the wrist. Can Assoc Radiol J 46:137, 1995.

357. Palmer WE, Rosenthal DI, Schoenberg OI, et al: Quantification of inflammation in the wrist with gadolinium-enhanced MR imaging and PET with 2-(F-18)-fluoro-2-deoxy-D-glucose. Radiology 196:647, 1995.

358. Miller TT, Potter HG, McCormack RR Jr: Benign soft tissue masses of the wrist and hand: MRI appearances. Skel Radiol 23:327, 1994.

359. Still JM, Kleinert HE: Anomalous muscles and nerve entrapment in the wrist and hand. Plast Reconstr Surg 52:394, 1973.

360. Sanger JFR, Krasniak CL, Matloub HS, et al: Diagnosis of an anomalous superficialis muscle in the palm by magnetic resonance imaging. J Hand Surg [Am] 16:98, 1991.

361. Gama C: Extensor digitorum brevis manus: A report on 38 cases and a review of the literature. J Hand Surg [Am] 8:578, 1983.

362. Pribyl CR, Moneim MS: Anomalous hand muscle found in the Guyon's canal at exploration for ulnar artery thrombosis: A case report. Clin Orthop 306:120, 1994.

363. Anderson MW, Benedetti P, Walter J, et al: MR appearance of the extensor digitorum manus brevis muscle: A pseudotumor of the hand. AJR 164:1477, 1995.

364. Zeiss J, Jakab E: MR demonstration of an anomalous muscle in a patient with coexistent carpal and ulnar tunnel syndrome: Case report and literature survey. Clin Imaging 19:102, 1995.

365. Hubbard LF: Metacarpophalangeal dislocations. Hand Clin 4:39, 1988.

366. Kaplan EB: Dorsal dislocation of the metacarpophalangeal joint of the index finger. J Bone Joint Surg [Am] 39:1081, 1957.

367. Sweterlitsch PR, Torg JS, Pollack H: Entrapment of a sesamoid in the index metacarpophalangeal joint: Report of two cases. J Bone Joint Surg [Am] 51:995, 1969.

368. Khuri SM, Fay JJ: Complete volar metacarpophalangeal joint dislocation of a finger. J Trauma 26:1058, 1986.

369. Vicar AJ: Proximal interphalangeal joint dislocations without fractures. Hand Clin 4:5, 1988.

370. Lubahn JD: Dorsal fracture dislocations of the proximal interphalangeal joint. Hand Clin 4:15, 1988.

371. Moberg E: Fractures and ligamentous injuries of the thumb and fingers. Surg Clin North Am 40:297, 1960.

372. Nance EP Jr, Kaye JJ, Milek MA: Volar plate fractures. Radiology 133:61, 1979.

373. Phillips JH: Irreducible dislocation of a distal interphalangeal joint: Case report and review of literature. Clin Orthop 154:188, 1981.

374. Rayan GM, Elias LS: Irreducible dislocation of the distal interphalangeal joint caused by long flexor tendon entrapment. Orthopedics 4:35, 1981.

375. Green DP, O'Brien ET: Fractures of the thumb metacarpal. South Med J 65:807, 1972.

376. Griffiths JC: Fractures at the base of the first metacarpal bone. J Bone Joint Surg [Br] 46:712, 1964.

377. Howard FM: Fractures of the basal joint of the thumb. Clin Orthop 220:46, 1987.

378. Pellegrini VD Jr: Fractures at the base of the thumb. Hand Clin 4:87, 1988.

379. Miller RJ: Dislocations and fracture dislocations of the metacarpophalangeal joint of the thumb. Hand Clin 4:45, 1988.

380. Yamanaka K, Yoshida K, Inoue H, Inoue A, Miyagi T: Locking of the metacarpophalangeal joint of the thumb. J Bone Joint Surg [Am] 67:782, 1985.

381. Margles SW: Intra-articular fractures of the metacarpophalangeal and proximal interphalangeal joints. Hand Clin 4:67, 1988.

382. McKerrell J, Bowen V, Johnston G, et al: Boxer's fractures—conservative or operative management. J Trauma 27:486, 1987.

383. Barton NJ: Fractures of the hand. J Bone Joint Surg [Br] 66:159, 1984.

384. DaCruz DJ, Slade RJ, Malone W: Fractures of the distal phalanges. J Hand Surg [Br] 13:350, 1988.

385. Stark HH, Gainor BJ, Ashworth CR, et al: Operative treatment of intra-articular fractures of the dorsal aspect of the distal phalanx of digits. J Bone Joint Surg [Am] 69:892, 1987.

386. Wehbe MA, Schneider LH: Mallet fractures. J Bone Joint Surg [Am] 66:658, 1984.

387. Street JM: Radiographs of phalangeal fractures: Importance of the internally rotated oblique projection for diagnosis. AJR 160:575, 1993.

388. Neviaser RJ, Wilson JN, Lievano A: Rupture of the ulnar collateral ligament of the thumb (gamekeeper's thumb): Correction by dynamic repair. J Bone Joint Surg [Am] 53:1357, 1971.

389. Coonrad RW, Goldner JL: A study of the pathological findings and treatment in soft-tissue injury of the thumb metacarpophalangeal joint with a clinical study of the normal range of motion in one thousand thumbs and a study of post mortem findings of ligamentous structures in relation to function. J Bone Joint Surg [Am] 50:439, 1968.

390. Campbell CS: Gamekeeper's thumb. J Bone Joint Surg [Br] 37:148, 1955.

391. Stener B: Displacement of the ruptured ulnar collateral ligament of the metacarpophalangeal joint of the thumb: A clinical and anatomical study. J Bone Joint Surg [Br] 44:869, 1962.

392. Sakellarides HT, DeWeese JW: Instability of the metacarpophalangeal joint of the thumb: Reconstruction of the collateral ligaments using the extensor pollicis brevis tendon. J Bone Joint Surg [Am] 58:106, 1976.

393. Schultz RJ, Fox JM: Gamekeeper's thumb: Result of skiing injuries. NY State J Med 73:2329, 1973.

394. Primiano GA: Skiers' thumb injuries associated with flared ski pole handles. Am J Sports Med 13:425, 1985.

395. van Dommelen BA, Zvirbulis RA: Upper extremity injuries in snow skiers. Am J Sports Med 17:751, 1989.

396. Winslet MC, Clarke NMP, Mulligan PJ: Breakdancer's thumb—partial rupture of the ulnar collateral ligament with a fracture of the proximal phalanx of the thumb. Injury 17:201, 1986.

397. Downey EF Jr, Curtis DJ: Patient-induced stress test of the first metacarpophalangeal joint: A radiographic assessment of collateral ligament injuries. Radiology 158:679, 1986.

398. Louis DS, Huebner JJ Jr, Hankin FM: Rupture and displacement of the ulnar collateral ligament of the metacarpophalangeal joint of the thumb: Preoperative diagnosis. J Bone Joint Surg [Am] 68:1320, 1986.

399. Linscheid RL: Arthrography of the metacarpophalangeal joint. Clin Orthop 103:91, 1974.

400. Resnick D, Danzig LA: Arthrographic evaluation of injuries of the first metacarpophalangeal joint: Gamekeeper's thumb. AJR 126:1046, 1976.

401. Hergan K, Mittler C: Sonography of the injured ulnar collateral ligament of the thumb. J Bone Joint Surg [Br] 77:77, 1995.

402. Noszian IM, Dinkhauser LM, Orthner E, et al: Ulnar collateral ligament: Differentiation of displaced and nondisplaced tears with US. Radiology 194:61, 1995.

403. O'Callaghan BI, Kohut G, Hoogewoud H-M: Gamekeeper thumb: Identification of the Stener lesion with US. Radiology 192:477, 1994.

404. Noszian I, Dinkhauser L, Csanady M: Der Skidaumen. Sonographische Abklarung retrahierter Rupturen. ROFO 160:340, 1994.

405. Hergan K, Mittler C, Oser W: Ulnar collateral ligament: Differentiation of displaced and nondisplaced tears with US and MR imaging. Radiology 194:65, 1994.

406. Hinke DH, Erickson SJ, Chamoy L, et al: Ulnar collateral ligament of the thumb: MR findings in cadavers, volunteers, and patients with ligamentous injury (Gamekeeper's thumb). AJR 163:1431, 1994.

407. Louis DS, Buckwalter KA: Magnetic resonance imaging of the collateral ligaments of the thumb. J Hand Surg [Am] 14:739, 1989.

408. Spaeth HJ, Abrams RA, Bock GW, et al: Gamekeeper thumb: Differentiation of nondisplaced and displaced tears of the ulnar collateral ligament with MR imaging. Work in progress. Radiology 188:553, 1993.

409. Yin Y, Wilson AJ, Gilula LA: Three-compartment wrist arthrography: Direct comparison of digital subtraction with nonsubtraction images. Radiology 197:287, 1995.

410. Yin YM, Evanoff B, Gilula LA, et al: Evaluation of selective wrist arthrography of contralateral asymptomatic wrists for symmetric ligamentous defects. AJR 166:1067, 1996.

411. Yin Y, Evanoff BA, Gilula LA, et al: Surgeons' decision making in patients with chronic wrist pain: Role of bilateral three-compartment wrist arthrography—prospective study. Radiology 200:829, 1996.

412. Weiss A-PC, Akelman E, Lambiase R: Comparison of the findings of triple-injection cinearthrography of the wrist with those of arthroscopy. J Bone Joint Surg [Am] 78:348, 1996.

413. Kihara H, Short WH, Werner FW, et al: The stabilizing mechanism of the distal radioulnar joint during pronation and supination. J Hand Surg [Am] 20:930, 1995.

414. Tan ABH, Tan SK, Yung SW, et al: Congenital perforations of the triangular fibrocartilage of the wrist. J Hand Surg [Br] 20:342, 1995.

415. Wright TW, Del Charco M, Wheeler D: Incidence of ligament lesions and associated changes in the elderly wrist. J Hand Surg [Am] 19:313, 1994.

416. Totterman SMS, Miller RJ, McCance SE, et al: Lesions of the triangular fibrocartilage complex: MR findings with a three-dimensional gradient-recalled-echo sequence. Radiology 199:227, 1996.

417. Oneson SR, Scales LM, Timins ME, et al: MR imaging interpretation of the Palmer classification of triangular fibrocartilage complex lesions. Radiographics 16:97, 1996.

418. Totterman SMS, Miller RJ: Scapholunate ligament: Normal MR appearance on three-dimensional gradient-recalled-echo images. Radiology 200:237, 1996.

419. Ruch DS, Poehling GG: Arthroscopic management of partial scapholunate and lunotriquetral injuries of the wrist. J Hand Surg [Am] 21:412, 1996.

420. Buul MMC, Broekhuizen TH, van Beek EJR, et al: Choosing a strategy for the diagnostic management of suspected scaphoid fracture: A cost-effectiveness analysis. J Nucl Med 36:45, 1995.

421. Smith DK, Murray PM: Avulsion fractures of the volar aspect of triquetral bone of the wrist: A subtle sign of carpal ligament injury. AJR 166:609, 1996.

422. Hashizume H, Asahara H, Nishida K, et al: Histopathology of Kienböck's disease. Correlation with magnetic resonance and other imaging techniques. J Hand Surg [Br] 21:89, 1996.

423. Oleaga L, Florencio MR, Ereno C, et al: Fibrolipomatous hamartoma of the radial nerve: MR imaging findings. Skeletal Radiol 24:559, 1995.

424. Glajchen N, Schweitzer M: MRI features in de Quervain's tenosynovitis of the wrist. Skeletal Radiol 25:63, 1996.

425. Sueyoshi E, Uetani M, Hayashi K, et al: Tuberculous tenosynovitis of the wrist: MRI findings in three patients. Skeletal Radiol 25:569, 1996.

426. Rubin DA, Kneeland JB, Kitay GS, et al: Flexor tendon tears in the hand: Use of MR imaging to diagnose degree of injury in a cadaver model. AJR 166:615, 1996.

427. Matloub HS, Dzwierzynski WW, Erickson S, et al: Magnetic resonance imaging scanning in the diagnosis of zone II flexor tendon rupture. J Hand Surg [Am] 21:451, 1996.

428. Parellada JA, Balkissoon ARA, Hayes CW, et al: Bowstring injury of the flexor tendon pulley system: MR imaging. AJR 167:347, 1996.

429. Calandruccio JH, Steichen JB: Magnetic resonance imaging for diagnosis of digital flexor tendon rupture after primary repair. J Hand Surg [Br] 20:289, 1995.

430. Drapé J-L, Silbermann-Hoffman O, Houvet P, et al: Complications of flexor tendon repair in the hand: MR imaging assessment. Radiology 198:219, 1996.

431. Vo P, Wright T, Hayden F, et al: Evaluating dorsal wrist pain: MRI diagnosis of occult dorsal wrist ganglion. J Hand Surg [Am] 20:667, 1995.

432. Drapé J-L, Idy-Peretti I, Goettmann S, et al: MR imaging of digital mucoid cysts. Radiology 200:531, 1996.

433. Haramati N, Hiller N, Dowdle J, et al: MRI of the Stener lesion. Skeletal Radiol 24:515, 1995.

434. Ryu J, Fagan R: Arthroscopic treatment of acute complete thumb metacarpophalangeal ulnar collateral ligament tears. J Hand Surg [Am] 20:1037, 1995.

435. Magee TH, Rowedder AM, Degnan GG: Intraosseous ganglia of the wrist. Radiology 195:517, 1995.

436. Timins ME, O'Connell SE, Erickson SJ, et al: MR imaging of the wrist: Normal findings that may simulate disease. Radiographics 16:987, 1996.

437. Oneson SR, Scales LM, Erickson SJ, et al: MR imaging of the painful wrist. Radiographics 16:997, 1996.

438. Zeiss J, Guilliam-Haidet L: MR demonstration of anomalous muscles about the volar aspect of the wrist and forearm. Clin Imag 20:219, 1996.

439. Nakamura R, Horii E, Imaeda T, et al: Criteria for diagnosing distal radioulnar joint subluxation by computed tomography. Skeletal Radiol 25:649, 1996.

440. Nakahara N, Uretani M, Hayashi K, et al: Gadolinium-enhanced MR imaging of the wrist in rheumatoid arthritis: Value of fat suppression pulse sequences. Skeletal Radiol 25:639, 1996.

No other aspect of orthopedic surgery has received greater attention than the hip and its disorders, and none presents greater therapeutic challenges. Whether it be developmental abnormalities in the neonate, synovitis and ischemic changes in the child, physeal injury in the adolescent, accidental trauma in the adult, osteoarthritis or insufficiency fractures in the elderly, or any of the other countless conditions that affect the hip, accurate assessment depends heavily on imaging techniques. Ultrasonography, bone scintigraphy, arthrography, CT scanning, and MR imaging have assumed increasing importance in recent years as supplements to routine radiography in the evaluation of disorders of the hip and pelvis. In this chapter, a summary is provided of the applications of these imaging methods to some of the more important processes that involve the hip and pelvis. The interested reader should refer also to other portions of this text that describe some of these processes in more detail.

ANATOMY

Osseous Anatomy

At the hip, the globular head of the femur articulates with the cup-shaped fossa of the acetabulum. This latter structure develops in fetal life from ossification of the ilium, ischium, and pubis. At birth, the acetabulum is cartilaginous, with a triradiate stem extending medially from its deep aspect, producing a Y-shaped physeal plate between ilium, ischium, and pubis. Continued ossification results in eventual fusion of these three bones.

The fully developed acetabular cavity is hemispherical and possesses an elevated bony rim (Fig. 15–1). This rim is absent inferiorly, the defect being termed the acetabular notch. A fibrocartilaginous labrum is attached to the bony rim, deepening the acetabular cavity. The acetabular floor above the notch, the acetabular fossa, is depressed and irregular. Between the rim and fossa is a smooth horseshoe-shaped articular lunate surface. A discontinuity in the medial aspect of the acetabular roof, termed the superior acetabular notch, appears to represent an accessory fossa in the apex of the acetabulum.[1]

The hemispherical head of the femur extends superiorly, medially, and anteriorly (Fig. 15–2). It is smooth except for a central roughened pit, the fovea, to which is attached the ligament of the head of the femur. The anterior surface of the femoral neck is intracapsular, as the capsular line extends to the intertrochanteric line; only the medial half of the posterior surface of the femoral neck is intracapsular, as the posterior attachment of the hip capsule does not extend to the intertrochanteric crest. The greater trochanter projects from the posterosuperior aspect of the femoral neck-shaft junction and is the site of attachment of numerous muscles, including the gluteus minimus, gluteus medius, and piriformis. The lesser trochanter is located at the posteromedial portion of the femoral neck-shaft

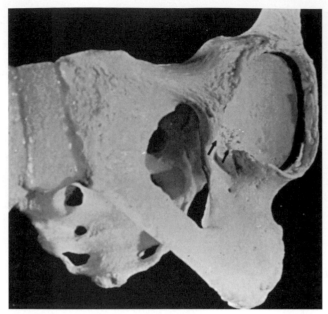

Figure 15–1
Acetabular cavity: Osseous anatomy (anterior). A metal marker (black strip) identifies the posterior acetabular rim. This rim is continuous except at the area of the acetabular notch inferiorly (arrows). (From Armbuster TG, et al: Radiology *128*:1, 1978.)

junction. The psoas major and iliacus muscles attach to it.

The acetabular angle, iliac angle, and angle of anteversion of the femoral neck are useful radiographic measurements, particularly in the young skeleton. The center-edge (CE) angle of Wiberg[2] is an indication of acetabular depth (Fig. 15–3). It refers to the angle formed by a perpendicular line through the midportion of the femoral head and a line from the femoral head center to the upper outer acetabular margin. The normal CE angle is reported to be 20 to 40 degrees, with an average of 36 degrees.[3] This angle may be slightly larger in women and in older persons.[4]

The pelvic radiograph also is useful in outlining certain normal lines and structures.[4, 5] The acetabular rim appears as an osseous ring surrounding the outer aspect of the acetabulum. The posterior acetabular rim can be identified on radiographs exposed in various obliquities, but the 15- to 30-degree anterior oblique projection offers optimal visualization. The anterior acetabular rim is visualized optimally in the 30- to 45- degree posterior oblique projection. The ilioischial line is formed by that portion of the quadrilateral surface of the ilium that is tangent to the x-ray beam; the iliopubic line is simply the inner margin of the ilium, which forms a continuous line with the inner superior aspect of the pubis. Two columns of bone produce an arch, with the acetabulum located in the concavity of the arch. The ilioischial or posterior column is a thick structure that includes a portion of the ilium and extends to the ischial tuberosity. The iliopubic or anterior column consists of a portion of ilium and pubis and extends superolaterally to the anterior inferior iliac spine.

The "teardrop" is a U-shaped shadow medial to the hip joint that has been used to detect abnormalities of acetabular depth,[6] thereby establishing a diagnosis of acetabular protrusion (Fig. 15–4). It has been compared to a pedicle of a vertebra in that its disappearance establishes that significant bone destruction has oc-

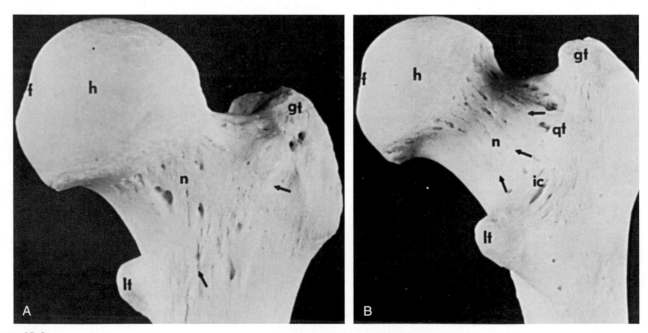

Figure 15–2
Proximal end of femur: Osseous anatomy.
  A Anterior aspect, neutral position. Observe the smooth femoral head (h), fovea (f), neck (n), greater trochanter (gt), and lesser trochanter (lt). The hip capsule attaches anteriorly to the intertrochanteric line (arrows).
  B Posterior aspect, neutral position. The same structures as in **A** are identified. The intertrochanteric crest (ic) and quadrate tubercle (qt) also are indicated. Arrows point to the site of capsular attachment.

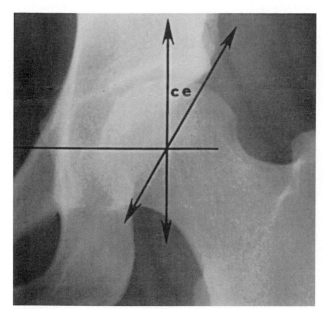

Figure 15–3
Center-edge (CE) angle of Wiberg. This is the angle formed by the intersection of a perpendicular line through the midpoint of the femoral head and a line from the femoral head center to the upper outer acetabular margin. The normal value for this angle is reported to be 20 to 40 degrees, with an average of 36 degrees. (From Armbuster TG, et al: Radiology *128*:1, 1978.)

curred.[7] The lateral aspect of the teardrop is the wall of the acetabular fossa, and the medial aspect is the anteroinferior margin of the quadrilateral surface. In the usual anteroposterior radiograph of the pelvis, the latter surface is parallel to the x-ray beam and is thereby projected as a typical "teardrop." The configuration of the teardrop varies in normal persons, however. Furthermore, it is affected significantly by positioning the patient in oblique projections.[4]

Differentiation of normal acetabular depth and acetabular protrusion (protrusio acetabuli) can be accomplished by careful analysis of plain films in adults.[4] The

acetabular line, which is the medial wall of the acetabulum, and the ilioischial line, which is a portion of the quadrilateral surface, are central structures whose relationships are little affected by minimal degrees of rotation. Although acetabular depth is a continuum from "shallow" to "normal" to "deep" to "protrusio acetabuli," available data[4] have led to the following conclusions:

1. Protrusio acetabuli is diagnosed when the acetabular line projects medial to the ilioischial line by 3 mm or more in men or by 6 mm or more in women. In children, 1 mm in boys and 3 mm in girls are the corresponding values.[8]
2. The teardrop configuration is affected by minor degrees of rotation and therefore cannot be used as an indicator of protrusio acetabuli.
3. Measurement of the CE angle of Wiberg adds little to the diagnosis of protrusio acetabuli.

The normal joint space on frontal radiographs can be analyzed in adults by dividing it into three segments: the superior, axial, and medial joint spaces.[4] The superior and axial joint space measurements usually are quite similar, but the medial joint space measurement normally is greater because it includes the acetabular fossa,[9, 10] which adds synovium and fat to the joint space. The average medial joint space is 9 mm in men and 8 mm in women. The average axial and superior joint spaces are 4 mm in both men and women.[11] Minor modifications of these measurements occur with advancing age of the person.[12]

Articular and Soft Tissue Anatomy

The femoral head is covered with articular cartilage, although a small area exists on its surface that is devoid of cartilage, to which attaches the ligament of the head of the femur (Fig. 15–5). The lunate surface is covered

Figure 15–4
The "teardrop."

A Anteroposterior tomogram. The teardrop (t) and femoral head (asterisk) are seen. The lateral wall of the teardrop is the wall of the acetabular fossa. The medial wall is the anteroinferior margin of the quadrilateral surface.

B On a cadaveric specimen, a metal marker has been placed on the teardrop. The quadrilateral surface is not visualized in this projection.

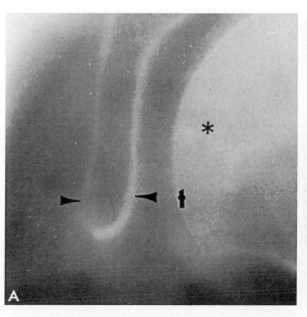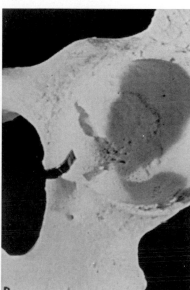

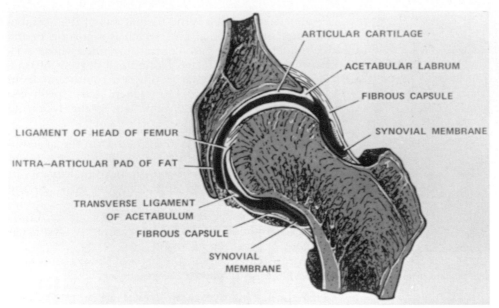

ARTICULAR CARTILAGE

ACETABULAR LABRUM

FIBROUS CAPSULE

SYNOVIAL MEMBRANE

LIGAMENT OF HEAD OF FEMUR

INTRA-ARTICULAR PAD OF FAT

TRANSVERSE LIGAMENT OF ACETABULUM

FIBROUS CAPSULE

SYNOVIAL MEMBRANE

Figure 15–5

Hip joint: Normal articular anatomy. Drawing of a coronal section through the hip.

with articular cartilage; the floor of the acetabular fossa within this surface does not contain cartilage but has a fibroelastic fat pad covered with synovial membrane.

A fibrous capsule encircles the joint and much of the femoral neck (Fig. 15–6). The capsule attaches proximally to the acetabulum, labrum, and transverse ligament of the acetabulum. Distally it surrounds the femoral neck; in front, it is attached to the trochanteric line at the junction of the femoral neck and shaft; above and below, it is attached to the femoral neck close to the junction with the trochanters; behind, the capsule extends over the medial two thirds of the neck. Because of these capsular attachments, the physeal plate of the femur is intracapsular and the physeal plates of the trochanters are extracapsular. The fibers of the fibrous capsule, although oriented longitudinally from pelvis to femur, also consist of a deeply situated circular group

of fibers termed the zona orbicularis. The fibrous capsule is strengthened by surrounding ligaments, including the iliofemoral, pubofemoral, and ischiofemoral ligaments. The external surface of the capsule is covered by musculature and separated anteriorly from the psoas major and iliacus by a bursa. In this area, the joint may communicate with the subtendinous iliac bursa (iliopsoas bursa) beneath the psoas major tendon through an aperture between the pubofemoral and iliofemoral ligaments.

The extensive synovial membrane of the hip extends from the cartilaginous margins of the femoral head over intracapsular portions of the femoral neck. It is reflected beneath the fibrous capsule and covers the acetabular labrum, the ligament of the head of the femur, and the fat pad in the acetabular fossa.

Important ligaments include the iliofemoral, pubo-

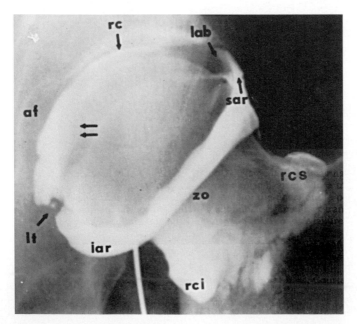

Figure 15–6

Hip joint: Normal articular anatomy—hip arthrogram. The recess capitus (rc) is a thin, smooth collection of contrast medium between apposing articular surfaces and is interrupted only where the ligamentum teres (double arrows) enters the fovea centralis of the femoral head. The ligamentum transversum (lt) is seen as a radiolucent defect adjacent to the inferior rim of the acetabulum. The ligamentum teres bridges the acetabular notch and effectively deepens the acetabulum. The inferior articular recess (iar) forms a pouch at the inferior base of the femoral head below the acetabular notch and ligamentum transversum. The superior articular recess (sar) extends cephalad around the acetabular labrum (lab). The acetabular labrum is seen as a triangular radiolucent area adjacent to the superolateral lip of the acetabulum. The zona orbicularis (zo) is a circumferential lucent band around the femoral neck, which changes configuration with rotation of the femur. The recess colli superior (rcs) and recess colli inferior (rci) are poolings of contrast material at the apex and base of the intertrochanteric line and are the most caudal extensions of the synovial membrane. (From Guerra J Jr, et al: Radiology *128*:11, 1978.)

femoral, and ischiofemoral ligaments, the ligament of the head of the femur, the transverse ligament of the acetabulum, and the acetabular labrum (Fig. 15–7). The strong iliofemoral ligament attaches proximally to the anterior inferior iliac spine and the adjoining part of the acetabular rim and distally to the intertrochanteric line on the femur. This ligament becomes taut in full extension of the hip. The pubofemoral ligament extends from the pubic part of the acetabular rim and the superior pubic ramus to the undersurface of the femoral neck, some of its fibers blending with the fibrous capsule. This ligament also becomes taut on hip extension. The ischiofemoral ligament is attached to the ischium below and behind the acetabulum and extends in a superolateral direction across the back of the femoral neck. Its fibers are continuous with those of the zona orbicularis or attach to the greater trochanter. This ligament, as the others, becomes taut in extension of the hip. The ligament of the head of the femur is a weak intra-articular ligament, which is attached to the

margin of the acetabular fossa and the transverse ligament of the acetabulum. It extends to a pit on the femoral head. Between these areas of attachment, this ligament is clothed by a synovial sheath. In some persons, the sheath alone is present, without the ligament, and in others, neither sheath nor ligament can be identified. The ligament is stretched when the thigh is flexed, adducted, and rotated laterally. The transverse ligament of the acetabulum is a portion of the acetabular labrum whose fibers extend across the acetabular notch. The acetabular labrum, the fibrocartilaginous rim about the acetabulum, is attached firmly to the bony rim and transverse ligament, is triangular on cross section, and has a free edge or apex that forms a smaller circle that closely embraces the femoral head.

Active movements of the hip are flexion, extension, adduction, abduction, circumduction, and medial and lateral rotation. Because of the close fit between acetabulum and femur and the intimacy of the acetabular labrum, the movements of the hip are restricted in

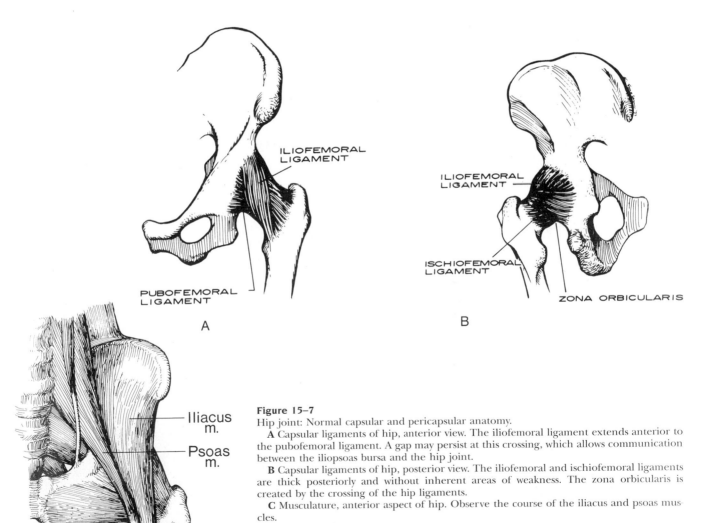

Figure 15–7
Hip joint: Normal capsular and pericapsular anatomy.
  A Capsular ligaments of hip, anterior view. The iliofemoral ligament extends anterior to the pubofemoral ligament. A gap may persist at this crossing, which allows communication between the iliopsoas bursa and the hip joint.
  B Capsular ligaments of hip, posterior view. The iliofemoral and ischiofemoral ligaments are thick posteriorly and without inherent areas of weakness. The zona orbicularis is created by the crossing of the hip ligaments.
  C Musculature, anterior aspect of hip. Observe the course of the iliacus and psoas muscles.

comparison to those of the glenohumeral joint. No accessory movements occur in the hip.

A number of periarticular fat planes have been described that can be recognized on radiographs and which, when disturbed, reportedly may indicate significant intra-articular disease (Fig. 15–8).[13–19]

Fat plane 1: On the pelvic surface of the acetabulum and pubis.
Fat plane 2: Medial to the femoral neck, extending to the lesser trochanter.
Fat plane 3: Lateral to the hip and extending to the greater trochanter.
Fat plane 4: Lateral to the hip and medial to fat plane 3, extending to the region of the greater trochanter.

Anatomic studies have revealed that fat plane 1 is medial to the obturator internus muscle[13, 20] and fat plane 2 is medial to the iliopsoas muscle.[20, 21] Fat plane 3 is between the gluteus medius (lateral) and the gluteus minimus (medial) muscles.[19–21] Fat plane 4 has been termed the "capsular" fat plane,[21] although more recent evidence suggests that this fat pad is not related to the joint capsule.[19, 20] The bulk of this fat plane is intermuscular, lying between the rectus femoris and tensor fasciae latae muscles.

Fat plane 2, the iliopsoas fat plane, is medial to the tendinous portion of the iliopsoas muscle. Anteriorly it blends with the fat of the femoral triangle just lateral to the femoral vessels. Posteriorly it reaches the superomedial portion of the hip capsule and inferomedial lip of the acetabulum. In its posterior course, it sends a fat plane laterally, posterior to the iliopsoas tendon. Here it makes intimate contact with the medial portion of the

hip capsule adjacent to the femoral neck. This represents a point of weakness between the iliofemoral and iliopubic ligaments of the hip capsule. It is here that the iliopsoas bursa originates, a space that potentially could allow decompression of a joint in cases of elevated intra-articular pressure.[20]

The iliopsoas bursa represents the largest and most important bursa about the hip. It is present in 98 per cent of hips and is located anterior to the joint capsule.[22] It may extend proximally and communicate with the joint space in approximately 15 per cent of normal hips[23, 24] through a gap between the iliofemoral and pubofemoral ligaments.[25] Extension of hip disease into this bursa has been recognized in a variety of articular diseases, occasionally producing a mass in the ilioinguinal region with possible obstruction of the femoral vein (see later discussion). One additional site that represents an inherent weak part of the hip capsule occurs at the crossing of the iliofemoral and iliopubic ligaments. At this site, fluid may extravasate into the fat plane of the obturator externus muscle.[20]

Bursae about the gluteus muscles also may be demonstrated anatomically and radiographically.[26] The bursa deep to the gluteus medius muscle is larger than that deep to the gluteus minimus muscle. Both bursae are intimate with the greater trochanter, and bursitis can lead to pain and soft tissue calcifications in this region.

Some of the muscles about the hip are shown in Figure 15–9.

Anatomy of Vessels and Nerves

The major arterial supply of the adult femoral head originates from the medial and lateral femoral circum-

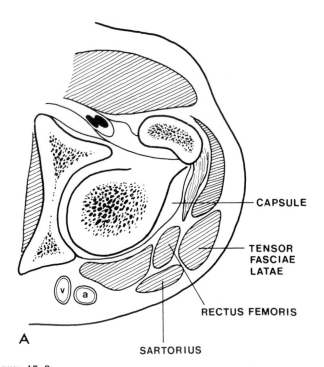

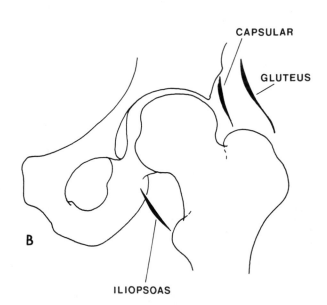

Figure 15–8
Periarticular fat planes.
  A A simplified schematic representation of a transverse section through the hip.
  B A drawing of three of the four fat planes that have been described.

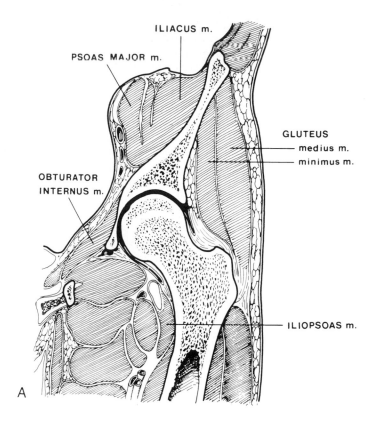

ILIACUS m.

PSOAS MAJOR m.

GLUTEUS
medius m.
minimus m.

OBTURATOR
INTERNUS m.

ILIOPSOAS m.

A

Figure 15–9
Hip joint: Normal muscle anatomy.
  A Musculature, coronal section of hip.
  B Musculature, transverse section of hip.
Anterior structures are located at the bottom
of the drawing.

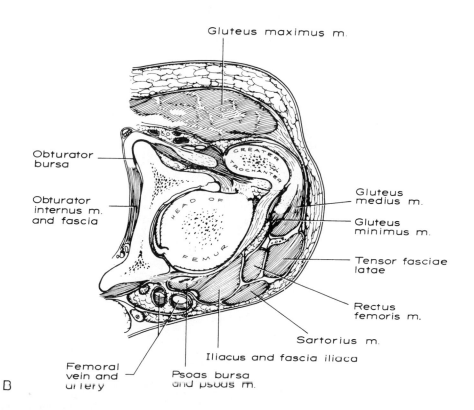

Gluteus maximus m.

Obturator
bursa

Obturator
internus m.
and fascia

GREATER
TROCHANTER

HEAD OF FEMUR

Gluteus
medius m.

Gluteus
minimus m.

Tensor fasciae
latae

Rectus
femoris m.

Sartorius m.

Iliacus and fascia iliaca

Femoral
vein and
artery

Psoas bursa
and psoas m.

B

flex arteries, which are branches of either the femoral artery or deep femoral artery (Fig. 15–10).[27] Additional vessels contributing to the blood supply of the hip are the obturator artery and the inferior and superior gluteal arteries. An extracapsular vascular ring at the base of the femoral neck is supplied posteriorly by a branch of the medial femoral circumflex artery and anteriorly by a branch of the lateral femoral circumflex artery. Ascending cervical branches arising from this vascular ring pierce the hip joint at the level of the capsular insertion, and, from there, continue along the synovial reflections on the femoral neck to enter the bone just below the articular cartilage of the femoral head.[27] The contribution to the blood supply of the femoral head provided by the artery of the ligamentum teres is variable.

The sciatic nerve exits the pelvis at the greater sciatic notch, intimate with the piriformis muscle. Some variation exists, however, in the relationship of these two structures (Fig. 15–11).

FUNCTION

In common with the glenohumeral joint, the hip is a ball-and-socket joint. As opposed to the glenohumeral joint, however, the hip is extremely stable. This stability relates to a number of factors, including the geometry of the femoral head and acetabulum, the presence of the acetabular labrum, the thickness and ligamentous condensations of the joint capsule, and the regional muscular anatomy.[27] The femoral head is deeply situated within the acetabulum; indeed, in any position of the hip, about 40 per cent of the femoral head is covered by the bony acetabulum. The acetabular labrum serves to deepen the acetabulum still further, such that almost 50 per cent of the femoral head is covered by the osteocartilaginous labral-acetabular complex (Fig. 15–12).[27] Longitudinally oriented capsular fibers are reinforced by very strong ligamentous condensations that are arranged in a circular and spiral fashion. As indicated earlier, important capsular ligaments include the iliofemoral, pubofemoral, and ischiofemoral ligaments. The pubofemoral ligament is believed to represent a checkrein against pathologic extension of the hip.[27]

In addition to having inherent stability, the joint between the acetabulum and the femoral head retains great mobility.[28] The hip can move in three planes, sagittal, frontal, and transverse, with the greatest motion occurring in the sagittal plane. To perform the activities of daily living in a normal fashion, hip flexion of at least 120 degrees, abduction of at least 20 degrees, and external rotation of at least 20 degrees are required.[29] Greater motion is required for participation in sporting activities.

During simple, one-legged standing, the force transmission across the hip is 2.6 times body weight.[28, 30] This transmission increases to about 3.3 times body weight during rapid walking and to about 5 times body weight during certain phases of running. The considerable force that is generated across the joint is resisted by a unique trabecular architecture found in the proximal portion of the femur (Fig. 15–13). Alterations in these trabeculae occurring in osteoporosis explain the vulnerability of the femoral neck to fracture.

IMAGING TECHNIQUES

A variety of imaging methods can be used as a supplement to routine radiography in the evaluation of disorders of the pelvis and hip. Bone scintigraphy is used most frequently to assess neoplastic (e.g., skeletal metastasis), infectious, and traumatic (e.g., femoral neck fractures) conditions, although MR imaging may be used as an alternative technique in some cases (see later discussion). Arteriography is especially useful in delineating sites of vascular injury accompanying pelvic trauma, although it may be used for other purposes as well (Fig. 15–14). Ultrasonography can be employed in the evaluation of muscle injury (see later discussion), and CT scanning has widespread clinical applications (see later discussion).

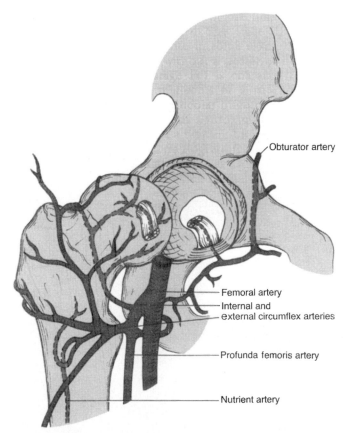

Obturator artery

Femoral artery

Internal and external circumflex arteries

Profunda femoris artery

Nutrient artery

Figure 15–10
Vascular supply to femoral head. (Reproduced with permission from Levin P: Hip dislocations. *In* BD Browner, JB Jupiter, AM Levine, et al [Eds]: Skeletal Trauma: Fractures, Dislocations, Ligamentous Injuries. Philadelphia, WB Saunders Co, 1992, p 1332.)

Arthrography

Many techniques exist for puncturing the hip joint. Some use a direct or angulated anterior approach,[31, 32]

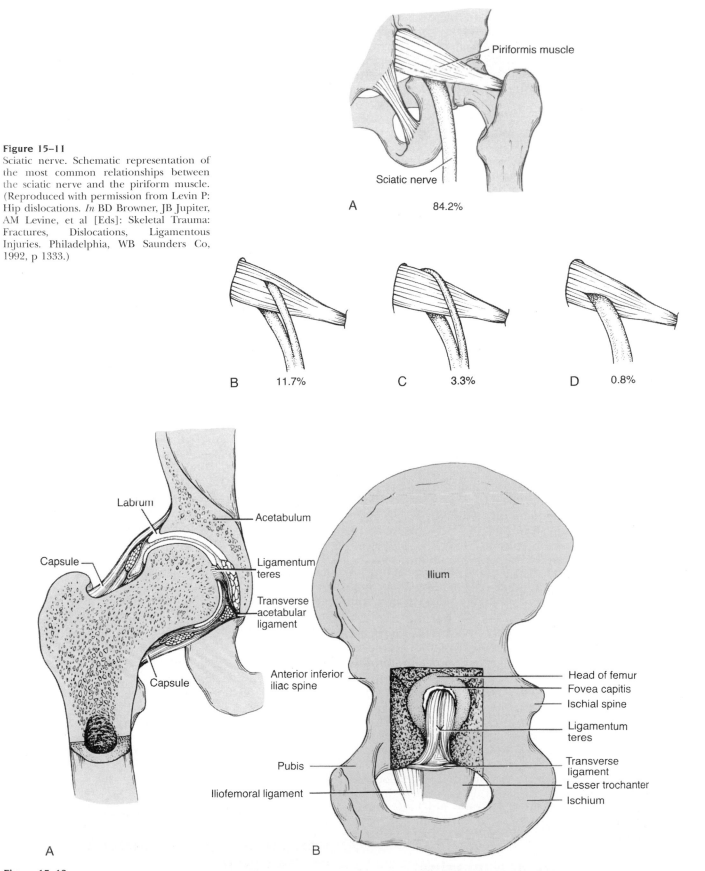

Figure 15–11
Sciatic nerve. Schematic representation of the most common relationships between the sciatic nerve and the piriform muscle. (Reproduced with permission from Levin P: Hip dislocations. *In* BD Browner, JB Jupiter, AM Levine, et al [Eds]: Skeletal Trauma: Fractures, Dislocations, Ligamentous Injuries. Philadelphia, WB Saunders Co, 1992, p 1333.)

Piriformis muscle

Sciatic nerve

A   84.2%

B   11.7%   C   3.3%   D   0.8%

Labrum

Capsule

Acetabulum

Ligamentum teres

Transverse acetabular ligament

Capsule

Ilium

Anterior inferior iliac spine

Head of femur
Fovea capitis
Ischial spine

Ligamentum teres

Pubis

Transverse ligament
Lesser trochanter

Iliofemoral ligament

Ischium

A   B

Figure 15–12
The relationship of the femoral head, labrum, and acetabulum. The labrum extends beyond the equator of the femoral head, increasing the degree of joint stability. (Reproduced with permission from Levin P: Hip dislocations. *In* BD Browner, JB Jupiter, AM Levine, et al [Eds]: Skeletal Trauma: Fractures, Dislocations, Ligamentous Injuries. Philadelphia, WB Saunders Co, 1992, p 1330.)

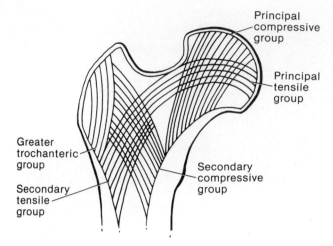

Figure 15–13
Anatomy of the bony trabeculae of the proximal femur. (Reproduced with permission from Gross ML, Nasser S, Finerman GAM: Hip and pelvis. *In* JC DeLee, D Drez Jr [Eds]: Orthopaedic Sports Medicine: Principles and Practice. Philadelphia, WB Saunders Co, 1994, p 1065.)

whereas others describe lateral,[33] superior,[34] or inferior[35, 36] approaches. Fluoroscopy is mandatory.[37] In infants and children, an anterolateral subphyseal plate site is ideal for contacting the bone.[37] This metaphyseal location is within the joint capsule yet distant from the femoral vessels, cartilaginous femoral head, and growth plate. Some arthrographers prefer an anteromedial or inferomedial approach.[38] Ten to 15 ml of radiopaque contrast medium is injected in adults. Approximately 1.5 to 2 ml of contrast medium is injected in infants and 5 to 8 ml in adolescents.[39] Some investigators prefer to document the intra-articular location of the needle tip by injecting a small amount of air; air emboli may complicate this testing strategy.[40]

In performing hip arthrography in patients with joint prostheses, subtraction arthrography frequently is necessary so that contrast material can be differentiated from the radiopaque acrylic cement that is used to fix the prosthesis in place.[41] Conventional or digital techniques can be used to create the subtracted images.[40, 42–44] In patients who have been treated with Girdlestone arthroplasty, intracapsular placement of the needle is best accomplished from an anterior approach with needle advancement to the midpoint of the intertrochanteric line.[45] Additional modifications with regard to hip arthrography include its supplementation with conventional tomography or CT scanning and the incorporation of pressure monitoring within the joint during or after the injection of the contrast material.[46–48]

The normal hip arthrogram in adults is shown in Figure 15–6. In children, similar arthrographic features are apparent.[37] The cartilaginous tissue around the immature femoral head is abundant, reflecting both articular cartilage and that portion of the femoral head that is not yet ossified.

Magnetic Resonance Imaging

The role of MR imaging in the analysis of hip disorders is well established. Imaging protocols have been suggested,[49, 50] although these vary from one institution to another and, ideally, should be tailored according to the specific indications for the examination.[393] Specific options relate to type of imaging sequence, choice of imaging plane or planes, selection of receiver coils, the need to image one or both hips, and the need for intravenous or intra-articular contrast agents. As at other anatomic sites, conventional or fast spin echo MR imaging sequences are used most commonly to examine the hip and pelvis. Typical parameters chosen for standard spin echo images include repetition times (TR) of 500 to 600 msec and echo times (TE) of about 20 msec for T1-weighted sequences and TR values of about 2000 msec and TE values of approximately 20 and 80 msec for proton density and T2-weighted sequences. In these sequences, thin sections (3 to 5 mm thick) and minimal interslice gaps generally are chosen. Three-dimensional Fourier transform (3DFT) gradient echo imaging allows acquisition of very thin (1 mm) sections. Short tau inversion recovery (STIR) MR images represent an effective screening technique for the assessment of fluid, hemorrhage, pus, or tumor in the marrow, joint, or soft tissues. STIR images are extremely sensitive in detecting a variety of pathologic processes (see later discussion). Fat suppression MR imaging, when combined with the intravenous (or intra-articular) administration of a gadolinium compound, also is effective and often is employed when evaluating neoplastic or infectious diseases (intravenous injection), abnormalities of articular cartilage or labrum, or possible intra-articular osteocartilaginous bodies (intra-articular injection).

In most instances, at least two imaging planes are used (i.e., coronal, sagittal, and transaxial) and, often, all three planes are employed (Plates 15–1 through 15–9). Oblique sagittal and transaxial planes (oriented along the axis of the femoral neck) have been advocated by some investigators.[49] When images of both hips are required (in instances of bilateral abnormalities or for comparison purposes), a body coil can be used with a field of view (FOV) of 32 to 40 cm. When imaging a single hip, a smaller FOV (20 to 24 cm) provides images with improved spatial resolution. Surface coils have been recommended as a method allowing more optimal visualization of the hip. As an example, surface coil imaging in the sagittal plane with a small FOV (18 to 20 cm) may improve the sensitivity of the MR imaging examination in cases of osteonecrosis of the femoral head. The use of flexible shoulder surface coils in an off-coronal plane parallel to the long axis of the femoral neck was emphasized in one report.[51] In pediatric patients, the smallest possible coil should be employed; in infants and small children, an extremity or head coil can be used.[49]

SPECIFIC ABNORMALITIES

Fractures and Dislocations of the Pelvis

In common with the situation in the skull and in the thoracic cage, the bony pelvis is intimate with vital inter-

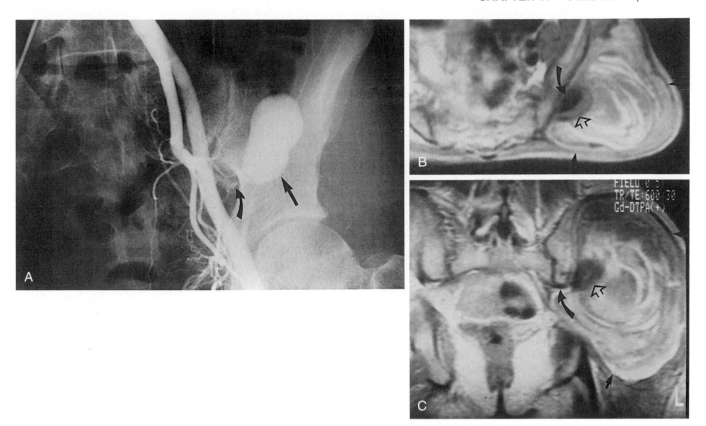

Figure 15–14

Arteriography: Aneurysm of the inferior gluteal artery. This 34 year old man developed bacterial endocarditis leading to septic embolization and a mycotic aneurysm.

A Arteriography reveals a large aneurysm (straight arrow) arising from the inferior gluteal artery (curved arrow).

B In a transaxial T1-weighted (TR/TE, 700/30) spin echo MR image, the aneurysm (open arrow) appears to contain a thrombus (curved arrow) and is surrounded by a large hematoma (straight solid arrows).

C After intravenous administration of a gadolinium contrast agent, a coronal T1-weighted (TR/TE, 600/30) spin echo MR image shows the inferior gluteal artery (curved arrow), the aneurysm (open arrow), and the hematoma (straight solid arrows).

nal organs and it is the evaluation of these organs that becomes mandatory in cases in which osseous or ligamentous disruption is apparent. Hemorrhage due to vascular injury of arteries (e.g., hypogastric and superior gluteal arteries and their branches) or veins, injury of the urinary tract (e.g., bladder and urethra), compression of peripheral nerves (e.g., the sacral plexus, sciatic nerve, and lumbosacral nerve roots), and disruption of viscera (e.g., liver and spleen) are among the significant complications of pelvic fractures and dislocations, the frequency of which depends on the site and the magnitude of the abnormal forces. Radiographic examinations directed at the detection of such complications are as fundamental to proper analysis of pelvic fractures and dislocations as are the radiographs of the bones themselves. With regard to the latter radiographs, adequate technique is made difficult owing to patient pain and discomfort and depends on the inclusion of specialized projections (including oblique radiographs and angled views)[52, 53] and CT (with or without three-dimensional display of image data). Furthermore, as the bony pelvis as a whole is a ringlike structure and, indeed, some of its components also are rings (e.g., pubic rami), it is common to encounter more than a single injury (in the form of a fracture, subluxation, or dislocation).

Fractures of the pelvis, which account for approximately 3 per cent of all fractures,[54] have been classified in a number of ways on the basis of such factors as sites of involvement, direction of force, and mechanisms of injury.[55–63] No system is ideal, as attention to both biomechanical and anatomic aspects (Fig. 15–15) is required. These biomechanics have been well outlined by Tile,[64, 65] whose book should be consulted by the interested reader and whose observations are summarized here.

The major forces acting on the pelvic ring are external rotation, lateral compression (internal rotation), vertical shear, and complex forces (Fig. 15–16).

External Rotation

External rotation may occur when a direct force is applied either to the posterior superior iliac spines (Fig. 15–16B) or to the anterior superior iliac spines or the femora (Fig. 15–16C). This mechanism of injury relates to disruptive forces in the sagittal plane and, sometimes, is referred to as anteroposterior compression. The pelvis is opened like a book, with diastasis of the symphysis pubis and disruption of the anterior sacroiliac and sacrospinous ligaments. In the absence of a shearing

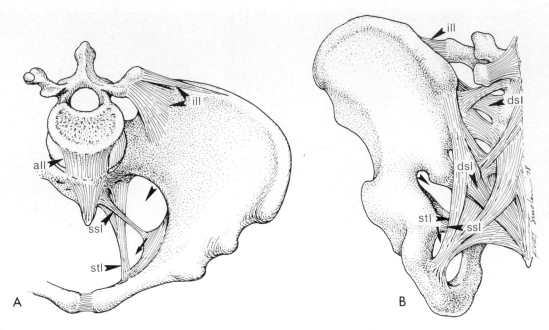

Figure 15–15
Pelvic-vertebral ligaments: Anatomy.

A Anterior aspect. Visualized structures are the iliolumbar ligament (ill) with two pelvic attachments, sacrospinous ligament (ssl), sacrotuberous ligament (stl), anterior longitudinal ligament (all), and greater (arrowhead) and lesser (arrow) sciatic foramina.

B Posterior aspect. Observe the iliolumbar ligament (ill), short and long dorsal sacroiliac ligaments (dsl), sacrotuberous ligament (stl), sacrospinous ligament (ssl), and greater (arrowhead) and lesser (arrow) sciatic foramina.

(From Warwick R, Williams P: Gray's Anatomy. 35th British Ed. Philadelphia, WB Saunders Co, 1973.)

force, the posterior ligaments usually remain intact so that no vertical displacement is seen.

Lateral Compression

A lateral compressive force applied to the iliac crest leads to internal rotation of the hemipelvis with disruption of the anterior portion of the sacrum and displacement of the anterior pubic rami (Fig. 15–16*D*). A similar force applied to the greater trochanter will produce disruption of the pubic rami and ipsilateral sacroiliac complex (Fig. 15–16*E*). A third pattern of lateral compression occurs when the forces are directed parallel to the trabeculae about the sacroiliac joint, causing impaction of bone (Fig. 15–16*F*). In general, these mechanisms are associated with compression of posterior pelvic structures and the absence of posterior ligamentous disruption.

Vertical Shear

Vertical shearing forces, acting perpendicular to the major trabecular pattern of the posterior pelvic complex, cause displacement of bone and disruption of soft tissues both anteriorly and posteriorly (Fig. 15–16*G*).

Complex Forces

Complex forces represent the combination of external rotation, lateral compression, and shear.

In this scheme, stability of the pelvic ring is considered to depend primarily on the integrity of its ligamentous structures, especially those located posteriorly (see Fig. 15–15). Instability is most characteristic of injuries resulting from vertical shear and complex forces. In severe forms of lateral compression (in which the lateral compressive forces on one side of the pelvis continue to the contralateral side as distracting forces with external rotation of the anterior portion of the pelvis) and of anteroposterior compression (in which all of the sacroiliac ligaments are disrupted), pelvic instability may result.[62] In other classification systems, stable fractures generally are considered to be those that either do not disrupt the osseous ring or disrupt it only in one place, and unstable fractures are those that disrupt the ring in two or more places. This latter approach is well suited to the conventional radiographic examination, which is able to identify directly only osseous elements and to assess indirectly ligamentous structures by delineating sites of diastasis. CT, although possessing superior contrast resolution, allows identification of sites of soft tissue hemorrhage but is unable to define the status of the pelvic ligaments precisely. CT does provide an exquisite cross-sectional display of the bony pelvis[66] and, combined with conventional radiography, can delineate cephalad or posterior displacement of the hemipelvis, which generally is considered a sign of instability.[55] MR imaging eventually may hold the key to the accurate analysis of both the osseous and the ligamentous structures of the pelvis.

A summary of injuries of the bony pelvis organized according to sites of involvement and the presence or absence of disruption of the pelvic ring is provided in Figure 15–17. This represents a slight modification

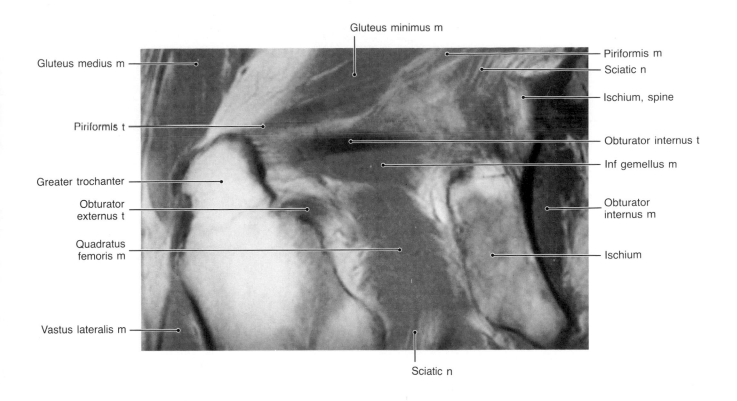

Gluteus minimus m

Gluteus medius m

Piriformis t

Greater trochanter

Obturator
externus t

Quadratus
femoris m

Vastus lateralis m

Piriformis m

Sciatic n

Ischium, spine

Obturator internus t

Inf gemellus m

Obturator
internus m

Ischium

Sciatic n

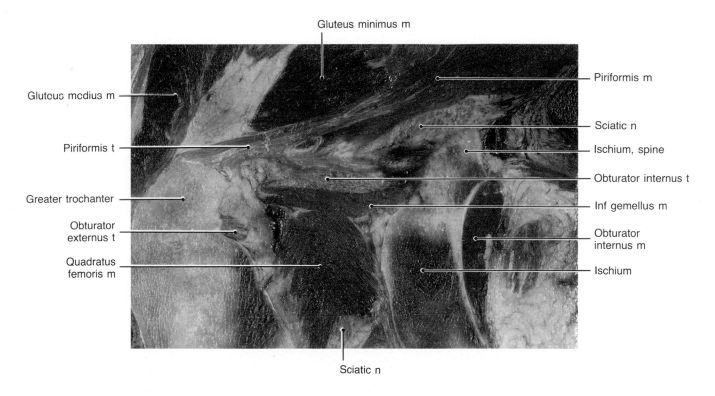

Gluteus minimus m

Gluteus medius m

Piriformis t

Greater trochanter

Obturator
externus t

Quadratus
femoris m

Piriformis m

Sciatic n

Ischium, spine

Obturator internus t

Inf gemellus m

Obturator
internus m

Ischium

Sciatic n

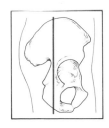

PLATE 15–1

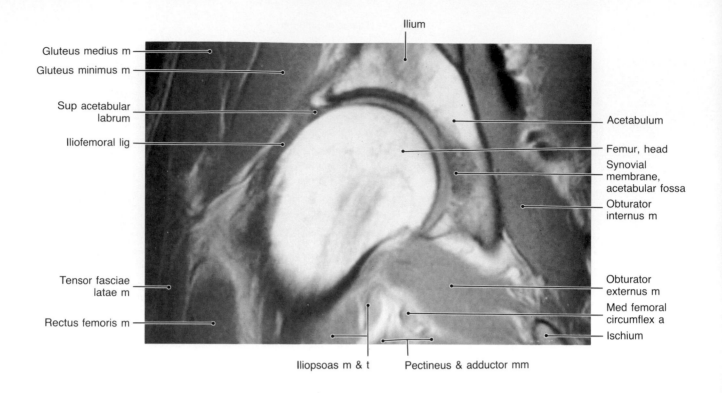

Gluteus medius m

Gluteus minimus m

Sup acetabular labrum

Iliofemoral lig

Ilium

Acetabulum

Femur, head

Synovial membrane, acetabular fossa

Obturator internus m

Tensor fasciae latae m

Rectus femoris m

Obturator externus m

Med femoral circumflex a

Ischium

Iliopsoas m & t

Pectineus & adductor mm

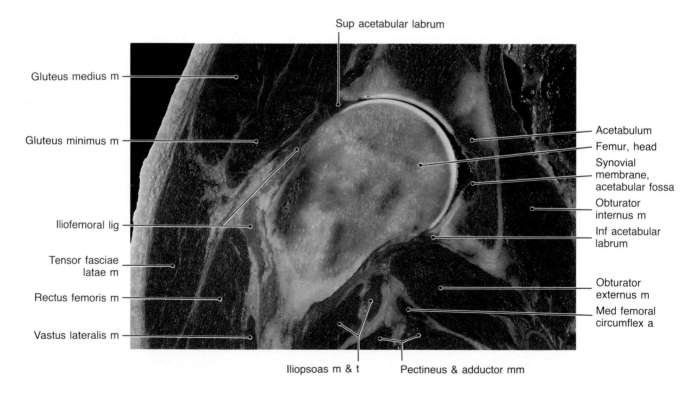

Sup acetabular labrum

Gluteus medius m

Gluteus minimus m

Iliofemoral lig

Tensor fasciae latae m

Rectus femoris m

Vastus lateralis m

Acetabulum

Femur, head

Synovial membrane, acetabular fossa

Obturator internus m

Inf acetabular labrum

Obturator externus m

Med femoral circumflex a

Iliopsoas m & t

Pectineus & adductor mm

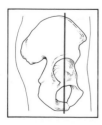

PLATE 15–2

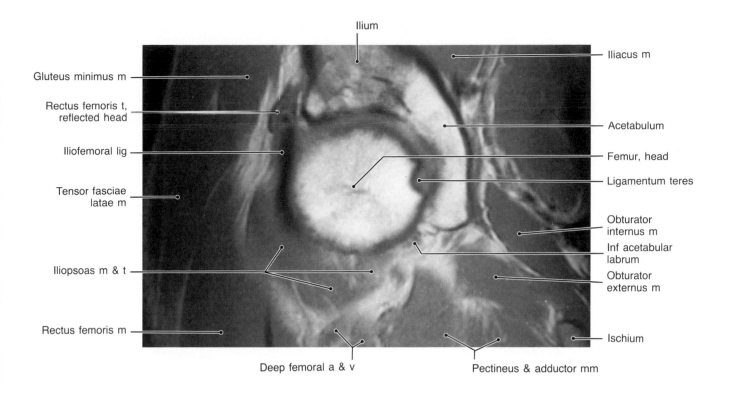

Ilium

Gluteus minimus m

Rectus femoris t, reflected head

Iliofemoral lig

Tensor fasciae latae m

Iliopsoas m & t

Rectus femoris m

Deep femoral a & v

Iliacus m

Acetabulum

Femur, head

Ligamentum teres

Obturator internus m

Inf acetabular labrum

Obturator externus m

Ischium

Pectineus & adductor mm

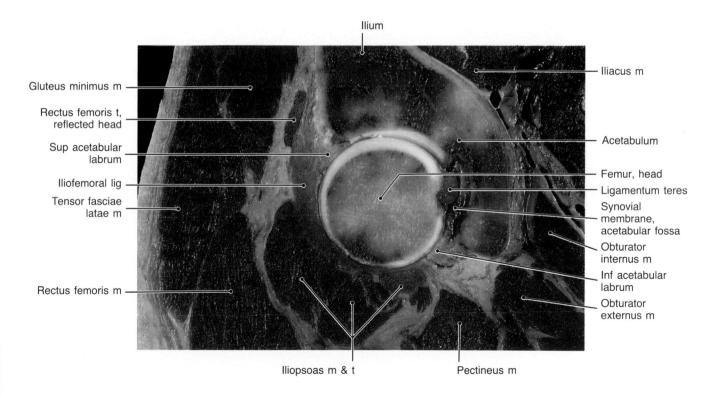

Ilium

Gluteus minimus m

Rectus femoris t, reflected head

Sup acetabular labrum

Iliofemoral lig

Tensor fasciae latae m

Rectus femoris m

Iliopsoas m & t

Pectineus m

Iliacus m

Acetabulum

Femur, head

Ligamentum teres

Synovial membrane, acetabular fossa

Obturator internus m

Inf acetabular labrum

Obturator externus m

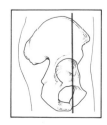

PLATE 15–3

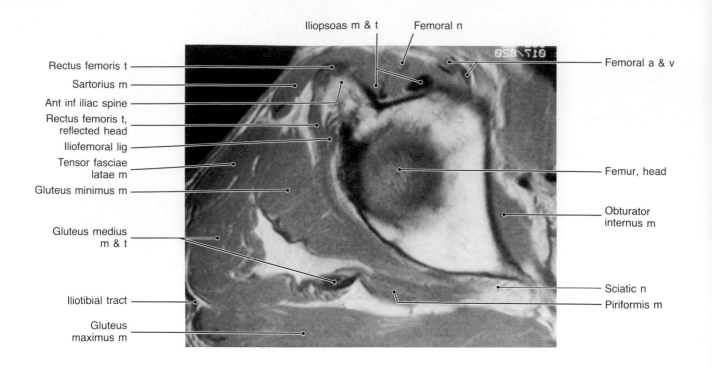

Iliopsoas m & t — Femoral n

Rectus femoris t

Sartorius m

Ant inf iliac spine

Rectus femoris t,
reflected head

Iliofemoral lig

Tensor fasciae
latae m

Gluteus minimus m

Gluteus medius
m & t

Iliotibial tract

Gluteus
maximus m

Femoral a & v

Femur, head

Obturator
internus m

Sciatic n

Piriformis m

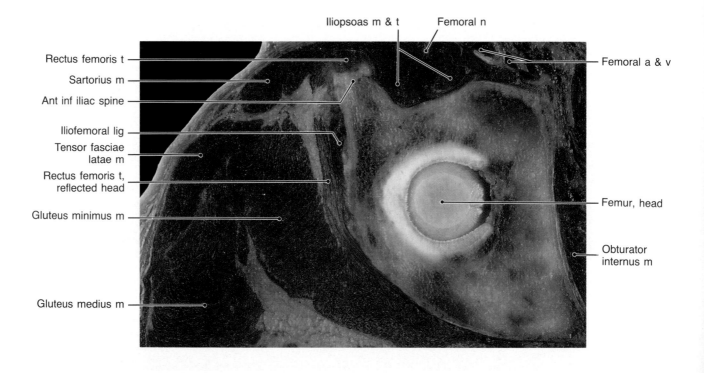

Iliopsoas m & t — Femoral n

Rectus femoris t

Sartorius m

Ant inf iliac spine

Iliofemoral lig

Tensor fasciae
latae m

Rectus femoris t,
reflected head

Gluteus minimus m

Gluteus medius m

Femoral a & v

Femur, head

Obturator
internus m

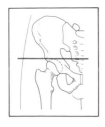

PLATE 15–4

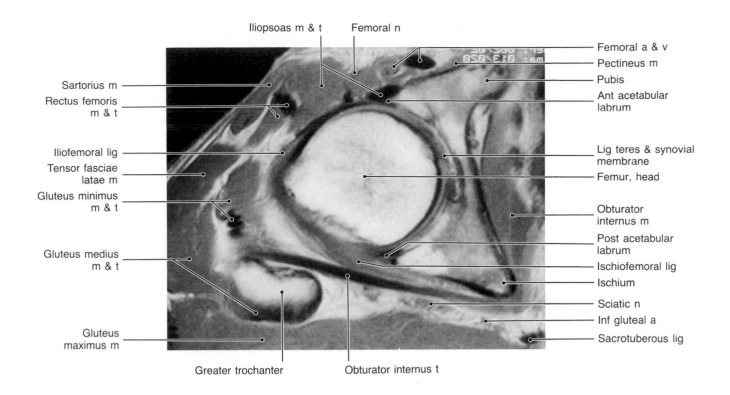

Iliopsoas m & t   Femoral n

Sartorius m

Rectus femoris
m & t

Iliofemoral lig

Tensor fasciae
latae m

Gluteus minimus
m & t

Gluteus medius
m & t

Gluteus
maximus m

Femoral a & v
Pectineus m
Pubis
Ant acetabular
labrum

Lig teres & synovial
membrane
Femur, head

Obturator
internus m

Post acetabular
labrum
Ischiofemoral lig
Ischium

Sciatic n
Inf gluteal a
Sacrotuberous lig

Greater trochanter   Obturator internus t

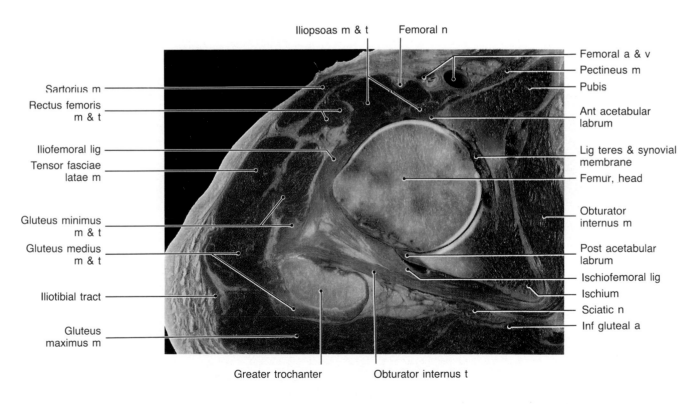

Iliopsoas m & t   Femoral n

Sartorius m

Rectus femoris
m & t

Iliofemoral lig

Tensor fasciae
latae m

Gluteus minimus
m & t

Gluteus medius
m & t

Iliotibial tract

Gluteus
maximus m

Femoral a & v
Pectineus m
Pubis

Ant acetabular
labrum

Lig teres & synovial
membrane
Femur, head

Obturator
internus m

Post acetabular
labrum
Ischiofemoral lig
Ischium
Sciatic n
Inf gluteal a

Greater trochanter   Obturator internus t

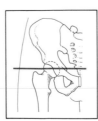

PLATE 15–5

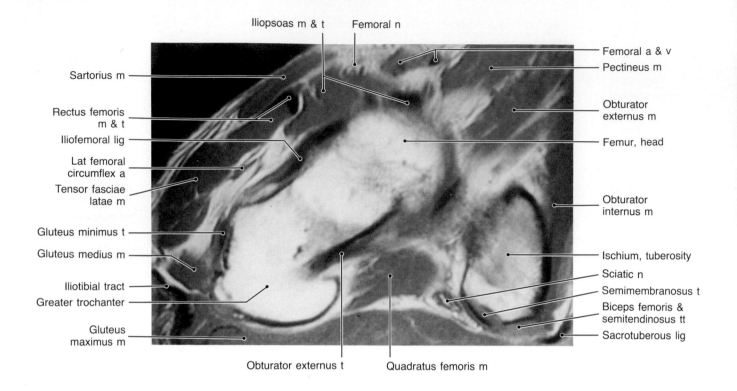

Iliopsoas m & t   Femoral n

Sartorius m

Rectus femoris m & t

Iliofemoral lig

Lat femoral circumflex a

Tensor fasciae latae m

Gluteus minimus t

Gluteus medius m

Iliotibial tract

Greater trochanter

Gluteus maximus m

Femoral a & v

Pectineus m

Obturator externus m

Femur, head

Obturator internus m

Ischium, tuberosity

Sciatic n

Semimembranosus t

Biceps femoris & semitendinosus tt

Sacrotuberous lig

Obturator externus t   Quadratus femoris m

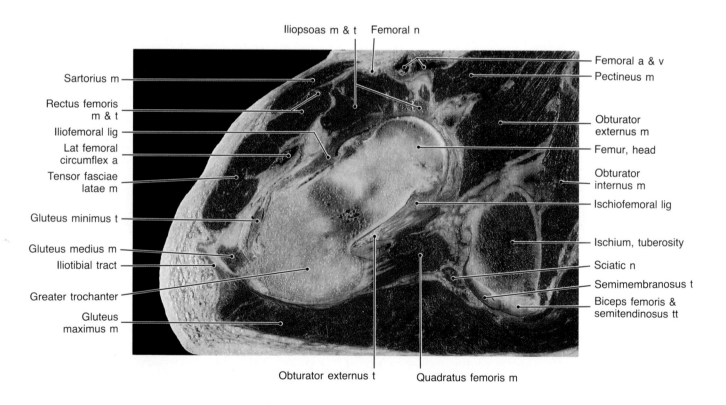

Iliopsoas m & t   Femoral n

Sartorius m

Rectus femoris m & t

Iliofemoral lig

Lat femoral circumflex a

Tensor fasciae latae m

Gluteus minimus t

Gluteus medius m

Iliotibial tract

Greater trochanter

Gluteus maximus m

Femoral a & v

Pectineus m

Obturator externus m

Femur, head

Obturator internus m

Ischiofemoral lig

Ischium, tuberosity

Sciatic n

Semimembranosus t

Biceps femoris & semitendinosus tt

Obturator externus t   Quadratus femoris m

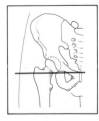

PLATE 15-6

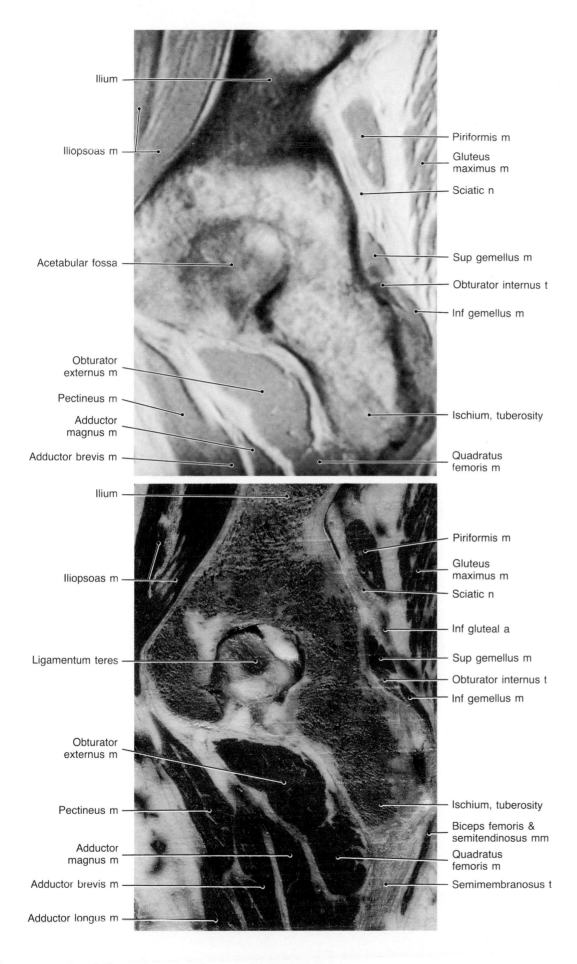

Ilium

Iliopsoas m

Acetabular fossa

Obturator
externus m

Pectineus m

Adductor
magnus m

Adductor brevis m

Piriformis m

Gluteus
maximus m

Sciatic n

Sup gemellus m

Obturator internus t

Inf gemellus m

Ischium, tuberosity

Quadratus
femoris m

Ilium

Iliopsoas m

Ligamentum teres

Obturator
externus m

Pectineus m

Adductor
magnus m

Adductor brevis m

Adductor longus m

Piriformis m

Gluteus
maximus m

Sciatic n

Inf gluteal a

Sup gemellus m

Obturator internus t

Inf gemellus m

Ischium, tuberosity

Biceps femoris &
semitendinosus mm

Quadratus
femoris m

Semimembranosus t

PLATE 15–7

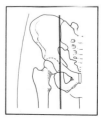

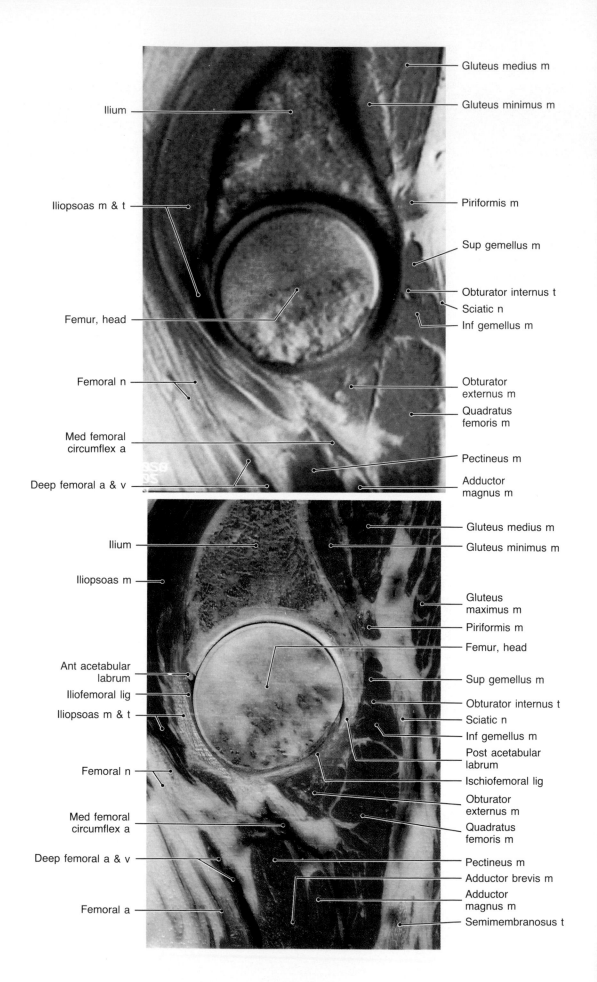

Gluteus medius m

Gluteus minimus m

Ilium

Iliopsoas m & t

Piriformis m

Sup gemellus m

Femur, head

Obturator internus t

Sciatic n

Inf gemellus m

Femoral n

Obturator externus m

Quadratus femoris m

Med femoral circumflex a

Pectineus m

Deep femoral a & v

Adductor magnus m

Ilium

Gluteus medius m

Gluteus minimus m

Iliopsoas m

Gluteus maximus m

Piriformis m

Femur, head

Ant acetabular labrum

Sup gemellus m

Iliofemoral lig

Obturator internus t

Iliopsoas m & t

Sciatic n

Inf gemellus m

Post acetabular labrum

Femoral n

Ischiofemoral lig

Obturator externus m

Med femoral circumflex a

Quadratus femoris m

Deep femoral a & v

Pectineus m

Adductor brevis m

Adductor magnus m

Femoral a

Semimembranosus t

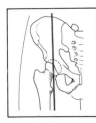

PLATE 15-8

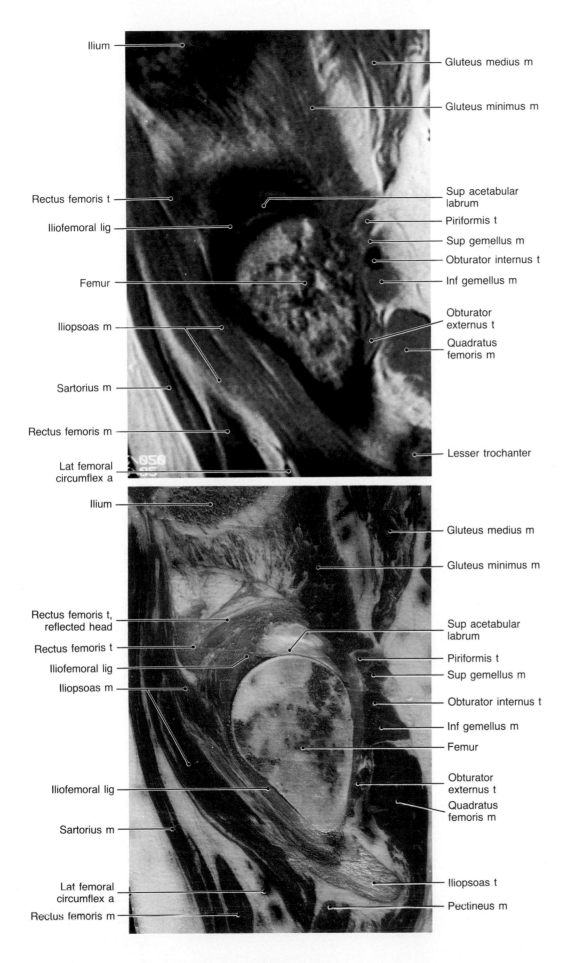

Ilium

Gluteus medius m

Gluteus minimus m

Rectus femoris t

Sup acetabular labrum

Iliofemoral lig

Piriformis t

Sup gemellus m

Obturator internus t

Femur

Inf gemellus m

Iliopsoas m

Obturator externus t

Quadratus femoris m

Sartorius m

Rectus femoris m

Lat femoral circumflex a

Lesser trochanter

Ilium

Gluteus medius m

Gluteus minimus m

Rectus femoris t, reflected head

Sup acetabular labrum

Rectus femoris t

Piriformis t

Iliofemoral lig

Sup gemellus m

Iliopsoas m

Obturator internus t

Inf gemellus m

Femur

Iliofemoral lig

Obturator externus t

Quadratus femoris m

Sartorius m

Lat femoral circumflex a

Iliopsoas t

Rectus femoris m

Pectineus m

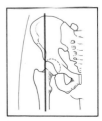

PLATE 15-9

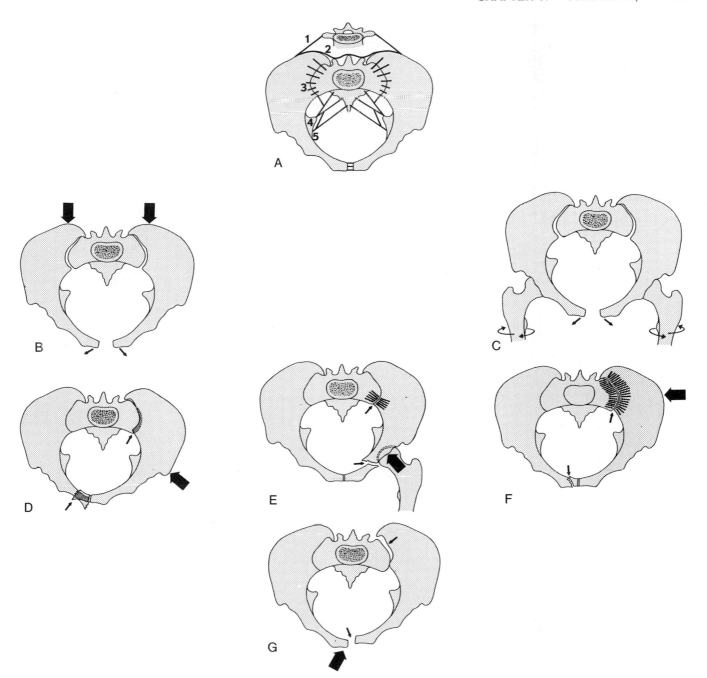

Figure 15–16
Fractures and dislocations of the pelvis: Biomechanical principles.

  A Normal situation. Schematic representation of the major ligamentous structures is shown. These include the iliolumbar ligaments (1), posterior (2) and anterior (3) sacroiliac ligaments, sacrospinous ligaments (4), and sacrotuberous ligaments (5).

  B External rotation forces. A direct blow to the posterior superior iliac spines (large arrows) leads to opening of the symphysis pubis (small arrows). Without the addition of a shearing force, the posterior ligamentous complex remains intact.

  C External rotation forces. External rotation of the femora (curved arrows) or direct compression against the anterior superior iliac spines also produces springing of the symphysis pubis (small arrows). Without the addition of a shearing force, the posterior ligamentous complex remains intact.

  D Lateral compression forces. A lateral compression force against the iliac crest (large arrow) causes the hemipelvis to rotate internally. The anterior portions of the sacrum and pubic rami (small arrows) are injured.

  E Lateral compression forces. A direct force against the greater trochanter (large arrow) leads to similar injuries to the pubic rami and ipsilateral sacroiliac joint ligamentous complex (small arrows).

  F Lateral compression forces. A force (large arrow) directed parallel to the trabeculae about the sacroiliac joint may produce impaction of bone posteriorly and disruption of the pubic rami (small arrows).

  G Vertical shearing forces. A shearing force (large arrow) crosses perpendicular to the main trabecular pattern and causes both anterior and posterior injuries (small arrows).

  (From Tile M: Fractures of the Pelvis and Acetabulum. Copyright 1984, Williams & Wilkins Co, Baltimore, p 22.)

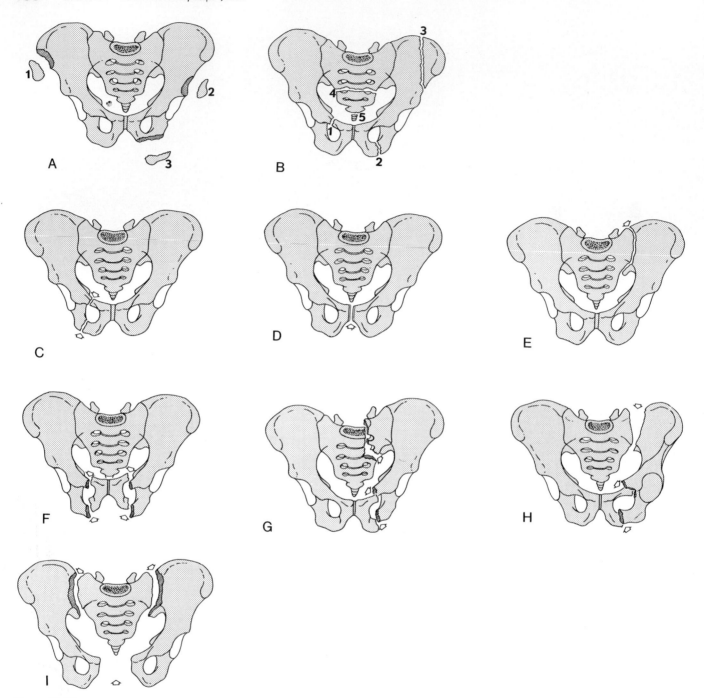

Figure 15–17

Fractures and dislocations of the pelvis: Classification system.

A Type I injury: Avulsion fractures. These may involve the anterior superior iliac spine (1), the anterior inferior iliac spine (2), or the ischial tuberosity (3).

B Type I injury: Fractures of a single pubis ramus or iliac wing (Duverney fracture). A single break in the superior or inferior pubic ramus (1, 2), certain fractures of the ilium (3), or some types of fractures of the sacrum (4) or coccyx (5) do not lead to disruption of the pelvic ring.

C Type II injury: Ipsilateral fractures of the pubic rami. Such fractures (open arrows) lead to a single break in the pelvic ring.

D Type II injury: Diastasis of the symphysis pubis. This injury (open arrow), or an isolated fracture of parasymphyseal bone, also leads to a single break in the pelvic ring.

E Type II injury: Subluxation of the sacroiliac joint. This subluxation (open arrow), or an isolated fracture near the sacroiliac joint, is an additional example of a single break in the pelvic ring.

F Type III injury: Straddle fracture. Note disruption of the pelvis in two places owing to bilateral vertical fractures involving both pubic rami (open arrows).

G Type III injury: Malgaigne fracture. Vertical fractures of both pubic rami on one side combined with a sacral fracture (open arrows) lead to disruption of the pelvic ring in two places.

H Type III injury: Malgaigne fracture. Similar vertical fractures of both pubic rami on one side combined with dislocation of the sacroiliac joint (open arrows) again produce disruption of the pelvic ring in two places.

I Complex injury: "Sprung" pelvis. Disruptions of the pelvic ring relate to bilateral dislocations of the sacroiliac joint and diastasis of the symphysis pubis (open arrows).

of the excellent analysis provided by Kane.[67] Other reference sources are available to the interested reader.[68–75, 77–83]

Complications

The mortality associated with all pelvic fractures is about 10 per cent, which in most cases relates to a variety of serious complications.[80] With regard to the complications of pelvic fractures and dislocations, four types deserve emphasis: hemorrhage, urinary tract injury, peripheral nerve injury, and remote injuries. The serious nature of the excessive bleeding that accompanies many of these fractures, particularly type III injuries, is underscored by the necessity for blood transfusions in almost 50 per cent of cases and the significant mortality that follows inadequate blood replacement.[81] Injuries to the urinary tract are associated most typically with symphyseal diastasis or fractures of the pubic rami, or both; urethral damage is somewhat more frequent than that of the bladder, the latter commonly being displaced upward by the accumulating blood. Urethral injuries predominate in men.[82] Microscopic or macroscopic hematuria after a pelvic fracture deserves immediate attention and may require specialized studies, including retrograde urethrography, cystography, or intravenous pyelography, or combinations of these. Of importance, a catheter should not be placed in the bladder until the extent of urethral damage is known.

Damage to the peripheral nerves occurs in approximately 10 per cent of patients after injuries of the bony pelvis, and this frequency increases in those with sacral fractures.[83] In addition to the bladder, other viscera that are injured in association with fractures and dislocations of the pelvis include the liver, spleen, testes, and bowel as well as the diaphragm.

Hip Dislocation

Dislocation of the femoral head with or without an acetabular fracture is an injury that usually follows considerable trauma and that may be associated with significant injury elsewhere in the body. Hip dislocations represent approximately 5 per cent of all dislocations. Hip dislocations generally are classified as anterior, posterior, and central, although other types such as luxatio erecta (in which the hip is flexed and the leg extends along the torso) are encountered rarely.[84] In general, forces producing hip dislocation are transmitted from one of three sources[27]: the anterior surface of the flexed knee striking an object, the sole of the foot with the ipsilateral knee extended, and the greater trochanter. Less commonly, a force may be applied to the posterior aspect of the pelvis with the ipsilateral foot or knee acting as the counterforce. Motor vehicle accidents represent the primary cause of hip dislocations. In one classic example, an unrestrained automobile driver sustains a posterior dislocation of the left hip and either a fracture-dislocation or anterior dislocation of the right hip (Fig. 15–18).[27] The precise type of injury, however, depends on such factors as the amount and direction of the applied force, the quality of the bone, and the

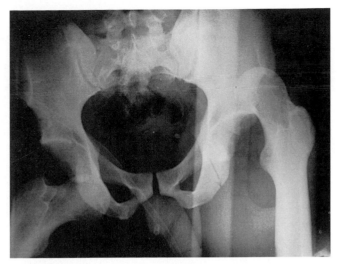

Figure 15–18

Hip dislocation. Observe a posterior dislocation of the left hip and an anterior dislocation of the right hip. In this case, the injuries resulted from a motorcycle accident. (Courtesy of T. Martin, M.D., and J. Spaeth, M.D., Albuquerque, New Mexico.)

position of the hip (particularly the degree of hip rotation) at the time of injury. As the femoral head exits the acetabulum, fractures of the femoral head may result from impaction or avulsive (i.e., at the site of attachment of the ligamentum teres) forces.

Anterior dislocation of the hip is a relatively rare type of dislocation, representing 5 to 10 per cent of all hip dislocations, and it relates to forced abduction and external rotation of the leg.[85, 86] If the hip is flexed, an anterior obturator dislocation occurs; if the hip is extended, a superoanterior (pubic) dislocation results. On radiographs, the abnormal position of the femoral head is readily apparent; on frontal radiographs, an anteriorly displaced femoral head typically moves inferomedially with the femur abducted and externally rotated, and a posteriorly displaced femoral head usually is located superolaterally with the femur adducted and internally rotated, although exceptions to these rules are encountered.[87] Thus, a superior anterior dislocation, sometimes termed a pubic dislocation, may simulate a posterior dislocation of the hip if only the frontal radiograph is analyzed. In anterior hip dislocations, associated fractures of the acetabular rim, greater trochanter, or femoral neck,[88, 89] or, more commonly, femoral head[90, 91] may be observed. A characteristic depression or flattening of the posterosuperior and lateral portion of the femoral head can be seen (Fig. 15–19).[92–94] Rarely, anterior dislocation of the hip may be recurrent.[95–97]

Posterior dislocation of the hip is more common (approximately 80 to 85 per cent of all hip dislocations) and may result from a dashboard injury in which the flexed knee strikes the dashboard during a head-on automobile collision.[85, 98–102] Motorcycle accidents provide another important source for this type of hip dislocation.[103] The leg is shortened, internally rotated, and adducted. Associated problems include knee trauma (e.g., patellar, tibial, or fibular fracture, or combinations of these fractures), femoral head or shaft fractures,[104, 105]

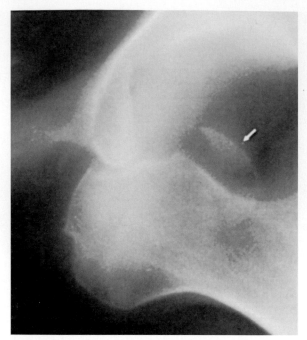

Figure 15–19
Anterior dislocation. Tomogram reveals an inferomedial position of the dislocated femoral head and a fracture fragment of the lateral portion of the head (arrow).

and sciatic nerve injury. The frequent occurrence of posterior acetabular rim fractures after posterior dislocation of the hip requires careful analysis of routine radiographs and the use of oblique and lateral projections.[5, 106] The posteriorly dislocated femoral head usually lies superior to the acetabulum on the frontal radiograph, although occasionally it may lie at the same level as the acetabulum. A persistently widened hip joint may indicate abnormally placed fragments or significant acetabular injury. CT scanning (Fig. 15–20) can be used to identify lipohemarthroses, small osseous fragments, deformity of the femoral head, and the extent of damage to the posterior acetabular rim.[107] Two types of femoral head fractures are seen: shear fractures, which involve principally the inferior and anterior portions of the femoral head, occurring in 7 to 10 per cent of posterior hip dislocations; and compression fractures, which involve mainly the anterior to inferomedial portion of the femoral head, occurring in 13 to 60 per cent of such dislocations and poorly seen on conventional radiographs.[94, 108–110] The Pipkin classification system sometimes is employed to describe the pattern of such fractures in cases of posterior dislocation of the hip (Figs. 15–21 and 15–22).[27] Additional complications of this injury are periarticular soft tissue calcification and ossification, acetabular labrum tears, acetabular fractures, osteonecrosis of the femoral head, and secondary degenerative joint disease.[111–115] Osteonecrosis may complicate as many as 25 per cent of posterior hip dislocations, especially when the injury is associated with a delay in diagnosis and treatment and a fracture of the posterior acetabular margin. Recurrent posterior dislocations of the hip have been described.[116–118]

Central acetabular fracture-dislocation usually results from a force applied to the lateral side of the trochanter and pelvis, with the stress applied through the femoral head. Various patterns of acetabular fracture complicate this injury (in fact, the injury is not really a true dislocation but, rather, relates to displacement of the femoral head accompanying a displaced acetabular fracture[27]), and hemorrhage into the pelvis also may be observed. Secondary degenerative joint disease is not infrequent.

Traumatic dislocation of the hip usually is encountered in adults, although children and infants also can be affected.[119–125] In the younger age group, dislocation almost always is posterior, although anterior dislocations are described.[126, 127] Entrapment of the acetabular labrum[126] or capsule[127] or the presence of osteocartilaginous fragments[128] may prevent adequate reduction. Such dislocation may be associated with ischemic necrosis of the femoral head[129, 130] or physeal injury,[131] and in the infant, traumatic displacement must be differentiated from developmental dysplasia of the hip.

Although the value of routine radiography and CT scanning is well established in assessment of hip dislocations, that of MR imaging is not clear. The identification of labral injuries (see later discussion) with MR imaging may represent one important application of the technique, particularly in cases in which hip instability persists, although such identification may require MR arthrography. In one study of 18 patients with posterior (14 patients) or anterior (4 patients) dislocation of the hip, MR imaging revealed joint effusions or hemarthroses in all cases, femoral head fractures or contusions in

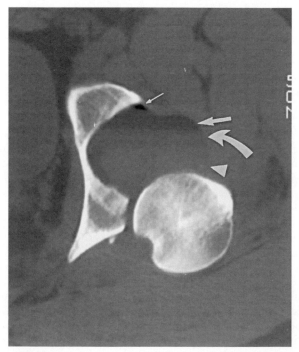

Figure 15–20
Hip dislocation: Lipohemarthrosis. Transaxial CT scanning shows a posterior dislocation of the left femoral head with a fracture of the posterior acetabular rim. Note four layers with three fluid levels. These consist of gas (small arrow), fat (large straight arrow), serum (large curved arrow), and the more cellular components of blood (arrowhead). (Courtesy of M. Mitchell, M.D., Halifax, Nova Scotia, Canada.)

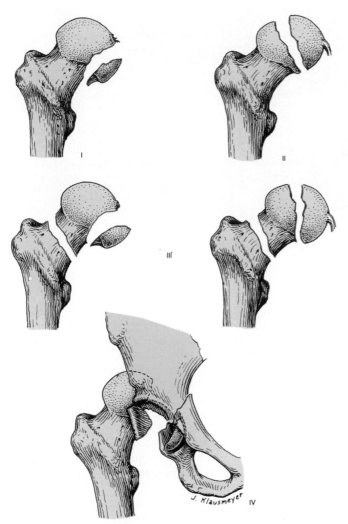

Figure 15–21

Pipkin's classification of femoral head fractures. Pipkin's type I is a fracture fragment below the ligamentum teres; type II is a fracture fragment above the ligamentum. Type III is either of these with an associated femoral neck fracture—a combination with a significantly poorer patient prognosis. Type IV is either of these with an associated acetabular fracture. (Reproduced with permission from Swiontkowski MF: Intracapsular hip fractures. *In* BD Browner, JB Jupiter, AM Levine, et al [Eds]: Skeletal Trauma: Fractures, Dislocations, Ligamentous Injuries. Philadelphia, WB Saunders Co, 1992, p. 1373.)

the majority of cases, and acetabular fractures in six patients.[132] Additional findings included muscle injuries of the gluteal region or of the posterior, anterior, or medial fascial compartments, iliofemoral ligament injuries, intra-articular osteocartilaginous bodies, labral tears, and entrapment of the ligamentum teres.[132] The identification of specific muscle injuries appears to be predictive of the type of hip dislocation that has occurred and may be of value in cases in which the diagnosis of such dislocation is otherwise not clear. Although MR imaging also may allow detection of acetabular fractures and injuries to the sciatic nerve, the technique appears inferior to CT scanning in the delineation of intra-articular fracture fragments.[133] Ultimately, arthroscopy of the hip, although technically demanding, may be the procedure of choice in the detection and treat-

ment of labral tears and intra-articular bodies.[134] MR imaging, however, is useful in detecting osteonecrosis of the femoral head occurring subsequent to hip dislocation.[394]

Fractures of the Proximal Portion of the Femur

The extraordinary amount of attention that has been directed toward the diagnosis and treatment of fractures of the femoral neck is indicative of the frequency and the potential seriousness of these injuries.[135] Although occurring as a stress fracture in the young athlete and as a pathologic fracture in patients with skeletal metastasis, Paget's disease, and other disorders, it is the occurrence of fractures of the proximal portion of the femur in elderly persons with osteopenia, particularly women with osteoporosis, that has received the greatest attention.[136–141] In the latter situation, the injuries are similar to insufficiency stress fractures, although a history of minor trauma usually is evident. Two major mechanisms of injury have been proposed in the production of femoral neck fractures: a fall producing a direct blow on the greater trochanter[142] and lateral rotation of the extremity.[143] Cyclic loading leading to microfractures that become complete after a minor torsional injury and, in young patients, major direct forces along the shaft of the femur with or without a rotational component are additional potential mechanisms of injury.[144] Nondisplaced fractures of the proximal portion of the femur may escape detection on initial routine radiographic examination. Diagnostic help is provided by MR imaging (Fig. 15–23) and bone scintigraphy (see discussion later in this chapter).

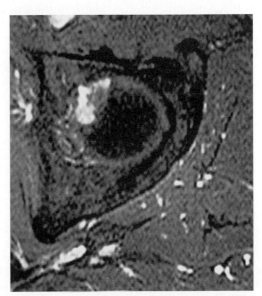

Figure 15–22

Hip dislocation with femoral head fracture. This transverse T1-weighted (TR/TE, 717/20), fat-suppressed spin echo MR image obtained after the intravenous administration of a gadolinium compound shows the anteromedial fracture of the femoral head as a region of high signal intensity. (Courtesy of C. Neumann, M.D., Palm Springs, California.)

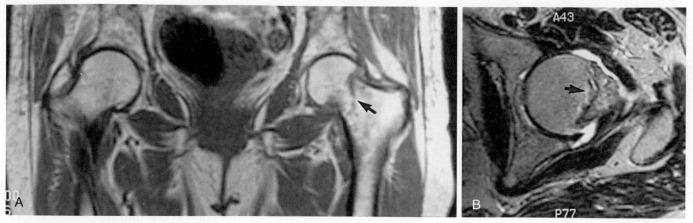

Figure 15–23
Fractures of the femoral neck: MR imaging. An intracapsular fracture (arrows) of the femoral neck is shown in a coronal T1-weighted (TR/TE, 800/16) spin echo MR image **(A)** and a transaxial fast spin echo (TR/TE, 4666/160) MR image **(B)**. Note the large joint effusion. (Courtesy of D. Berthoty, M.D., Las Vegas, Nevada.)

No universally accepted classification system of fractures of the proximal portion of the femur exists. Anatomic designations, including subcapital, transcervical, basicervical, intertrochanteric, and subtrochanteric, frequently are used to define the location of the fracture and can be modified to include intracapsular fractures (those in the subcapital and transcervical regions) and extracapsular fractures (those in the basicervical and trochanteric regions). Subcapital fractures occur immediately beneath the articular surface of the femoral head; transcervical fractures pass across the middle of the femoral neck; basicervical fractures occur at the base of the femoral neck; intertrochanteric fractures are located in a line between the greater and lesser trochanters; and subtrochanteric fractures occur subjacent to this.[144] Difficulty in fracture classification based on this anatomic scheme relates to the inability to differentiate clearly between subcapital and transcervical fractures, between basicervical and intertrochanteric fractures, and between intertrochanteric and subtrochanteric fractures in instances in which radiographs are suboptimal, fracture lines are subtle, or marked rotation or angulation occurs at the fracture site.[145, 146]

Intracapsular fractures, which are approximately twice as frequent as those in the trochanteric region,[147] also may be classified according to the direction of the fracture angle or the degree of displacement of the fracture fragments.[148] The former system, which was developed by Pauwels,[149] uses three categories of fracture based on its angle with the horizontal: type I is a fracture that is oriented at 30 degrees from the horizontal; type II is one that is oriented at 50 degrees from the horizontal; and type III is oriented at 70 degrees from the horizontal.[144] The belief that the shearing forces encountered in the more vertical fractures (e.g., type III) led to nonunion was the stimulus for this classification system, but the radiographic accuracy in the detection of the fracture angle subsequently has been challenged.[150] Classification of intracapsular fractures according to the degree of displacement on prereduction radiographs commonly is referred to as the Garden system.[148, 150] Four types of fractures are identified: type I fractures are incomplete or impacted; type II fractures are complete and without osseous displacement; type III fractures also are complete but with partial displacement of the fracture fragments commonly associated with shortening and external rotation of the distal fragments; and type IV fractures are complete with total displacement of the fracture fragments.[144] It is the type III or IV fracture that is associated with significant complications and technical failures. Difficulty in this latter classification system relates to disagreement regarding the alignment (type IV fracture) or malalignment (type III fracture) of the trabeculae of the femoral head with those of the acetabulum.[151]

Several complications of intracapsular fractures of the femoral neck deserve emphasis. It generally is believed that, under normal circumstances, these fractures will reveal evidence of healing in the first 6 to 12 months. Delayed union and nonunion are not uncommon, and the latter occurs in approximately 5 to 25 per cent of cases.[152–154] Factors predisposing to nonunion include advancing age of the patient, osteoporosis, posterior comminution of the fracture, inadequate reduction, and poor internal fixation technique.[144] The frequency of ischemic necrosis of the femoral head varies from 10 to 30 per cent, increasing in cases with moderate or severe displacement of the fracture fragments or with persistent motion at the fracture site owing to poor stabilization.[155] Measurement of intracapsular pressure in patients with femoral neck fractures reveals elevated values related to hemarthrosis, although the role of the elevated pressure in the pathogenesis of osteonecrosis is not agreed on.[156–159] Furthermore, it should be noted that the vascular insult to the femoral head may occur not only at the time of fracture but also after attempts at reduction or internal fixation. Bone scintigraphy (Fig. 15–24) has been used not only in the initial diagnosis of the fracture but also as a means for detection of osteonecrosis (and other complications) that influences the eventual clinical outcome.[160–165] MR imaging has been employed for these same purposes (see Fig. 15–24) (see later discussion),[166–168] although routine radiography still remains important in the assessment of post-

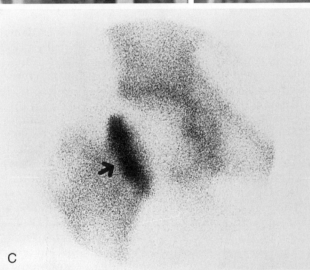

Figure 15–24
Fractures of the femoral neck: Osteonecrosis of the femoral head.

A, B This 60 year old man developed osteonecrosis of the femoral head after a femoral neck fracture that had been treated with an intramedullary nail. Coronal (TR/TE, 400/17) **(A)** and sagittal (TR/TE, 550/17) **(B)** T1-weighted spin echo MR images show the region of osteonecrosis (open arrows) and the nail insertion site (solid arrows).

C Anterior pinhole bone scintigraphy of the right hip in a second patient shows a large photon deficient area involving the entire femoral head and a sharply defined, extremely intense bandlike region in the femoral neck (arrow) at the site of fracture. (Reproduced with permission from Y. W. Bahk: Combined Scintigraphic and Radiographic Diagnosis of Bone and Joint Diseases. New York, Springer-Verlag, 1994, p. 154.)

traumatic osteonecrosis. The resulting radiographic abnormalities are typical, appearing as early as 3 months and as late as 3 years after the fracture, and consisting primarily of increased radiodensity of the femoral head[169] as well as irregularity of the articular surface and subchondral radiolucent areas. Late segmental collapse of the necrotic bone is inconstant but, when present, leads to significant clinical manifestations and a propensity to develop osteoarthritis.[170, 171]

Additional complications of intracapsular femoral neck fractures include posttraumatic thromboembolic phenomena[144] and postoperative osteomyelitis and septic arthritis.[172]

Intertrochanteric fractures also predominate in elderly patients (Fig. 15–25), with a somewhat higher frequency in women (unlike the overwhelming female predilection observed in intracapsular femoral neck fractures). Osteopenia, usually osteoporosis, is common at the site of fracture, leading to the vulnerability of this

femoral region to minor trauma. Direct or indirect forces resulting from a fall constitute the typical mechanism of injury.[173, 174] Fracture comminution is common, leading to multiple fragments of bone, which may include the greater trochanter, the lesser trochanter, or both. The radiographic analysis is complicated by this comminution as well as by the typical displacement and rotation that occur.

As in the case of intracapsular fractures of the femoral neck, no uniform classification system exists for intertrochanteric fractures. Available systems are based on stability versus instability or the ease by which fracture reduction can be accomplished.[175–178] As has been emphasized by DeLee,[144] a stable fracture (approximately 50 per cent of cases) is characterized by the absence of comminution of the medial cortices of the proximal and distal fragments and of displacement of the lesser trochanter. Unstable intertrochanteric fractures (approximately 50 per cent of cases) occur in two situations[144]: fractures

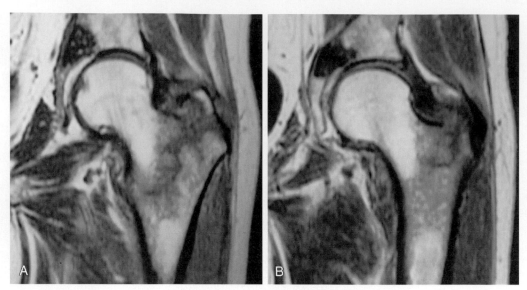

Figure 15–25
Fractures of the femoral neck: Intertrochanteric fractures. Two examples are shown in coronal T1-weighted (TR/TE, 600/12) spin echo MR images. In **A**, the fracture line extends almost completely across the neck. In **B**, the fracture line extends only partially across the neck. In both cases, marrow edema also is present.

with reversed obliquity with a marked tendency toward medial displacement of the femoral shaft owing to adductor muscle pull or to comminution of the greater trochanter and adjacent posterolateral surface of the shaft; and fractures with absence of contact between the proximal and distal fragments owing to comminution or medial and posterior displacement of fracture fragments.

Complications of intertrochanteric fractures include varus displacement both in nonsurgically treated injuries and in those associated with failure of internal reduction, secondary subcapital fractures (after internal fixation of intertrochanteric fractures), laceration of adjacent vessels (a rare finding), nonunion (which is an uncommon occurrence owing to the fact that these fractures occur in cancellous bone with good blood supply), and ischemic necrosis of the femoral head (which also is uncommon, appearing in less than 1 per cent of cases).[144, 179, 180]

Isolated fractures of the greater trochanter in adults are infrequent and generally relate to injury (avulsion or direct blow) of the bone after a fall, particularly in elderly persons. Differentiation of a fracture of the greater trochanter from one that also involves the proximal portion of the femur (i.e., intertrochanteric fracture) may require tomographic imaging techniques. Furthermore, as fractures of the greater trochanter usually are not displaced to a significant extent, their detection also may necessitate tomography. MR imaging in patients with radiographically evident fractures that appear to be isolated to the greater trochanter reveals several patterns of abnormality: Fracture lines may be detected within the greater trochanter alone; true intertrochanteric fractures may be delineated; or trochanteric fractures may extend incompletely across the femoral neck (Fig. 15–26).

Fractures isolated to the lesser trochanter also are unusual and may represent the initial manifestation of skeletal metastasis. Avulsion injuries of the lesser trochanter are seen more typically in children and adolescents.

Fractures of the femur that commence immediately below the trochanter are considered subtrochanteric,[176, 181, 182] although some of these fractures extend into the trochanteric region, making precise classification difficult. Some classification systems do not separate trochanteric and subtrochanteric fractures, whereas others deal solely with those in the subtrochanteric region[176] or emphasize the configuration of the fracture line.[182] The precise location of the fracture is of more than academic interest, as those that occur more distally are associated with a greater frequency of nonunion or delayed union and implant failure.[144] Problems of fracture union are indicative of the tendency for cortical comminution in cases of subtrochanteric fractures, and surgical failures are reflective of the considerable biomechanical stress in this region of the femur.

Approximately 5 to 30 per cent of fractures of the proximal portion of the femur occur in the subtrochanteric region, the reported frequency varying according to the criteria used to designate a fracture as subtrochanteric. These fractures occur in older patients with relatively minor injuries and in younger patients with major trauma. Pathologic or insufficiency fractures (Fig. 15–27) also are not infrequent in this region of the femur and are typical of Paget's disease.

Fractures of the Acetabulum

Although the acetabulum represents a portion of the bony pelvis, it also is an essential component of the hip; therefore, a discussion of acetabular fractures is appropriate here owing to their association with hip dislocations as well as their modification of proper function of the joint. The classic description of acetabular

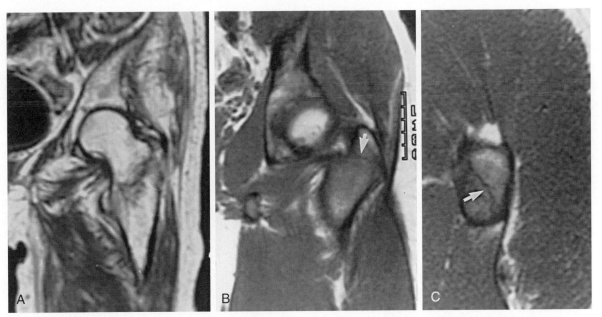

Figure 15–26

Fractures of the femoral neck: Trochanteric versus intertrochanteric fractures. MR imaging can be used effectively in this differentiation.

   A In this case, a coronal T1-weighted (TR/TE, 500/16) spin echo MR image reveals a nondisplaced intertrochanteric fracture. (Courtesy of D. Goodwin, M.D., Hanover, New Hampshire.)

   B, C In a second case, coronal (TR/TE, 600/17) **(B)** and sagittal (TR/TE 500/10) **(C)** T1-weighted spin echo MR images show an isolated greater trochanteric fracture (arrows). (Courtesy of D. Witte, M.D., Memphis, Tennessee.)

fracture belongs to Judet and his colleagues,[5] who devised a classification system based on the specific sites of fracture and emphasized the need for a complete radiographic examination, including oblique projections. Although these radiographs remain important, more recent modifications in imaging protocols for the injured acetabulum have been proposed in which CT

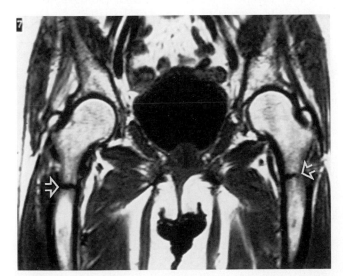

Figure 15–27

Fractures of the proximal portion of the femur: subtrochanteric fractures—insufficiency fractures. In this 48 year old woman with systemic lupus erythematosus, insufficiency fractures occurred in both femora. A coronal T1-weighted (TR/TE, 500/20) spin echo MR image reveals these fractures as linear areas of low signal intensity (arrows). More diffuse regions of decreased signal intensity about the fractures represent foci of bone marrow edema. (Courtesy of A. Motta, M.D., Cleveland, Ohio.)

plays an important role.[183–190] The role of MR imaging in the assessment of acetabular fractures is not clear, although preliminary data have been encouraging (Fig. 15–28).[133] With any imaging system, the delineation of four bony landmarks remains fundamental to proper assessment of the extent of injury: the anterior acetabular rim, the posterior acetabular rim, the iliopubic (anterior) column, and the ilioischial (posterior) column. Furthermore, with CT, additional features, including the integrity of the acetabular dome and quadrilateral surface as well as the presence of intra-articular osseous fragments and associated fractures of the bony pelvis, can be determined readily (Fig. 15–29).

   Although a complete discussion of acetabular fractures is beyond the scope of the current chapter, a few points deserve emphasis. These fractures result from the impact of the femoral head against the central regions of the acetabulum or its rims, especially the posterior rim in association with a posterior dislocation of the hip. Isolated fractures of the anterior or superior portion of the acetabular rim are unusual. The precise location of the force depends on a number of factors, including the degree of flexion or extension, adduction or abduction, and internal or external rotation of the thigh with respect to the bony pelvis, and such factors account for a spectrum of injuries that encompasses pure dislocations of the hip, fractures of the acetabulum, and combinations of the two.[191] The number of categories that have been used to describe the resultant acetabular fractures has varied,[5, 192] although the need to identify the acetabular rims and osseous columns in the assessment of these fractures remains unchallenged. Fractures may involve the anterior or posterior column alone, or a transverse fracture may involve both of these columns.

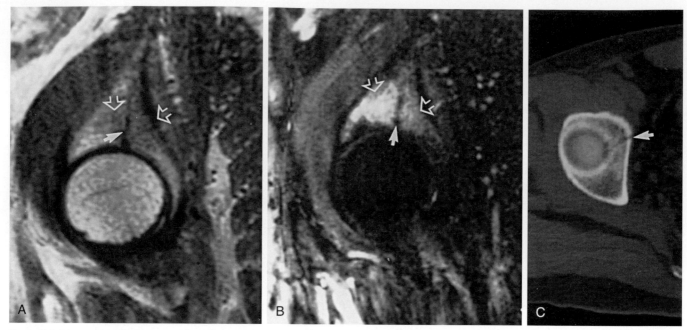

Figure 15–28
Acetabular fractures: MR imaging and CT scanning. In a 44 year old man, sagittal proton density–weighted (TR/TE, 2100/30) spin echo **(A)** and fast spin echo STIR (TR/TE, 4500/39; inversion time, 160 msec) **(B)** MR images show a nondisplaced fracture (arrows) of the acetabulum, surrounded by marrow edema (arrowheads). With transaxial CT scanning **(C)**, the fracture line is evident (arrow). (Courtesy of B.Y. Yang, M.D. Taipei, Taiwan.)

Although displacement of fracture fragments is not uncommon, leading to obvious radiographic abnormalities,[193–197] nondisplaced or occult fractures of the acetabulum present diagnostic difficulties on both the clinical and the radiographic examination,[193] and acetabular fractures in children, although rare, may involve the triradiate cartilage, compounding this difficulty.[198] The complications of acetabular fractures include osteoarthritis of the hip (in cases in which incongruity of the articular surface exists), ischemic necrosis of the femoral head (in cases in which there is an associated posterior dislocation of the hip), heterotopic ossification,[199] and hemorrhage as well as urinary tract, bowel, and peripheral nerve injury (particularly in cases in which there are multiple pelvic fractures).

Fractures of the Femoral Diaphysis

As the femoral shaft represents the strongest portion of the longest and most resilient bone in the human body, it is not surprising that its fracture requires violent force and that associated musculoskeletal injuries, blood loss, and shock are common. Motor vehicle accidents and those involving pedestrians struck by a moving vehicle are frequent causes of such injuries. Femoral shaft fractures may be classified as simple (with transverse, oblique, or spiral components), segmental, or comminuted.[200, 201] Although transverse or oblique fractures of the femoral diaphysis are very common, comminuted fractures with one or more butterfly fragments also are encountered regularly, as are segmental fractures, leading to therapeutic difficulties.[202–207]

Fractures and dislocations in the ipsilateral leg occur in 10 to 20 per cent of femoral diaphysis fractures. Such injuries include hip dislocations, fractures of the neck or supracondylar region of the femur, tibial or patellar fractures, and ligamentous disruptions of the knee. Occult fractures about the hip (e.g., acetabular fractures), posterior dislocations of the hip, and femoral neck fractures may escape detection on initial radiographs confined to the region of the femoral shaft.[208, 209] Occult injuries of the knee occur in 5 to 15 per cent of femoral shaft fractures and, in adolescents, may include physeal injuries in the distal femur or proximal tibia that subsequently may lead to physeal growth arrest.[210]

Complications of femoral shaft fractures include arterial injuries (more common in cases of supracondylar fractures of the femur), malunion (rotational or angular deformity and femoral shortening), refracture (occurring in as many as 9 per cent of cases), fat embolization, and sequelae of associated cranial or visceral injuries (Table 15–1).[209]

Labral Abnormalities

Abnormalities of the acetabular labrum occur both in children and in adults. Those associated with developmental dysplasia of the hip in infants and in young children are discussed later in this chapter.

A spectrum of abnormalities of the acetabular labrum and adjacent bone appears to relate to either acute injury or chronic stress in adolescents and adults. The labral abnormalities may take the form of acute tears, chronic deformation and cyst formation, or degeneration. The osseous abnormalities include cyst formation

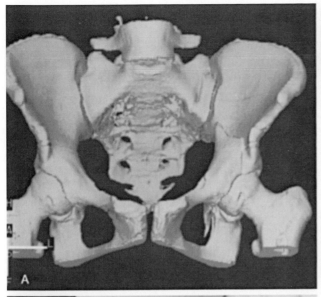
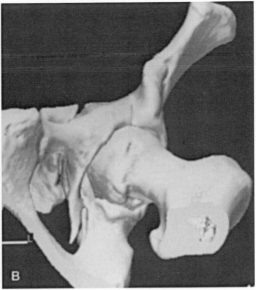
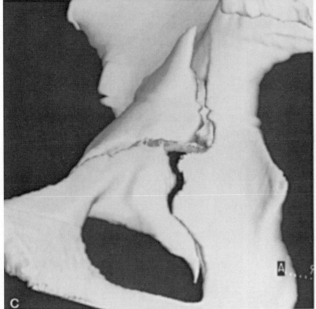

Figure 15–29
Acetabular fractures: CT scanning. Three-dimensional images derived from transaxial CT data show, in vivid fashion, a comminuted fracture of the acetabulum with involvement primarily of the iliopubic column.

Table 15–1. FRACTURES OF THE FEMORAL SHAFT

Site	Characteristics	Complications
Any level	Major violence with associated injuries of femur, tibia, patella, acetabulum, hip, and knee Open or closed Spiral, oblique, or transverse fracture with possible butterfly fragment and comminution	Refracture Peroneal nerve injury owing to skeletal traction Vascular injury (femoral artery) Thrombophlebitis Nonunion (1 per cent of cases), malunion, or delayed union Infection Fat embolization (approximately 10 per cent of cases)
Proximal	Associated with osteoporosis and Paget's disease Less common than midshaft fractures Commonly extend into subtrochanteric region	Malalignment Nonunion
Middle	Most common site Transverse fracture is most typical	
Distal and supracondylar	Less common than midshaft fractures	Malalignment Arterial injury

or fragmentation. In instances in which bone changes are evident, routine radiography is positive, although differentiation of avulsion fractures of the acetabular margin and accessory ossicles (such as the os acetabulum) may be difficult.[211, 212] In instances in which abnormalities are isolated to the acetabular labrum, other imaging methods (such as arthrography, CT arthrography, and MR imaging) may be necessary. In the following discussion, labral tears and cystic degeneration of the labrum are considered separately, although overlap exists between these two categories of abnormality.

Labral Tears

Although tears of the acetabular labrum occurring in association with irreducible traumatic posterior dislocation of the hip in adults were described in 1957 by Paterson[213] and in 1959 by Dameron,[214] and those occurring with falls in elderly patients were described in 1977 by Altenberg,[215] the report in 1986 by Dorrell and Catterall[216] was the first to emphasize the association of acetabular labral tears in adult patients with developmental dysplasia of the hip. In this report, 12 hips in 11 patients ranging in age from 13 to 47 years were affected, and initial clinical manifestations included local pain and aching. In all patients, radiographic evidence of acetabular dysplasia was evident. Additional radiographic findings included subchondral cysts in the acetabulum and a relatively rapid appearance of osteoarthritis of the hip (Fig. 15–30). Standard arthrography revealed evidence of a labral tear in every patient, manifested as an opacified channel extending into the labrum after the introduction of radiopaque contrast material into the hip. The authors concluded that uncovering of the femoral head in patients with developmental dysplasia of the acetabulum leads to mechanical deformation and subsequent degeneration of the labral tissues. In the same year, Suzuki and coworkers,[217] using

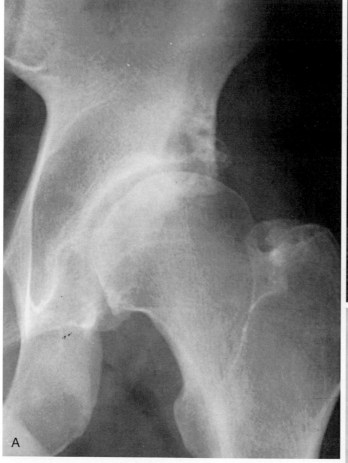

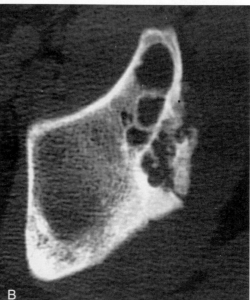

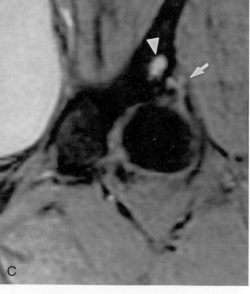

Figure 15–30

Acetabulum and acetabular labrum: Developmental dysplasia associated with intraosseous ganglion cysts and labral tears. Mild flattening of the acetabular roof and uncovering of the femoral head, with subchondral cystic changes in the acetabulum and joint space loss, are evident in the routine radiograph **(A)**. A transaxial CT scan **(B)** documents the extent of the acetabular cysts. A coronal MPGR (TR/TE, 650/15; flip angle, 25 degrees) MR image **(C)** reveals high signal intensity in the ganglion cyst (arrowhead) of the acetabulum and in a labral tear (arrow).

hip arthroscopy, identified rupture of the posterior or posterosuperior portion of the acetabular labrum in five adolescents and young adults who had hip pain and no evidence of hip dysplasia or arthrographic abnormalities.

In 1988, Ikeda and associates[218] described arthroscopically evident tears involving mainly the posterosuperior portion of the acetabular labrum in seven adolescents or young adults whose routine radiographs were normal. A history of developmental dysplasia of the hip was apparent in only one of these patients. Pain, especially during physical activity and on passive flexion and medial rotation of the hip, was a constant clinical manifestation. Arthrography in some patients showed abnormal shape of the acetabular labrum, characterized by enlargement and a rounded contour, but the actual tears were not opacified. In 1991, Klaue and associates[219] described an *acetabular rim syndrome* occurring mainly in young adults that was associated with growing pain and locking of the hip. Routine radiography in many cases showed subtle or obvious findings of acetabular dysplasia. In some patients, conventional arthrography or computed arthrotomography revealed hypertrophy, displacement, or truncation of the acetabular labrum but no evidence of labral tears. In 6 of 29 cases, CT showed cysts (or ganglia) in the periacetabular soft tissues or intraosseous cysts (or ganglia) in the acetabular roof. At surgery, in all cases, a tear of the acetabular labrum was apparent, involving the anterosuperior quadrant of the acetabular rim and resembling a bucket-handle tear of a meniscus in the knee. The authors speculated that in cases of acetabular dysplasia, abnormal forces generated in the acetabular rim lead to degenerative abnormalities of the bone, labrum, and adjacent soft tissues. They postulated further that cyst formation within the limbus (i.e., labrum) is analogous to cystic degeneration of a knee meniscus.

Cystic Degeneration of the Labrum and Ganglion Cysts

The concept of cystic deformation of the acetabular labrum, as described by Klaue and collaborators,[219] had been identified earlier in reports by Ueo and Hamabuchi[220] in 1984 and Matsui and colleagues[221] in 1988, and the association of acetabular ganglia and adjacent soft tissue ganglia had been reported by McBeath and Neidhart[222] in 1976 and by Lagier and associates[223] in 1984. Ueo and Hamabuchi[220] reported two adult patients with developmental dysplasia of the acetabulum and chronic hip pain who revealed a deformed cartilaginous labrum due to ganglion cyst formation; and in the report of Matsui and coworkers,[221] a similar lesion was detected in a single young adult. Arthrography in all three patients in these two reports revealed an enlarged and deformed acetabular labrum.

Haller and coworkers[224] and Silver and associates[225] have described seven and three adult patients, respectively, with labral tears, acetabular dysplasia, osteoarthritis of the hip, acetabular ganglion cysts, or para-acetabular soft tissue ganglia, or combinations of these findings. In both reports, gas adjacent to and within the acetabulum represented a diagnostic clue that was evident on routine radiographs and CT. In two patients reported by Haller and collaborators,[224] spin echo MR images showed the soft tissue ganglion cysts adjacent to the labrum; they appeared as well-defined masses of low signal intensity on T1-weighted spin echo MR images and of high signal intensity on T2-weighted spin echo MR images. Haller and associates[224] indicated possible pathogeneses of these ganglia: abnormal pressure on the lateral portion of the acetabulum that leads to the formation of an intraosseous ganglion cyst, which breaks through the outer edge of the bone, creating a soft tissue ganglion; or elevated intra-articular pressure, which forces synovial fluid through a labral tear and, subsequently, into the soft tissues, producing a ganglion cyst.

The data in all of these reports of acetabular labral tears and adjacent ganglia generate a number of important observations (Figs. 15–31, 15–32, and 15–33):

1. Tears of the acetabular labrum occur not only in infants but also in young adults and, rarely, in elderly persons.

2. In adults, these labral tears may or may not be associated with long-standing dysplastic changes of the acetabulum.

3. Ganglion cysts in the acetabulum or adjacent to the acetabular labrum, or in both locations, may be associated with dysplastic acetabuli, with labral tears, or with both findings.

4. Routine radiography may show gas within the osseous and para-articular ganglion cysts.

5. Opacification of the labral tears may be seen during hip arthrography or computed arthrotomography.

6. MR imaging and CT scanning are effective techniques for the detection of the ganglion cysts.

7. A number of unrelated disorders can lead to clinical manifestations affecting the acetabular rim (Table 15–2.)

The role of MR imaging in the assessment of the torn acetabular labrum is not clear. Indeed, the relative value of MR imaging when compared to other techniques such as CT arthrography and arthroscopy[76, 395] in this assessment is not known, nor is it clear whether or not MR arthrography is required.[227, 396] To clarify these issues, Hodler and associates[226] studied 12 cadaveric hip joints (derived from patients who were elderly at the time of death) using T1-weighted spin echo and three-dimensional spoiled GRASS (gradient recalled acquisition in the steady state [SPGR]) MR imaging sequences obtained both before and after intra-articular injection of gadolinium contrast material. The imaging findings

Table 15–2. ACETABULAR RIM SYNDROME

Tears or cystic degeneration, or both, of the acetabular labrum
Para-acetabular ganglion cysts
Hydroxyapatite crystal deposition
Avulsion fractures
Os acetabuli

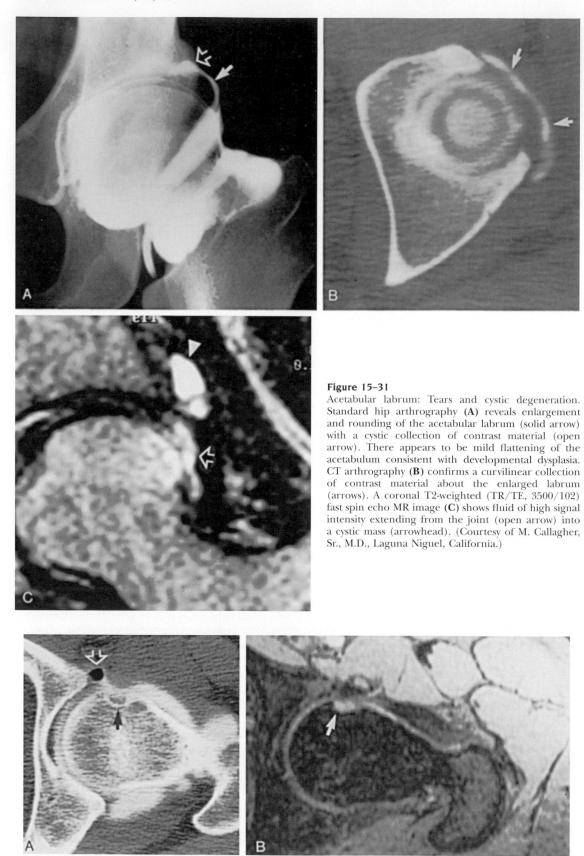

Figure 15–31
Acetabular labrum: Tears and cystic degeneration. Standard hip arthrography **(A)** reveals enlargement and rounding of the acetabular labrum (solid arrow) with a cystic collection of contrast material (open arrow). There appears to be mild flattening of the acetabulum consistent with developmental dysplasia. CT arthrography **(B)** confirms a curvilinear collection of contrast material about the enlarged labrum (arrows). A coronal T2-weighted (TR/TE, 3500/102) fast spin echo MR image **(C)** shows fluid of high signal intensity extending from the joint (open arrow) into a cystic mass (arrowhead). (Courtesy of M. Callagher, Sr., M.D., Laguna Niguel, California.)

Figure 15–32
Acetabular labrum: Tears and cystic degeneration. In this 23 year old woman, a transaxial CT arthrographic image (obtained by injection of radiopaque contrast material only) **(A)** shows a cystic lesion containing gas (open arrow) and subtle erosion (solid arrow) of the anterior surface of the femoral head. A transaxial 3DFT gradient recalled acquisition in the steady state (GRASS) MR image (TR/TE, 60/11; flip angle, 10 degrees) **(B)** shows the site of bone erosion (solid arrow) with adjacent high signal intensity. (Courtesy of S. K. Brahme, M.D., La Jolla, California.)

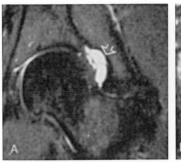
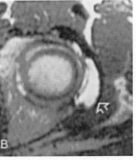

Figure 15-33

Acetabular labrum: Tears and cystic degeneration. In a 39 year old woman, a coronal STIR MR image (TR/TE, 4000/17; inversion time, 150 msec) **(A)** shows a cystic collection of high signal intensity (open arrow) within the labrum. A transaxial T2-weighted (TR/TE, 2100/70) spin echo MR image **(B)** reveals the posterolateral location of the cystic lesion (open arrow). (Courtesy of S. K. Brahme, M.D., La Jolla, California.)

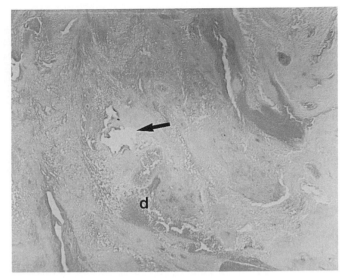

Figure 15-35

Acetabular labrum: Intralabral degeneration. A photomicrograph (H&E stain, ×40) shows extensive degeneration (d) within the substance of the labrum. Some areas with vacuolation and focal cavitation are evident (arrow). (Reproduced with permission from Hodler J, et al: AJR *165*:887, 1995. Copyright 1995, American Roentgen Ray Society.)

were correlated with the results of histologic analysis. Delineation of the labrum from the adjacent joint capsule with MR imaging was far easier on arthrographic images than on standard images (Fig. 15-34). Intralabral eosinophilic, mucoid, or vacuolar degeneration was observed commonly with histologic assessment (Fig. 15-35), and such degeneration was associated with regions of increased signal intensity on MR images (Fig. 15-36). Increased signal intensity at the base of the labrum also was frequent (see Fig. 15-36) and was correlated with histologically evident cartilage degeneration (Fig. 15-37), the presence of fissures at the transitional zone between the fibrocartilage of the labrum and the subchondral bone, or partial detachment of the labrum from the bone (Fig. 15-38). Gross detachment of the labrum was rarely observed on the MR images (Fig. 15-39). The authors concluded that delineation of the acetabular labral complex (and its abnormalities) is improved when intra-articular administration of a gadolinium compound is used as an adjunct to the MR imaging examination.

A similar conclusion was reached by Czerny and co-workers[227] in a study of 56 patients with chronic hip pain and a strong clinical suspicion of labral pathology. These investigators used an extensive classification system to categorize the MR imaging features of labral abnormality (Fig. 15-40). When findings on three-dimensional gradient echo images obtained both before and after intra-articular gadolinium contrast agent administration were compared and were correlated with surgical observations available in almost 50 per cent of

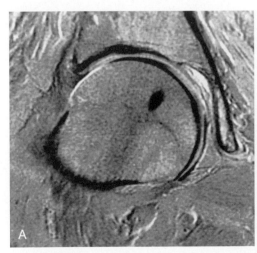
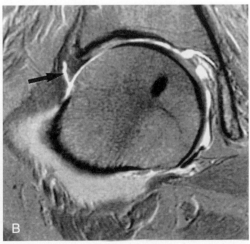

Figure 15-34

Acetabular labrum: Normal appearance with MR imaging and MR arthrography. A normal recess exists between the labrum and the joint capsule. With standard MR imaging, in this case a coronal T1-weighted (TR/TE, 600/15) spin echo MR image **(A),** the recess may be collapsed, making difficult the discrimination of the labrum from the capsular tissue. With gadolinium contrast agent injected in the joint, the recess (arrow) may be identified, as in this coronal T1-weighted (TR/TE, 600/15) spin echo MR image **(B).** (Reproduced with permission from Hodler J, et al: AJR *165*:887, 1995. Copyright 1995, American Roentgen Ray Society.)

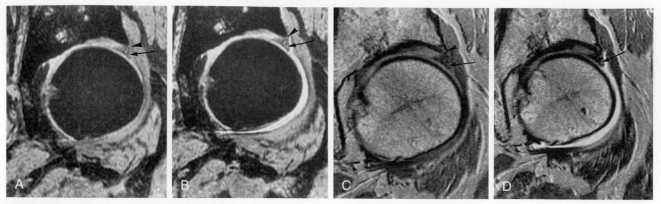

Figure 15–36

Acetabular labrum: Intralabral degeneration. Labral degeneration generally is delineated on MR images as areas of increased signal intensity. These areas are present in all sequences (arrows). An increase in signal intensity at the base of the labrum often correlates with histologically evident fissures (arrowheads), seen as an area of surface irregularity at the interface of the labral fibrocartilage and subchondral bone.

A Coronal fat-suppressed spoiled GRASS (SPGR) (TR/TE, 60/10; flip angle, 30 degrees) MR image.

B Coronal SPGR MR arthrogram (with a gadolinium contrast agent) at the same level as in **A** and with the same imaging parameters.

C Coronal T1-weighted (TR/TE, 600/15) spin echo MR image.

D Coronal T1-weighted spin echo MR arthrogram (with a gadolinium contrast agent) at the same level and with the same imaging parameters as in **C**.

(Reproduced with permission from Hodler J, et al: AJR *165*:887, 1995. Copyright 1995, American Roentgen Ray Society.)

the patients, the superiority of the arthrographic studies in the detection and characterization of labral abnormalities was evident (Figs. 15–40 and 15–41).

Although the data derived from these studies support the application of MR arthrography to the analysis of the acetabular labrum, CT arthrography may reveal similar information. Furthermore, standard MR imaging combined with leg traction and intravenous administration of a gadolinium compound has been found to be useful in delineating acetabular labral tears,[397] and in some studies,[228] hip arthroscopy has been shown to be an effective technique in the diagnosis of a variety of intra-articular causes of pain, including labral abnormalities. Arthroscopy has also been used to classify labral tears into several categories, including traumatic, degen-

erative, congenital, and idiopathic.[395] Whichever diagnostic method is chosen, the occurrence of labral alterations in asymptomatic persons, as has been verified in the glenohumeral joint, ultimately may limit the clinical usefulness of the examination.[417]

Synovial Abnormalities

Synovitis

The involvement of the hip in a variety of articular disorders is well known. Systemic diseases, such as rheu-

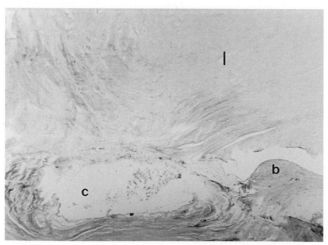

Figure 15–37

Acetabular labrum: Intralabral degeneration. A photomicrograph (H&E, ×40) demonstrates cystic degeneration (c) at the base of the labrum (l). b, Bone. (Reproduced with permission from Hodler J, et al: AJR *165*:887, 1995. Copyright 1995, American Roentgen Ray Society.)

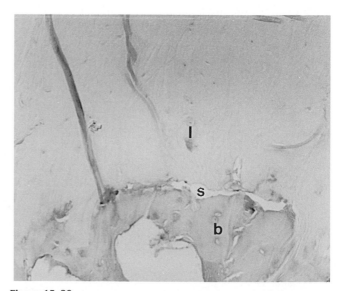

Figure 15–38

Acetabular labrum: Partial labral detachment. A photomicrograph (H&E, ×40) depicts separation (s) of the labrum (l) from the underlying bone (b). (Reproduced with permission from Hodler J, et al: AJR *165*:887, 1995. Copyright 1995, American Roentgen Ray Society.)

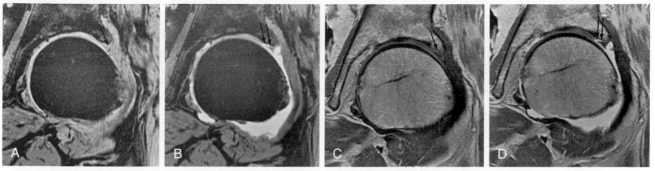

Figure 15–39

Acetabular labrum: Partial labral detachment. Increased signal intensity at the base of the labrum (single arrows) in standard MR images (**A, C**) suggests labral detachment, but the extent of the detachment (double arrows) is shown more accurately with MR arthrography employing a gadolinium compound (**B, D**).

  A Coronal fat-suppressed spoiled GRASS (SPGR) (TR/TE, 60/10; flip angle, 30 degrees) MR image.
  B Coronal SPGR MR arthrogram at the same level and with the same parameters as in **A**.
  C Coronal T1-weighted (TR/TE, 600/15) spin echo MR image.
  D Coronal T1-weighted spin echo MR arthrogram at the same level and with the same parameters as in **C**.
  (Reproduced with permission from Hodler J, et al: AJR *165*:887, 1995. Copyright 1995, American Roentgen Ray Society.)

matoid arthritis and the seronegative spondyloarthropathies, and localized processes, such as septic arthritis, pigmented villonodular synovitis, and idiopathic synovial (osteo)chondromatosis, may affect this joint. In some cases, routine radiography allows precise diagnosis, although data provided by clinical assessment, other imaging methods, and, occasionally, joint aspiration or examination of synovial tissue may be required.

Contrast opacification of the hip may allow more accurate diagnosis of some of these articular disorders (Fig. 15–42). In idiopathic synovial (osteo)chondromatosis or pigmented villonodular synovitis, the extent of synovial and capsular abnormality can be determined arthrographically.[229, 230] This is important not only in outlining the severity of the disorder but also in establishing the correct diagnosis when plain films are not conclusive. In patients with septic arthritis, hip arthrography provides a technique for aspiration and culture and also a means for evaluating cartilaginous, osseous, and synovial abnormalities. In infants and young children, this method allows differentiation of septic arthritis with dislocation of the femoral head from osteomyelitis with epiphyseal separation. Hip arthrography also provides information regarding the origin and nature of intra-articular and para-articular radiodense areas.

As in other regions of the body, bone scintigraphy can be used to assess articular disease in the hip. The examination is sensitive but lacks specificity. Its role includes confirmation of the presence of an abnormality when results of conventional radiography are negative, demonstration of the anatomic distribution of the disease, and evaluation of the activity of the process.[231] Bone scintigraphy also allows detection of osseous abnormalities, such as stress fractures and ischemic necrosis, that can produce clinical manifestations simulating those of arthritis.

Ultrasonography represents a useful technique for the detection of intra-articular fluid (Fig. 15–43), especially in children, and therefore can be applied to the assessment of such conditions as transient synovitis.

CT scanning may be used to assess the extent of bone

involvement in a variety of diseases that involve the synovial membrane (Fig. 15–44).

MR imaging provides information regarding the extent of synovial disease in the hip that is not apparent on routine radiographs (Fig. 15–45). Typical examples of such disease include septic arthritis (Fig. 15–46), pigmented villonodular synovitis,[232] and idiopathic synovial (osteo)chondromatosis.[233] Abnormal collections of joint fluid also may be detected.[234] As in other locations, such as the knee, however, the differentiation of synovial inflammatory tissue and a joint effusion using MR imaging may require the intravenous administration of gadolinium compounds. As the assessment of the arthritic hip in the immature skeleton often necessitates analysis of the developing chondroepiphysis, MR imaging is superior to routine radiography.[49, 235]

Synovial Cysts

With any process of the hip that leads to elevation of intra-articular pressure, escape of fluid from the joint through a number of anatomic pathways serves to decompress the joint. Typically, the fluid passes into a surrounding synovial sac which, with distention, can be seen or palpated. These synovial cysts also can be assessed with imaging methods, including ultrasonography, CT, arthrography, computed arthrotomography, and MR imaging. Of all the potential locations of synovial cysts about the hip, the iliopsoas bursa deserves special emphasis.

Iliopsoas Bursal Distention

Opacification of the iliopsoas bursa may be noted during hip arthrography. Although this is apparent in 15 per cent of normal hips,[236] communication of the hip and iliopsoas bursa in the presence of intra-articular diseases such as osteoarthritis, rheumatoid arthritis, pigmented villonodular synovitis, infection, calcium pyrophosphate dihydrate crystal deposition disease, and idiopathic synovial (osteo)chondromatosis may lead to

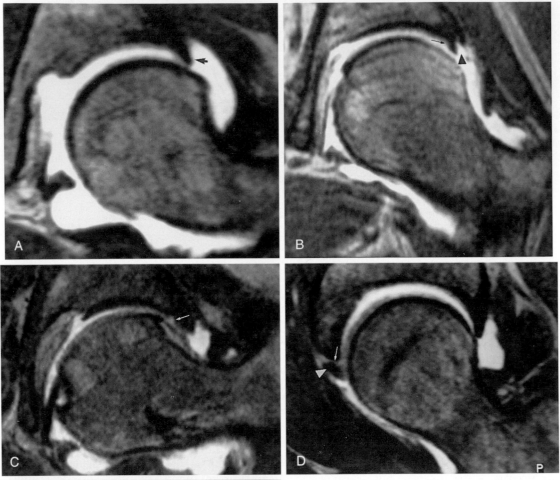

Figure 15–40

Acetabular labrum: Patterns of tear and detachment. Three-dimensional gradient echo (TR/TE, 30/9; flip angle, 45 degrees) MR images obtained after the intra-articular administration of a gadolinium compound show normal appearance of labrum **(A)** and various stages of labral abnormalities **(B–F).** (See Czerny C, et al: Radiology 200:225, 1996.)

A Normal labrum, coronal oblique plane. The labrum (arrow) is clearly seen, is triangular in shape and smooth, and contains no internal areas of higher signal intensity. No sulcus or notch is evident between the labrum and the acetabulum.

B Stage IA abnormality, coronal oblique plane. The labrum, smaller than in **A,** contains a small focus (arrow) of intermediate signal intensity, consistent with minimal degeneration. Note the labral recess (arrowhead).

C Stage IIB abnormality, coronal oblique plane. The labrum is thickened, with a collection of contrast material in the labrum consistent with a tear (arrow). The labral recess is small.

D Stage IIIA abnormality, sagittal oblique plane. A linear collection of contrast material (arrow) separates the labrum (arrowhead) from the anterior portion of the acetabulum, indicating a labral detachment, or avulsion.

E Stage IIIB abnormality, coronal oblique plane. The labrum (arrowhead) is thickened with centrally located abnormalities of signal intensity, and the collection of contrast agent (arrow) indicates that the labrum is detached from the acetabulum.

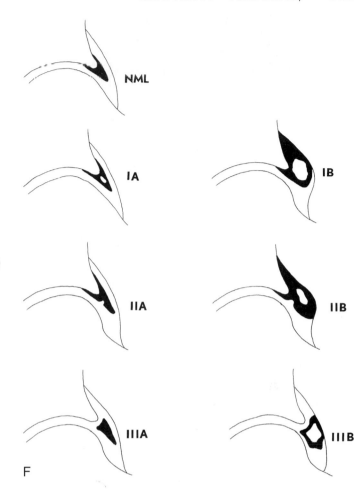

Figure 15–40 *Continued*
F Staging system. NML, Normal.
(Courtesy of C. Czerny, M.D., and J. Kramer, M.D., Vienna, Austria.)

bursal enlargement, producing a mass in the ilioinguinal region that may simulate a hernia and cause obstruction of the femoral vein.[237, 238]

The iliopsoas bursa (also termed the iliopectineal, iliofemoral, iliac, or subpsoas bursa) is the most important of the 15 or more synovium-lined bursae that have been described about the hip. Measuring approximately 3 to 7 cm long and 2 to 4 cm wide and extending from the inguinal ligament to the lesser trochanter of the femur, the iliopsoas bursa is present in about 98 per cent of adults. It communicates with the hip joint via an aperture ranging in diameter from 1 mm to 3 cm, and enlargement of this channel in the 15 per cent of normal adults who possess this aperture or creation of a communicating pathway in those adults who do not is an expected consequence of virtually any disease process of the hip that leads to an elevation of intra-articular pressure. This phenomenon is somewhat less frequent in children, owing to a decreased prevalence of normal communication between the iliopsoas bursa and the hip.

The iliopsoas bursa is bounded anteriorly by the iliopsoas muscle and posteriorly by the pectineal eminence and the thin portion of the capsule of the hip joint.[239] Its lateral border is the iliofemoral ligament and its medial border is the cotyloid ligament; its superior border is the inguinal ligament and its inferior border is the pubofemoral ligament.[239] When distended, a painless or painful soft tissue mass is created, possibly accompanied by shortening of the stride related to avoidance of hyperextension, flexion of the hip and knee with external rotation of the thigh, weakness of the extremity, and point tenderness inferior to the inguinal ligament and 2 cm lateral to the femoral artery. The mass itself may compress the adjacent neurovascular structures, rarely causing secondary venous obstruction with distal edema, or displace pelvic organs, or it may become secondarily infected or traumatized or induce an abducted gait. In the absence of a clear-cut history of arthritis, the patient with an enlarged iliopsoas bursa initially may be evaluated by a general surgeon, who easily may misinterpret the mass and its associated symptoms and signs as evidence of an inguinal hernia, aneurysm of the femoral artery, undescended testicle, varices, adenopathy, or solid neoplasm. Arteriographic evaluation may lead to inadvertent puncture of the bursa or, at the time of operation, the enlarged synovium-lined structure may present a puzzle to the surgeon, who was anticipating some other disease process.[240] Accurate preoperative diagnosis is provided by arthrography of the hip (which may be combined with CT), direct opacification of the bursa, ultrasonography, MR imaging, or CT alone (Fig. 15–47).[239, 241–244]

With regard to the imaging strategy that is used to evaluate suspected iliopsoas bursal distention or other synovial cysts about the hip, ultrasonography should be

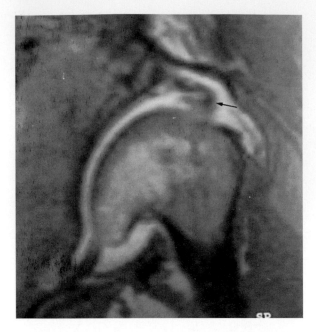

Figure 15–41
Acetabular labrum: Developmental dysplasia associated with labral abnormalities. After the intra-articular injection of a gadolinium compound, a coronal MR image shows developmental dysplasia of the hip and a displaced and deformed acetabular labrum (arrow) containing abnormal internal signal intensity. (Courtesy of J. Kramer, M.D., Vienna, Austria.)

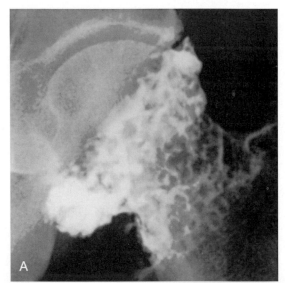

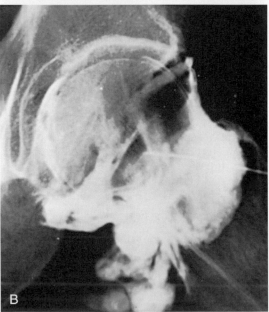

Figure 15–42
Synovial disorders: Arthrography.

A Idiopathic synovial (osteo)chondromatosis. Arthrography reveals multiple filling defects within the opacified hip joint that, at surgery, represented noncalcified cartilaginous bodies. (Courtesy of G. Greenway, M.D., Dallas, Texas.)

B Pigmented villonodular synovitis. Arthrography reveals an enlarged and irregular joint cavity with small, medial collections or pools of contrast material.

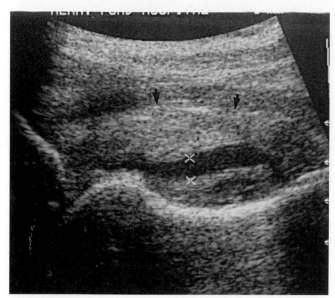

Figure 15–43
Synovial disorders: Ultrasonography. A sonogram of the hip in the sagittal plane demonstrates anechoic fluid (x markers) surrounded by hyperechoic synovial proliferative tissue (arrows) anterior to the proximal portion of the femur. (Courtesy of M. van Holsbeeck, M.D. Detroit, Michigan, and J. Jacobson, M.D., San Diego, California.)

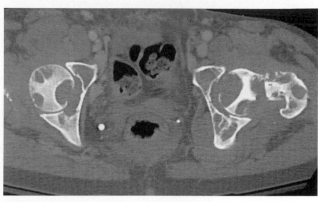

Figure 15–44
Synovial disorders: CT scanning. In a patient with chronic renal disease being maintained on hemodialysis, amyloidosis has led to destructive lesions about both hips, as shown in this transaxial image. A pathologic fracture of the femoral neck is evident on the left side. (Courtesy of E. Pike, M.D., T. Pope, M.D., and L. Rogers, M.D., Winston-Salem, North Carolina.)

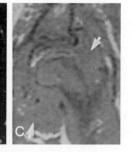

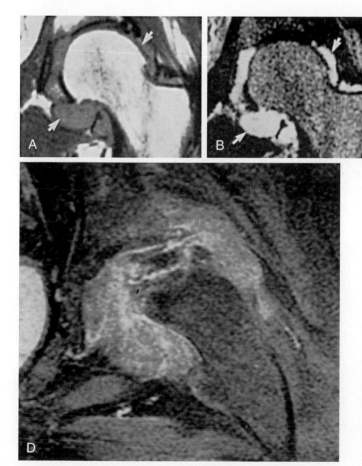

Figure 15–45
Synovial disorders: MR imaging.

A, B Idiopathic synovial (osteo)chondromatosis. Coronal proton density–weighted (TR/TE, 2000/20) **(A)** and T2-weighted (TR/TE, 2000/80) **(B)** spin echo MR images show joint distention (arrows) in this 37 year old man with an 8 month history of hip pain. In **A,** the intra-articular process is of low signal intensity; in **B,** it is of high signal intensity. The MR imaging findings simulate those of a joint effusion.

C Septic arthritis. In this child with hematogenous osteomyelitis of the femur and septic arthritis of the hip, a coronal T1-weighted (TR/TE, 500/30) spin echo MR image shows destruction of the femoral capital epiphysis and acetabulum and a mass (arrows) of low signal intensity.

(Courtesy of T. Mattsson, M.D., Riyadh, Saudi Arabia.)

D Septic arthritis. In a coronal SPGR MR image (TR/TE, 240/4; flip angle, 70 degrees), obtained immediately after the intravenous injection of a gadolinium compound, note massive distention of the hip joint with lateral displacement and fragmentation of the femoral head. (Courtesy of S.K. Brahme, M.D., La Jolla, California.)

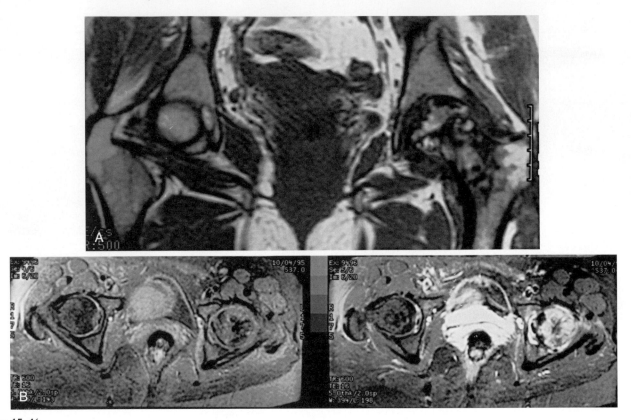

Figure 15–46
Septic arthritis: MR imaging.

A A coronal T1-weighted (TR/TE, 500/10) spin echo MR image shows distention of the left hip joint and abnormal signal intensity in the femoral epiphysis and metaphysis. The signal intensity of the fat in the acetabular fossa is altered.

B Transaxial T1-weighted (TR/TE, 600/16) spin echo MR images obtained with fat suppression alone (left) and with fat suppression after the intravenous administration of a gadolinium compound (right) show findings of septic arthritis and osteomyelitis. In the right image, note enhancement of signal intensity in the femoral head, acetabulum, and joint.

(Courtesy of D. Salonen, M.D., Toronto, Ontario, Canada.)

performed after conventional radiography in the setting of a probable groin mass or other suggestive clinical manifestations. If a nonpulsatile fluid collection without Doppler sonographic evidence of flow is demonstrated, this technique then can be used for diagnostic aspiration of its contents. Fluid analysis should distinguish a

synovial cyst or iliopsoas bursitis from a lymphocele, abscess, or hematoma. Subsequent injection of contrast material into the bursa or cyst may opacify the hip joint, confirming the diagnosis; if not, hip arthrography, CT, or MR imaging may be desirable for delineation of potential articular communication if surgery is being

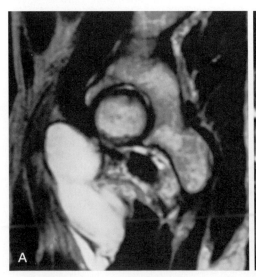

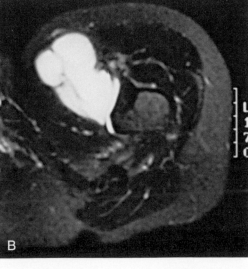

Figure 15–47
Iliopsoas bursal distention: MR imaging.

A A sagittal fast spin echo MR image (TR/TE, 5200/91) shows a fluid-filled cystic mass of high signal intensity anterior to the hip joint.

B A transaxial fat-suppressed fast spin echo MR image (TR/TE, 4350/88) reveals the distended iliopsoas bursa.

(Courtesy of S.K. Brahme, M.D., La Jolla, California.)

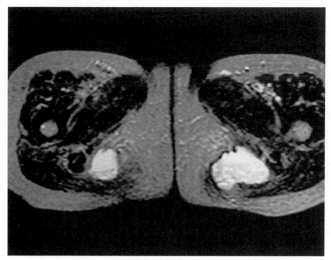

Figure 15-48
Trochanteric bursitis: MR imaging. A transaxial T2-weighted (TR/TE, 1500/90) spin echo MR image shows evidence of bilateral trochanteric bursitis. (Courtesy of J. Dillard, M.D., San Diego, California.)

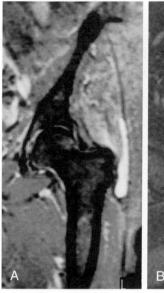
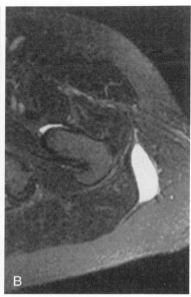

Figure 15-49
Trochanteric and perigluteal bursitis: MR imaging. Several bursae exist about the greater trochanter and gluteal muscles. Inflammation and fluid accumulation lead to increased signal intensity on gradient echo (**A**) and fat-suppressed fast spin echo (TR/TE, 4600/80) (**B**) MR images. (**A,** Courtesy of E. Bosch, M.D., Santiago, Chile; **B,** courtesy of D. Salonen, M.D., Toronto, Ontario, Canada.)

contemplated. The results of conservative management can be followed noninvasively with either ultrasonography or CT. In general, arteriography and lymphangiography have no place in the present-day diagnosis of suspected disease of synovial origin about the hip joint.

Iliopsoas Bursitis

The synovium lining the iliopsoas bursa can be involved in a variety of processes, including rheumatoid arthritis and infection. Typically, such involvement is associated with abnormality in the adjacent hip, particularly when communication between the two structures is evident. As in diseases of the subacromial-subdeltoid, prepatellar, and olecranon bursae, isolated involvement of the iliopsoas bursa may occur, however.[245] CT, MR imaging, and ultrasonography are the best techniques for further evaluation of an inflamed and distended iliopsoas bursa.[246]

Other Types of Bursitis

Inflammation of the ischial bursa may result from acute injury or chronic stress. Clinical manifestations resemble those associated with injury to the hamstring muscles. Trochanteric bursitis leads to tenderness about the greater trochanter of the femur, which may be accentuated by adduction and external rotation of the hip. Such bursitis may relate to strenuous activity, irritation caused by the adjacent iliotibial tract, and foot deformities. MR imaging can be used to assess these types of bursitis (Figs. 15-48, 15-49, and 15-50).

Infectious involvement of bursae about the hip also

Figure 15-50
Trochanteric bursitis: MR imaging. Coronal T1-weighted spin echo (**A**) and STIR (**B**) MR images show an inflamed bursa (arrows) and reactive intraosseous edema (arrowheads). (Courtesy of J. Rivera, M.D., Oklahoma City, Oklahoma.)

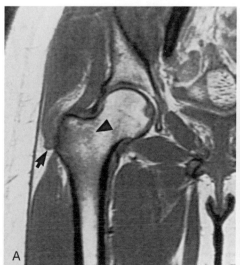
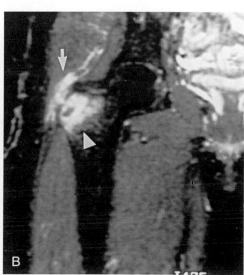

may be encountered. Tuberculosis is an important cause of inflammation of the trochanteric, ischial, and subgluteal bursae (Figs. 15–51 and 15–52).

Intra-Articular Osteocartilaginous Bodies

As in other anatomic locations, intra-articular osteocartilaginous bodies in the hip may result from any process that leads to disintegration of the articular surface. Such processes include osteoarthritis, crystal deposition diseases, neuropathic osteoarthropathy, and injury (e.g., fracture-dislocation of the hip). If the bodies become free in the articular space, they may migrate to distant locations, including the region of the acetabular fossa. In addition to routine radiography, conventional tomography, CT scanning, CT arthrography, MR imaging, or MR arthrography may be used to detect intra-articular osteocartilaginous bodies in the hip (Fig. 15–53).

Cartilage Abnormalities

Cartilage Degeneration

The evaluation of cartilage loss in the hip joint with imaging methods frequently relies on routine radiography. Although characteristic patterns of such loss allow accurate diagnosis of a number of conditions that affect

the hip, the detection of small degrees of cartilage destruction in this location is not possible with routine radiography. Indeed, damage to articular cartilage can only be estimated on conventional radiographs related to the presence and distribution of joint space loss and other secondary signs, such as bone sclerosis and osteophytosis. The role of routine radiographs of the hip obtained with the patient standing is not clear, although this technique has been used extensively to evaluate cartilage loss in the knee. Ultrasonography is not effective as a means of detecting cartilage damage in the hip. Arthrotomographic methods may provide some information regarding this detection, but these methods generally are considered insensitive.

Although the value of MR imaging in assessing cartilage lesions in the knee has been investigated thoroughly (see Chapter 16), the evaluation of similar lesions in the hip using MR imaging has received little attention. Li and coworkers[247] employed standard spin echo MR images in 10 patients with clinically and radiographically documented osteoarthritis of the hip. From data provided by transaxial and coronal images, these investigators developed a grading system based on the extent of cartilage and bone involvement. Grade 1 abnormalities were characterized by nonhomogeneity of the high signal intensity in the articular cartilage; grade 2 abnormalities were characterized by such nonhomogeneity and discontinuity of the high signal intensity in

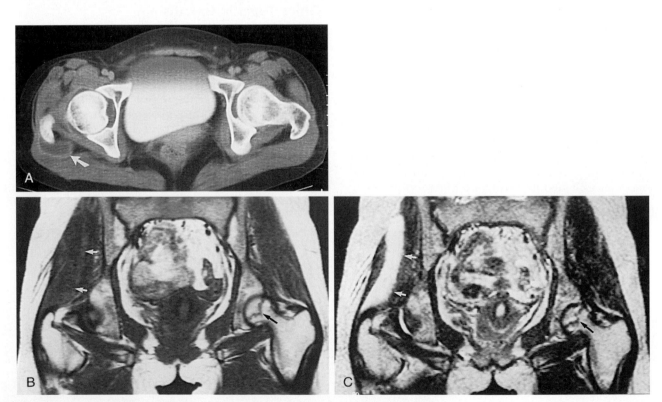

Figure 15–51

Tuberculosis bursitis: Trochanteric bursa (MR imaging). This 22 year old woman developed pain and swelling about the greater trochanter on the right. Routine radiographs (not shown) were normal.

    A After intravenous administration of a contrast agent, transaxial CT reveals a cystic mass with an enhancing thin wall (arrow).

    B A coronal T1-weighted (TR/TE, 450/17) spin echo MR image shows the extent of the fluid-filled mass (white arrows). Osteonecrosis of the left femoral head also is evident (black arrow).

    C On a coronal T2-weighted (TR/TE, 1800/80) spin echo MR image, note high signal intensity within the inflamed bursa (white arrows), a joint effusion in the right hip, absence of osteomyelitis, and osteonecrosis of the left femoral head (black arrow).

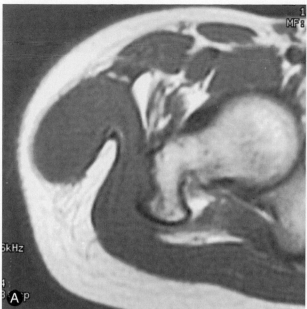

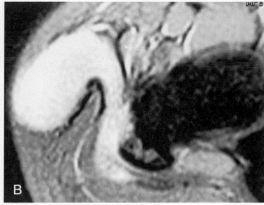

Figure 15–52

Tuberculous bursitis: Trochanteric bursa (MR imaging). Transaxial T1-weighted (TR/TE, 400/17) spin echo **(A)** and MPGR (TR/TE, 600/20; flip angle, 25 degrees) **(B)** MR images show tuberculous involvement of the trochanteric bursa with subjacent bone erosion. (Courtesy of S. Jaovisidha, M.D., Bangkok, Thailand.)

the articular cartilage, blurring of the adjacent trabeculae, and overall loss of signal intensity in the marrow of the femoral head and neck; grade 3 alterations included those of grade 2 and, in addition, irregularities of the cortical outlines of the femoral head and acetabulum, a zone of intermediate signal intensity between the acetabulum and the femoral head, and regions of intermediate signal intensity surrounded by a rim of low signal intensity in the femoral head; and grade 4 abnormalities represented all of the previous changes plus deformity of the femoral head. These authors concluded that a grading system based on MR imaging findings was more useful than one based on routine radiographic findings in cases of mild to moderate osteoarthritis of the hip.

Although these results suggest a role for MR imaging in the detection of cartilage loss in the hip, the deficiencies of standard MR imaging in the analysis of chondral lesions in the knee has been well documented (see Chapter 16). Furthermore, the results of an additional study by Hodler and associates[248] emphasized the deficiencies of one particular MR imaging sequence in the detection of cartilage lesions in the acetabulum and femoral head (Fig. 15–54). In this investigation, femoral heads and acetabula derived from 10 cadavers were imaged with a T1-weighted fat-suppressed (ChemSat) spin echo MR imaging sequence in both the coronal and sagittal planes (using a send-receive extremity coil, a 12 cm field of view, and two excitations), and the thickness of the articular cartilage in numerous locations in the femoral head and acetabulum as measured by MR images was compared with that detected on gross inspection of the specimens. The highest correlation between the two measurement methods was found for femoral cartilage, particularly in regions where the femoral cartilage was applied directly to acetabular cartilage. Significant inconsistencies were noted in the measurements derived from inspection and from MR imaging, however, leading the authors to conclude that fat-suppression spin echo MR images were not suffi-

ciently accurate to be of clinical value (Fig. 15–55). As is indicated in the section on cartilage lesions in the knee (see Chapter 16), a number of newer MR imaging sequences and methods may hold more promise for the detection of chondral loss.

In more advanced cases of arthritis, standard MR imaging does allow assessment of cartilage and subchondral bone abnormalities (Figs. 15–56 and 15–57).

Idiopathic Chondrolysis

Chondrolysis is a well recognized complication of slipped capital femoral epiphysis. The reports of Jones in 1971[249] and Moule and Golding in 1974[250] focused attention on the occurrence of chondrolysis of the hip joint in adolescent girls, particularly blacks, who did not have slipped capital femoral epiphyses. Subsequent investigators confirmed the presence of this entity, noting its occasional appearance not only in black female adolescents but also in men, Hispanics, other whites, and Native Americans and in persons over the age of 20 years.[251–257] Monoarticular disease of the hip is typical, and clinical findings include pain, stiffness, restriction of motion, and the absence of a history of trauma. Radiographs outline periarticular osteoporosis, joint space narrowing that usually is diffuse or maximal on the weight-bearing surface, and irregularity and erosion of the subchondral bone. In addition, slight enlargement and alteration in the shape of the femoral head, an increase in width and periosteal bone formation of the femoral neck, narrowing of the growth plate, and mild protrusio acetabuli may be evident. The last-mentioned feature is reminiscent of that seen in primary protrusio acetabuli (Otto pelvis), and differentiating between the two conditions may be difficult.[256] Joint aspiration usually confirms the absence of an effusion or of organisms, and arthrography may demonstrate the irregularity and narrowing of the chondral surface (Fig. 15–58). Pathologic examination outlines changes in car-

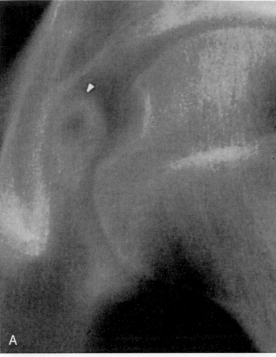

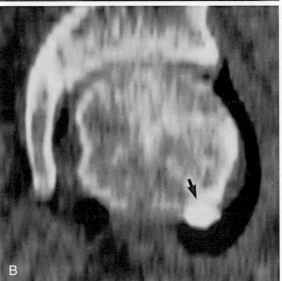

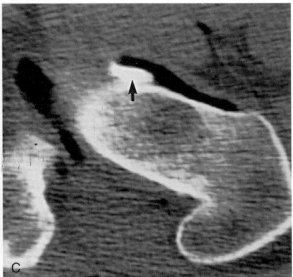

Figure 15–53
Intra-articular osteochondral bodies: Conventional and computed tomography.
A Note an osseous body (arrowhead) in the acetabular fossa.
B, C In a second patient, computed arthrotomography in the coronal (**B**) and transaxial (**C**) planes shows an intra-articular body (arrows).

tilage that are identical to those that occur in chondrolysis complicating slipped capital femoral epiphysis, including replacement of the deep layers of the articular cartilage, thinning of the superficial layers, and absence of widespread synovial inflammation. Some degree of villous formation, nodular lymphoid hyperplasia in the subsynovial areas, and perivascular infiltrates of lymphocytes, plasma cells, and monocytes may be noted. Fibrinoid necrosis and granulomas are not seen. The adjacent bone is osteoporotic, and cystic areas may be filled with synovium. Osteonecrosis also has been reported.[253]

Later stages of the process can be associated with obliteration of the articular space, cysts, osteophytes, and deformity.

Major alternatives in differential diagnosis include juvenile chronic arthritis and infection. Monoarticular involvement of the hip is somewhat unusual in juvenile chronic arthritis, although its clinical and radiologic features can simulate those in idiopathic chondrolysis of the hip. Similarly, infection can lead to an identical radiographic picture, necessitating joint aspiration and culture of the fluid in all suspected cases of chondrolysis. Additional diagnostic considerations are transient osteoporosis of the hip, ischemic necrosis of the femoral head, primary protrusio acetabuli, and pigmented villonodular synovitis.

Bone Abnormalities

Many localized and generalized diseases of bone may involve the acetabulum or proximal portion of the fe-

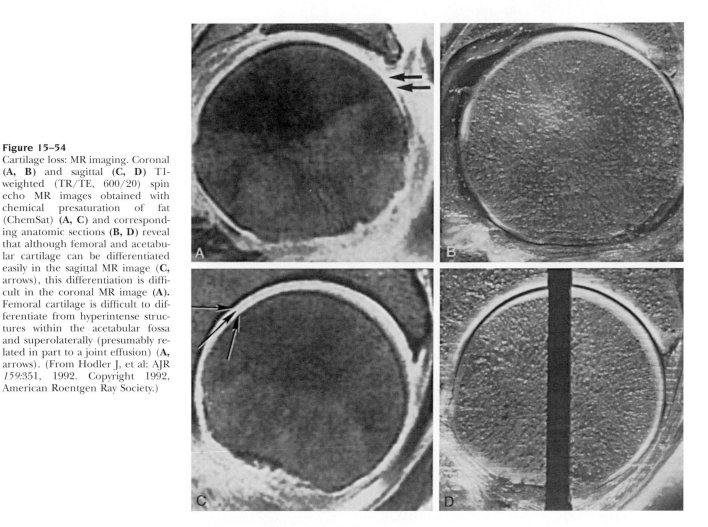

Figure 15–54
Cartilage loss: MR imaging. Coronal **(A, B)** and sagittal **(C, D)** T1-weighted (TR/TE, 600/20) spin echo MR images obtained with chemical presaturation of fat (ChemSat) **(A, C)** and corresponding anatomic sections **(B, D)** reveal that although femoral and acetabular cartilage can be differentiated easily in the sagittal MR image (**C**, arrows), this differentiation is difficult in the coronal MR image (**A**). Femoral cartilage is difficult to differentiate from hyperintense structures within the acetabular fossa and superolaterally (presumably related in part to a joint effusion) (**A**, arrows). (From Hodler J, et al: AJR *159*:351, 1992. Copyright 1992, American Roentgen Ray Society.)

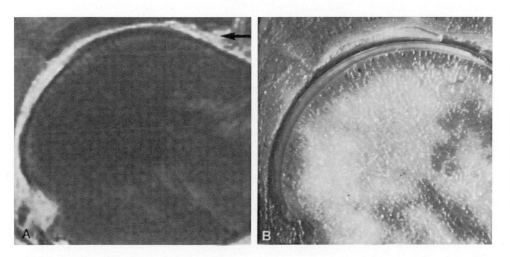

Figure 15–55
Cartilage loss: MR imaging. A coronal T1-weighted (TR/TE, 600/20) spin echo MR image obtained with chemical presaturation of fat (ChemSat) **(A)** and a corresponding anatomic section **(B)** reveal difficulty in differentiation between superolateral femoral cartilage and parts of the labrum (arrow), capsule, and surrounding soft tissue. (From Hodler J, et al: AJR *159*:351, 1992. Copyright 1992, American Roentgen Ray Society.)

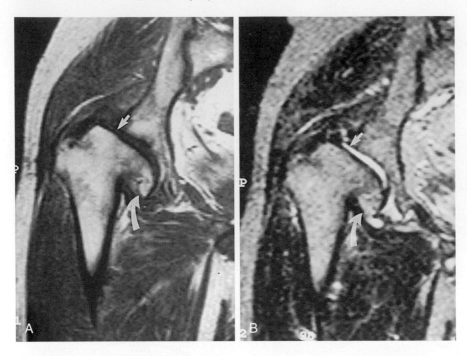

Figure 15–56

Cartilage loss: MR imaging. Legg-Calvé-Perthes disease with secondary osteoarthritis. Coronal T1-weighted (TR/TE, 500/15) **(A)** and T2-weighted (TR/TE, 2000/90) **(B)** spin echo MR images reveal chronic sequelae of Legg-Calvé-Perthes disease in a 35 year old man. Osteophytosis (curved arrows), flattening of the femoral head, and cartilage loss (straight arrows) are evident, the last finding being more evident in **B** owing to the presence of joint fluid of high signal intensity.

mur. Classic examples include Paget's disease, fibrous dysplasia, intraosseous lipoma, and slipped capital femoral epiphysis (Fig. 15–59). Several additional conditions are of importance in any discussion of hip disorders.

Osteonecrosis

The causative factors leading to ischemic necrosis of bone are diverse and include trauma (Fig. 15–60), corticosteroid medications, sickle cell anemia and other hemoglobinopathies, Gaucher's disease, alcoholism, pancreatitis, and radiation; furthermore, in many cases, a specific etiologic factor cannot be identified (idiopathic osteonecrosis). Although the site of osteonecrosis in any patient varies according to its precise cause, the femoral head, femoral condyles, and humeral head commonly are involved. The predilection for involvement of the

femoral head relates to the vulnerability of a blood supply, which includes arteries that extend beneath the capsule of the hip joint.

A desire to identify a sensitive method for detection of osteonecrosis of the femoral head has led to extensive investigation of a number of imaging methods, and the sensitivity of many of these techniques has been found wanting. Routine radiography, conventional tomography, and CT scanning are not reliable in the diagnosis of early osteonecrosis of the femoral head, although the two tomographic methods are useful in defining the extent of bone collapse. Scintigraphy using bone-seeking radiopharmaceutical agents is sensitive to early changes of osteonecrosis, but the scintigraphic findings lack specificity. Single photon emission computed tomography (SPECT) improves the sensitivity but does not improve the specificity of the radionuclide examina-

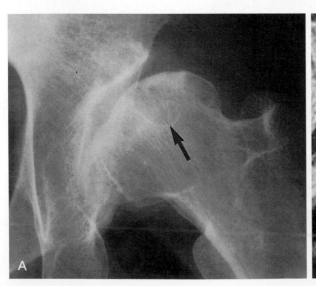

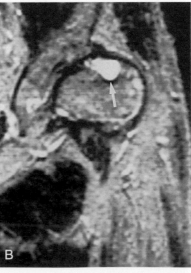

Figure 15–57

Cartilage loss and subchondral bone abnormalities: MR imaging. Developmental dysplasia of the hip with secondary osteoarthritis. In a 32 year old man, routine radiograph **(A)** reveals a dysplastic acetabulum, lateral subluxation and flattening of the femoral head, and subchondral cysts (arrow). In a coronal T2-weighted (TR/TE, 2500/80) spin echo MR image **(B),** the cyst is of high signal intensity (arrow).

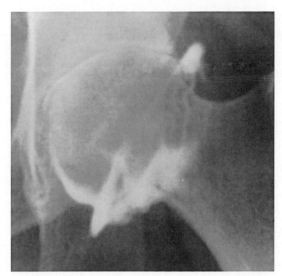

Figure 15–58
Idiopathic chondrolysis of the hip: Arthrography. In this teenage girl with clinical and radiographic manifestations of idiopathic chondrolysis, hip arthrography reveals diffuse loss of acetabular and femoral cartilage.

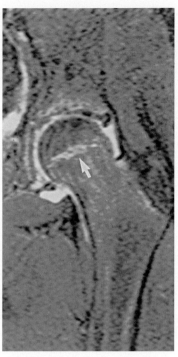

Figure 15–59
Slipped capital femoral epiphysis: MR imaging. A coronal STIR MR image (TR/TE, 2000/30; inversion time, 140 msec) in a 13 year old girl with an acute epiphysiolysis reveals high signal intensity about the physis (arrow) and a joint effusion. (Courtesy of S. Eilenberg, M.D., San Diego, California.)

tion. MR imaging appears best suited to the detection of the early stages of ischemic necrosis of bone (Table 15–3). Although MR imaging abnormalities occur early in the course of osteonecrosis and, in some situations, may be evident within days after an ischemic event, these abnormalities are somewhat variable in their time of occurrence. They depend on alterations of the fat cells in the bone marrow. Ischemic changes first become evident in hematopoietic cells, becoming apparent 6 to 12 hours after the ischemic event, and then are observed in the osteocytes, osteoblasts, and osteoclasts, occurring within 2 days of the ischemic event. Fat cells are more resistant to ischemia, surviving for 2 to 5 days after the insult. Furthermore, initial changes in the fat cells may not lead to an alteration in MR imaging signal characteristics. An inflammatory and hyperemic response in via-

ble tissue adjacent to the devascularized regions produces a reactive interface about the osteonecrotic areas that is associated with increased vascularity, inflammation, granulation tissue, and fibrosis. MR imaging is sensitive to the presence of this reactive interface.

No uniform agreement exists regarding the choice of imaging plane or specific sequence when MR imaging is applied to the evaluation of osteonecrosis of the femoral head. Most authors use and prefer the coronal plane,

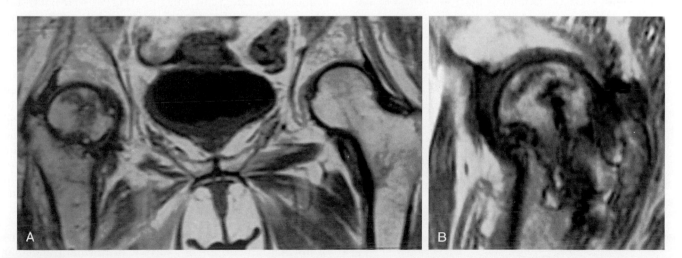

Figure 15–60
Posttraumatic osteonecrosis: MR imaging. T1-weighted (TR/TE, 516/12) coronal (**A**) and sagittal (**B**) spin echo MR images show a subcapital fracture of the femoral neck with resulting osteonecrosis of the right femoral head. Note the serpentine configuration of the area of signal intensity abnormality in the femoral head.

Table 15–3. PROPOSED STAGING SYSTEM FOR OSTEONECROSIS OF THE FEMORAL HEAD

		Imaging Manifestations		
Stage	Clinical Manifestations	*Routine Radiography*	*Radionuclide Scanning*	*MR Imaging*
0	− (patient at risk)	−	−	−
IA	±	−	±	+
IB	±	−	+	+
II	±	Osteopenia, cysts, bone sclerosis*	+	+
IIIA	+	Crescent sign with no subchondral collapse	+	+
IIIB	+	Crescent sign with subchondral collapse and normal joint space	+	+
IV	+	Stage IIIB and joint spacing narrowing	+	+

−, absent or negative; ±, present or absent, positive or negative; +, present or positive.
*Includes cases of segmental infarct.

perhaps related to the fact that anatomic features of the proximal end of the femur are best recognized in this plane. The coronal plane is ideally suited to the analysis of the subchondral bone of the femoral head, although transaxial images may add supplemental data to this analysis. Sagittal images, particularly when combined with the application of surface coils and small fields of view, appear to increase the sensitivity of MR imaging in the diagnosis of early disease. In the sagittal plane, the fovea centralis of the femoral head, a normal anatomic finding, may be misinterpreted as a site of osteonecrosis, however.

The MR imaging characteristics of osteonecrosis of the femoral head are variable. Factors that may predispose a femoral head to osteonecrosis and that may be identified on MR images include increased amounts of fatty marrow in the trochanters and the presence of a sealed-off physeal scar.[258] Although a joint effusion may be an initial abnormality, the finding lacks specificity and may be seen even in asymptomatic persons. A diffuse pattern of bone marrow edema, identical to that of transient bone marrow edema (see later discussion), may be identified in the early stages of the process. Subsequently, a more focal process within the femoral head allows a more specific diagnosis (Figs. 15–61 and 15–62). The area of ischemic marrow may be surrounded by a reactive interface that is characterized by low signal intensity on T1-weighted spin echo MR images and an outer margin of low signal intensity and an inner margin of high signal intensity on T2-weighted spin echo MR images (Fig. 15–63). This pattern, often designated a double line sign, is virtually diagnostic of osteonecrosis.[259] The involved segment of the femoral head may extend to the subchondral bone plate or, less commonly, it may occur at a distance from it. The central region within the infarcted area initially may reveal signal characteristics of normal fat but, with chronicity, its signal characteristics may change, resembling those of fluid, hemorrhage, or fibrosis. Staging the ischemic process on the basis of these changing patterns of signal intensity has been attempted (Fig. 15–64; Table 15–4), but the prognostic significance of this type of staging system is not clear.[259–261] Although quantifying the extent of femoral head involvement with MR imaging in cases of osteonecrosis as a means to determine the likelihood of subchondral bone collapse also has been attempted,[398–400] the value of this method is not proved.

Modifications of MR imaging methods may be used successfully in the initial diagnosis and subsequent monitoring of osteonecrosis of the femoral head; these modifications include STIR imaging (Fig. 15–64*F*), fat-suppression techniques (Fig. 15–64*D*), and the intravenous administration of gadolinium compounds. Although the last of these may lead to different patterns of enhancement of signal intensity in early and advanced stages of the disease process,[262] the added benefit of contrast administration is not clear and, generally, standard spin echo images are sufficient. Successful application of spin echo imaging in cases of osteonecrosis of the femoral head usually requires (1) imaging in more than one plane (coronal, transaxial, or sagittal) and, in some cases, in all three planes, (2) the use of surface coils to allow detection of early disease, and (3) the inclusion of at least one T2-weighted spin echo MR imaging sequence to allow assessment of the healing of the process. Improper diagnosis of osteonecrosis on the basis of MR images may relate to misinterpretation of regions of normal hematopoietic marrow, of normal trabecular groups, or of normal synovial herniation pits in the proximal portion of the femur as abnormal findings. Furthermore, diagnostic difficulty may be encountered

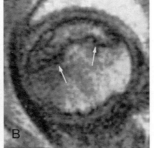

Figure 15–61
Osteonecrosis: MR imaging.
  A A sagittal T1-weighted (TR/TE, 966/12) spin echo MR image shows a curvilinear region of low signal intensity (arrows) representing osteonecrosis of the femoral head.
  B A sagittal T1-weighted (TR/TE, 800/20) spin echo MR image in a second patient reveals a large area of osteonecrosis of the femoral head manifest as a serpentine line of low signal intensity (arrows) with a central zone whose signal intensity is similar to that of fat.

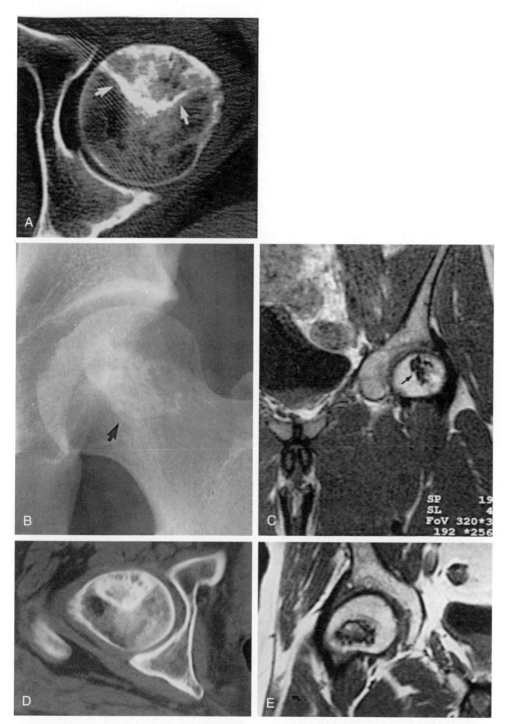

Figure 15–62

Spontaneous osteonecrosis of the femoral head: Segmental type (routine radiography, CT scanning, and MR imaging).

A In this 55 year old man, a transaxial CT scan shows a wedge-shaped lesion (arrows) with its base situated on the anterior femoral surface. Note the sclerotic margins of this osteonecrotic region.

B, C A segmental infarct (arrows) of the femoral head is shown with routine radiography **(B)** and a coronal T1-weighted (TR/TE, 500/15) spin echo MR image **(C).**

D, E In a 47 year old man, note the segmental infarct of the femoral head displayed with transaxial CT scanning **(D)** and a coronal T1-weighted (TR/TE, 644/25) spin echo MR image **(E).** (Courtesy of T. Hughes, M.D., Christchurch, New Zealand.)

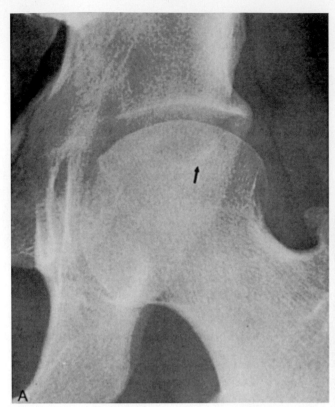

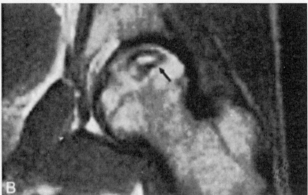

Figure 15–63

Osteonecrosis (MR imaging, double line sign). In this patient with sickle cell anemia, direct radiographic magnification (**A**) reveals a subtle sclerotic zone (arrow), which corresponds in position to an area in **B** characterized by a peripheral region of decreased signal intensity and a central region of increased signal intensity (arrow) on the coronal T2-weighted spin echo display. (Courtesy of L. Rogers, M.D., Winston-Salem, North Carolina.)

when a second process (other than osteonecrosis) also involves the hip (Fig. 15–65).

MR imaging may be a useful technique in the assessment of the response of the osteonecrotic femoral head to operative intervention,[245, 247] especially core decompression (Table 15–5). Considerable controversy exists regarding the efficacy of this therapeutic technique, and opposing points of view have been well summarized by Colwell[401] and Hungerford.[402] The rationale for performing core decompression is the belief that the basic causative factor in osteonecrosis of the femoral head is intraosseous hypertension. Therefore, core biopsy might seem a logical and rational therapeutic approach, serving to decompress the bone and thereby improving its blood flow,[402] a procedure that would be more effective in the earlier stages of osteonecrosis, prior to the occurrence of irreversible cellular injury or death. Opponents of this treatment option cite flaws in the basic hypothesis: there is no clear indication that venous stasis plays any major role in ischemic necrosis of the femoral head secondary to trauma; the analogy of metaphyseal bone representing the same type of closed space as a soft tissue compartment is not accurate, owing to the presence of intraosseous arteries and veins that allow for significant changes in flow rates mediated by neurologic pathways; multiple disorders of the femoral head, including osteoarthritis, have increased venous pressure as part of their pathologic process, and they have not been treated successfully by core decompression; and it has not been shown that venous pressure that is decreased by core decompression remains decreased for any extended time period.[401] Although proponents of core decompression recognize inconsistent and, sometimes, nonbeneficial results of this procedure in some reported series of patients with osteonecrosis of the femoral head, they cite technical factors involved in the surgery or improper choice of candidates for the procedure, or both, as being responsible for such results. Although many authors have concluded that core decompression may not be effective,[403, 404] the procedure continues to enjoy some popularity.

MR imaging accomplished at variable times after core decompression of osteonecrotic femoral heads occasionally may reveal changing patterns of involvement.[405] Ischemic lesions may decrease in size, although this is not seen uniformly and is more likely to occur when initial lesions are small. Patterns of bone marrow edema also may resolve after surgery. Most typically, however, little change in the MR imaging abnormalities is seen, and the signal intensity characteristics of the necrotic zone remain constant.[405]

Table 15–4. OSTEONECROSIS OF THE FEMORAL HEAD: CLASSIFICATION OF SIGNAL INTENSITY CHARACTERISTICS OF CENTRAL PORTION OF NECROTIC AREA

Category	T1-Weighted Sequences	T2-Weighted Sequences	Suggested Cause
A	↑	→	Fat
B	↑	↑	Blood
C	↓	↑	Fluid
D	↓	↓	Fibrous tissue

↑, high; →, intermediate; ↓, low.
Data from Mitchell DG, et al: Radiology *162*:709, 1987.

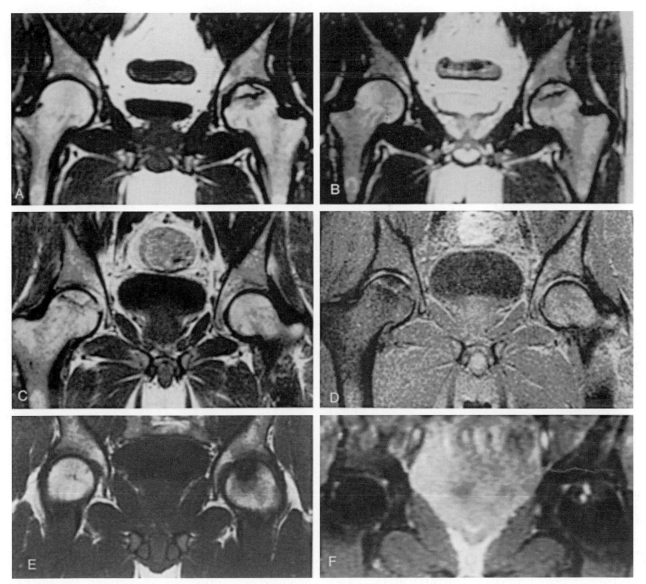

Figure 15–64

Osteonecrosis: MR imaging. Classification system.

A, B Type A pattern. Coronal T1-weighted (TR/TE, 600/20) **(A)** and T2-weighted (TR/TE, 2500/70) **(B)** spin echo MR images reveal an area of osteonecrosis in the left femoral head in which a serpentine region of low signal intensity surrounds a central region whose signal characteristics are identical to those of fat.

C, D Type A pattern. Coronal T1-weighted (TR/TE, 600/20) **(C)** and coronal T1-weighted (TR/TE, 650/20) fat-suppressed (ChemSat) **(D)** spin echo MR images show osteonecrosis of the right femoral head. In **C,** note the central region displaying signal intensity characteristics of fat surrounded by a curvilinear zone of low signal intensity. In **D,** suppression of the fat signal within the central zone is evident, and a peripheral region of higher signal intensity is seen.

E, F Type C pattern. On the coronal T1-weighted (TR/TE, 600/20) spin echo image **(E),** the area of osteonecrosis in the left femoral head is of low signal intensity. It was of high signal intensity on a T2-weighted image (not shown) and on a short tau inversion recovery (STIR) image (TR/TE, 2200/15; inversion time, 160 msec) **(F).**

Although the application of MR imaging to the detection of ischemic necrosis at skeletal sites other than the femoral head has received far less attention, there is little doubt concerning its efficacy. Ischemic changes in the humeral head, about the knee, in the talus, in the diametaphyseal regions of tubular bones, and in other skeletal locations, whether occurring spontaneously, as a result of trauma, or as a complication of an underlying systemic disease process, can be assessed with MR imaging. The basic MR imaging characteristics in these situations are similar or identical to those seen in cases of

osteonecrosis of the femoral head, and the MR imaging examination provides greater sensitivity in diagnosis than routine radiography and bone scintigraphy. Furthermore, in some instances, the MR imaging findings are specific for the diagnosis of osteonecrosis, clarifying the nature of routine radiographic changes that may be misinterpreted as evidence of infection or neoplasm. The MR imaging changes that occur in association with diametaphyseal infarction vary according to the stage of the process. Early infarcts may be of intermediate to high signal intensity on T1-weighted sequences and of

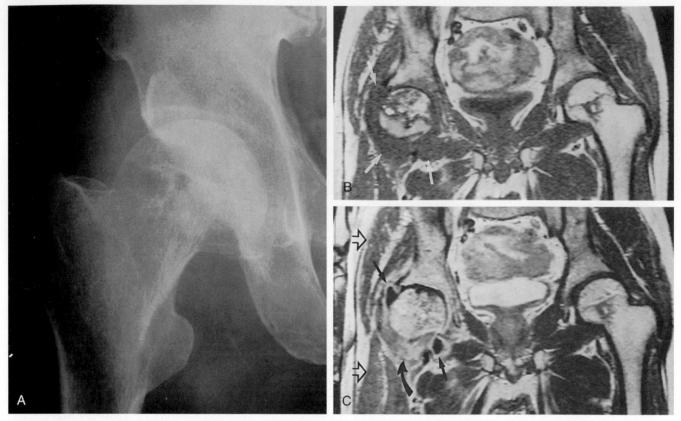

Figure 15–65
Spontaneous osteonecrosis of the femoral head (routine radiography and MR imaging, associated septic arthritis of the hip).
  A In a 44 year old man, routine radiography reveals subtle increase in radiodensity of the femoral head and a joint effusion.
  B A coronal T1-weighted (TR/TE, 400/17) spin echo MR image shows bilateral osteonecrosis of the femoral heads and distention of the right hip joint (arrows).
  C After intravenous gadolinium administration, a coronal T1-weighted (TR/TE, 400/17) spin echo MR image reveals enhancement of signal intensity in the inflamed synovial membrane (closed arrows), joint fluid of low signal intensity, and periarticular enhancement of signal intensity (open arrows).

high signal intensity on T2-weighted sequences; chronic infarcts typically are of low signal intensity on both T1- and T2-weighted images. In both instances, a serpentine zone of low signal intensity, representing bone sclerosis or fibrosis, may surround the necrotic region. Diagnostic difficulty may be encountered in the detection of infarction in hyperplastic marrow when only T1-weighted spin echo MR images are employed because

both may have the same low signal intensity. T2-weighted spin echo MR images and the intravenous administration of a gadolinium compound may be helpful diagnostically in this particular situation. Diffusely distributed infarcts in a tubular bone also may lead to diagnostic difficulty, the MR imaging abnormalities resembling those of infection, tumor, or stress fracture.
  Several other techniques have been used to diagnose

Table 15–5. SOME SURGICAL METHODS OF TREATMENT OF ISCHEMIC NECROSIS OF THE FEMORAL HEAD

Method	Rationale
Drilling or forage	Multiple drill holes in the femoral head and neck to establish channels for revascularization
Core decompression	Coring device to create large and small channels from trochanteric region to femoral head, allowing decompression of elevated intraosseous pressure
Free bone grafts with cancellous or cortical bone	Placement of cortical bone (for mechanical support) or cancellous bone (for rapid incorporation) into channels in the femoral head and neck
Vascularized bone grafts with attached muscle pedicle	Same as for free bone grafts except living rather than dead bone is used
Osteochondral allograft	Replacement of collapsed portion of the articular surface with allograft
Osteotomy: Varus or valgus	Shift of femoral head in acetabulum to provide new weight-bearing area
Rotational	Rotation of femoral head in acetabulum to provide new weight-bearing area
Electrical stimulation	Use of electrical current to induce bone formation
Arthroplasty	Replacement of abnormal femoral head (and acetabulum) with prothesis

osteonecrosis. Functional exploration of bone is regarded by some investigators as a simple and safe method that is indispensable for diagnosis in the early stages of ischemic necrosis of bone.[406] This method has been well summarized by Ficat,[407] whose analysis is included here. Measurement of the *pressure in the bone marrow* in the femoral head can be accomplished with the introduction of a cannula placed in the intertrochanteric region under local anesthesia; the normal baseline pressure is approximately 20 mm Hg and values above 30 mm Hg are regarded as abnormal.[407] A stress test used in conjunction with this pressure determination is provided by the injection of 5 ml of isotonic saline solution into the bone; a normal response is an elevation of bone marrow pressure of less than 10 mm Hg above the baseline level.[407] *Oxygen saturation* of greater than 85 per cent in a specimen of blood removed through the cannula is indirect evidence of circulatory failure.

Intramedullary phlebography is accomplished by the injection of contrast material directly into the intertrochanteric region of the femur. The normal venogram is characterized by the absence of pain and the presence of rapid opacification of efferent vessels, especially the ischial and circumflex veins, without any diaphyseal reflux or stasis; in ischemic necrosis of the femoral head, a painful injection is followed by reflux in the diaphysis and intramedullary stasis for 15 minutes after the procedure.[407]

The final stage of functional exploration of bone is the *core biopsy*, in which a hollow trephine is introduced into the femoral neck from an opening in the greater trochanter and advanced into the subchondral regions of the femoral head; a second channel is made with a smaller trephine in a different direction.[407] Arlet and Durroux[408] have classified the degrees of histologic alterations in the core biopsy into four types; lesser degrees of involvement are accompanied by necrosis of the hematopoietic or fatty elements, and greater degrees are accompanied by medullary and trabecular necrosis.

The value of some of these tests in the diagnosis of ischemic necrosis of the femoral head, as well as of other sites, has been examined in a number of articles. Robinson and coworkers,[409] in a study of 23 hips that were suspected of having early-stage disease, found that 78 per cent of the femoral heads had MR imaging changes of osteonecrosis, 61 per cent had positive findings by bone marrow pressure studies and intramedullary venography, and 83 per cent revealed histologic evidence of osteonecrosis. In an analysis of 41 patients with known or suspected osteonecrosis of the femoral head, Stulberg and colleagues[410] reported the following values for sensitivity, specificity, positive predictive value, and negative predictive value: bone scintigraphy—83, 83, 96, and 48 per cent; SPECT—91, 78, 94, and 70 per cent; MR imaging—87, 83, 96, and 55 per cent; intraosseous pressure measurements—80, 60, 95, and 25 per cent; and core biopsy—88, 100, 100, and 25 per cent. Zizic and coworkers[411] studied 42 patients with ischemic necrosis of bone about the hip, shoulder, and knee. Hemodynamic studies were performed on the contralateral, asymptomatic joint. Thirty-six of 48 joints

had increased bone marrow pressure and of these, 15 (42 per cent) developed histologic or radiographic evidence of osteonecrosis. In none of the 12 bones with normal bone marrow pressure did ischemic necrosis occur. Intraosseous venography also was significantly predictive for ischemic necrosis, both alone and in conjunction with bone marrow pressure measurements.

Transient Bone Marrow Edema

An understanding of this process requires a review of a previously described condition involving the proximal portion of the femur, designated transient demineralization (i.e., osteoporosis) of the hip in 1959 by Curtiss and Kincaid.[263] Although early reports emphasized the occurrence of this condition in the left femoral head of women in the third trimester of pregnancy, transient osteoporosis about the hip has proved to be more common in men than in women, affecting either the right side or the left side, and occasionally migrating from one side to the other. Early reports also suggested that the diagnosis was based on the presence of osteopenia of the femoral head, an intact joint space, the absence of bone erosions or collapse, and increased accumulation of bone-seeking radionuclide agents. Although the relationships of transient osteoporosis about the hip, reflex sympathetic dystrophy (Sudeck's atrophy), and regional migratory osteoporosis remain controversial,[264] numerous reports have documented the occurrence of pain, restricted motion, and a limp in patients with transient osteoporosis about the hip, leading to its general acceptance as a disease entity.

The application of MR imaging to the assessment of transient osteoporosis about the hip was reported in 1988 by Wilson and collaborators.[265] Their findings, which consisted of altered signal intensity in the marrow of the femoral head and neck, were interpreted as evidence of bone marrow edema (Figs. 15–66 and 15–67). Biopsy specimens indicated the presence of normal marrow and bone and the absence of osteonecrosis. Although the histologic data reported in this study did not confirm the presence of marrow edema, such histologic confirmation (Fig. 15–68) was provided in a study of 10 hips in nine patients reported by Hofman and coworkers[266] in 1993. Furthermore, in this latter study, elevation of the pressure within the involved bone marrow and abnormalities seen during intraosseous venography were documented in five patients, and histologic evidence of bone death was absent.

The association of transient pain and limitation of motion in the hip, radiographically evident osteopenia, and an MR imaging pattern consistent with bone marrow edema appears definite on the basis of results from many reported investigations. What also appears definite is the presence of identical marrow findings on MR imaging examinations of painful hips in patients whose routine radiographs do not reveal osteopenia. This is not surprising, owing to the relative insensitivity of conventional radiography in the detection of minor to moderate degrees of bone loss. Therefore, the designation of transient bone marrow edema appears to be more comprehensive than that of transient osteoporosis about

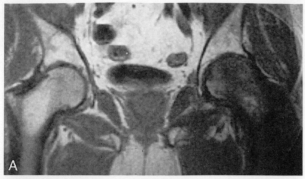

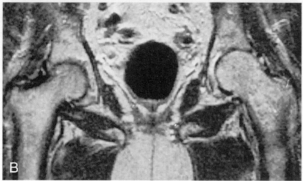

Figure 15–66

Transient bone marrow edema: MR imaging. This patient complained of left hip pain of several months' duration. Routine radiographs were normal, and bone scintigraphy was not performed.

A A coronal T1-weighted (TR/TE, 930/26) spin echo MR image reveals low signal intensity replacing the normal signal of the bone marrow in the left femoral head and neck. The acetabulum appears normal, as does the opposite hip.

B A coronal T2-weighted (TR/TE, 2000/80) spin echo MR image reveals increased signal intensity in the left femoral head and neck. The signal intensity is slightly greater than that on the opposite side. A very small joint effusion is present. The pain and MR imaging abnormalities diminished over a period of 3 months.

the hip. In some instances, the pattern of marrow edema may migrate from one segment of the femoral head to another (Fig. 15–69).

The relationship between transient bone marrow edema and osteonecrosis of the femoral head, however, is not clear (Table 15–6).[267, 268] On the basis of their observations, Hofman and coworkers[266] concluded that the bone marrow edema syndrome was an initial phase of nontraumatic ischemic necrosis of the femoral head. Supporters of this idea point to the fact that in cases of proved osteonecrosis, the typical focal changes on MR images sometimes are preceded by diffuse abnormalities characteristic of bone marrow edema; skeptics argue that this is not surprising, because the reparative phase of osteonecrosis is associated with inflammation, hyperemia, marrow congestion, a decrease in fat, and an increase in interstitial fluid.[269] Similarly, supporters call attention to the study by Turner and associates,[270] who reported five patients with hip pain and evidence of marrow edema on MR imaging examinations who subsequently developed biopsy-proved marrow and bone necrosis, and skeptics emphasize the characteristic MR imaging findings seen in most patients with osteonecrosis of the femoral head, which allow its differentiation from bone marrow edema.

Vande Berg and collaborators[262] provide further insight into this controversy. These authors emphasized that careful analysis of the diffuse pattern of marrow abnormality that may occur in some patients with osteonecrosis of the femoral head reveals features different from those of bone marrow edema (Fig. 15–70). High spatial resolution T2-weighted spin echo MR images in cases of osteonecrosis showed the lesion to be inhomogeneous and associated with crescent-shaped subchondral marrow areas of low signal intensity. Furthermore, intravenous contrast-enhanced MR images showed intense enhancement within the entire lesion except in the subchondral bone areas, suggesting that the necrotic zone was limited to very small portions of the marrow. These authors concluded that collapse of the subchondral bone in cases of transient bone marrow edema is indicative of epiphyseal fractures rather than osteonecrosis.

As indicated by Solomon,[269] whatever the answer to this puzzle, it is important to recognize the difference between bone marrow edema without osteonecrosis and that with osteonecrosis. The former is a hypervascular, usually self-limiting disorder, whereas the latter is unequivocally ischemic.

Occult Fractures

As indicated in Chapter 8, various types of fracture in the pelvis and about the hip may lead to only minor radiographic abnormalities or may escape radiographic detection altogether. These include some acute fractures, trabecular microfractures, and stress fractures (i.e., fatigue and insufficiency fractures). The occurrence of insufficiency fractures of the sacrum, innominate bone, and proximal portion of the femur is well recognized in patients with osteoporosis or renal osteodystrophy and in those who have undergone radiation therapy. Classic radiographic features of such fractures include linear zones of increased radiodensity, although patchy bone sclerosis, producing a speckled pattern, is equally characteristic (Figs. 15–71 and 15–72). The application of other imaging methods, such as bone scintigraphy (Fig. 15–73) and MR imaging (Figs. 15–73, 15–74, and 15–75), to the detection of these fractures, especially those of the femoral neck, has received a great deal of attention.

Scintigraphy using bone-seeking radiopharmaceutical agents is useful in the initial diagnosis of a fracture of the femoral neck and in the determination of the risk for subsequent osteonecrosis of the femoral head. Bone scintigraphy has proved to be more sensitive than routine radiography in confirming a femoral neck fracture.[271] Although it has been widely accepted that, in the elderly patient, a traumatic fracture might not be detected with bone scintigraphy for 2 or 3 days after the injury,[272–274] Holder and associates[275] found that patients of all ages, regardless of the time after injury, can undergo bone scintigraphy as soon as they are evaluated. Although their results eliminate one of the deficiencies of radionuclide bone scanning in the assessment of femoral neck fractures, the scintigraphic abnormalities are not specific and they provide little data regarding

Text continued on page 525

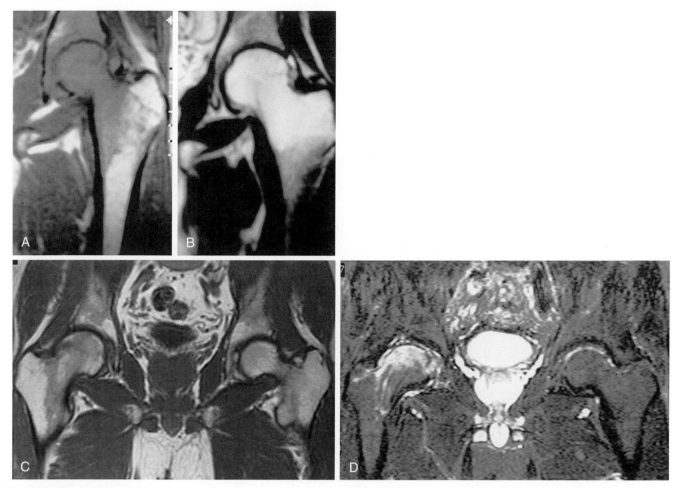

Figure 15–67

Transient bone marrow edema: MR imaging.

A, B Coronal T1-weighted (TR/TE, 645/25) **(A)** and T2-weighted (TR/TE, 2832/110) **(B)** spin echo MR images reveal classic features of this condition, affecting the proximal portion of the femur. Note low signal intensity of the marrow in **A** and high signal intensity of the marrow in **B**. (Courtesy of T. Claudice-Engle, M.D., Stanford, California.)

C, D In a second patient, a coronal T1-weighted (TR/TE, 550/20) spin echo MR image **(C)** shows abnormally low signal intensity of the bone marrow in the right femoral head and neck. The adjacent acetabular marrow is normal. A coronal T2-weighted (TR/TE, 2000/80) spin echo MR image obtained with fat suppression **(D)** reveals high signal intensity of the involved marrow. Bilateral joint effusions, more prominent in the right hip, are evident. (Courtesy of S. Eilenberg, M.D., San Diego, California.)

Table 15–6. TRANSIENT BONE MARROW EDEMA OF THE HIP VERSUS OSTEONECROSIS OF THE FEMORAL HEAD

	Transient Bone Marrow Edema	**Osteonecrosis**
Patient age, y	20-50	20-40
Patient sex	Male/female, 3/1	Equal distribution by sex
Predisposing factors	Generally none; pregnancy in women	Many, including hemoglobinopathies, Gaucher's disease, Caisson disease, excessive alcohol intake, corticosteroid administration, trauma
Distribution	Unilateral, but may later involve other hip or other joints in lower extremity	Bilateral in more than 50 per cent of patients
Imaging abnormalities		
Routine radiography	Negative or osteopenia	Negative or variable findings including bone sclerosis, cysts, and collapse
Bone scintigraphy	Increased radionuclide uptake in femoral head, often diffuse	Increased radionuclide uptake in femoral head, often focal in superior portion, ± photopenic areas
MR imaging	Diffuse abnormalities of femoral head and neck, low signal intensity in T1-weighted images and high signal intensity in T2-weighted images; rarely, focal abnormalities perhaps related to subchondral collapse of femoral head	Focal abnormalities of femoral head, low signal intensity in T1-weighted images and variable signal intensity in T2 weighted images; rarely, diffuse abnormalities of femoral head and neck related to marrow edema
Prognosis	Spontaneous resolution in 1–3 months	Variable but progressive in 75 per cent of patients
Treatment	Restricted weight-bearing	Variable but operative intervention often chosen

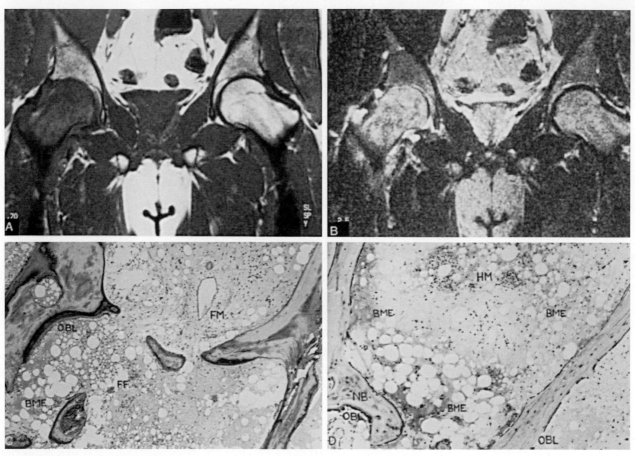

Figure 15–68

Transient bone marrow edema: MR imaging and histology.

A, B Coronal T1-weighted (TR/TE, 700/15) **(A)** and T2-weighted (TR/TE, 2500/90) **(B)** spin echo MR images reveal characteristic features of transient bone marrow edema. In **A,** note low signal intensity in the marrow of the right femoral head and neck with normal signal intensity in the adjacent acetabulum. The opposite femur and acetabulum also are normal. In **B,** note high signal intensity in the involved marrow in the right femur and a large joint effusion. The altered signal intensity extends to the base of the femoral neck. Again, the acetabula and left femur appear normal. (Courtesy of J. Kramer, M.D., Vienna, Austria.)

C, D Photomicrographs derived from undecalcified sections of material obtained from the affected marrow of the right femur are shown. In **C,** note dark gray osteoid seams with the trabecular surfaces partly covered by active osteoblasts (OBL). Homogeneous material is seen in the marrow cavity, representing marrow edema (BME), fat cell fragmentation (FF), or fibrous marrow regeneration (FM) (trichrome Goldner stain, ×60). In **D,** trabeculae are partly covered by active osteoblasts (OBL), leading to new bone formation (NB). The homogeneous extracellular material now is dark or basophilic, with marrow edema (BME) between fat cells and remnants of hematopoietic marrow (HM) (Giemsa stain, ×60). (From Hoffmann S, et al: J Bone Joint Surg [Br] 75:210, 1993.)

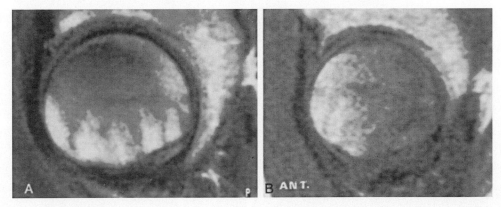

Figure 15–69

Transient bone marrow edema: Migrating MR imaging abnormalities. This 46 year old man had clinical and radiographic evidence of transient osteoporosis of the hip.

A A sagittal T1-weighted (TR/TE, 475/20) spin echo MR image obtained 2 months after the onset of pain shows a decrease in signal intensity in the anterior and superior portions of the femoral head (A, anterior; P, posterior).

B Three months later, a similar sagittal spin echo MR image (TR/TE, 475/20) now reveals that the region of low signal intensity is located in the posterior part of the femoral head (ANT, anterior).

(From Hauzeur JP, et al: J Rheumatol *18*:1211, 1991.)

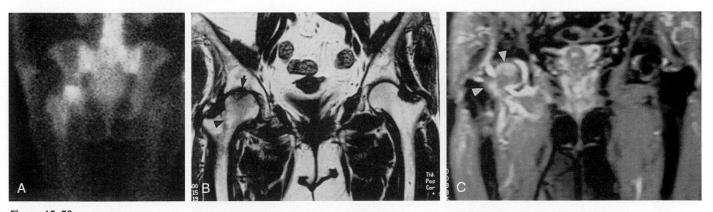

Figure 15–70

Osteonecrosis: MR imaging, diffuse marrow abnormalities.

A A bone scan shows intense activity in a portion of the right femoral head and lesser but abnormal accumulation of the radionuclide in the right femoral neck.

B A coronal T1-weighted (TR/TE, 500/15) spin echo MR image documents a focal abnormality (arrow) in the femoral head and marrow edema of low signal intensity extending into the femoral neck (arrowhead).

C A coronal fast spin echo STIR MR image (TR/TE, 3500/19; inversion time, 140 msec) confirms abnormality characterized by high signal intensity in the femoral head and neck (arrowheads) and a joint effusion.

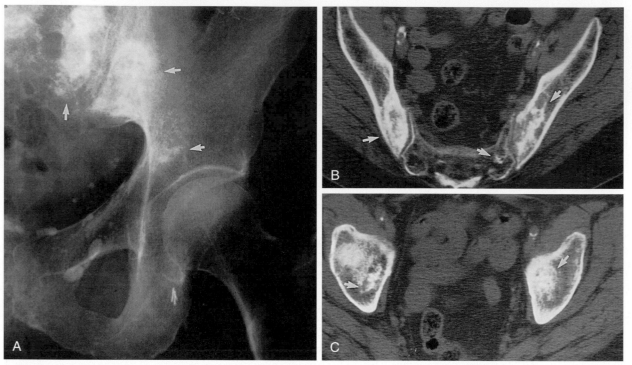

Figure 15–71
Occult fractures: Insufficiency fractures of the pelvis after irradiation. Routine radiograph **(A)** and CT scans **(B,C)** show patchy areas of bone sclerosis (arrows) about the sacroiliac joints and acetabula, which are typical of these fractures.

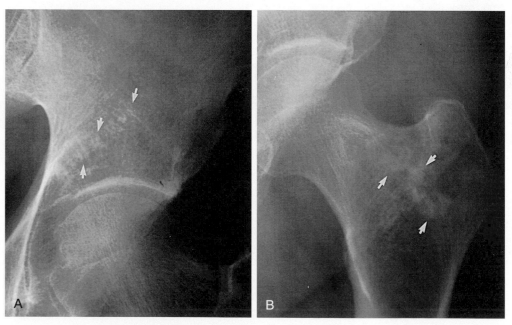

Figure 15–72
Occult fractures: Insufficiency fractures of the pelvis and femoral neck—routine radiography.

A This speckled pattern (arrows) about the acetabulum is characteristic.

B In a second patient, note patchy bone sclerosis (arrows) aligned with tensile trabeculae of the femoral neck.

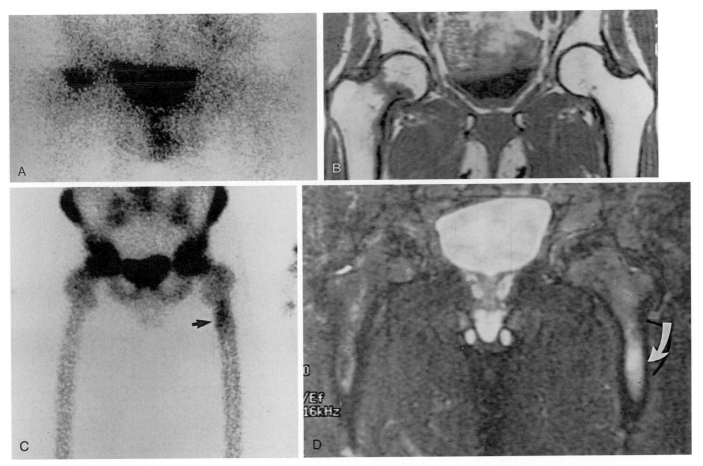

Figure 15–73

Occult fractures: Insufficiency fractures and stress reaction of the femoral neck. Bone scintigraphy and MR imaging.

A, B Although initial radiographs were normal in this 75 year old woman who had fallen, bone scintigraphy **(A)** reveals increased accumulation of radionuclide in the right femoral neck. A coronal T1-weighted (TR/TE, 600/20) spin echo MR image **(B)** clearly shows the fracture of the right femoral neck.

C, D In a second patient with thigh pain, a bone scan **(C)** shows uptake (arrow) of radionuclide in the proximal femur. A coronal STIR (TR/TE, 4000/51; inversion time 150 msec) MR image **(D)** shows high signal intensity in this same region (arrow). The findings are those of a stress reaction, or thigh splints, which was confirmed by biopsy of the lesion.

the morphology of the fracture. The interest in using MR imaging in this clinical setting, therefore, is understandable. The MR imaging examination appears to be equally sensitive and far more specific in the detection of fractures of the femoral neck.[276-279] A negative MR imaging examination effectively eliminates the diagnosis of such fractures. Furthermore, in some cases, the MR images indicate other bone or soft tissue injuries that have produced clinical manifestations simulating those of fractures of the femoral neck.[279] This examination may not allow determination of the viability of the femoral head after these fractures[166]; however, it can be tailored in such a fashion that imaging time is limited and costs are competitive with those of other advanced imaging methods.[168] A coronal T1-weighted spin echo MR imaging sequence, requiring approximately 7 minutes, may be sufficient.[168]

The MR imaging characteristics of a nondisplaced fracture of the femoral neck on T1-weighted spin echo MR sequences are a well-defined linear zone of low signal intensity that may be surrounded by a broader and poorly defined zone of low signal intensity consis-

tent with marrow edema.[280] On T2-weighted spin echo MR images, the fracture line may remain of low signal intensity, but the edematous zone demonstrates high signal intensity. STIR images are very sensitive to the detection of these fractures, which appear as broad bands of high signal intensity within the normal, low signal intensity bone marrow; however, these images are less specific, as the fracture line itself may not be identifiable.[412] The use of fat suppression in combination with the intravenous administration of gadolinium compounds represents an additional sensitive MR imaging method for the detection of occult fractures of the femoral neck. A variety of MR imaging sequences also can be used to evaluate other subtle fractures, including stress fractures, of the pelvis (Fig. 15–76). CT, however, is a superior method for the assessment of complex fractures and fracture-dislocations about the hip.

Posttraumatic Osteolysis

Prominent osteolysis about a fracture site or occurring after other types of injury is encountered in numerous

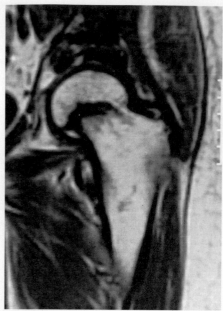

Figure 15–74
Occult fractures: Insufficiency fractures of the femoral neck—MR imaging. In a patient with lymphoma receiving corticosteroid medication, a coronal T1-weighted (TR/TE, 600/17) spin echo MR image shows a linear zone of low signal intensity extending almost completely across the femoral neck. (Courtesy of D. Witte, M.D., Memphis, Tennessee.)

skeletal locations, of which the distal portion of the clavicle is the best known (see Chapter 12). In the pubic or ischial rami or parasymphyseal bone, exaggerated resorption of bone about a fracture, with or without associated sclerosis, can simulate the appearance of a malignant process.[281–285] Furthermore, the pathologist may misinterpret the exuberant cartilage and disorderly membranous bone formation of a rapidly forming primary callus as evidence of a chondrosarcoma or other malignancy, thus compounding the diagnostic dilemma. Such fractures occur as a result of either direct trauma or, frequently, chronic stress in an osteopenic skeleton

(insufficiency fractures), sometimes in combination with similar fractures of the sacrum. The cause of osteolysis about these ramus fractures is not known, although instability, particularly in single ramus fractures, should not be a factor. As no impaction of bone occurs in these latter fractures, perhaps a lack of sound, direct bone contact is an explanation for the excessive osteolysis and delayed union.[286]

Prominent posttraumatic osteolysis also has been noted in the ulna, radius, and carpal bones. In the femoral neck, resorption and rotation at the fracture site can produce a radiographic picture that may be misinterpreted as a malignant process.[287, 288]

Synovial Herniation Pits

A commonly encountered aperture, designated a herniation pit, is seen in the anterior surface of the femoral neck (Fig. 15–77).[289] Ingrowth of fibrous and cartilaginous elements occurs through a perforation in the cortex in a roughened reaction area of sclerotic bone, resulting in unilateral or bilateral, small, rounded radiolucent areas in the anterolateral aspect of the femoral neck.[289, 290] Although the lucent regions generally are stable, they may rarely disappear spontaneously.[413] They also may enlarge in persons of all ages, perhaps related to changing mechanics such as pressure and the abrasive effect of the overlying hip capsule and anterior muscles.[291] Such enlargement, which may occur rapidly,[291] is evident more frequently in patients with a history of athletic physical activity.[289, 291] Bone scintigraphy, although typically negative in persons with herniation pits, occasionally may be positive with increased accumulation of the radiopharmaceutical agent.[291, 292] MR imaging generally shows a focus of low signal intensity on T1-weighted spin echo MR images and high signal intensity, consistent with that of fluid, on T2-weighted spin echo images (Figs. 15–78 and 15–79).[291, 293] CT scanning confirms the anterior location of the cyst, thinning of the adjacent femoral cortex, small cortical perforations in some cases, and the pres-

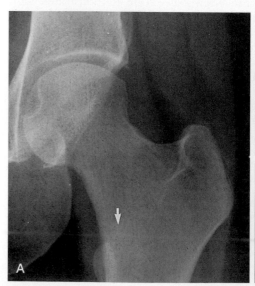

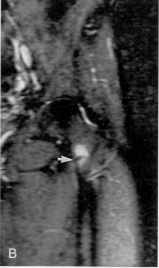

Figure 15–75
Occult fractures: Fatigue fractures of the femoral neck. MR imaging. In a 30 year old female runner, a routine radiograph **(A)** reveals subtle sclerosis (arrow) at the base of the femoral neck. The coronal STIR MR image (TR/TE, 3666/17; inversion time, 150 msec) **(B)** reveals the fracture line (arrow) and surrounding marrow edema.

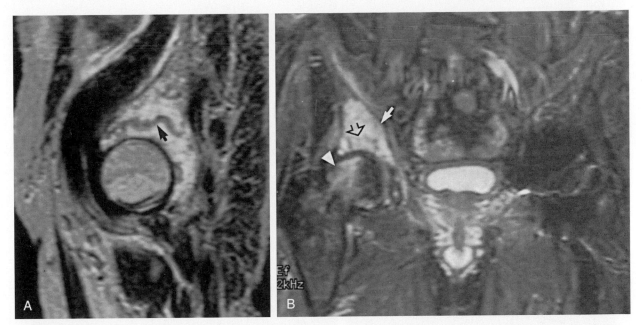

Figure 15–76
Osteoporosis: Insufficiency fracture—acetabulum (MR imaging). This patient had a history of carcinoma of the prostate treated with radiation therapy and developed bilateral osteonecrosis of the femoral heads. A total joint replacement of the left hip was performed. Progressive right hip pain led to an MR imaging examination.

A A sagittal fast spin echo (TR/TE, 4600/102) MR image of the right hip shows an insufficiency fracture of the acetabulum (arrow) manifested as an irregular linear region of low signal intensity surrounded by marrow edema of high signal intensity. In this image, the right femoral head appears normal.

B A coronal STIR MR image (TR/TE, 4000/52; inversion time, 150 msec) reveals abnormally high signal intensity of the marrow in the right acetabulum (solid arrow) and femoral head (arrowhead). The insufficiency fracture of the acetabulum is visible (open arrow). Signal void in the left hip relates to the previous surgery. Plain films (not shown) confirmed that the right femoral head was the site of osteonecrosis.

ence of a well-defined margin to the cyst (see Figs. 15–78 and 15–79).

Osteomyelitis

In common with other skeletal regions, the bones about the hip may be involved in osteomyelitis. Such involvement generally relates to one of two possible mechanisms: hematogenous spread of infection or spread of infection from a contiguous contaminated source, usually the skin and subcutaneous tissues. In both situations, the primary roles of MR imaging are to detect abnormalities prior to those appearing on routine radiographs and to delineate the full extent of the process (Figs. 15–80 and 15–81). Conventional spin echo sequences may be supplemented by additional, more sensitive ones, including STIR sequences and fat-suppression sequences obtained after the intravenous injection of a gadolinium-containing compound. Although bone abscesses may be well delineated with MR imaging, sequestered fragments of bone often are better demonstrated with CT scanning.

Bone Tumors and Tumor-Like Lesions

Although a variety of bone tumors and tumor-like lesions are encountered in the pelvis about the hip (Table 15–7), a few deserve emphasis.

Osteoid osteomas are not infrequent in the femoral neck. A subperiosteal location is typical. As bone sclerosis often is not prominent, these lesions may escape

detection when routine radiographs alone are used. CT scanning and MR imaging (Figs. 15–82 and 15–83) are equally sensitive when compared with bone scintigraphy in the identification of these lesions, and, with MR imaging, an accompanying joint effusion related to lymphoreticular synovial proliferation may be evident.

Simple bone cysts are commonly found in the proximal metaphysis of the femur in the immature skeleton. Their fluid contents lead to typical changes in signal intensity in MR images, and enhancement of signal intensity in the wall of the cysts is observed after intravenous administration of a gadolinium compound. A similar lesion occurring in the femoral neck is an intraosseous lipoma, whose fat content can be confirmed with either CT scanning or MR imaging. Other benign lesions also occur in this same region (Fig. 15–84).

Of the malignant bone tumors occurring about the hip, skeletal metastasis, plasma cell myeloma, lymphoma, osteosarcoma (Fig. 15–85), and chondrosarcoma (Fig. 15–86) are seen most frequently. Although the accompanying MR imaging features in these tumors are not specific, the technique does allow accurate assessment of the osseous and soft tissue extent of the lesions.

Legg-Calvé-Perthes Disease

MR imaging is useful for the assessment of a variety of causes of hip pain in the child, including Legg-Calvé-Perthes disease. In some children with hip pain, MR imaging may reveal findings consistent with transient

Text continued on page 532

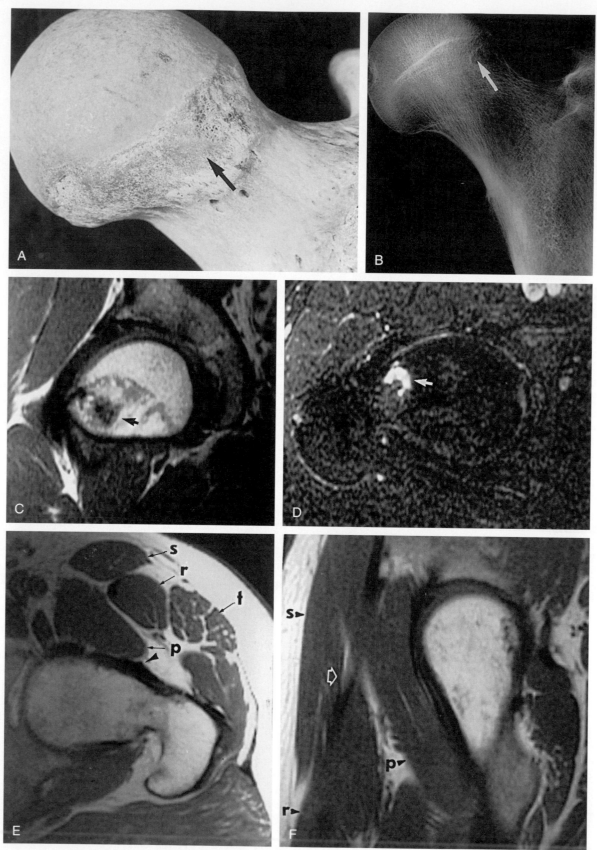

Figure 15–77
See legend on opposite page

Figure 15–78
Synovial herniation pit of the femoral neck. This Olympic runner developed increasing pain in the left hip, as well as a stress fracture of the right ischium. Biopsy of the femoral neck lesion revealed tissue with histologic features compatible with those of a herniation pit.

A Observe the well-defined osteolytic lesion in the femoral neck.

B A transaxial CT scan confirms its anterior location, with thinning and buckling of the adjacent cortex.

C A coronal T1-weighted (TR/TE, 300/16) spin echo MR image reveals a lesion whose signal intensity is similar to that of muscle.

D High signal intensity of the lesion is evident on a transaxial fast spin echo MR image (TR/TE, 4000/102).

(Courtesy of A.G. Bergman, M.D., Stanford, California.)

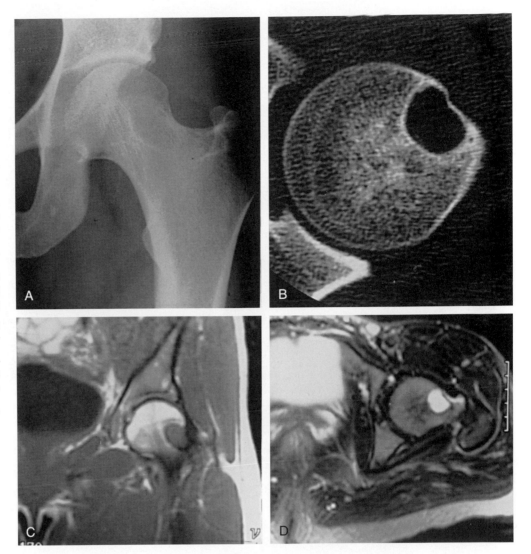

Figure 15–77
Synovial herniation pit of the femoral neck.

   A, B In a femoral specimen, a photograph **(A)** of the anterior surface of the femur shows a region (arrow), designated the reaction area, that resembles a plaque and has slightly elevated margins. A routine radiograph **(B)** of the specimen reveals a small herniation pit (arrow) beneath the reaction area.

   C, D In a 30 year old man, the herniation pit (arrows) is of low signal intensity in a coronal T1-weighted (TR/TE, 500/12) spin echo MR image **(C)** and of high signal intensity in a transaxial fat-suppressed fast spin echo (TR/TE, 3000/84) MR image **(D)**. (Courtesy of S.K. Brahme, M.D., La Jolla, California.)

   E, F The normal relationships of various muscles and supporting structures to the anterior surface of the femoral neck are shown in a transaxial T1-weighted (TR/TE, 400/20) spin echo MR image **(E)** and a sagittal T1-weighted spin echo MR image **(F)**, both obtained with the hip in neutral position. Labeled structures are the iliopsoas muscle (p), iliofemoral ligament (arrowhead), rectus femoris muscle and tendon (r), sartorius muscle (s), and tensor fascia latae (t). The open arrow in **F** indicates the position of the tendon of the rectus femoris muscle. The movement of some of these structures across the femoral neck as the hip moves may be important in the pathogenesis of synovial herniation pits.

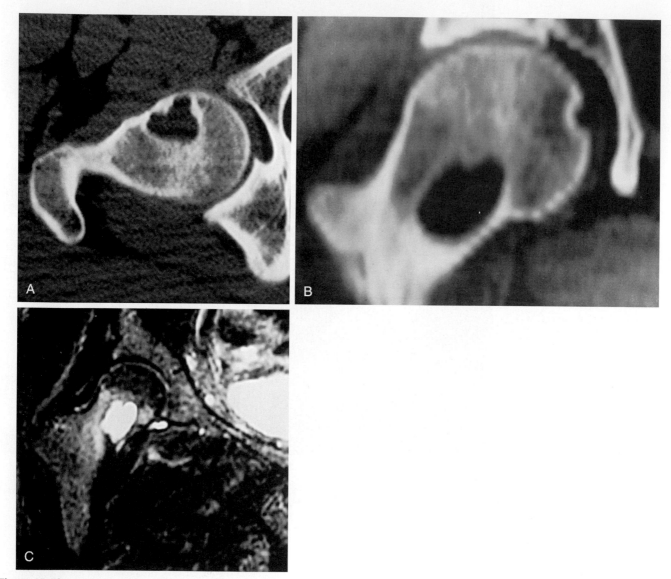

Figure 15–79
Synovial herniation pit of the femoral neck.
   A, B In a 35 year old woman, transaxial **(A)** and reformatted coronal **(B)** CT scans reveal a well-defined osteolytic lesion with thinning of the adjacent cortex.
   C A coronal fat-suppressed fast spin echo MR image (TR/TE, 3200/95) shows a lesion of high signal intensity, with surrounding marrow edema.
   (Courtesy of D. Goodwin, M.D., Hanover, New Hampshire.)

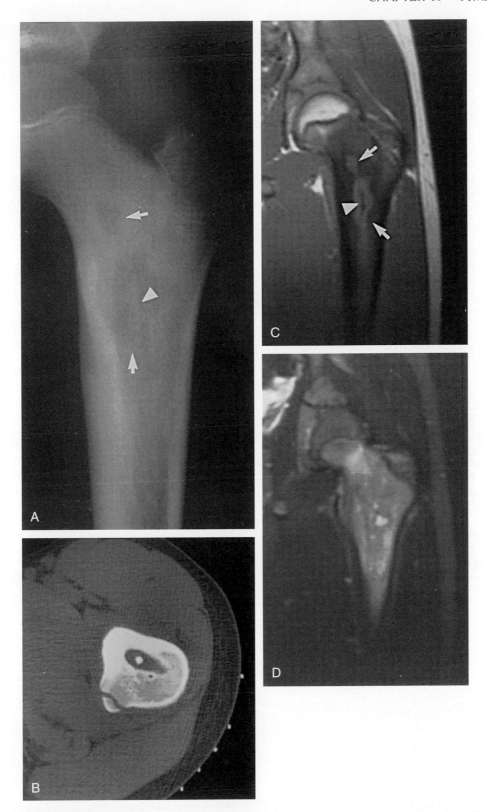

Figure 15–80

Osteomyelitis: CT scanning and MR imaging.

A In this 9 year old girl, the routine radiograph reveals a multifocal abscess (arrows) in the proximal portion of the femur containing a sequestrum (arrowhead) and surrounded by sclerotic bone.

B A transaxial CT scan shows the abscess and sequestered bone.

C In a coronal T1-weighted (TR/TE, 666/11) spin echo MR image, the abscess (arrows) and sequestrum (arrowhead) are identified. Note the extent of marrow abnormality.

D In a coronal fat-suppressed fast spin echo MR image (TR/TE, 2800/80), the abnormal marrow has high signal intensity, with a circular focus of even higher signal intensity.

(Courtesy of D. Witte, M.D., Memphis, Tennessee.)

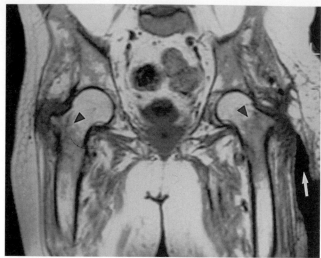

Figure 15–81

Pressure sores with osteomyelitis: MR imaging. In a 46 year old paraplegic man, bilateral pressure sores developed in the buttock, one of which is well shown on this coronal T1-weighted (TR/TE, 666/12) spin echo MR image (arrow). Note evidence of osteomyelitis involving both femoral trochanters and adjacent marrow (arrowheads).

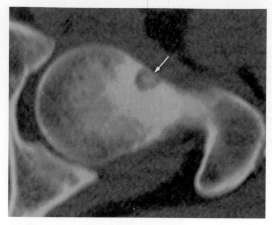

Figure 15–82

Osteoid osteoma: CT scanning. The partially calcified nidus (arrow) of an osteoid osteoma and surrounding bone sclerosis are shown effectively in a transaxial CT scan.

bone marrow edema, characterized by decreased signal intensity in the femoral head on T1-weighted spin echo images and normal or increased signal intensity on T2-weighted spin echo images. As such findings in adults occasionally are followed by those of ischemic necrosis of bone, transient bone marrow edema of the femoral head in a child may be a precursor to Legg-Calvé-Perthes disease, although this potential association is not proved. In children with transient synovitis of the hip, MR findings include evidence of a joint effusion; similar findings occur in patients with septic arthritis of the hip.

In Legg-Calvé-Perthes disease, MR imaging reveals a number of findings, including thickening of both the acetabular cartilage and the cartilage of the femoral head, physeal irregularity and transphyseal bone bridging, loss of containment of the femoral head within the acetabulum, changes of signal intensity in the marrow and epiphyseal cartilage, synovial inflammation and, ultimately in some cases, secondary osteoarthritis (Figs. 15–87 and 15–88). The role of intravenous administration of a gadolinium compound in the MR imaging assessment of hip involvement in this disease is not clear.

Developmental Abnormalities

Developmental Dysplasia of the Hip

Developmental dysplasia of the hip (DDH) is a disease with extremely variable morphologic patterns. Although detection of DDH at birth by appropriate neonatal clinical and imaging examinations and immediate inception of treatment are desirable, the diagnosis is missed in many children.[294–297] The most reliable methods for diagnosing DDH in the neonatal period are clinical: the Ortolani and Barlow maneuvers.[298] Despite routine application of these tests, a 0.1 to 0.2 per cent prevalence of late diagnosis exists among infants found to be normal in the neonatal period.[299–303]

Selection of appropriate imaging techniques in patients with DDH depends on age and differs for diagnostic versus management situations. Ultrasonography generally is preferred over conventional radiography among children under 1 year of age. Contrast arthrography[304] and CT[305] are indicated for preoperative planning. MR imaging also is a useful method, but its specific role remains to be completely established. In this short discussion, only ultrasonography, CT scanning, and MR imaging are considered.

Table 15–7. TUMORS AND TUMOR-LIKE LESIONS OF BONE: FREQUENCY OF INVOLVEMENT OF BONES IN THE PELVIS AND ABOUT THE HIP

Lesion	Frequency, %*
Enostosis	35
Osteoid osteoma	30
Osteoblastoma	5
Osteosarcoma	5
Enchondroma	5
Periosteal chondroma	4
Chondroblastoma	10
Chondromyxoid fibroma	7
Osteochondroma	10
Chondrosarcoma	25
Nonossifying fibroma	3
Desmoplastic fibroma	12
Fibrosarcoma	10
Giant cell tumor	8
Malignant fibrous histiocytoma	10
Lipoma	10
Hemangioma	4
Hemangiopericytoma	15
Hemangioendothelioma	15
Neurofibroma/neurilemoma	5
Simple bone cyst	22
Aneurysmal bone cyst	15
Adamantinoma	1
Ewing's sarcoma	30

*Approximate figures, based on analysis of major reports containing the greatest number of cases.

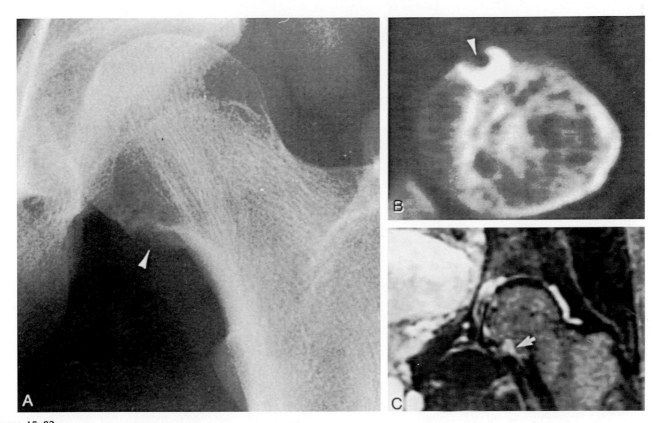

Figure 15–83
Osteoid osteoma: CT scanning and MR imaging.

A The routine radiograph reveals subtle osseous irregularity (arrowhead) in the superomedial aspect of the femoral neck.

B A transaxial CT scan shows the subsynovial osteoid osteoma (arrowhead).

(**A, B,** Courtesy of P. VanderStoep, M.D., St. Cloud, Minnesota.)

C In a different patient, a coronal T2-weighted (TR/TE, 1500/70) spin echo MR image reveals an osteoid osteoma (arrow) in the femoral neck and a joint effusion.

(**C,** Courtesy of W. Peck, M.D., Orange, California.)

Real-time ultrasonographic systems, when compared with older static B-mode units, have provided increasingly accurate images of the infant hip as well as valuable information concerning function.[306–309] The advantages to this method include the following: (1) ultrasonography provides detailed depiction of the cartilaginous femoral head and its relationship to the bony and cartilaginous acetabulum; (2) patients in spica casts, Pavlik harnesses, and braces can be evaluated to ensure concentric reduction; (3) hip motion can be studied dynamically, documenting subluxation, dislocation, and reduction as they occur; and (4) exposure to ionizing radiation and sedation are avoided.[310–315]

Just as the clinical diagnosis of DDH relies on the detection of hip instability using the Barlow and Ortolani maneuvers, the real-time sonographic evaluation of the hip should include dynamic techniques to elicit and record hip instability.[316] Motion and stability of the hip are evaluated on both transverse and longitudinal scans. In the transverse plane with the hip flexed, gentle force is exerted on the femur in an attempt to displace the cartilaginous head posteriorly (Fig. 15–89). Although no movement should occur in the absence of DDH, normal infants may demonstrate sufficient capsular laxity to permit minor degrees of posterior subluxation

during the first week of life.[317, 318] This phenomenon should resolve within the first month after birth.

Acetabular dysplasia, which results from hip instability and is an anticipated consequence of untreated subluxation or dislocation, is evaluated optimally in the coronal plane.[319] The sonographic features of dysplasia include (1) present or past untreated hip instability; (2) thick echogenic acetabular labrum; (3) thick joint capsule; (4) shallow acetabulum with rounding of the superior margin; and (5) occasional demonstration of a pulvinar and thickened ligamentum teres.

Correlation of sonographic results with clinical findings, other available imaging studies, and long-term patient follow-up has demonstrated high sensitivity and specificity for dynamic ultrasonography of the neonatal hip.[320, 321] The value of real-time ultrasonography in diagnosis and follow-up of DDH is well established, and this method currently should be considered the imaging method of choice for documenting the condition objectively and monitoring the effectiveness of treatment.[322–328]

CT scanning usually can provide accurate documentation of the adequacy of a reduction in DDH.[329–331] CT provides a clear image of the reduction in the transverse plane, so that anterior or posterior subluxation

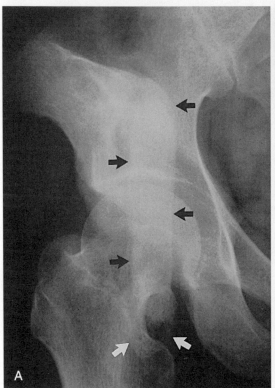

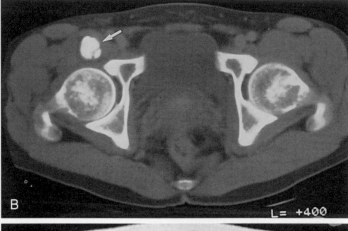

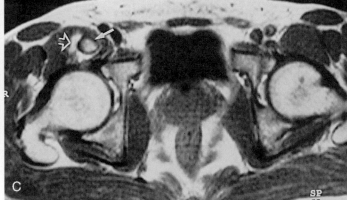

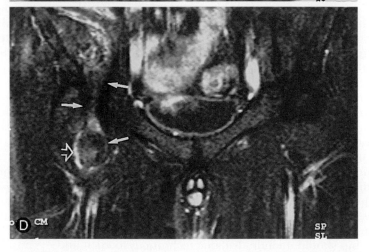

Figure 15–84

Benign bone tumors and tumor-like lesions: MR imaging.

A–D Solitary osteochondroma. In a 38 year old man, a routine radiograph **(A)** reveals an unusually long osteochondroma that arose from the ilium and extended inferiorly across the hip joint (arrows). Transaxial CT scan **(B)** reveals a portion of the ossified lesion (arrow) in the region of the iliopsoas muscle. A transaxial T1-weighted (TR/TE, 600/15) spin echo MR image **(C)** reveals fatty marrow (solid arrow) in the osteochondroma and surrounding fat deposition (open arrow). A coronal fat-suppressed T1-weighted (TR/TE, 570/15) spin echo MR image obtained after intravenous administration of a gadolinium contrast agent **(D)** shows the osseous lesion (solid arrows) and enhanced signal intensity in the cartilaginous cap (open arrow). An osteochondroma, benign in appearance, was documented histologically after surgical resection of the lesion.

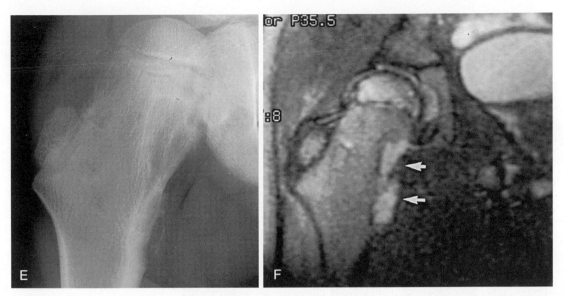

Figure 15–84 *Continued*

E, F Ollier's disease. The channel-like radiolucent regions of the femoral neck (**E**) are typical of cartilaginous foci. The coronal fast spin echo STIR (TR/TE, 4000/38; inversion time, 100 msec) MR image (**F**) reveals high signal intensity in these foci (arrows). (Courtesy of U. Mayer, M.D., Klagenfurt, Austria.)

of the femoral head can be detected readily with as few as one slice.[332, 333] Pulvinar hypertrophy, contracture of the iliopsoas tendon, and intra-articular osteocartilaginous bodies preventing relocation also can be demonstrated.[334, 335] CT allows direct measurement of acetabular anteversion.[336] CT, particularly with three-dimensional analysis, is extremely useful in characterizing the abnormal acetabular morphology of untreated and postoperative DDH (Fig. 15–90).[337–340]

MR imaging offers great promise in the evaluation of DDH, owing to its excellent depiction of unmineralized tissues, including cartilage, its direct multiplanar im-

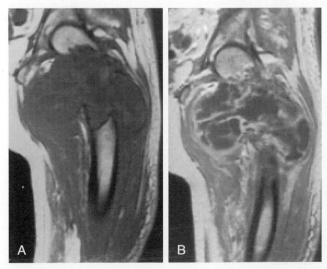

Figure 15–85

Conventional osteosarcoma: MR imaging. Coronal T1-weighted (TR/TE, 700/15) spin echo MR images obtained before (**A**) and after (**B**) the intravenous injection of a gadolinium-based contrast agent reveal a tumor of low signal intensity in the femur and adjacent soft tissue with inhomogeneous enhancement of signal intensity in **B**. (Courtesy of J. Kramer, M.D., Vienna, Austria.)

aging capabilities, its lack of need for ionizing radiation, and its high sensitivity in the early detection of ischemic necrosis of bone.[341, 342] Three-dimensional image reconstruction of data derived by MR imaging also can be accomplished using sophisticated software and hardware.[343] MR imaging can accurately depict the most important determinants of stability in the neonatal hip.[344–346] These include femoral head shape, acetabular shape, position of the labrum, invagination of the joint capsule by the iliopsoas tendon, degree of femoral and acetabular anteversion, and position of the transverse acetabular ligament.[347, 348] Femoral anteversion can be measured using MR imaging by obtaining an additional transaxial image through the femoral condyles.[349] Additional structures, including the ligamentum teres, the fat pad within the acetabular fossa, and various portions of the joint capsule, also are demonstrated by MR imaging.[344]

T1-weighted spin echo MR images provide adequate contrast between bone, cartilage, ligaments, and adjacent soft tissues. Coronal images are optimal for depicting the clinically important structures of the acetabular roof, including the labrum. Transaxial images are best suited for demonstrating the anterior and posterior structures of the joint. Routine use of both planes permits exact determination of the spatial relationship between the acetabulum and femoral head.[350, 351] The application of rapid scanning techniques, such as gradient echo and fast spin echo imaging, allows the acquisition of scans in multiple hip positions within a reasonable time period, which partially overcomes the difficulty in obtaining dynamic images with MR imaging in young children (Figs. 15–91 and 15–92). MR imaging, however, should not be used for initial diagnosis or evaluation of routine DDH but rather should be reserved for complicated cases in which initial treatment has been unsuccessful.[344]

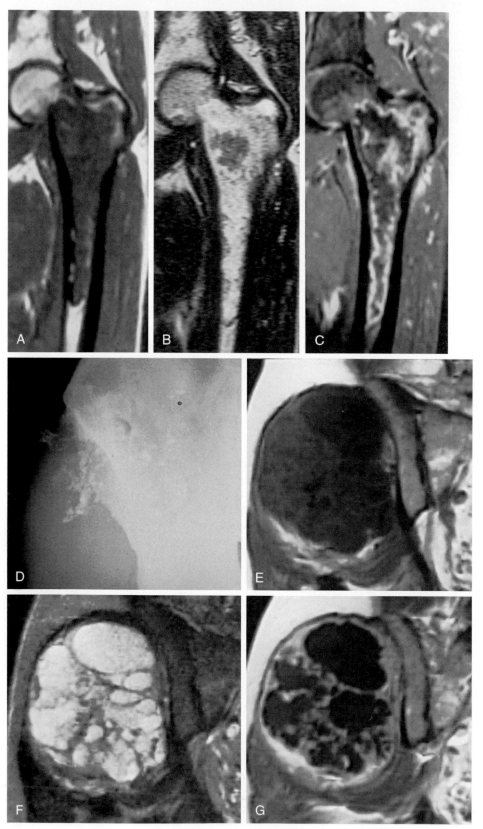

Figure 15–86
Conventional chondrosarcoma, MR imaging.

A–C Central type. A coronal T1-weighted (TR/TE, 500/16) spin echo MR image (**A**) demonstrates the tumor of low signal intensity involving the femoral neck and shaft. In the coronal plane, with T2 weighting (TR/TE, 4000/102), the tumor is inhomogeneous but mainly of high signal intensity (**B**). A coronal, fat-suppressed, intravenous gadolinium-enhanced T1-weighted (TR/TE, 600/16) spin echo MR image (**C**) shows irregular enhancement of signal intensity in the tumor.

(Courtesy of D. Goodwin, M.D., Hanover, New Hampshire.)

D–G Peripheral type. Routine radiograph (**D**) reveals a calcified lesion extending from the ilium. Note the large size of the tumor and its low signal intensity in a coronal T1-weighted (TR/TE, 700/15) spin echo MR image (**E**). In a coronal T2-weighted (TR/TE, 2500/90) spin echo MR image (**F**), the tumor is lobulated, is mainly of high signal intensity, and contains septations of low signal intensity. Following the intravenous administration of a gadolinium compound, a coronal T1-weighted (TR/TE, 700/15) spin echo MR image (**G**) shows irregular enhancement of signal intensity in portions of the tumor.

(Courtesy of J. Kramer, M.D., Vienna, Austria.)

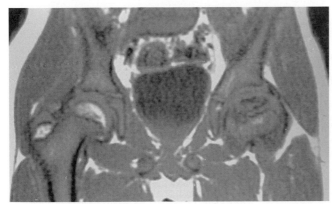

Figure 15–87

Legg-Calvé-Perthes disease: MR imaging. A coronal T1-weighted (TR/TE, 400/15) spin echo MR image shows involvement of the left hip. Findings include an irregular ossification center with abnormally low signal intensity of the left femoral head and prominent cartilage in the adjacent acetabulum. (Courtesy of D. Goodwin, M.D., Hanover, New Hampshire.)

Proximal Femoral Focal Deficiency

Proximal femoral focal deficiency (PFFD) is the term applied to a spectrum of conditions characterized by partial absence and shortening of the proximal portion of the femur.[352–359] Although some cases of PFFD are associated with other skeletal defects, including aplasia of the cruciate ligaments of the knee,[360] this disorder usually is an isolated occurrence, appearing in a unilateral fashion in 90 per cent of patients. A variety of classification systems have been suggested on the basis of presence and location of the femoral head and neck.[352, 358, 359] The designation of a specific type of PFFD in an individual patient may require both radiography and arthrography.[361, 362] The role of MR imaging in the classification of the disorder is promising (Fig. 15–93) but not entirely clear.

Infantile Coxa Vara

The term coxa vara indicates a neck-shaft angle that is less than 120 degrees despite the variation of normal values that occurs in different age groups. Coxa vara may accompany various processes, including PFFD, osteogenesis imperfecta, renal osteodystrophy, rickets, and fibrous dysplasia.[362] Infantile or developmental coxa vara is a designation of a proximal femoral deformity that usually becomes apparent in the first few years of life. The condition is unilateral in 60 to 75 per cent of cases.[363] Clinically, the affected child has a painless lurching gait or, in the case of bilateral involvement, a "duck-waddle" gait.[364–369]

Radiographs reveal a decrease in the femoral shaft-neck angle and a medially located triangular piece of bone in the neck adjacent to the head. The growth plate itself is widened, and its alignment is more vertical than normal. MR imaging reveals a widened growth plate with expansion of cartilage mediodistally between the capital femoral epiphysis and metaphysis.[370]

Primary Protrusion of the Acetabulum

Protrusio acetabuli can appear in the absence of any recognizable cause, and, in such a case, it is termed primary acetabular protrusion. The primary variety is sometimes referred to as Otto pelvis.[371] A failure of ossification[372, 373] or premature fusion[374] of the Y cartilage has been offered as a possible etiologic factor. The deformity also may be the direct result of a failure of normal acetabular remodeling.[375] Primary acetabular protrusion usually affects both hips and is much more frequent in women than in men. With progressive protrusion deformity, the femoral head assumes an intrapelvic location, and the joint space may be normal, narrowed, or obliterated.

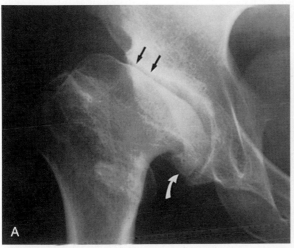 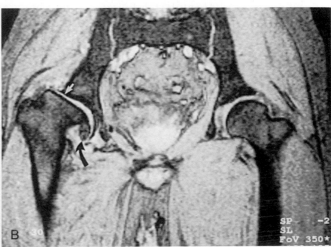

Figure 15–88

Legg-Calvé-Perthes disease: MR imaging.

A In this adult, routine radiography shows a deformed and flattened femoral head containing a medial osteophyte (curved arrow), a broad and short femoral neck, and a narrowed joint space (straight arrows).

B This coronal fast low angle shot (FLASH) MR image (TR/TE, 400/10; flip angle, 30 degrees) shows these same findings (arrows). Compare to the opposite side.

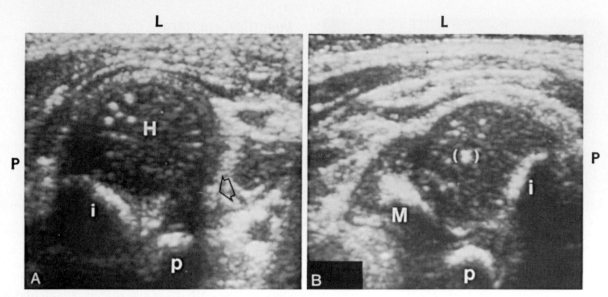

Figure 15–89
Developmental dysplasia of the hip: Ultrasonography.
  A Transaxial image of right subluxatable hip after stress. The femoral head (H) has subluxated posteriorly and laterally with respect to acetabulum.
  B Contralateral normal left hip for comparison. More advanced maturation of the femoral head ossific nucleus (parentheses) is evident.
  i, Ischium; p, pubis; arrow, echogenicity within acetabular fossa; L, lateral; P, posterior; M, femoral metaphysis.

Multiple Epiphyseal Dysplasias

A detailed discussion of multiple epiphyseal dysplasias is beyond the scope of this text. Radiographs reveal characteristic irregularity and flattening of epiphyseal ossification centers. Arthrography, CT scanning, or a combination of the two methods can be used to assess the status of the cartilaginous portions of the femoral head and the relationship between the femoral epiphysis and the acetabulum. With MR imaging, normal signal intensity is observed in the marrow of the femoral heads in most cases, allowing differentiation of multiple epiphyseal dysplasias from Legg-Calvé-Perthes disease.[49] Diagnostic difficulties are encountered, however, owing to some variability and heterogeneity in the signal intensity

secondary to the irregular ossification of the femoral heads that occurs in epiphyseal dysplasias and occasional reports that indicate the occurrence of osteonecrosis of the femoral heads in patients with these dysplasias.[49]

Meyer's Dysplasia

Meyer's dysplasia represents either a mild localized epiphyseal dysplasia limited to the femoral capital epiphyses or a normal variant of ossification.[376–378] Most cases are discovered as an incidental finding on hip or pelvic radiographs obtained for other reasons. Radiographic studies reveal delayed ossification of the femoral heads. As the femoral capital epiphyses begin to ossify, granular

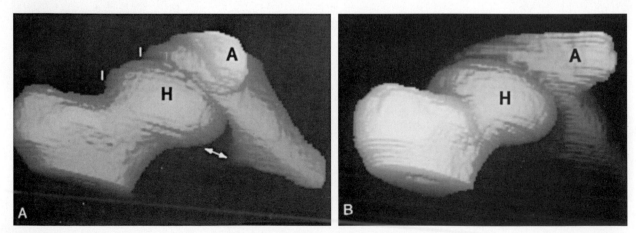

Figure 15–90
Developmental dysplasia of the hip (DDH): CT scanning—three-dimensional CT scan in untreated DDH. Anterior **(A)** and right anterior oblique **(B)** images reveal an aspherical femoral head (H) with diminished lateral coverage (vertical lines), as well as femoral-acetabular (A) incongruence (double-headed arrow).

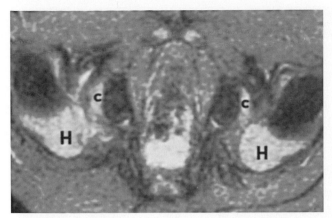

Figure 15–91
Developmental dysplasia of the hip (DDH): MR imaging in bilateral DDH. Transaxial gradient echo image (TR/TE, 100/25; flip angle, 40 degrees) reveals posterior dislocation of both femoral heads (H). c, Triradiate cartilage. (Courtesy of A. Poznanski, M.D., Chicago, Illinois.)

foci or multiple irregular centers develop with an abnormal flattened appearance. As growth continues, serial radiographic studies reveal a return to the normal hemispherical shape of the femoral heads. Unlike the case with osteonecrosis, the changes are bilaterally symmetric in 50 per cent of cases, no predilection for the superior aspect of the femoral heads is seen, the density of the epiphyses is not increased, and the children usually are younger. In Meyer's dysplasia, all three phases of the radionuclide bone scan (blood flow, blood pool, static) are normal, and the signal intensity of the multiple foci in the femoral head are normal on all MR imaging sequences. These imaging methods allow definitive exclusion of an ischemic process such as Legg-Calvé-Perthes disease.

Soft Tissue Abnormalities

Snapping Hip Syndrome

A variety of causes have been implicated in the hip pain associated with an audible snapping. Intra-articular abnormalities, including single or multiple osteocartilaginous bodies, typically result in a faint sound associated with true femoral-acetabular motion; extra-articular causes often are characterized by a loud snap and, in some cases, a sudden jump of the fascia lata or gluteus maximus over the greater trochanter as the hip moves in a well-delineated fashion.[379] Other proposed causes have included slipping of the iliopsoas tendon over the iliopectineal eminence,[380] of the tendon of the long head of the biceps femoris muscle over the ischial tuberosity, and of the iliofemoral ligaments over the anterior portion of the hip capsule.[381]

Several studies[379, 382–384, 414] have confirmed that subluxation of the iliopsoas tendon is one cause of a snapping hip. Iliopsoas bursography,[382, 385, 415] iliopsoas tenography,[383] or hip arthrography in which the iliopsoas bursa also is opacified[379] confirms the changing position of the iliopsoas tendon and its displacement over the iliopectineal line during flexion and extension of the hip. An abrupt change in the position of the tendon coincident with the audible sound and palpable snap is observed. Ultrasonography also can be used to provide a correct diagnosis.[416]

Calcific Tendinitis and Bursitis

Calcium hydroxyapatite crystal deposition may involve tendons and bursae throughout the body. In the hip, pelvis, and thigh, calcific deposits are frequent in the gluteal insertions into the greater trochanter and in the surrounding bursae, where they appear as single or multiple cloudlike linear, triangular, or circular radio-

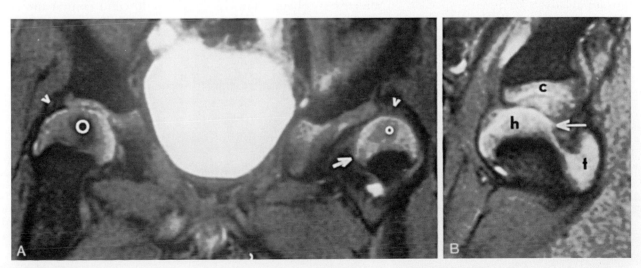

Figure 15–92
Developmental dysplasia of the hip: Gradient echo MR imaging.
  A Coronal image (TR/TE, 100/25) reveals lateral subluxation of the left femur (arrow), and a secondary ossification center that is delayed in development (O > o). Both acetabular labra are in the normal everted position (arrowheads).
  B Sagittal image (TR/TE, 100/25) demonstrates mild anterior subluxation of the femoral head (arrow). Note the continuity between the cartilaginous femoral head (h) and the greater trochanter (T). c, Triradiate cartilage.

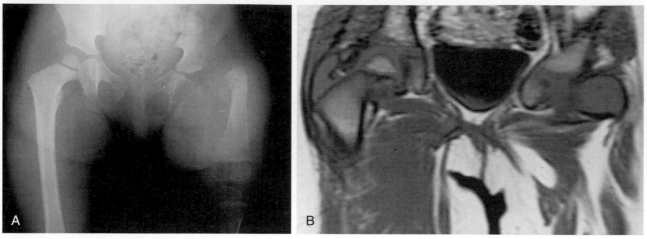

Figure 15-93
Proximal femoral focal deficiency (PFFD): MR imaging. Routine radiography **(A)** and a coronal T1-weighted (TR/TE, 800/11) spin echo MR image **(B)** in a 4 year old girl show absence of ossification in the proximal portion of the left femur. The unossified cartilage in the femoral epiphysis and metaphysis is well shown in **B**. (Courtesy of J. Spaeth, M.D., Albuquerque, New Mexico.)

dense areas (Fig. 15-94). These radiodense regions also may be observed adjacent to the acetabular margin, lesser trochanter, and lateral and medial aspects of the proximal end of the femur. They may relate to other tendinous structures, such as the piriformis, rectus femoris (Fig. 15-95), vastus lateralis, adductor magnus, and biceps femoris tendons.[418] Differentiation among these sites of calcification is difficult, as is differentiation between painful calcification about the acetabulum and os acetabuli. At any of these locations, subjacent erosion of bone may be observed.[386, 387]

Large, tumor-like calcifications about the hip may be encountered in patients with chronic renal disease or collagen vascular disorders (Fig. 15-96).

Muscle and Soft Tissue Injury

Muscular and myotendinous injuries about the pelvis and hip are relatively frequent, especially in athletes.

The pelvic ring and proximal portion of the femur are the sites of origin or insertion for several major muscle groups (Fig. 15-97): the insertion of the abdominal muscles on the iliac wing; the origin of the gluteal muscles from the ilium and their insertion in the proximal portion of the femur; the origin of the adductor muscles from the pubis; the origin of the hamstring muscles from the ischial tuberosity; and the insertion of the iliopsoas muscle in the lesser trochanter.[28] The types of injury vary in the severity (e.g., partial or complete tears of the muscle) and according to the age of the patient (e.g., apophyseal avulsion injuries may be seen in the adolescent) (see Chapter 10). Typical examples of athletic injuries include iliopsoas tendon strains caused by forceful contraction of the iliopsoas muscle when the thigh is fixed or in an extended position, as in soccer players; strains of the aponeurosis of the external oblique muscle caused by forceful contracture of the

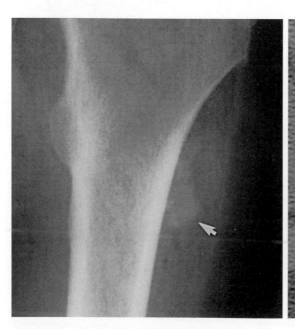

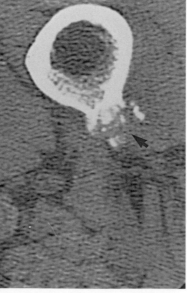

Figure 15-94
Calcific tendinitis: CT scanning. Note calcification (arrows) in the tendon of the gluteus maximus muscle in a routine radiograph **(A)** and transaxial CT scan **(B)**. Subjacent cortical erosion is evident in **B**. (Courtesy of G. Bock, M.D., Winnipeg, Manitoba, Canada.)

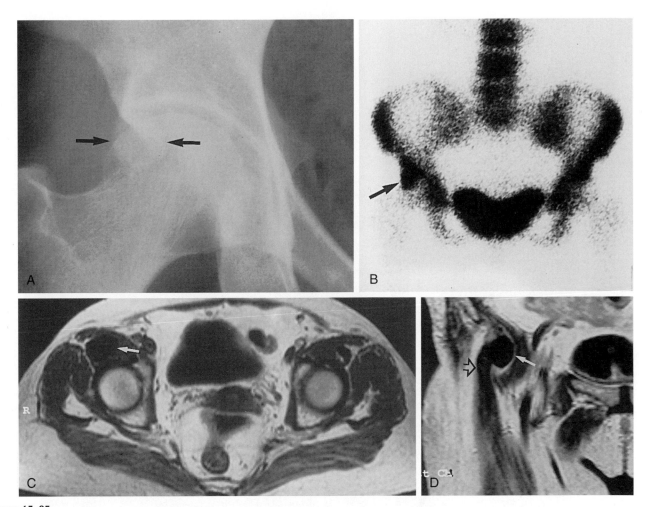

Figure 15–95
Calcific tendinitis: Bone scintigraphy and MR imaging. Hip pain developed in this 55 year old woman.
   A Routine radiograph shows circular calcification (arrows) adjacent to the acetabulum.
   B With bone scintigraphy, increased accumulation of the radionuclide is evident (arrow).
   C A transverse T1-weighted (TR/TE, 500/15) spin echo MR image reveals the site of calcification as a region of low signal intensity (arrow).
   D After intravenous administration of a gadolinium contrast agent, a coronal T1-weighted (TR/TE, 500/15) spin echo MR image shows enhancement of signal intensity (solid arrow) about the calcific focus, which is located in the tendon of the rectus femoris muscle (open arrow).

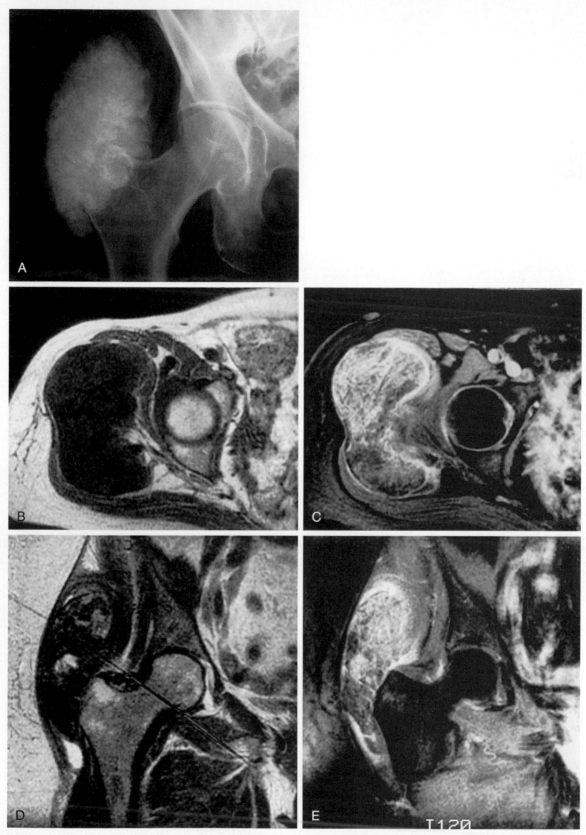

Figure 15–96
See legend on opposite page

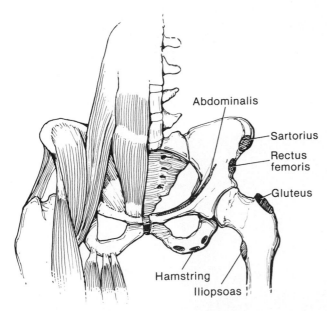

Figure 15–97

Anterior view of the pelvis showing muscular origins and insertions. (Reproduced with permission from Gross ML, Nasser S, Finerman GAM: Hip and pelvis. *In* JC DeLee, D Drez [Eds]: Orthopaedic Sports Medicine: Principles and Practice. Philadelphia, WB Saunders Co. 1994, p. 1063.)

abdominal muscles while the trunk is forced to the contralateral side, as in American football and hockey players; and adductor muscle injuries ("pulled groin") caused by forceful external rotation of an abducted leg, as in soccer and hockey players.[28] Of the adductor muscles, the gracilis muscle is particularly vulnerable because it spans two joints (i.e., hip and knee), and these muscles may be injured in long distance runners. At any of these sites, ultrasonography and MR imaging represent effective diagnostic techniques (Figs. 15–98 and 15–99).

The hamstring muscles (i.e., semimembranosus, semitendinosus, and biceps femoris muscles) arise as a conjoined tendon at the posterolateral aspect of the ischial tuberosity, except for the short head of the biceps femoris muscle, which originates at the posterior aspect of the middle and distal thirds of the femur.[388] In addition, a portion of the adductor magnus muscle functions as a hip extensor and acts as a hamstring muscle.[389] Injuries to the hamstring muscles usually occur at the proximal end (as opposed to their distal insertions

about the knee), involving the tendon itself or the myotendinous junction. They are often seen in athletes, including American football and baseball players. In adolescents, routine radiography may show avulsion of portions of the ischial apophysis or the entire apophysis. MR imaging may reveal damage to the conjoined tendon or muscle, information that may be useful for the referring physician who is contemplating conservative (the usual therapeutic choice) or surgical management.[388]

The quadriceps group is composed of four muscles in the anterior aspect of the thigh that insert distally as a conjoined tendon into the proximal portion of the patella. Of these muscles, the rectus femoris muscle is unique as it spans the hip joint. The other three muscles (i.e., vastus medialis, vastus intermedius, and vastus lateralis) do not cross the hip joint. Strains of the quadriceps musculature relate to excessive contraction and are encountered in American football and basketball players and track and field athletes. A typical site of injury is at the insertion site of the rectus femoris muscle into the quadriceps tendon, and the injury leads to thigh pain and a mass (e.g., hematoma). Myositis ossificans (i.e., posttraumatic heterotopic bone formation) may complicate this injury.

Myonecrosis (Fig. 15–100) and decubitus ulcers (Fig. 15–101) occur in debilitated persons who maintain a single position for long periods of time. With MR imaging, myonecrosis is associated with findings that resemble those of pyomyositis. Soft tissue hematomas (Fig. 15–102) may relate to direct injury, as sustained from a fall.

Neurovascular Entrapment Syndromes

As indicated in Chapter 11, several types of nerve entrapment syndromes occur about the hip. Examples of these include the piriformis syndrome (entrapment of the sciatic nerve by the piriformis muscle), entrapment of the obturator nerve in the obturator canal (which may accompany an obturator hernia or osteitis pubis), and entrapment of the femoral nerve in the inguinal region of the pelvis (which relates to many different causes, including tumors, abscesses, aneurysms, and bleeding).

The adductor canal syndrome is characterized by entrapment of the superficial femoral artery in the adductor canal (Hunter's canal).[390] This aponeurotic canal (Fig. 15–103) is located in the middle third of the thigh

Text continued on page 548

Figure 15–96

Soft tissue calcification: MR imaging, periarticular tumoral deposits in chronic renal disease.

A The routine radiograph shows a large tumor-like region of soft tissue calcification about the greater trochanter.

B A transverse T1-weighted (TR/TE, 350/11) spin echo MR image reveals a mass of low signal intensity displacing the gluteal muscles.

C A transverse spoiled GRASS (SPGR) MR image (TR/TE, 449/3; flip angle, 70 degrees) obtained with fat suppression after intravenous administration of gadolinium contrast agent shows irregular enhancement of signal intensity within the mass.

D A coronal fast spin echo MR image (TR/TE, 3000/91) demonstrates inhomogeneous but mainly low to intermediate signal intensity in the mass. Small fluid collections of high signal intensity are evident.

E A coronal SPGR MR image (TR/TE, 299/2; flip angle, 70 degrees) obtained with fat suppression after the intravenous administration of gadolinium contrast agent again shows irregular enhancement of signal intensity within the mass. Its location is consistent with a peritrochanteric bursa but, without the routine radiograph, an erroneous diagnosis of a soft tissue tumor might be considered.

(Courtesy of S. K. Brahme, M.D., San Diego, California.)

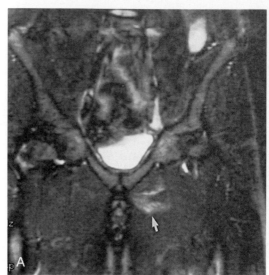
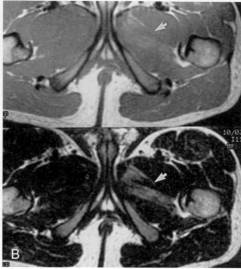

Figure 15–98

Muscle strain: MR imaging. An adductor muscle strain (grade 1) is characterized by regions of high signal intensity (arrows) on a coronal fast spin echo STIR (TR/TE, 5000/51; inversion time, 150 msec) MR image (**A**) and on transaxial proton density–weighted (TR/TE, 3600/13) (**B**, top image) and T2-weighted (TR/TE, 3600/104) (**B**, bottom image) spin echo MR images.

Figure 15–99

Muscle tear: Ultrasonography. Longitudinal scans of the abnormal (**A**) and normal (**B**) thighs, with the anterior aspect of the thighs at the top of the images and the cephalad aspect of the body to the left, reveal a complete tear (arrow) of the rectus femoris muscle (arrowheads) in **A** and a normal rectus femoris muscle (arrowheads) in **B**. The abnormal muscle is retracted proximally. (Courtesy of J. Jacobson, M.D., San Diego, California.)

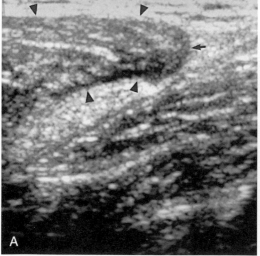
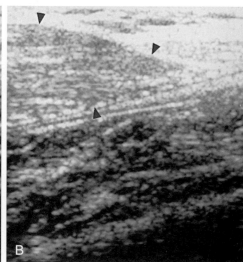

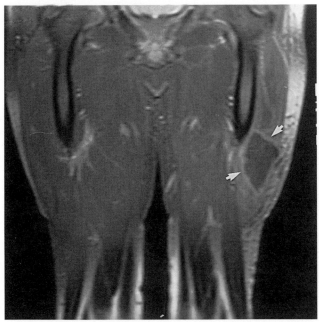

Figure 15–100
Myonecrosis. On a coronal T1-weighted (TR/TE, 400/11) spin echo MR image, obtained with fat suppression and after intravenous administration of a gadolinium contrast agent, peripheral enhancement of signal intensity (arrows) about the necrotic focus is evident. Subcutaneous edema also is noted.

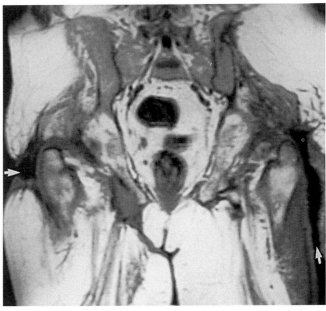

Figure 15–101
Decubitus ulcers. This coronal T1-weighted (TR/TE, 666/12) spin echo MR image of a 41 year old paraplegic man shows bilateral decubitus ulcers (arrows) with sinus tracts extending from the skin to the greater trochanter of both femora.

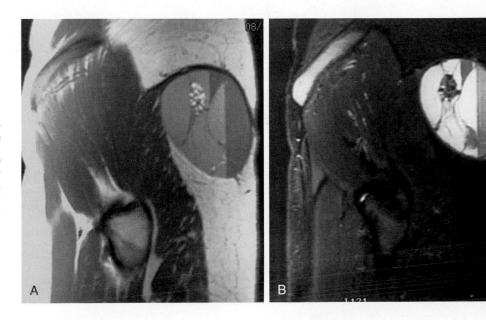

Figure 15–102
Soft tissue hematoma. Sagittal T1-weighted (TR/TE, 500/16) (**A**) and fast spin echo STIR (TR/TE, 6500/51; inversion time, 150 msec) (**B**) MR images in a 15 year old girl who had sustained a fall show a buttock hematoma with fluid levels. (Courtesy of D. Witte, M.D., Memphis, Tennessee.)

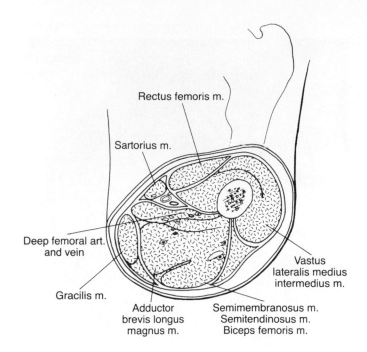

Figure 15–103
Adducter canal: Anatomy. (Reproduced with permission from Brunet ME, Hontas RB: The thigh. In JC DeLee, D Drez Jr [Eds]: Orthopaedic Sports Medicine: Principles and Practice. Philadelphia, WB Saunders Co, 1994, p 1109.)

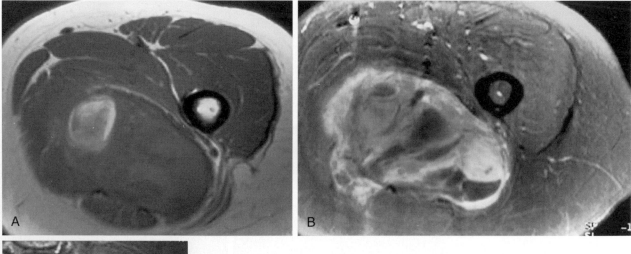

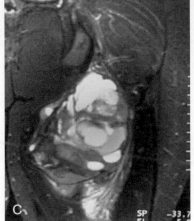

Figure 15–104
Synovial sarcoma: MR imaging. The extent of this tumor in the thigh is well shown in a transverse T1-weighted (TR/TE, 690/14) spin echo MR image **(A)**, a transaxial fat-suppressed, gadolinium-enhanced T1-weighted (TR/TE, 820/12) spin echo MR image **(B)**, and a coronal fat-suppressed fast spin echo (TR/TE, 6846/60) MR image **(C)**. (Courtesy of T. Learch, M.D., Los Angeles, California.)

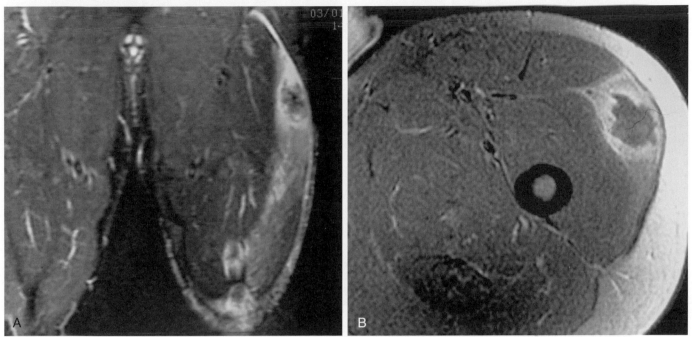

Figure 15–105
Nodular fasciitis: MR imaging. This superficial lesion of the thigh is inhomogeneous in signal intensity in a coronal fast spin echo STIR (TR/TE, 6000/39; inversion time, 150 msec) MR image **(A)**. The transaxial fat-suppressed, gadolinium-enhanced T1-weighted (TR/TE, 700/11) spin echo MR image **(B)** shows a central, nonenhanced region and peripheral enhancement. (Courtesy of B. Edwards, M.D. and D. Witte, M.D., Memphis, Tennessee.)

Figure 15–106
Neurofibromatosis: MR imaging. A coronal T2-weighted (TR/TE, 2000/80) spin echo MR image demonstrates an elongated and lobulated neurofibroma of high signal intensity involving the sciatic nerve. Although not shown in this image, a smaller tumor was present on the opposite side. (Courtesy of A. G. Bergman, M.D., Stanford, California.)

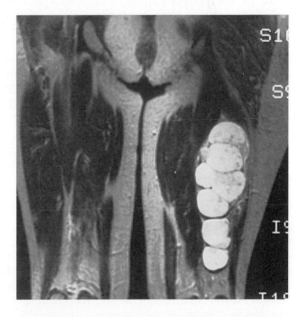

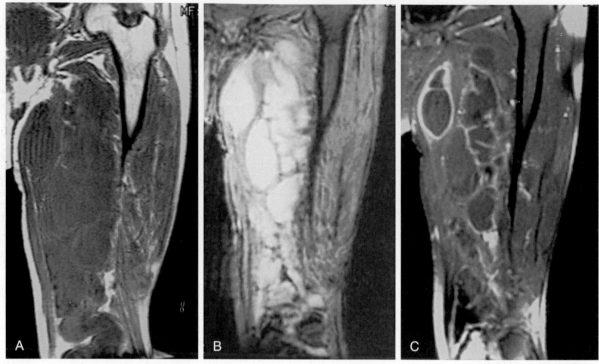

Figure 15–107

Echinococcosis: MR imaging. A large soft tissue mass, composed of individual cystic lesions, is shown in a coronal T1-weighted (TR/TE, 600/12) spin echo MR image (**A**), a coronal MPGR (TR/TE, 740/18; flip angle, 15 degrees) MR image (**B**), and a coronal T1-weighted (TR/TE, 440/18) spin echo MR image obtained after the intravenous injection of a gadolinium compound (**C**). Note enhancement of signal intensity in the wall of the cysts in **C**. (Courtesy of E. Bosch, M.D., Santiago, Chile.)

and is bounded anterolaterally by the vastus medialis muscle, medially by the sartorius muscle, and posterolaterally by the adductor longus muscle. The femoral artery, femoral vein, and saphenous nerve pass through this space.[390] The precise cause of the syndrome is not clear, although an abnormal musculotendinous band arising from the adductor muscle or direct injury to the artery has been implicated.[391] Entrapment of the saphenous nerve at this site also may occur.[392] Typically, affected patients are young, athletic, and otherwise healthy. Exertional claudication of the leg is evident, and accurate diagnosis can be provided by Doppler sonographic studies or arteriography.[390]

Soft Tissue Tumors and Infections

The thigh is a common site for a variety of soft tissue tumors, both benign and malignant, including lipomas, liposarcomas, malignant fibrous histiocytomas, synovial sarcomas (Fig. 15–104), hemangiomas, nodular fasciitis (Fig. 15–105), and neurogenic neoplasms (Fig. 15–106). The MR imaging features generally lack specificity and, further, differentiation of many benign and malignant soft tissue tumors is not possible using MR imaging. Indeed, some types of infectious processes produce soft tissue masses simulating neoplasms (Fig. 15–107). As with bone tumors, MR imaging is effective in delineating the full extent of neoplastic and infectious processes of soft tissue, and intravenous administration of a gadolinium compound represents an effective imaging strategy.

Other Abnormalities

Sacroiliac Joint Sprain

Although numerous strong ligaments support the sacroiliac joint, including the anterior and posterior sacroiliac, interosseous, and sacrotuberous ligaments, stretching and tearing of these ligaments may occur, particularly in certain situations[28]: sudden violent contraction of the hamstring or abdominal muscles; sudden torsion; a severe, direct blow to the buttocks; or forceful straightening from a crouched position. Local pain or pain radiating to the back, thigh, and groin is noted. The diagnosis may be confirmed on physical examination using specific provocative tests, such as compression of the iliac wings, that induce pain.[28] The role of imaging methods in the assessment of these sprains appears limited.

SUMMARY

Abnormalities of the pelvis and hip are common and include major injuries (dislocations and fractures), occult injuries (stress fractures and labral tears), osteonecrosis of the femoral head, transient bone marrow edema, cartilage degeneration and chondrolysis, synovial abnormalities (including synovial cysts and iliopsoas bursal enlargement), developmental abnormalities, and soft tissue, tendon, and muscle disorders. Routine radiography represents the most important imaging method applied to the initial assessment of these disorders, although arthrography, ultrasonography, CT scanning, and MR imaging are required in certain situations, both for improved diagnosis and in treatment planning.

REFERENCES

1. Johnstone WH, Keats TE, Lee ME: The anatomic basis for the superior acetabular roof notch: "Superior acetabular notch." Skel Radiol 8:25, 1982.
2. Wiberg G: Studies on dysplastic acetabula and congenital subluxation of the hip joint—with special reference to the complication of osteoarthritis. Acta Chir Scand Suppl 58:1, 1939.
3. Hooper JC, Jones EW: Primary protrusion of the acetabulum. J Bone Joint Surg [Br] 53:23, 1971.
4. Armbuster TG, Guerra J Jr, Resnick D, et al: The adult hip: An anatomic study. I. The bony landmarks. Radiology 128:1, 1978.
5. Judet R, Judet J, Letournal E: Fractures of the acetabulum: Classification and surgical approaches for open reduction—preliminary report. J Bone Joint Surg [Am] 46:1615, 1964.
6. Goodman SB, Adler SJ, Fyhrie DP, et al: The acetabular teardrop and its relevance to acetabular migration. Clin Orthop 236:199, 1988.
7. Bowerman JW, Sena JM, Chang R: The teardrop shadow of the pelvis: Anatomy and clinical significance. Radiology 143:659, 1982.
8. Gusis SE, Babini JC, Garay SM, et al: Evaluation of the measurement methods for protrusio acetabuli in normal children. Skel Radiol 19:279, 1990.
9. Stein MG, Barmeir E, Levin J, et al: The medial acetabular wall: Normal measurements in different population groups. Invest Radiol 17:476, 1982.
10. Rubenstein J, Kellam J, McGonigal D: Cross-sectional anatomy of the adult bony acetabulum. Can Assoc Radiol J 33:137, 1982.
11. Pogrund H, Bloom R, Mogle P: The normal width of the adult hip joint: The relationship to age, sex, and obesity. Skel Radiol 10:10, 1983.
12. Gregorczyk A, Pospula W, Golda W: Radiological and computed tomographic studies of the width of the normal hip joint in men aged 30–60 years. Röntgenblatter 43:141, 1990.
13. Hefke HW, Turner VC: The obturator sign as the earliest roentgenographic sign in the diagnosis of septic arthritis and tuberculosis of the hip. J Bone Joint Surg 24:857, 1942.
14. Jorup S, Kjellberg SR: The early diagnosis of acute septic osteomyelitis, periostitis and arthritis and its importance in the treatment. Acta Radiol (Diagn) 30:316, 1948.
15. Drey L: A roentgenographic study of transitory synovitis of the hip joint. Radiology 60:588, 1953.
16. Bartley O, Chidekel N: Roentgenologic changes in postoperative septic osteoarthritis of the hip joint. Acta Radiol (Diagn) 4:113, 1966.
17. Lewis MS, Norman A: The earliest signs of postoperative hip infection. Radiology 104:325, 1972.
18. Brown I: A study of the "capsular" shadow in disorders of the hip in children. J Bone Joint Surg [Br] 57:175, 1975.
19. Reichmann S: Roentgenologic soft tissue appearances in hip disease. Acta Radiol (Diagn) 6:167, 1967.
20. Guerra J Jr, Armbuster TG, Resnick D, et al: The adult hip: An anatomic study. II. The soft-tissue landmarks. Radiology 128:11, 1978.
21. Lange M: Die Erleichterung der Frühdiagnose der Koxitis durch bisher wenig beachtete Veränderungen im Röntgenbild. Z Orthop Chir 48:90, 1927.
22. Armstrong P, Saxton H: Iliopsoas bursa. Br J Radiol 45:493, 1972.
23. Chandler SB: The iliopsoas bursa in man. Anat Rec 58:235, 1934.
24. Staple TW: Arthrographic demonstration of the iliopsoas bursa extension of the hip joint. Radiology 102:515, 1972.
25. Last RJ: Anatomy: Regional and Applied. 5th Ed. London, Churchill Livingstone, 1972, p. 211.
26. Weston WJ: The bursae deep to gluteus medius and minimus. Australas Radiol 14:325, 1970.
27. Levin P: Hip dislocations. In BD Browner, JB Jupiter, AM Levine, et al (Eds): Skeletal Trauma: Fractures, Dislocations, Ligamentous Injuries. Philadelphia, WB Saunders Co, 1992, p. 1329.
28. Gross ML, Nasser S, Finerman GAM: Hip and pelvis. In JC DeLee, D Drez Jr (Eds): Orthopaedic Sports Medicine: Principles and Practice. Philadelphia, WB Saunders Co, 1994, p. 1063.
29. Johnson RC, Schmidt GL: Hip motion measurements for selected activities of daily living. Clin Orthop 72:205, 1970.
30. Morris JM: Biomechanical aspects of the hip joint. Orthop Clin North Am 2:33, 1971.
31. Heubelin GW, Greene GS, Conforti VP: Hip joint arthrography. AJR 68:736, 1952.
32. Kenin A, Levine J: A technique for arthrography of the hip. AJR 68:107, 1952.
33. Kilcoyne RF, Kaplan P: The lateral approach for hip arthrography. Skel Radiol 21:239, 1992.
34. Mitchell GP: Arthrography in congenital displacement of the hip. J Bone Joint Surg [Br] 45:88, 1963.
35. Astley R: Arthrography in congenital dislocation of the hip. Clin Radiol 18:253, 1967.
36. Schwartz AM, Goldberg MJ: The medial adductor approach to arthrography of the hip in children. Radiology 132:483, 1979.
37. Ozonoff MB: Controlled arthrography of the hip: A technic of fluoroscopic monitoring and recording. Clin Orthop 93:260, 1973.
38. Strife JL, Towbin R, Crawford A: Hip arthrography in infants and children: The inferomedial approach. Radiology 152:536, 1984.
39. Crawford AH, Carothers TA: Hip arthrography in the skeletally immature. Clin Orthop 162:54, 1982.
40. Newberg AH, Wetzner SM: Digital subtraction arthrography. Radiology 154:238, 1985.
41. Salvati EA, Ghelman B, McLaren T, et al: Subtraction technique in arthrography for loosening of total hip replacement fixed with radiopaque cement. Clin Orthop 101:105, 1974.
42. Resnick D, Kerr R, André M, et al: Digital arthrography in the evaluation of painful joint prostheses. Invest Radiol 19:432, 1984.
43. Walker CW, FitzRandolph RL, Collins DN, et al: Arthrography of painful hips following arthroplasty: Digital versus plain film subtraction. Skel Radiol 20:403, 1991.
44. Kelcz F, Peppler WW, Mistretta CA, et al: K-edge digital subtraction arthrography of the painful hip prosthesis: A feasibility study. AJR 155:1053, 1990.
45. Swan JS, Braunstein EM, Capello W: Aspiration of the hip in patients treated with Girdlestone arthroplasty. AJR 156:545, 1991.
46. Cone RO, Yaru N, Resnick D, et al: Intracapsular pressure monitoring during arthrographic evaluation of painful hip prostheses. AJR 141:885, 1983.
47. Hendrix RW, Wixson RL, Rana NA, et al: Arthrography after total hip arthroplasty: A modified technique used in the diagnosis of pain. Radiology 148:647, 1983.
48. Razzano CD, Nelson CL, Wilde AH: Arthrography of the adult hip. Clin Orthop 99:86, 1974.
49. Gabriel H, Fitzgerald SW, Myers MT, et al: MR imaging of hip disorders. Radiographics 14:763, 1994.
50. Stutley JE, Conway WF: Magnetic resonance imaging of the pelvis and hips. Orthopedics 17:1053, 1994.
51. Do-Dai DD, Youngberg RA: MRI of the hip with a shoulder surface coil in off-coronal plane. J Comput Assist Tomogr 19:336, 1995.
52. Resnik CS, Stackhouse DJ, Shanmuganathan K, et al: Diagnosis of pelvic fractures in patients with acute pelvic trauma: Efficiency of plain radiographs. AJR 158:109, 1992.
53. Edeiken-Monroe BS, Browner BD, Jackson H: The role of standard roentgenograms in the evaluation of instability of pelvic ring disruption. Clin Orthop 240:63, 1989.
54. Weil GC, Price EM, Rusbridge HW: The diagnosis and treatment of fractures of the pelvis and their complications. Am J Surg 44:108, 1939.
55. Pennal GF, Tile M, Waddell JP, et al: Pelvic disruption: Assessment and classification. Clin Orthop 151:12, 1980.
56. Watson-Jones R: Dislocations and fracture-dislocations of the pelvis. Br J Surg 25:773, 1938.
57. Huttinen VM, Slatis P: Fractures of the pelvis: Trauma mechanism, types of injury, and principles of treatment. Acta Chir Scand 137:576, 1971.
58. Conolly WB, Hedberg EA: Observations on fractures of the pelvis. J Trauma 9:104, 1969.
59. Looser KG, Crombie HD Jr: Pelvic fractures: An anatomic guide to severity of injury. Am J Surg 132:638, 1976.
60. Trunkey DD, Chapman MW, Lim RC Jr, et al: Management of pelvic fractures in blunt trauma injury. J Trauma 14:912, 1974.
61. Young JWR, Burgess AR, Brumback RJ, et al: Pelvic fractures: Value of plain radiography in early assessment and management. Radiology 160:445, 1986.
62. Young JWR, Resnick CS: Fracture of the pelvis: Current concepts of classification. AJR 155:1169, 1990.
63. Dalal SA, Burgess AR, Siegel JH, et al: Pelvic fracture in multiple trauma: Classification by mechanism is key to pattern of organ injury, resuscitative requirements, and outcome. J Trauma 29:981, 1989.
64. Tile M: Fractures of the Pelvis and Acetabulum. Baltimore, Williams & Wilkins Co, 1984.
65. Tile M: Pelvic ring fractures: Should they be fixed? J Bone Joint Surg [Br] 70:1, 1988.
66. Gill K, Bucholz RW: The role of computerized tomographic scanning in the evaluation of major pelvic fractures. J Bone Joint Surg [Am] 66:34, 1984.
67. Kane WJ: Fractures of the pelvis. In CA Rockwood Jr, DP Green (Eds): Fractures in Adults. 2nd Ed. Philadelphia, JB Lippincott Co, 1984, p. 1093.
68. Rankin LM: Fractures of the pelvis. Ann Surg 106:266, 1937.
69. Fountain SS, Hamilton RM, Jameson RM: Transverse fractures of the sacrum: A report of six cases. J Bone Joint Surg [Am] 59:486, 1977.
70. Montana MA, Richardson ML, Kilcoyne RF, et al: CT of sacral injury. Radiology 161:499, 1986.
71. Sabiston CP, Wing PC: Sacral fractures: Classification and neurologic implications. J Trauma 26:1113, 1986.
72. Jackson H, Kam J, Harris JH Jr, et al: The sacral arcuate lines in upper sacral fractures. Radiology 145:35, 1982.

73. Northrop CH, Eto RT, Loop JW: Vertical fracture of the sacral ala: Significance of non-continuity of the anterior superior sacral foraminal line. AJR *124*:102, 1975.
74. Shild H, Muller HA, Klose K, Ahlers J, Huwel N: Anatomie, Rontgenologie und Klinik der Sakrumfrakturen. ROFO *134*:522, 1981.
75. Balseiro J, Brower AC, Ziessman HA: Scintigraphic diagnosis of sacral fractures. AJR *148*:111, 1987.
76. Byrd JWT: Labral lesions: An elusive source of hip pain. Case reports and literature review. Arthroscopy *12*:603, 1996.
77. Berg PM: Acute pelvic disruption, the bucking horse injury. Orthop Trans *3*:271, 1979.
78. Peltier LF: Complications associated with fractures of the pelvis. J Bone Joint Surg [Am] *47*:1060, 1965.
79. Holdsworth FW: Dislocations and fracture-dislocations of the pelvis. J Bone Joint Surg [Br] *30*:461, 1948.
80. Failinger MS, McGanity PLJ: Unstable fractures of the pelvic ring. J Bone Joint Surg [Am] *74*:781, 1992.
81. Hauser CW, Perry JF Jr: Massive hemorrhage from pelvic fractures. Minn Med *49*:285, 1966.
82. Colapinto V: Trauma to the pelvis: Urethral injury. Clin Orthop *151*:46, 1980.
83. Huittinen VM, Slatis P: Nerve injury in double vertical pelvic fractures. Acta Chir Scand *138*:571, 1972.
84. Eddy RJ, Connell DG: Luxatio erecta of the hip. AJR *151*:412, 1988.
85. Epstein HC: Traumatic dislocations of the hip. Clin Orthop *92*:116, 1973.
86. Zamani MH, Saltzman DI: Bilateral traumatic anterior dislocation of the hip: Case report. Clin Orthop *161*:203, 1981.
87. Bassett LW, Gold RH, Epstein HC: Anterior hip dislocation: Atypical superolateral displacement of the femoral head. AJR *141*:385, 1983.
88. Sadler AH, DiStefano M: Anterior dislocation of the hip with ipsilateral basicervical fracture: A case report. J Bone Joint Surg [Am] *67*:326, 1985.
89. Korovessis P, Droutsas P, Spastris P, et al: Anterior dislocation of the hip associated with fracture of the ipsilateral greater trochanter: A case report. Clin Orthop *253*:164, 1990.
90. Scham SM, Fry LR: Traumatic anterior dislocation of the hip with fracture of the femoral head. Clin Orthop *62*:133, 1969.
91. Yandow DR, Austin CW: Femoral defect after anterior dislocation. J Comput Assist Tomogr *7*:1112, 1983.
92. Dussault RG, Beauregard G, Fauteaux P, et al: Femoral head defect following anterior hip dislocation. Radiology *135*:627, 1980.
93. DeLee JC, Evans JA, Thomas J: Anterior dislocation of the hip and associated femoral-head fractures. J Bone Joint Surg [Am] *62*:960, 1980.
94. Tehranzadeh J, Vanarthros W, Pais MJ: Osteochondral impaction of the femoral head associated with hip dislocation: CT study in 35 patients. AJR *155*:1049, 1990.
95. Dall D, Macnab I, Gross A: Recurrent anterior dislocation of the hip. J Bone Joint Surg [Am] *52*:574, 1970.
96. Haddad RJ Jr, Drez D: Voluntary recurrent anterior dislocation of the hip: A case report. J Bone Joint Surg [Am] *56*:419, 1974.
97. Guyer B, Levinsohn EM: Recurrent anterior dislocation of the hip: Case report with arthrographic findings. Skel Radiol *10*:262, 1983.
98. Larson CB: Fracture dislocations of the hip. Clin Orthop *92*:147, 1973.
99. Whitehouse GH: Radiological aspects of posterior dislocation of the hip. Clin Radiol *29*:431, 1978.
100. Canale ST, Manugian AH: Irreducible traumatic dislocations of the hip. J Bone Joint Surg [Am] *61*:7, 1979.
101. Epstein HC: Posterior fracture-dislocations of the hip; Long-term follow-up. J Bone Joint Surg [Am] *56*:1103, 1974.
102. Smith GR, Loop JW: Radiologic classification of posterior dislocations of the hip: Refinement and pitfalls. Radiology *119*:569, 1976.
103. Yang R-S, Tsuang Y-H, Hang Y-S, et al: Traumatic dislocation of the hip. Clin Orthop *265*:218, 1991.
104. Butler JE: Pipkin type-II fractures of the femoral head. J Bone Joint Surg [Am] *63*:1292, 1981.
105. Klasen JH, Binnendik B: Fracture of the neck of the femur associated with posterior dislocation of the hip. J Bone Joint Surg [Br] *66*:45, 1984.
106. Quackenbush D, DiDonato R, Butler D: A modified lateral projection for anterior and posterior lips of the acetabulum. Radiology *125*:536, 1977.
107. Calkins MS, Zych G, Latta L, et al: Computed tomography evaluation of stability in posterior fracture dislocation of the hip. Clin Orthop *227*:152, 1988.
108. Richardson P, Young JWR, Porter D: CT detection of cortical fracture of the femoral head associated with posterior hip dislocation. AJR *155*:93, 1990.
109. Hougaard K, Lindequist S, Nielsen LB: Computerised tomography after posterior dislocation of the hip. J Bone Joint Surg [Br] *69*:556, 1987.
110. Hougaard K, Thomsen PB: Traumatic posterior fracture-dislocation of the hip with fracture of the femoral head or neck, or both. J Bone Joint Surg [Am] *70*:233, 1988.
111. Hougaard K, Thomsen PB: Coxarthrosis following traumatic posterior dislocation of the hip. J Bone Joint Surg [Am] *69*:679, 1987.
112. Proctor H: Dislocations of the hip joint (excluding "central" dislocation) and their complications. Injury *5*:1, 1973.
113. Paterson I: The torn acetabular labrum: A block to reduction of a dislocated hip. J Bone Joint Surg [Br] *39*:306, 1957.
114. Dameron TB Jr: Bucket-handle tear of acetabular labrum accompanying posterior dislocation of the hip. J Bone Joint Surg [Am] *41*:131, 1959.
115. Connolly JF: Acetabular labrum entrapment associated with a femoral-head fracture-dislocation: A case report. J Bone Joint Surg [Am] *56*:1735, 1974.
116. Rashleigh-Belcher HJC, Cannon SR: Recurrent dislocation of the hip with a "Bankart-type" lesion. J Bone Joint Surg [Br] *68*:398, 1986.
117. Graham B, Lapp RA: Recurrent posttraumatic dislocation of the hip: A report of two cases and review of the literature. Clin Orthop *256*:115, 1990.
118. Provenzano MP, Holmes PF, Tullos HS: Atraumatic recurrent dislocation of the hip: A case report. J Bone Joint Surg [Am] *69*:938, 1987.
119. Hovelius L: Traumatic dislocation of the hip in children: Report of two cases. Acta Orthop Scand *45*:746, 1974.
120. Hammelbo T: Traumatic hip dislocation in childhood: A report of three cases. Acta Orthop Scand *47*:546, 1976.
121. Schlonsky J, Miller PR: Traumatic hip dislocations in children. J Bone Joint Surg [Am] *55*:1057, 1973.
122. Gaul RW: Recurrent traumatic dislocation of the hip in children. Clin Orthop *90*:107, 1973.
123. Petterson H, Theander G, Danielsson L: Voluntary habitual dislocation of the hip in children. Acta Radiol (Diagn) *21*:303, 1980.
124. Barquet A: Traumatic hip dislocation in childhood: A report of 26 cases and a review of the literature. Acta Orthop Scand *50*:549, 1979.
125. Hougaard K, Thomsen PB: Traumatic hip dislocation in children: Follow up of 13 cases. Orthopedics *12*:375, 1989.
126. Shea KP, Kalamchi A, Thompson GH: Acetabular epiphysis-labrum entrapment following traumatic anterior dislocation of the hip in children. J Pediatr Orthop *6*:215, 1986.
127. Cinats JG, Moreau MJ, Swersky JF: Traumatic dislocation of the hip caused by interposition in a child: A case report. J Bone Joint Surg [Am] *70*:130, 1988.
128. Barrett IR, Goldberg JA: Avulsion fracture of the ligamentum teres in a child: A case report. J Bone Joint Surg [Am] *71*:438, 1989.
129. Barquet A: Avascular necrosis following traumatic hip dislocation in childhood: Factors of influence. Acta Orthop Scand *53*:809, 1982.
130. Barquet A: Natural history of avascular necrosis following traumatic hip dislocation in childhood: A review of 145 cases. Acta Orthop Scand *53*:815, 1982.
131. Fiddian NJ, Grace DL: Traumatic dislocation of the hip in adolescence with separation of the capital epiphysis: Two case reports. J Bone Joint Surg [Br] *65*:148, 1983.
132. Laorr A, Greenspan A, Anderson MW, et al: Traumatic hip dislocation: Early MRI findings. Skel Radiol *24*:239, 1995.
133. Potter HG, Montgomery KD, Heise CW, et al: MR imaging of acetabular fractures: Value in detecting femoral head injury, intraarticular fragments, and sciatic nerve injury. AJR *163*:881, 1993.
134. Villar R: Hip arthroscopy. J Bone Joint Surg [Br] *77*:517, 1995.
135. Koval KJ, Zuckerman JD: Functional recovery after fracture of the hip. J Bone Joint Surg [Am] *76*:751, 1994.
136. Lender M, Makin M, Robin G, et al: Osteoporosis and fractures of the neck of the femur: Some epidemiologic considerations. Isr J Med Sci *12*:596, 1976.
137. Vose GP, Lockwood RM: Femoral neck fracturing: Its relationship to radiographic bone density. J Gerontol *20*:300, 1965.
138. Stevens J, Freeman PA, Nordin BEC, et al: The incidence of osteoporosis in patients with femoral neck fracture. J Bone Joint Surg [Br] *44*:520, 1962.
139. Lowell JD: Fractures of the hip. N Engl J Med *274*:1480, 1966.
140. Nilsson BE: Spinal osteoporosis and femoral neck fracture. Clin Orthop *68*:93, 1970.
141. Horiuchi T, Tokuyama H, Igarashi M, et al: Spontaneous fractures of the hip in the elderly. Orthopedics *11*:1277, 1988.
142. Linton P: On different types of intracapsular fractures of the femoral neck. Acta Chir Scand *90*(Suppl 86):1, 1944.
143. Backman S: The proximal end of the femur. Acta Radiol *146*(Suppl):1, 1957.
144. DeLee JC: Fractures and dislocations of the hip. *In* CA Rockwood Jr, DP Green (Eds): Fractures in Adults. 2nd Ed. Philadelphia, JB Lippincott Co, 1984, p. 1211.
145. Kenerman L, Marcuson RW: Intracapsular fractures of the neck of the femur. J Bone Joint Surg [Br] *52*:514, 1970.
146. Askin SR, Bryan RS: Femoral neck fractures in young adults. Clin Orthop *114*:259, 1976.
147. Alffram PA: An epidemiologic study of cervical and trochanteric fractures of the femur in an urban population: Analysis of 1,664 cases with special reference to etiologic factors. Acta Orthop Scand *65*(Suppl):11, 1964.
148. Garden RS: Stability and union in subcapital fractures of the femur. J Bone Joint Surg [Br] *46*:630, 1964.
149. Pauwels F: Der Schenkenholsbruck, ein mechanisches Problem: Grundlagen des Heilungsvorganges. Prognose und kausale Therapie. Stuttgart, Beilageheft zur Zeitschrift fur Orthopaedische Chirurgie, Ferdinand Enke, 1935.
150. Garden RS: Reduction and fixation of subcapital fractures of the femur. Orthop Clin North Am *5*:683, 1974.
151. Fransden PA, Anderson E, Madsen F, et al: Garden's classification of femoral neck fractures: An assessment of inter-observer variation. J Bone Joint Surg [Br] *70*:588, 1988.

152. Barnes R, Brown JT, Garden RS, et al: Subcapital fractures of the femur. J Bone Joint Surg [Br] 58:2, 1976.

153. Barr JS: Experiences with a sliding nail in femoral neck fractures. Clin Orthop 92:63, 1973.

154. Arnold WD, Lyden JP, Minkoff J: Treatment of intracapsular fractures of the femoral neck. J Bone Joint Surg [Am] 56:254, 1974.

155. Sevitt S: Avascular necrosis and revascularization of the femoral head after intracapsular fractures. J Bone Joint Surg [Br] 46:270, 1964.

156. Melberg P-E, Körner L, Lansinger O: Hip joint pressure after femoral neck fracture. Acta Orthop Scand 57:501, 1986.

157. Stromqvist B, Nilsson LT, Egund N, et al: Intracapsular pressures in undisplaced fractures of the femoral neck. J Bone Joint Surg [Br] 70:192, 1988.

158. Crawford EJP, Emery RJH, Hansell DM, et al: Capsular distension and intracapsular pressure in subcapital fractures of the femur. J Bone Joint Surg [Br] 70:195, 1988.

159. Holmberg S, Dalen N: Intracapsular pressure and caput circulation in nondisplaced femoral neck fractures. Clin Orthop 219:124, 1987.

160. Holder LE, Schwarz C, Wernicke PG, et al: Radionuclide bone imaging in the early detection of fractures of the proximal femur (hip): Multifactorial analysis. Radiology 174:509, 1990.

161. Fairclough J, Colhoun E, Johnston D, et al: Bone scanning for suspected hip fractures. A prospective study in elderly patients. J Bone Joint Surg [Br] 69:251, 1987.

162. Strömqvist B, Hansson LI, Nilsson LT, et al: Prognostic precision in postoperative 99mTc-MDP scintimetry after femoral neck fracture. Acta Orthop Scand 58:494, 1987.

163. Alberts KA, Dahlborn M, Ringertz H: Sequential scintimetry after femoral neck fracture. Acta Orthop Scand 58:217, 1987.

164. Hirano T, Taguchi A, Suzuki R, et al: Correlation of 99mTc-MDP scintimetry and histology in cervical hip fracture. Acta Orthop Scand 58:33, 1987.

165. Alberts KA: Prognostic accuracy of preoperative and postoperative scintimetry after femoral neck fracture. Clin Orthop 250:221, 1990.

166. Speer KP, Spritzer CE, Harrelson JM, et al: Magnetic resonance imaging of the femoral head after acute intracapsular fracture of the femoral neck. J Bone Joint Surg [Am] 72:98, 1990.

167. Rizzo PF, Gould ES, Lyden JP, et al: Diagnosis of occult fractures about the hip: Magnetic resonance imaging compared with bone-scanning. J Bone Joint Surg [Am] 75:395, 1993.

168. Quinn SF, McCarthy JL: Prospective evaluation of patients with suspected hip fracture and indeterminate radiographs: Use of T1-weighted MR images. Radiology 187:469, 1993.

169. Bayliss AP, Davidson JK: Traumatic osteonecrosis of the femoral head following intracapsular fracture: Incidence and earliest radiological features. Clin Radiol 28:407, 1977.

170. Phemister DB: Fractures of the neck of the femur, dislocation of the hip and obscure vascular disturbances producing aseptic necrosis of the head of the femur. Surg Gynecol Obstet 59:415, 1934.

171. Catto MA: The histological appearances of late segmental collapse of the femoral head after transcervical fracture. J Bone Joint Surg [Br] 47:777, 1965.

172. Barr JS: Diagnosis and treatment of infections following internal fixation of hip fractures. Orthop Clin North Am 5:847, 1974.

173. Cleveland M, Bosworth DM, Thompson FR: Intertrochanteric fractures of the femur. J Bone Joint Surg 29:1049, 1947.

174. Cleveland M, Bosworth DM, Thompson FR, et al: A ten year analysis of intertrochanteric fractures of the femur. J Bone Joint Surg [Am] 41:1399, 1959.

175. Evans EM: The treatment of trochanteric fractures of the femur. J Bone Joint Surg [Br] 31:190, 1949.

176. Boyd HB, Griffin LL: Classification and treatment of trochanteric fractures. Arch Surg 58:853, 1949.

177. Herrlin K, Strömberg T, Lidgren L, et al: Trochanteric fractures: Classification and mechanical stability in McLaughlin, Ender and Richard osteosynthesis. Acta Radiol Diagn 29:189, 1988.

178. Sernbo I, Johnell O, Gentz C-F, et al: Unstable intertrochanteric fractures of the hip: Treatment with Ender pins compared with a compression hip-screw. J Bone Joint Surg [Am] 70:1297, 1988.

179. Mariani EM, Rand JA: Subcapital fractures after open reduction and internal fixation of intertrochanteric fractures of the hip: Report of three cases. Clin Orthop 245:165, 1989.

180. Søballe K, Christensen F: Laceration of the superficial femoral artery by an intertrochanteric fracture fragment: A case report. J Bone Joint Surg [Am] 69:781, 1987.

181. Fielding JW, Magliata HJ: Subtrochanteric fractures. Surg Gynecol Obstet 122:555, 1966.

182. Seinsheimer F: Subtrochanteric fractures of the femur. J Bone Joint Surg [Am] 60:300, 1978.

183. Sauser DD, Billimoria PE, Rouse GA, et al: CT evaluation of hip trauma. AJR 135:269, 1980.

184. Shirkhoda A, Brashear HR, Staab EV: Computed tomography of acetabular fractures. Radiology 134:683, 1980.

185. Mack LA, Harley JD, Winquist RA: CT of acetabular fractures: Analysis of fracture patterns. AJR 138:407, 1982.

186. Harley JD, Mack LA, Winquist RA: CT of acetabular fractures: Comparison with conventional radiography. AJR 138:413, 1982.

187. Walker RH, Burton DS: Computerized tomography in assessment of acetabular fractures. J Trauma 22:227, 1982.

188. Rafii M, Firooznia H, Golimbu C, et al: The impact of CT in clinical management of pelvic and acetabular fractures. Clin Orthop 178:228, 1983.

189. Tillie B, Fontaine Ch, Stahl P, et al: The place of computed tomography in the diagnosis and treatment of acetabular fractures: A review of 88 cases. Fr J Orthop Surg 1:13, 1987.

190. Martinez CR, Di Pasquale TG, Helfet DL, et al: Evaluation of acetabular fractures with two- and three-dimensional CT. Radiographics 12:227, 1992.

191. Knight RA, Smith H: Central fractures of the acetabulum. J Bone Joint Surg [Am] 40:1, 1958.

192. Letournel E: Acetabulum fractures: Classification and management. Clin Orthop 151:81, 1980.

193. Rogers LF, Novy SB, Harris NF: Occult central fractures of the acetabulum. AJR 124:96, 1975.

194. Dunn AW, Russo CL: Central acetabular fractures. J Trauma 13:695, 1973.

195. Nerubay J, Glancz G, Katznelson A: Fractures of the acetabulum. J Trauma 13:1050, 1973.

196. Lansinger O: Fractures of the acetabulum: A clinical, radiological and experimental study. Acta Orthop Scand (Suppl) 165:7, 1977.

197. Lovelock JE, Monaco P: Central acetabular fracture dislocations: An unusual complication of seizures. Skel Radiol 10:91, 1983.

198. Weisel A, Hecht HL: Occult fracture through the triradiate cartilage of the acetabulum. AJR 134:1262, 1980.

199. Bosse MJ, Poka A, Reiner CM, et al: Heterotopic ossification as a complication of acetabular fracture: Prophylaxis with low-dose irradiation. J Bone Joint Surg [Am] 70:1231, 1988.

200. Winquist RA, Hansen ST Jr: Comminuted fractures of the femoral shaft treated by intramedullary nailing. Orthop Clin North Am 11:633, 1980.

201. Winquist RA, Hansen ST Jr, Clawson DK: Closed intramedullary nailing of femoral fractures. J Bone Joint Surg [Am] 66:529, 1984.

202. Hooper GJ, Lyon DW: Closed unlocked nailing for comminuted femoral fractures. J Bone Joint Surg [Br] 70:619, 1988.

203. Brumback RJ, Reilly JP, Poka A, et al: Intramedullary nailing of femoral shaft fractures. I. Decision-making errors with interlocking fixation. J Bone Joint Surg [Am] 70:1441, 1988.

204. Brumback RJ, Uwagie-Ero S, Lakatos RP, et al: Intramedullary nailing of femoral shaft fractures. II. Fracture-healing with static interlocking fixation. J Bone Joint Surg [Am] 70:1453, 1988.

205. Franklin JL, Winquist RA, Benirschke SK, et al: Broken intramedullary nails. J Bone Joint Surg [Am] 70:1463, 1988.

206. Lhowe DW, Hansen ST: Intramedullary nailing of open fractures of the femoral shaft. J Bone Joint Surg [Am] 70:812, 1988.

207. Christie J, Court-Brown C, Kinninmonth AWG, et al: Intramedullary locking nails in the management of femoral shaft fractures. J Bone Joint Surg [Br] 70:206, 1988.

208. Daffner RH, Riemer BL, Butterfield SL: Ipsilateral femoral neck and shaft fractures: An overlooked association. Skel Radiol 20:251, 1991.

209. Rogers LF: Radiology of Skeletal Trauma. 2nd Ed. New York, Churchill Livingstone, 1992.

210. Hresko MT, Kasser JR: Physeal arrest about the knee associated with nonphyseal fractures in the lower extremity. J Bone Joint Surg [Am] 71:698, 1989.

211. Caudle RJ, Crawford AH: Avulsion fracture of the lateral acetabular margin: A case report. J Bone Joint Surg [Am] 70:1568, 1988.

212. Ponseti IV: Growth and development of the acetabulum in the normal child: Anatomical, histological, and roentgenographic studies. J Bone Joint Surg [Am] 60:575, 1978.

213. Paterson I: The torn acetabular labrum: A block to reduction of a dislocated hip. J Bone Joint Surg [Br] 39:306, 1957.

214. Dameron TB: Bucket-handle tear of the acetabular labrum accompanying posterior dislocation of the hip. J Bone Joint Surg [Am] 41:131, 1959.

215. Altenberg AR: Acetabular labrum tears: A cause of hip pain and degenerative osteoarthritis. South Med J 70:174, 1977.

216. Dorrell JH, Catterall A: The torn acetabular labrum. J Bone Joint Surg [Br] 68:400, 1986.

217. Suzuki S, Awaya G, Okada Y, et al: Arthroscopic diagnosis of ruptured acetabular labrum. Acta Orthop Scand 57:513, 1986.

218. Ikeda T, Awaya G, Suzuki S, et al: Torn acetabular labrum in young patients: Arthroscopic diagnosis and management. J Bone Joint Surg [Br] 70:13, 1988.

219. Klaue K, Durnin CW, Ganz R: The acetabular rim syndrome: A clinical presentation of dysplasia of the hip. J Bone Joint Surg [Br] 73:423, 1991.

220. Ueo T, Hamabuchi M: Hip pain caused by cystic deformation of the labrum acetabulare. Arthritis Rheum 27:947, 1984.

221. Matsui M, Ohzono K, Saito S: Painful cystic degeneration of the limbus in the hip: A case report. J Bone Joint Surg [Am] 70:448, 1988.

222. McBeath AA, Neidhart DA: Acetabular cyst with communicating ganglion. A case report. J Bone Joint Surg [Am] 58:267, 1976.

223. Lagier R, Seigne JM, Mbakop A: Juxta-acetabular mucoid cyst in a patient with osteoarthritis of the hip secondary to dysplasia. Int Orthop (SICOT) 8:19, 1984.

224. Haller J, Resnick D, Greenway G, et al: Juxtaacetabular ganglionic (or synovial) cysts: CT and MR features. J Comput Assist Tomogr 13:976, 1989.

225. Silver DAT, Cassar-Pullicino VN, Morrissey BM, et al: Gas-containing ganglia of the hip. Clin Radiol 46:257, 1992.
226. Hodler J, Yu JS, Goodwin D, et al: MR arthrography of the hip: Improved imaging of the acetabular labrum with histologic correlation in cadavers. AJR 165:887, 1995.
227. Czerny C, Hofmann S, Neuhold A, et al: Lesions of the acetabular labrum: Accuracy of MR imaging and MR arthrography in detection and staging. Radiology 200:225, 1996.
228. Edwards DJ, Lomas D, Villar RN: Diagnosis of the painful hip by magnetic resonance imaging and arthroscopy. J Bone Joint Surg [Br] 77:374, 1995.
229. Cardinal E, Dussault RG, Kaplan PA: Imaging and differential diagnosis of masses within a joint. Can Assoc Radiol J 45:363, 1994.
230. Murphy WA, Siegel MJ, Gilula LA: Arthrography in the diagnosis of unexplained chronic hip pain with regional osteopenia. AJR 129:283, 1977.
231. Brower AC, Kransdorf MJ: Imaging of hip disorders. Radiol Clin North Am 28:955, 1990.
232. Sharafuddin MJA, Sundaram M, McDonald D: Progression from simple joint effusion to extensive pigmented villonodular synovitis of the hip within 2 years: Demonstration with MR imaging. AJR 165:742, 1995.
233. Hermann G, Abdelwahab IF, Klein M, et al: Synovial chondromatosis. Skel Radiol 24:298, 1995.
234. Beltran J, Caudill JL, Herman LA, et al: Rheumatoid arthritis: MR imaging manifestations. Radiology 165:153, 1987.
235. Yulish BS, Lieberman JM, Newman AJ, et al: Juvenile rheumatoid arthritis: Assessment with MR imaging. Radiology 165:149, 1987.
236. Armstrong P, Saxton H: Iliopsoas bursa. Br J Radiol 45:493, 1972.
237. Warren R, Kaye JJ, Salvati EA: Arthrographic demonstration of an enlarged iliopsoas bursa complicating osteoarthritis of the hip—a case report. J Bone Joint Surg [Am] 57:413, 1975.
238. O'Connor DS: Early recognition of iliopectineal bursitis. Surg Gynecol Obstet 57:674, 1933.
239. Steinbach LS, Schneider R, Goldman AB, et al: Bursae and abscess cavities communicating with the hip: Diagnosis using arthrography and CT. Radiology 156:303, 1985.
240. Chaiamnuay P, Davis P: An unusual case of inguinal swelling. Arthritis Rheum 27:239, 1984.
241. Weinreb JC, Cohen JM, Maravilla KR: Iliopsoas muscles: MR study of normal anatomy and disease. Radiology 156:435, 1985.
242. Penkava RR: Iliopsoas bursitis demonstrated by computed tomography. AJR 135:175, 1980.
243. Peters JC, Coleman BG, Turner ML, et al: CT evaluation of enlarged iliopsoas bursa. AJR 135:392, 1980.
244. Janus CL, Hermann G: Enlargement of the iliopsoas bursa: Unusual cause of cystic mass on pelvic sonogram. J Clin Ultrasound 10:133, 1982.
245. Fortin L, Belanger R: Bursitis of the iliopsoas: Four cases with pain as the only clinical indicator. J Rheumatol 22:1971, 1995.
246. Helfgott SA: Unusual features of iliopsoas bursitis. Arthritis Rheum 31:1331, 1988.
247. Li KC, Higgs J, Aisen AM, et al: MRI in osteoarthritis of the hip: Gradations of severity. Magn Res Imaging 6:229, 1988.
248. Hodler J, Trudell D, Pathria MN, et al: Width of the articular cartilage of the hip: Quantification by using fat-suppression spin-echo MR imaging in cadavers. AJR 159:351, 1992.
249. Jones BS: Adolescent chondrolysis of the hip joint. S Afr Med J 45:196, 1971.
250. Moule NJ, Golding JSR: Idiopathic chondrolysis of the hip. Clin Radiol 25:247, 1974.
251. Wenger DR, Mickelson MR, Ponseti IV: Idiopathic chondrolysis of the hip: Report of two cases. J Bone Joint Surg [Am] 57:268, 1975.
252. Duncan JW, Schranz JL, Nasca RJ: The bizarre stiff hip: Possible idiopathic chondrolysis. JAMA 231:382, 1975.
253. Sivanantham M, Kutty MK: Idiopathic chondrolysis of the hip: Case report with a review of the literature. Aust NZ J Surg 47:229, 1977.
254. Duncan JW, Nasca R, Schrantz J: Idiopathic chondrolysis of the hip. J Bone Joint Surg [Am] 61:1024, 1979.
255. Bleck EE: Idiopathic chondrolysis of the hip. J Bone Joint Surg [Am] 65:1266, 1983.
256. Hughes AW: Idiopathic chondrolysis of the hip: A case report and review of the literature. Ann Rheum Dis 44:268, 1985.
257. van der Hoeven H, Keessen W, Kuis W: Idiopathic chondrolysis of the hip. A distinct clinical entity? Acta Orthop Scand 60:661, 1989.
258. Jiang C-C, Shih TTF: Epiphyseal scar of the femoral head: Risk factor of osteonecrosis. Radiology 191:409, 1994.
259. Mitchell DG, Rao VM, Dalinka MK, et al: Femoral head avascular necrosis: Correlation of MR imaging, radiographic staging, radionuclide imaging, and clinical findings. Radiology 162:709, 1987.
260. Mitchell DG, Joseph PM, Fallon M, et al: Chemical-shift MR imaging of the femoral head: An in vitro study of normal hips and hips with avascular necrosis. AJR 148:1159, 1987.
261. Lang P, Jergesen HE, Moseley ME, et al: Avascular necrosis of the femoral head: High field strength MR imaging with histologic correlation. Radiology 169:517, 1988.
262. Vande Berg BE, Malghem JJ, Labaisse MA, et al: MR imaging of avascular necrosis and transient marrow edema of the femoral head. RadioGraphics 13:501, 1993.
263. Curtiss PH Jr, Kincaid WE: Transient demineralization of the hip in pregnancy: A report of three cases. J Bone Joint Surg [Am] 41:1327, 1959.
264. Doury P: Bone-marrow oedema, transient osteoporosis, and algodystrophy. J Bone Joint Surg [Br] 76:993, 1994.
265. Wilson AJ, Murphy WA, Hardy DC, et al: Transient osteoporosis: transient bone marrow edema? Radiology 167:757, 1988.
266. Hofman S, Engel A, Neuhold A, et al: Bone marrow oedema syndrome and transient osteoporosis of the hip: An MRI-controlled study of treatment by core decompression. J Bone Joint Surg [Br] 75:210, 1993.
267. Richardson ML: Can MR imaging distinguish between transient osteoporosis of the femoral head and osteonecrosis? AJR 162:1244, 1994.
268. Guerra JJ, Steinberg ME: Distinguishing transient osteoporosis from avascular necrosis of the hip. J Bone Joint Surg [Am] 77:616, 1995.
269. Solomon L: Bone-marrow oedema syndrome. J Bone Joint Surg [Br] 75:175, 1993.
270. Turner DA, Templeton AC, Selzer PM, et al: Femoral capital osteonecrosis: MR finding of diffuse marrow abnormalities without focal lesions. Radiology 171:135, 1989.
271. Fairclough J, Colhoun E, Johnston D, et al: Bone scanning for suspected hip fractures: A prospective study in elderly patients. J Bone Joint Surg [Br] 69:251, 1987.
272. Matin P: The appearance of bone scans following fractures, including immediate and long-term studies. J Nucl Med 20:1227, 1979.
273. Matin P: Bone scintigraphy in the diagnosis and management of traumatic injury. Semin Nucl Med 13:104, 1983.
274. Slavin JD, Mathews J, Spencer RP: Bone imaging in the diagnosis of fractures of the femur and pelvis in the sixth to tenth decades. Clin Nucl Med 11:328, 1986.
275. Holder LE, Schwarz C, Wernicke PG, et al: Radionuclide bone imaging in the early detection of fractures of the proximal femur (hip): Multifactorial analysis. Radiology 174:509, 1990.
276. Rizzo PF, Gould ES, Lyden JP, et al: Diagnosis of occult fractures about the hip: Magnetic resonance imaging compared with bone-scanning. J Bone Joint Surg [Am] 75:395, 1993.
277. Haramati N, Staron RB, Barax C, et al: Magnetic resonance imaging of occult fractures of the proximal femur. Skel Radiol 23:19, 1994.
278. Feldman F, Staron R, Zwass A, et al: MR imaging; its role in detecting occult fractures. Skel Radiol 23:439, 1994.
279. Bogost GA, Lizerbram EK, Crues JV III: MR imaging in evaluation of suspected hip fracture: Frequency of unsuspected bone and soft-tissue injury. Radiology 197:263, 1995.
280. Deutsch AL, Mink JH, Waxman AD: Occult fractures of the proximal femur: MR imaging. Radiology 170:113, 1989.
281. Hall FM, Goldberg RP, Kasdon EJ, et al: Post-traumatic osteolysis of the pubic bone simulating a malignant lesion. J Bone Joint Surg [Am] 66:121, 1984.
282. Hall FM: Post-traumatic pubic osteolysis simulating malignancy. J Bone Joint Surg [Am] 66:975, 1984.
283. McGuigan LE, Edmonds JP, Painter DM: Pubic osteolysis. J Bone Joint Surg [Am] 66:127, 1984.
284. Casey D, Mirra J, Staple TW: Parasymphyseal insufficiency fractures of the os pubis. AJR 142:581, 1984.
285. Ghezail M, Leroux JL, Chertok P, et al: Pubic post-fracture osteolysis simulating a malignancy. Clin Exp Rheumatol 9:635, 1991.
286. Goergen TG, Resnick D, Riley RR: Post-traumatic abnormalities of the pubic bone simulating malignancy. Radiology 126:85, 1978.
287. Roback DL: Posttraumatic osteolysis of the femoral neck. AJR 134:1243, 1980.
288. Newberg AH, Howe JG: Posttraumatic osteolysis vs. fracture. AJR 135:1317, 1980.
289. Pitt MJ, Graham AR, Shipman JH, et al: Herniation pit of the femoral neck. AJR 138:1115, 1982.
290. Angel JL: The reaction area of the femoral neck. Clin Orthop 32:130, 1964.
291. Crabbe JP, Martel W, Matthews LS: Rapid growth of femoral herniation pit. AJR 159:1038, 1992.
292. Thomason CB, Silverman ED, Walter RD, et al: Focal bone tracer uptake associated with a herniation pit of the femoral neck. Clin Nucl Med 8:304, 1983.
293. Nokes SR, Vogler JB, Spritzer CE, et al: Herniation pits of the femoral neck: Appearance at MR imaging. Radiology 172:231, 1989.
294. Davies SJM, Walker G: Problems in the early recognition of hip dysplasia. J Bone Joint Surg [Br] 66:474, 1984.
295. Mackenzie IG, Wilson JG: Problems encountered in the early diagnosis and management of congenital dislocation of the hip. J Bone Joint Surg [Br] 63:38, 1981.
296. Williamson DM, Glover SD, Benson MK: Congenital dislocation of the hip presenting after the age of three years: A long-term review. J Bone Joint Surg [Br] 71:745, 1989.
297. Walker JM: Morphological variants in the human fetal hip joint: Their significance in congenital hip disease. J Bone Joint Surg [Am] 62:1073, 1980.
298. Summers BN, Turner A, Wynn-Jones CH: Presentation of congenital hip dysplasia. J Bone Joint Surg [Br] 70:63, 1988.
299. Macnicol MF: Results of a 25-year screening programme for neonatal hip instability. J Bone Joint Surg [Br] 72:1057, 1990.

300. Yngve D, Gross R: Late diagnosis of hip dislocation in infants. J Pediatr Orthop 10:777, 1990.
301. Burger BJ, Burger JD, Bos CFA, et al: Neonatal screening and staggered early treatment for congenital dislocation or dysplasia of the hip. Lancet 336:1549, 1990.
302. Catford JC, Bennet GC, Wilkinson JA: Congenital hip dislocation: An increasing and still uncontrolled disability? Br Med J 285:1527, 1982.
303. Morrissy RT, Cowie GH: Congenital dislocation of the hip: Early detection and prevention of late complications. Clin Orthop 222:79, 1987.
304. Drummond DS, O'Donnell J, Breed A, et al: Arthrography in the evaluation of congenital dislocation of the hip. Clin Orthop 243:148, 1989.
305. Harcke HT: Imaging in congenital dislocation and dysplasia of the hip. Clin Orthop 281:22, 1992.
306. Emerson DS, Brown DL, Mabie BC: Prenatal sonographic diagnosis of hip dislocation. J Ultrasound Med 7:687, 1988.
307. Boal DKB, Schwenkter EP: The infant hip: Assessment with real-time US. Radiology 157:667, 1985.
308. Berman L, Catterall A, Meire HB: Ultrasound of the hip: A review of the applications of a new technique. Br J Radiol 59:13, 1986.
309. Novick G, Ghelman B, Schneider M: Sonography of the neonatal and infant hip. AJR 141:639, 1983.
310. Clarke NMP, Harcke HT, McHugh P, et al: Real-time ultrasound in the diagnosis of congenital dislocation and dysplasia of the hip. J Bone Joint Surg [Br] 67:406, 1985.
311. Clarke MNP: Sonographic clarification of the problems of neonatal hip instability. Clin Orthop 6:527, 1986.
312. Keller MS, Chawla HS: Sonographic delineation of the neonatal acetabular labrum. J Ultrasound Med 4:501, 1985.
313. Keller MS, Chawla HS, Weiss AA: Real-time sonography of infant hip dislocation. Radiographics 6:447, 1986.
314. Harcke HT, Lee MS, Sinning L, et al: Ossification center of the infant hip: Sonographic and radiographic correlation. AJR 7:317, 1986.
315. Boal DKB, Schwentker EP: Assessment of congenital hip dislocation with real-time ultrasound: A pictorial essay. Clin Imaging 15:77, 1991.
316. Berman L, Hollingdale J: The ultrasound appearance of positive hip instability tests. Clin Radiol 38:117, 1987.
317. Sosnierz A, Karel M, Maj S, et al: Ultrasound appearance of the hip joint in newborns during the first week of life. J Clin Ultrasound 19:971, 1991.
318. Keller MS, Weltin GG, Rattner Z, et al: Normal instability of the hip in the neonates: US standards. Radiology 169:733, 1988.
319. Morin C, Harcke HT, MacEwen GD: The infant hip: Real-time US assessment of acetabular development. Radiology 157:673, 1985.
320. Zieger M: Ultrasonography of the infant hip. II. Validity of the method. Pediatr Radiol 16:488, 1986.
321. Berman L, Klenerman L: Ultrasound screening for hip abnormalities: Preliminary findings in 1001 neonates. Br Med J 293:719, 1986.
322. Bialik V, Reuveni A, Pery M, et al: Utrasonography in developmental displacement of the hip: A critical analysis of our results. J Pediatr Orthop 9:154, 1989.
323. Bick U, Muller-Leisse C, Troger J: Ultrasonography of the hip in preterm neonates. Pediatr Radiol 20:331, 1990.
324. Gardiner HM, Clarke NMP, Dunn PM: A sonographic study of the morphology of the preterm neonatal hip. J Pediatr Orthop 10:663, 1990.
325. Jones DA, Powell N: Ultrasound and neonatal hip screening: A prospective study of "high risk" babies. J Bone Joint Surg [Br] 72:457, 1990.
326. Tonnis D, Storch K, Ulbrich HJ: Results of newborn screening for CDH with and without sonography and correlation of risk factors. J Pediatr Orthop 10:145, 1990.
327. Harcke HT, Grissom LE: Performing dynamic sonography of the infant hip. AJR 155:837, 1990.
328. Engesaeter LB, Wilson DJ, Nag D, et al: Ultrasound and congenital dislocation of the hip: The importance of dynamic assessment. J Bone Joint Surg [Br] 72:197, 1990.
329. Edelson JG, Hirsch M, Weinberg H, et al: Congenital dislocation of the hip and computerised axial tomography. J Bone Joint Surg [Br] 66:472, 1984.
330. Helms CA, Goodman PC, Jeffrey RB Jr: Use of computed tomography in congenital dislocation of the hip. J Comput Assist Tomogr 7:363, 1983.
331. Peterson HA, Klassen RA, Hoffman AD: The use of computerised tomography in dislocation of the hip and femoral neck anteversion in children. J Bone Joint Surg [Br] 63:198, 1981.
332. Hernandez RJ: Concentric reduction of the dislocated hip: Computed tomographic evaluation. Radiology 150:266, 1984.
333. Hernandez J, Poznanski AK: CT evaluation of pediatric hip disorders. Orthop Clin North Am 16:513, 1985.
334. Hernandez RJ, Tachdjian MO, Dias LS: Hip CT in congenital dislocation: Appearance of tight iliopsoas tendon and pulvinar hypertrophy. AJR 139:335, 1982.
335. Simons GW, Flatley TJ, Sty JR, et al: Intra-articular osteocartilaginous obstruction to reduction of congenital dislocation of the hip: Report of three cases. J Bone Joint Surg [Am] 70:760, 1988.
336. Browning WH, Rosenkrantz H: Computed tomography in congenital hip dislocation: The role of acetabular anteversion. J Bone Joint Surg [Am] 64:27, 1982.
337. Lang P, Genant HK, Steiger P, et al: Three-dimensional digital displays in congenital dislocation of the hip: Preliminary experience. J Pediatr Orthop 9:532, 1989.
338. Lee DY, Choi IH, Lee CK, et al: Assessment of complex hip deformity using three-dimensional CT image. J Pediatr Orthop 11:13, 1991.
339. Lafferty CM, Sartoris DJ, Tyson R, et al: Acetabular alterations in untreated congenital dysplasia of the hip: Computed tomography with multiplanar reformation and three-dimensional analysis. J Comput Assist Tomogr 10:84, 1986.
340. Azuma H, Taneda H, Igarashi H, et al: Preoperative and postoperative assessment of rotational acetabular osteotomy for dysplastic hips in children by three-dimensional surface reconstruction computed tomography imaging. J Pediatr Orthop 10:33, 1990.
341. Bos CFA, Bloem JL: Treatment of dislocation of the hip, detected in early childhood, based on magnetic resonance imaging. J Bone Joint Surg 71:1523, 1989.
342. Bos CFA, Bloem JL, Obermann WR, et al: Magnetic resonance imaging in congenital dislocation of the hip. J Bone Joint Surg [Br] 70:174, 1988.
343. Lang P, Steiger P, Genant HK, et al: Three-dimensional CT and MR imaging in congenital dislocation of the hip: Clinical and technical considerations. J Comput Assist Tomogr 12:459, 1988.
344. Johnson ND, Wood BP, Jackman KV: Complex infantile and congenital hip dislocation: Assessment with MR imaging. Radiology 168:151, 1988.
345. Toby BE, Koman LA, Bechtold RE: Magnetic resonance imaging of pediatric hip disease. J Pediatr Orthop 5:665, 1985.
346. Fisher R, O'Brien TS, Davis KM: Magnetic resonance imaging in congenital dysplasia of the hip. J Pediatr Orthop 11:617, 1991.
347. Hughes JR: Intrinsic obstructive factors in congenital dislocation of the hip: The role of arthrography. In MO Tachdjian (Ed): Congenital Dislocation of the Hip. New York, Churchill Livingstone, 1982, p. 227.
348. Tachdjian MO: Treatment after walking age. In MO Tachdjian (Ed): Congenital Dislocation of the Hip. New York, Churchill Livingstone, 1982, p. 344.
349. Hernandez RJ: Evaluation of congenital hip dysplasia and tibial torsion by computed tomography. J Comput Tomogr 7:101, 1983.
350. Krasny R, Prescher A, Botschek A, et al: MR-anatomy of infant hips: Comparison to anatomical preparations. Pediatr Radiol 21:211, 1991.
351. Johnson ND, Wood BP, Noh KS, et al: MR imaging anatomy of the infant hip. AJR 153:127, 1989.
352. Goldman AB, Schneider R, Wilson PD Jr: Proximal focal femoral deficiency. Can Assoc Radiol J 29:101, 1972.
353. Levinson ED, Ozonoff MB, Royen PM: Proximal femoral focal deficiency (PFFD). Radiology 125:197, 1977.
354. Lange DR, Schoenecker PL, Baker CL: Proximal femoral focal deficiency: Treatment and classification in forty-two cases. Clin Orthop 135:15, 1978.
355. Panting AL, Williams PF: Proximal femoral focal deficiency. J Bone Joint Surg [Br] 60:46, 1978.
356. Fixsen JA, Lloyd-Roberts GC: The natural history and early treatment of proximal femoral dysplasia. J Bone Joint Surg [Br] 56:86, 1974.
357. Gupta DKS, Gupta SK: Familial bilateral proximal femoral focal deficiency: Report of a kindred. J Bone Joint Surg [Am] 66:1470, 1984.
358. Kalamchi A, Cowell HR, Kim KI: Congenital deficiency of the femur. J Pediatr Orthop 5:129, 1985.
359. Gillespie R, Torode IP: Classification and management of congenital abnormalities of the femur. J Bone Joint Surg [Br] 65:557, 1983.
360. Johansson E, Aparisi T: Missing cruciate ligament in congenital short femur. J Bone Joint Surg [Am] 65:1109, 1983.
361. Hillmann JS, Mesgarzadeh M, Revesz G, et al: Proximal femoral focal deficiency: Radiologic analysis of 49 cases. Radiology 165:769, 1987.
362. Calhoun JD, Pierret G: Infantile coxa vara. AJR 115:561, 1972.
363. Weinstein JN, Kuo KN, Millar EA: Congenital coxa vara: A retrospective review. J Pediatr Orthop 4:70, 1984.
364. Babb FS, Ghormley RK, Chatterton CC: Congenital coxa vara. J Bone Joint Surg [Am] 31:115, 1949.
365. Hark FW: Congenital coxa vara. Am J Surg 80:305, 1950.
366. Johanning K: Coxa vara infantum. I. Clinical appearance and aetiological problems. Acta Orthop Scand 21:273, 1951.
367. Zadek I: Congenital coxa vara. Arch Surg 30:62, 1935.
368. Golding FC: Congenital coxa vara. J Bone Joint Surg [Br] 30:161, 1948.
369. Fisher FL, Waskowitz WJ: Familial developmental coxa vara. Clin Orthop 86:2, 1972.
370. Bos CFA, Sakkers RJB, Bloem JL, et al: Histological, biochemical, and MRI studies of the growth plate in congenital coxa vara. J Pediatr Orthop 9:660, 1989.
371. Otto AW, Ein Becken: Mit Hagelformig aus gedehnten Pfannen. In Neue seltene Beobachtungen zur Anatomie, Physiologie, und Pathologie gehörig. Berlin, August Rücker, 1824.
372. Eppinger H: Pelvis-Chrobak: Coxarthrolisthesis-Becken (Festschir R Chrobak). Beitr Geb Gynakol 2:176, 1903.
373. Golding FC: Protrusio acetabuli (central luxation). Br J Surg 22:56, 1934.
374. Gilmour J: Adolescent deformities of the acetabulum and investigation into the nature of protrusio acetabuli. Br J Surg 26:670, 1939.
375. Alexander C: The aetiology of primary protrusio acetabuli. Br J Radiol 38:567, 1965.
376. Meyer J: Dysplasia epiphysealis capitis femoris: A clinico-radiological syndrome and its relationship to Legg-Calvé-Perthes' disease. Acta Orthop Scand 34:183, 1964.
377. Harrison S: Dysplasia epiphysealis capitis femoris. Clin Orthop 80:118, 1971.

378. Brower AC: The osteochondroses. Orthop Clin North Am *14*:99, 1983.
379. Lyons JC, Peterson LFA: The snapping iliopsoas tendon. Mayo Clin Proc *59*:327, 1984.
380. Nunziata A, Blumenfeld I: Cadeva a resorte: A proposito de una variedad. Prensa Med Argent *38*:1997, 1951.
381. House AJG: Orthopaedists and ballet. Clin Orthop *89*:52, 1972.
382. Schaberg JE, Harper MC, Allen WC: The snapping hip syndrome. Am J Sports Med *12*:361, 1984.
383. Silver SF, Connell DG, Duncan CP: Case report 550. Skel Radiol *18*:327, 1989.
384. Staple TW, Jung D, Mork A: Snapping tendon syndrome: Hip tenography with fluoroscopic monitoring. Radiology *166*:873, 1988.
385. Harper MC, Schaberg JE, Allen WC: Primary iliopsoas bursography in the diagnosis of disorders of the hip. Clin Orthop *221*:238, 1987.
386. Fritz P, Bardin T, Laredo J-D, et al: Paradiaphyseal calcific tendinitis with cortical bone erosion. Arthritis Rheum *37*:718, 1994.
387. Mizutani H, Ohba S, Mizutani M, et al: Calcific tendinitis of the gluteus maximus tendon with cortical bone erosion: CT findings. J Comput Assist Tomogr *18*:310, 1994.
388. Brandser EA, El-khoury GY, Kathol MH, et al: Hamstring injuries: Radiographic, conventional tomographic, CT, and MR imaging characteristics. Radiology *197*:257, 1995.
389. Pomeranz SJ, Heidt RS Jr: MR imaging in the prognostication of hamstring injury. Radiology *189*:897, 1993.
390. Brunet ME, Hontas RB: The thigh. *In* JC DeLee, D Drez Jr (Eds): Orthopaedic Sports Medicine: Principles and Practice. Philadelphia, WB Saunders Co, 1994, p. 1086.
391. Verta MJ, Vitello J, Fuller J: Adductor canal compression syndrome. Arch Surg *119*:345, 1984.
392. Romanoff ME, Cory PC, Kalenak A, et al: Saphenous nerve entrapment at the adductor canal. Am J Sports Med *17*:478, 1989.
393. Conway WF, Totty WG, McEnery KW: CT and MR imaging of the hip. Radiology *198*:297, 1996.
394. Poggi JJ, Callaghan JJ, Spritzer CE, et al: Changes on magnetic resonance images after traumatic hip dislocation. Clin Orth Rel Res *319*:249, 1995.
395. Lage LA, Patel JV, Villar RN: The acetabular labral tear: An arthroscopic classification. Arthroscopy *12*:269, 1996.
396. Petersilge CA, Haque MA, Petersilge WJ, et al: Acetabular labral tears: Evaluation with MR arthrography. Radiology *200*:231, 1996.
397. Nishii T, Nakanishi K, Sugano N, et al: Acetabular labral tears: Contrast-enhanced MR imaging under continuous leg traction. Skeletal Radiol *25*:349, 1996.
398. Koo K-H, Kim R: Quantifying the extent of osteonecrosis of the femoral head. A new method using MRI. J Bone Joint Surg [Br] *77*:875, 1995.
399. Holman AJ, Gardner GC, Richardson ML, et al: Quantitative magnetic resonance imaging predicts clinical outcome of core decompression for osteonecrosis of the femoral head. J Rheumatol *22*:1929, 1995.
400. Sugano N, Masuhara K, Nakamura N, et al: MRI of early osteonecrosis of the femoral head after transcervical fracture. J Bone Joint Surg [Br] *75*:253, 1996.
401. Colwell CW Jr: The controversy of core decompression of the femoral head for osteonecrosis. Arthritis Rheum *32*:797, 1989.
402. Hungerford DS: Response: The role of core decompression in the treatment of ischemic necrosis of the femoral head. Arthritis Rheum *32*:801, 1989.
403. Hopson CN, Siverhus SW: Ischemic necrosis of the femoral head: Treatment by core decompression. J Bone Joint Surg [Am] *70*:1048, 1988.
404. Saito S, Ohzono K, Ono K: Joint-preserving operations for idiopathic avascular necrosis of the femoral head: Results of core decompression, grafting and osteotomy. J Bone Joint Surg [Br] *70*:78, 1988.
405. Chan TW, Dalinka MK, Steinberg ME, et al: MRI appearance of femoral head osteonecrosis following core decompression and bone grafting. Skel Radiol *20*:103, 1991.
406. Zizic TM, Marcoux C, Hungerford DS, et al: The early diagnosis of ischemic necrosis of bone. Arthritis Rheum *29*:1177, 1986.
407. Ficat RP: Idiopathic bone necrosis of the femoral head: Early diagnosis and treatment. J Bone Joint Surg [Br] *67*:3, 1985.
408. Arlet J, Durroux R: Diagnostic histologique précoce de l'osteonécrose aseptique de la tête fémorale par le forage-biopsie. *In* Premier Symposium International de Circulation Osseouse, Toulouse, Paris, Inserm, 1973.
409. Robinson HJ Jr, Hartleben PD, Lund G, et al: Evaluation of magnetic resonance imaging in the diagnosis of osteonecrosis of the femoral head: Accuracy compared with radiographs, cone biopsy, and intraosseous pressure measurements. J Bone Joint Surg [Am] *71*:650, 1989.
410. Stulberg BN, Levine M, Bauer TW, et al: Multimodality approach to osteonecrosis of the femoral head. Clin Orthop *240*:181, 1989.
411. Zizic TM, Lewis CG, Marcoux C, et al: The predictive value of hemodynamic studies in preclinical ischemic necrosis of bone. J Rheumatol *16*:1559, 1989.
412. May DA, Purins JL, Smith D: MR imaging of occult traumatic fractures and muscular injuries of the hip and pelvis in elderly patients. AJR *166*:1075, 1996.
413. Lerais JM, Jacob D, Thibaud JC, et al: Disparition spontanée d'une lacune sous-corticale du col fémoral. J Radiol *76*:593, 1995.
414. Taylor GR, Clarke NMP: Surgical release of the "snapping iliopsoas tendon." J Bone Joint Surg [Br] *77*:881, 1995.
415. Vaccaro JP, Sauser DD, Beals RK: Iliopsoas bursa imaging: Efficacy in depicting abnormal iliopsoas tendon motion in patients with internal snapping hip syndrome. Radiology *197*:853, 1995.
416. Cardinal E, Buckwalter KA, Capello WN, et al: US of the snapping iliopsoas tendon. Radiology *198*:521, 1996.
417. Lecouvet FE, Vande Berg BC, Malghem J, et al: MR imaging of the acetabular labrum: Variations in 200 asymptomatic hips. AJR *167*:1025, 1996.
418. Sarkar JS, Haddad FS, Crean SV, et al: Acute calcific tendinitis of the rectus femoris. J Bone Joint Surg [Br] *78*:814, 1996.

Although assessment of internal derangements of the knee begins with clinical evaluation including careful physical examination, imaging is fundamental to accurate diagnosis of many of these derangements. Typically, routine radiography is the first imaging method employed. The subsequent use of other imaging techniques is determined on the basis of the specific information that is needed. In this chapter, an analysis is provided of the indications, methodologies, and findings related to the evaluation of a number of knee disorders using routine and advanced imaging procedures with emphasis given to MR imaging.

ANATOMY

The knee joint is the largest and most complicated joint in the human body. In this joint, three functional spaces exist: the medial femorotibial space, the lateral femoro-

tibial space, and the patellofemoral space. In the following discussion, general anatomic features of the joint are summarized initially. A more detailed analysis of the anatomy and function of individual structures, such as the menisci and ligaments, is contained in subsequent sections of this chapter that deal with the imaging of each of them.

Osseous Anatomy

The lower end of the femur contains a medial and lateral condyle, separated posteriorly by an intercondylar fossa or notch (Fig. 16–1). The medial condyle is larger than the lateral condyle and possesses a superior prominence called the adductor tubercle for attachment of the tendon of the adductor magnus muscle. Below this tubercle is a ridge, the medial epicondyle. The lateral condyle possesses a similar protuberance,

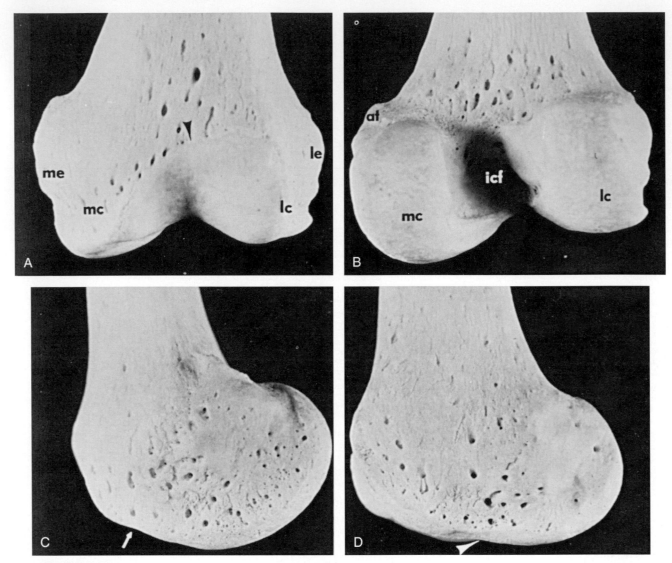

Figure 16–1

Distal femur: Osseous anatomy. Anterior **(A)** and posterior **(B)** aspects. Observe the medial (mc) and lateral (lc) condyles, medial (me) and lateral (le) epicondyles, adductor tubercle (at), patellar surface (arrowhead), and intercondylar fossa (icf). Medial **(C)** and lateral **(D)** aspects. On the medial aspect, observe the groove (arrow) that separates the anterior and middle thirds of the distal end of the femur. On the lateral aspect, there is a groove (arrowhead) that divides the femoral surface approximately in half.

the lateral epicondyle. The intercondylar fossa, between the condyles, stretches from the intercondylar line posteriorly to the lower border of the patellar surface anteriorly. The patella, the largest sesamoid bone of the body, is embedded within the tendon of the quadriceps femoris. It is oval, with a pointed apex on its inferior surface. The ligamentum patellae (patellar tendon), a continuation of the quadriceps tendon, is attached to the apex and adjacent bone of the patella.

Articular surfaces of the femur, tibia, and patella are not congruent. The articular surface of the femur comprises the condylar areas (femorotibial spaces) and the patellar surface (patellofemoral space). A shallow groove is present between each condylar surface and the patellar surface. As viewed from below, the outline of the femoral condylar surfaces generally conforms to that of the tibial articular surfaces. The surface on the lateral femoral condyle appears circular, whereas that

on the medial femoral condyle is large and oval, elongated in an anteroposterior direction, with concavity extending laterally.

The tibial articular surfaces are the cartilage-clothed condyles, each with a central hollow and peripheral flattened area (Fig. 16–2). Between the condyles is the intercondylar area. The articular surface of the medial tibial condyle is oval, with its long axis in the sagittal plane, whereas the articular surface of the lateral tibial condyle is circular and smaller than the medial condyle.

Articular Anatomy

The adjacent articular surfaces of the tibia and femur are more closely fitted together by the presence of the medial and lateral menisci (Fig. 16–3). The medial meniscus is nearly semicircular, with a broadened or wid-

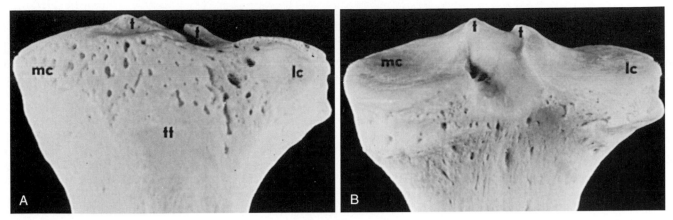

Figure 16–2
Proximal tibia: Osseous anatomy. Anterior **(A)** and posterior **(B)** aspects. Structures include the tibial tuberosity (tt), tubercles (t) of the intercondylar eminence, medial condyle (mc), and lateral condyle (lc).

ened posterior horn. The anterior end of the medial meniscus is attached to the intercondylar area of the tibia anterior to the attachment of the anterior cruciate ligament. The posterior end of the medial meniscus is attached to the intercondylar area of the tibia between the attachments of the posterior cruciate ligament and

lateral meniscus. The peripheral aspect of the medial meniscus is attached to the fibrous capsule and tibial collateral ligament. The lateral meniscus, which is of relatively uniform width throughout, resembles a ring. Its anterior aspect is attached to the intercondylar eminence of the tibia behind and lateral to the anterior

Figure 16–3
Knee joint: Normal anatomy. Menisci and cruciate ligaments. Drawings of tibial articular surfaces without **(A)** and with **(B)** the addition of soft tissue structures. Note the medial condyle (mc), lateral condyle (lc), intercondylar eminences (ie), anterior intercondylar area (a), and posterior intercondylar area (p). Soft tissue structures are the medial meniscus (mm), lateral meniscus (lm), posterior cruciate ligament (pcl), posterior meniscofemoral ligament (pml), and anterior cruciate ligament (acl).

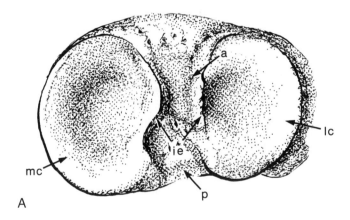

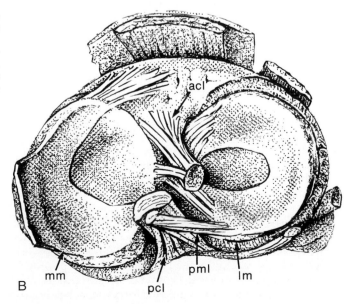

cruciate ligament. Its posterior portion is attached to the intercondylar eminence of the tibia just anterior to the attachment of the medial meniscus. The lateral meniscus is grooved posteriorly by the popliteus tendon and its accompanying tendon sheath. Meniscofemoral ligaments, both anterior and posterior, represent attachments of the posterior horn of the lateral meniscus.

The articular surface of the patella is oval and contains an osseous vertical ridge that divides it into a smaller medial area and a larger lateral area. This patellar ridge fits into a corresponding groove on the anterior surface of the femur. The patellar articulating surface is subdivided still further by two poorly defined horizontal ridges of bone into three facets on either side. One additional vertical ridge of bone separates a narrow elongated facet on the medial border of the articular surface. Contact between these various patellar articular facets and the femur varies, depending on the position of the knee. In full flexion, the most medial facet of the patella contacts the lateral portion of the medial femoral condyle, and the superior aspect of the lateral patellar facet contacts the anterior part of the lateral condyle. With extension of the knee, the middle facet of the patella becomes intimate with the lower portion of the femoral patellar surface, and in full extension, only the lowest patellar articular facets contact the femur. During forced extension of the joint, the patella has a tendency to be displaced laterally, which is prevented by the action of adjacent musculature and the prominence of the lateral patellar surface of the femur.

Capsular and Synovial Anatomy

The fibrous capsule of the knee joint is not a complete structure. Rather, the knee is surrounded by tendinous expansions, which reinforce the capsule. Between the capsule or tendinous expansions and synovial lining are various intra-articular structures, including ligaments and fat pads.

Anteriorly, the fibrous capsule is absent above and over the patellar surface. The ligamentous sheath in this area is composed mainly of a tendinous expansion from the rectus femoris and the vastus musculature, which descends to attach around the superior half of the bone. Superficial fibers continue to descend onto the strong ligamentum patellae. This structure, which represents the continuation of the quadriceps muscle, is attached above to the apex of the patella and below to the tibial tuberosity. Adjacent fibers, the medial and lateral patellar retinacula, pass from the osseous margins of the patella to the tibial condyles. Superficial to these tendinous structures are the expansions of the fascia lata. Above the patella, deficiency of the fibrous capsule creates a suprapatellar bursa, which freely communicates with the articular cavity.

Posteriorly, capsular fibers extend from the femoral surface above the condyles and the intercondylar line to the posterior border of the tibia. This portion of the capsule is strengthened by the oblique popliteal ligament, which is derived from the semimembranosus tendon. Additional posterior reinforcement relates to the arcuate popliteal ligament, which emerges from the fibular head to blend with the capsular fibers.

Laterally, capsular fibers run from the femoral to the tibial condyles. In this area, the fibular collateral ligament is found, which is attached above to the lateral epicondyle of the femur and below to the fibular head. There is a space between capsular fibers and the fibular collateral ligament through which extend genicular vessels and nerves.

Medially, the capsule is strengthened by tendinous expansions from sartorius and semimembranosus muscles. These fibers pass upward to the tibial collateral ligament, which is attached above to the medial epicondyle of the femur and below to the medial tibial condyle and shaft. One or more bursae may separate the tibial collateral ligament from the fibrous capsule. On its deep surface, the fibrous capsule connects the menisci and adjacent tibia, a connection termed the coronary ligament.

The tibial and fibular collateral ligaments reinforce the medial and lateral sides of the joint. They are taut in joint extension, and in this position, they prevent rotation of the knee.

The synovial membrane of the knee joint is the most extensive in the body and can be divided conveniently into several parts (Fig. 16–4).[1]

1. *Central portion.* This extends between the patella and the patellar surface of the femur to the cruciate ligaments (Fig. 16–5). This portion lies between femoral and tibial condyles and, in addition, above and below the menisci. An infrapatellar fat pad below the patella, located deep to the patellar ligament, presses the synovial membrane posteriorly. In this area, a vertical infrapatellar synovial fold runs from the synovial surface of the fat pad to the intercondylar fossa. Horizontal alar synovial folds run from each side of the infrapatellar synovial fold.

2. *Suprapatellar synovial pouch.* This cavity, which develops separately from the knee joint but eventually communicates with it, extends vertically above the patella between the quadriceps muscle anteriorly and the femur posteriorly.

3. *Posterior femoral recesses.* These recesses lie behind the posterior portion of each femoral condyle, deep to the lateral and medial heads of the gastrocnemius muscle (Fig. 16–6). Single or multiple bursae may be located between the muscular portions and the fibrous capsule and may communicate with the articular cavity. The medial and lateral posterior femoral recesses are separated by a thick central septum formed by a broad synovial fold around the cruciate ligaments, which may be continuous with the infrapatellar synovial fold.

4. *Subpopliteal recess.* A small synovial cul-de-sac lies between the lateral meniscus and the tendon of the popliteus, which may communicate with the superior tibiofibular joint in 10 per cent of adults.[2]

Numerous additional bursae may be found about the knee.[1, 3] These include the subcutaneous prepatellar and subfascial prepatellar bursae anterior to the patella; deep infrapatellar bursa between the upper tibia and ligamentum patellae; anserine bursa between the tibial

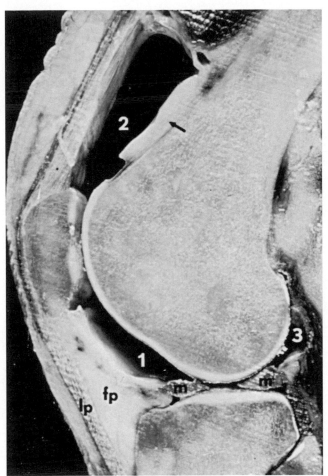

Figure 16–4
Knee joint: Normal anatomy: Various parts of the joint. A photograph of a sagittal section of an air-distended knee joint outlining ligamentum patellae (lp), infrapatellar fat pad (fp), and menisci (m). The joint can be divided into a central portion (1), suprapatellar pouch (2), and posterior femoral recesses (3). Note fatty tissue (arrow), which is pressed against the anterior aspect of the femur.

collateral ligament and tendons of the sartorius, gracilis, and semitendinosus muscles; and bursae between the semimembranosus tendon and tibial collateral ligament, and between the biceps tendon and fibular collateral ligament.

Anatomy of Supporting Structures

The supporting structures of the knee are numerous and complex, consisting of capsular thickenings, ligaments, tendons, and retinacula. As is discussed in detail later in this chapter, these structures can be classified according to location as follows:

1. Medial supporting structures, which include the superficial and deep portions of the medial collateral ligament, pes anscrinus tendons, and patellar retinaculum (as well as other structures).

2. Lateral supporting structures, which include the biceps femoris muscle and tendon, iliotibial tract, fibu-

lar collateral ligament, oblique popliteal ligament, lateral capsular ligament, meniscofemoral ligaments, and patellar retinaculum (as well as other structures).

3. Anterior supporting structures, which include the patellar tendon, patellofemoral ligaments, and quadriceps muscle and tendon (as well as other structures).

4. Central supporting structures, which include the anterior and posterior cruciate ligaments.

FUNCTION

In addition to its large size and complex anatomy, the knee possesses little inherent stability. It exists between the two longest tubular bones of the body, the femur and tibia, which underscores the considerable leverage that it must endure; its articular surfaces are not very congruent; and its range of motion is great. In large part, stability of the knee depends on surrounding powerful ligaments and strong muscles that bind the bones together.[4]

The knee is not a true hinge joint. It has six degrees of freedom: flexion, extension, internal rotation, external rotation, abduction, and adduction.[5] Indeed, classic movements of flexion and extension are made more complex in the knee, being combined with a shift in the axis around which the movements occur owing to the spiral profiles of the femoral condyles; this axis shifts upward and forward during extension of the leg on the thigh and downward and backward during flexion.[4]

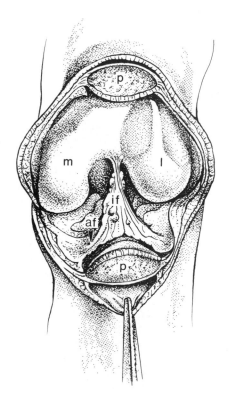

Figure 16–5
Knee joint: Normal anatomy, central portion. The patella (p) has been divided to expose the joint interior. Observe the medial (m) and lateral (l) femoral condyles and alar folds (af) of synovium, which converge to form the infrapatellar fold (if) or ligamentum mucosum.

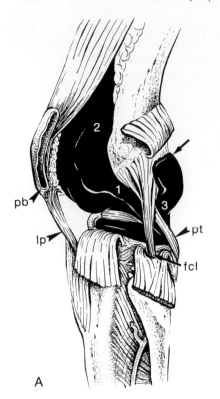

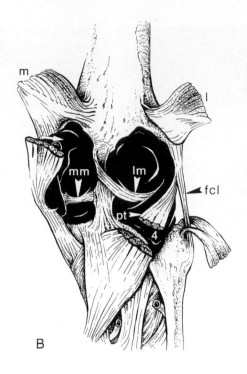

A

B

Figure 16–6

Knee joint: Normal anatomy, suprapatellar synovial pouch and posterior femoral recesses.

A Lateral aspect. Distended joint is indicated in black. Observe the central portion (1), suprapatellar pouch (2), and posterior femoral recesses (3). The prepatellar bursa (pb), ligamentum patellae (lp), fibular collateral ligament (fcl), and popliteus tendon (pt) are indicated. The lateral head of the gastrocnemius muscle has been turned up, exposing a communicating bursa (arrow).

B Posterior aspect. The distended joint is indicated in black. The medial (m) and lateral (l) heads of the gastrocnemius muscle have been sectioned. Note the bursa (arrow) beneath the lifted medial head, medial meniscus (mm), lateral meniscus (lm), popliteus tendon (pt), fibular collateral ligament (fcl), and subpopliteal recess (4).

Furthermore, rotational movements accompany flexion and extension of the knee: with the foot on the ground, the final 30 degrees of extension is inevitably associated with some medial rotation of the femur and the first few degrees of flexion with a corresponding degree of lateral rotation; with the foot off the ground, extension of the knee is associated with lateral rotation of the tibia and flexion with medial rotation of this bone.[4] The movements of flexion and extension of the knee also are accompanied by changes in the precise points of contact and contact areas of the articular surfaces of the femur and tibia and by shifting of the menisci. The movements of rotation at the knee joint, which are small in comparison to those of flexion and extension, are divided into two types: conjunct rotations, which are an integral part of the movements of flexion and extension; and adjunct rotations, which can occur independently of flexion and extension.[4] Conjunct medial rotation of the femur on the tibia occurs in the later stages of knee extension and serves to lock the joint in full extension, a position in which maximum congruence, compression, and contact area of the articular surfaces and maximum spiralization and tautening of the ligaments are evident.[4] With the foot on the ground, initial flexion of the fully extended knee results in lateral rotation of the femur, unlocking the joint. The popliteus muscle appears to play an important function during this movement, exerting a downward and backward force at its site of attachment to the lateral condyle of the femur and a backward force on the posterior horn of the lateral meniscus (preventing its compression between the articular surfaces).

In the extended position, both cruciate ligaments, both collateral ligaments, the oblique posterior liga-ment, and the posterior aspect of the joint capsule (as well as the fascia and skin) are taut, abduction and adduction of the knee are prevented, and the anterior parts of the menisci are compressed between the femoral condyles and the tibia; when the knee is flexed, the fibular collateral ligament and the posterior part of the tibial collateral ligament are relaxed, the cruciate ligaments and anterior part of the tibial collateral ligament remain taut, the posterior parts of the menisci are compressed between the femoral condyles and tibia, and a limited amount of abduction and adduction of the knee is possible.[4] The cruciate ligaments are taut in all positions of the joint, serving to bond together the femur and the tibia; forward gliding of the tibia on the femur is prevented by the anterior cruciate ligament and backward gliding of the tibia on the femur is prevented by the posterior cruciate ligament.

The muscles producing the various movements of the knee include the following[4]: Flexion—biceps femoris, semitendinosus, and semimembranosus, assisted by the gracilis, sartorius, and popliteus muscles (and, with the foot on the ground, the gastrocnemius and plantaris muscles); extension—quadriceps femoris, assisted by the tensor fasciae latae; medial rotation of the flexed leg—popliteus, semimembranosus, and semitendinosus, assisted by the sartorius and gracilis muscles; and lateral rotation of the flexed leg—biceps femoris alone.

IMAGING TECHNIQUES

The value of a number of imaging techniques, including routine radiography, scintigraphy, ultrasonography, arthrography, CT scanning, CT arthrography, and MR imaging, in assessing disorders of the knee is addressed in detail throughout this chapter as well as in other parts of this text. A few introductory comments regarding some of these methods are included here.

Routine Radiography

Although investigations have indicated that two views (anteroposterior and lateral) are adequate in the assessment of most disorders of the knee,[6] complete evaluation of patients with knee effusions after acute trauma may require additional views to ensure that occult fractures are not overlooked.[7, 8] In patients with knee trauma, a crosstable lateral projection should be added to the examination,[9] allowing demonstration of fat-fluid levels, indicative of fractures with release of medullary fat into the articular cavity.

Various techniques have been described for adequate evaluation of the patellofemoral joint. Original descriptions suggested using the prone position with acute knee flexion (the sunrise view). This degree of knee flexion results in the patella's becoming deeply situated within the intercondylar fossa. As most cases of subluxation of the patella occur with lesser degrees of knee flexion, this view is not ideal.[10] Hughston[11] suggested that a view obtained with the patient prone and the knee flexed to 50 or 60 degrees was a more suitable technique for visualization of the patellofemoral joint. Subsequently, some investigators described techniques in which the patient was examined supine.[12, 13] Merchant and coworkers[14] proposed a technique in which the patient is positioned supine on the table with the leg flexed 45 degrees over the end of the table. Radiographs also can be obtained at various degrees of knee flexion, perhaps providing a more accurate appraisal of the patellofemoral area.[15–17]

Weight-bearing radiography of the knee is particularly helpful in the evaluation of degenerative joint disease, providing a more accurate assessment of the articular space.[18–21] Radiography performed during varus and valgus stress of the knee allows evaluation of ligament instability.[22] Stress radiography is especially useful in the assessment of the cruciate ligaments.[23]

On routine radiographs, the shallow grooves in the distal articular surface of the femur can be recognized.[24–27] The groove on the medial condyle appears as a sulcus at the junction of the anterior and middle thirds of the articular surface on lateral radiographs. In the same projection, the groove on the lateral condyle is located at the center of the articular surface and is generally more prominent. Blumensaat's line is identified as a condensed linear shadow on the lateral radiograph representing tangential bone in the intercondylar fossa.[28, 29] The location and appearance of Blumensaat's line is extremely sensitive to changes in knee position.[25]

In the lateral projection of a mildly flexed knee, the collapsed suprapatellar pouch creates a sharp vertical radiodense line between an anterior fat pad superior to the patella (anterior suprapatellar fat) and a posterior fat pad in front of the distal supracondylar region of the femur (prefemoral fat pad) (Fig. 16–7). This line

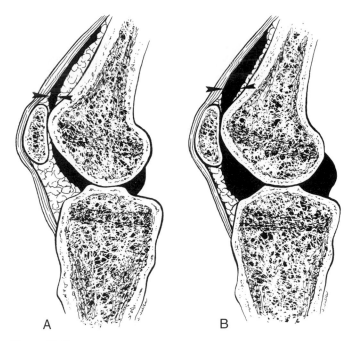

Figure 16–7
Knee joint: Radiographic anatomy.
  A In normal situations, the collapsed suprapatellar pouch (arrowheads) creates a radiodense area (arrows) that generally is less than 5 mm in width but may be between 5 and 10 mm in width.
  B In the presence of intra-articular fluid, distention of the pouch (arrowheads) creates a radiodense region of increased thickness with blurred margins (arrows).

generally is less than 5 mm wide, but it may be between 5 and 10 mm. Shadows of increased thickness suggest the presence of intra-articular fluid.[30–32] Distortion of soft tissue planes[30, 33] with the production of a piriform mass[34] in this projection and displacement of fat planes about the suprapatellar pouch on frontal projections[35] are additional but less sensitive signs of knee effusions. Axial radiographs reveal abnormal radiodensity in the medial patellofemoral compartment in such cases.[32] Intra-articular fluid in the knee also may cause displacement of the ossified fabella.[36] In lateral projections, a thin layer of extrasynovial fat hugs the femoral condyles posteriorly.[37]

Arthrography

Despite the challenge presented by arthroscopy and newer imaging techniques such as CT and MR imaging, the role of arthrography is most established for abnormalities of the knee.[38–41] Single contrast examination using air and oxygen[42] or radiopaque substances[43, 44] has been replaced, in large part, by double contrast examination using air and radiopaque contrast material.[45–63] In recent years computed arthrotomography (or CT alone) has been introduced in the evaluation of chondromalacia of the patella, cruciate ligament injuries, and even meniscal abnormalities.

It is imperative that most of the intra-articular fluid be aspirated.[64] When considerable intra-articular fluid is present, contrast coating of the menisci is less than ideal, and subtle tears will be missed. The presence of wear particles in the synovial fluid, consisting of cartilaginous fragments, is strongly indicative of significant intra-articular pathologic processes.[65-67] The addition of intra-articular epinephrine (0.2 ml of 1:1000 solution) may enhance meniscal visualization by causing vasoconstriction of synovial vessels, decreasing both the amount of contrast material absorbed from the joint cavity and the amount of intra-articular fluid formed.

Magnetic Resonance Imaging

Historical Review and Perspective

Many of the early descriptions of MR imaging of the knee represented general overviews of the subject. Later, the investigations became more focused, examining various pathologic conditions (e.g., meniscal tears, cruciate ligament disruptions, patellofemoral disorders). Although it is impossible to do justice to all of the investigations that have dealt with MR imaging of the knee, a brief review is required.

The reports in 1983 by Kean and coworkers[68] and Moon and associates,[69] and in 1984 by Li and collaborators[70] were the first to describe the potential of MR imaging in assessing the knee. Although primitive by today's standards, they served as a stimulus for subsequent investigation. In 1985, Reicher and coworkers[71, 72] provided further evidence of this potential, using close imaging-pathologic correlation in cadaveric knees and imaging-arthroscopic correlation in knees of symptomatic patients. The foundation having been laid and the potential clearly in sight, the deluge of investigations dealing with MR imaging of the knee began.[73-97] MR imaging was touted early on as a noninvasive diagnostic method that could compete favorably with standard arthrography in the analysis of knee disorders; subsequently, MR imaging became regarded as superior to standard arthrography and as a substitute for, or, at the very least, a complement to diagnostic arthroscopy of the knee. With technical advances in the field, MR images of the knee became sharper and the findings more definite. Three-dimensional gradient echo imaging,[98, 99] reformatted or reconstructed multiplanar images,[100] and innovative and faster MR imaging methods[101] for assessing the knee all were given attention. Furthermore, as many of the MR imaging abnormalities were seen more easily in the presence of a knee effusion, the added benefit of using intra-articular administration of gadolinium compounds was studied. The work of Hajek and coworkers[102, 103] in 1987 gave birth to the concept of gadolinium-enhanced MR arthrography of the knee (and other joints), and the technique remains popular in certain parts of the United States and Europe.[104]

That MR imaging has invaded the territory once held firm by conventional arthrography is certain. In many institutions in which MR imaging is available, knee arthrography rarely is employed, being reserved for patients who are claustrophobic, who have certain types of metallic implants in whom MR imaging is contraindi-

cated, or who are too large to be placed on the MR imaging table. Is MR imaging needed as a supplement to clinical assessment in an age in which diagnostic and therapeutic arthroscopy is being used increasingly? There are no easy answers to this question. Boden and associates,[105] in an analysis of the financial impact of the diagnostic methods used to evaluate the acutely injured knee, concluded that arthroscopy is more cost effective than MR imaging if 78 per cent or more of the scanned patients eventually undergo arthroscopy. Ruwe and collaborators,[106] in another study addressing the issue of cost effectiveness, indicated that the results of MR imaging of the knee in 53 of 103 patients averted a potentially unnecessary diagnostic arthroscopy, resulting in a net savings of $103,700. As might be expected, the first of these two investigations was accomplished by orthopedic surgeons and published in a journal devoted to arthroscopy, and the second, although resulting from the combined efforts of both orthopedic surgeons and radiologists, was published in a diagnostic radiology journal. Spiers and coworkers,[107] in a study of 58 patients with suspected internal derangements of the knee, indicated the advantages and disadvantages of MR imaging and concluded that MR imaging studies on all patients scheduled for knee arthroscopy would lead to a modest increase in the cost of treatment but one that represented "a small price to pay for a reduction in the morbidity associated with arthroscopy, and the liberation of theatres and surgeons for other work." Noble[108] emphasized the need to avoid unnecessary arthroscopy, indicating that the results of MR imaging of the knee in some patients augment the clinical judgment, "leaving the arthroscope to bring about a practical solution for the patient's demonstrable (and verified) problem."

Few would argue that a diagnostic test, such as MR imaging, is not indicated if the treatment will not be affected by the result, no matter what that result might be.[109] Identification of the correct therapeutic method, however, requires the attention of a highly skilled and often specialized orthopedic surgeon. Such a physician is expected to be able to determine whether or not the results of an MR imaging examination of the knee will affect treatment of the patient. With less skilled physicians, this type of determination may not be possible, and MR imaging may represent an effective means of identifying the problem and, thereby, influencing the decision as to the appropriateness of surgical intervention. Proper interpretation of MR images requires the attention of a highly skilled and often specialized radiologist. Furthermore, owing to the occurrence of positive findings on MR images of the knee in asymptomatic persons,[110] the results of the MR imaging examination must be correlated with those derived from careful clinical assessment and other imaging methods.[1110, 1111]

When analyzing the cost effectiveness of MR imaging of the knee, several additional factors deserve consideration. The procedure is far more likely to be cost effective when it is used as a supplement to careful clinical evaluation that indicates a strong possibility of an internal derangement of the knee. It is far less likely to be cost effective when it is used as a substitute for careful clinical evaluation or routine radiography, or both. Furthermore, owing to variations in the cost of the MR imaging examination among different institutions, what is cost effective at one facility may not be cost effective at a second. Indeed, two obvious modern trends in MR imaging are the use of rapid sequences and the employment of shortened imaging protocols. Such protocols, which have been shown to be valuable in the initial identification of occult fractures, often rely on a single imaging plane and the utilization of sensitive methods such as short tau inversion recovery (STIR) MR imaging. The expense of these tailored examinations compares favorably to that of alternative diagnostic methods such as bone scintigraphy and to that of delayed and repeated assessments when a correct diagnosis is not made initially. Furthermore, less costly "extremity only" MR imaging systems have been introduced in recent years. Some imaging techniques, however, clearly are less expensive than MR imaging. Among these, routine radiography and ultrasonography should be stressed.[111] If the diagnostic information required is likely to be evident with either of these methods, that technique should be employed first. The advantages of routine radiography are well known. Those of ultraso-

nography include its wide availability, lack of invasiveness, and ability to provide functional information; the disadvantages of ultrasonography include its operator dependence and limited acceptance by referring physicians.

Technical Considerations

Spin echo MR imaging remains the most commonly employed method for assessing disorders of the knee. Typically, sagittal and coronal MR images are obtained (Fig. 16–8), the sagittal images often being acquired in the plane of the anterior cruciate ligament (see later discussion). Transaxial MR images also are used, although they have limited value in the diagnosis of meniscal tears. The transaxial images may be acquired with either spin echo or gradient echo methods. There is no uniform agreement regarding the type of spin echo sequences that should be obtained in the coronal and sagittal planes. Typically, in one of these (usually the sagittal plane), proton density and T2-weighted spin echo MR images are acquired, and in the other (usually the coronal plane), T1-weighted spin echo MR images

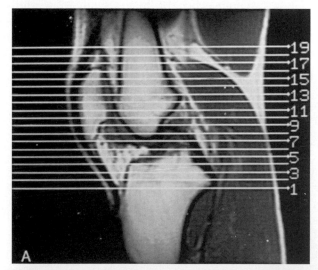

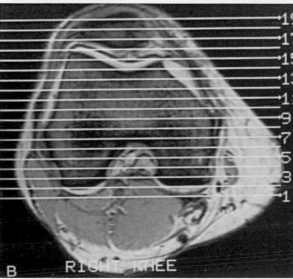

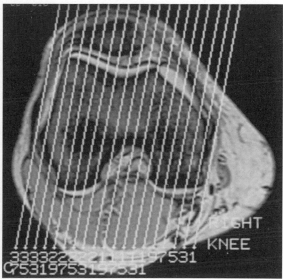

Figure 16–8

MR imaging of the knee: Technical considerations. Three MR imaging planes usually are used to evaluate the knee: sagittal (oblique), coronal, and transaxial planes. Various methods may be used to provide the MR images in these three planes. One method is illustrated here. From a sagittal T1-weighted (TR/TE, 400/12) spin echo localizer image **(A)**, transaxial MR images may be programmed. The transaxial images may consist of multiplanar gradient recalled (MPGR) MR images (TR/TE, 450/15; flip angle, 60 degrees) from which the coronal **(B)** and sagittal oblique **(C)** MR images may be programmed. The sagittal oblique MR images are oriented in an anteromedial to posterolateral direction in order to allow better visualization of the anterior cruciate ligament.

are obtained. The value of coronal T2-weighted spin echo MR images in the evaluation of the collateral ligaments of the knee is addressed later in this chapter.

The sagittal plane is regarded as most important in assessment of the menisci. Although the menisci also are visualized in the coronal plane, supportive rather than new data regarding the integrity of the menisci usually are derived from the coronal MR images.[112] In cases of discoid menisci or meniscal cysts, MR images in the coronal plane may provide additional information.[113] High contrast, narrow window width MR images (meniscal windowing) in both the coronal and sagittal planes frequently are employed. These images may be useful in determining the nature and extent of regions of intermediate signal intensity within the menisci, although their usefulness is not agreed on.[114] In both the coronal and sagittal planes, moderately thin slices (approximately 3 or 4 mm) obtained in a contiguous fashion or with a small interslice gap (approximately 1 mm) are sufficient.

Both the sagittal and coronal imaging planes are fundamental to analysis of the cruciate ligaments, although the sagittal plane is the more valuable of the two. The coronal plane allows careful assessment of the collateral ligaments and iliotibial tract. The transaxial images are essential in the diagnosis of patellofemoral abnormalities (including subluxation and chondromalacia) and,

when combined with sagittal images, are required for full evaluation of the quadriceps and patellar tendons. Articular cartilage assessment relies on analysis of images in all three planes.

In recent years, two-dimensional fast spin echo sequences, which allow more rapid acquisition of image data than standard spin echo sequences, especially for T2-weighted images, have been used in many institutions as the primary MR imaging method for the assessment of the menisci and other structures in the knee.[115, 116] Although image contrast with this technique is similar to that of standard spin echo images, subtle differences exist (see Chapter 1), including some blurring of normally sharp anatomic margins in the fast spin echo proton density images. In one study, such blurring (as well as other factors) led to decreased sensitivity of fast spin echo sequences (with conventional spin echo sequences used as the gold standard) in the detection of meniscal tears of the knee.[117] Fast spin echo techniques, however, are useful for the evaluation of articular cartilage owing, in part, to the heavy T2 weighting (which can be obtained in a reasonable amount of time) combined with magnetization transfer effects in the cartilage.[118] When coupled with fat-suppression methodology, fast spin echo MR images (with T2 weighting) are sensitive to the presence of marrow abnormalities and, in the traumatized knee, to the detection of trabecular

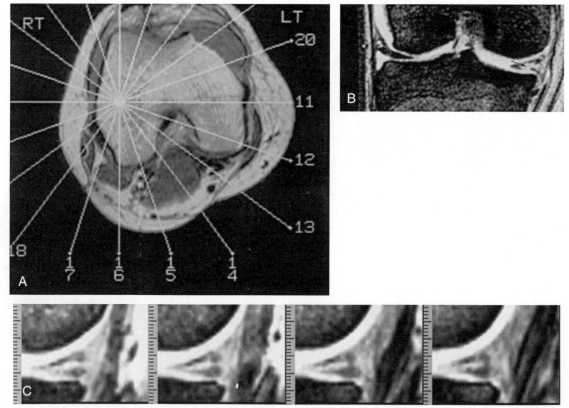

Figure 16–9

MR imaging of the knee: Technical considerations. Radial imaging of the menisci. From data supplied from transaxial MR images, radial sections of the menisci (**A**) can be programmed, which provide an arthrogram-like analysis of the menisci, as shown in a MPGR MR image (TR/TE, 400/12; flip angle, 15 degrees) (**B**). In this patient, a tear of the medial meniscus (arrow) is present. In a different patient, multiple radial images (**C**) with similar factors reveal a tear of the medial meniscus. (C, Courtesy of N. Chafetz, M.D., Torrance, California.)

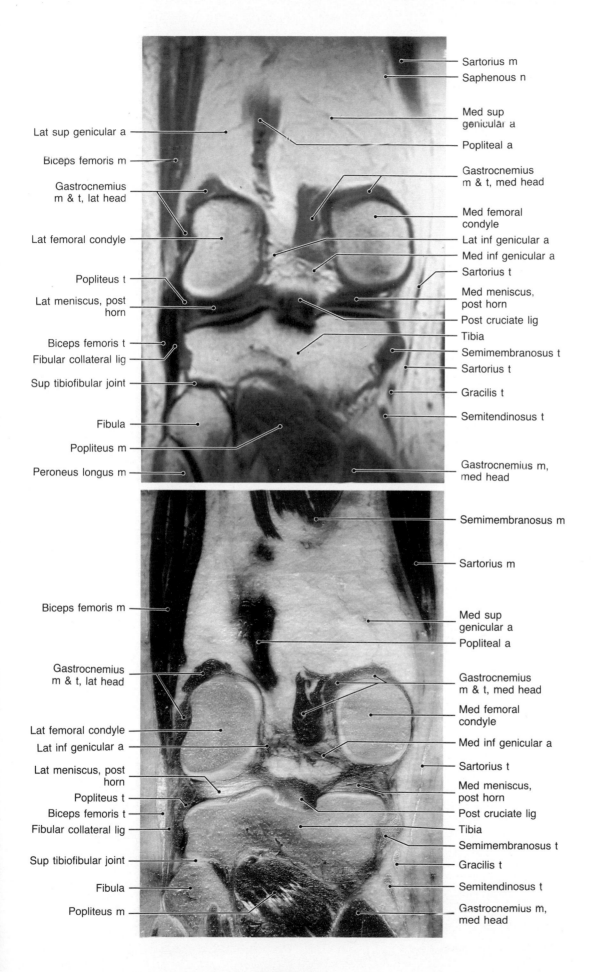

Sartorius m
Saphenous n

Med sup genicular a
Popliteal a

Lat sup genicular a
Biceps femoris m
Gastrocnemius m & t, lat head

Gastrocnemius m & t, med head

Med femoral condyle

Lat femoral condyle

Lat inf genicular a
Med inf genicular a
Sartorius t

Popliteus t
Lat meniscus, post horn

Med meniscus, post horn
Post cruciate lig

Biceps femoris t
Fibular collateral lig

Tibia
Semimembranosus t
Sartorius t

Sup tibiofibular joint

Gracilis t

Fibula
Popliteus m

Semitendinosus t

Peroneus longus m

Gastrocnemius m, med head

Semimembranosus m

Sartorius m

Biceps femoris m

Med sup genicular a
Popliteal a

Gastrocnemius m & t, lat head

Gastrocnemius m & t, med head

Med femoral condyle

Lat femoral condyle
Lat inf genicular a

Med inf genicular a

Lat meniscus, post horn
Popliteus t

Sartorius t

Biceps femoris t

Med meniscus, post horn
Post cruciate lig

Fibular collateral lig

Tibia
Semimembranosus t

Sup tibiofibular joint

Gracilis t

Fibula
Popliteus m

Semitendinosus t

Gastrocnemius m, med head

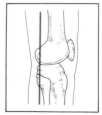

PLATE 16–1

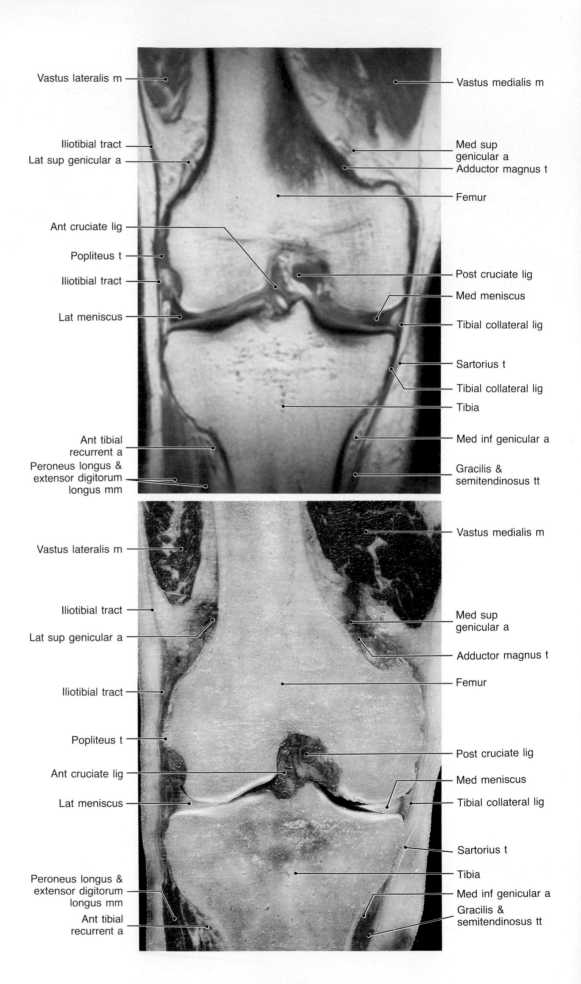

Vastus lateralis m

Vastus medialis m

Iliotibial tract

Lat sup genicular a

Med sup genicular a

Adductor magnus t

Femur

Ant cruciate lig

Popliteus t

Iliotibial tract

Post cruciate lig

Med meniscus

Tibial collateral lig

Lat meniscus

Sartorius t

Tibial collateral lig

Tibia

Ant tibial recurrent a

Med inf genicular a

Peroneus longus & extensor digitorum longus mm

Gracilis & semitendinosus tt

Vastus medialis m

Vastus lateralis m

Iliotibial tract

Lat sup genicular a

Med sup genicular a

Adductor magnus t

Iliotibial tract

Femur

Popliteus t

Post cruciate lig

Ant cruciate lig

Med meniscus

Lat meniscus

Tibial collateral lig

Sartorius t

Tibia

Peroneus longus & extensor digitorum longus mm

Med inf genicular a

Gracilis & semitendinosus tt

Ant tibial recurrent a

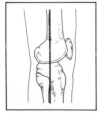

PLATE 16-2

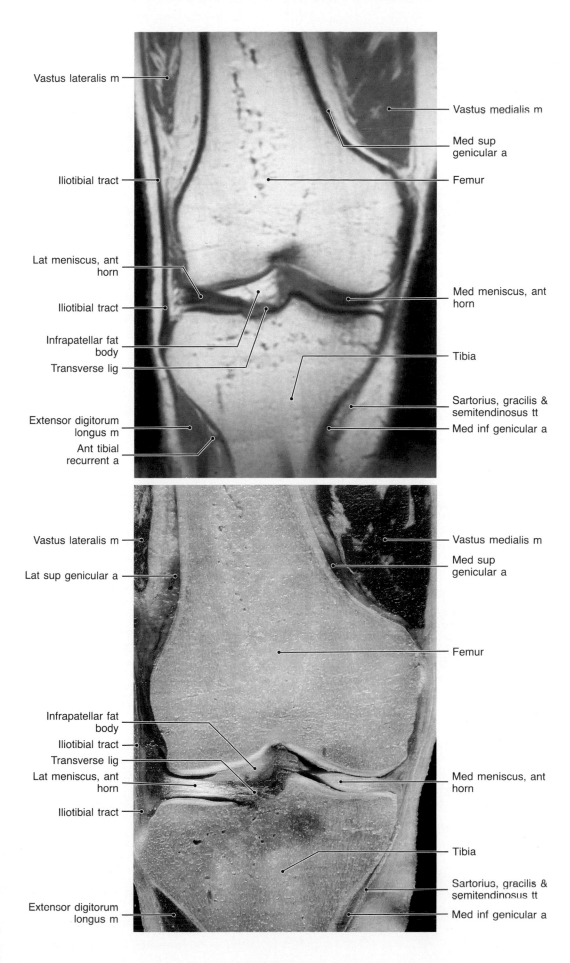

Vastus lateralis m

Iliotibial tract

Lat meniscus, ant horn

Iliotibial tract

Infrapatellar fat body

Transverse lig

Extensor digitorum longus m

Ant tibial recurrent a

Vastus medialis m

Med sup genicular a

Femur

Med meniscus, ant horn

Tibia

Sartorius, gracilis & semitendinosus tt

Med inf genicular a

Vastus lateralis m

Lat sup genicular a

Infrapatellar fat body

Iliotibial tract

Transverse lig

Lat meniscus, ant horn

Iliotibial tract

Extensor digitorum longus m

Vastus medialis m

Med sup genicular a

Femur

Med meniscus, ant horn

Tibia

Sartorius, gracilis & semitendinosus tt

Med inf genicular a

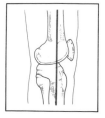

PLATE 16–3

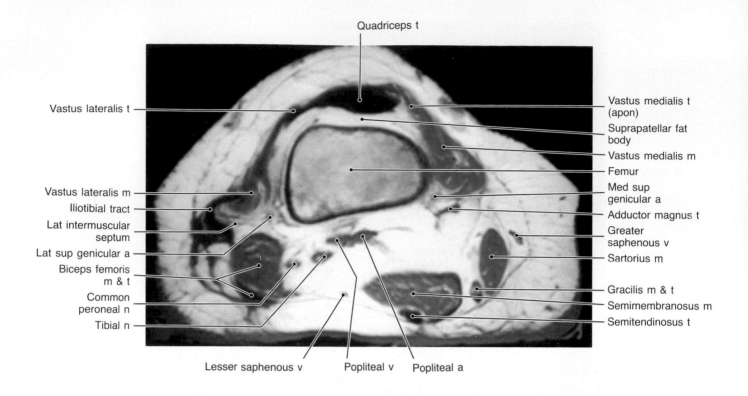

Quadriceps t

Vastus lateralis t

Vastus medialis t (apon)

Suprapatellar fat body

Vastus medialis m

Femur

Med sup genicular a

Adductor magnus t

Greater saphenous v

Sartorius m

Vastus lateralis m

Iliotibial tract

Lat intermuscular septum

Lat sup genicular a

Biceps femoris m & t

Common peroneal n

Tibial n

Gracilis m & t

Semimembranosus m

Semitendinosus t

Lesser saphenous v   Popliteal v   Popliteal a

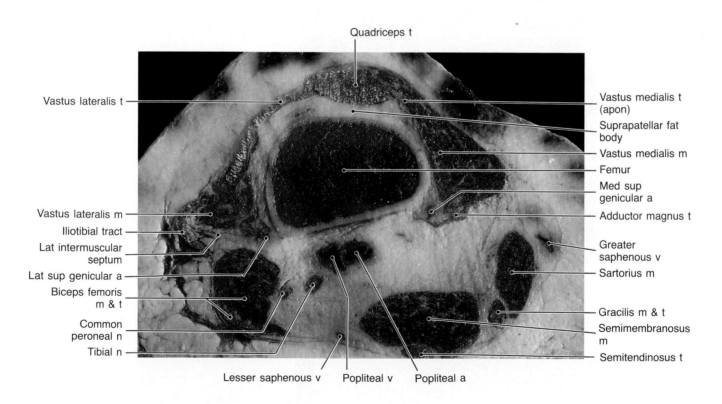

Quadriceps t

Vastus lateralis t

Vastus medialis t (apon)

Suprapatellar fat body

Vastus medialis m

Femur

Med sup genicular a

Adductor magnus t

Greater saphenous v

Sartorius m

Vastus lateralis m

Iliotibial tract

Lat intermuscular septum

Lat sup genicular a

Biceps femoris m & t

Common peroneal n

Tibial n

Gracilis m & t

Semimembranosus m

Semitendinosus t

Lesser saphenous v   Popliteal v   Popliteal a

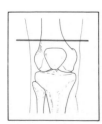

PLATE 16-4

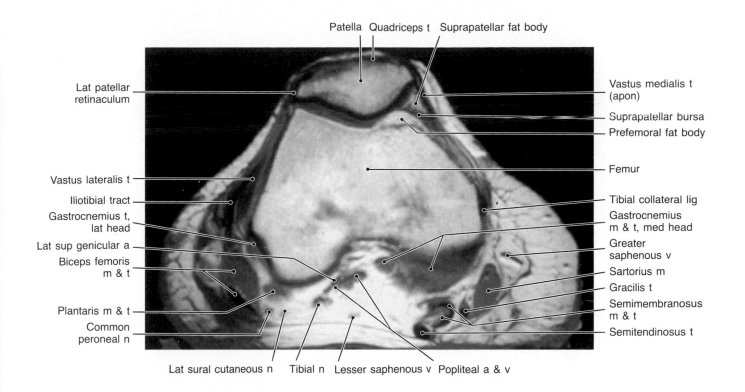

Patella Quadriceps t Suprapatellar fat body

Lat patellar
retinaculum

Vastus medialis t
(apon)

Suprapatellar bursa

Prefemoral fat body

Femur

Vastus lateralis t

Iliotibial tract

Gastrocnemius t,
lat head

Lat sup genicular a

Biceps femoris
m & t

Plantaris m & t

Common
peroneal n

Tibial collateral lig

Gastrocnemius
m & t, med head

Greater
saphenous v

Sartorius m

Gracilis t

Semimembranosus
m & t

Semitendinosus t

Lat sural cutaneous n Tibial n Lesser saphenous v Popliteal a & v

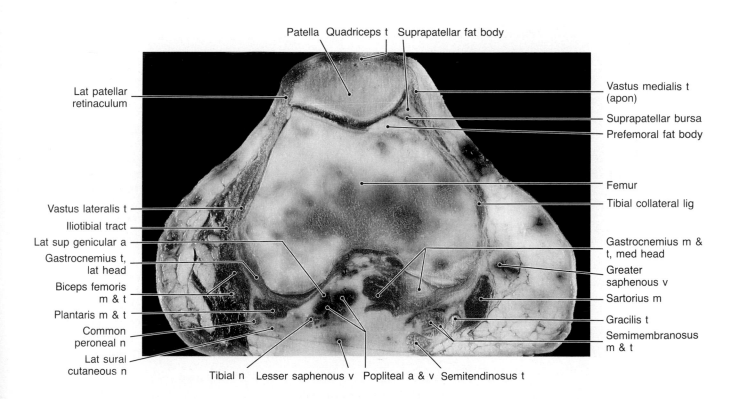

Patella Quadriceps t Suprapatellar fat body

Lat patellar
retinaculum

Vastus medialis t
(apon)

Suprapatellar bursa

Prefemoral fat body

Femur

Tibial collateral lig

Vastus lateralis t

Iliotibial tract

Lat sup genicular a

Gastrocnemius t,
lat head

Biceps femoris
m & t

Plantaris m & t

Common
peroneal n

Lat sural
cutaneous n

Gastrocnemius m &
t, med head

Greater
saphenous v

Sartorius m

Gracilis t

Semimembranosus
m & t

Tibial n Lesser saphenous v Popliteal a & v Semitendinosus t

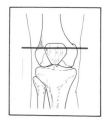

PLATE 16–5

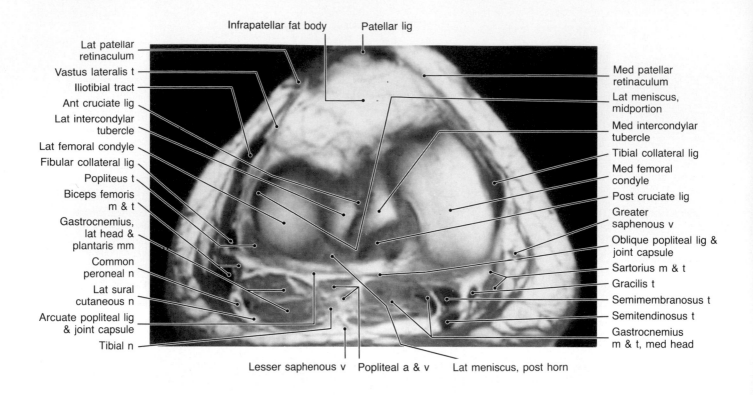

Lat patellar retinaculum
Vastus lateralis t
Iliotibial tract
Ant cruciate lig
Lat intercondylar tubercle
Lat femoral condyle
Fibular collateral lig
Popliteus t
Biceps femoris m & t
Gastrocnemius, lat head & plantaris mm
Common peroneal n
Lat sural cutaneous n
Arcuate popliteal lig & joint capsule
Tibial n

Infrapatellar fat body
Patellar lig

Med patellar retinaculum
Lat meniscus, midportion
Med intercondylar tubercle
Tibial collateral lig
Med femoral condyle
Post cruciate lig
Greater saphenous v
Oblique popliteal lig & joint capsule
Sartorius m & t
Gracilis t
Semimembranosus t
Semitendinosus t
Gastrocnemius m & t, med head

Lesser saphenous v   Popliteal a & v   Lat meniscus, post horn

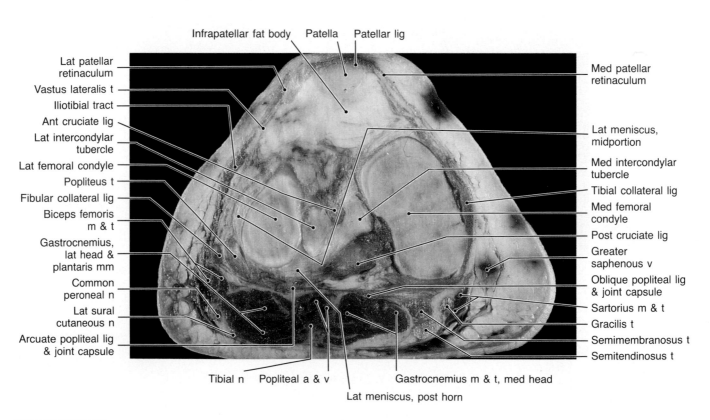

Lat patellar retinaculum
Vastus lateralis t
Iliotibial tract
Ant cruciate lig
Lat intercondylar tubercle
Lat femoral condyle
Popliteus t
Fibular collateral lig
Biceps femoris m & t
Gastrocnemius, lat head & plantaris mm
Common peroneal n
Lat sural cutaneous n
Arcuate popliteal lig & joint capsule

Infrapatellar fat body   Patella   Patellar lig

Med patellar retinaculum
Lat meniscus, midportion
Med intercondylar tubercle
Tibial collateral lig
Med femoral condyle
Post cruciate lig
Greater saphenous v
Oblique popliteal lig & joint capsule
Sartorius m & t
Gracilis t
Semimembranosus t
Semitendinosus t

Tibial n   Popliteal a & v   Gastrocnemius m & t, med head
Lat meniscus, post horn

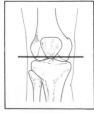

PLATE 16-6

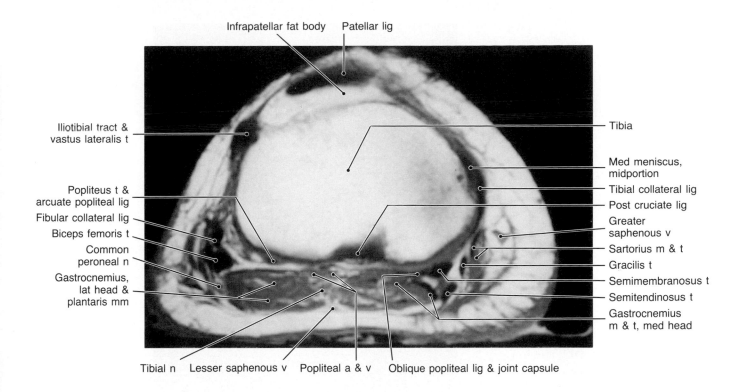

Infrapatellar fat body   Patellar lig

Iliotibial tract &
vastus lateralis t

Popliteus t &
arcuate popliteal lig

Fibular collateral lig

Biceps femoris t

Common
peroneal n

Gastrocnemius,
lat head &
plantaris mm

Tibia

Med meniscus,
midportion

Tibial collateral lig

Post cruciate lig

Greater
saphenous v

Sartorius m & t

Gracilis t

Semimembranosus t

Semitendinosus t

Gastrocnemius
m & t, med head

Tibial n   Lesser saphenous v   Popliteal a & v   Oblique popliteal lig & joint capsule

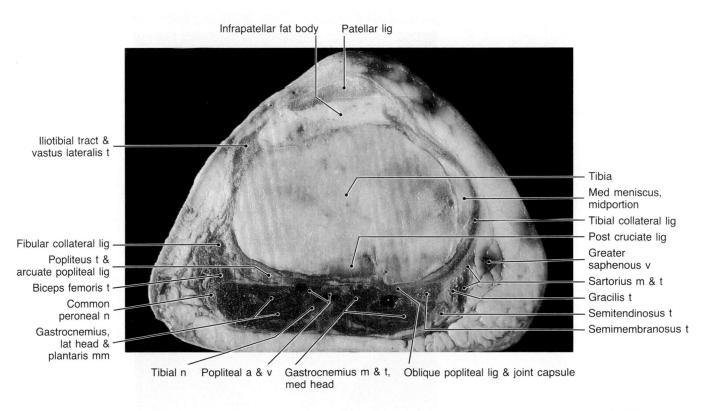

Infrapatellar fat body   Patellar lig

Iliotibial tract &
vastus lateralis t

Fibular collateral lig

Popliteus t &
arcuate popliteal lig

Biceps femoris t

Common
peroneal n

Gastrocnemius,
lat head &
plantaris mm

Tibia

Med meniscus,
midportion

Tibial collateral lig

Post cruciate lig

Greater
saphenous v

Sartorius m & t

Gracilis t

Semitendinosus t

Semimembranosus t

Tibial n   Popliteal a & v   Gastrocnemius m & t,   Oblique popliteal lig & joint capsule
                               med head

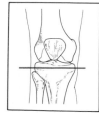

PLATE 16-7

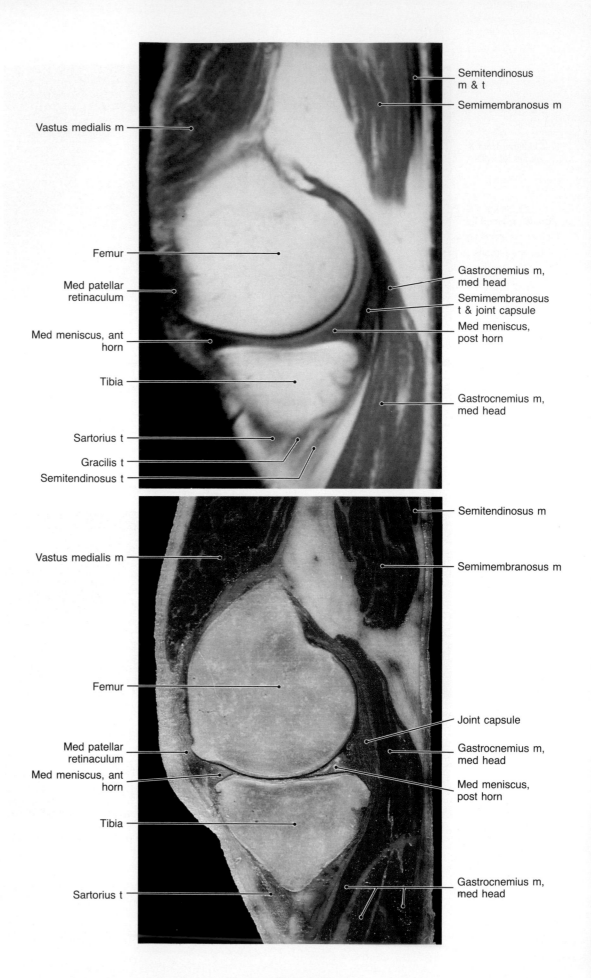

Semitendinosus
m & t

Semimembranosus m

Vastus medialis m

Femur

Gastrocnemius m,
med head

Med patellar
retinaculum

Semimembranosus
t & joint capsule

Med meniscus, ant
horn

Med meniscus,
post horn

Tibia

Gastrocnemius m,
med head

Sartorius t

Gracilis t

Semitendinosus t

Semitendinosus m

Vastus medialis m

Semimembranosus m

Femur

Joint capsule

Med patellar
retinaculum

Gastrocnemius m,
med head

Med meniscus, ant
horn

Med meniscus,
post horn

Tibia

Sartorius t

Gastrocnemius m,
med head

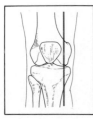

PLATE 16-8

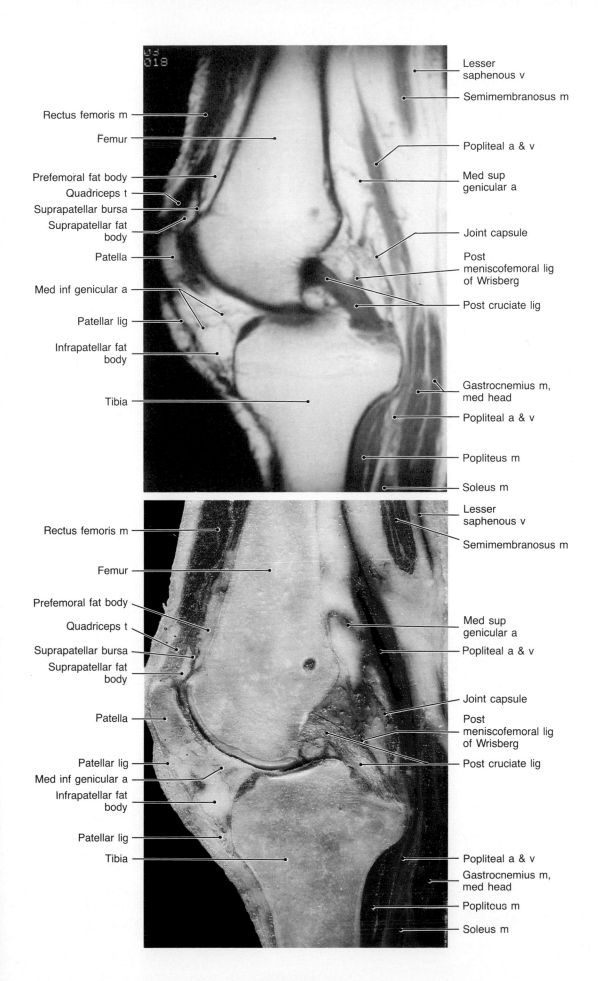

Rectus femoris m

Femur

Prefemoral fat body

Quadriceps t

Suprapatellar bursa

Suprapatellar fat body

Patella

Med inf genicular a

Patellar lig

Infrapatellar fat body

Tibia

Lesser saphenous v

Semimembranosus m

Popliteal a & v

Med sup genicular a

Joint capsule

Post meniscofemoral lig of Wrisberg

Post cruciate lig

Gastrocnemius m, med head

Popliteal a & v

Popliteus m

Soleus m

Rectus femoris m

Femur

Prefemoral fat body

Quadriceps t

Suprapatellar bursa

Suprapatellar fat body

Patella

Patellar lig

Med inf genicular a

Infrapatellar fat body

Patellar lig

Tibia

Lesser saphenous v

Semimembranosus m

Med sup genicular a

Popliteal a & v

Joint capsule

Post meniscofemoral lig of Wrisberg

Post cruciate lig

Popliteal a & v

Gastrocnemius m, med head

Popliteus m

Soleus m

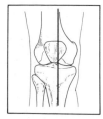

PLATE 16-9

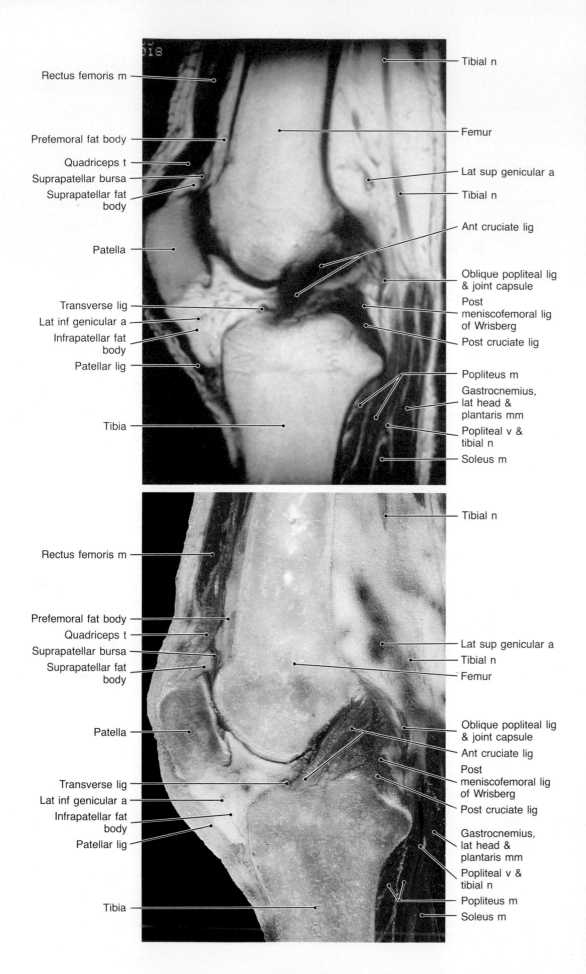

Rectus femoris m

Prefemoral fat body

Quadriceps t
Suprapatellar bursa
Suprapatellar fat body

Patella

Transverse lig
Lat inf genicular a
Infrapatellar fat body
Patellar lig

Tibia

Tibial n

Femur

Lat sup genicular a
Tibial n

Ant cruciate lig

Oblique popliteal lig & joint capsule
Post meniscofemoral lig of Wrisberg
Post cruciate lig

Popliteus m
Gastrocnemius, lat head & plantaris mm
Popliteal v & tibial n
Soleus m

Tibial n

Rectus femoris m

Prefemoral fat body
Quadriceps t
Suprapatellar bursa
Suprapatellar fat body

Patella

Transverse lig
Lat inf genicular a
Infrapatellar fat body
Patellar lig

Tibia

Lat sup genicular a
Tibial n
Femur

Oblique popliteal lig & joint capsule
Ant cruciate lig
Post meniscofemoral lig of Wrisberg
Post cruciate lig

Gastrocnemius, lat head & plantaris mm
Popliteal v & tibial n
Popliteus m
Soleus m

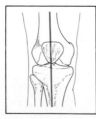

PLATE 16–10

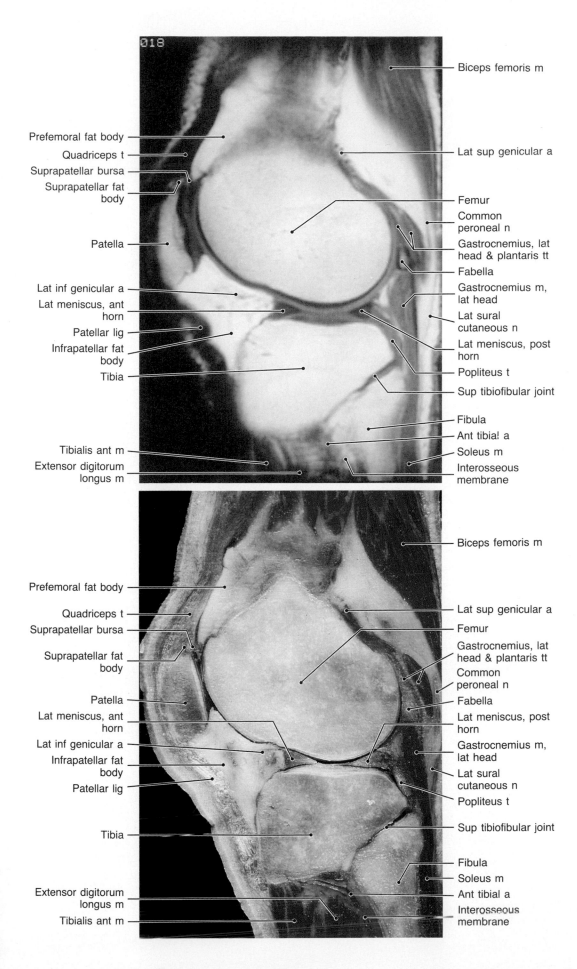

Biceps femoris m

Prefemoral fat body

Quadriceps t

Suprapatellar bursa

Suprapatellar fat body

Lat sup genicular a

Femur

Common peroneal n

Gastrocnemius, lat head & plantaris tt

Fabella

Patella

Gastrocnemius m, lat head

Lat inf genicular a

Lat sural cutaneous n

Lat meniscus, ant horn

Patellar lig

Lat meniscus, post horn

Infrapatellar fat body

Popliteus t

Tibia

Sup tibiofibular joint

Fibula

Ant tibia! a

Tibialis ant m

Soleus m

Extensor digitorum longus m

Interosseous membrane

Biceps femoris m

Prefemoral fat body

Quadriceps t

Lat sup genicular a

Suprapatellar bursa

Femur

Gastrocnemius, lat head & plantaris tt

Suprapatellar fat body

Common peroneal n

Fabella

Patella

Lat meniscus, post horn

Lat meniscus, ant horn

Gastrocnemius m, lat head

Lat inf genicular a

Infrapatellar fat body

Lat sural cutaneous n

Patellar lig

Popliteus t

Tibia

Sup tibiofibular joint

Fibula

Soleus m

Extensor digitorum longus m

Ant tibial a

Tibialis ant m

Interosseous membrane

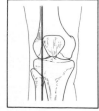

PLATE 16-11

microfractures. Similar sensitivity to marrow abnormalities is provided by STIR or fast spin echo STIR MR imaging.[119, 120]

Gradient recalled MR images also have been used to assess the knee. Such images are obtained most commonly in the transaxial plane, although gradient recalled MR images in the coronal plane can be used to assess ligamentous abnormalities or meniscocapsular separations if small flip angles are employed. Radial imaging can be coupled with gradient recalled MR sequences, providing cross-sectional images perpendicular to the long axis of the meniscus (Fig. 16–9). Radial imaging is best accomplished by programming separately appropriate imaging planes for the medial meniscus and for the lateral meniscus.[113] In one study,[121] the simultaneous analysis of sagittal spin echo MR images and multiplanar gradient recalled (MPGR) radial images led to a slight improvement in sensitivity and specificity in the diagnosis of meniscal tears. Radial MR images increase the conspicuity of meniscal tears but at the expense of anatomic detail.[121] One additional problem that arises with radial imaging of the knee is the presence of a signal void in the center of the images, representing the location of the axis of rotation.[113]

Three-dimensional Fourier transformation (3DFT) gradient echo MR imaging of the knee also has been employed in the assessment of the menisci and other intra-articular structures.[86, 89, 98, 99, 122–124] The advantages of this technique relate to the rapid acquisition of extremely thin (approximately 1 mm) contiguous slices of the knee. Reported data indicate high accuracy in the detection of meniscal tears, although the assessment of the cruciate ligaments and the bone marrow may be less accurate than with standard spin echo images. With three-dimensional MR imaging, meniscal tears may be delineated in the transaxial plane (Fig. 16–10),[123, 124] in addition to the standard coronal and sagittal planes. Furthermore, imaging data acquired in one plane may be reconstructed in another, and three-dimensional re-

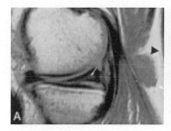
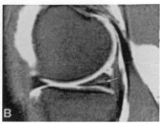

Figure 16–11

MR imaging of the knee: Technical considerations—MR arthrography of the menisci. An initial sagittal proton density–weighted (TR/TE, 2200/20) spin echo MR image **(A)** shows altered signal intensity (arrow) in the posterior horn of the medial meniscus. It is not certain if the region of altered signal intensity extends to the inferior surface of the meniscus. A posterior synovial cyst (arrowhead) also is evident. A sagittal T1-weighted (TR/TE, 650/20) spin echo MR image obtained with chemical presaturation of fat (ChemSat) and after the intra-articular administration of a gadolinium compound **(B)** shows fluid of high signal intensity in the joint and in the synovial cyst, but there is no increase in the signal intensity in the meniscus (arrow). The findings suggest that a meniscal tear is not present.

formatting procedures allow creation of images with apparent depth that then can be rotated in any direction.[113]

The intravenous administration of a gadolinium compound combined with immediate MR imaging (typically T1-weighted fat-suppressed spin echo imaging sequences) is most useful in the analysis of infectious and neoplastic disorders,[125, 126] although this method also can be beneficial in the assessment of synovial inflammatory processes (see later discussion) and, if imaging is delayed after gadolinium contrast agent administration, can provide an arthrographic effect owing to the leakage of the contrast agent from the synovium into the joint fluid.[1112] Such leakage is more prominent and occurs more rapidly if the extremity is exercised.

MR arthrography has a limited role in the evaluation of the knee, although this role may be expanded in instances of persistent or recurrent clinical manifestations after meniscectomy or meniscal repair (see later discussion). Occasionally, when the extent of increased signal intensity within the meniscus is not clear, and specifically, when it is not certain if the altered signal intensity extends to the surface of the meniscus, MR arthrography using gadolinium compounds (or saline solution) may prove useful (Fig. 16–11). The accumulation of contrast agent within the meniscus is strong evidence that a tear is present, a finding that may be accentuated when fat suppression MR imaging methods also are used.

Additional MR imaging techniques applied to the analysis of disorders of the knee (and other joints) include magnetization transfer, particularly in evaluation of the articular cartilage (see later discussion), first-pass contrast imaging, especially in cases of tumor, and dynamic motion studies, generally used to evaluate the patellofemoral joint (see later discussion).

Important anatomic landmarks about and within the knee shown in standard spin echo MR images are shown in Plates 16–1 to 16–11.

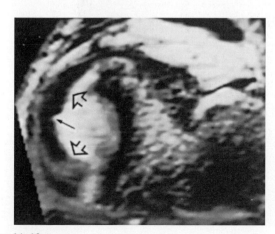

Figure 16–10

MR imaging of the knee: Technical considerations—three-dimensional Fourier transform (3DFT) gradient recalled acquisition in the steady state (GRASS) MR image (TR/TE, 34/15; flip angle, 60 degrees) of the menisci. In this example, a radial tear (solid arrow) of the medial meniscus (open arrows) is evident. (Courtesy of S. Eilenberg, M.D., San Diego, California.)

SPECIFIC ABNORMALITIES

Synovial Abnormalities

Joint Effusion

In normal joints, including the knee, fluid is present in small quantities sufficient to coat the numerous folds of the synovial membrane and to pool in one or more joint recesses. In the normal state, there never is sufficient volume of fluid to distend the joint or to separate redundant surfaces of the synovium.[127] The intra-articular pressure within a normal joint may be a negative one in comparison to ambient atmospheric pressure.[127] The accumulation of abnormal amounts of joint fluid leads to separation of adjacent synovial surfaces, distortion of the joint capsule, and elevation of intra-articular pressure. With large amounts of joint fluid, rupture of the synovial contents or the creation or enlargement of an opening between the joint and a surrounding synovial sac with distention of that sac (i.e., synovial cyst) may occur.

The precise amount of fluid that may be present in a normal knee joint is not clear. What is clear, however, is that such fluid may move from one portion of the joint to another during passive or active movement of the knee, the pattern of flow being guided by the location of intra-articular pressure gradients and physiologic compartmentation.[128] Physiologic compartmentation of a joint is defined as a synovial cavity that is anatomically continuous but is hydraulically divided into separate compartments at physiologic pressures.[129] Pathologic compartmentation of the knee joint may result as a consequence of synovial plicae (see later discussion).

Although abnormal amounts of joint fluid in the knee may be palpated clinically, such fluid also can be detected with several different imaging methods, including routine radiography, ultrasonography, CT, and MR imaging. As indicated earlier, the lateral radiograph of the knee is the most sensitive of all routine radiographic projections in the detection of a joint effusion. Enlargement of the normally collapsed suprapatellar recess is appreciated radiographically on the lateral projection, owing to abnormal separation between a fat body above the patella and the prefemoral fat body. A measurement of 10 mm between these fat bodies is considered definitely abnormal, and between 5 and 10 mm is considered possibly abnormal. An abnormal measurement can result not only from joint fluid but also from an intra-articular mass or hypertrophy of the synovial membrane. A recent study employing MR imaging has indicated that approximately 4 or 5 ml of fluid in the knee joint is required before an effusion can be detected with conventional radiography.[130]

MR imaging is extremely sensitive to the presence of intra-articular fluid (Fig. 16–12). Such fluid is of low signal intensity on T1-weighted spin echo MR images and of high signal intensity on T2-weighted spin echo MR images and on many gradient echo images. Modifications in these patterns of signal intensity occur in the presence of a hemarthrosis. Furthermore, the differentiation of joint fluid and synovial inflammatory tissue may require additional MR imaging techniques (see later discussion). The precise distribution of joint fluid in the knee as detected with MR imaging depends on the size of the effusion, the position of the knee during the examination, and anatomic and pathologic factors such as the presence of synovial plicae and synovial cysts. Schweitzer and coworkers,[130] in a study of cadaveric knees, indicated that sagittal MR images allowed detec-

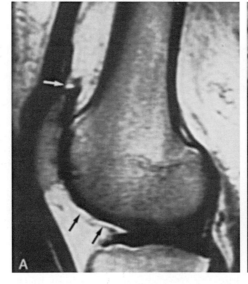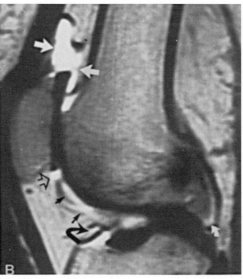

Figure 16–12

Joint effusion: MR imaging. Sagittal T1-weighted (TR/TE, 600/20) spin echo MR images obtained after the intra-articular instillation of 1 ml (**A**) and 15 ml (**B**) of a gadolinium compound show patterns of distribution of fluid in a cadaveric knee joint. In **A,** a small amount of fluid is seen adjacent to the femoral condyle (black arrows) and a tiny amount of fluid is evident in the suprapatellar pouch or recess (white arrow). In **B,** increased fluid is seen in the suprapatellar recess (straight white arrows). Small amounts of fluid are seen distending a superior vertical cleft in Hoffa's infrapatellar fat body (open arrow), filling a horizontally oriented inferior cleft (curved black arrow), extending between the femoral condyle and the infrapatellar fat body (straight solid black arrows), and extending posteriorly about the cruciate ligaments (curved white arrow). (From Schweitzer ME, et al: *AJR 159*:361, 1992.)

tion of as little as 1 ml of fluid, such fluid collecting about the condyles of the femur. Kaneko and collaborators,[131] reviewing MR imaging examinations of 300 traumatized knees, noted the common occurrence of fluid in the central portion of the joint and in the suprapatellar recess, and the infrequent occurrence of fluid in the posterior femoral or subpopliteal regions of the knee. No reported data currently indicate that the precise patterns of distribution of fluid in the knee depend on the specific internal derangements present.

The detection of a knee effusion with MR imaging is aided by differences in the signal intensity of fluid and that of adjacent soft tissue structures. In particular, in the region of the suprapatellar recess and of the anteroinferior portion of the joint, the synovial membrane is intimate with three fat bodies: the anterior and posterior (or prefemoral) suprapatellar fat bodies and the infrapatellar (or Hoffa's) fat body. These fat bodies are intracapsular but extrasynovial. The presence of a bland knee effusion (defined as one that results from trauma or an internal derangement) typically does not lead to distortion of the interface between these fat bodies and the adjacent fluid; the presence of a proliferative effusion (defined as one associated with synovial proliferation) may lead to scalloping, truncation, or displacement of these fat bodies and obscuration of the interface between them and the adjacent fluid (Fig. 16–13).[132]

Hemarthrosis and Lipohemarthrosis

A hemarthrosis may result from an injury or a number of articular processes, including pigmented villonodular synovitis, hemophilia and other bleeding disorders, intra-articular tumors (e.g., synovial hemangioma), neuropathic osteoarthropathy, crystal deposition diseases, and renal osteodystrophy. Posttraumatic hemarthrosis of the knee generally is considered a manifestation of serious ligamentous injury, particularly in adults.[133-135, 1113] A joint effusion appearing within the first few hours after trauma usually is related to a hemarthrosis; nonbloody effusions typically appear 12 to 24 hours after injury.[136, 137] One factor leading to posttraumatic hemarthrosis is a subtle increase in vascular permeability, caused by mechanisms other than gross disruption of vessels.[138]

No reliable routine radiographic features of a hemarthrosis exist. In cases of chronic and recurrent hemarthroses, as in pigmented villonodular synovitis or hemophilia, increased radiodensity of the distended joint due to intrasynovial hemosiderin deposition occasionally may be evident. In such cases, CT may reveal a thickened synovial membrane and increased attenuation values in the hemosiderin-laden synovial membrane.

MR imaging allows a specific diagnosis in some types of hemarthrosis. Although acute hemorrhagic effusions may have signal intensity characteristics similar to those of normal synovial fluid, subacute and chronic hemarthrosis may reveal high signal intensity on both T1-weighted and T2-weighted spin echo MR images. A fluid level representing a layering phenomenon between serum (above) and sediment (below) also may be seen. In cases of chronic hemarthroses, hemosiderin deposition within the synovial membrane leads to regions of low signal intensity in both T1- and T2-weighted spin echo MR images and, especially, in gradient echo images (Fig. 16–14).

The identification of lipid material in synovial fluid by histochemical and microscopic techniques and by imaging methods has diagnostic utility in the injured patient.[139-142] The discovery of intra-articular fat, in combination with bone marrow spicules, is reliable evidence of an intra-articular fracture, the fat being released from the marrow after cortical violation. Frequently, however, a hemorrhagic effusion containing fat may be observed in patients without fracture, probably related to cartilaginous or ligamentous injury.[143, 144] As fat also is present in the synovium, it is possible that damage to the synovium alone can release fat into the synovial fluid.[144] Other sources of lipids in the synovial fluid include the rich vascular bed between the joint and the intra-capsular fat

Figure 16–13

Bland versus proliferative knee effusion: MR imaging.

A Bland effusion. A sagittal T1-weighted (TR/TE, 600/20) spin echo MR image in a patient with a large, bland effusion (curved arrows) shows fluid extending into the normal recesses (solid straight arrows) in the infrapatellar fat body. The interfaces (arrowheads) between the fluid and the adjacent fat bodies are well defined.

B Proliferative effusion. In a patient with pigmented villonodular synovitis, a sagittal proton density–weighted (TR/TE, 1800/19) spin echo MR image shows distortion and displacement (arrows) of the infrapatellar fat body.

(From Schweitzer ME, et al: AJR *160*:823, 1993.)

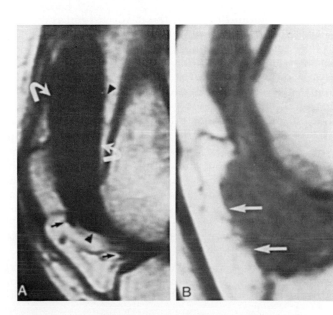

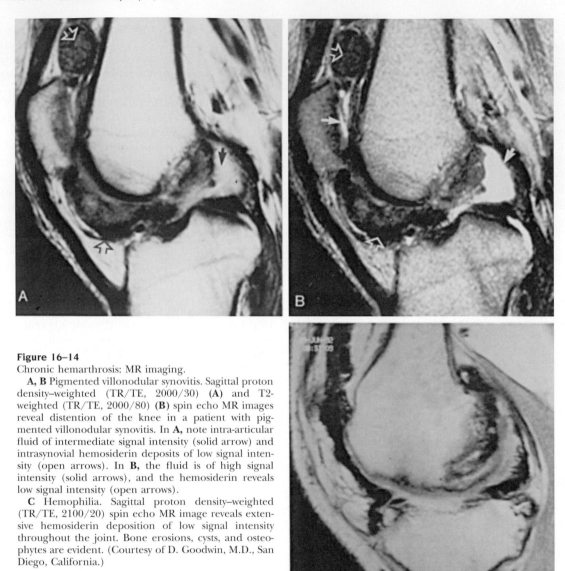

Figure 16–14
Chronic hemarthrosis: MR imaging.

A, B Pigmented villonodular synovitis. Sagittal proton density–weighted (TR/TE, 2000/30) **(A)** and T2-weighted (TR/TE, 2000/80) **(B)** spin echo MR images reveal distention of the knee in a patient with pigmented villonodular synovitis. In **A,** note intra-articular fluid of intermediate signal intensity (solid arrow) and intrasynovial hemosiderin deposits of low signal intensity (open arrows). In **B,** the fluid is of high signal intensity (solid arrows), and the hemosiderin reveals low signal intensity (open arrows).

C Hemophilia. Sagittal proton density–weighted (TR/TE, 2100/20) spin echo MR image reveals extensive hemosiderin deposition of low signal intensity throughout the joint. Bone erosions, cysts, and osteophytes are evident. (Courtesy of D. Goodwin, M.D., San Diego, California.)

pads. The amount of fat in the synovial fluid is directly proportional to the severity of the joint injury.[143, 145]

The detection of a lipohemarthrosis can be accomplished with several different imaging methods (Figs. 16–15 and 16–16). Routine radiographic examination employing horizontal beam technique allows the demonstration of a fat-blood fluid level after injury to the joint.[142, 146–148] Although this finding is observed most often in the knee (in the region of the suprapatellar recess), it also may be noted in other joints, such as the elbow, hip, ankle, and glenohumeral joint. In the knee, lipohemarthrosis may accompany fractures of the tibial plateau, proximal portion of the fibula, patella, or distal portion of the femur, as well as soft tissue injury to cartilage, ligaments, fat pads, or synovium.[149] Small amounts of fat and blood in the knee may not be sufficient to produce a fat-blood fluid level on cross-table radiography, however. Furthermore, a single fluid level detected with horizontal beam technique is not entirely diagnostic of a lipohemarthrosis; a hemarthrosis alone can produce such a level owing to separation of serum and sediment.[1114] Occasionally, routine lateral films of the knee taken without horizontal beam technique in patients with significant intra-articular fat allow visualization of the capsule as a linear structure of water density outlined on both sides by fat.[150]

The value of ultrasonography in the detection of a lipohemarthrosis is not clear. In one study of patients with fractures about the knee, shoulder, and hip, supplemented with data derived from an in vitro experimental model, ultrasonography was shown to be reliable in the identification of lipohemarthroses.[151] Initial examination obtained within minutes after immobilization of the injured region revealed a two-band appearance, representing a fat-blood level. Subsequent examination obtained hours after such immobilization showed a three-band appearance, related to layers composed of fat, serum, and erythrocytes.

Transaxial images provided by CT also demonstrate a lipohemarthrosis as a fat-blood fluid level.[152] This tech-

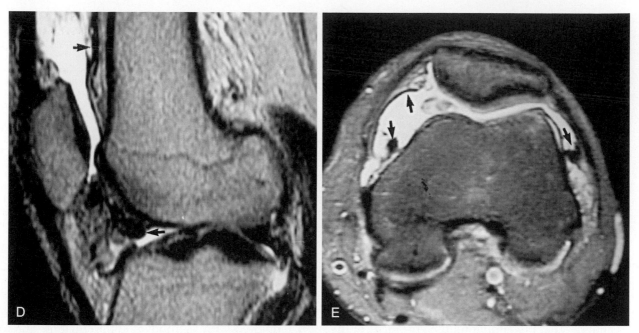

Figure 16–14 *Continued*
D, E Pigmented villonodular synovitis. Hemosiderin deposition of low signal intensity in the synovial membrane (arrows) is shown in a sagittal T2-weighted (TR/TE, 2100/80) spin echo MR image **(D)** and in a transaxial fat-suppressed fast spin echo (TR/TE, 3693/17) MR image **(E)**.

nique appears to be more sensitive than routine radiography, but MR imaging probably is the most sensitive method that allows detection of a lipohemarthrosis. The characteristics of a lipohemarthrosis on MR images are relatively complex.[153] Fat droplets in the knee in the supine patient appear as foci of high signal intensity on T1-weighted coronal spin echo MR images and of intermediate signal intensity on T2-weighted coronal spin echo MR images. In the transaxial and sagittal planes, four distinct signal intensity bands may be evident[153]: a superior band representing floating fat, a central band containing serum, an inferior band of dependent erythrocytes, and a thin band representing chemical shift artifact at the interface of serum and fat.

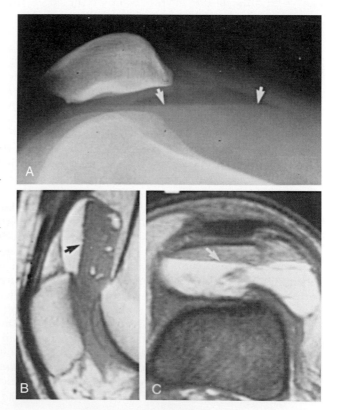

Figure 16–15
Lipohemarthrosis: Routine radiography and MR imaging.
  A Routine radiography. In a patient with a tibial plateau fracture, a cross-table radiograph (obtained with horizontal beam technique) shows a fluid level (arrows) between fat (above) and blood (below).
  B, C MR imaging. In a patient with an avulsion at the tibial site of attachment of the anterior cruciate ligament, a sagittal T1-weighted (TR/TE, 886/15) spin echo MR image **(B)** and a transaxial MPGR MR image (TR/TE, 424/18; flip angle, 20 degrees) **(C)** show a fluid level (arrows) indicative of a lipohemarthrosis. In **B**, the upper layer, representing fat, is of high signal intensity, and the lower layer, representing blood, is of low signal intensity, although it contains regions of high signal intensity, indicative of fat, probably entrapped in blood clots. In **C**, the upper layer is of intermediate signal intensity, again representing fat, and the lower layer is of high signal intensity and contains regions of intermediate signal intensity representing blood.

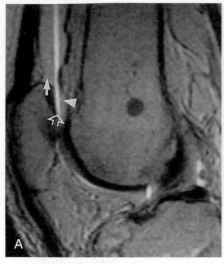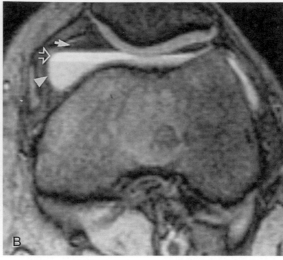

Furthermore, the relative signal intensities of the serum and precipitate vary, depending on the chronicity of the bleed and the specific pulse sequence chosen.

Synovitis

The differentiation of synovial inflammatory tissue and joint fluid is important to the physician who is treating patients with rheumatoid arthritis and related disorders. With most imaging methods, including routine radiography and CT, such differentiation is not possible. MR imaging holds promise in this area (Figs. 16–17 and 16–18).

In 1990, Kursunoglu-Brahme and coworkers[154] reported results in the examination of the knee in 14 patients with classic rheumatoid arthritis, with MR images obtained both before and immediately after the intravenous administration of gadopentetate dimeglumine. T1-weighted and T2-weighted spin echo MR images obtained prior to administration of a gadolinium compound demonstrated identical signal intensity characteristics in both the effusion and the inflamed synovial membrane. The intravenous administration of the gadolinium compound, however, allowed distinction between effusion and abnormal synovium, with the effusion remaining of low signal intensity and the synovium demonstrating enhancement and increased signal intensity on T1-weighted spin echo MR images. Two years later, Singson and Zalduondo[155] reported that standard spin echo MR images (i.e., those obtained without the intravenous administration of gadolinium compounds) could be used for the same purpose. They indicated that thickened synovium was of intermediate signal intensity on T1-weighted spin echo MR images compared with the lower signal intensity of joint effusion. In eight of 12 knees with significant joint effusions and thickened synovium, the abnormal synovium had an intermediate signal intensity on T2-weighted spin echo MR images relative to the high signal intensity of the joint effusion, although in the other four knees, the increased signal intensity of the abnormal synovium was identical to that of the articular fluid.

If intravenous injection of gadolinium compounds is employed as a method of differentiating abnormal synovium and joint fluid, it becomes mandatory to obtain MR images immediately after their injection.[156] The delayed enhancement of joint fluid after intravenous gadolinium contrast agent administration is well documented.[157, 158] A faster rate and greater degree of enhancement of joint fluid occurs in knees that are exercised than in those at rest, presumably related to an increased rate of transsynovial flow and more rapid diffusion in the exercised knees.[158, 1112] A peripheral rim of enhancing joint fluid in delayed MR images may be misinterpreted as enhanced, thickened synovium; thus, noninflammatory joint effusions may mistakenly be diagnosed as synovitis.[158] In rheumatoid arthritis, it also is possible that enhancement of the signal intensity of the joint fluid occurs at a more rapid rate, leading to further diagnostic difficulty.

Advances related to improved discrimination between synovium and joint fluid (as well as among cartilage, synovium, and joint fluid) have included the application of fat-suppressed imaging and saturation transfer techniques (the latter altering the signal intensity through effects on cross relaxation, or magnetization transfer, between the aqueous and macromolecular components of tissue).[159] Some of these techniques are addressed later in this chapter in a discussion of cartilage imaging.

In the later stages of synovial inflammatory diseases, including juvenile-onset or adult-onset rheumatoid arthritis, septic arthritis, and the seronegative spondyloarthropathies, MR imaging provides useful information regarding the severity of the process and the extent of cartilaginous and osseous destruction (Figs. 16–19, 16–20, and 16–21).

Synovial Plicae

The term synovial plicae refers to remnants of synovial tissue that in early development originally divided the joint into three separate compartments, and that may be found normally in the adult knee.[160–168] Usually of no consequence, these structures may become pathologi-

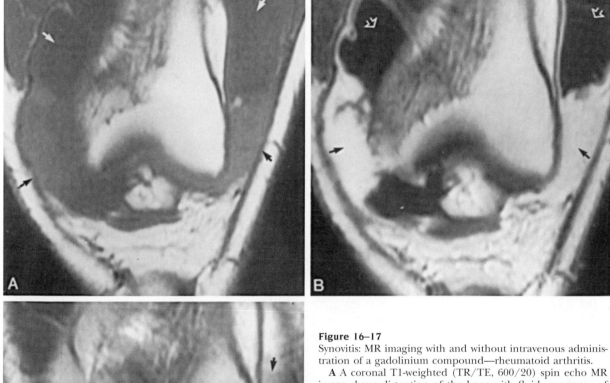

Figure 16–17

Synovitis: MR imaging with and without intravenous administration of a gadolinium compound—rheumatoid arthritis.

A A coronal T1-weighted (TR/TE, 600/20) spin echo MR image shows distention of the knee with fluid or pannus of inhomogeneous low signal intensity (arrows).

B An identical T1-weighted (TR/TE, 600/20) spin echo MR image obtained immediately after the intravenous administration of a gadolinium compound reveals pannus of high signal intensity (solid arrows) and joint fluid of low signal intensity (open arrows).

C An identical T1-weighted (TR/TE, 600/20) spin echo MR image obtained in a delayed fashion after the intravenous administration of a gadolinium compound reveals regions of intermediate signal intensity (arrows) throughout the joint.

(Courtesy of S.K. Brahme, M.D., La Jolla, California.)

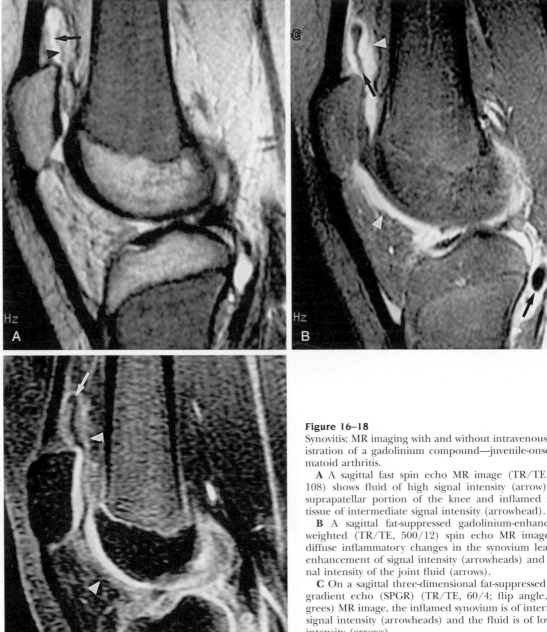

Figure 16–18

Synovitis: MR imaging with and without intravenous administration of a gadolinium compound—juvenile-onset rheumatoid arthritis.

A A sagittal fast spin echo MR image (TR/TE, 3500/108) shows fluid of high signal intensity (arrow) in the suprapatellar portion of the knee and inflamed synovial tissue of intermediate signal intensity (arrowhead).

B A sagittal fat-suppressed gadolinium-enhanced T1-weighted (TR/TE, 500/12) spin echo MR image shows diffuse inflammatory changes in the synovium leading to enhancement of signal intensity (arrowheads) and low signal intensity of the joint fluid (arrows).

C On a sagittal three-dimensional fat-suppressed spoiled gradient echo (SPGR) (TR/TE, 60/4; flip angle, 60 degrees) MR image, the inflamed synovium is of intermediate signal intensity (arrowheads) and the fluid is of low signal intensity (arrows).

(Courtesy of V. Gylys-Morin, M.D., Cincinnati, Ohio.)

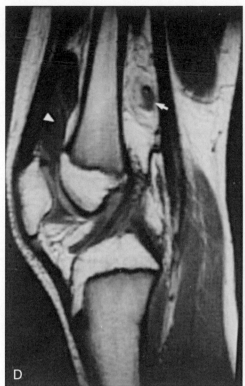

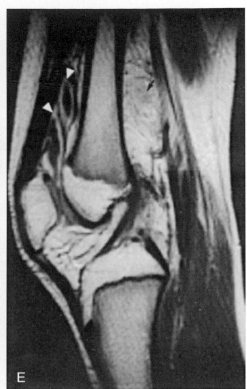

Figure 16–18 *Continued*

D, E In a second patient, initial unenhanced T1-weighted sagittal spin echo MR image (TR/TE, 560/26) **(D)** shows a large effusion (arrowhead) and lymph node (arrow). The joint fluid is of low signal intensity. After intravenous administration of gadolinium tetraazacyclododecanetetraacetic acid (DOTA), a repeat T1-weighted spin echo sagittal MR image (TR/TE, 560/26) **(E)** reveals enhancement of portions of the suprapatellar and cruciate regions (arrowheads), consistent with synovial inflammatory tissue, and of the lymph node (arrow). Note that some unenhanced joint fluid remains, especially in the suprapatellar recess.

(Reproduced with permission from Hervé-Somma CMP, et al: *Radiology 182*:93, 1992.)

cally thickened and lead to symptoms mimicking arthritis, injuries involving the meniscus, and other common internal derangements of the knee. In addition, persistence of these structures in their embryonic form, as complete septa, may cause a variety of intra-articular compartmental syndromes.

The synovial cavity of the adult knee is the most extensive and complex in the body, and it represents in its final form the end result of a sequence of developmental steps that have been studied extensively. In the embryo of 7 weeks' gestation, the tibial and femoral cartilages are separated by unchondrified blastema, which becomes thinned to form a discrete disc or intermediate zone.[169] As the joint continues to grow, and

prior to the development of the fibrous joint capsule, adjacent mesenchyme becomes incorporated into an intra-articular position. This embryonic mesenchyme gives rise to the menisci and cruciate ligaments at approximately 8 weeks of development.[169] It generally is agreed that cavities are not seen in the previously solid embryonic synovial mesenchyme until approximately 9 weeks of embryogenesis. Originally, three compartments are partitioned by septa of embryonic synovium: a superior femoropatellar compartment and two inferior femorotibial compartments.[170] These primitive cavities enlarge by proliferation of the lining tissue and extend into the middle portion of the blastemal intermediate zone. At this time, the cavities are irregular in outline

Figure 16–19

Synovitis: MR imaging—rheumatoid arthritis.

A This coronal T1-weighted (TR/TE, 500/14) spin echo MR image shows severe destruction of cartilage and bone. Fluid or pannus, or both, fills the joint cavity. The menisci and cruciate and medial collateral ligaments also are destroyed.

B On a sagittal fat-suppressed fast spin echo MR image (TR/TE, 3000/120), note joint fluid, synovial thickening, and cystlike regions of bone destruction.

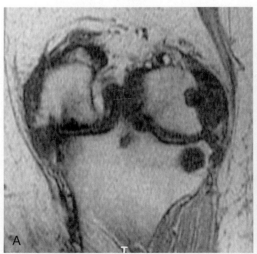

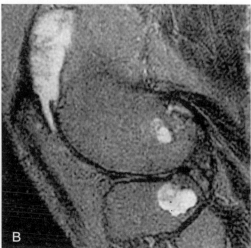

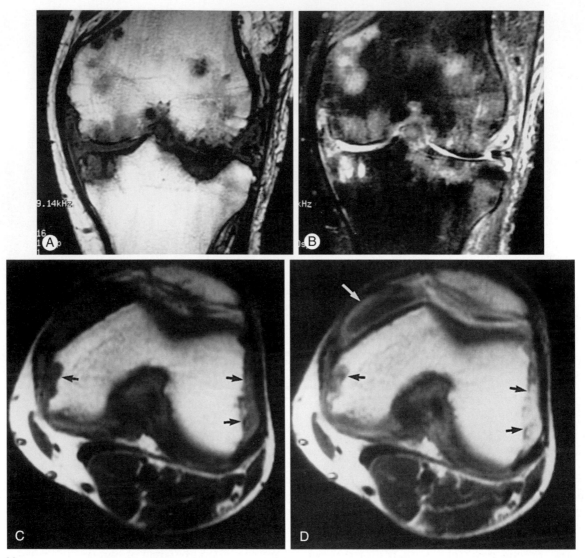

Figure 16–20
Synovitis: MR imaging—septic arthritis.

A, B Coronal T1-weighted (TR/TE, 600/20) spin echo **(A)** and fat-suppressed fast spin echo (TR/TE, 3000/21) **(B)** MR images demonstrate severe central and marginal bone destruction, cartilage loss, meniscal destruction, and a joint effusion. *Mycobacterium avium* was the causative agent. (Courtesy of C. Beaulieu, M.D., and A.G. Bergman, M.D., Stanford, California.)

C, D In this patient with tuberculous arthritis, a transaxial T1-weighted (TR/TE, 600/30) spin echo MR image **(C)** reveals fluid or synovial inflammatory tissue, or both, of low signal intensity in the knee and marginal erosions of bone (arrows). Immediately after the intravenous administration of a gadolinium compound, an identical MR image (TR/TE, 600/30) **(D)** reveals enhancement of signal intensity in the synovial membrane (white arrow) and in the tissue about the sites of bone erosion (black arrows).

and frequently contain strands of tissue, and their lining bears little resemblance to the typical synovial tissue of the adult.[169] Progressive involution of these mesenchymal septa leads to the formation of a single joint space by approximately 12 weeks.[169] Persistence of any portion of these embryonic partitions constitutes a synovial plica. These synovial remnants can be encountered in 18 to 60 per cent of adult knees, a frequency that largely may reflect the diligence and persistence of the examiner.[164, 165]

The three most commonly encountered plicae are classified according to the partitions from which they took origin, as suprapatellar, medial patellar, and infrapatellar (Fig. 16–22). Of these, the infrapatellar plica is most frequent, followed by the suprapatellar plica and

then the medial plica.[165] Rarely, a lateral patellar plica is observed.[171] Each of these septa varies widely in size and shape, and various combinations may exist simultaneously. Their identification can be accomplished by arthrography,[162, 172–174] computed arthrotomography,[175, 176] MR imaging, or arthroscopy,[167, 168, 177–181] depending on their location and size.

The suprapatellar plica, or plica synovialis suprapatellaris, represents a remnant of the embryonic septum that divides the suprapatellar cavity from the medial and lateral joint compartments. This synovial fold may vary widely in the adult and most commonly takes one of the following three forms: (1) an intact septum completely dividing the suprapatellar pouch from the remainder of the knee; (2) an intact septum except for a variably

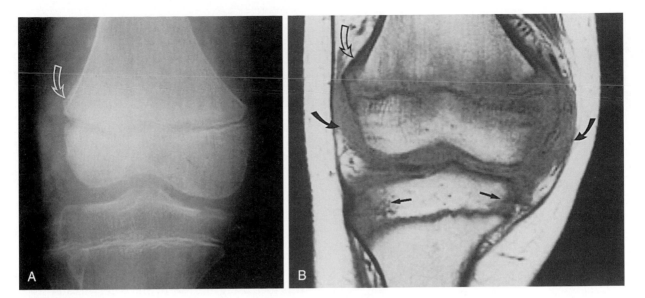

Figure 16–21
Synovitis: MR imaging—Septic arthritis.
  A In a 10 year old boy, a routine radiograph shows widening and indistinctness of the femoral physis and periostitis (open arrow).
  B A coronal T1-weighted (TR/TE, 600/15) spin echo MR image reveals articular and periarticular soft tissue involvement (solid curved arrows), involvement of the marrow in the tibial epiphysis (solid straight arrows), femoral involvement, and periosteal reaction (open arrow).

sized, centrally placed diaphragm known as the porta; and (3) a variably sized, crescent-shaped fold arising medially from the undersurface of the quadriceps tendon above the level of the patella and extending inferiorly to insert along the medial edge of the knee joint (Fig. 16–23).[170]

On double contrast arthrograms, the suprapatellar plica is best visualized on the lateral view with the knee in full extension. This position allows for complete distention of the suprapatellar pouch. The plica is seen as a thin, delicate fold obliquely crossing the suprapatellar pouch to insert near the patella. On fluoroscopy, it is readily pliable, moving easily with flexion and extension of the knee. With computed arthrotomography, this plica most commonly appears as a fine line parallel to the medial wall of the joint.[175] With MR imaging, it is seen more easily when there is fluid in the joint.

The medial patellar plica has been referred to variously as a wedge, a band, or a shelf.[159] This synovial remnant has its origin on the medial wall of the knee

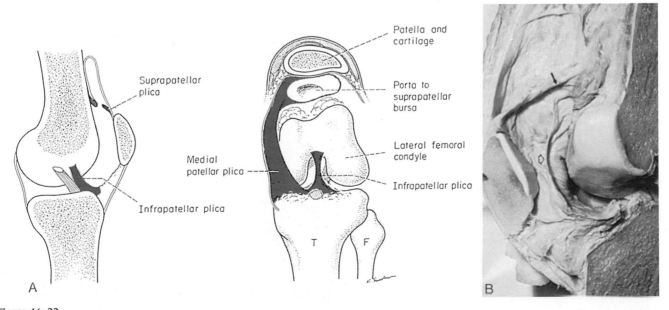

Figure 16–22
Synovial plicae: Classification.
  A A schematic drawing depicts the three most commonly encountered synovial plicae.
  B A sagittal section through the knee demonstrates the suprapatellar plica (solid arrow) and the medial patellar plica (open arrow).
  (From Deutsch AL, et al: Radiology *141*:627, 1981.)

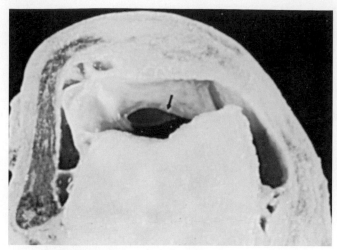

Figure 16–23

Synovial plicae: Suprapatellar plicae—anatomy. A transverse section through the suprapatellar pouch in a cadaver demonstrates the plica and prominent porta (arrow). (From Deutsch AL, et al: Radiology *141*:627, 1981.)

joint, near the suprapatellar plica, and courses obliquely downward relative to the patella to insert into the synovium, which covers the infrapatellar fat pad (Fig. 16–24). Its inner edge may be rounded, sharp, or smooth, or it may contain small fenestrations.[159] Its configuration varies with knee position, lying transverse to the femur with the knee extended and parallel to the axis of the femur with the joint flexed.

Arthrographic demonstration of the medial patellar plica depends on careful technique and the inclusion of axial views of the patellofemoral compartment.[173, 182, 183] On the axial projections, this plica is seen as a flat, lucent region lying just anterior to the medial femoral condyle in the medial aspect of the patellofemoral joint. In an almost lateral projection, with the knee in slight internal rotation, the medial patellar plica appears as a stringlike radiolucent line superimposed on the superior part of the medial femoral condyle, extending from

the suprapatellar bursa to the infrapatellar fat pad.[182] Computed arthrotomography delineates the location and the thickness of this plica.[175, 176] With MR imaging, the medial patellar plica is seen on transaxial and sagittal images when fluid is present in the joint (Fig. 16–25).

The infrapatellar plica, or ligamentum mucosum, represents a vestige of the membranous partition that once separated the medial and lateral embryonic compartments of the knee.[162] It often is fan-shaped, with a narrow femoral margin in the intercondylar notch, widening as it descends through the inferior joint space to attach distally to the inferior and medial aspects of the patellar articular cartilage (see Fig. 16–5). From there the plica continues as two fringe-like alar folds to cover the infrapatellar fat and separate the synovium from the ligamentum patellae.[184] Its course parallels that of the anterior cruciate ligament, which is located just posterior to it. The course and position of the plica change with increasing flexion of the knee because the site of insertion into the intercondylar fossa is displaced. On rare occasions, the infrapatellar plica may be double, or it may persist into adult life as an intact septum, although more commonly it is encountered as a fenestrated septum or series of fibrous bands in the adult knee.[159, 184]

The infrapatellar plica can be identified on double contrast arthrography on both the lateral and the intercondylar views. Because of their anatomic relationship, the infrapatellar plica may easily be confused with the anterior cruciate ligament, resulting in an incorrect diagnosis in patients with complete disruption of the anterior cruciate ligament.[185]

Symptomatic plicae most commonly are encountered in what has been referred to as the plica syndrome.[159, 160, 164, 166, 186] In this syndrome, the medial patellar plica, which normally exists as a fine, thin, flexible fold of synovium of little clinical significance, becomes pathologically thickened and symptomatic.[177–180, 187–192] Infrapatellar plicae also may become thickened, leading to flexion contractures of the knee,[1115] although pathologic abnormalities related to medial plicae are far more com-

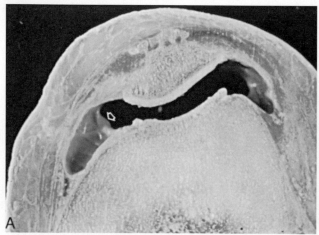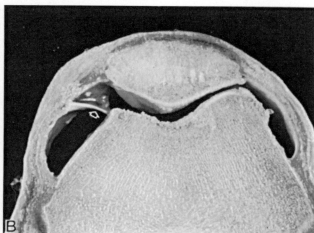

Figure 16–24

Synovial plicae: Medial patellar plicae—anatomy. Transverse sections through cadaveric knee joints at the level of the patella demonstrate medial patellar plicae (arrows). (From Deutsch AL, et al: Radiology *141*:627, 1981.)

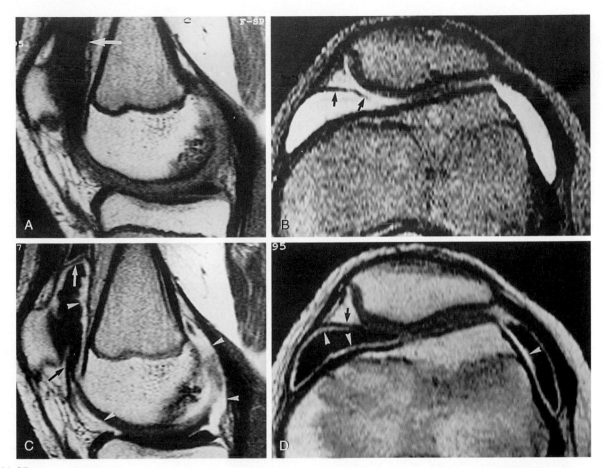

Figure 16–25

Juvenile chronic arthritis with synovial plicae: MR imaging.

A A sagittal T1-weighted (TR/TE, 600/15) spin echo MR image shows distention of the suprapatellar pouch (arrow).

B A transaxial T2-weighted (TR/TE, 2000/90) spin echo MR image reveals fluid or fluid and pannus of high signal intensity and a medial patellar plica (arrows).

C Immediately after the intravenous injection of a gadolinium compound, a sagittal T1-weighted (TR/TE, 600/15) spin echo MR image shows thickened synovium (arrowheads) of high signal intensity and a medial patellar plica (black arrow) of low signal intensity. Note also a suprapatellar plica (white arrow) with adjacent inflamed synovium.

D A transaxial T1-weighted (TR/TE, 600/15) spin echo MR image obtained after intravenous gadolinium administration again shows the thickened synovium (arrowheads) and medial patellar plica (arrow).

mon. Among the postulated factors in the initiation of a traumatic synovitis leading to secondary abnormalities within the plicae are trauma, strenuous exercise, osteochondritis dissecans, injuries to the meniscus, and intra-articular osteocartilaginous bodies. Regardless of the inciting event, when inflammation exists with edema and thickening, fibrous repair may result in increasing collagenization and progressive loss of elasticity.[164] With continued thickening, the plica becomes relatively unpliable and no longer glides normally but snaps against the underlying femoral condyle. Repeated irritation and abrasion result in erosive changes of the articular cartilage of the condyle or even the patella.[176, 187, 188]

The diagnosis may be suspected from the history and physical examination. Classically, the patient relates an episode of blunt or twisting trauma followed by the development of a joint effusion. Excessive stress precipitates a dull, aching pain medial to the patella, which is aggravated by flexion. A clicking sensation without locking or giving way is another common clinical complaint. A palpable or audible snap may occur on knee move-

ment, and a symptomatic plica may be palpated as a tender, bandlike structure parallel to the medial border of the patella. In some cases, a pathologic plica may simulate primary monoarticular arthritis.[190] Alternatively, in rheumatoid arthritis and in other conditions in which a chronic synovial inflammatory process is present, the plicae may become irregularly thickened. The thickened medial plica may be visualized with CT arthrography or MR imaging (Fig. 16–26).

Although much recent attention has focused on the plica syndrome, these embryonic remnants may manifest themselves in another clinically significant manner. Both the suprapatellar and infrapatellar plicae may persist in their entirety and lead to complete compartmentalization of the knee joint. Failure of the suprapatellar partition to involute may produce an entirely separate suprapatellar bursa.[160, 162, 191, 193] Clinically, the bursa may be manifested as a mass in the suprapatellar area, which is cystic or rubbery and firm on palpation.[160, 170] This may be recognized on double contrast arthrography by the appearance of either a small suprapatellar space

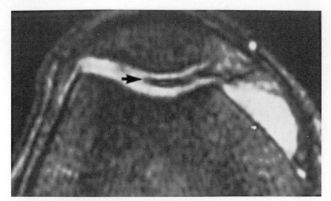

Figure 16–26

Synovial plicae: Plica syndrome. A thickened medial patellar plica (arrow) is well shown on a transaxial short tau inversion recovery (STIR) MR image (TR/TE, 1650/25; inversion time, 160 msec).

or an extrinsic compression on the suprapatellar pouch.[162, 193] CT or CT arthrography may be of value in further characterizing the nature of the mass and its relation to the knee joint. MR imaging also may display the mass (Figs. 16–27 and 16–28).[194] Documentation of a separate bursa is of considerable importance in planning an optimal surgical approach; in this regard, a case has been described in which osteocartilaginous bodies in a separate suprapatellar bursa could not be located by using an infrapatellar surgical incision.[170] Documentation of a separate bursa also is important in the management of penetrating wounds with acute suppurative bursitis, in which rupture of the partitioning membrane may contaminate the joint unnecessarily.[170] Furthermore, diffuse synovial processes such as pigmented villonodular synovitis may affect not the entire joint but the sequestered suprapatellar bursa.[195]

Persistence of the infrapatellar plica in its entirety will divide the knee joint into separate medial and lateral compartments.[196] This finding may occur in patients who have had a history of previous trauma with healed supracondylar fractures.[162] This fact suggests that trauma may initiate either fibrous thickening and hypertrophy of the infrapatellar plica or intra-articular fibrosis, leading to abnormal compartmentalization of the joint. Similar compartmentalization has been identified in hereditary onycho-osteoarthrodysplasia (the nail-patella syndrome).[162] The probable relation, however, between anomalies of the patella and aberrations in joint development remains incompletely understood.[197]

Periarticular Synovial and Ganglion Cysts

Minor variations in histologic features and inconsistencies in terminology have led to great confusion regarding the classification of synovial cysts and other periarticular fluid collections. The existence of numerous bursae about the knee[1, 3, 37, 198, 199] further complicates the classification of fluid-filled cystic lesions in this location. Although such cysts occurring in the popliteal fossa that communicate with the joint usually are referred to as synovial cysts or Baker's cysts, cysts in this region that do not communicate with the joint and those in other locations about the knee that may or may not communicate with the joint are described using a variety of terms, such as noncommunicating synovial cysts, ganglion cysts, meniscal cysts, and juxta-articular myxomas. Subtle differences in the histologic features of the lesions or in their contents may allow an experienced pathologist to differentiate among these many fluid-filled cysts, although no uniformly accepted classification system exists. In this section, a discussion of some of the more typical synovial and ganglion cysts occurring about the knee is presented. Cystic lesions that generally communicate with an abnormal meniscus (i.e., meniscal cysts) and special forms of bursitis are considered later in this chapter.

Synovial cysts about the knee are most frequent in the popliteal region, where communication between the joint and normal posterior bursae can be identified.[198, 200, 201] The most commonly involved bursa is the gastrocnemiosemimembranosus bursa,[202, 203] located posterior to the medial femoral condyle between the tendons of the gastrocnemius and semimembranosus muscles, with an additional portion anterior to the medial head of the gastrocnemius muscle. The anterior limit of this bursa abuts on the posterior surface of the joint capsule and is relatively thin.[204] Communication between the bursa and the knee joint occurs in 35 to 55 per cent of cadavers[198, 204] and increases in frequency with advancing age. This communication occurs via a transverse slit, usually between 15 to 20 mm long.[204] The opening may be covered with a fibrous membrane in approximately 70 per cent of cases.[204]

Swelling of this posterior bursa is termed a Baker's cyst.[205, 206] The cause of such cysts is not entirely clear, and various theories have been proposed: (1) herniation of the synovial membrane of the knee through a weak area in the posterior joint capsule; (2) rupture of the posterior joint capsule with extravasation of fluid into the soft tissues and secondary encapsulation; and (3) rupture of the posterior joint capsule, producing communication with a normally occurring posterior bursa. Of these theories, the third theory seems most probable,[198, 200, 207, 208] as direct observation rarely has documented a synovial herniation from the knee into a normal bursa or a popliteal cyst completely separated from the articular cavity.

The presence of a slit between articular cavity and posterior bursa may be responsible for a ball-valve mechanism that has been noted in conjunction with synovial cysts[209–211]; fluid introduced into a cyst may not enter the joint cavity (Fig. 16–29). Because of this one-way directional flow, arthrography rather than bursography is more accurate in defining the extent of a cyst and its connection with a neighboring joint. This ball-valve mechanism, however, is not present invariably. Rauschning and collaborators[203] have divided popliteal cysts into those with a true one-way valve (approximately 50 per cent of cases) and those in which unimpeded flow of fluid occurs in both directions; strong positive correlation was found between the presence of a valve mechanism and the absence of articular disorders and between the absence of a valve mechanism and the presence of joint effusions and disease.

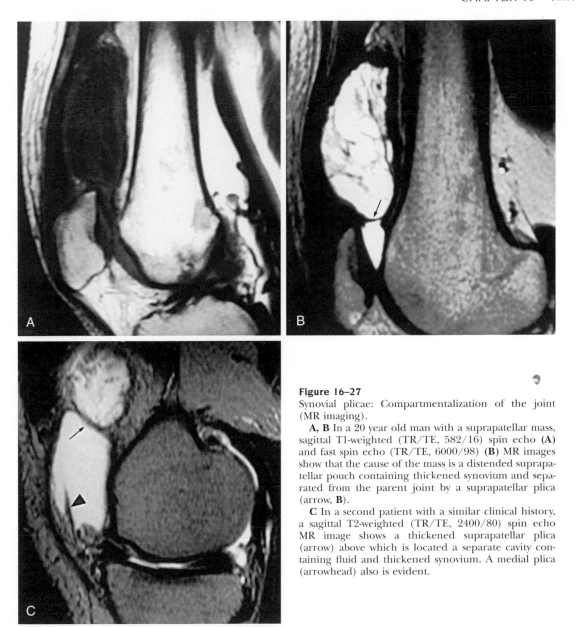

Figure 16–27
Synovial plicae: Compartmentalization of the joint (MR imaging).

A, B In a 20 year old man with a suprapatellar mass, sagittal T1-weighted (TR/TE, 582/16) spin echo **(A)** and fast spin echo (TR/TE, 6000/98) **(B)** MR images show that the cause of the mass is a distended suprapatellar pouch containing thickened synovium and separated from the parent joint by a suprapatellar plica (arrow, **B**).

C In a second patient with a similar clinical history, a sagittal T2-weighted (TR/TE, 2400/80) spin echo MR image shows a thickened suprapatellar plica (arrow) above which is located a separate cavity containing fluid and thickened synovium. A medial plica (arrowhead) also is evident.

In addition to the gastrocnemiosemimembranosus bursa, a second posterior bursa is located beneath the popliteal tendon, which communicates less frequently with the joint. A third posterior bursa exists between the medial head of the gastrocnemius muscle and the distal end of the biceps muscle. A weak point occurs laterally beneath the popliteal tendon, which may represent an extended popliteal tendon sheath. Furthermore, communication may exist between the knee and proximal tibiofibular joint cavity in 10 per cent of adults. Occasionally, anterior, medial, and lateral synovial cysts also may be observed.[212–217] In fact, synovial cysts may extend simultaneously in more than one direction.[218]

Any of these synovial cysts may enlarge, producing a mass with or without pain. Rupture of a cyst is associated with soft tissue extravasation of fluid contents. Ruptures occurring posteriorly can simulate thrombophlebitis,[219] and, in fact, the two conditions can coexist.[220–224] Giant synovial cysts can extend into the calf, ankle, heel, and thigh.[225–229]

Conventional radiography usually provides nonspecific evidence of a synovial cyst. A joint effusion and a soft tissue mass are evident in some cases, although the latter abnormality may be difficult to distinguish from normal soft tissue structures. Occasionally, intrabursal osteocartilaginous bodies or radiolucent collections, calcification in the bursal wall, or bone erosions are seen.[230–235]

Arthrography of the knee is an accurate method of diagnosing synovial cysts,[236–241] although some investigators also recommend sonographic[242–254] or isotopic[255–258] examination in this clinical situation. Computed tomography appears of little value in diagnosing these cysts in most cases, although this examination is useful in the evaluation of a suspected synovial cyst when its position is atypical or when it is not opacified on arthrogra-

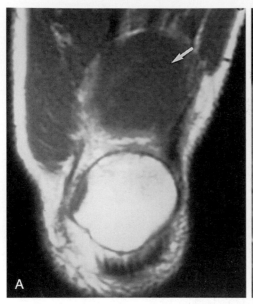

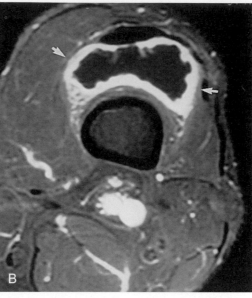

Figure 16–28
Synovial plicae: Compartmentalization of the joint (MR imaging).

A A coronal T1-weighted (TR/TE, 666/16) spin echo MR image shows a circumscribed mass (arrow) of low signal intensity above the patella.

B A transverse fat-suppressed T1-weighted (TR/TE, 650/16) spin echo MR image obtained after the intravenous injection of a gadolinium compound reveals inflamed synovium (arrows) of high signal intensity surrounding the fluid of low signal intensity. These findings represent synovial inflammation in a sequestered suprapatellar portion of the knee joint.

(Courtesy of C. Chen, M.D., Kaohsiung, Taiwan.)

phy.[259–262] Assessment of such cysts with MR imaging may provide information regarding the degree of synovial inflammation (see later discussion).

The arthrographic appearance of an abnormal synovial cyst will vary.[263] In most instances, a well-defined, lobulated structure filled with air and radiopaque contrast material will be revealed. It may have an irregular surface related to hypertrophy of its synovial lining. Alternatively, the entire cyst or a portion of it may rupture.[264, 265]

MR imaging is effective in the demonstration of intact

as well as ruptured popliteal cysts.[266–270] In one study, however, only a 5 per cent prevalence of such cysts was detected in a retrospective analysis of 1000 consecutive MR imaging examinations of the knee performed in patients referred for evaluation of internal derangement, leading the authors to conclude that the reported higher prevalence of popliteal cysts detected with arthrography may relate to distention of normal, collapsed bursae.[271] The typical appearance of a popliteal cyst is a well-defined mass of variable size with signal intensity characteristics of fluid, located between the

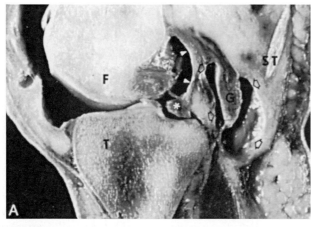

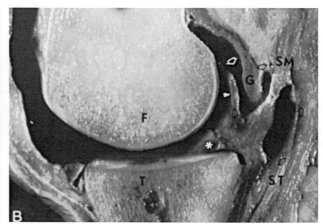

Figure 16–29
Synovial cysts: Anatomy of the posterior bursae—photographs and a photomicrograph of sagittal sections through the knee of a cadaveric specimen.

A Sagittal section through the knee at the level of the medial femoral condyle near the intercondylar notch. F, Femur; T, tibia; asterisk, posterior horn of medial meniscus. The anterior margin of the band of tissue directly posterior to the medial femoral condyle is the knee joint capsule (arrowheads). The posterior margin of this same band of tissue is the anterior margin of the gastrocnemiosemimembranosus bursa (arrows), which lies anterior to the medial head of the gastrocnemius muscle (G). The semimembranosus muscle is not seen in this section. The semitendinosus muscle (ST) is seen more posteriorly, with the posterior margin of the bursa (arrows) apposed to it.

B A sagittal section through the medial femoral condyle 1 cm medial to **A.** A transverse slit (white arrow) represents communication between the knee joint and the gastrocnemiosemimembranosus bursa (black arrows). The opening is cranially oriented and arises about 2 cm inferiorly to the most superior aspect of the posterior joint capsule. The semimembranosus muscle (SM) courses obliquely posterior to the medial head of the gastrocnemius muscle (G). The semitendinosus muscle (ST) forms the posterior margin of the gastrocnemiosemimembranosus bursa. Arrowhead, Knee joint capsule; asterisk, posterior horn of medial meniscus.

(From Guerra J Jr, et al: AJR *136:*593, 1981. Copyright 1981, American Roentgen Ray Society.)

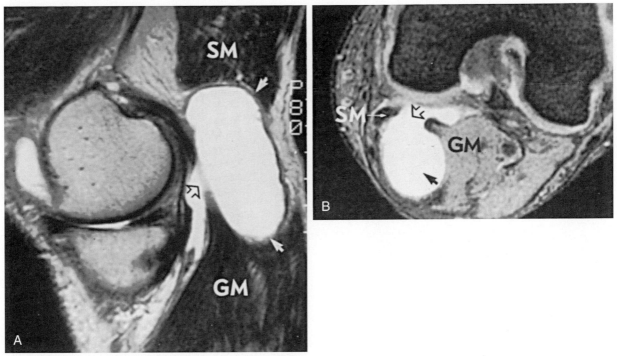

Figure 16–30
Synovial cysts: MR imaging.

A A sagittal T2-weighted (TR/TE, 4000/76) fast spin echo MR image shows a channel (open arrow) leading from the joint into a large synovial cyst (solid arrows) located between the semimembranosus muscle (SM) and medial head of the gastrocnemius muscle (GM).

B A transaxial MPGR MR image (TR/TE, 500/11; flip angle, 15 degrees) shows the channel (open arrow) and the synovial cyst (solid arrow) located between the semimembranosus tendon (SM) and the medial head of the gastrocnemius muscle and its tendon (GM).

(Courtesy of S.K. Brahme, M.D., La Jolla, California.)

tendons of the medial head of the gastrocnemius muscle and the semimembranosus muscle (Fig. 16–30). Changes in these signal intensity characteristics may indicate hemorrhage[272] or intrabursal osteocartilaginous bodies (Fig. 16–31). The relationship of the cyst to nearby arteries and veins and the documentation of cyst dissection or rupture are easily accomplished with MR imaging (Figs. 16–32, 16–33, and 16–34).

Figure 16–31
Synovial cysts: MR imaging. Intrabursal bodies (arrow) are evident in a sagittal fast spin echo MR image (TR/TE, 4500/18).

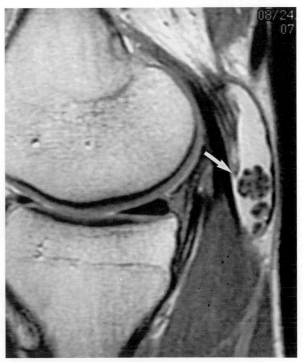

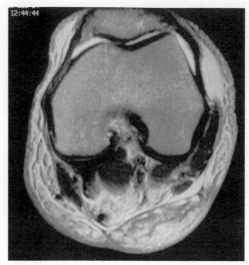

Figure 16–32
Synovial cyst: MR imaging—cyst rupture. On a transaxial T2-weighted (TR/TE, 3400/95) spin echo MR image, fluid of high signal intensity is present about the knee, particularly posteriorly and laterally, and in the joint. The extra-articular fluid had resulted from rupture of a popliteal cyst.

Any inflammatory, degenerative, traumatic, or neoplastic condition that produces a knee effusion can lead to synovial cyst formation. These conditions include rheumatoid arthritis, degenerative joint disease, gout, pigmented villonodular synovitis, and idiopathic synovial (osteo)chondromatosis, as well as other localized or systemic articular conditions. In the absence of any obvious cause, the radiologist must search diligently for meniscal abnormality. Synovial cysts may be noted in children with juvenile chronic polyarthritis[273] or on a

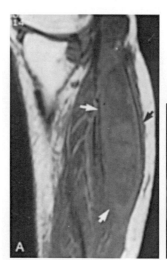
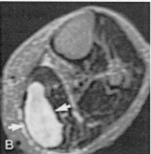

Figure 16–33
Synovial cysts: MR imaging—cyst dissection.
A A sagittal T1-weighted (TR/TE, 800/20) spin echo MR image shows a large mass (arrows) in the posterior aspect of the knee and calf with low inhomogeneous signal intensity. It begins at the level of the joint.
B A transaxial T2-weighted (TR/TE, 2000/80) spin echo MR image shows the mass (arrows) of inhomogeneous signal intensity superficial to the medial head of the gastrocnemius muscle.
(Courtesy of T. Broderick, M.D., Orange, California.)

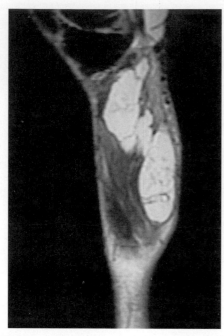

Figure 16–34
Synovial cysts: MR imaging—cyst dissection. This sagittal fast spin echo STIR MR image (TR/TE, 3650/34; inversion time, 150 msec) shows a large septated synovial cyst extending from the knee medially and inferiorly into the calf.

familial basis.[274] In children, popliteal cysts appear to have a much better prognosis than in adults, and the frequency of noncommunicating cysts is higher. Surgical removal of synovial cysts without treatment of the underlying articular disease process rarely is successful, as the cyst will recur.[275]

The differential diagnosis of synovial cysts about the knee includes a variety of neoplasms of soft tissue or bone origin,[276–278] thrombophlebitis and hematomas,[279, 280] varicose and focally dilated veins, aneurysms, and other conditions. The simultaneous occurrence of synovial cysts and some of these disorders is well known, especially with regard to venous thrombosis, thrombophlebitis, and cystic degeneration of the popliteal artery (see later discussion).[281–283]

Ganglion cysts classically contain a jelly-like viscous fluid, are loculated or septated, may arise within muscle bundles or be attached to a tendon sheath, and may or may not communicate with a joint. Those occurring about the knee usually are located close to the proximal tibiofibular joint and fibular head (Figs. 16–35 and 16–36), where they may lead to compression of the common peroneal nerve.[284–288] Ganglion cysts in this location (and other locations) may be multiple (Fig. 16–37), extend into the adjacent bone (Fig. 16–38), contain gas, and migrate for considerable distances within the fascial planes. Owing to the proximal extent of the fascia of the anterior compartment of the leg and the relatively distal origin of the muscles of the lateral compartment, ganglia arising from the proximal tibiofibular joint have a tendency to extend into the anterior (rather than the lateral) compartment and, in rare instances, may cause the anterior compartment syndrome.[289] Ultrasonogra-

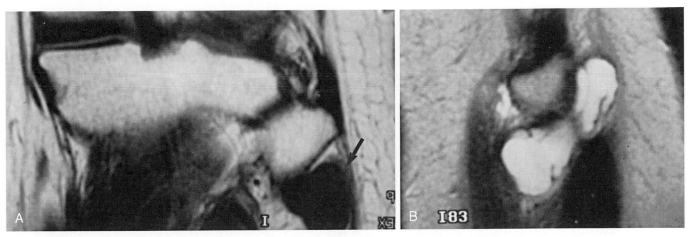

Figure 16-35

Periarticular ganglion cysts: MR imaging. This 36 year old man developed a mass in the lateral aspect of the knee and a tingling sensation in the foot, findings that were related to a ganglion cyst arising from the common peroneal nerve.

A A coronal T1-weighted (TR/TE, 500/21) spin echo MR image shows the cyst (arrow) of low signal intensity adjacent to the head and neck of the fibula.

B A sagittal fast spin echo MR image (TR/TE, 4066/95) reveals the ganglion of high signal intensity wrapping itself about the fibular neck. (Courtesy of S. Eilenberg, M.D., San Diego, California.)

phy, CT, and MR imaging can be used in their assessment.[284, 285, 290]

Pes Anserinus Ganglion Cysts and Bursitis

Cystic lesions may arise close to the tibial insertion site of the pes anserinus tendons, where they have been referred to as ganglion cysts, juxta-articular bone cysts, and pes anserine (anserinus) bursitis.[291-294] The condition may be acute or chronic, and it may occur in isolation or in association with rheumatoid arthritis, osteoarthritis, or other forms of joint disease. The term pes anserinus refers to the conjoined tendons of the sartorius, semitendinosus, and gracilis muscles. This structure is reminiscent of a goose's webbed foot (i.e., from Latin *pes*, foot, and *anserinus*, goose).[294] A bursa exists just deep to the pes anserinus, which may become acutely or chronically inflamed and enlarged. In this location, erosion of the medial tibial margin and periosteal bone proliferation in the form of broad spicules extending perpendicular to the external surface of the cortex may be evident. In some instances the resulting outgrowths simulate osteochondromas or are accompanied by subperiosteal extension of the cystic lesions (i.e., subperiosteal ganglion cysts) (Fig. 16-39).[295] As in other sites, ganglion cysts near the pes anserinus tendons may

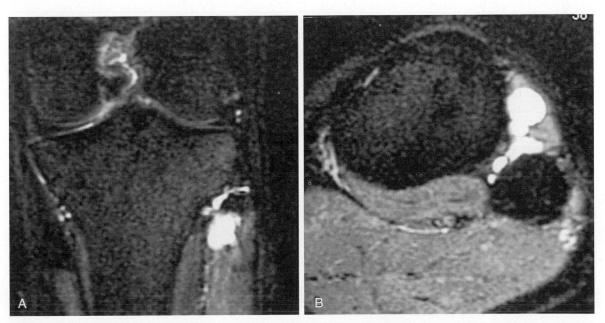

Figure 16-36

Periarticular ganglion cysts: MR imaging. As shown on coronal (TR/TE, 3000/38; inversion time, 160 msec) **(A)** and transaxial (TR/TE, 4000/36; inversion time, 160 msec) **(B)** STIR MR images, a lobulated ganglion cyst extends anteriorly from the proximal tibiofibular joint. (Courtesy of R. Kerr, M.D., Los Angeles, California.)

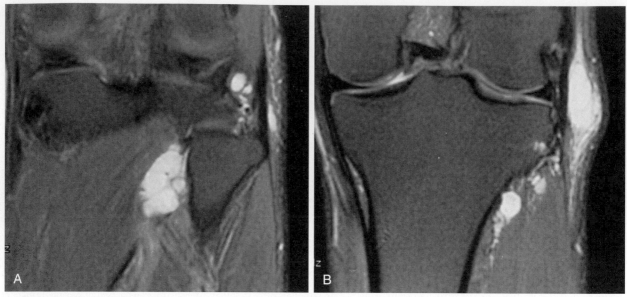

Figure 16–37

Periarticular ganglion cysts: MR imaging. Coronal fat-suppressed fast spin echo MR images (TR/TE, 2800/34), with **A** being located more posterior than **B,** show multiple ganglion cysts located near the proximal tibiofibular joint and extending anterolaterally. (Courtesy of M. Hueffle, M.D., Reno, Nevada.)

be diagnosed using ultrasonography (Fig. 16–40), cystography, CT scanning (Fig. 16–41), or MR imaging (Fig. 16–42). Usually, although not invariably,[293] the signal intensity characteristics of the lesion on various MR imaging sequences are those of fluid.

Intra-Articular Ganglion Cysts

Ganglion cysts arising within the knee joint are encountered infrequently. These cysts arise most typically at two specific sites: the alar folds that cover the infrapatellar fat body, and the cruciate ligaments. Intra-articular ganglion cysts arising from the alar folds were described in 1972 by Muckle and Monahan.[296] These cysts may present as knee pain similar to that of a torn meniscus, joint fullness, or an effusion. They generally are seen as well-defined and smooth masses during conventional arthrography or computed arthrotomography and, with MR images, the signal intensity abnormalities of the

lesions are those of fluid (Fig. 16–43). Localized nodular synovitis of the knee may have a similar arthrographic appearance, although if the nodular lesion contains hemosiderin, it will reveal a different pattern of signal intensity on the MR imaging examination.

Ganglion cysts arising from the anterior or posterior cruciate ligament were noted during routine necropsy in 1924 by Caan.[297] They were described further in reports by Sjovall[298] in 1942 and Levine[299] in 1948. More modern descriptions have been given by Chang and Rose,[300] Yasuda and Majima,[301] and Kaempffe and D'Amato.[302] In 1990, Brown and Dandy,[303] in a retrospective analysis of the results of 6500 arthroscopic examinations of the knee, noted the occurrence of 38 cases in which an intra-articular ganglion cyst was found. Of these, 28 ganglia arose from the tibial insertion site of the anterior cruciate ligament and one from its femoral insertion site, and six arose from the tibial insertion site of the posterior cruciate ligament. All contained

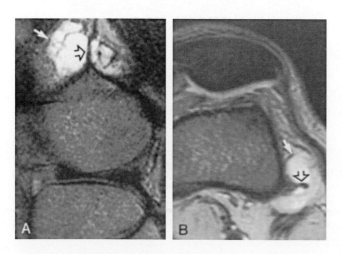

Figure 16–38

Subperiosteal ganglion cysts: MR imaging. Ganglion cysts arising close to the surface of a bone can lead to distinctive bone spiculation. This feature is demonstrated (open arrows) in a sagittal T2-weighted (TR/TE, 2200/80) spin echo MR image **(A)** and a transaxial MPGR MR image (TR/TE, 267/15; flip angle, 25 degrees) **(B)** with regard to a ganglion cyst (solid arrows) involving the lateral surface of the distal portion of the femur.

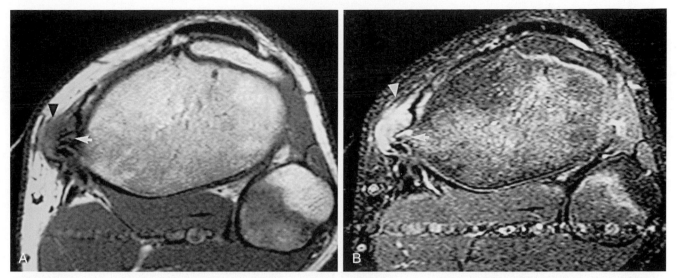

Figure 16–39

Pes anserinus ganglion cysts (bursitis): Osteochondroma-like proliferation. Transaxial T1-weighted (TR/TE, 583/20) spin echo **(A)** and STIR (TR/TE, 2000/30; inversion time, 140 msec) **(B)** MR images show the fluid-filled mass (arrowheads) with subjacent bone proliferation (arrows). (Courtesy of S. Eilenberg, M.D., San Diego, California.)

clear fluid, and their average diameter was 5 mm (range, 3 to 8 mm). The clinical manifestations of these ganglion cysts were similar to those of other internal derangements of the knee, and none of the lesions recurred after arthroscopic excision.[304]

Routine radiography in such cases may reveal pressure erosion of the femoral condyles, best seen on tunnel views. Ultrasonography may allow detection of a mass that is intimate with the cruciate ligaments (Fig. 16–44). CT also may show an intercondylar soft tissue mass in close proximity to one or both cruciate ligaments (Fig. 16–45A). The MR imaging features consist of a well-defined mass applied to the surface of the anterior cruciate ligament (Fig. 16–45B) or posterior cruciate ligament (Figs. 16–46 and 16–47) with signal intensity characteristics of fluid.[305] These MR imaging findings allow a specific diagnosis in most cases.[306] In

some cases, however, determining the precise origin of the ganglion cyst either by MR imaging or by arthroscopy is difficult. One reported cyst appeared to arise from a chondral fracture of the medial femoral condyle and then extended through the synovial lining of the posterior cruciate ligament.[307] Furthermore, localized nodular synovitis also may lead to a mass lesion arising from a cruciate ligament.[1116]

Of related interest, McLaren and coworkers[308] noted the presence of intraosseous cystic lesions at or near the tibial insertion site of the anterior cruciate ligament, posterior cruciate ligament, or both ligaments, in approximately 1 per cent of 1710 knees evaluated with MR imaging. The lesions generally were solitary, and all were spherical and well marginated (Fig. 16–48). The

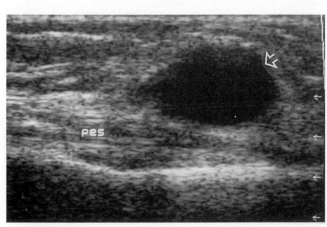

Figure 16–40

Pes anserinus ganglion cysts (bursitis): Ultrasonography. Coronal sonogram demonstrates anechoic bursal fluid (arrow) adjacent to the pes anserinus. (Courtesy of M. van Holsbeeck, M.D., Detroit, Michigan, and J. Jacobson, M.D., San Diego, California.)

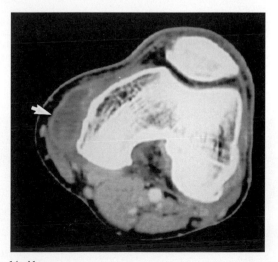

Figure 16–41

Pes anscrinus ganglion cysts (bursitis): CT scanning. This transverse scan was obtained after intravenous administration of contrast agent and shows the cystic lesion with increased peripheral attenuation (arrow). (Courtesy of B.Y. Yang, M.D., Taipei, Taiwan.)

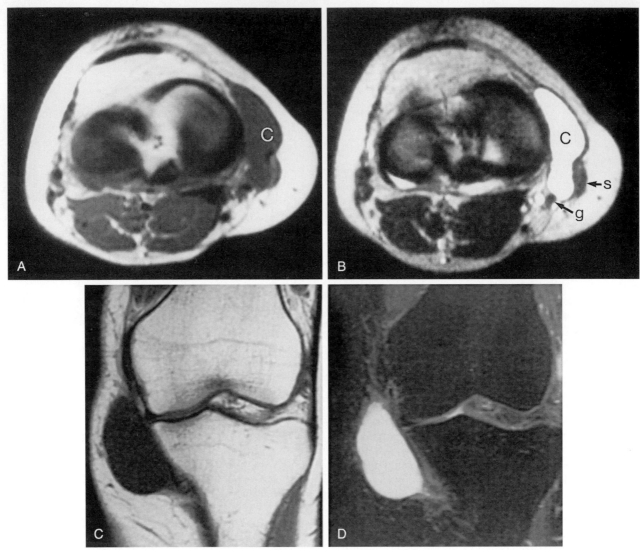

Figure 16–42
Pes anserinus ganglion cysts (bursitis): MR imaging. **A, B** Transaxial T1-weighted (TR/TE, 700/30) **(A)** and T2-weighted (TR/TE, 2000/85) **(B)** spin echo MR images show the ganglion cyst (C) and its relationship to the sartorius (s) and gracilis (g) tendons.

C, D In a second patient, a coronal T1-weighted (TR/TE, 400/20) spin echo MR image **(C)** and a coronal STIR MR image (TR/TE, 2500/40; inversion time, 160 msec) **(D)** show a large, fluid-filled mass adjacent to the anteromedial portion of the tibia.

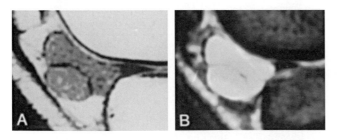

Figure 16–43
Intra-articular ganglion cysts: MR imaging. Alar folds. Sagittal T1-weighted (TR/TE, 500/20) **(A)** and MPGR MR images (TR/TE, 550/25; flip angle, 25 degrees) **(B)** show a septated ganglion cyst located anteriorly and extending into the infrapatellar fat body. (Courtesy of J. Schils, M.D., Cleveland, Ohio.)

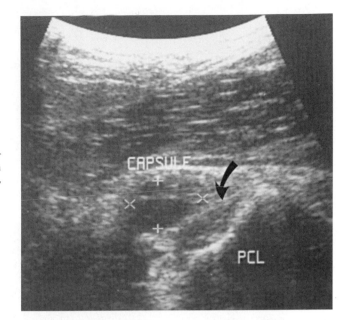

Figure 16–44
Intra-articular ganglion cysts: Ultrasonography. A sonogram of the posterior aspect of the knee in the sagittal plane demonstrates the anechoic ganglion cyst (white markers) adjacent to the posterior cruciate ligament (PCL, black arrow) and tibial cortex.

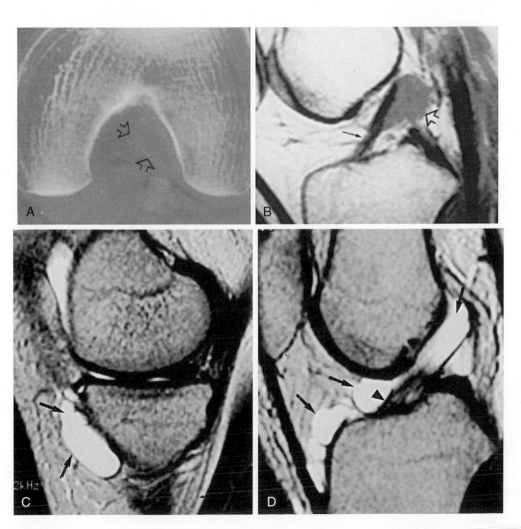

Figure 16–45
Intra-articular ganglion cysts: CT scanning and MR imaging. Anterior cruciate ligament.

A, B A transaxial CT scan (**A**) reveals a well-defined lesion (open arrows) containing fluid (of low attenuation) adjacent to the inner aspect of the lateral femoral condyle close to the site of attachment of the anterior cruciate ligament. A sagittal proton density–weighted (TR/TE, 1200/30) spin echo MR image (**B**) confirms the presence of the mass (open arrow) adjacent to the anterior cruciate ligament (solid arrow).

C, D In a second patient, sagittal fast spin echo (TR/TE, 4000/99) MR images, with **C** medial to **D**, show a large ganglion cyst (arrows) that has originated from the anterior cruciate ligament (arrowhead, **D**). (Courtesy of S. Fernandez, M.D., Mexico City, Mexico.)

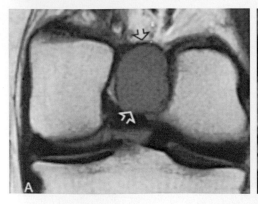

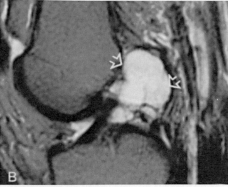

Figure 16-46

Intra-articular ganglion cysts: MR imaging—posterior cruciate ligament. A coronal T1-weighted (TR/TE, 800/25) spin echo MR image (**A**) and a sagittal T2-weighted (TR/TE, 2000/80) spin echo MR image (**B**) show the large ganglion cyst (open arrows) which arose from the posterior cruciate ligament.

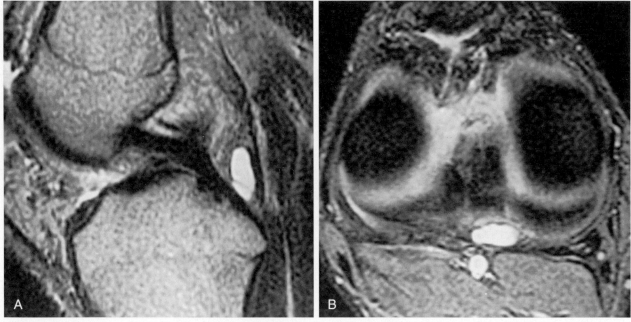

Figure 16-47

Intra-articular ganglion cysts: MR imaging—posterior cruciate ligament. Sagittal T2-weighted (TR/TE, 2000/85) spin echo (**A**) and transverse MPGR (TR/TE, 800/20; flip angle, 20 degrees) (**B**) MR images show the ganglion cyst of high signal intensity located just posterior to the tibial insertion of the posterior cruciate ligament. (Courtesy of D. Goodwin, M.D., Hanover, New Hampshire.)

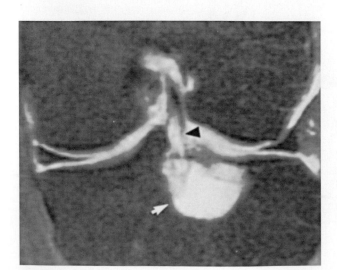

Figure 16-48

Intraosseous ganglion cysts: MR imaging—anterior cruciate ligament. A coronal proton density–weighted (TR/TE, 2850/18) fast spin echo MR image obtained with chemical presaturation of fat (ChemSat) shows a large lesion (arrow) in the tibia close to the site of attachment of the anterior cruciate ligament (arrowhead). Surgical confirmation of the nature of this lesion was not obtained. (Courtesy of G. Applegate, M.D., Van Nuys, California.)

signal intensity characteristics of the intraosseous cysts were typical of a fluid-filled structure surrounded by a rim of sclerotic bone or fibrous tissue. The cruciate ligaments were normal in almost all cases, and no soft tissue masses were evident. Although histologic confirmation of the nature of the lesions was not obtained, the authors speculated that they were intraosseous ganglia. They further noted the presence of a soft tissue mass adjacent to a similar intraosseous cystic lesion in one additional patient, consistent with the presence of both extraosseous and intraosseous ganglion cysts.

Bursitis

Any of the bursae about the knee may become inflamed, leading to the accumulation of bursal fluid (Fig. 16–49). Prepatellar bursitis (housemaid's knee), deep or superficial infrapatellar bursitis, pes anserinus bursitis, and bursitis involving a suprapatellar recess that is isolated from the remaining portion of the knee by a suprapatellar plica are typical examples. Ultrasonography[309] and MR imaging represent the two most effective imaging methods for diagnosis of these conditions. With MR imaging, bursal fluid is of high signal intensity on T2-weighted spin echo images (Fig. 16–50) as well as on STIR images. Hemorrhage within an involved bursa may lead to more complex patterns of signal intensity.[1117] Prepatellar bursitis may result from chronic stress, as may occur in wrestling or with prolonged kneeling, infection (Figs. 16–51 and 16–52), or synovial inflammatory diseases such as rheumatoid arthritis or gout (Fig. 16–53). Rheumatoid nodules and gouty tophi (Fig. 16–54) may lead to a prepatellar soft tissue mass, although the imaging characteristics of these lesions usually differ from those of fluid. The differential diagnosis

of prepatellar and anterior soft tissue masses also includes hematomas, xanthomas and other tumors, and varicosities (Figs. 16–55 and 16–56).

Hoffa's Disease

Hoffa's disease is a term that has been applied to traumatic and inflammatory changes occurring in the infrapatellar fat body.[310–314] This rare condition is seen in young athletic persons in whom pain, swelling, and limitation of joint motion may occur as a result of a single injury or repetitive trauma. The fat body hypertrophies and may become entrapped between the femur and the tibia when the flexed knee is extended suddenly. Initial inflammatory abnormalities later may lead to fibrosis in the fat pad. MR imaging reveals alterations in signal intensity in the infrapatellar fat body (Figs. 16–57 and 16–58), which acutely indicate fluid and chronically resemble those related to scarring after knee arthroscopy. Open or arthroscopic surgery may be required.[314]

Rarely, acute injuries to the infrapatellar fat body may lead to rupture of the overlying synovial fold and hemarthrosis.[315]

Tumors and Tumor-Like Lesions

A number of tumors and tumor-like lesions may arise from the synovium or capsule of the knee joint or nearby intra-articular tissue. These lesions include pigmented villonodular synovitis and localized nodular synovitis, idiopathic synovial (osteo)chondromatosis, synovial hemangioma, intracapsular and capsular chondroma, synovial chondrosarcoma, synovial lipoma, and lipoma arborescens (see Chapters 5 and 6). In some of

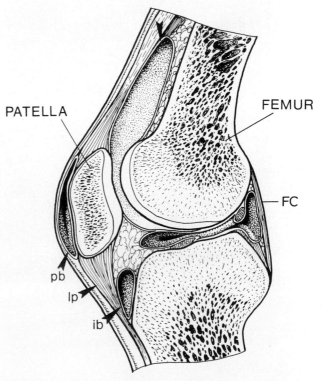

Figure 16–49
Bursa about the knee: Normal anatomy. Drawing of sagittal section shows femur, patella, tibia, fibrous capsule (FC), prepatellar bursa (pb), deep infrapatellar bursa (ib), ligamentum patellae (lp), and suprapatellar pouch (arrowhead).

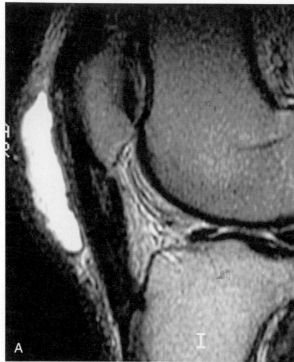

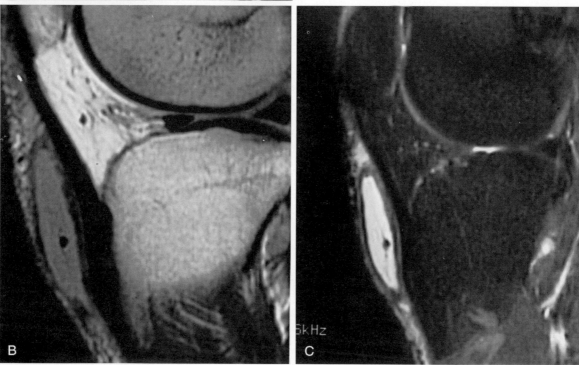

Figure 16–50
Bursitis: MR imaging
A Prepatellar bursitis. A sagittal T2-weighted (TR/TE, 2200/80) spin echo MR image shows the fluid-filled bursa and a thickened and partially torn patellar tendon.
B, C Superficial infrapatellar bursitis. Sagittal proton density–weighted (TR/TE, 2000/32) spin echo (**B**) and fast spin echo STIR (TR/TE, 3300/36; inversion time, 150 msec) (**C**) MR images demonstrate the distended fluid-filled bursa.
(Courtesy of D. Goodwin, M.D., Hanover, New Hampshire.)

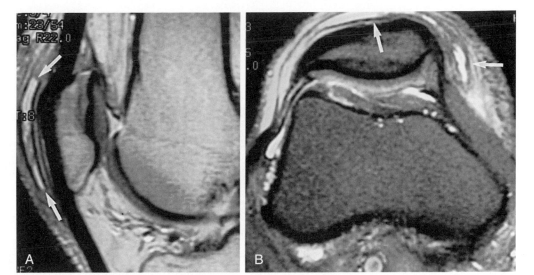

Figure 16–51
Bursitis: MR imaging—septic prepatellar bursitis. Sagittal fast spin echo (TR/TE, 4900/17) **(A)** and transaxial fat-suppressed fast spin echo (TR/TE, 3000/38) **(B)** MR images reveal the bursa (arrows) filled with fluid or pannus, or both, and surrounded by extensive soft tissue edema.

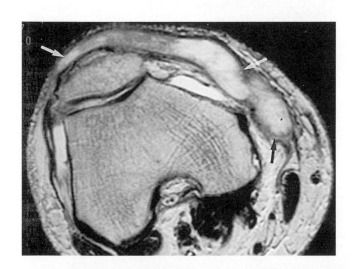

Figure 16–52
Bursitis: MR imaging—septic prepatellar bursitis. Staphylococcal infection developed in this 50 year old man. A transaxial T2-weighted (TR/TE, 3000/85) fast spin echo MR image reveals the extent of bursal infection (arrows), adjacent soft tissue edema, and a joint effusion. (Courtesy of D. Salonen, M.D., Toronto, Ontario, Canada.)

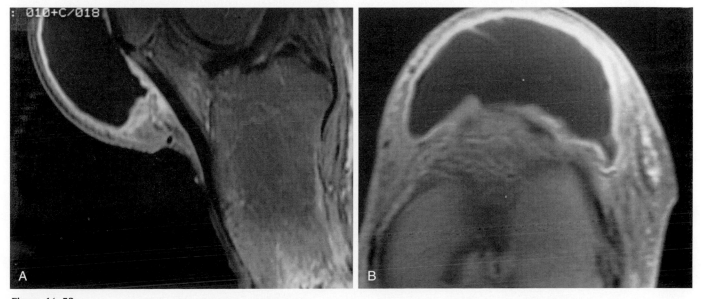

Figure 16–53
Bursitis: MR imaging—gouty prepatellar bursitis. Sagittal (TR/TE, 600/12) **(A)** and transaxial (TR/TE, 800/12) **(B)** fat-suppressed T1-weighted spin echo MR images obtained after intravenous administration of a gadolinium compound show enhancement of signal intensity in the wall of a fluid-filled bursa. Urate crystals were recovered from the fluid.

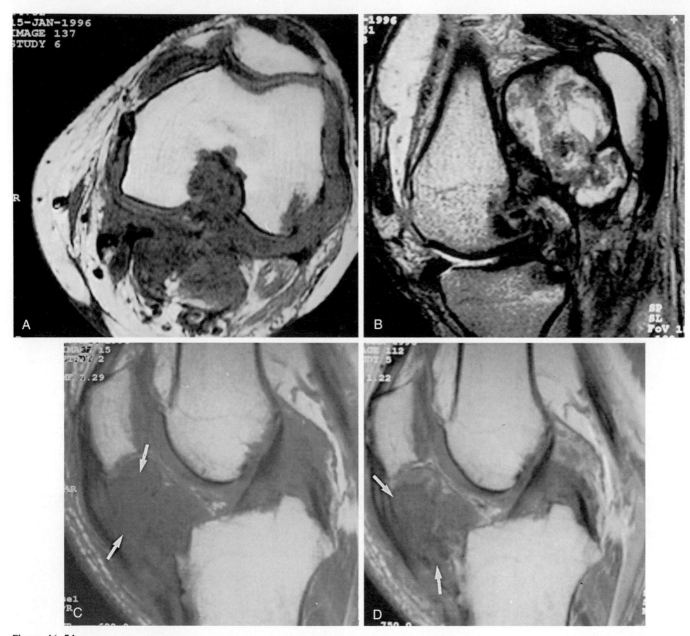

Figure 16–54

Prepatellar and anterior soft tissue masses: Gouty arthritis, MR imaging.

A, B In a 53 year old man, gouty involvement of the knee is shown in transaxial T1-weighted (TR/TE, 600/15) **(A)** and sagittal T2-weighted (TR/TE, 3000/119) **(B)** spin echo MR images. Findings include a large joint effusion tophaceous material of low signal intensity, especially in a popliteal cyst, and bone erosions. (Courtesy of D. Witte, M.D., Memphis, Tennessee.)

C, D Gouty involvement of the knee is shown in a 44 year old man on a sagittal T1-weighted (TR/TE, 690/15) spin echo MR image **(C)** and a similar image (TR/TE, 750/15) after intravenous administration of a gadolinium compound **(D).** Note a large tophaceous mass (arrows) beneath the patella with slight contrast enhancement of signal intensity. Similar enhancement has occurred about the cruciate ligaments. (Courtesy of J. Kramer, M.D., Vienna, Austria.)

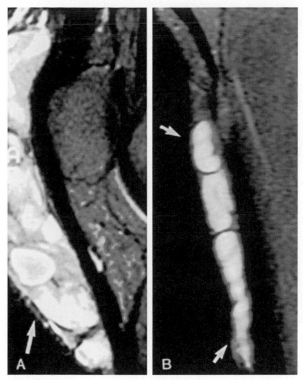

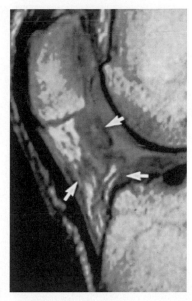

Figure 16–57
Hoffa's disease: MR imaging. This male adolescent had undergone several arthroscopic procedures in which resection of a medial patellar plica and an enlarged and inflamed infrapatellar fat body had been accomplished. He had recurrent anterior knee pain. A sagittal proton density–weighted (TR/TE, 2700/20) spin echo MR image shows serpentine and irregular areas of low signal intensity (arrows) in the deep infrapatellar fat body. Repeat arthroscopy confirmed inflammation of the fat pad and adjacent synovial membrane. (Courtesy of G. Bock, M.D., and P. Major, M.D., Winnipeg, Manitoba, Canada.)

Figure 16–55
Prepatellar and anterior soft tissue masses.
  A Prepatellar hematoma. A sagittal T2-weighted (TR/TE, 2433/80) spin echo MR image shows a large, septated mass of high signal intensity, representing a hematoma, anterior to the patella (arrow). (Courtesy of S. Eilenberg, M.D., San Diego, California.)
  B Varicosities. A similar sagittal T2-weighted spin echo MR image shows a septated mass of high signal intensity (arrows), which corresponded to clinically evident varicose veins.

these lesions, imaging abnormalities may allow a specific diagnosis.

With pigmented villonodular synovitis, a monoarticular process of the knee in a young adult associated with a radiodense joint effusion, preservation of joint space, and well-defined bone erosions and cysts is typical. The conventional arthrogram in diffuse pigmented villonodular synovitis reveals an enlarged synovial cavity, an irregular synovial outline with pooling of contrast material, and nodular filling defects.[316–318] MR imaging shows synovial proliferation with regions of persistently low signal intensity, consistent with hemosiderin deposition

Figure 16–56
Prepatellar soft tissue masses. This xanthoma (arrows) shows moderate enhancement of signal intensity after intravenous administration of a gadolinium compound, as shown on this sagittal T1-weighted (TR/TE, 680/15) spin echo MR image.

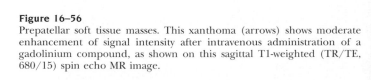

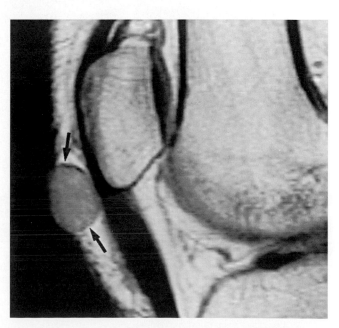

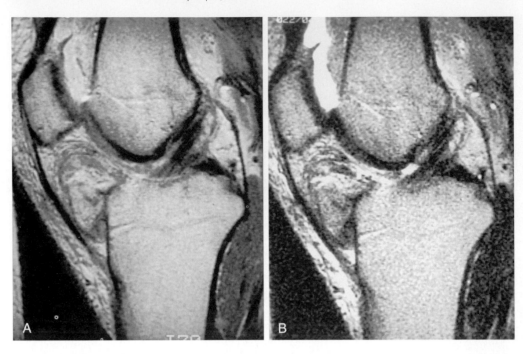

Figure 16–58
Hoffa's disease: MR imaging. These sagittal proton density–weighted (TR/TE, 4900/20) **(A)** and T2-weighted (TR/TE, 4900/100) **(B)** fast spin echo MR images reveal distortion of morphology and alterations in signal intensity in the infrapatellar fat body. Note curvilinear regions of persistently low signal intensity with other regions of high signal intensity. (Courtesy of C. Gundry, M.D., Minneapolis, Minnesota.)

(Figs. 16–59 and 16–60).[319, 320] Localized (pigmented or nonpigmented) nodular synovitis is not uncommon in the knee, leads to a soft tissue mass generally in the anterior aspect of the joint, and may produce symptoms similar to those of an internal derangement.[321, 322] With MR imaging, a mass generally of intermediate to low signal intensity is evident (Fig. 16–61). The findings are not specific, however (Fig. 16–62).

In idiopathic synovial (osteo)chondromatosis, par-tially calcified intra-articular and intrasynovial bodies may or may not be evident on routine radiographs (Fig. 16–63). Conventional arthrography shows an enlarged synovial cavity and multiple small, sharply defined filling defects.[323, 324] The nodular lesions in this condition are of variable size but usually are better defined arthrographically than those of pigmented villonodular synovitis. MR imaging characteristics of idiopathic synovial (osteo)chondromatosis are variable, depending on the

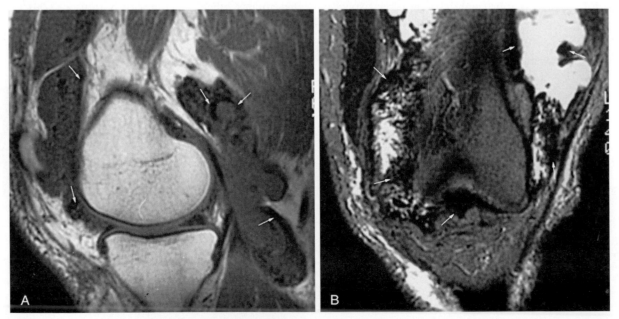

Figure 16–59
Pigmented villonodular synovitis: MR imaging. In a 56 year old man, a sagittal T1-weighted (TR/TE, 600/12) spin echo MR image **(A)** shows massive distention of the joint, both anterior and posteriorly (including a synovial cyst). Regions of very low signal intensity (arrows) in the synovial lining of the joint and cyst are recognizable. A coronal T2-weighted (TR/TE, 2700/80) spin echo MR image **(B)** through the anterior portion of the joint reveals fluid of high signal intensity and hemosiderin deposits of low signal intensity (arrows). (Courtesy of G. Greenway, M.D., Dallas, Texas.)

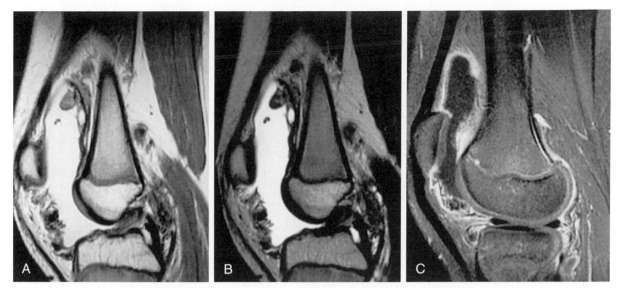

Figure 16–60

Pigmented villonodular synovitis: MR imaging. In a 14 year old boy, sagittal proton density–weighted (TR/TE, 4000/19) **(A)** and T2-weighted (TR/TE, 4000/95) **(B)** spin echo MR images show fluid of high signal intensity and intrasynovial hemosiderin deposits of low signal intensity. After the intravenous administration of a gadolinium compound, a sagittal fat-suppressed T1-weighted (TR/TE, 400/12) spin echo MR image **(C)** documents enhancement of signal intensity in the synovial membrane. Some deposits of hemosiderin are evident as regions of low signal intensity. (Courtesy of V. Gylys-Morin, M.D., Cincinnati, Ohio.)

presence or absence of calcification or ossification within the bodies (Figs. 16–64 and 16–65).[325]

Hemangiomas of the synovium occur most frequently in the knee. Initial radiographs may reveal soft tissue masses, calcified phleboliths, and a hemophilia-like arthropathy with osteoporosis and epiphyseal enlargement.[326] Conventional arthrography may reveal single or multiple radiolucent defects, and arteriography will outline hypervascular tumors.[327] MR imaging shows the extent of the lesions, which have variable signal intensity (Figs. 16–66, 16–67, and 16–68).[328]

Intracapsular and capsular chondromas are associated with masses of variable size that may calcify (Fig. 16–69). An infrapatellar location is most typical, and erosion of the lower portion of the patella and displacement of the patellar tendon may be evident. Either inhomogeneous or homogeneous signal intensity may be noted on MR imaging examinations (Figs. 16–70 and 16–71). Synovial chondrosarcomas are extremely rare, occur most often in the knee, may or may not be related to idiopathic synovial (osteo)chondromatosis, reveal bizarre calcification, and are accompanied by inhomogeneity of signal intensity on MR images (Fig. 16–72).

Lipoma arborescens is a rare intra-articular lesion of unknown cause, most commonly located in the knee, consisting of focal deposits of fat beneath the swollen synovial lining.[329] Arthrography reveals numerous moderately well defined defects of variable size.[330, 331] The fatty nature of the process can be determined accurately with CT or MR imaging (Figs. 16–73 and 16–74).[332–336] Rarely, true lipomas may produce filling defects in the opacified knee during arthrography.[337] Once again, MR imaging provides evidence regarding the fatty nature of the process.

Numerous other tumors and tumor-like lesions may affect the knee. These include metastasis, lymphomas (Fig. 16–75), and neurogenic tumors.[338]

Meniscal Abnormalities

Anatomic Considerations

The menisci of the knee are composed of fibrocartilage and are located between the articular surfaces of the condyles of the femur and the tibial plateaus (Fig. 16–76). They serve to deepen and enlarge the articular surfaces of the proximal portion of the tibia and, thereby, to better accommodate the condyles of the femur. The two menisci are not identical in shape. The lateral meniscus appears as a circular structure and, in comparison to the medial meniscus, covers more of the articular surface of the tibia. Its width is relatively constant from its anterior to posterior portions. The lateral meniscus has a loose peripheral attachment and, posteriorly, is separated from the capsule by the popliteus tendon and its sheath. Therefore, the lateral meniscus normally is more mobile than the medial meniscus. The meniscofemoral ligaments are intimate with the posterior horn of the lateral meniscus (see later discussion). The shape of the medial meniscus is semicircular, and its width is greater posteriorly than anteriorly. The width of its central portion varies. Peripherally, the medial meniscus is firmly attached to the joint capsule, particularly in its midportion, in the region of the medial (tibial) collateral ligament. The tibial attachment of the meniscus often is referred to as the coronary ligament. The medial meniscus has no direct attachments to any muscle, but indirect capsular connections to the semimembranosus muscle may provide some retraction of its posterior horn.[339]

Text continued on page 605

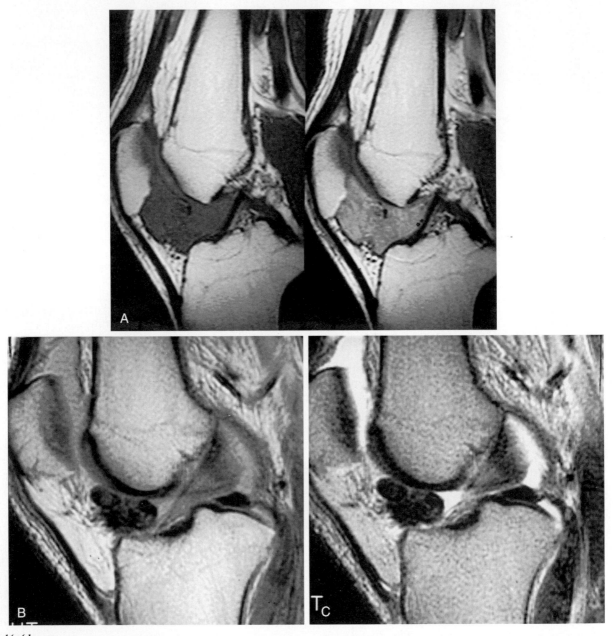

Figure 16–61

Localized nodular synovitis: MR imaging.

A Sagittal T1-weighted (TR/TE, 583/16) spin echo MR images obtained before (left) and after (right) intravenous administration of a gadolinium compound show involvement of the anterior portion of the joint, with invasion of the infrapatellar fat body. Moderate enhancement of signal intensity in the lesion is seen in the right image.

B, C In a second patient, sagittal proton density–weighted (TR/TE, 2100/20) **(B)** and T2-weighted (TR/TE, 2100/60) **(C)** spin echo MR images reveal a mass of low signal intensity in the anterior aspect of the joint.

(Courtesy of D. Berthoty, M.D., Las Vegas, Nevada.)

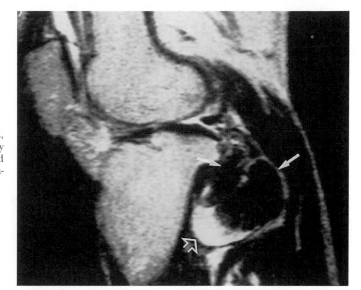

Figure 16–62
Tuberculous synovitis: MR imaging. A sagittal T2-weighted (TR/TE, 2000/85) spin echo MR image reveals fluid of high signal intensity (open arrow) and an inflammatory mass of low signal intensity (solid arrows). The appearance of the mass simulates that of localized nodular synovitis.

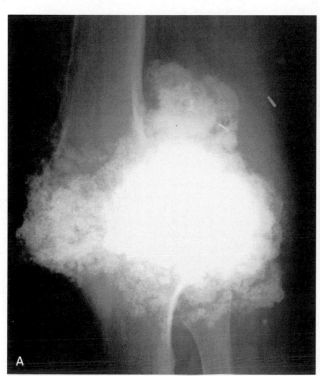

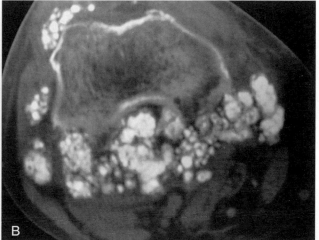

Figure 16–63
Idiopathic synovial (osteo)chondromatosis: Routine radiography and CT scanning. This patient had undergone surgical treatment for idiopathic synovial (osteo)chondromatosis, but the condition recurred, leading to extensive calcification and ossification of intrasynovial cartilaginous nodules, as shown on a routine radiograph **(A)** and CT scan **(B).** (Courtesy of R Kerr, M.D., Los Angeles, California.)

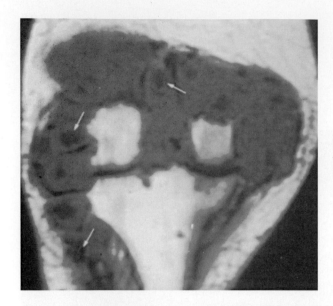

Figure 16–64

Idiopathic synovial (osteo)chondromatosis: MR imaging. A coronal T1-weighted (TR/TE, 600/15) spin echo MR image shows fluid of intermediate signal intensity throughout the knee. Note many foci of low signal intensity (arrows), indicative of calcified bodies.

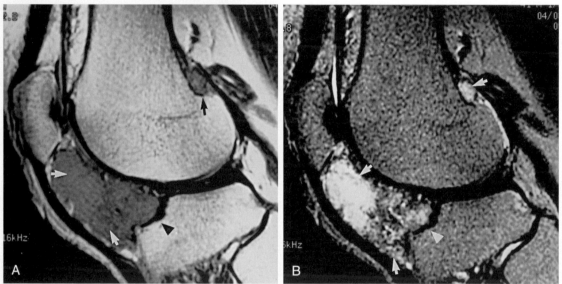

Figure 16–65

Idiopathic synovial (osteo)chondromatosis: MR imaging. Sagittal proton density–weighted (TR/TE, 2150/17) **(A)** and T2-weighted (TR/TE, 2150/80) **(B)** spin echo MR images show a mass occupying the anterior and posterior portions of the knee (arrows). The mass is of intermediate signal intensity in **A** and inhomogeneous but mainly of high signal intensity in **B.** Note displacement of the patellar tendon and erosion (arrowheads) of the tibia. (Courtesy of D. Levey, M.D., Corpus Christi, Texas.)

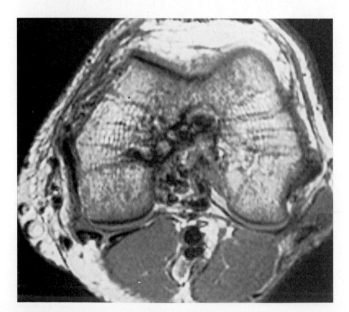

Figure 16–66

Synovial and soft tissue hemangioma: Klippel-Trenaunay-Weber syndrome. MR imaging. This transaxial proton density–weighted (TR/TE, 2700/22) spin echo MR image in a 16 year old boy shows regions of signal void in the intercondylar notch of the femur and soft tissues.

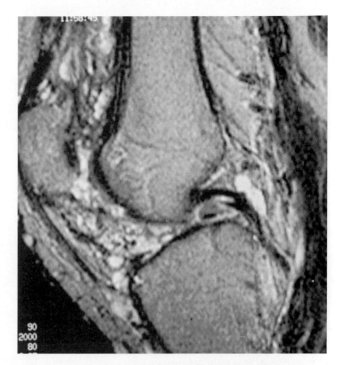

Figure 16–67
Synovial hemangioma: MR imaging. In this patient with a diffusely swollen knee and adjacent varicosities, a sagittal T2-weighted (TR/TE, 2000/80) spin echo MR image shows inhomogeneous signal intensity in and around the joint, with circular and channel-like regions of high signal intensity.

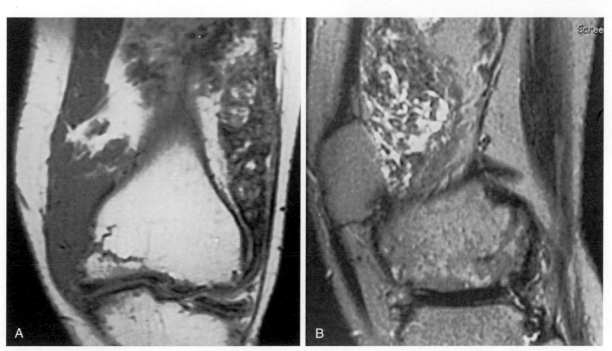

Figure 16–68
Synovial and soft tissue hemangiomas: MR imaging. In a 30 year old patient with the Klippel-Trenaunay Weber syndrome, coronal T1-weighted (TR/TE, 500/19) spin echo (**A**) and sagittal fast spin echo (TR/TE, 4500/105) (**B**) MR images show diffuse involvement of the knee with a process of inhomogeneous signal intensity. Serpentine structures, regions of signal void, and areas of high signal intensity are noted in **A,** and some areas of low signal intensity persist in **B.** (Courtesy of J. Hodler, M.D., Zurich, Switzerland.)

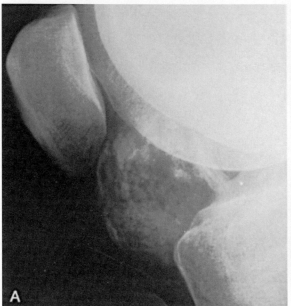

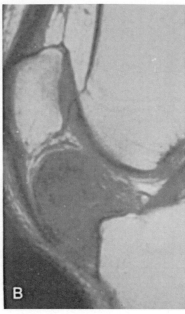

Figure 16–69

Intracapsular chondroma: MR imaging. In this 55 year old man, a mass developed below the patella that interfered with his swinging of a golf club. The routine radiograph **(A)** reveals an ossified mass below the patella within the infrapatellar fat body. A sagittal T1-weighted (TR/TE, 500/20) spin echo MR image **(B)** shows a mass of inhomogeneous but mainly low signal intensity displacing the patellar tendon. It had inhomogeneous high signal intensity on T2-weighted spin echo MR images (not shown). It was excised easily. (Courtesy of B. Sosnow, M.D., Phoenix, Arizona.)

Figure 16–70

Intracapsular chondroma: MR imaging. A sagittal proton density–weighted (TR/TE, 2500/20) spin echo MR image **(A)** and a sagittal MPGR MR image (TR/TE, 1200/15; flip angle, 70 degrees) **(B)** reveal a large, partly ossified mass in the region of the deep infrapatellar fat body. The mass contains foci whose signal intensity is that of marrow fat. Note erosion of the lower portion of the patella and anterior displacement of the patellar tendon.

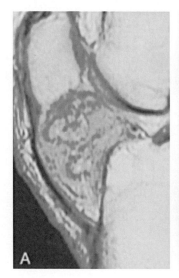

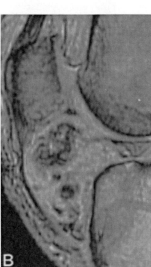

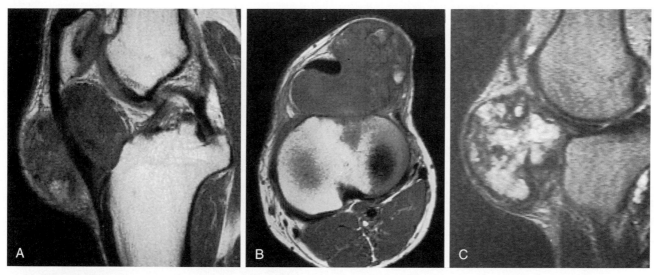

Figure 16–71
Intracapsular chondroma: MR imaging. This 40 year old man developed progressive swelling in the anterior aspect of the knee over a 2 year period after an injury.

A, B Sagittal **(A)** and transaxial **(B)** T1-weighted (TR/TE, 760/17) spin echo MR images show a mass of predominantly low signal intensity (with foci of high signal intensity compatible with ossified bodies containing marrow) wrapped about the patellar tendon.

C A sagittal T2-weighted (TR/TE, 2200/90) spin echo MR image reveals mainly high signal intensity within the mass.

(Courtesy of D. Witte, M.D., Memphis, Tennessee.)

Figure 16–72
Synovial chondrosarcoma: MR imaging. A sagittal T1-weighted (TR/TE, 867/12) spin echo MR image **(A)** and a sagittal STIR MR image (TR/TE, 2500/40; inversion time, 160 msec) **(B)** show the large mass involving the posterior aspect of the knee and posterior soft tissues. The lesion is inhomogeneous but mainly of high signal intensity in **B.** At surgery, the tumor was adherent to the posterior capsule of the knee joint. The final histologic diagnosis was extraskeletal myxoid chondrosarcoma or synovial chondrosarcoma. (Courtesy of G. Greenway, M.D., Dallas, Texas.)

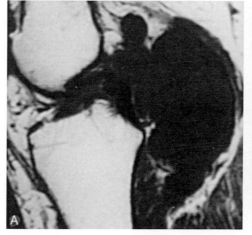
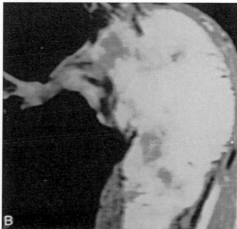

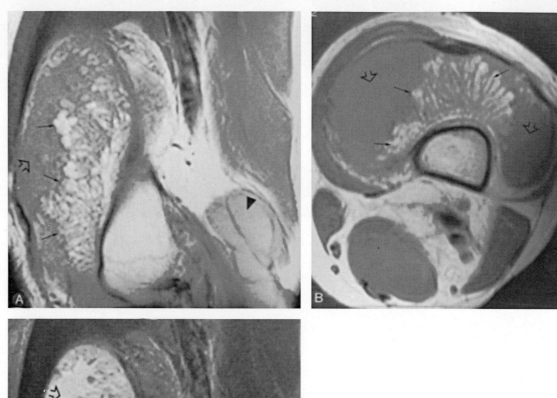

Figure 16–73
Lipoma arborescens: MR imaging.

A–C Sagittal **(A)** and transaxial **(B)** proton density–weighted (TR/TE, 2000/20) spin echo MR images and a sagittal T2-weighted (TR/TE, 2000/80) spin echo MR image **(C)** show fatty infiltration of the synovial membrane (solid arrows) associated with a fluid-filled joint (open arrows) and a posterior synovial cyst (arrowheads). Note that the signal intensity of the involved synovium is identical to that of fat. (Courtesy of M. Schweitzer, M.D., Philadelphia, Pennsylvania.)

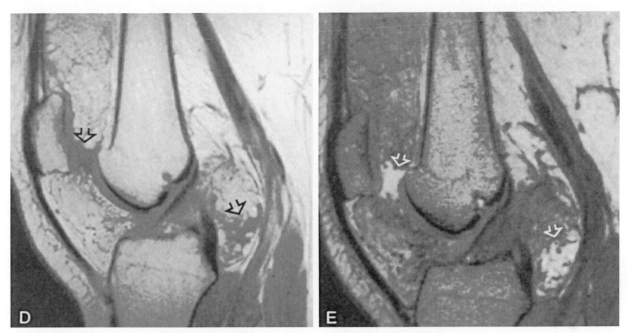

Figure 16–73 *Continued*
D, E In a second patient, sagittal proton density–weighted (TR/TE, 1000/15) spin echo **(D)** and 3DFT gradient recalled (TR/TE, 31/10; flip angle, 40 degrees) **(E)** MR images show massive enlargement of the knee joint with a process that is mainly lipomatous. The signal intensity of the infiltrative process primarily is that of fat, although fluid collections (arrows) also are apparent. The popliteal vessels are displaced. (Courtesy of T. Hughes, M.D., Christchurch, New Zealand.)

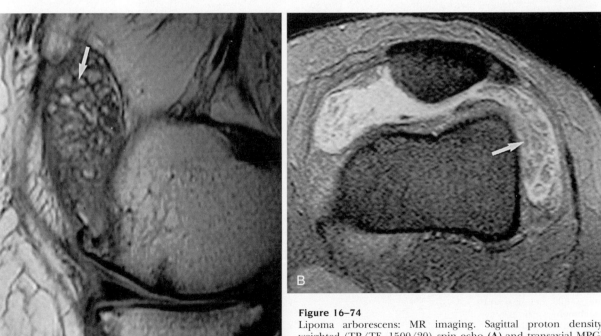

Figure 16–74
Lipoma arborescens: MR imaging. Sagittal proton density–weighted (TR/TE, 1500/20) spin echo **(A)** and transaxial MPGR (TR/TE, 500/13; flip angle, 20 degrees) **(B)** MR images show fatty infiltration of the synovial membrane (arrows) and joint fluid. (Courtesy of A.O. Motta, M.D., Cleveland, Ohio.)

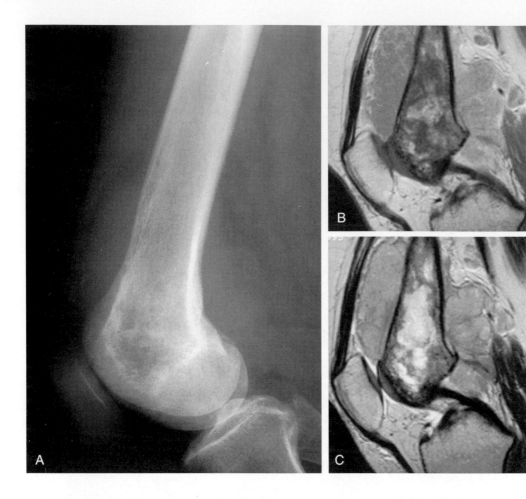

Figure 16–75
Lymphoma: MR imaging.

A A lateral radiograph reveals mottled osteolysis in the distal portion of the femur and a surrounding soft tissue mass.

B, C Sagittal T1-weighted (TR/TE, 600/15) (**B**) and T2-weighted (TR/TE, 5000/85) (**C**) spin echo MR images (**C** is obtained with fast spin echo technique) show osseous, articular, and soft tissue involvement. In **B,** the tumor is of intermediate to low signal intensity. In **C,** tumor in the femur shows high signal intensity and that in the joint and posterior soft tissues (including perivascular regions) is of intermediate signal intensity.

Figure 16–76
Menisci of the knee: Normal anatomy. Coronal section (on left) and view of the upper portion of the tibia (on right). A, anterior; P, posterior. Visualized structures are the medial meniscus (1), lateral meniscus (2), medial collateral ligament (3), fibular collateral ligament (4), anterior cruciate ligament (5), posterior cruciate ligament (6), transverse ligament of the knee (7), and meniscofemoral ligament of Wrisberg (arrow). Observe the relatively large posterior horn of the medial meniscus and its firm attachment to the medial collateral ligament and the more circular configuration of the lateral meniscus, with its relatively uniform size.

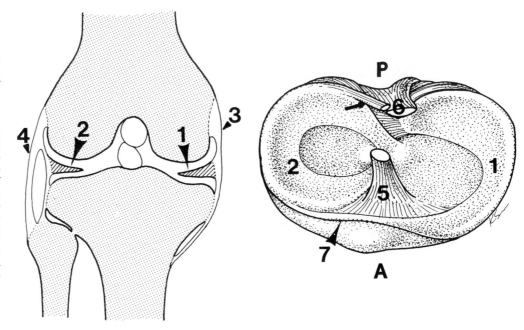

The posterior fibers of the anterior horn of the medial meniscus are intimate with the transverse (geniculate) ligament of the knee, which connects the anterior horns of both menisci.[340] This ligament is of variable thickness and lies in the frontal plane anterior to the capsule of the knee joint, in the posterior portion of Hoffa's infrapatellar fat body.[341] In one anatomic study, the transverse ligament was present in 64 per cent of specimens.[342] It can be recognized regularly on MR images (Fig. 16–77) and, occasionally, on lateral radiographs.

The meniscofemoral ligaments are accessory ligaments of the knee that extend from the posterior horn of the lateral meniscus to the lateral aspect of the medial femoral condyle.[340] As they extend across the knee, they are intimate with portions of the posterior cruciate ligament.[343–345] The anterior meniscofemoral ligament, or ligament of Humphrey, passes in front of the posterior cruciate ligament, and the posterior meniscofemoral ligament, or ligament of Wrisberg, passes behind the posterior cruciate ligament. The prevalence of these ligaments is not clear, and their size varies. In an investigation of 92 knees derived from 46 cadavers, the posterior meniscofemoral ligament was present in 76 per cent of specimens and the anterior meniscofemoral ligament in 50 per cent of specimens, and an identical pattern of both meniscofemoral ligaments in both knees of a single donor was evident in about 12 per cent of the cadavers.[342] The reported prevalence of one or the other of the two meniscofemoral ligaments in a single knee is 70 to 100 per cent,[343, 345] and the reported prevalence of both ligaments in a single knee is 6 to 80 per cent. As a general guide, the ligament of Humphrey probably is present in at least one third of knees, the ligament of Wrisberg probably is present in at least one third of knees, and both ligaments are present in

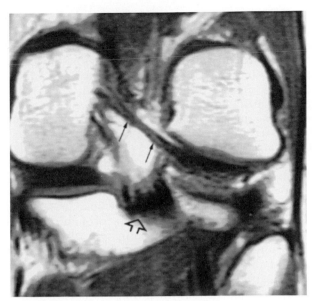

Figure 16–78
Posterior meniscofemoral ligament (ligament of Wrisberg): MR imaging. A coronal T1-weighted (TR/TE, 650/20) spin echo MR image shows the posterior meniscofemoral ligament (solid arrows) extending from the region of the posterior horn of the lateral meniscus to the medial femoral condyle. The tibial attachment site of the posterior cruciate ligament is seen (open arrow).

approximately 6 to 20 per cent of knees. The meniscofemoral ligaments are well demonstrated in coronal and sagittal MR images (Figs. 16–77 and 16–78), in which they may have an appearance simulating that of a tear of either the posterior cruciate ligament or the posterior horn of the lateral meniscus (see later discussion). The precise function of these ligaments also is not clear. The ligaments become taut when the knee is flexed, and this flexion leads to anterior and medial movement of the posterior horn of the lateral meniscus while the meniscus as a whole rotates backward and outward.[345] These movements appear to provide increased congruity between the meniscotibial socket and the lateral femoral condyle.[340, 343, 344] Shortening of the ligament of Wrisberg in association with absence of a posterior tibial attachment of the lateral meniscus may disturb the meniscal kinetics and may represent one causative factor of a discoid lateral meniscus (see later discussion).

Water represents approximately 75 per cent of the wet content of the meniscus. The dry content of the meniscus is composed of about 75 per cent collagen, 8 to 13 per cent noncollagenous proteins, and 1 per cent hexosamine.[339, 346, 347] The collagen fibers within the meniscus are oriented primarily in a circumferential fashion, thereby resisting the loads applied to them by the femur.[339, 348] Radially oriented fibers also are present, however, which may prevent longitudinal splitting of the structure resulting from undue compression.[339] Elastin fibers, accounting for approximately 0.6 per cent of the dry weight of the meniscus, connect the collagen fibers in a bridgelike fashion,[349] and they may contribute to recovery after its deformation.[339]

The vascular supply to the medial and lateral menisci originates predominantly from the superior and inferior

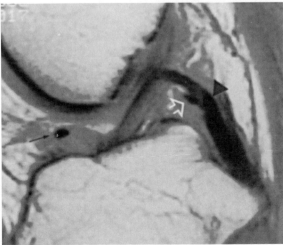

Figure 16–77
Transverse (geniculate) ligament of the knee and anterior meniscofemoral ligament (ligament of Humphrey): MR imaging. A sagittal proton density–weighted (TR/TE, 2000/20) spin echo MR image shows the transverse ligament (solid arrow) and anterior meniscofemoral ligament (open arrow) adjacent to the posterior cruciate ligament (arrowhead). The anterior cruciate ligament also is seen. (Courtesy of S. K. Brahme, M.D., La Jolla, California.)

branches of both the medial and lateral genicular arteries.[340] These vessels give rise to a perimeniscal capillary plexus within the synovial and capsular tissues of the knee that reaches the entire meniscus at the time of birth and in the first and second years of life but, after that, supplies only the peripheral border of the meniscus at its attachment to the joint capsule.[340] The central and major portion of the menisci is avascular, deriving its nutrition from the synovial fluid (Fig. 16–79).[350]

The functions of the menisci of the knee have been the subject of intense investigation, the results of which have been summarized by Renström and Johnson.[339] These functions appear to include load transmission, shock absorption, stress reduction, promotion of joint congruity, joint stabilization, limitation of extremes of flexion and extension of the knee, and articular lubrication and nutrition. Investigators have confirmed that the menisci transmit between 30 and 70 per cent of the load applied across the knee, that the lateral meniscus transmits a load equal to or greater than the load transmitted by the medial meniscus, that the posterior horns of the menisci transmit more of the load than the anterior horns, and that the distribution of the load depends on the degree of flexion of the joint.[339] The effects of partial or total meniscectomy on ipsilateral compartmental contact areas and contact pressures and on the transmission of force across the knee may be profound,[351] although the contribution of such meniscectomy to the development of osteoarthritis of the knee remains controversial. The menisci also are im-

portant in reducing the shock that is applied to the articular cartilage and subchondral bone of the knee.[352] Meniscectomy reduces the shock absorption capacity of the normal knee by 20 per cent.[340, 353] Similarly, meniscectomy leads to a significant increase in the stress applied to the knee.[354, 355] By filling in the space between the femur and the tibia, the menisci increase the congruency of the knee joint. By deepening the articular surface of the tibial plateaus, they also stabilize the joint. During the final phases of extension of the knee, the menisci are forced anteriorly, and their anterior position blocks further extension of the joint; conversely, the posterior horns are driven far posteriorly in full flexion of the knee and assist in preventing further flexion.[339] During knee motion, the medial meniscus translates on the tibial plateau between 2 and 5 mm and the lateral meniscus, untethered by its collateral ligament, is more mobile, its excursion being estimated at between 9 and 11 mm.[356] The anterior horns of the menisci are more mobile than the posterior horns of the menisci.[356] Finally, the menisci may contribute to joint lubrication by reducing the space available for distribution of the fluid that is expressed from the articular cartilage during weight-bearing, and they may assist in compressing the synovial fluid into the articular cartilage, aiding in joint nutrition.[339]

Pathologic Considerations

Although the vast majority of meniscal lesions are considered traumatic, other processes (developmental, in-

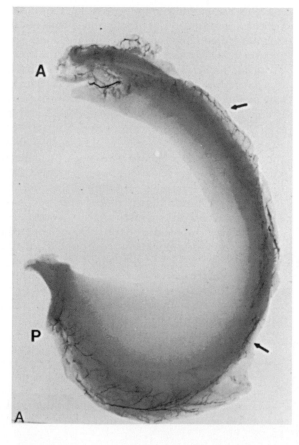

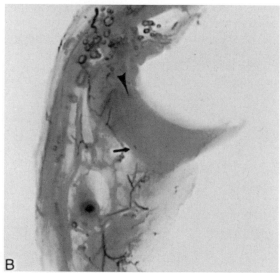

Figure 16–79

Menisci of the knee: Normal vascular anatomy.

A Medial meniscus. Note the peripheral arterial blood supply (arrows) and the avascular inner zone. A, Anterior; P, posterior.

B Medial meniscus. A cross section shows a blood vessel in the central zone of the meniscus (arrow) and absence of blood supply in the superior (arrowhead) and inferior surfaces of the meniscus. (From Danzig L, et al: Clin Orthop *172*:271, 1983.)

flammatory, infectious, neoplastic, metabolic, and degenerative) also affect these structures.[357, 358] The discoid meniscus is the most important of the developmental processes and is discussed later in this chapter. Rheumatoid arthritis, the seronegative spondyloarthropathies, juvenile chronic arthritis, and septic arthritis are among the inflammatory processes that involve the knee, including the menisci. Generally, owing to their fibrocartilaginous nature, the menisci are more resistant than articular cartilage to the detrimental effects of these processes. Aggressive inflammatory tissue, or pannus, however, can lead to significant changes of the menisci, related to enzymatic destruction and interference with proper nutrition. The peripheral portions of the menisci appear more vulnerable than the central portions,[358] although the entire meniscus may be affected. Pigmented villonodular synovitis and idiopathic synovial (osteo)chondromatosis are additional synovial processes that directly or indirectly alter meniscal integrity. All of these processes are discussed elsewhere in this book.

Crystal deposition diseases, particularly those related to calcium pyrophosphate dihydrate (CPPD) and calcium hydroxyapatite (HA) crystal accumulation, affect the menisci. Both of these disorders lead to cartilage calcification (i.e., chondrocalcinosis) that can be detected pathologically and with imaging methods. Diffuse calcification in more than one meniscus and, frequently, in the medial and lateral menisci of both knees in a middle-aged or elderly person is virtually pathognomonic for CPPD crystal deposition. Alkaptonuria, which is associated with alterations in the metabolism of tyrosine and the accumulation of homogentisic acid and its derivatives in the body tissues, can lead to abnormal pigmentation of the menisci of the knee and structural joint change (i.e., ochronotic arthropathy).

The association of meniscal abnormalities and degenerative disease is complex. The occurrence of degenerative alterations in the menisci, with or without intrameniscal crystal deposition, and osteoarthritis in the same knee is well recognized.[359, 360] The prominent role played by the menisci in maintaining joint stabilization—promoting joint congruence, stress reduction, and shock absorption—suggests that any damage to these structures may be detrimental to the adjacent articular cartilage. Furthermore, the importance of the menisci in promoting joint lubrication and nutrition of the articular cartilage is recognized. Meniscal damage interferes with these functions. Arthroscopic surgery with more limited resection or even repair of meniscal tears is a recent trend that underscores the value of maintaining as much meniscal tissue as possible in an attempt to prevent subsequent deterioration of the articular cartilage and, eventually, osteoarthritis of the knee.

Meniscal Degeneration

Changes in the composition of the menisci of the knee have been observed with advancing age, although it is difficult to determine which changes are age-related alone and which occur as a consequence of other age-related phenomena such as osteoarthritis and CPPD crystal deposition disease. In association with osteoarthritis of the knee, the prevalence of horizontal cleavage lesions of the meniscus increases; in one study consisting of 100 random necropsy examinations, the prevalence of such lesions rose from 18.4 per cent in knees without evidence of osteoarthritis to 61.5 per cent in those with severe osteoarthritis.[361] In animal models in which osteoarthritis of the knee was created by ligamentous resection, profound changes in the menisci occur, characterized by initial evidence of small vertical and horizontal tears and subsequent evidence of extensive disruption.[362] Significant alterations in water content, proteoglycans, and other matrix proteins in the menisci of the knee accompany naturally occurring or experimentally induced osteoarthritis (as well as rheumatoid arthritis).[347] Calcium HA crystal deposition, representing a dystrophic phenomenon, and CPPD crystal accumulation increase with advancing age, and either or both of these crystals can lead to an inflammatory response that, in turn, could evoke or activate proteases and catabolic factors, thus initiating or accelerating meniscal degeneration.[347] Whatever their cause, degenerative changes in the menisci of the knee are common in middle-aged and elderly persons, especially those with osteoarthritis. Such degenerative changes may predispose to tears of the menisci, owing to a decrease in their elasticity.[361] Whether degenerative meniscal abnormalities are an essential prerequisite for meniscal tears, however, is not clear, as the histologic distinction between acute tears, progressive wear and tear, and degeneration of the meniscus may not be possible.[363]

Degenerative changes of the menisci may lead to imaging abnormalities that often are characteristic and, yet, that occasionally lead to diagnostic problems. On routine radiographs, gas may accumulate within the substance of a chronically fragmented and degenerative meniscus. The gas, representing nitrogen, leads to a thick, radiolucent shadow, often in a compartment of the knee that also reveals evidence of osteoarthritis (joint space narrowing and bone sclerosis). This type of vacuum phenomenon should be differentiated from a thin, curvilinear collection of gas that may accumulate between the articular surfaces of the femur and the tibia. Gas within the meniscus is a sign of a pathologic process and is reminiscent of the vacuum phenomenon occurring in a degenerative intervertebral disc; gas within the knee joint itself is not a sign of a pathologic process but, rather, its detection generally eliminates the possibility of a large joint effusion. Both types of gas collection may be identified with CT. On MR images of the knee, however, intrameniscal or intra-articular gas produces a signal void that may simulate the appearance of a torn (or calcified) meniscus or other type of intra-articular abnormality (Fig. 16–80).[364]

Meniscal calcification related to calcium HA or CPPD crystal deposition may occur in association with meniscal degeneration. On routine radiographs, the correct diagnosis is made easily and, based on the pattern and extent of the calcific deposits, a distinction between these two types of crystals often is possible. With MR imaging, however, the meniscal calcification may be overlooked completely, and its signal void may lead to obscuration of other meniscal findings (Fig. 16–81).

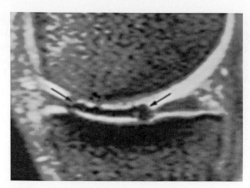

Figure 16–80

Meniscal or intra-articular gas: MR imaging. A signal void (arrows) related to gas in the knee joint, as demonstrated in this sagittal MPGR MR image (TR/TE, 500/11; flip angle, 30 degrees), may lead to diagnostic difficulty in the interpretation of meniscal integrity with MR imaging. (Courtesy of C. Hayes, M.D., Richmond, Virginia.)

With any imaging method, meniscal calcification should be differentiated from a discrete focus of ossification within the meniscus, the meniscal ossicle (see later discussion).

The presence of mucinous and myxoid degeneration (and other forms of degeneration) in a variety of intraarticular structures, such as the rotator cuff and glenoid labrum of the shoulder and the triangular fibrocartilage complex of the wrist, has received considerable attention, owing to its effect on the signal intensity of those structures during the MR imaging examination. The menisci of the knee participate in these types of degeneration. Thus, in elderly patients, differentiation of clinically significant meniscal tears and clinically insignificant meniscal degeneration with MR imaging may become problematic. The diagnosis of a meniscal tear on the basis of MR imaging is related, in part, on the presence of characteristic changes in signal intensity (see later discussion), but similar changes in signal intensity also are observed with extensive meniscal degeneration (Fig. 16–82). Therefore, although the exclusion of a tear of the meniscus in an older person may be accomplished reliably with MR imaging, the documentation of such a tear, as opposed to meniscal degeneration, may not be possible with this imaging method.[365]

Meniscal Tears

Although meniscal tears may be discovered incidentally, they may have a variety of clinical manifestations, foremost of which are knee pain and disability. The nerve supply to the meniscus is similar to the vascular supply, with the peripheral portion of the meniscus being innervated most richly.[366] In adults, invagination of the innervated synovium into the tear, particularly in cases of chronic tear, may generate pain.[361, 364] The pain may lead to a feeling of instability of the joint that often is reported by the patient. Further disability may result from displacement of portions of the torn meniscus, such as occurs with a bucket-handle meniscal tear, because the displaced fragment becomes lodged between the ipsilateral femoral condyle and tibial plateau. Associated injuries, which may include medial collateral and anterior cruciate ligament disruption, amplify the clinical manifestations of meniscal tears.

Pathogenesis. Two categories of meniscal tears commonly are identified: traumatic and degenerative. Traumatic tears are believed to result from excessive application of force to a normal meniscus. As load is applied to the knee, the meniscus is forced toward the periphery. Radial displacement is resisted by hoop stress, which converts axial load into tensile strain.[356] When the strain exceeds the capacity of the meniscus to deform, a tear is created. Degenerative tears are believed to result from normal forces acting on a degenerated structure.[358] Traumatic tears usually are vertical tears that may propagate in a longitudinal or transverse direction and commonly involve the thin edge of the meniscus. Vertical transverse tears appear to be less common than vertical longitudinal tears and characteristically involve the middle third of the lateral meniscus.[358] Degenerative tears are horizontal cleavage lesions that typically occupy the posterior half of the menisci.[358, 367]

In young persons, especially athletes, a single traumatic episode is responsible for the majority of meniscal lesions. The precise mechanisms leading to injury of the meniscus have been well summarized by Crues and Stoller.[368] Meniscal injuries frequently result from twisting strains applied to the knee when it is either slightly

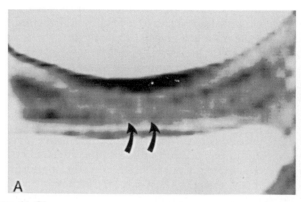
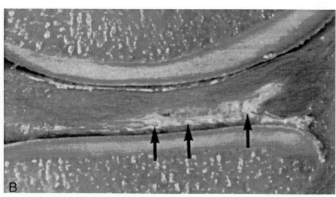

Figure 16–81

Meniscal calcification: MR imaging. A sagittal T1-weighted (TR/TE, 500/20) spin echo MR image photographed with meniscal windowing **(A)** reveals inhomogeneities in the signal intensity of the medial meniscus (arrows) that simulate those of a tear. A corresponding anatomic section **(B)** confirms the presence of calcium deposition (arrows) and the absence of a tear. (From Hodler J, et al: Radiology *184*:221, 1992.)

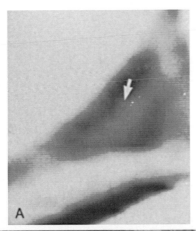

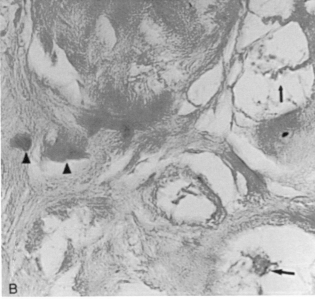

Figure 16–82
Meniscal degeneration: MR imaging. A sagittal T1-weighted (TR/TE, 500/20) spin echo MR image photographed with meniscal windowing **(A)** reveals increased signal intensity in the lateral meniscus (arrow), which corresponds to sites of mucoid (arrows) and eosinophilic (arrowheads) degeneration shown histologically (×100) **(B)**. (From Hodler J, et al: Radiology *184:*221, 1992.)

flexed or fully extended. In full extension, the stability of the knee joint is increased; therefore, meniscal tears resulting from injury during full extension often are accompanied by ligamentous injuries or fractures of the tibial plateau.[368, 369] In some instances, the peripheral portion of the meniscus becomes detached from the joint capsule over a variable length. In either situation, displacement of a portion of the meniscus (in cases of meniscal tear) or of the entire meniscus (in cases of meniscal detachment) may occur during subsequent flexion or rotation of the joint.

Degenerative tears occur more commonly in older persons and in association with osteoarthritis of the knee. The degenerative changes in the meniscus include fibrillation, fibrochondrocyte necrosis and proliferation, and loss of normal staining properties of the matrix proteins. These alterations apparently make the meniscus more vulnerable to normal stress, and the cumula-

tive effects of the stress eventually lead to loss of meniscal integrity.

The categorization of a meniscal tear as traumatic or degenerative generally is based on analysis of the clinical history, the age of the patient, and the gross morphology of the meniscus at the time of arthroscopy or open surgery. Imaging abnormalities, particularly those derived from arthrography or MR imaging, provide information regarding the type of meniscal tear. In some instances, however, it is not possible to separate degenerative and traumatic tears of the meniscus on the basis of clinical, imaging, and gross pathologic findings. Even microscopic analysis of the meniscal tissue may not allow such separation.

Classification. No uniformly accepted classification system exists for meniscal tears. Most systems of classification emphasize the direction of the tear. Tears can be described as longitudinal, radial, vertical, or horizontal, and as complete, incomplete, or complex.[357] With most types of tears, the medial meniscus is involved more frequently than the lateral meniscus, and the posterior horn of the medial meniscus and the anterior horn of the lateral meniscus are affected most commonly.

Longitudinal tears are the most frequent type encountered. Such tears may occur in a vertical direction (Fig. 16–83A) dividing the meniscus into inner and outer segments, or in a horizontal direction (Fig. 16–83B), dividing the meniscus into an upper and lower segment, resembling a fish mouth.[357] Vertical longitudinal tears are more common in the medial meniscus than in the lateral meniscus (approximately 3 to 1), and they may involve the peripheral or central portion of the meniscus. They vary in length, being isolated to the posterior horn, midportion, anterior horn, or various combinations of these. When a large part of the meniscus is affected, the inner fragment may be displaced into the central part of the joint, a phenomenon termed a bucket-handle tear. Horizontal longitudinal tears represent the cleavage lesions common in older persons and in degenerated menisci. These tears may extend in a slightly oblique direction, exiting on the superior or inferior surface of the meniscus. Such tears involve either the medial or lateral meniscus or both menisci, and they may be accompanied by a meniscal cyst (see later discussion).

A radial tear is a special type of vertical tear that involves the inner margin of the meniscus (Fig. 16–83C). This tear is most frequent in the middle third of the lateral meniscus and, in either meniscus, may extend outwardly for a variable distance in any direction. Such tears sometimes extend anterolaterally or posterolaterally, being referred to as parrot beak or flap tears and, when extensive, they divide the meniscus into an anterior and posterior portion. Radial tears and flap tears transect the longitudinal cords of collagen in the meniscus, require a great force or a meniscus with a compromised integrity, and are uncommon (approximately 5 to 10 per cent of meniscal tears).[356]

Although optimally being able to differentiate among these various types of tears on the basis of imaging abnormalities would be helpful, this commonly is not

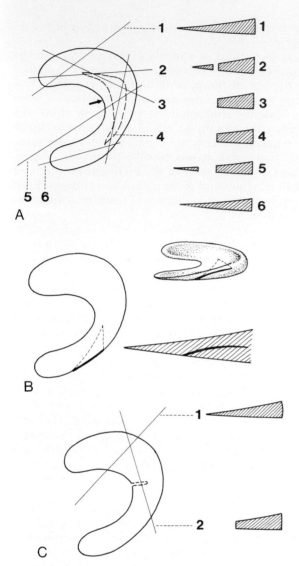

A

B

C

Figure 16–83
Meniscal tears: Classification.

  A Longitudinal vertical tears (with displacement). The medial meniscus is viewed from above with the posterior horn located superiorly. The longitudinal vertical tear can be seen and the inner fragment is displaced centrally (arrow). The arthrographic appearance as well as the appearance in radial sections obtained with MR imaging will depend on the specific site of the tear. A view of the posterior aspect of the meniscus (1) will be normal. Slightly more anteriorly (2) a vertical tear will be apparent with minimal displacement of the fragment. At positions 3 and 4, an amputated meniscal shadow will be apparent. At position 5, significant displacement of the inner fragment will be observed. The anterior horn of the meniscus (6) will appear normal.

  B Longitudinal horizontal tears. The medial meniscus is viewed from above (drawing on left), in front (drawing on top right), and in longitudinal section (drawing on bottom right). The extent and appearance of the tear can be appreciated.

  C Radial tear. The medial meniscus is viewed from above, with its posterior horn located superiorly. A radial tear is evident on the inner contour of the meniscus. Some arthrographic views or MR imaging views (with radial sections) (1) will appear normal, whereas others passing through the tear (2) will reveal a blunted, contrast-coated (i.e., with arthrography) inner meniscal shadow.

possible. Many tears are complex, demonstrating features of more than one type of lesion. More significant from an imaging standpoint is the accurate diagnosis of a tear, its proper localization to the medial, lateral, or both menisci, and documentation of displacement of any meniscal fragments. Differentiation between traumatic and degenerative tears also is not possible on many occasions. Acute traumatic tears in young persons often lead to rounded and smooth margins, and chronic degenerative tears in older persons commonly are associated with frayed, fibrillated, and irregular margins.[357] The localization of a tear to the peripheral portion of the meniscus has therapeutic importance, owing to the possibility of spontaneous healing of this tear (see later discussion). Tears in this region may appear hemorrhagic on gross inspection, an appearance related to the prominent vascular supply to the peripheral portion of the meniscus.

  Clinical Abnormalities. The clinical diagnosis of a meniscal tear relies on careful questioning of the patient and physical examination. A history of pain and a slowly developing joint effusion are helpful clues, but

neither finding is diagnostic of a meniscal tear. In cases of a bucket-handle tear of the meniscus, locking of the knee may be reported by the patient, but this likewise is not a pathognomonic finding. Pain and tenderness on palpation of the meniscal margin near the site of tear may be elicited. A positive McMurray test, characterized by an audible snap or pop as an abnormal meniscus extends over a bone protuberance, lends support to the clinical diagnosis of a meniscal tear, but a negative McMurray test does not eliminate the possibility of such a tear.[368]

  The reported accuracy in diagnosis of meniscal tears based on results of analysis of the patient's history and physical examination has varied.[369, 370, 1118] This accuracy appears to be greater for medial than for lateral meniscus tears. A diagnostic accuracy of approximately 90 per cent for tears of the medial meniscus and of approximately 70 per cent for tears of the lateral meniscus may be possible when experienced orthopedic surgeons are assessing the knee. In the hands of less experienced physicians, however, a far lower diagnostic accuracy usually is apparent and, independent of the level of experience of the examiner, determination of the precise location, type, and extent of the tear usually is not possible on the basis of the clinical history and physical examination.[368] An interest in the value of imaging studies in the assessment of menisci, therefore, is understandable, although such studies should be regarded as a supplement to, rather than a replacement for, careful clinical assessment.[1119, 1195]

Ultrasonographic Abnormalities. Despite recent interest in the application of ultrasonography to the detection of meniscal tears,[371–373] the technique rarely is employed for this purpose. In one cadaveric study,[371] ultrasonography proved useful in demonstrating even small meniscal tears, and the type of tear could be assessed in some cases. In general, however, it is difficult to study the entire meniscus with ultrasonography, and the results depend to a great extent on the experience of the examiner. Although the use of an intra-articular transducer is an interesting extension of sonographic technique,[372] this method requires a skin incision and, therefore, is invasive.

Scintigraphic Abnormalities. Bone scintigraphy has been employed in a limited fashion for the diagnosis of meniscal tears.[374, 375] Even when combined with SPECT, bone scintigraphy is at best a moderately sensitive method, and it lacks specificity.

CT Abnormalities. The use of standard CT (i.e., without the introduction of intra-articular contrast material) in the assessment of the menisci of the knee has been studied.[376–381] The reported sensitivity of CT has varied from 63 to 96 per cent, the reported specificity from 81 to 93 per cent, and the reported accuracy from 84 to 91 per cent.[377, 379] In one study, CT was found to be more efficacious than MR imaging (performed with a 0.5 Tesla magnet) in meniscal evaluation,[378] and in another study, CT was found accurate in the diagnosis of a bucket-handle tear of the meniscus (using arthroscopy as the standard) in 49 of 53 patients (92.5 per cent).[380] This method requires thin (2 or 3 mm) contiguous or overlapping transaxial images and angulation of the gantry so that the sections are parallel to the tibial plateau. Diagnostic difficulty arises in cases in which a nondisplaced horizontal tear of the meniscus is oriented parallel to the transaxial imaging plane. In comparison to arthrography, CT of the meniscus is noninvasive, can be used to assess both knees, and is not a physician-intensive examination (as the study can be performed within 20 to 25 min by experienced technologists). Disadvantages of the CT examination, when compared with arthrography, are its higher cost, degradation of the images owing to patient movement, poor visualization of the menisci as a result of a hemarthrosis, difficulty in imaging horizontal tears of the meniscus and meniscocapsular separations, and findings related to meniscal degeneration that simulate those of a meniscal tear.[381] Furthermore, modern MR imaging allows more detailed analysis of the knee menisci and other intra-articular and periarticular structures, albeit at a slightly higher cost.

Arthrographic Abnormalities. With regard to the normal arthrographic appearance of the menisci, the medial meniscus is identified as a sharply defined, soft tissue triangular shadow (Fig. 16–84). Its posterior horn usually is large, averaging 14 mm wide.[382] Its midportion is somewhat smaller, whereas the anterior horn usually is the smallest portion of the medial meniscus, averaging 6 mm wide.[382] Occasionally, the anterior horn may be larger than the midportion of the medial meniscus. The peripheral surface of the medial meniscus is firmly attached to the medial collateral ligament. Certain normal recesses about the medial meniscus produce focal pouchlike collections of air and contrast material.[383, 384] A superior recess frequently is present above the posterior horn of the medial meniscus. A posterior inferior recess is less common, although the presence of such a recess beneath the anterior horn of the medial meniscus is more frequent. These inferior recesses beneath the medial meniscus generally are small, and some authori-

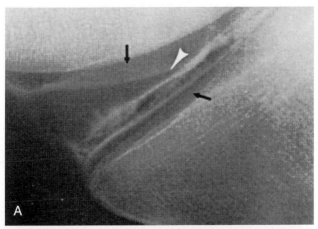

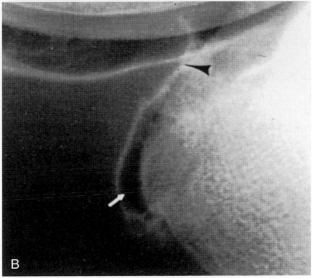

Figure 16–84

Normal medial meniscus: Arthrography.

A Posterior horn of the medial meniscus. This segment is relatively large, extending for a considerable distance into the articular cavity (arrowhead). The adjacent articular recesses are small. The articular cartilage (arrows) is smooth.

B Anterior horn of the medial meniscus. The size of this segment is variable (arrowhead). An inferior recess is visualized (solid arrow).

ties regard recesses that are greater than 2 mm in size as abnormal.[385] The anterior part of the medial meniscus is covered with the base of the infrapatellar fat pad, making evaluation of this region more difficult.

The lateral meniscus normally is more circular in configuration than the medial meniscus. It too is projected as a sharply defined triangular radiodense area surrounded by air and contrast material (Fig. 16–85). It changes little in size from its anterior to its posterior horn, averaging 10 mm wide.[386] Inferior recesses are frequent beneath both the anterior and the posterior horns of the lateral meniscus. The anterior horn is attached to the capsule, but the posterior horn of the lateral meniscus is separated from the capsule by the synovial sheath of the popliteus tendon. This sheath fills with air and contrast material and overlies the peripheral portion of the posterior horn of the lateral meniscus, producing variable arthrographic find-

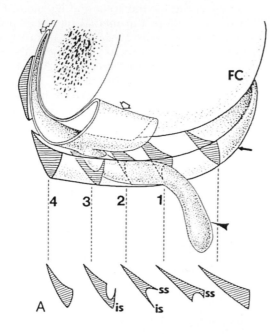

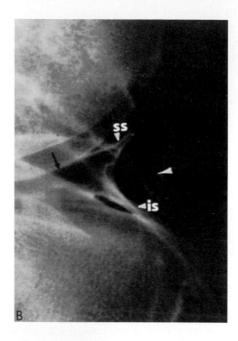

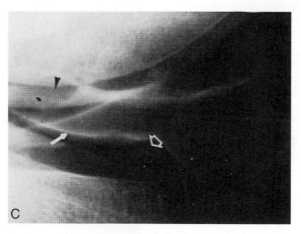

Figure 16–85

Normal lateral meniscus: Arthrography.

 A Diagrammatic representation of the posterolateral aspect of the knee joint demonstrates relationships of the lateral meniscus (solid arrow) and popliteus tendon sheath (arrowhead). The most posterior aspect of the femoral condyle (FC) and synovial reflection (open arrow) are indicated. The popliteus muscle originates posteriorly and inferiorly on the tibia and extends obliquely, anteriorly, and superiorly to insert on the lateral aspect of the femur. The popliteus tendon enters the joint close to the posterior and lateral aspects of the meniscus and passes through an oblique tunnel. Anteroinferior and posterosuperior to the intra-articular portion of the popliteus tendon are recesses, which fill with contrast medium during arthrography. Two bands of connective tissue, termed struts or fascicles, connect the posterior horn of the lateral meniscus to the joint capsule around the popliteal tendon sheath. Classically, (1) the more posterior aspect of the lateral meniscus will reveal an intact superior strut (ss); (2) a slightly more anterior section will reveal both superior strut (ss) and inferior strut (is); (3) a more anterior section will reveal only an inferior strut (is); and (4) a still further anterior section (midportion of the lateral meniscus) will depict an intact meniscus with no visible popliteal tendon sheath.

 B Posterior aspect of the lateral meniscus (section 2). In this arthrogram observe the popliteus tendon sheath (arrowhead), lateral meniscus (arrow), superior strut (ss), and inferior strut (is).

 C Anterior horn of the lateral meniscus. In this arthrogram the meniscus (solid arrow) is well shown. Observe the articular cartilage (arrowhead) and prominent recess (open arrow).

ings.[384, 387-390] Two delicate bands of connective tissue, termed struts or fascicles, connect the posterior horn of the lateral meniscus to the joint capsule around the popliteal tendon sheath. In any one view of this portion of the lateral meniscus, two struts may be observed with the intervening sheath, one strut may be apparent in conjunction with the sheath, or the sheath may be observed without visualization of either strut. Classically, however, arthrography of the most posterior aspect of the lateral meniscus will reveal an intact superior strut; a slightly more anterior view will reveal both struts; and a more anterior projection will reveal an inferior strut. The variability in appearance of the fascicles or struts of the lateral meniscus combined with the presence of an overlying air-filled tendon sheath makes difficult the evaluation of the posterior horn of the lateral meniscus. Narrowing, compression, or absence of the popliteus tendon sheath, however, may indicate tears of the lateral menisci, discoid menisci, adhesive capsulitis, prior surgery, or a rare congenital abnormality.[391]

Arthrography remains a highly accurate technique for the evaluation of a number of meniscal abnormalities, including tears. The arthrographic appearance of meniscal tears in both adults[392-396] and children[397-399] has been well described. A classification of types of meniscal tears has been used,[392] although specification of a particular type of tear during arthrography often is impossible and, even when possible, may have little clinical significance. The location of the tear in one aspect of the meniscus is of greater significance. In cases of vertical longitudinal (concentric) tears, a vertical radiodense line extending through the meniscus will be observed (Fig. 16–86). The inner fragment may be displaced, producing a bucket-handle tear, and may lodge in the central portion of the articulation, where it may or may not be identified during arthrography.[400] A vertical tear along the inner contour of the meniscus (radial tear) will produce a contrast medium-coated inner meniscal margin and a blunted meniscal shadow (Fig. 16–87). With a horizontal meniscal tear, a radiopaque line of contrast material is apparent overlying the meniscal shadow, extending to the superior or inferior surface (Fig. 16–88). The meniscus may lose its wedge-shaped configuration.

MR Imaging Abnormalities

Technical Considerations. Many of the technical aspects of MR imaging of the knee (including the menisci) are addressed earlier in this chapter. Some important points are summarized here.

1. Diagnostic images can be obtained on magnets with field strengths ranging from 0.3 to 1.5 Tesla. In general, the higher field strength systems provide high quality images in a shorter period of time, as low field strength systems must employ more signal averages to generate equivalent information.

2. The meniscal examination relies on the use of a surface coil, often a dedicated knee coil. Most such coils are cylindrical, fitting about the knee and providing a homogeneous imaging volume. In some instances, such

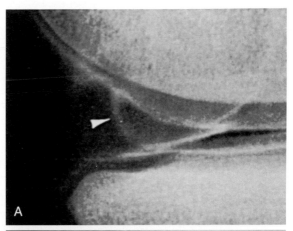

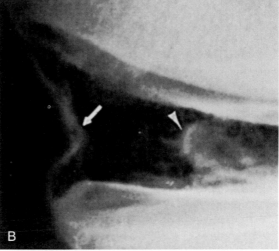

Figure 16–86
Vertical longitudinal (concentric) meniscal tears: Arthrography. Two examples are shown. In **A,** contrast material coats the tear (arrowhead) in the medial meniscus. In **B,** the tear (arrow) of the medial meniscus is associated with central displacement (arrowhead) of its inner portion.

as after an acute injury, a flexible surface coil may be used as a replacement for a rigid extremity coil.[401]

3. Spin echo MR imaging remains the most popular of the techniques used to study the menisci. The choice of conventional versus fast spin echo sequences is controversial. Some studies have suggested inferiority of fast spin echo MR images (when compared to conventional ones) in the diagnosis of meniscal tears due to such factors as image blurring.[117, 402]

4. Although gradient echo MR imaging has been employed in the analysis of the menisci, it is less popular than spin echo MR imaging. With gradient echo techniques, either two-dimensional or three-dimensional sequences are possible, radial imaging provides data similar to those of routine arthrographic projections, and (with three-dimensional gradient echo sequences) image reconstructions in various planes and three-dimensional image renderings are possible.[403]

5. The sagittal and coronal imaging planes are fundamental to assessment of the menisci. Although sagittal images generally provide more information than coronal images, both planes usually are employed. Typically,

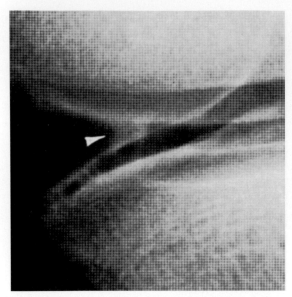

Figure 16–87
Vertical radial meniscal tears: Arthrography. Note the radial tear (arrowhead) of the medial meniscus in the arthrogram.

sagittal and coronal spin echo MR images are obtained with slice thicknesses varying from 3 to 4 mm, fields of view ranging from 120 to 160 mm, and imaging matrices ranging from 256 × 192 to 256 phase-encoding steps.[401] Lower imaging matrices (such as 256 × 128) are associated with truncation artifacts. Short echo time (TE) sequences are preferable for meniscal imaging; T1-weighted and proton density–weighted images are superior to T2-weighted images in the assessment of intrameniscal signal intensity.

6. The value of high contrast, narrow window photographic technique (i.e., meniscal windowing) is not agreed on. Although such technique highlights altered patterns of intrameniscal signal intensity, perhaps improving accuracy in the diagnosis of subtle meniscal tears, a potential danger exists owing to the possible choice of a specific window setting that exaggerates intrameniscal signal intensity such that a meniscal tear

is diagnosed when one is not present. Strict supervision of MR imaging photography is essential to accurate interpretation of the menisci whether conventional window widths or meniscal windowing is used.

7. The role of MR arthrography (using gadolinium or iodinated contrast agents or saline solution) in the evaluation of the menisci appears to be limited. Its major application, if any, is in the assessment of recurrent meniscal pathologic lesions in a patient in whom prior repair of a meniscal tear or partial resection of a meniscus has been employed (see later discussion). A second potential application of MR arthrography is in the further assessment of altered intrameniscal signal intensity when it is not clear if the meniscal surface has been violated. Other applications of MR arthrography include evaluation of nonmeniscal abnormalities (see later discussion).

Normal Menisci. Two aspects of the MR imaging appearance of the normal meniscus are morphology and internal signal intensity.

As with arthrography, the normal morphology of the meniscus is characterized by a triangular appearance and a sharp central tip.[97, 404] This appearance is apparent in both coronal and sagittal planes (Fig. 16–89). In the sagittal plane, the anterior and posterior horns of the menisci unite in peripheral sections, forming a structure that is shaped like a bow-tie.[78] In central sections, the menisci normally have a rhomboid shape. In the coronal plane, far posterior sections show the menisci as broad and elongated structures extending far into the central portion of the joint. The medial (tibial) collateral ligament is seen adjacent to the midportion of the medial meniscus, with an interface apparent between it and the outer portion of the meniscus. In both the sagittal and coronal images, the course of the popliteus tendon and its sheath and their intimacy with the posterior horn of the lateral meniscus are evident.

Although classic morphologic changes (e.g., blunting of the tip of the meniscus, displacement of a portion of the meniscus, an interrupted appearance of the meniscus, and an abnormality in the size of a segment of the meniscus) occur in the presence of a meniscal tear, normal morphologic variations in the menisci exist that

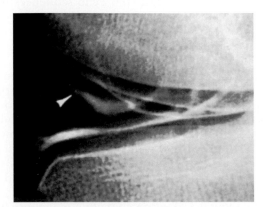

Figure 16–88
Horizontal meniscal tears: Arthrography. An arthrogram in a patient with a horizontal tear of the medial meniscus. Note the tear (arrowhead), which is filled with contrast material.

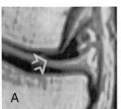 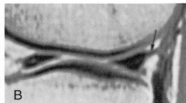

Figure 16–89
Normal lateral meniscus of the knee: MR imaging.
A In a coronal proton density–weighted (TR/TE, 2000/20) spin echo MR image, note the normal appearance of the lateral meniscus (open arrow). It is of uniform low signal intensity. Its fascicles are seen.
B A sagittal proton density–weighted (TR/TE, 2000/30) spin echo MR image reveals the anterior and posterior horns of the lateral meniscus. The lateral meniscus is of low signal intensity and its morphology is normal. Note the superior fascicle (arrow) of the lateral meniscus.

can lead to diagnostic difficulty. Some of these variations relate to normal anatomic structures, physiologic changes in the shape of the meniscus, and artifacts of the MR imaging examination itself. The normal anatomic structures that may simulate the appearance of a meniscal tear include the following:

1. *Transverse ligament of the knee.* The transverse ligament of the knee extends between the convex portions of the anterior horns of the medial and lateral menisci. Its size varies, and it may be absent in some persons. This ligament usually is identified on sagittal MR images of the knee and occasionally can be detected on coronal images as well. Its course can be traced on sequential sagittal MR images of the central portion of the knee (Fig. 16–90). As it separates from the menisci, particularly the medial meniscus, the space between it and the meniscus may be misinterpreted as evidence of a meniscal tear.

2. *Lateral inferior genicular artery.* The lateral inferior genicular artery is closely applied to the anterior portion of the lateral meniscus.[87] The space between this vessel and the meniscus may be misinterpreted as evidence of a meniscal tear.

3. *Popliteus tendon.* The popliteus tendon and its synovial sheath course between the posterior horn of the lateral meniscus and the joint capsule. An area of intermediate signal intensity between the posterior horn of the lateral meniscus and the popliteus tendon on sagit-

tal MR images may be misinterpreted as evidence of a tear (see Fig. 16–90). This area extends in an oblique fashion from anterior above to posterior below and differs in orientation from the usual tear of the posterior horn of the lateral meniscus.

4. *Meniscofemoral ligaments.* The meniscofemoral ligaments extend from the posterior horn of the lateral meniscus to the medial condyle of the femur. The anterior branch, or ligament of Humphrey, is directed in an oblique craniomedial orientation, anterior to the posterior cruciate ligament; the posterior branch, or ligament of Wrisberg, has a similar orientation but passes posterior to the posterior cruciate ligament.[405] The relatively high signal intensity of the loose connective tissue between either one of these ligaments and the most medial part of the posterior horn of the lateral meniscus may be misinterpreted as evidence of a meniscal tear.[405–407] As in most cases of meniscal pseudotears, analysis of sequential MR images allows proper interpretation (Fig. 16–91).

5. *Capsular attachment.* The junctional region between the posterior portion of the medial meniscus and the joint capsule contains peripheral vessels whose signal intensity leads to tissue inhomogeneity that can simulate the appearance of a meniscocapsular detachment.[406] Less conspicuity of this region of increased signal intensity on gradient echo MR images may be useful in differentiating the normal situation from such detachment.[406]

6. *Bursa of the medial collateral ligament.* The bursa of the medial collateral ligament is present in more than 90 per cent of cadaveric knees.[408] This bursa separates the peripheral region of the midportion of the medial meniscus and the medial collateral ligament. Fluid collections accompanying bursitis lead to increased signal intensity in this junctional region that simulates the appearance of meniscocapsular separation.[409, 1120]

Physiologic changes in the shape of the meniscus may be observed during the MR imaging examination, and the resulting appearance may simulate that of a meniscal tear. The medial meniscal flounce is one example of these changes (Fig. 16–92).[410] The flounce, which is observed regularly during knee arthrography, results from traction on the peripheral portion of the medial meniscus that occurs during tibial rotation, leading to waviness or folding of the inner edge of the medial meniscus. A similar phenomenon occurs during MR imaging in the presence of a joint effusion and joint laxity (related to ligamentous injury), when the tibia is rotated for positioning within the magnet.[410] The resulting appearance during the MR imaging examination may resemble that of a meniscal tear.[411]

Certain artifacts produced during the MR imaging examination may simulate the features of a meniscal tear.

1. *Volume averaging.* As indicated previously, problems in interpretation of meniscal integrity are encountered at the site of attachment of the meniscus to the capsule. A concavity filled with periarticular fat and neurovascular structures exists in this junctional region.[87, 406] Sagittal images through the periphery of the meniscus often

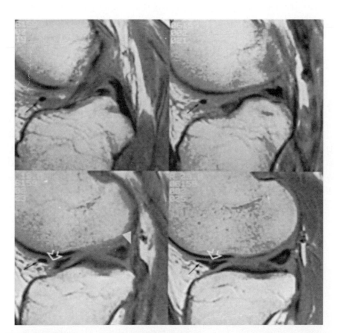

Figure 16–90
Pseudotears of the menisci: Transverse ligament of the knee and popliteus tendon. Four sagittal proton density–weighted (TR/TE, 2000/20) spin echo MR images show the course of the transverse ligament of the knee (solid arrows) from its most central position (top left) to its most lateral position (bottom right). As it approaches the anterior horn of the lateral meniscus, a space of intermediate signal intensity (open arrows) between it and the meniscus may be misinterpreted as evidence of a meniscal tear. Posteriorly, the popliteus tendon (arrowhead) separates the posterior horn of the lateral meniscus and the joint capsule. This region also may be misinterpreted as evidence of a meniscal tear.

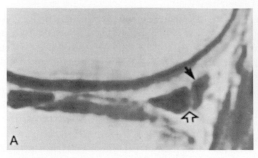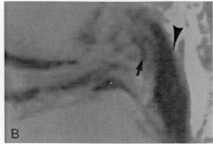

Figure 16–91

Pseudotears of the menisci: Anterior meniscofemoral ligament (ligament of Humphrey). Two sagittal proton density–weighted (TR/TE, 2300/30) spin echo MR images photographed with meniscal windowing reveal the course of the anterior meniscofemoral ligament. In **A,** the more lateral image, note the ligament (solid arrow) adjacent to the posterior horn of the lateral meniscus with a space (arrowhead) between them that may be misinterpreted as evidence of a meniscal tear. In **B,** a central image, the anterior meniscofemoral ligament (solid arrow) is located anterior to the posterior cruciate ligament (arrowhead).

demonstrate a linear artifact of high signal intensity within the normal meniscus (of low signal intensity) due to volume averaging of these junctional tissues and the meniscus. A similar appearance sometimes is seen in the most posterior coronal MR images of the menisci (Fig. 16–93).

2. Truncation artifact. Truncation artifacts result from the use of Fourier transform methods to construct MR images of high contrast boundaries, such as between the articular cartilage and the meniscus.[412] Truncation artifacts appear as a series of lines of high and low signal intensity, adjacent and parallel to these boundaries. Such a line of high signal intensity within the low signal intensity of the meniscus may simulate the appearance of a meniscal tear. In the knee, truncation artifacts affecting the meniscus have been reported to be most prominent when the acquisition matrix is 128 × 256 and the 128 pixel (phase-encoded) axis is in a superoinferior orientation; acquisition of images using a 192 × 256 or 256 × 256 matrix or with anteroposterior orientation of the 128 pixel axis results in a diminution

of these artifacts.[412] Truncation artifacts within the meniscus may be accentuated when meniscal windowing is used, and they may be accompanied by similar artifacts within the subchondral bone plate of the tibia. When superimposed on the meniscus, truncation artifacts tend to be subtle, uniform in thickness, and parallel to the surfaces of the menisci, approximately 2 pixels distant from the articular cartilage.[412] They may extend beyond the boundaries of the menisci.

3. *Magic angle phenomenon.* The magic angle phenomenon is a manifestation of the anisotropic behavior of collagen on MR imaging. It may lead to increased signal intensity in meniscal segments that are oriented at approximately 55 degrees relative to the main magnetic field on short echo time (TE) MR images. This phenomenon has led to difficulty in the assessment of the upsloping medial segment of the posterior horn of the lateral meniscus (Fig. 16–94). In one study, increased signal intensity was observed in this segment in about 75 per cent of examinations.[413]

The second aspect of the MR imaging characteristics of the normal meniscus relates to its internal signal intensity. Although the menisci commonly are described as structures of uniformly low signal intensity, this de-

Figure 16–92

Pseudotears of the menisci: Meniscal flounce. This sagittal fast spin echo MR image (TR/TE, 4633/17) shows a meniscal flounce involving the inner margin of the posterior horn of the medial meniscus. A waviness of the meniscal contour is apparent (arrow).

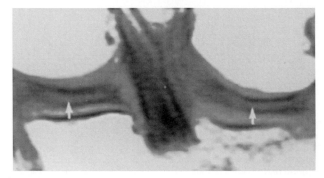

Figure 16–93

Pseudotears of the menisci: Volume averaging. Linear regions of intermediate signal intensity (arrows) normally may be evident at the peripheral portions of the medial and lateral menisci. Here they are seen in the posterior portions of both menisci in a coronal T1-weighted (TR/TE, 650/20) spin echo MR image photographed with meniscal windowing.

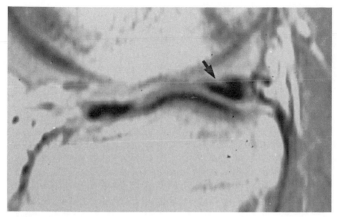

Figure 16-94
Pseudotears of the menisci: Magic angle phenomenon. In this sagittal proton density–weighted (TR/TE, 2300/25) spin echo MR image, filmed with meniscal windowing, note increased signal intensity (arrow) in the upsloping medial segment of the posterior horn of the lateral meniscus.

scription is misleading and not accurate. Regions of intermediate signal intensity commonly are encountered within the menisci of asymptomatic persons, and misinterpretation of these regions as tears has led to unnecessary arthroscopy during which the grossly normal appearance of the meniscus has been documented.

In 1987, Stoller and colleagues[83] provided the first full description of the inhomogeneous signal intensity that may be seen in normal menisci. In a cadaver study using close MR imaging–histologic correlation, they developed a grading system based on the appearance and extent of the areas of higher intrameniscal signal intensity that, with minor modifications, is used today. This grading system recognized three patterns of intrameniscal signal (Fig. 16–95):

Grade 1: One or several punctate regions of intermediate signal intensity not contiguous with an articular surface of the meniscus (the capsular margin of the meniscus is not considered an articular surface).

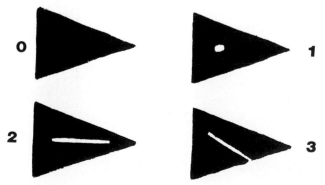

Figure 16-95
Grades of intrameniscal signal intensity. The meniscus may appear of uniform low signal intensity (grade 0); it may contain one or several circular foci of intermediate signal intensity (grade 1), or a linear region of intermediate signal intensity that does not extend to an articular surface (grade 2); or it may reveal linear or irregular regions of intermediate signal intensity that extend to the articular surface (grade 3).

Grade 2: Linear regions of intermediate signal intensity without extension to the articular surface of the meniscus.

Grade 3: Regions of intermediate signal intensity with extension to an articular surface of the meniscus.

Correlation of the grades of intrameniscal signal intensity and histologic findings confirmed the existence of increasing amounts of degenerative changes within the menisci with grades 1 and 2 imaging findings and evidence of fibrocartilaginous tears in the menisci with grade 3 imaging findings.[83] The primary pattern of degenerative alteration was mucinous change, appearing as discrete foci in menisci with grade 1 signal intensity and as linear bands in menisci with grade 2 signal intensity. In menisci with grade 3 signal intensity, degenerative alterations were accompanied by distinct cleavage planes with or without macroscopically evident extension to the articular surface of the meniscus.

The occurrence of mucinous and myxoid changes within the meniscus as a consequence of aging is well documented.[365, 414] Thus, intrameniscal regions of intermediate signal intensity detected on MR images of the knee may progress with advancing age of the patient, leading to diagnostic difficulty in the interpretation and clinical significance of grade 3 signal intensity in middle-aged and elderly persons.[365] The appearance of extensive regions of intermediate signal intensity within the menisci of asymptomatic persons in the fourth through sixth decades of life and beyond is well recognized. These degenerative abnormalities may predispose the meniscus to structural failure. In one study, patients with documented meniscal tears had evidence of a more advanced degree of meniscal degeneration in the opposite, asymptomatic knee than did members of an age-matched normal control population or patients with nonmeniscal knee disorders.[414] Degenerative changes predominate in the posterior segment of the medial meniscus, the most common site of meniscal tear.

Despite the diagnostic problems encountered caused by age-related meniscal degeneration, the grading system proposed by Stoller and coworkers[83] is useful clinically. This system relies on the occurrence of grade 3 signal intensity within the meniscus in cases of meniscal tear (Fig. 16–96). Differentiation between grade 2 signal intensity, which may extend close to the articular surface of the meniscus, and grade 3 signal intensity, which

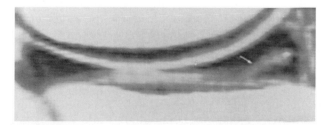

Figure 16-96
Meniscal tears: Grade 3 intrameniscal signal intensity. A sagittal proton density–weighted (TR/TE, 2000/20) spin echo MR image photographed with meniscal windowing shows a linear region of intermediate signal intensity (arrow) extending to the inferior surface of the posterior horn of the medial meniscus.

violates this surface, obviously becomes important, as the first pattern generally is regarded as evidence of degenerative changes that cannot be detected at the time of arthroscopy and the second pattern is considered evidence of a meniscal tear that can be found and treated at the time of arthroscopy. In clinical practice, a great deal of time is spent trying to interpret correctly the intrameniscal signal intensity as evidence of a grade 2 or grade 3 pattern. The general consensus emphasizes caution in "overcalling" the extent of intrameniscal signal intensity and in using photographic maneuvers during meniscal windowing to create an illusion of violation of the meniscal surface. The wisdom of this philosophy is underscored by the results of studies by Kaplan and coworkers[415] and by De Smet and collaborators.[416] In the first of these two investigations, an analysis of MR images of the knee in 142 consecutive patients revealed 20 patients (14 per cent) in whom it was difficult to decide if the region of intermediate signal intensity extended to the meniscal surface. In 17 of 20 patients, the posterior horn of the lateral meniscus was involved. In 13 of 20 patients who underwent arthroscopy or arthrotomy, no meniscal tears were found. The authors concluded that a meniscal tear is unlikely when the focus of altered intrameniscal signal intensity does not involve the meniscal surface unequivocally. De Smet and associates,[416] in an assessment of MR imaging findings in the knees of 200 consecutive patients, found that more than 90 per cent of menisci with abnormal signal intensity contacting the surface on more than one image were torn, but only 55 per cent of medial menisci and 30 per cent of lateral menisci with such signal intensity patterns on a single MR image were torn. The authors concluded that the presence of regions of intermediate signal intensity within the meniscus that contact the surface of the meniscus on only one image should lead to the diagnosis of a possible tear rather than a definite tear.

To determine the prognosis in patients with grade 2 intrameniscal signal intensity, Dillon and collaborators[417] performed a prospective study of this pattern of signal intensity in patients with intact anterior cruciate ligaments. In 27 menisci in 22 patients in whom the initial MR imaging examination showed evidence of grade 2 changes in one or both menisci that had been proved at arthroscopy not to be torn, subsequent evaluation using MR imaging after a period of 11 to 41 months showed an unchanged pattern of signal intensity in 18 of 27 menisci, decreased intrameniscal signal intensity in six menisci, and increased intrameniscal signal intensity in only three menisci. These data support the conclusion that grade 2 patterns of signal intensity within the meniscus generally are stable for at least 1 year to several years.

The effects of physiologic exercise on the patterns of intrameniscal signal intensity have been studied, with inconsistent results. Kursunoglu-Brahme and coworkers,[418] evaluating MR images of the knee in 10 healthy subjects before and immediately after 30 min of continuous jogging, found subtle increases in intrameniscal signal intensity (as well as joint effusions) in five of their subjects. It was suggested that the changes in signal intensity occurred as a result of imbibition of water by meniscal proteoglycans in association with the presence of joint fluid. Shellock and collaborators[419, 420] performed MR imaging examinations of the knee in healthy long distance runners and found no increased prevalence of meniscal degeneration or tears in these persons and that none demonstrated an increase in intrameniscal signal intensity or an increase in joint fluid when comparison was made between MR images obtained before and after competition. MR imaging examinations of the knee in asymptomatic collegiate and professional (American) football and basketball players have shown a high prevalence of signal intensity patterns consistent with meniscal degeneration or tear[421] and a progression of these patterns on sequential examinations.[422]

An expanded classification system of intrameniscal signal intensity was described by Mesgarzadeh and colleagues (Fig. 16–97).[406] Although these authors included the categories of grade 1 and grade 2 signal intensity as described by Stoller and coworkers,[83] they classified short and truncated menisci as grade 3 and grade 4 abnormalities, respectively. They further divided the previously described category of grade 3 signal intensity into three new grades: intermediate signal intensity extending to only one surface of the meniscus (grade 5), signal intensity extending to both meniscal surfaces (grade 6), and an irregular pattern of intermediate signal intensity within the meniscus that may or may not extend to the meniscal surface (grade 7). Arthroscopically proved meniscal tears occurred in 2 per cent of menisci with grade 1 signal intensity, 5 per cent of menisci with grade 2 signal intensity, 23 per cent of menisci with grade 3 signal intensity, 71 per cent of menisci with grade 4 signal intensity, 85 per cent of menisci with grade 5 signal intensity, 95 per cent of menisci with grade 6 signal intensity, and 82 per cent of menisci with grade 7 signal intensity. These results indicate that reliance on the presence of violation of the meniscal surface in the diagnosis of meniscal tears will result in a definite but small percentage of false-negative MR im-

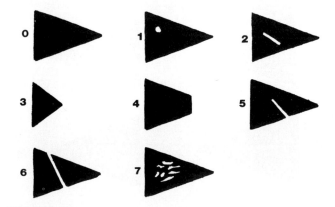

Figure 16–97

Grading of intrameniscal signal intensity and meniscal morphology: Expanded classification system. A grade 0 pattern consists of a meniscus that is of homogeneous low signal intensity. Grades 1 and 2 patterns are similar to those previously illustrated. Additional grades (3, 4, 5, 6, and 7) are described in the text. (Modified from Mesgarzadeh M, et al: Radiographics *13*:489, 1993.)

aging examinations, that violation of both meniscal surfaces as opposed to one is a more definite sign of a meniscal tear, and that correct interpretation of the significance of a short and truncated meniscus as seen on MR images is difficult, particularly in patients who have had previous meniscal surgery. The assessment of the significance of grade 7 signal intensity also is difficult (Fig. 16–98). When the altered signal intensity reaches the surface of the meniscus, the diagnosis of a tear in menisci with grade 7 signal intensity becomes more definite; when it does not reach the meniscal surface, prominent meniscal degeneration appears to be highly likely, particularly in older persons. Such meniscal degeneration may be interpreted as evidence of a meniscal tear during arthroscopy if the meniscus is probed vigorously.

Although most patients who reveal altered signal intensity within the meniscus that does not extend to the meniscal surface do not have a torn meniscus, one exception to this rule deserves emphasis. Prominent areas of intermediate signal intensity confined to the substance of a discoid meniscus may indicate extensive cavitation of that meniscus, which often is regarded as evidence of an intrameniscal tear at the time of arthroscopy (see later discussion).

Torn Menisci. Once the many variations of signal intensity that characterize the grossly intact meniscus are mastered, diagnosis of meniscal tears on MR images becomes straightforward. Most reports have indicated that the sensitivity, specificity, and accuracy of MR imaging in the detection of meniscal tears is close to or even greater than 85 to 90 per cent.[80, 82, 91, 423–425, 1121] Much lower values for the sensitivity, specificity, and accuracy of MR imaging in such detection have been reported, however, which may reflect variations in sample size[426] or observer bias.[1122] Other factors that potentially may explain discrepancies in reported results of MR imaging of the menisci include differences in study populations, technical variations, and observer performance. Furthermore, there is no true standard by which

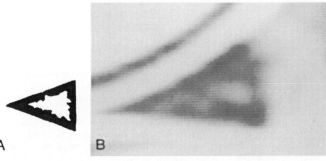

Figure 16–98
Intrameniscal signal intensity: Diagnostic difficulty. The presence of extensive regions of intermediate signal intensity within a meniscus that do not extend to the articular surface, as demonstrated diagrammatically (**A**) and in a sagittal proton density–weighted (TR/TE, 2000/20) spin echo MR image photographed with meniscal windowing (**B**), creates some diagnostic difficulty. A significant percentage of patients with such intrameniscal signal intensity are found to have a meniscal tear at the time of arthroscopic surgery.

to measure the accuracy of the MR imaging findings. Arthroscopy, which has been used as the standard in most reports dealing with noninvasive imaging studies of the knee, is not without limitations.[427] Not all segments of the posterior horns of the menisci can be visualized directly with arthroscopy; probing of the meniscus rather than direct visualization is used as an arthroscopic test for some tears of the inferior (tibial) surface of the meniscus, and the level of expertise varies among orthopedic surgeons performing arthroscopy (just as it varies among radiologists interpreting MR imaging examinations of the knee).

Assessment of certain parts of the menisci with MR imaging may be difficult.[428, 429] One such region is the free, or inner, edge of each meniscus, where small tears may be obscured by volume averaging artifacts, leading to a false-negative MR imaging examination. Similarly, meniscal tears may be overlooked during MR imaging in trouble spots such as the posterior horn of the lateral meniscus where normal structures obscure meniscal detail. Tears in this location are not uncommon in patients with associated injuries of the anterior cruciate ligament.[430] The chance of missing a large (and potentially unstable) meniscal tear in any location is unlikely if the MR images are interpreted by an experienced observer. False-positive results on MR images of the menisci often relate to some of the normal anatomic variations described earlier. Additional causes of false-positive results relate to distortion of meniscal contour or alterations in meniscal signal intensity occurring in association with severe meniscal degeneration or extensive calcification. Analysis of meniscal abnormalities also is made more difficult when gas is present in the joint or in the meniscus (Fig. 16–99).

The two MR imaging criteria for diagnosis of the meniscal tear are intrameniscal signal intensity that extends to a meniscal surface and abnormal meniscal morphology (Fig. 16–100).[431] The sagittal plane and T1-weighted and proton density–weighted spin echo MR images are more valuable in this diagnosis than the coronal and transaxial planes and T2-weighted spin echo MR images. Although some meniscal tears will fill with fluid and appear as regions of high signal intensity on T2-weighted spin echo images (Fig. 16–101), most do not.

Alterations in morphology of torn menisci take several forms. The inner portion of the meniscus may appear blunted on coronal or sagittal MR images. The meniscus may have a normal triangular shape but appear too small (Fig. 16–102). As an example of this, the width of the posterior horn of the medial meniscus normally is greater than the width of the anterior horn of the medial meniscus; when sagittal MR images display a posterior horn of the medial meniscus that is equal in size to or smaller than its anterior horn, a tear should be suspected even if the meniscal contour appears normal. Diagnosis of tears of the free edge of the meniscus often requires careful analysis of both the sagittal and coronal MR images so that subtle blunting or poor definition of the involved portion of the meniscus is recognized. An abrupt change of contour or focal deformity of the meniscus (Fig. 16–103), designated the notch sign,[411] is

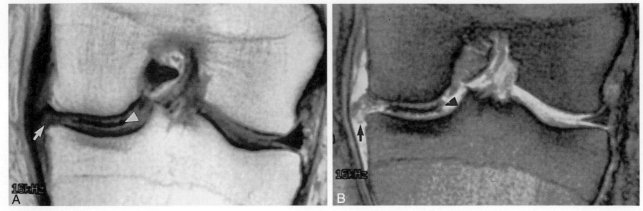

Figure 16–99
Meniscal tears: Associated vacuum phenomenon. On coronal T1-weighted (TR/TE, 600/18) spin echo **(A)** and MPGR (TR/TE, 549/12; flip angle, 30 degrees) **(B)** MR images, a torn and partially extruded medial meniscus (arrows) is associated with a meniscal cyst. Note the curvilinear region of signal void (arrowheads), more evident in **B,** indicative of gas within the joint. (Courtesy of S. Eilenberg, M.D., San Diego, California.)

an important indicator of a meniscal tear, but it can be simulated by the normal meniscal flounce (see previous discussion). The notch sign is a more definite indicator of meniscal tear when it is accompanied by abnormalities of intrameniscal signal intensity.

Radial tears of the menisci may be difficult to recognize.[431, 432] Such tears are oriented perpendicular to the long circumferential axis of the meniscus, may be full thickness (extending from the apex to the peripheral portion of the meniscus) or partial thickness, and may be straight (true radial tear) or obliquely oriented (parrot beak or flap tear).[432] The MR imaging findings vary according to the specific type of tear that is present, but such findings include complete absence of visualization of the meniscus on at least one image and blunting of the apex of the meniscus. Especially

difficult is the diagnosis of a full thickness radial tear that occurs at or adjacent to the tibial attachments of the meniscus. Subtle subluxation of the meniscus results. As one example, in the normal situation it is extremely unusual for no meniscal shadow to be seen on a sagittal image 3 mm thick medial to the tibial attachment of the posterior cruciate ligament; when no such meniscal shadow is seen, a radial tear at the tibial attachment site with meniscal subluxation should be considered.[432]

Bucket-handle tears of the meniscus are associated with characteristic MR imaging abnormalities (Figs. 16–104 and 16–105).[433] This term is derived from the appearance of the tear, in which the inner displaced meniscal fragment resembles a handle and the peripheral nondisplaced portion of the meniscus has the appearance of a bucket.[434] Bucket-handle tears usually are

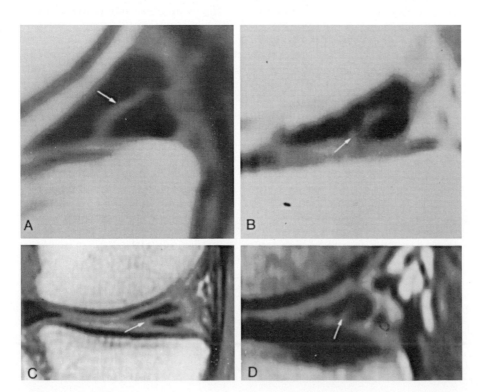

Figure 16–100
Meniscal tears: Abnormalities of intrameniscal signal intensity and meniscal morphology. Sagittal proton density–weighted (TR/TE, 2000/20) spin echo MR images.

A Posterior horn of the medial meniscus. A grade 3 pattern of intrameniscal signal intensity (arrow) is evident.

B Posterior horn of the medial meniscus. A grade 3 pattern of intrameniscal signal intensity (arrow) and irregularity of the inferior meniscal surface are seen.

C Posterior horn of the medial meniscus. A grade 3 pattern of intrameniscal signal intensity (arrow) and altered meniscal morphology are evident.

D Posterior horn of the lateral meniscus. A grade 3 pattern of intrameniscal signal intensity (arrow) and an irregular inferior and inner meniscal surface are seen.

Figure 16–101

Meniscal tears: Abnormalities of intrameniscal signal intensity and meniscal morphology. Sagittal proton density–weighted (TR/TE, 2200/20) spin echo MR images **(A, C)** and sagittal T2-weighted (TR/TE, 2200/60) spin echo MR images **(B, D)**.

A, B Posterior horn of the medial meniscus. Note the grade 3 pattern of intrameniscal signal intensity (arrows), which increases further in signal intensity in **B**. The superior portion of the meniscus is irregular.

C, D Posterior horn of the medial meniscus. Note the grade 3 pattern of intrameniscal signal intensity (arrows), which reveals a further increase in signal intensity in **D**.

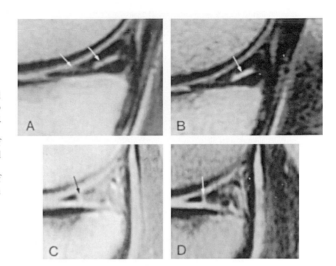

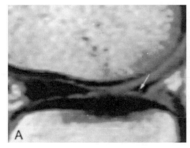
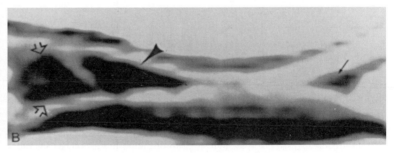

Figure 16–102

Meniscal tears: Abnormalities of meniscal morphology. Posterior horn of the lateral meniscus. Sagittal proton density–weighted (TR/TE, 1000/20) spin echo MR images obtained without **(A)** and with **(B)** meniscal windowing show an abnormally small posterior horn of the lateral meniscus (solid arrows). A bucket-handle tear of the posterior portion of the lateral meniscus is present, with a more central fragment displaced anteriorly (open arrows), lying in front of the anterior horn of the lateral meniscus (arrowhead). (Courtesy of A. Nemcek, M.D., Chicago, Illinois.)

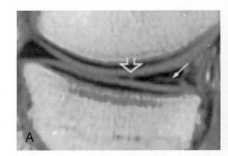
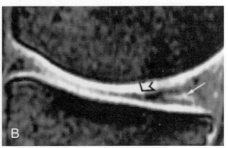

Figure 16–103

Meniscal tears: Abnormalities of intrameniscal signal intensity and meniscal morphology. Posterior horn of the medial meniscus. A sagittal proton density–weighted (TR/TE, 2200/20) spin echo MR image **(A)** and a sagittal 3DFT SPGR MR image (TR/TE, 58/10; flip angle, 60 degrees) obtained with chemical presaturation of fat (ChemSat) **(B)** show altered intrameniscal signal intensity (solid arrows) with a further increase in signal intensity in **B** and an irregular notch (open arrows) in the superior surface of the meniscus.

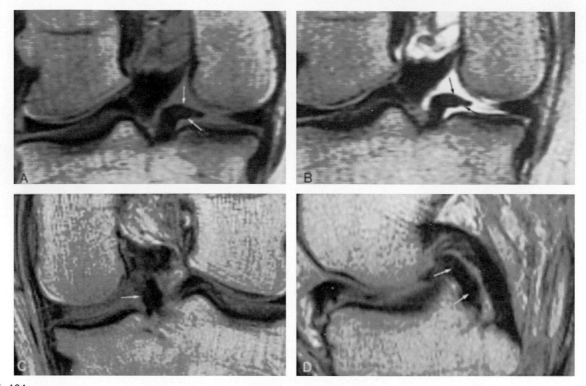

Figure 16–104

Meniscal tears: Bucket-handle tears.

A, B Medial meniscus. Coronal proton density–weighted (TR/TE, 2500/20) **(A)** and T2-weighted (TR/TE, 2500/60) **(B)** spin echo MR images reveal a bucket-handle tear of the medial meniscus with central displacement (arrows) of the inner portion of the meniscus.

C, D Medial meniscus. Coronal proton density–weighted (TR/TE, 1750/20) **(C)** and sagittal proton density–weighted (TR/TE, 3000/20) **(D)** spin echo MR images reveal a bucket-handle tear of the medial meniscus with central displacement (arrows) of the inner portion of the meniscus. In **D,** the meniscal fragment is located in front of the posterior cruciate ligament.

(Courtesy of R. Stiles, M.D., Atlanta, Georgia.)

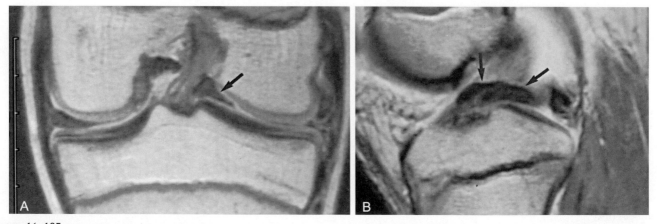

Figure 16–105

Meniscal tears: Bucket-handle tears. Coronal T1-weighted (TR/TE, 800/20) **(A)** and sagittal proton density–weighted (TR/TE, 4000/26) **(B)** spin echo MR images show a bucket-handle tear of the lateral meniscus with central displacement of the inner meniscal fragment (arrows). The appearance in **B** simulates that of a tear of the anterior cruciate ligament. (Courtesy of D. Levey, M.D., Corpus Christi, Texas.)

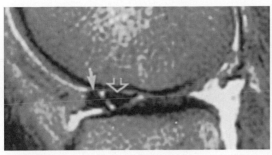

Figure 16–106
Meniscal tears: Flipped meniscus sign—lateral meniscus. A sagittal T2-weighted (TR/TE, 2000/70) spin echo MR image reveals that the posterior horn of the lateral meniscus is not visualized posteriorly but rather is seen anteriorly (solid arrow), located in front of the anterior horn of the lateral meniscus (open arrow). (Courtesy of J. Kirkham, M.D., Minneapolis, Minnesota.)

observed in young adults and in the medial meniscus, and they may be associated with a history of locking of the knee joint. MR imaging findings include a foreshortened and blunted meniscus with central displacement of its inner fragment.[434, 435] As the peripheral nondisplaced component of the meniscus also may appear relatively normal, recognition of the displaced inner portion of the meniscus is important.[434] In cases of bucket-handle tears of the medial meniscus, the displaced fragment typically appears as a band of low signal intensity extending across the joint and projecting over the medial tibial eminence.[434] On sagittal MR images, the displaced fragment often lies in front of, below, and parallel to the posterior cruciate ligament. The resulting appearance, sometimes designated the double posterior cruciate ligament sign,[433] may simulate that of the normal meniscofemoral ligament of Humphrey or a tear of the anterior cruciate ligament.

Bucket-handle tears involving the lateral meniscus (and, perhaps, a few involving the medial meniscus) may have a different appearance on MR images. This appearance, designated the flipped meniscus sign,[436] relates to displacement of a posteriorly located fragment of the meniscus that is still attached to the central portion of the meniscus (Fig. 16–106). The fragment may flip, or invert, and become located on top of the anterior horn of the involved meniscus. On sagittal images, the flipped meniscal fragment may be located anterior to the anterior horn of the meniscus with a cleavage plane between the two.[437] In such cases, a tear or nonvisualization of the posterior horn of the meniscus and an increase in height of the anterior meniscal contour are helpful diagnostic clues.[436] The predilection for the lateral meniscus may relate to its greater mobility.

Wright and colleagues[433] evaluated the sensitivity of MR imaging in the detection of displaced meniscal fragments using three diagnostic signs: double posterior cruciate ligament sign, the flipped meniscus sign, and a fragment in the intercondylar notch. The double posterior cruciate ligament sign was present in 53 per cent of medial and none of the lateral bucket-handle tears; the flipped meniscus sign was noted in 44 per cent of the medial and 29 per cent of the lateral bucket-handle

tears; and an intercondylar meniscal fragment was present in 66 per cent of the medial and 43 per cent of the lateral bucket-handle tears. Overall, MR imaging proved to be more sensitive in detecting fragments in large rather than small bucket-handle meniscal tears.

Meniscocapsular Separation

Meniscocapsular separation refers to disruption of the meniscal attachment to the joint capsule. The posterior horn of the medial meniscus is involved most frequently, perhaps related to its solid adherence to the capsule. Once separated, the mobility of the medial meniscus is increased, and subsequent tears of this structure probably are uncommon. Surgical repair of meniscocapsular separations is a therapeutic option,[438] underscoring the importance of correct diagnosis.

The principles related to the diagnosis of meniscocapsular separation are the same whether the lesion is detected arthrographically or with MR imaging. The presence of fluid between the peripheral portion of the posterior horn of the medial meniscus and the joint capsule is the most important finding on either type of examination. With arthrography, the fluid represents a portion of the injected contrast material; with MR imaging, the fluid is derived from a portion of a joint effusion, and it is observed best in sagittal T2-weighted spin echo images or gradient echo images (in the steady state) employing small to moderate flip angles. The fluid may collect in the entire interface between the meniscus and capsule or in a portion of this interface, particularly its inferior portion (Fig. 16–107). Uncovering of the tibial articular cartilage, owing to central displacement of the medial meniscus, does not appear to be a reliable sign of meniscocapsular separation. The role of MR imaging using intra-articular or intravenous administration of gadolinium compounds in establishing this diagnosis is not clear. At present, arthrography appears to be equally sensitive to or more sensitive than MR imaging in establishing a diagnosis of a meniscocapsular separation, although prominent perimeniscal recesses can have a similar appearance. Another type of lesion occurring at the periphery of the medial meniscus, disruption of the meniscotibial (coronary) ligament

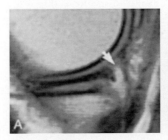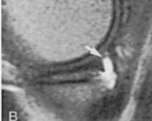

Figure 16–107
Meniscocapsular separation: MR imaging. Medial meniscus. Sagittal proton density–weighted (TR/TE, 2000/30) (**A**) and T2-weighted (TR/TE, 2000/80) (**B**) spin echo MR images reveal fluid (arrows) between the posterior portion of the medial meniscus and the joint capsule. Diagnostic difficulty arises, however, as a similar appearance can be seen with a meniscal cyst or fluid in a bursa that is intimate with the posterior oblique fibers of the medial collateral ligament.

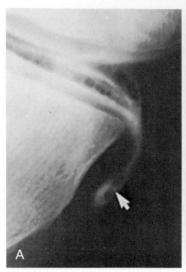
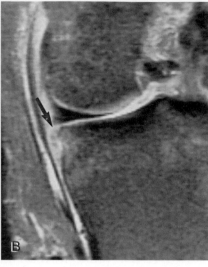

Figure 16–108

Meniscotibial (coronary) ligament tear: Arthrography and MR imaging.

A Arthrography. Observe elevation of the medial meniscus with an abnormal collection of contrast material extending inferiorly (arrow).

B MR imaging. A coronal fat-suppressed fast spin echo MR image (TR/TE, 4000/16) in a second patient reveals disruption of the meniscotibial ligament (arrow) with marrow and periligamentous edema.

(Courtesy of C. Chen, M.D., Taipei, Taiwan.)

that normally connects the meniscus to the tibia, also can be established with MR imaging or arthrography (Figs. 16–108 and 16–109).[439]

The differential diagnosis of a meniscocapsular separation includes normal recesses that may appear above or below the peripheral portion of the meniscus, a large joint effusion displacing the meniscus, a longitudinal vertical tear through the periphery of the meniscus, and bursitis beneath the tibial collateral ligament (Fig. 16–110).[409, 1120]

Meniscal Cysts

Meniscal cysts are multiloculated collections of mucinous material of unknown cause that occur at the periphery of the meniscus and, therefore, appear as a focal mass or swelling at the joint line. These cysts may occur in parameniscal soft tissue (parameniscal cysts) or within the substance of the meniscus (intrameniscal cysts).[440] They also are referred to as ganglion cysts or juxta-articular myxomas. They appear to be uncommon lesions, observed in approximately 1 per cent of menis-

cectomies.[441] Although reports have indicated that meniscal cysts on the lateral side of the knee are three to seven times more frequent than those on the medial side,[442–449] meniscal cysts on the medial side are being reported frequently,[450, 451] particularly on MR imaging examinations.[290] Medial meniscal cysts tend to be larger than those on the lateral side,[443] and they are more often asymptomatic.[452] The most common location of meniscal cysts is adjacent to the middle third of the lateral meniscus.[453] Meniscal cysts usually occur in young adult men with an average age of 30 years, but they have been reported in patients as young as 5 years and as old as 80 years.[443]

The precise cause of meniscal cysts is not clear. They have been reported in association with other disorders, such as calcium pyrophosphate dihydrate crystal deposition disease and rheumatoid arthritis.[453] Most observers believe that these cysts are traumatic, although degenerative or congenital factors also may be important. Many, if not most, meniscal cysts are associated with myxoid degeneration and horizontal cleavage tears of the adjacent meniscus that extend into the parameniscal

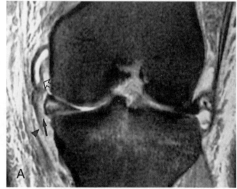
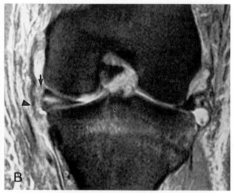

Figure 16–109

Meniscocapsular separation and meniscotibial (coronary), meniscofemoral, and medial collateral ligament tear: MR imaging. Coronal fat-suppressed fast spin echo (TR/TE, 3950/18) MR images, with **A** slightly anterior to **B**, show a medial meniscal tear, meniscocapsular separation (solid arrows), meniscofemoral (open arrow) and meniscotibial ligament tears, and disruption of the medial collateral ligament (arrowheads), findings that were confirmed during arthroscopy. The anterior cruciate ligament was also torn, evident in the MR images by its absence. Soft tissue edema is seen.

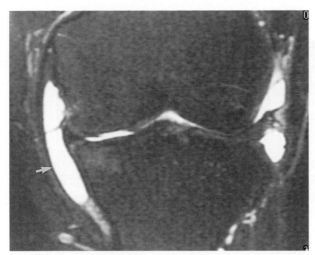

Figure 16–110

Medial collateral ligament bursitis: MR imaging. Observe fluid (arrow) between the superficial and deep portions of the medial collateral ligament in a coronal fat-suppressed fast spin echo (TR/TE, 4000/102) MR image. The appearance should not be mistaken for a meniscocapsular separation or a meniscal cyst.

region.[443–445, 452, 454] Fluid from the joint extending into a horizontal tear of the meniscus and subsequently into the cystic lesion is one explanation for their occurrence. Pathologically, cysts are septated lesions containing clear, bloody, or gelatinous fluid that has a high protein content and histochemically is similar if not identical to synovial fluid.[443, 453] Some cysts at the periphery of the meniscus are not accompanied by meniscal tears, however, and their pathogenesis may relate to a compression injury to the meniscal periphery with degenerative changes that extend into the soft tissue rather than centrally, leaving an apparently undamaged meniscus.[1123, 1124]

In addition to swelling at the joint line, patients with meniscal cysts may experience pain and limitation of motion, perhaps related to the presence of an underlying meniscal tear. Irritation of the common peroneal nerve in cases of lateral meniscal cysts may be noted.[443, 455] On physical examination, a soft tissue mass is palpable. Meniscal cysts on the lateral side of the knee often are smaller, and they may be located anterior or posterior to the fibular collateral ligament. Such cysts may be palpated posteriorly adjacent to the tendons of the popliteus muscle and the biceps femoris muscle or anteriorly near the iliotibial band.[443] On the medial side of the knee, meniscal cysts may dissect through the joint capsule and even the medial collateral ligament and, in such cases, may enlarge, appear mobile, and dissect into the soft tissues for considerable distances.[443]

Although the diagnosis of a meniscal cyst often is made clinically, imaging studies may be used to evaluate the lesion further. On routine radiography, gas formation or erosion of bone, in addition to a mass, may be observed.[456–458] Calcified bodies in the cyst also may be noted.[459] CT typically reveals a well-defined mass containing fluid that often communicates with the adjacent meniscus.[460] Ultrasonography confirms the cystic nature of the lesion and, in some cases, cystic degeneration of

the adjacent meniscus.[461] Standard arthrography may reveal contrast material extending from the joint into a horizontal tear of the meniscus and, from there, pooling in a cystic mass at the periphery of the torn meniscus. Such communication may be more apparent on delayed radiographs after arthrography.[462] Meniscal cysts also may lead to distortion of the adjacent meniscus on arthrographic examination.[463] On MR images, an ovoid mass of variable size containing fluid is seen (Figs. 16–111, 16–112, 16–113, and 16–114).[290, 440, 443] Although high signal intensity of the cyst on T2-weighted spin echo MR images is typical, it is not invariable.[440] The cyst may extend either anteriorly or posteriorly, and an associated meniscal tear may be evident. Meniscal cysts also may be diagnosed and treated arthroscopically.[443–445, 451] Treatment strategies generally include cyst decompression and partial meniscectomy (in cases of associated meniscal tear), although cyst extirpation and peripheral meniscal repair also have been employed (in cases in which a meniscal tear has not been apparent).[1123]

Discoid Menisci

A discoid meniscus has an altered shape. It is broad and disclike rather than semilunar, although intermediate varieties of discoid menisci have been described (Fig. 16–115).[464] These include slab (flat, circular meniscus), biconcave (biconcave disc, thinner in its central portion), wedge (large but normally tapered meniscus), anterior (enlarged anterior horn), forme fruste (slightly enlarged meniscus), and grossly torn (too deformed for accurate classification) types. A discoid lateral meniscus[465–471] is much more common than a discoid medial meniscus.[472–481]

The reported frequency of discoid lateral menisci varies from 0 to 2.7 per cent,[464, 482] although occasionally a higher frequency, determined by arthrography in children[483] or by direct inspection during meniscectomy,[466, 469, 484] is cited. The usual age of patients at the time of clinical presentation is between 15 and 35 years, and men are affected more frequently. These patients commonly have symptoms of a torn cartilage. Bilateral discoid menisci[485, 1125] and a familial occurrence of an abnormal meniscal shape[486] also have been noted.

Three basic theories have been set forth to explain the occurrence of a discoid lateral meniscus: embryologic, developmental, and congenital. An embryologic explanation for discoid menisci remains theoretical. During development, undifferentiated mesenchymal tissue exists between the cartilaginous precursors of bone.[487] This tissue subsequently cavitates, producing an articular cavity. In some joints, a portion of the mesenchyme exists as fibrocartilaginous discs or menisci. In knee development, under normal circumstances, undifferentiated mesenchyme evolves into fetal cartilage, which by the 10th week is semilunar in shape, closely resembling the adult meniscus. This normal sequence of embryologic development, therefore, does not contain a stage in which either the medial or the lateral meniscus is of discoid shape; the appearance of such a meniscus in a child or adult cannot occur

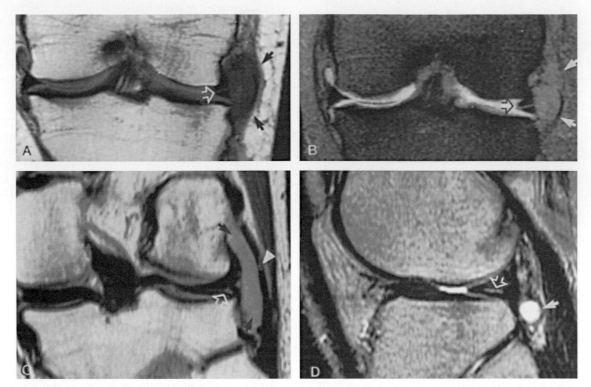

Figure 16–111

Meniscal cysts: MR imaging—lateral meniscus.

A, B A coronal T1-weighted (TR/TE, 800/12) spin echo MR image **(A)** and a coronal T1-weighted (TR/TE, 750/20) spin echo MR image obtained with chemical presaturation of fat (ChemSat) **(B)** show a mass (solid arrows) adjacent to the midportion of the lateral meniscus. Note a grade 3 pattern of signal intensity (open arrows) in the meniscus, consistent with a horizontally oriented meniscal tear.

C, D In a second patient, a coronal proton density–weighted (TR/TE, 2200/20) spin echo MR image **(C)** and a sagittal T2-weighted (TR/TE, 2200/80) spin echo MR image **(D)** show a meniscal cyst (solid arrows) associated with a horizontal tear of the lateral meniscus (open arrows). Note that the cyst displaces the lateral (fibular) collateral ligament (arrowhead).

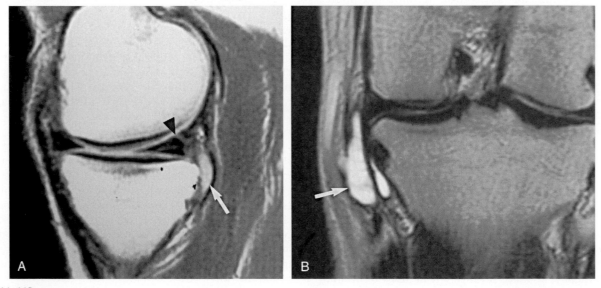

Figure 16–112

Meniscal cysts: MR imaging—medical meniscus. A large meniscal cyst (arrows) associated with a tear (arrowhead) of the posterior horn of the medial meniscus is well shown on a sagittal proton density–weighted (TR/TE, 2000/32) spin echo **(A)** and a coronal fast spin echo (TR/TE, 3300/100) **(B)** MR image. Observe the intimate relationship of the cyst and superficial portion of the medial collateral ligament in **B**. (Courtesy of D. Goodwin, M.D., Hanover, New Hampshire.)

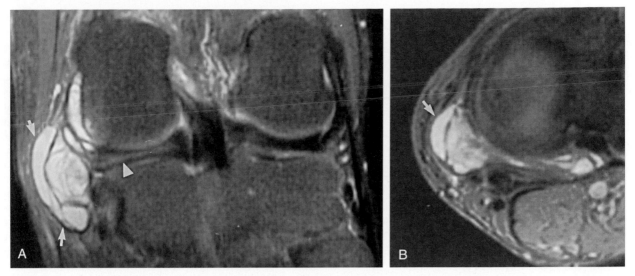

Figure 16–113

Meniscal cysts: MR imaging—medial meniscus. A large septated meniscal cyst (arrows) is shown in a coronal fat-suppressed fast spin echo (TR/TE, 4700/18) MR image **(A)** and in a transaxial MPGR (TR/TE, 650/14; flip angle, 15 degrees) MR image **(B).** The accompanying meniscal tear (arrowhead) was better seen in other images. (Courtesy of D. Goodwin, M.D., Hanover, New Hampshire.)

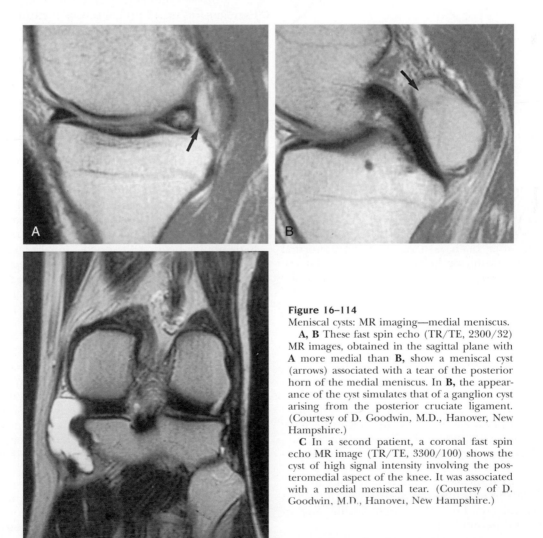

Figure 16–114

Meniscal cysts: MR imaging—medial meniscus.

A, B These fast spin echo (TR/TE, 2300/32) MR images, obtained in the sagittal plane with **A** more medial than **B,** show a meniscal cyst (arrows) associated with a tear of the posterior horn of the medial meniscus. In **B,** the appearance of the cyst simulates that of a ganglion cyst arising from the posterior cruciate ligament. (Courtesy of D. Goodwin, M.D., Hanover, New Hampshire.)

C In a second patient, a coronal fast spin echo MR image (TR/TE, 3300/100) shows the cyst of high signal intensity involving the posteromedial aspect of the knee. It was associated with a medial meniscal tear. (Courtesy of D. Goodwin, M.D., Hanover, New Hampshire.)

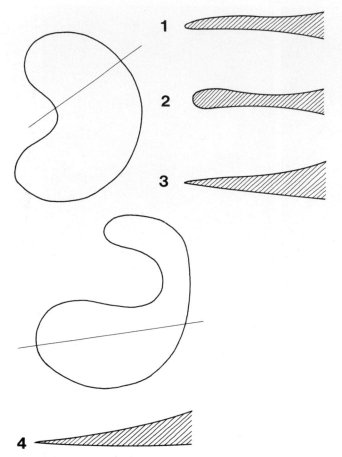

Figure 16–115
Discoid menisci: Classification system. Types of discoid menisci include the slab type (1), biconcave type (2), wedge type (3), and anterior type (4).

through persistence of a fetal stage. Of interest, however, is the demonstration of discoid menisci as normal findings in various vertebrates.

Kaplan[467] has postulated that the discoid lateral meniscus is acquired after birth as a result of an abnormal attachment of its posterior horn to the tibial plateau. He suggested that a primary abnormality of the inferior strut or fascicle will leave a lateral meniscus attached posteriorly only by the meniscofemoral ligament (ligament of Wrisberg) and eventually will produce a discoid meniscus because of repetitive abnormal mediolateral and anteroposterior movement of the meniscus, with subsequent enlargement and thickening of meniscal tissue. Other investigators have noted that this strut frequently is poorly visualized or definitely abnormal in many patients with discoid lateral menisci, observations that lend support to Kaplan's theory. Investigations have documented that a complete type of discoid lateral meniscus with intact ligamentous attachments, which generally is asymptomatic, also exists.

The third theory indicates the importance of congenital factors and is supported by the occurrence of discoid menisci in several members of a single family, and in twins, fetuses, and neonates.[488]

No single classification system exists for discoid menisci. Some systems divide these menisci into complete and incomplete forms (referring to the degree of meniscal interposition between the tibial plateau and femoral condyle in the presence of intact meniscal attachments) and the Wrisberg ligament type, in which the posterior attachment site of the lateral meniscus is altered. Evidence suggests that incomplete and complete discoid menisci are symptomatic only when torn and that the Wrisberg ligament type is associated with a snapping knee.[471] Many authors believe that a discoid lateral meniscus with normal posterior attachments does not require surgical treatment unless it is torn.[471, 488] Some authorities believe that all discoid menisci undergo cystic mucoid degeneration,[489] although this is not accepted uniformly.[488] The Wrisberg ligament type discoid meniscus is believed to be associated with meniscal hypermobility, although the precise movement of such a meniscus during flexion and extension of the knee is not agreed on. Furthermore, some authors view the hypermobile meniscus as one in which a posterior capsular tear has occurred and not one related to a developmental alteration in the capsular attachment of the lateral meniscus.[488] Although reports of long-term follow-up examinations of the knee in children who have had a discoid meniscus excised have indicated good to excellent results,[490] no consensus regarding the optimal method of treatment of this condition exists.

Discoid menisci may be discovered incidentally or associated with clinical manifestations that include pain and a snapping knee. Torn discoid menisci lead to pain, swelling, and locking of the knee, findings in common with all meniscal tears. The classic clinical finding, the snapping knee, may be absent in cases in which the discoid meniscus possesses normal capsular attachments. Accurate diagnosis depends on the results of arthroscopic examination, arthrography, or MR imaging.

Initial plain films in patients with discoid menisci generally are unrewarding, although widening of the articular space in the ipsilateral compartment of the knee documented by weight-bearing radiography, a high fibular head, a "cupped" tibial plateau,[491] and an abnormally shaped lateral malleolus have been observed in patients with discoid lateral menisci. A discoid medial meniscus may be associated with irregularity of the medial margin of the proximal tibial epiphysis.[492] An association of discoid lateral menisci and osteochondritis dissecans of the lateral femoral condyle also has been noted.[493] Arthrography reveals the abnormally large and elongated meniscus, frequently extending to the intercondylar notch. The margins of the body of the meniscus are relatively parallel rather than converging. An associated meniscal tear frequently is observed.[494]

MR imaging has been used to confirm the existence of either an intact or a torn discoid meniscus.[431, 495–499] This can be accomplished by analysis of both sagittal and coronal MR images (Fig. 16–116). Observations based on sagittal images relate to the number of consecutive scans that reveal a bow-tie appearance of the meniscus, in which the anterior and posterior horns of the meniscus still are connected or continuous. This number is directly related to the width of the meniscus; an enlarged meniscus is compatible with the diagnosis of a

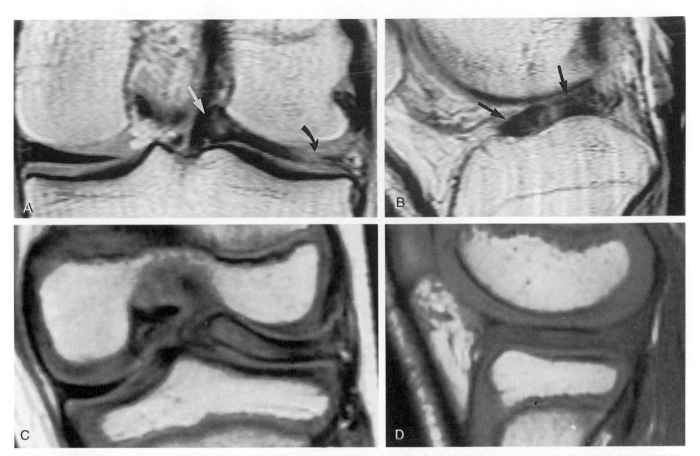

Figure 16–116

Discoid menisci: MR imaging.

A, B Lateral meniscus. Coronal (**A**) and sagittal (**B**) proton density–weighted (TR/TE, 2700/20) spin echo MR images show a discoid lateral meniscus extending into the central aspect of the joint (straight arrows), containing a tear (curved arrow).

C, D Lateral meniscus. Coronal proton density–weighted (TR/TE, 3300/15) (**C**) and sagittal T1-weighted (TR/TE, 630/15) (**D**) spin echo MR images reveal a lateral discoid meniscus with extensive intrameniscal cavitation (i.e., tear) manifested as a region of intermediate signal intensity.

(Courtesy of J. Kramer, M.D., Vienna, Austria.)

Illustration continued on following page

discoid meniscus, although no precise dimensions are available for normal menisci. The average transverse diameter of the lateral meniscus appears to be approximately 11 or 12 mm; the visualization of a bow-tie appearance on three or more contiguous sagittal sections that are 5 mm thick, an abnormally thickened bow-tie, or the presence of both of these findings is evidence of a discoid lateral meniscus.[496] Similarly, the presence of two adjacent peripheral 5 mm thick sagittal sections demonstrating equal or nearly equal meniscal height is suggestive of this diagnosis.[496] Similar diagnostic rules apply to the analysis of the sagittal MR images in cases of discoid medial meniscus. In the coronal plane, the abnormal shape of the meniscus, involving the entire meniscus or a portion of it, is identified more readily. Importantly, however, the normal central attachments of the menisci produce a pseudodiscoid appearance on the most anterior and posterior coronal images.

The MR imaging criteria for diagnosing a tear of a discoid meniscus are similar (but not identical) to those used to diagnose a tear in a nondiscoid meniscus. The presence of extensive intermediate signal intensity within a discoid meniscus, however, should be interpre-

ted cautiously. Such a finding in a nondiscoid meniscus usually is considered evidence of mucinous or myxoid change without a tear, unless the region of altered signal intensity extends to the surface of the meniscus. In a discoid meniscus, cavitation or intrasubstance tears may present as areas of intermediate signal intensity that do not violate the meniscal surface (see Fig. 16–116). The likelihood of such intrasubstance tears, which may not be identified during arthroscopy, increases if extensive intrameniscal signal intensity is associated with flattening of the meniscus.[498]

MR imaging allows analysis of the capsular attachments of the posterior horn of the lateral meniscus. As alterations in the morphology of the meniscofemoral ligament of Wrisberg and similar alterations or absence of other capsular structures, such as the posterior coronary ligament,[500] may be responsible for discoid menisci or altered movement of the lateral meniscus, analysis of these structures should be accomplished on MR images. One case of a discoid lateral meniscus associated with an abnormally short and thick ligament of Wrisberg has been described in which the MR images allowed a correct diagnosis.[345]

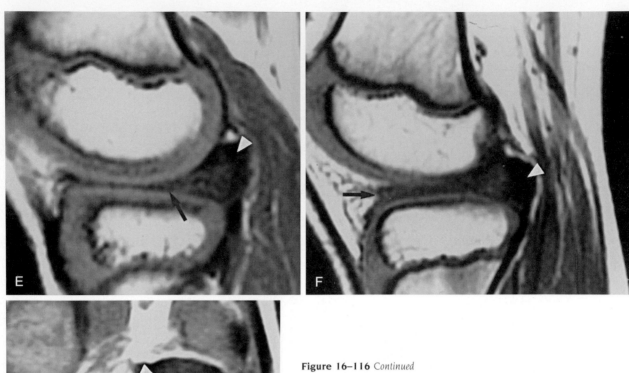

Figure 16–116 *Continued*
E–G Lateral meniscus. Sagittal **(E, F)** and coronal **(G)** T1-weighted (TR/TE, 600/14) spin echo MR images show a discoid lateral meniscus (arrows) with cyst-like enlargement of the posterior horn (arrowheads). (Courtesy of S. Fernandez, M.D., Mexico City, Mexico.)

Discoid menisci are but one of a variety of anomalies that lead to alterations in meniscal shape, size, or attachment sites. In general, such variations are more common on the lateral side of the knee. They include aplasia or hypoplasia of an entire meniscus or a portion of it (sometimes in association with hypoplasia of the cruciate ligaments), meniscal attachment sites to the femoral condyles or cruciate ligaments, absent fixation of the transverse ligament to the tibial plateau, and ring-shaped menisci.[1126–1128]

Meniscal Ossicles

Meniscal ossicles represent foci of ossification within the menisci. They rarely are observed in the human knee,[501–506] although they are a normal finding in the knees of certain rodents[507] and of several types of small and large animals.[508] Ossicles represent hyaline cartilage enclosing lamellar and cancellous bone and marrow. They should be differentiated from meniscal calcifications, which are frequent and relate to calcium pyrophosphate dihydrate crystal deposition in many cases.[509] The origin of meniscal ossicles in humans is controversial; some investigators believe they are vestigial structures,[503, 507] whereas others suggest they are acquired after trauma.[501, 506, 510] Reports have indicated an association of meniscal ossicles with longitudinal tears of the medial meniscus in which the origin of the ossicles appeared to be an avulsion at the tibial site of attachment of the posterior horn of the medial meniscus.[511, 512] Thinning of adjacent articular cartilage also may be seen.[513] Patients with knee ossicles may be asymptomatic or have local pain and swelling.[514]

Initial films reveal ossification of variable shape in the anterior or posterior portion of either the medial or the lateral meniscus (Fig. 16–117). The most common site is the posterior horn of the medial meniscus. Thus, the radiodense region generally is located centrally within the articular space. Arthrography confirms the location of the ossification within the meniscus.[505] The meniscus itself may be normal, contain associated tears,[501–503, 511] or be discoid in type.[512]

MR imaging also may be used to diagnose or confirm the existence of a meniscal ossicle (Figs. 16–118, 16–119, and 16–120).[513, 515, 516] As the ossicle may contain bone marrow, the signal intensity characteristics of fat may be seen within the ossicle.[517] The ossicle likewise may reveal low signal intensity on all MR imaging sequences. MR

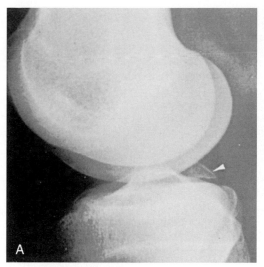
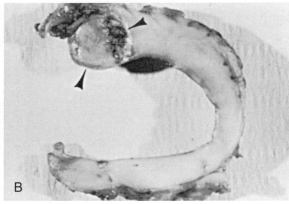

Figure 16–117
Meniscal ossicles: Routine radiography. This 20 year old man injured his knee playing basketball and, during the next year, noted pain, clicking, and popping.
 A The lateral radiograph reveals a bone fragment (arrowhead) in the distribution of the posterior horn of the medial meniscus.
 B In a different patient, an ossicle (arrowheads) in the posterior horn of the medial meniscus is evident. (Courtesy of G. Greenway, M.D., Dallas, Texas.)

imaging allows precise localization of the ossicle to the meniscus and provides evidence of any associated meniscal tear.

Meniscal ossicles must be differentiated from other causes of articular radiodense shadows, particularly intra-articular osteochondral fragments. These latter fragments are not centrally located, may move in location from one examination to another, or may appear in the joint recesses. If a meniscal ossicle produces considerable symptoms, requiring meniscectomy, radiography of the removed meniscus will document the intrameniscal location of the ossification.

Postoperative Menisci

Significant changes in the surgical management of meniscal abnormalities in the knee are the consequence of two major factors: (1) the increasing awareness that the menisci have weight-bearing capacity and transmit an important component of the load during daily physical activities,[518, 519] and (2) the current popularity of arthroscopic surgery. Meniscectomy is no longer considered a harmless operation, because of the documentation of progressive damage of the articular cartilage after removal of the meniscus,[520–524] although similar

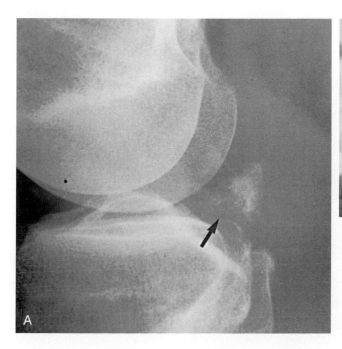
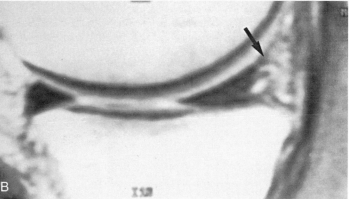

Figure 16–118
Meniscal ossicles: MR imaging. In a 50 year old man, a routine radiograph (**A**) and a sagittal proton density–weighted (TR/TE, 4100/23) spin echo MR image (**B**), photographed with meniscal windowing, reveal the ossicle (arrows) in the posterior horn of the medial meniscus. Note the high signal intensity in the ossicle in **B**, indicative of fatty marrow. (Courtesy of D. Artenian, M.D., Fresno, California.)

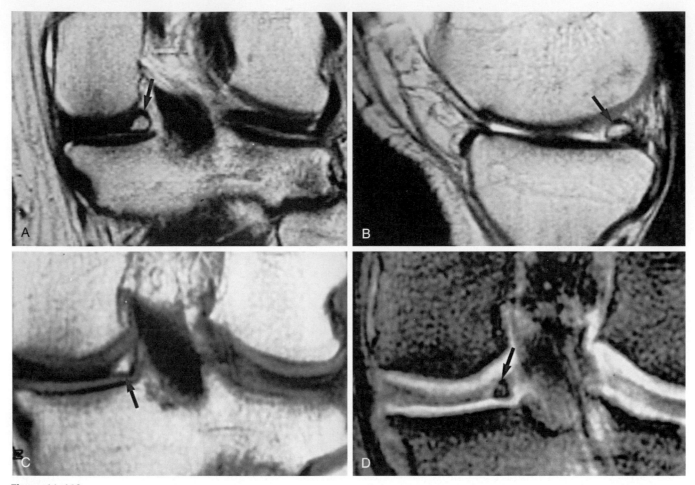

Figure 16–119
Meniscal ossicles: MR imaging.

A, B A meniscal ossicle containing fatty marrow (arrows) is present in a torn posterior horn of the medial meniscus, as shown on coronal T2-weighted (TR/TE, 4000/85) **(A)** and sagittal proton density–weighted (TR/TE, 4000/17) **(B)** spin echo MR images. (Courtesy of A. Newberg, M.D., Boston, Massachusetts.)

C, D In a second patient, a meniscal ossicle containing fatty marrow (arrows) is present in the posterior horn of the medial meniscus (which was torn), as shown on coronal T1-weighted (TR/TE, 600/18) spin echo **(C)** and MPGR (TR/TE, 549/12; flip angle, 30 degrees) **(D)** MR images. (Courtesy of S. Eilenberg, M.D., San Diego, California.)

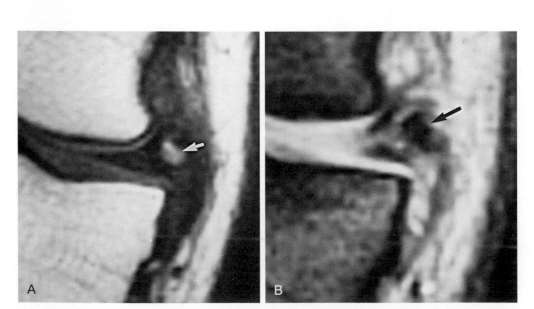

Figure 16–120
Meniscal ossicles: MR imaging. In a 47 year old man, a meniscal ossicle containing fatty marrow (arrows) is present in a torn lateral meniscus, as shown on coronal T1-weighted (TR/TE, 300/20) spin echo **(A)** and MPGR (TR/TE, 380/20; flip angle, 30 degrees) **(B)** MR images. (Courtesy of P. Kindynis, M.D., Geneva, Switzerland.)

degenerative changes are encountered when a severely torn meniscus is left in place,[525] and osteoarthritis also may develop after open or arthroscopic partial meniscectomies.[526] The advocacy of partial rather than total meniscectomy appeared to represent a philosophy midway between one that recommended complete removal of all damaged menisci and one that suggested a conservative approach to all meniscal injuries. Although partial and even total meniscectomies still are performed, the development and refinement of arthroscopic techniques have led to the choice of meniscal repair or meniscal reconstruction (i.e., meniscal transplantation) rather than meniscal resection as a better means to maintain meniscal function and, ultimately, to preserve the integrity of the knee joint. To understand the philosophy behind this choice, the interested reader needs to review the details of meniscal healing, regeneration, and remodeling. These are well summarized by Arnoczky,[340] some of whose observations are repeated here.

Meniscal Healing, Regeneration, and Remodeling. The peripheral portion of the meniscus possesses a vascular zone that supports a reparative response to injury similar to that observed in other connective tissues.[527] Inflammatory cell infiltration within a fibrin clot follows an injury to the peripheral portion of the meniscus. Subsequently, fibrovascular scar tissue appears in the injured region, becoming continuous with the adjacent normal meniscal fibrocartilage.[340] In experimental situations, peripheral meniscal tears that also involve the adjacent synovial tissue heal through the development of this scar tissue within 10 weeks of the injury.[527] This tissue may be weaker than the normal meniscus, however. Conversion of the scar tissue to normal-appearing fibrocartilage may require months, a fact that explains persistent alterations in intrameniscal signal intensity that are seen when MR imaging is employed to study the process of spontaneous healing of meniscal tears.[528] These results support the current rationale regarding surgical repair of peripheral meniscal injuries.[340, 529, 530] The success of these repairs relates to the vascular nature of the meniscus on either side or both sides of the tear. Tears involving the central, avascular portion of the meniscus are incapable of repair unless modifications of surgical technique, such as vascular access channels, synovial pedicle flaps, and synovial abrasion, are employed.[340, 527, 531] In general, tears known to be definitely capable of repair are traumatic, are within the vascular zone of the meniscus, and have caused minimum damage to the meniscal body fragment; such tears most commonly are longitudinal and vertical, are peripheral or nearly peripheral, and are 1 cm long or longer.[532] Tears that may be suitable for repair are those in the avascular zone or in an area in which the vascularity is in doubt; repair of these tears requires healing-enhancement techniques such as rasping of the superior and inferior fringes and the insertion of a fibrin clot.[532] Tears that are not suitable for repair include those with moderate or severe damage of the meniscus and complete radial tears; partial or complete meniscectomy is required for treatment in such cases.

In experimental studies in animals, regeneration of a meniscus-like structure after total meniscectomy has been observed.[533, 534] Such regeneration may depend on bleeding from incised perimeniscal vessels that results in an organized clot, cellular proliferation within the clot, and synthesis of a fibrous connective tissue.[340] Owing to the presence of joint motion, a transformation of this fibrous tissue to fibrocartilage may occur over a period of months.[340] The vascular synovial tissue in cases of total meniscectomy and the vascular peripheral meniscal tissue in cases of partial meniscectomy appear to be instrumental in the process of meniscal regeneration.[534] Whether a similar process of meniscal regeneration occurs in humans is a controversial matter, although regeneration of a meniscus-like structure, considerably smaller than a normal meniscus, has been demonstrated in long-term follow-up evaluations in some patients undergoing total meniscectomies.[535] Thus, after total (rather than partial) meniscectomies in humans, regeneration of the peripheral portion of the meniscus appears possible. Despite this evidence, most orthopedic surgeons believe partial meniscectomy is the preferred operation if meniscal removal is considered.[340] Remodeling (rather than regeneration) in the avascular zone of the meniscus may occur after partial meniscectomy, probably related to extrameniscal accretion of new tissue adjacent to the meniscectomy site.[536] The ability of the human meniscus to regenerate or remodel has led to attempts to identify implant material, such as collagen-based scaffolds, that will accelerate the processes.

Meniscal Reconstruction and Transplantation. In the last decade, synthetic, autogenous, and allograft substitutes for the torn meniscus have been used.[537, 538] The ideal candidate for meniscal reconstruction is a young patient who already has undergone complete meniscectomy, particularly on the lateral side. Other candidates for the procedure are those with ligamentous instability and with unreparable or previously removed menisci.[538] The most commonly used meniscal replacement substitutes are fresh, frozen, or cryopreserved meniscal allografts. There are two prerequisites for long-term survival of human meniscal allografts: The viability of meniscal chondrocytes must persist after cryopreservation and transplantation; and the viable cells must synthesize collagen, which ensures the integrity of the extracellular matrix, so that the meniscal allograft can perform its biomechanical function.[537] Precise surgical techniques are required, and many such techniques are described.[538] Meniscal implants must be chosen that are of the correct size; this can be accomplished through measurements derived from routine radiographs of cadaveric knees from which the meniscal allografts will be derived.[1129]

The two most commonly employed methods of postoperative assessment of meniscal transplantation are arthroscopy and MR imaging.[539] Changes in signal intensity within the meniscal allograft are observed for 6 to 12 months after the surgery,[540] although the significance of the findings is not clear. Detachment and displacement of the allograft, as well as its fragmentation and degeneration, can be identified with either MR imaging or arthroscopy.[539, 1130]

Meniscal transplantation surgery is in its infancy. Ultimately, the success of the procedure will be judged on the basis of its ability to prevent (or at least slow down) the occurrence of cartilage degeneration or osteoarthritis in the knee.

Partial Meniscectomy and Total Meniscectomy. Despite recent interest in meniscal repair or reconstruction, partial and total meniscectomies still are employed in the treatment of some meniscal tears. Results after partial meniscectomy accomplished by open or arthroscopic surgery have been promising[541–543] and depend on the type and location of the meniscal tear and the integrity of the remaining portions of the joint. Retention of the peripheral one third of the meniscus provides stress protection to the outer and middle regions of the ipsilateral compartment of the knee, and its salvage then appears to be physiologically sensible. Spontaneous healing of a tear in the peripheral (or central) portion of the meniscus[544, 545] occurs from an ingrowth of connective tissue and is consistent with anatomic studies indicating a relatively abundant vascular supply to the outer meniscal substance.[546] A peripheral vascular synovial fringe extends a short distance over both the femoral and the tibial surfaces of the menisci, except in the posterolateral region of the lateral meniscus, but it does not contribute any vessels to the meniscal stroma[527]; a vascular response originating from the perimeniscal vessels and peripheral synovial fringe is fundamental to the production of a fibrovascular scar at the site of a torn meniscus, emphasizing that the outer blood supply to the meniscus is sufficient to effect a reparative process in those meniscal lesions with which it communicates.[527]

A total meniscectomy involves the removal of the entire meniscus from its capsular attachment. A partial meniscectomy may involve the removal of the anterior two thirds of the abnormal meniscus, deliberately leaving the posterior horn in place; or, alternatively, the torn portion of the meniscus may be removed, leaving the remainder of the meniscus intact. After complete meniscectomy, fibrous regeneration of the meniscus occurs within 6 weeks to 3 months.[547] The regenerated meniscus is thinner and narrower than a normal meniscus, with a decreased surface area and diminished mobility. Tears through regenerated menisci, although reported,[548, 549] are rare.

Routine Radiography and Arthrography. Plain film radiographic findings after meniscectomy may include flattening of the ipsilateral femoral condyle, a bone outgrowth projecting inferiorly from the margin of the femoral condyle at the meniscectomy site, and joint space narrowing. Arthrographic evaluation after complete or partial meniscectomy may reveal a retained fragment, a regenerated meniscus, or a tear of the opposite meniscus.[550–553]

During arthrography, the retained posterior horn after incomplete meniscectomy resembles a normal posterior horn, although it may be irregular or contain an obvious tear. After removal of the inner fragment of a bucket-handle tear, the retained peripheral fragment appears as a truncated shadow with rough, irregular surfaces.[551] With regeneration of the meniscus, a small triangular shadow resembling an equilateral or isosceles triangle is observed, varying from 2 to 7 mm in width.[551] It possesses smooth, well-defined margins but is not associated with adjacent normal recesses at the meniscocapsular junction. Arthrographic findings in cases of tears of the opposite meniscus are no different from those associated with meniscal tears in patients who have not undergone meniscectomy. The torn meniscus may have been overlooked on preoperative imaging examinations or may have occurred after surgery.

MR Imaging. Despite considerable interest in the role of MR imaging in the assessment of the menisci after partial meniscectomy or meniscal repair, the value of this technique remains unclear, and its diagnostic superiority in comparison to standard arthrography remains unproved.[554] A spectrum of MR imaging findings consisting of altered intrameniscal signal intensity and contour alterations is seen after partial meniscectomy or surgical repair of a torn meniscus, and sorting out what is clinically significant from what is not is difficult.[555] Smith and Totty[556] used MR imaging to evaluate 40 patients who had had partial meniscectomies and correlated the appearance of the menisci on MR images with arthroscopic findings, which were available for 23 menisci. They emphasized the spectrum of MR imaging appearances of the meniscal remnants and cautioned against applying the classic diagnostic criteria of meniscal tears in the assessment of the postoperative knee. The authors concluded that although standard MR imaging criteria can be used to diagnose tears in postoperative menisci that do not reveal marked contour irregularity (Fig. 16–121), the diagnosis of tears in meniscal segments revealing marked contour irregularity is far more difficult, as such irregularity can be a normal postoperative finding. They further indicated that tears occurring through meniscal remnants with severe contour irregularity may not be detectable with MR imaging unless displacement of the fragment is evident.

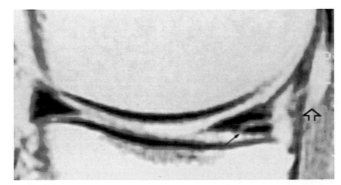

Figure 16–121

Postoperative menisci: Meniscal tear after partial meniscectomy. This patient developed recurrent symptoms after a partial meniscectomy for a torn medial meniscus. A sagittal proton density–weighted (TR/TE, 2000/20) spin echo MR image photographed with meniscal windowing shows a pattern of grade 3 intrameniscal signal intensity (solid arrow) as well as a meniscal cyst (open arrow). Both were confirmed at arthroscopy.

Kent and coworkers[557] emphasized the slow healing response that may follow meniscal surgery and noted that regions of altered signal intensity within the meniscal remnant on MR images can lead to diagnostic problems, particularly if a history of previous meniscal surgery is not known at the time of image interpretation. The persistence of altered signal intensity within meniscal remnants (as well as within torn menisci that are treated conservatively) also was emphasized by Deutsch and colleagues[558]; in this study, MR imaging examinations were obtained before and after therapy in 17 patients with arthroscopically confirmed meniscal tears who were treated either conservatively or operatively (meniscal repair). Follow-up MR imaging examinations, obtained 3 to 27 months after the initial studies, revealed persistent intrameniscal signal intensity (grade 3) that was unchanged from that on the initial examinations. In three patients, second-look arthroscopy was employed, and these procedures confirmed that grade 3 intrameniscal signal intensity can be observed in repaired menisci that appear intact (i.e., no new or recurrent tear) at the time of subsequent arthroscopic examination. The authors concluded that such intrameniscal signal intensity is not diagnostic of a meniscal retear. Farley and collaborators[559] arrived at conclusions similar to those of Deutsch and colleagues[558] with regard to the lack of clinical significance of grade 3 intrameniscal signal intensity in T1-weighted and proton density–weighted spin echo MR images in previously repaired menisci. These investigators noted, however, that a further increase in the intrameniscal signal intensity on T2-weighted spin echo images, with a resultant signal intensity identical to that of fluid, might be helpful in the diagnosis of a retorn meniscus. The specificity of this finding was 92 per cent, but its sensitivity was only 60 per cent. Although these authors indicated that a fluid-filled meniscal remnant, a tear at a location other than that of the repair site, and a displaced meniscal fragment all might be used to diagnose a tear in a meniscus that previously had been repaired, they concluded that standard arthrography might be a better procedure for the assessment of the symptomatic, previously repaired meniscus.

The previously cited studies differed in their methodology, but they all indicate the difficulty encountered in the MR imaging analysis of the repaired or partially resected meniscus.[1131] In the absence of a displaced tear, the presence of fluid collections within the meniscus appears to represent the most reliable MR imaging finding of a retear (Fig. 16–122). The fluid is derived from the joint space and, therefore, the finding would be expected to be more common in patients who have sizeable joint effusions. The diagnostic value of standard arthrography in this clinical setting is based primarily on the intrameniscal extension of fluid after an iatrogenic effusion produced by the injection of contrast material into the joint. MR arthrography using gadolinium compounds[560] or saline solution shares many of the advantages of standard arthrography in the diagnosis (or exclusion) of a retorn meniscus. With MR arthrography, the most definite sign of a retorn meniscus is the presence of contrast material within the meniscus (Figs.

16–123 and 16–124). The absence of such contrast material is consistent with (but not diagnostic of) the absence of a new tear (Fig. 16–125). Whether the added expense of this procedure, when compared with standard arthrography, is warranted in this clinical situation remains unproved.

One interesting imaging strategy in the assessment of the postoperative meniscus is to employ standard arthrography initially with either iodinated contrast material alone or iodinated contrast material mixed with a small amount of a gadolinium-containing agent. If this examination is not conclusive, the patient can be moved immediately to the MR imaging suite. Depending on the composition of the injected contrast agent (or agents), T1-weighted (if both iodinated and gadolinium contrast material has been injected) or T2-weighted (if iodinated contrast material alone has been used) spin echo sequences then are obtained (Fig. 16–126). The safety of mixing gadolinium compounds and iodinated contrast agents, however, is not proved.

MR imaging examinations, as well as quantitative bone mineral analysis,[561] reveal changes in the subchondral bone in the proximal portion of the tibia and in the distal portion of the femur in patients undergoing partial or complete meniscectomies.[1132, 1133] Similar abnormalities have been observed after arthroscopic laser meniscectomy.[1134] These changes may reflect the effects of redistribution of stress, osteoarthritis, or even osteonecrosis (Fig. 16–127).

Abnormalities of the Medial Supporting Structures

Anatomic Considerations

The gross anatomy of the supporting structures on the medial side of the knee (Fig. 16–128) often is discussed according to the depth of the tissue, in the form of layers.[562, 563] The most superficial of three layers is represented by fascia that covers the quadriceps mechanism, invests the sartorius tendon, and continues on as the deep fascia of the leg. It rarely is torn with injury. The second layer is the superficial portion of the medial collateral ligament (also called the tibial collateral ligament or superficial medial ligament), which is separated from the first layer at the tibial tuberosity by the gracilis and semitendinosus tendons. The superficial portion of the medial collateral ligament is approximately 10 to 11 cm long. It is composed of two bundles of fibers, one vertical and one oblique. The vertical fibers originate from the femoral epicondyle and insert in the proximal portion of the tibia, posterior to the pes anserinus tendons. The oblique fibers, often designated the posterior oblique ligament, also originate in the femoral epicondyle and insert in the posteromedial aspect of the proximal portion of the tibia, inferior to the articular surface (Fig. 16–129). The superficial portion of the medial collateral ligament has no meniscal attachment and is able to slide posteriorly over the proximal portion of the tibia during flexion of the knee.[562] The third layer is the capsule of the knee joint, which attaches to the margins of the joint.[563] The capsule is thin anteriorly,

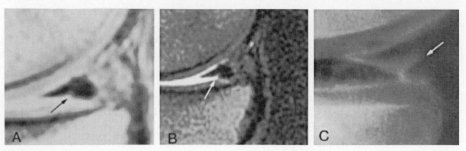

Figure 16–122

Postoperative menisci: Meniscal tear after partial meniscectomy. A sagittal proton density–weighted (TR/TE, 2000/30) spin echo MR image photographed with meniscal windowing **(A)** and a sagittal T2-weighted (TR/TE, 2000/80) spin echo MR image **(B)** reveal findings suggesting a tear in the posterior horn of the medial meniscus. In **A,** note irregularity (arrow) of the inferior margin of the meniscus. In **B,** a small amount of fluid (arrow) is present at the site of meniscal tear. Arthrography **(C)** confirms the presence of such a tear (arrow).

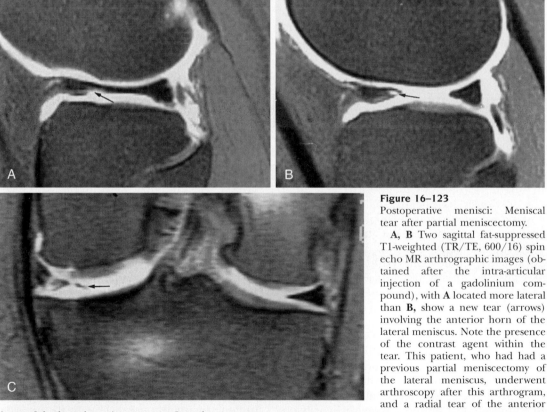

Figure 16–123

Postoperative menisci: Meniscal tear after partial meniscectomy.

A, B Two sagittal fat-suppressed T1-weighted (TR/TE, 600/16) spin echo MR arthrographic images (obtained after the intra-articular injection of a gadolinium compound), with **A** located more lateral than **B,** show a new tear (arrows) involving the anterior horn of the lateral meniscus. Note the presence of the contrast agent within the tear. This patient, who had had a previous partial meniscectomy of the lateral meniscus, underwent arthroscopy after this arthrogram, and a radial tear of the anterior horn of the lateral meniscus was confirmed.

C In a patient who had had repairs of medial meniscal and anterior cruciate ligament tears, a coronal fat-suppressed T1-weighted (TR/TE, 650/13) spin echo MR image (with a gadolinium compound in the joint) shows a recurrent, partially displaced medial meniscal tear (arrow), confirmed arthroscopically.

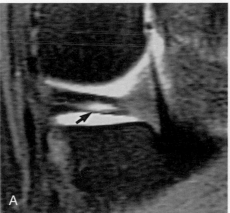
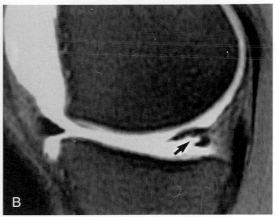

Figure 16–124
Postoperative menisci: Meniscal tear after partial meniscectomy. Coronal **(A)** and sagittal **(B)** fat-suppressed T1-weighted (TR/TE, 750/16) spin echo MR images obtained after the intra-articular injection of a gadolinium compound show contrast material (arrows) collecting within the tear of the medial meniscus.

providing little stability to the joint, it holds the meniscal rim to the tibia (i.e., the coronary ligament) and to a lesser extent to the femur, and it thickens beneath the superficial portion of the medial collateral ligament to form the deep portion of this ligament (also designated the deep medial ligament, deep collateral ligament, or middle capsular ligament).[562] The superficial and deep portions of the medial collateral ligament are intimate with a bursa that allows movement between the two. This bursa is shaped like an inverted U; a superficial arm is elliptical and is located between the semimembranosus tendon and the ligament and a deep arm is triangular and located between the semimembranosus tendon and the medial tibial condyle.[564] The deep portion of the medial collateral ligament is divided into meniscofemoral and meniscotibial ligaments, which extend from the medial meniscus to the femur and tibia, respectively.

Although this description is useful, the three layers of tissue on the medial side of the knee usually are not identified together at any one anatomic site (with the exception of the region of the superficial portion of the medial collateral ligament). Furthermore, some of these layers may appear to merge in certain anatomic regions.

One such region is the posteromedial corner of the knee, in which the second and third layers merge. In this region, an obliquely oriented band of fibers, often designated the posterior oblique ligament or the oblique portion of the tibial collateral ligament,[562, 565, 566] extends to the tibia, the fibers being reinforced by the semimembranosus muscle and its tendon.[563, 565, 567] The fibers in the posterior oblique ligament are tight with the knee extended and lax with the knee flexed; the fibers in the vertical segment of the superficial portion of the medial collateral ligament are tight throughout knee flexion (Fig. 16–130). The posterior oblique ligament, therefore, must be activated or "dynamized" in knee flexion through the pull of the semimembranosus muscle.[568] This dynamization is important for two reasons: Most injuries of the athlete's knee occur with the joint flexed 45 to 90 degrees; and the pull of the semimembranosus muscle also causes the posterior horn of the medial meniscus to move more posteriorly, preventing its entrapment.[568]

The supporting structures in the medial side of the knee also can be divided into three segments on the basis of their position in an anteroposterior plane: anterior third, middle third, and posterior third. The ante-

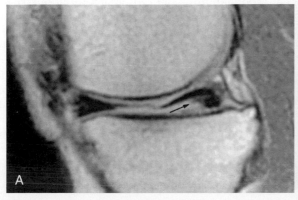
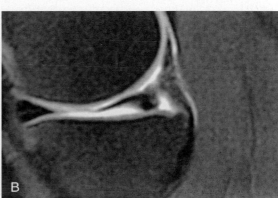

Figure 16–125
Postoperative menisci: Meniscal deformity (but no tear) after partial meniscectomy.
    A A sagittal proton density–weighted (TR/TE, 2400/30) spin echo MR image reveals irregularity (arrow) of the inferior surface of the posterior horn of the medial meniscus consistent with postoperative changes.
    B A sagittal fat-suppressed T1-weighted (TR/TE, 556/17) spin echo MR image obtained after the intra-articular injection of a gadolinium compound fails to reveal contrast material entering the deformed meniscus.
    (Courtesy of S. Eilenberg, M.D., San Diego, California.)

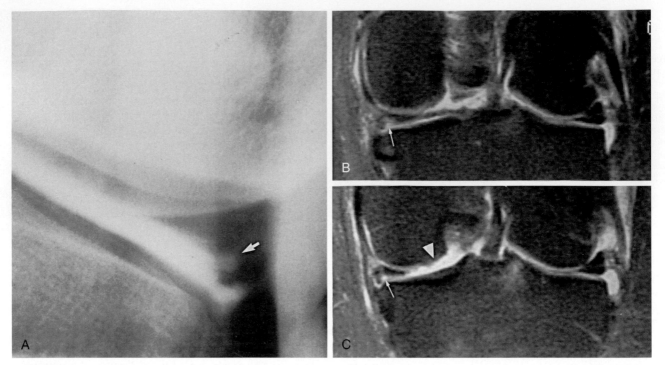

Figure 16–126

Postoperative menisci: Meniscal tear after meniscal repair. This patient had had a repair of a torn medial meniscus approximately 1 year previously and developed recurrent knee pain.

A An arthrographic image obtained after the intra-articular injection of iodinated contrast material alone shows a tear (arrow) involving the inferior surface of the posterior horn of the medial meniscus. A synovial cyst also is seen.

B,C The patient immediately underwent an MR imaging examination. These two coronal fat-suppressed proton density–weighted (TR/TE, 3000/18) fast spin echo MR images, with **B** located slightly posterior to **C**, show the iodinated contrast material entering the tear (arrows). Note loss of femoral articular cartilage (arrowhead) in the medial femorotibial compartment.

rior third of these supporting structures includes the anterior portion of the joint capsule with its reinforcement from the retinaculum of the vastus medialis muscle. The middle third consists of the superficial portion of the medial collateral ligament (i.e., tibial collateral ligament) and the deep portion of the medial collateral ligament (i.e., meniscofemoral and meniscotibial ligaments). The posterior third consists of the posterior oblique ligament with contributing fibers from the vastus medialis, adductor magnus, and semimembranosus muscles.

Pathologic Considerations

The medial supporting structures of the knee, particularly the superficial portion of the medial collateral ligament, act as the primary restraint to limit valgus angulation at the knee.[569–571] Medial structures also serve as the primary restraints to internal rotation of the tibia; if the superficial and deep portions of the medial collateral ligament are sectioned, increased tibial rotation occurs with the knee in either flexion or extension.[570, 571] The medial supporting structures are major secondary restraints to anterior displacement of the tibia.[570, 572] Although deficiencies confined to the medial supporting structures may lead to pure (straight) lateral instability of the knee, such deficiencies commonly are combined with deficiencies of the cruciate ligaments that allow a rotational component as well.[573–575] Thus,

deficiencies in various components of the medial supporting structures, either alone or in combination with deficiencies in other supporting structures, may lead to straight medial, straight anterior, straight posterior, anteromedial, and combined patterns of knee instability (see later discussion).

The medial supporting structures of the knee are injured more frequently than the lateral supporting structures. Indeed, the medial collateral ligament is the most commonly injured ligament about the knee.[568] Most of the major injuries to the medial capsuloligamentous complex are the result of a valgus stress, often produced by a blow to the lateral aspect of the lower portion of the thigh or the leg near the knee (e.g., clipping injury in American football players). The extent of the injury depends on whether the valgus forces occur alone or in combination with rotational forces. Pure valgus injuries lead to damage of the tibial collateral ligament with or without damage to the posterior oblique ligament; valgus injuries combined with rotational forces lead initially to damage to the posterior oblique ligament and, possibly, the anterior cruciate ligament and subsequently to damage to the tibial collateral ligament.[576] Rotational forces also may lead to injury of the medial meniscus. O'Donoghue's triad of injury consists of tears of the anterior cruciate ligament, medial collateral ligament, and the medial meniscus,[577] an injury that is particularly frequent in American football players.[578]

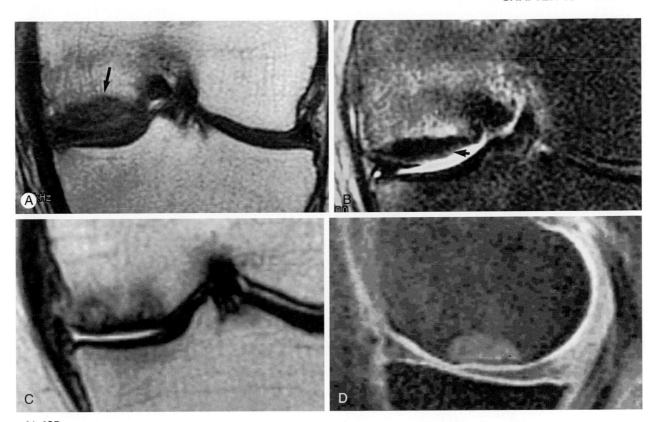

Figure 16–127

Postoperative menisci: Osteonecrosis.

A, B This 82 year old woman underwent arthroscopy with laser treatment of a torn medial meniscus. Knee pain recurred. Coronal T1-weighted (TR/TE, 300/20) spin echo **(A)** and T2-weighted (TR/TE, 4000/92) fat-suppressed fast spin echo **(B)** MR images show findings in the medial femoral condyle that are consistent with osteonecrosis. In **A,** a focal area of low signal intensity (arrow) involves the subchondral region of the condyle. In **B,** the subchondral region again shows low signal intensity (arrow), although surrounding marrow and soft tissue edema is seen, of high signal intensity. Note deformity of the medial meniscus in **B,** consistent with postoperative changes. (Courtesy of P. Kindynis, M.D., Geneva, Switzerland.)

C, D In a second patient who had had a medial meniscectomy, osteonecrosis of the medial femoral condyle is shown in coronal fast spin echo (TR/TE, 3360/105) **(C)** and sagittal three-dimensional fat-suppressed FLASH (TR/TE, 47/11; flip angle, 60 degrees) **(D)** MR images. Fluid in the medial joint space in **D** creates an appearance simulating that of a normal medial meniscus. (Courtesy of J. Kramer, M.D., Vienna, Austria.)

Medial Collateral Ligament Injuries

Tears of the medial collateral ligament may be classified as acute, subacute, or chronic; or according to their severity, varying from a ligament sprain (grade I) to partial (grade II) or complete (grade III) ruptures.

Clinical Abnormalities. Although the pattern and distribution of injury to the knee may be defined by a carefully obtained history, physical examination is fundamental to accurate diagnosis of an injury to the medial collateral ligament. A rapidly (less than 2 hours) developing joint effusion after an injury to the knee usually indicates a hemarthrosis, which typically relates to a collateral ligament sprain, a tear of the anterior cruciate ligament, a tear of the peripheral portion of a meniscus, or an osteochondral fracture; absence of joint swelling may indicate capsular disruption of such a degree that the fluid extravasates into the soft tissues surrounding the knee.[573] Localized edema and tenderness are good indicators of the site of disruption of the medial collateral ligament, although complete disruption of the medial ligaments of the knee may occur without significant pain, effusion, or difficulty in walk-ing.[573] One important physical finding relates to the response of the knee to the application of valgus stress. Valgus stress testing is performed with the knee in full extension and in 30 degrees of flexion. The extent of opening of the medial side of the injured knee in comparison to the opposite (uninjured) side is used as a measure of damage to the medial collateral ligament. When such opening occurs during the application of valgus stress to the fully extended knee, damage involving the deep and superficial portions of the medial collateral ligament, including the posterior oblique ligament, is likely; if severe instability is demonstrated during this stress test, damage to the cruciate ligaments also is probable.[576] If the knee is stable in full extension, the semimembranosus corner of the knee is not damaged significantly. If positive results are obtained when valgus stress is applied to the slightly flexed knee, damage to the deep and superficial portions of the medial collateral ligament and, possibly, to the anterior fibers of the posterior oblique ligament has occurred.[576] As subtle widening of the medial side of the knee during valgus stress testing is presumed on the basis of comparison with the contralateral uninjured knee, evidence of abnormality of the contralateral medial collateral ligament

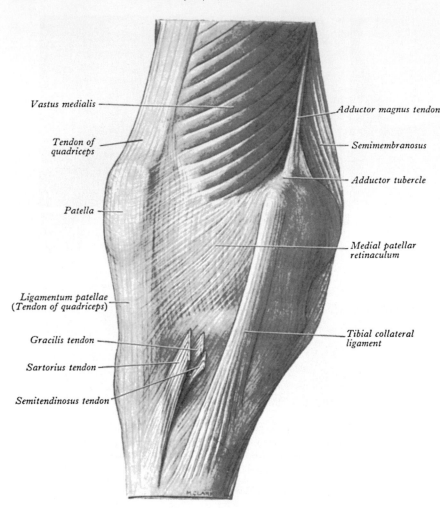

Vastus medialis

Tendon of
quadriceps

Patella

Ligamentum patellae
(Tendon of quadriceps)

Gracilis tendon

Sartorius tendon

Semitendinosus tendon

Adductor magnus tendon

Semimembranosus

Adductor tubercle

Medial patellar
retinaculum

Tibial collateral
ligament

Figure 16–128
Medial supporting structures: Anatomic considerations. (From Williams PL, Warwick R [Eds]: Gray's Anatomy. 35th British edition. Philadelphia, WB Saunders Co, 1973, p 453.)

in animals sustaining unilateral injuries (an effect that is largely unexplained) may have clinical relevance to humans.[579]

Routine Radiographic Abnormalities. Routine radiographic abnormalities associated with acute injuries to the medial collateral ligament of the knee include medial soft tissue swelling with or without a joint effusion, rarely an avulsion fracture at the sites of insertion of the ligament, and evidence of associated injuries, such as a fracture of the lateral tibial plateau that may be comminuted, displaced, or depressed. An avulsion of the intercondylar eminence of the tibia indicates an accompanying injury to the anterior cruciate ligament. In cases of chronic injury to the medial collateral ligament, ligamentous calcification or ossification may occur (i.e., Pellegrini-Stieda syndrome).

Arthrographic Abnormalities. Recent tears of the medial collateral ligament may be documented by conventional arthrography. Contrast material introduced into the joint space will extravasate into the adjacent soft tissues. A linear radiodense region may indicate a contrast-coated outer margin of the medial collateral ligament. An elevated meniscus and an enlarged synovial fold between the tibial margin and meniscus may indicate a tear of the coronary ligament.[439]

Two limitations are related to the arthrographic assessment of injuries to the medial collateral ligament. The examination must be performed within the first 24 to 48 hours after injury, because sealing of the synovial membrane after this time may prevent extravasation of contrast material. Furthermore, injuries involving only the superficial portion of the medial collateral ligament (with sparing of the deep portion of this ligament) are not demonstrated on the arthrographic examination.

Ultrasonographic Abnormalities. Although not commonly applied for this purpose, ultrasonography can be used to diagnose incomplete or complete ruptures of the medial collateral ligaments (Fig. 16–131).

MR Imaging Abnormalities
Normal Medial Collateral Ligament. Although parts of the medial collateral ligament can be seen in MR images in the transaxial and sagittal planes, the coronal plane best displays this ligament (Fig. 16–132). In the coronal plane, the medial collateral ligament appears as a smooth structure of low signal intensity that extends from the medial epicondyle of the femur above to the proximal metaphysis of the tibia below. In its lowest portion, the ligament may be separated from the tibial cortex by medial inferior genicular vessels. At the level of the joint line, the medial collateral ligament is sepa-

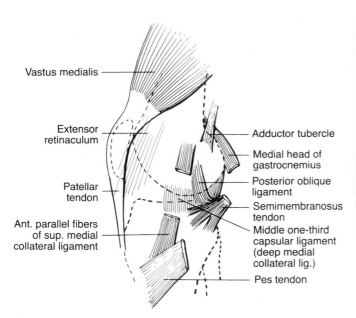

Figure 16–129
Medial supporting structures: Anatomic considerations. A section of the superficial medial collateral ligament has been removed to expose the middle third of the capsular ligament (deep medial collateral) and the posterior oblique ligament. (From Linton RC, Indelicato PA: Medial ligament injuries. *In* JC DeLee, D Drez Jr [Eds]: Orthopaedic Sports Medicine: Principles and Practice. Philadelphia, WB Saunders Co, 1994, p 1262.)

rated from the periphery of the medial meniscus by a bursa and surrounding fat. This junctional tissue should not be misinterpreted as evidence of a meniscocapsular separation. The normal junctional tissue frequently reveals signal intensity characteristics that are indicative of

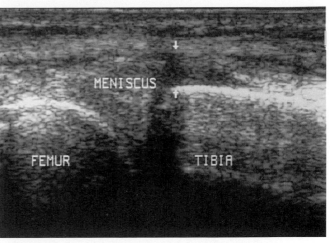

Figure 16–131
Medial collateral ligament injuries: Ultrasonography. Coronal sonogram of the medial aspect of the knee demonstrates focal discontinuity of the medial collateral ligament between the meniscus and the tibia (arrows). (Courtesy of M. van Holsbeeck, M.D., Detroit, Michigan, and J. Jacobson, M.D., San Diego, California.)

fat and, in such cases, misinterpretation of the normal appearance is not likely. In other instances, however, fluid within the bursa is identified between the medial collateral ligament and the medial meniscus or, more posteriorly, about the tendon of the semimembranosus muscle. This may be a normal finding or represent bursitis.[564, 1120] Although similar fluid collections may occur with capsular and ligamentous injuries in the medial side of the knee, other findings indicative of

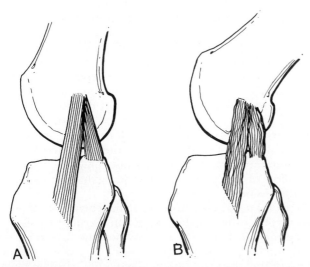

Figure 16–130
Medial supporting structures: Anatomic considerations.
  A Knee in extension with the posterior fibers of the medial ligaments tight.
  B Knee in flexion with the posterior fibers of the medial ligaments loose.
  (From Linton RC, Indelicato PA: Medial ligament injuries. *In* JC DeLee, D Drez Jr [Eds]: Orthopaedic Sports Medicine: Principles and Practice. Philadelphia, WB Saunders Co, 1994, p 1263.)

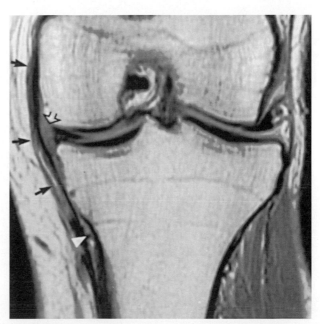

Figure 16–132
Normal medial collateral ligament: MR imaging. A coronal T1-weighted (TR/TE, 800/20) spin echo MR image shows the course of the vertical fibers of the superficial portion of the medial collateral ligament (solid arrows). Note that this portion of the ligament is separated (open arrow) from the medial meniscus (which is torn in this case). The medial inferior genicular vessels are seen (arrowhead).

trauma, including distortion of the signal intensity characteristics of the adjacent subcutaneous fat, also will be evident. Furthermore, large joint effusions resulting from any cause can lead to bowing or even displacement of the medial supporting structures of the knee.

Abnormal Medial Collateral Ligament. Injuries of the medial collateral ligament vary in severity and include sprains, partial tears, and complete tears. The proximal portions of the ligament are involved more frequently than the distal portions. The MR imaging characteristics depend on the severity of the injury and its acute or chronic nature,[580-585] although accurate classification of the severity of the injury on the basis of MR imaging findings is difficult. With acute injuries, subcutaneous edema or hemorrhage and, in some cases, a joint effusion are evident; with chronic injuries, such edema and hemorrhage are not apparent.

Sprains of the medial collateral ligament may lead to slight contour irregularity or thickening of the ligament, but there is no discontinuity of its fibers. In acute sprains, subcutaneous edema is an associated finding, but the signal intensity of the ligament usually is normal (Fig. 16–133). Partial tears of the medial collateral ligament lead to discontinuity of some of its fibers which, in acute injuries, is associated with increased signal intensity (particularly in T2-weighted spin echo and gradient echo MR images) within the substance of the liga-

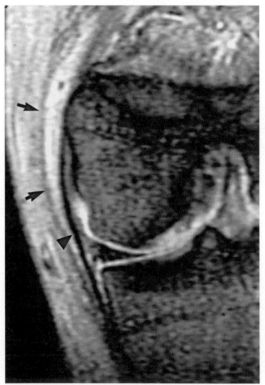

Figure 16–133
Injuries of the medial collateral ligament: MR imaging—sprain. A coronal MPGR (TR/TE, 350/15; flip angle, 25 degrees) MR image shows high signal intensity in the subcutaneous tissues (arrows), consistent with edema, and an apparently intact medial collateral ligament (arrowhead).

ment (Fig. 16–134) and in the subcutaneous tissues. Complete tears of the medial collateral ligament are associated with frank discontinuity of all of its fibers. In the acute stage, hemorrhage and edema within the ligament and subcutaneous tissues also are evident (Figs. 16–135 and 16–136). In the chronic stage, MR imaging may reveal foci of intraligamentous ossification (Pelligrini-Stieda syndrome) (Fig. 16–137).

Although the main diagnostic criteria of an injury to the medial collateral ligament relate to its appearance in the MR images, a spectrum of associated abnormalities produce additional MR imaging changes that can be helpful diagnostically.[582] Bone infractions in the lateral or medial femoral condyle, in the lateral or medial tibial plateau, or both medially and laterally, may be observed, appearing as regions of low signal intensity on T1-weighted spin echo MR images and of high signal intensity on T2-weighted MR images.[583] Fat suppression and STIR MR imaging techniques increase the conspicuity of the bone infractions. Associated tears of one or both cruciate ligaments and, less commonly, of the fibular collateral ligament also may be evident, and the lateral meniscus or medial meniscus may be injured.

Semimembranosus Tendon Abnormalities

The posteromedial corner of the knee is anatomically complex and functionally important. Portions of the joint capsule and semimembranosus tendon are intimate in this area, and the region sometimes is designated the semimembranosus corner of the knee.[576] The capsular attachments of the semimembranosus tendon merge with the oblique fibers of the superficial portion of the medial collateral ligament and, as indicated previously, sometimes are designated the posterior oblique ligament of the knee. The semimembranosus tendon is regarded as having five arms of insertion[562]: a direct attachment to the posteromedial portion of the tibia just below the joint line; a slightly anterior attachment to the tibia just beneath the superficial fibers of the medial collateral ligament; an attachment of its sheath to the posteromedial portion of the capsule; an attachment to the oblique popliteal ligament; and a distal attachment to the superficial fibers of the medial collateral ligament. The semimembranosus corner of the knee, or posterior oblique ligament, may be important in abolishing any valgus laxity in the extended knee.[576] The semimembranosus tendon also may contribute to activation of the posterior oblique ligament (see previous discussion).

Many injuries of the posteromedial corner of the knee also involve other medial supporting structures, as well as the medial meniscus, and any peripheral tear of the posterior horn of the medial meniscus usually includes a tear of the posterior oblique ligament.[576] Isolated avulsion injuries involving this corner of the knee presumably are rare. Identification of a small bone fragment adjacent to the posteromedial portion of the tibia is consistent with an avulsion injury, but its site of origin usually is not clear. One report has indicated the MR imaging findings of apparent avulsion injuries at or near the tibial sites of attachment of the semimembranosus

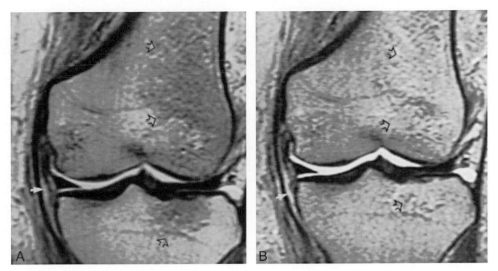

Figure 16–134

Injuries of the medial collateral ligament: MR imaging—partial tear. Coronal proton density–weighted (TR/TE, 2500/20) **(A)** and T2-weighted (TR/TE, 2500/60) **(B)** spin echo MR images show altered signal intensity superficial to and within the substance of the medial collateral ligament (solid arrows), with a higher signal intensity in **B.** Marrow edema (open arrows) in the lateral portions of the femur and tibia indicates the presence of bone bruises. A joint effusion is present.

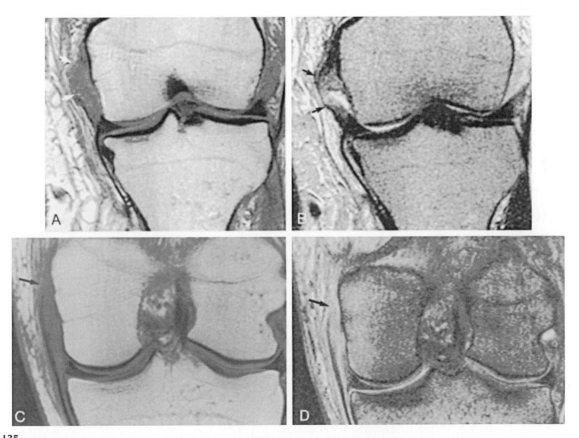

Figure 16–135

Injuries of the medial collateral ligament: MR imaging—complete tear.

A, B Coronal proton density–weighted (TR/TE, 1500/12) **(A)** and T2-weighted (TR/TE, 1500/80) **(B)** spin echo MR images show complete disruption (arrows) of the fibers of the medial collateral ligament. Note the increase in signal intensity in the ligament and soft tissues in **B.** A joint effusion is present. Additional injuries in this patient included tears of the lateral meniscus and anterior cruciate ligament. (Courtesy of V. Chandnani, M.D., Honolulu, Hawaii.)

C, D In a second patient, coronal T1-weighted (TR/TE, 550/20) spin echo **(C)** and MPGR (TR/TE, 600/15; flip angle, 40 degrees) **(D)** MR images reveal complete disruption (arrows) of the fibers of the medial collateral ligament. The menisci and anterior cruciate ligament appear normal. Fluid and edema are evident about the torn ligament.

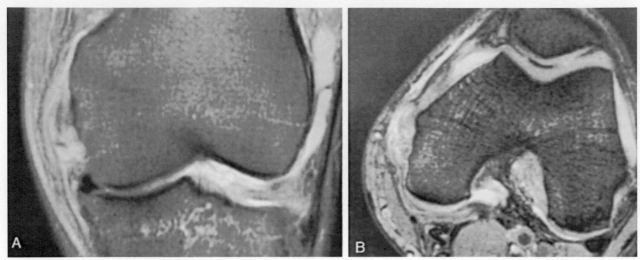

Figure 16–136
Injuries of the medial collateral ligament: MR imaging—complete tear. Coronal fast spin echo MR image with fat suppression (TR/TE, 4000/18) **(A)** and a transaxial MPGR MR image (TR/TE, 400/16; flip angle, 30 degrees) **(B)** show a poorly demarcated elongated area of high signal intensity adjacent to the medial femoral condyle, consistent with a tear of the medial collateral ligament. The anterior portion of the medial patellar retinaculum appears intact. (Courtesy of H. Pavlov, M.D., New York, New York.)

tendon in two patients who also had tears of the anterior cruciate ligament and posterior horn of the medial meniscus.[586] Surgical findings in these two cases were not described. A case with similar MR imaging findings was reported by Vanek.[587] Associated injuries again included a tear of the medial meniscus and a rupture of the anterior cruciate ligament. On the basis of additional cadaveric data, Vanek proposed that the injury was not an avulsion fracture at the site of attachment of the semimembranosus tendon but was produced by varus and external rotation forces on a flexed knee. As such, it was evidence of anterior subluxation of the medial tibial plateau occurring as a result of rupture of the anterior cruciate ligament.

Abnormalities of the Lateral Supporting Structures

Anatomic Considerations

As on the medial side of the knee, the anatomy of lateral supporting structures can be considered in the form of layers (according to the depth of the tissues)[562, 588] (Fig. 16–138) or in terms of their position in an anteroposterior plane.[574] Three layers of tissue can be defined[562]: superficial, intermediate, and deep. The superficial layer is composed of the deep fascia of the thigh and calf, including the condensed portion known as the iliotibial tract. The iliotibial tract extends along the lateral portion of the knee and inserts in the proximal, anterolateral surface of the tibia at Gerdy's tubercle. This tract has functionally important capsular and bone attachments that have been referred to as the anterolateral ligament of the knee; some fibers of the iliotibial tract are continuous with those of the vastus lateralis tendon and aponeurosis, forming the lateral patellar retinaculum (Fig. 16–139).[562, 589–591] The biceps femoris tendon lies just deep to the superficial layer; its main distal attachment is to the head and styloid process of the fibula, although some of its fibers attach to Gerdy's tubercle, blend with the crural fascia of the leg, and extend around the lateral (fibular) collateral ligament.[562]

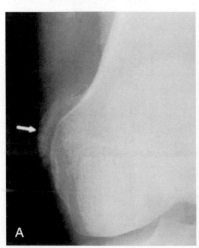
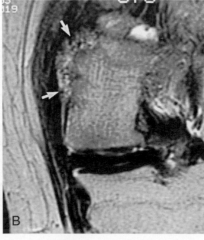

Figure 16–137
Ossification of ligaments: Pellegrini-Stieda syndrome.
  A This pattern of ossification (arrow) is typical of this syndrome.
  B In a different patient, a coronal fast spin echo MR image (TR/TE, 3800/126) shows the area of ossification (arrows) at the femoral attachment site of the medial collateral ligament.

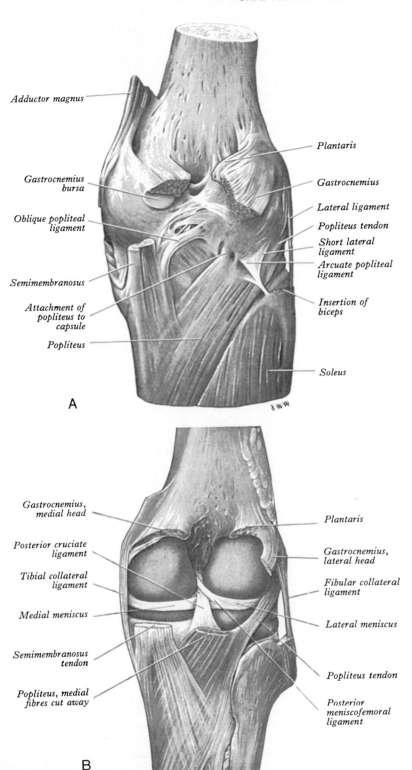

Figure 16–138
Posterolateral corner of the knee: Anatomic considerations. Drawings of the superficial (**A**) and deep (**B**) structures in the posterior aspect of the knee are shown. See text for details. (From Williams PL, Warwick R [Eds]: Gray's Anatomy. 36th British edition. Edinburgh, Churchill Livingstone, 1980, pp. 452, 453.)

The second layer consists of the retinaculum of the patella and the patellofemoral ligaments (see later discussion).[588] The third and deepest layer is composed of the capsule of the knee joint and the lateral (fibular) collateral ligament.[562] The lateral collateral ligament extends from the lateral epicondyle of the femur to the proximal lateral surface of the fibular head. It is taut when the knee is extended and loose when the knee is flexed, and it serves as the primary restraint to varus stress at the knee.[569] The deepest layer passes along the posterior portion of the lateral meniscus, comprising the coronary ligament (which is longer than the coronary ligament of the medial meniscus, and thus accounts for the increased mobility of the lateral meniscus), and terminates as the arcuate ligament. The arcuate ligament extends from the styloid process of the

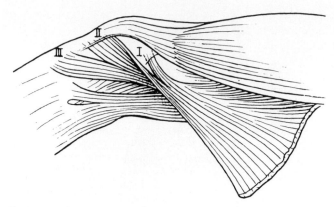

Figure 16-139

Iliotibial tract: Anatomic considerations. The three insertion sites of this tract are shown. Part I of the iliotibial tract blends into the intermuscular septum and inserts on the supracondylar tubercle (Kaplan's fibers). The insertions at the patella and the patellar ligament (part II) as well as Gerdy's tubercle (part III) also are shown. (From Jakob RP, Hassler H, Stäubli HU: Acta Orthop Scand Suppl *191*:6, 1981.)

fibular head to the posterior portion of the joint capsule (near the termination of the oblique popliteal ligament), and it is intimate with the junction of the popliteus muscle and its tendon.[562] A portion of the joint capsule forms the fabellofibular ligament (in cases in which a fabella is present). The popliteus muscle originates in the posterior surface of the proximal portion of the tibia, attaches to the posterior horn of the lateral meniscus and to the arcuate ligament, and terminates in the lateral femoral condyle, distal and posterior to the attachment site of the lateral collateral ligament.[562, 592, 593] An attachment of the popliteus tendon to the proximal portion of the fibula also may be evident, designated the popliteofibular ligament.[1135] The anatomy of the posterolateral corner of the knee (see Fig. 16-138) is complex and not agreed on.[594] Some authors refer to this region simply as the arcuate complex (composed of the arcuate ligament, the lateral collateral ligament, the popliteus muscle and tendon, and the tendon of the lateral head of the gastrocnemius muscle).[574, 595]

Hughston and coworkers[574] divide the lateral supporting structures into the anterior third, middle third, and posterior third of the knee. The structures in the anterior third include the capsular ligament, extending posteriorly from the lateral borders of the patella and patellar tendon to the anterior border of the iliotibial tract, reinforced by the lateral retinaculum of the quadriceps tendon. The structures in the middle third are the iliotibial tract and the capsular ligament deep to it, and this segment extends posteriorly as far as the lateral collateral ligament. Structures in the posterior third, including both capsular and noncapsular ligaments, are designated the arcuate complex of the knee (see previous discussion), and are reinforced by the lateral head of the gastrocnemius muscle and the biceps femoris and popliteus muscles.

Pathologic Considerations

The lateral supporting structures tend to be more substantial and stronger than the medial supporting structures and, in the course of the gait cycle, are subjected to greater forces. The lateral supporting structures restrain varus angulation at the knee and external rotation of the tibia. The relative contributions of each of these supporting structures in these functions is not clear. The lateral collateral ligament acts as a primary restraint to limit such varus angulation, although deep posterolateral structures provide considerable restraint as a secondary stabilizer. Injuries involving both the lateral collateral ligament and these deep posterolateral structures are associated with greater varus instability than those confined to the lateral collateral ligament.[596] No individual lateral supporting structure appears to act as the primary restraint to external rotation of the tibia; rather, the components of the posterolateral corner of the knee (consisting of the lateral collateral ligament, arcuate ligament, posterior portion of the lateral capsule, and popliteus tendon) function in concert as a complex to limit such external rotation.[596] The lateral supporting structures also act as secondary restraints to limit anterior and posterior motion at the knee. The effect of any one structure in this regard appears to be small, but together the lateral collateral ligament and deep posterolateral structures serve as a major secondary restraint to posterior displacement at the knee from full extension to 30 degrees of flexion.[596]

Injuries to the lateral supporting structures of the knee may be combined with other injuries such as those to the cruciate ligaments. The effects of deficiency of various combinations of knee ligaments and other supporting structures have been studied in vitro, and the data are summarized by Shoemaker and Daniel.[596] Disruptions of both the lateral collateral ligament and deep posterolateral structures yield increases in varus angulation at the knee and external rotation of the tibia and, in addition, minor anteroposterior instability. Combined disruption of the anterior cruciate ligament and deep posterolateral structures without injury to the lateral collateral ligament leads to an increase in anterior movement at the knee without evidence of accentuated external rotation of the tibia or varus angulation of the knee (owing to the restraint provided by the intact lateral collateral ligament). When the anterior cruciate ligament, lateral collateral ligament, and deep posterolateral structures are all incompetent, anterior and varus instability at the knee and exaggerated external rotation of the tibia are seen. Combined injury to the posterior cruciate ligament, lateral collateral ligament, and deep posterolateral structures allows increases in posterior movement, varus angulation, and external rotation of the tibia.

Hughston and collaborators[574] identified six types of lateral instability patterns of the knee encountered in clinical practice: (1) anterolateral rotary instability caused by disruption of the middle third of the lateral capsular ligament and accentuated by other tears, particularly a tear of the anterior cruciate ligament; (2) posterolateral rotary instability caused by a tear of the arcuate complex; (3) combined anterolateral and posterolateral rotary instability caused by disruption of all the lateral capsular ligaments with or without a tear of the iliotibial tract, with an intact posterior cruciate ligament; (4) combined anterolateral and anteromedial rotary instability caused by tears of the middle thirds of the medial and lateral capsular ligaments with an intact posterior cruciate ligament; (5) combined posterolateral, anterolateral, and anteromedial rotary instability caused by tears of both the lateral and the medial ligaments; and (6) straight lateral instability caused by tears of the lateral ligaments and the posterior cruciate ligament. Although this classification system furthered the understanding of knee instability and still is used today, it was not without problems. Differentiation between translational and rotational instabilities was arbitrary and the identification of the posterior cruciate ligament as the anatomic rotational center of the knee has been challenged.[591] Recent cadaveric studies have indicated that injury to the posterolateral structures of the knee frequently results in poorly understood patterns of instability that cannot be classified by the system of Hughston and coworkers.[591]

The lateral instability patterns are less frequent than those on the medial side of the knee, although eventually they may be more disabling. Initially, however, clinical findings associated with injuries to the supporting structures in the lateral side of the knee may be subtle and often unrecognized.[574] Acutely, pain and swelling may be evident, the severity of the findings being influenced by the location and extent of the injury. With time, instability of the knee may prevent the patient from participating in sports or even walking. A number of tests administered during physical examination can be employed to check the integrity of the lateral supporting structures as well as of the cruciate ligaments, which also may be injured. Many of these tests rely on the presence or absence, as well as the pattern, of motion that occurs when stress is applied to the injured knee. These tests, which include the anterior and posterior drawer tests and the adduction and abduction stress tests, are accomplished with varying degrees of flexion or extension of the knee. The results of such testing often allow an accurate diagnosis as to which specific ligaments are injured.[574]

Lateral Collateral Ligament Injuries

Routine radiography in cases of injury to the lateral collateral ligament of the knee generally does not reveal specific findings. Focal soft tissue swelling may be evident in some cases. Furthermore, as the lateral collateral ligament along with the tendon of the biceps femoris muscle attaches to the fibular head and styloid process, avulsion fractures of this portion of the fibula may be seen. The fragment is of variable size and may be large, although it usually is displaced only minimally. Rarely, significant proximal migration or even entrapment of the fragment in the lateral compartment of the knee is present. Standard arthrography is not useful in the diagnosis of injuries to the lateral collateral ligament, and the value of CT is restricted to detection of avulsion fractures of the proximal portion of the fibula.

MR imaging represents an effective technique for assessment of the integrity of the lateral collateral ligament and the adjacent tendon of the biceps femoris

muscle (Fig. 16–140A–C).[597] These structures can be identified on sagittal, coronal, and transaxial MR images. In posterior MR images in the coronal plane, the normal biceps femoris muscle is seen in the lateral aspect of the leg, above the knee. Its tendon is straight, is of low signal intensity, and attaches to the head and styloid process of the fibula. In coronal images just anterior to those that display the biceps femoris muscle and tendon, the lateral collateral ligament is seen arising from the fibula and extending superiorly and anteriorly to attach to the epicondyle in the distal portion of the femur. It, too, is of low signal intensity. In far lateral MR images in the sagittal plane, a V-shaped region of low signal intensity can be identified. The anterior limb of this region is the lateral collateral ligament, and the posterior limb is the tendon of the biceps femoris muscle. They join in the region of the proximal portion of the fibula. Because of the oblique course of the normal lateral collateral ligament, it may not be seen in its entirety in any single coronal or sagittal MR image. An oblique coronal image may show the structures of the posterolateral corner of the knee more optimally (Fig. 16–140D–L).[1136]

Disruption of the lateral collateral ligament, of the tendon of the biceps femoris muscle, or of both structures is recognized on MR images as an interruption or waviness of these tendons or regions of high signal intensity on T2-weighted spin echo MR images within or adjacent to these tendons (Figs. 16–141, 16–142, and 16–143).[582, 598] Associated injuries of other lateral supporting structures or the cruciate ligaments also may be evident (Fig. 16–144). In dislocations of the knee, injuries of lateral, medial, and cruciate ligaments are encountered.

Popliteus Muscle and Tendon Injuries

As indicated earlier, the popliteus muscle and tendon contribute significantly to the integrity of the posterolateral region of the knee. The precise role of the popliteus muscle and tendon is not certain, but these structures may initiate and maintain internal rotation of the tibia with respect to the femur and contribute to prevention of forward displacement of the femur in relation to the tibia during the initial stages of knee flexion.[599] It also has been suggested that the popliteus muscle acts to withdraw, and thereby protect, the lateral meniscus during flexion and rotation of the knee,[599, 1137] although some anatomic studies have failed to document a major attachment of the popliteus tendon to the lateral meniscus.[600] Injuries to the popliteus muscle and tendon may occur in association with injuries to other lateral supporting structures of the knee or, rarely, as an isolated phenomenon.[599, 601–603, 1138] Such isolated injuries may involve sudden external rotation of the tibia when the knee is partially flexed and bearing weight.[601, 603] Clinical findings include an acute hemarthrosis, lateral tenderness, and rarely, injury to the posterior tibial nerve.[601] Avulsion fractures of the femur may be seen with routine radiography, and an abnormal course or an abnormal signal intensity within the popliteus tendon or hem-

Text continued on page 654

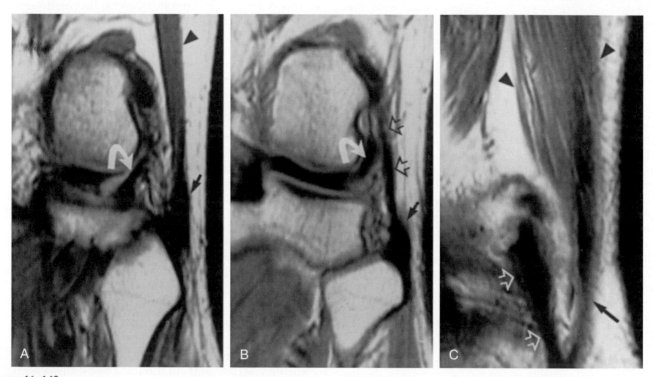

Figure 16–140

Normal lateral collateral ligament and biceps femoris muscle and tendon: MR imaging.

A, B Two consecutive coronal proton density–weighted (TR/TE, 2200/20) spin echo MR images show the normal appearance of the biceps femoris muscle (arrowhead) and its tendon (solid straight arrows), and the lateral collateral ligament (open arrows). In **A,** the more posterior image, the biceps femoris muscle and tendon are seen extending lateral to the joint and inserting into the proximal portion of the fibula. In **B,** the lateral collateral ligament extends from the fibula superiorly to insert into the femur. The popliteus tendon (curved arrows) is identified.

C A sagittal proton density–weighted (TR/TE, 2200/20) spin echo MR image of the lateral aspect of the knee shows the biceps femoris muscle (arrowheads) and its tendon (solid arrow) and the lateral collateral ligament (open arrows). Note the V-like pattern created at the junction of the biceps femoris tendon and lateral collateral ligament.

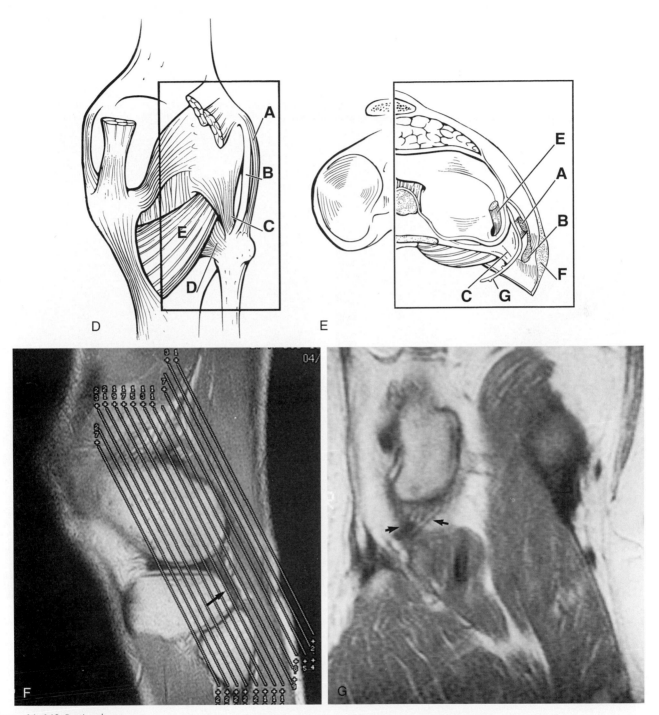

Figure 16–140 *Continued*

D, E The normal anatomy of the posterolateral corner of the knee is shown in posterior **(D)** and transverse **(E)** views. Structures include the following: A, lateral collateral ligament; B, fabellofibular ligament; C, arcuate ligament; D, fibular head origin of the popliteus muscle; E, popliteal muscle belly and tendon; F, biceps femoris muscle and tendon; G, inferior lateral geniculate artery.

F As shown on this sagittal proton density–weighted (TR/TE, 2000/20) spin echo MR image, a coronal oblique plane is chosen in an externally rotated knee that is parallel to the course of the long axis of the popliteal tendon (arrows).

G This coronal oblique proton density–weighted (TR/TE, 2000/20) spin echo MR image reveals the arcuate ligament (arrows).

Illustration continued on following page

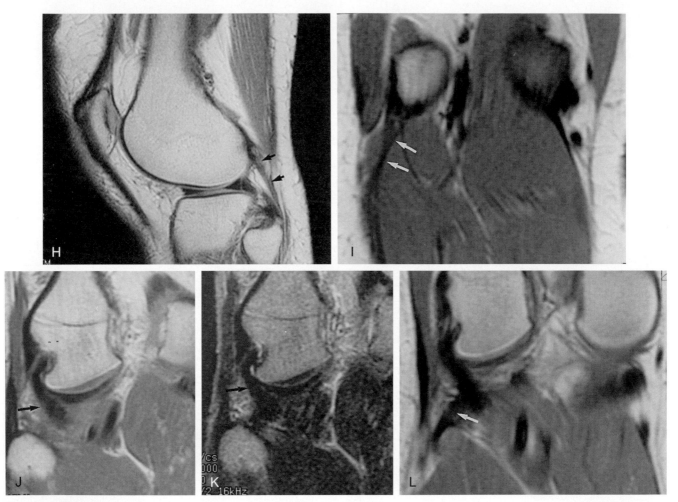

Figure 16–140 *Continued*

H, I Sagittal **(H)** and coronal oblique **(I)** proton density–weighted (TR/TE, 2000/20) spin echo MR images show the fabellofibular ligament (arrows, **H**), which extends from the styloid process of the fibula to the fabella (arrows, **I**).

J, K Coronal oblique proton density–weighted (TR/TE, 2000/20) **(J)** and T2-weighted (TR/TE, 2000/80) **(K)** spin echo MR image show the normal appearance of the popliteal tendon (arrows).

L The fibular origin (arrow) of the popliteal muscle is evident on a coronal oblique proton density–weighted (TR/TE, 2000/20) spin echo MR image.

(D–L, From Yu JS, et al: Radiology *198*:199, 1996.)

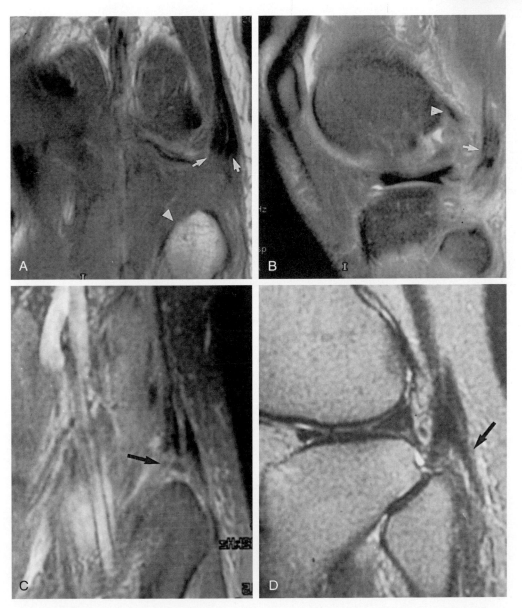

Figure 16–141
Injuries of the lateral collateral ligament and biceps femoris muscle and tendon: MR imaging. A coronal T2-weighted (TR/TE, 2500/80) spin echo MR image reveals complete disorganization in the posterolateral region of the knee. Although the fibular head (F) is seen, the tendon of the biceps femoris muscle and the lateral collateral ligament are not identifiable. A joint effusion is seen. Note high signal intensity within the biceps femoris muscle (arrows). An injury of the anterior cruciate ligament also was present in this patient.

Figure 16–142
Injuries of the lateral collateral ligament and biceps femoris muscle and tendon: MR imaging.

A, B In this 26 year old man with knee instability and signs of peroneal nerve injury after a fall, a coronal T1-weighted (TR/TE, 600/10) spin echo MR image **(A)** reveals avulsion of the biceps femoris tendon (arrows) from the fibular head (arrowhead). The lateral collateral ligament is not identified. The sagittal fat-suppressed fast spin echo (TR/TE, 2700/21) MR image **(B)** again shows the avulsed tendon of the biceps femoris muscle (arrow) and only a small proximal portion of the lateral collateral ligament (arrowhead).

(Courtesy of S. Eilenberg, M.D., San Diego, California.)

C, D In a second patient, disruption of the biceps femoris tendon (arrows) is evident in coronal fat-suppressed fast spin echo (TR/TE, 4000/36) **(C)** and sagittal fast spin echo (TR/TE, 5400/108) **(D)** MR images.

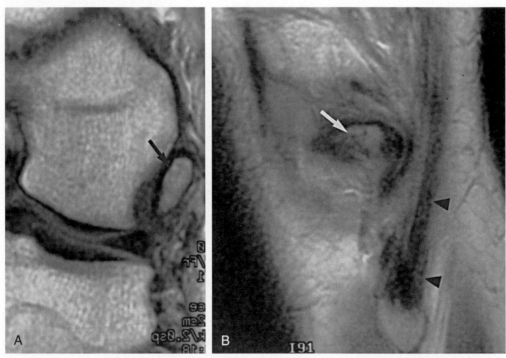

Figure 16–143
Injuries of the lateral collateral ligament: MR imaging. In a 21 year old man with a remote injury to the knee, an avulsion fracture (arrows) at the femoral insertion of the lateral collateral ligament is seen on a coronal T1-weighted (TR/TE, 600/10) spin echo MR image **(A)** and on a sagittal fat-suppressed fast spin echo (TR/TE, 2700/21) MR image **(B).** Note the intact biceps femoris tendon (arrowheads) in **B.** (Courtesy of S. Eilenberg, M.D., San Diego, California.)

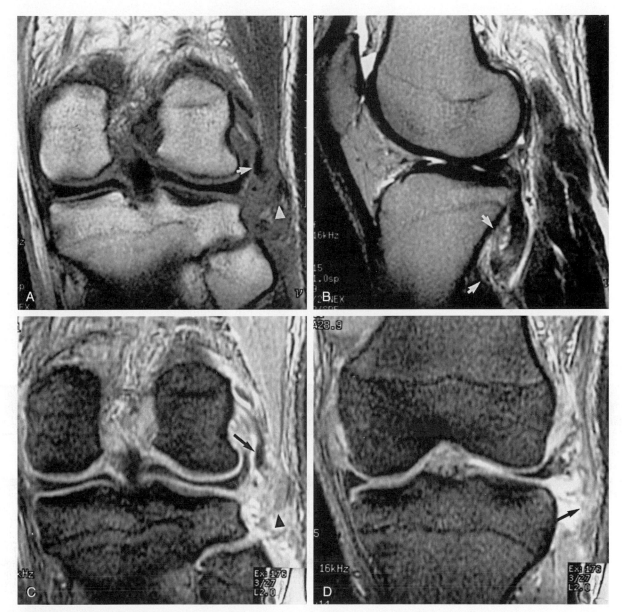

Figure 16–144

Injuries of the lateral collateral ligament, biceps femoris muscle and tendon, iliotibial tract, and popliteus muscle: MR imaging. This 21 year old man developed severe knee instability after a recent injury. Although not shown in these images, the anterior cruciate ligament also was disrupted.

A The coronal T1-weighted (TR/TE, 749/18) spin echo MR image shows avulsion of the biceps femoris tendon (arrowhead) and waviness of the lateral collateral ligament (arrow).

B On a sagittal fast spin echo (TR/TE, 4466/90) MR image, note abnormal signal intensity and morphology of the popliteus muscle (arrows), a joint effusion, and soft tissue edema.

C A coronal MPGR (TR/TE, 500/15; flip angle, 25 degrees) MR image of the posterior aspect of the joint again shows avulsion of the biceps femoris tendon (arrowhead) and an abnormal lateral collateral ligament (arrow). Note the high signal intensity in the adjacent soft tissues.

D More anteriorly, a coronal MPGR (TR/TE, 500/15; flip angle; 25 degrees) MR image shows disruption of the iliotibial tract (arrow), lateral displacement of the lateral meniscus, and lateral and, to a lesser extent, medial soft tissue edema. The anterior cruciate ligament appears abnormal, although this was more evident in other images.

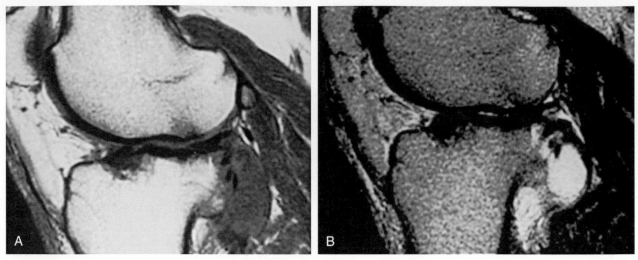

Figure 16–145
Injuries of the popliteus muscle: MR imaging. Coronal proton density–weighted (TR/TE, 2000/20) **(A)** and T2-weighted (TR/TE, 2000/80) **(B)** spin echo MR images show an enlarged popliteus muscle with high signal intensity in **B.** The findings are consistent with an intramuscular hematoma. Note anterior translation of the tibia with respect to the femur, indicating a tear of the anterior cruciate ligament. (Courtesy of M. Schweitzer, M.D., Philadelphia, Pennsylvania.)

orrhage in the popliteus muscle may be seen with MR imaging (Figs. 16–144 and 16–145).[604]

Iliotibial Tract Abnormalities

Injuries to the iliotibial tract usually are combined with injuries to other lateral supporting structures of the knee. Rarely, they may occur as an isolated phenomenon. Avulsion injuries occur at the tibial insertion site of the iliotibial tract (i.e., Gerdy's tubercle), resulting in a small fragment of bone that is difficult to detect in standard frontal and lateral projections of the knee but may be seen in oblique projections. As the iliotibial tract can be well evaluated on coronal MR images of the knee, MR imaging can be employed to detect traumatic abnormalities involving this structure. The normal iliotibial tract is observed on coronal MR images as a structure of low signal intensity traversing the lateral portion of the thigh, extending across the lateral aspect of the knee, and inserting in Gerdy's tubercle in the tibia (Fig. 16–146). Discontinuity of this structure and edema in the tibia adjacent to the site of its attachment may be observed when this tract is injured (Figs. 16–147 and 16–148).

The *iliotibial tract friction syndrome* is related to intense physical activity, as occurs in American football players, cyclists, or long distance runners, that leads to abnormal contact at the iliotibial tract and the lateral femoral epicondyle.[605–607] With knee extension, the iliotibial tract (or band) lies anterior to the lateral epicondyle of the femur; with knee flexion, it passes over the lateral condyle. A bursa develops in this location and becomes inflamed in patients with this syndrome. Predisposing factors may include tightness of the iliotibial tract in athletes, genu varum, tibial torsion, and foot pronation. Pain occurs in the lateral aspect of the thigh and knee, particularly with 30 degrees of flexion of the knee.[607] Although the diagnosis of this syndrome can be established on the basis of clinical findings, similar clinical

manifestations occur in association with injuries to the lateral ligaments of the knee or lateral meniscus. In one report, MR imaging produced evidence of the iliotibial tract friction syndrome due to the presence of fluid collections or edema adjacent to the iliotibial tract (Fig.

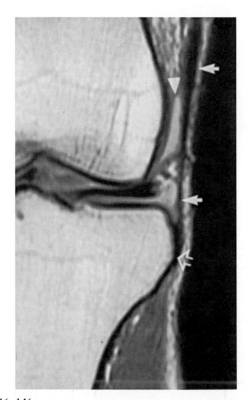

Figure 16–146
Normal iliotibial tract: MR imaging. A coronal proton density–weighted (TR/TE, 2000/20) spin echo MR image shows the iliotibial tract (solid arrows) attaching to Gerdy's tubercle (open arrow) in the tibia. A small joint effusion is evident, just medial to the iliotibial tract (arrowhead).

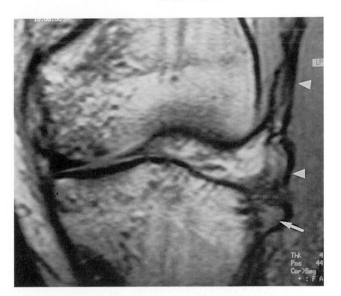

Figure 16–147
Iliotibial tract abnormalities: MR imaging. An avulsion fracture (arrow) of Gerdy's tubercle with laxity of the iliotibial tract (arrowheads) and bone bruises in the medial femoral condyle and tibial plateau is shown on a coronal proton density–weighted (TR/TE, 1950/20) spin echo MR image. This patient also sustained injuries to the posterolateral corner of the knee and anterior cruciate ligament.

16–149).[608] The MR imaging findings, however, resemble those of a joint effusion with fluid accumulating in the suprapatellar bursa.[1196] Conservative treatment generally is sufficient.

Other Lateral Capsular Ligament Injuries

A characteristic and important injury involves an avulsion fracture of the tibial rim that occurs at the site of attachment of the lateral capsular ligament of the knee. Described in 1879 (before the discovery of x-rays) by Segond,[609] this fracture results from forces of internal rotation and varus stress at the knee and is known simply as the Segond fracture. The resulting bone fragment is overlooked easily unless the lateral margin of the tibia is analyzed carefully on the anteroposterior and tunnel radiographic views of the knee (Fig. 16–150). An elliptically shaped piece of bone, measuring up to 10 mm long, occurs at the joint line or just proximal to it, and the donor site in the tibia reveals an irregular surface. The location of the Segond fracture is posterior and slightly proximal to Gerdy's tubercle, the insertion site of the iliotibial tract and, therefore, the fracture should not be misinterpreted as evidence of an injury to the iliotibial tract. With healing, the avulsed fragment may unite with the lateral tibial margin, creating a bone excrescence below the joint line that simulates the appearance of an osteophyte (Fig. 16–151).[610]

Although subtle and seemingly innocent, this lateral tibial rim fracture is indicative of anterolateral instability of the knee, which may become chronic and disabling if the fracture is not recognized and treated appropriately in the acute stage. A high association of the Segond fracture occurs with injuries to the anterior cruciate ligament (75 to 100 per cent of cases) and tears of the menisci (60 to 70 per cent of cases).[588, 611] Conversely, a Segond fracture occurs in approximately 10 per cent of patients with injuries to the anterior cruciate ligament.[612]

The MR imaging findings of the Segond fracture also are chracteristic (Fig. 16–152).[613] The dominant finding is marrow edema adjacent to the site of fracture (Fig.

Figure 16–148
Iliotibial tract abnormalities: MR imaging. This patient sustained an acute injury of the knee that resulted in disruption of most of the major lateral supporting structures. Two coronal MPGR (TR/TE, 600/25; flip angle, 40 degrees) MR images, with **A** located posterior to **B,** show disruption of the iliotibial tract (arrows), soft tissue edema, a bone bruise in the medial femoral condyle, and a joint effusion. (Courtesy of P. Tirman, M.D., San Francisco, California.)

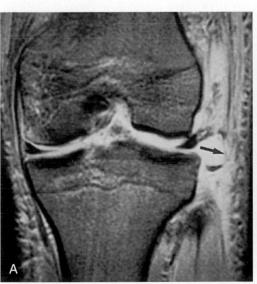

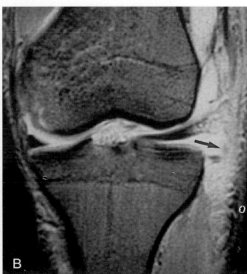

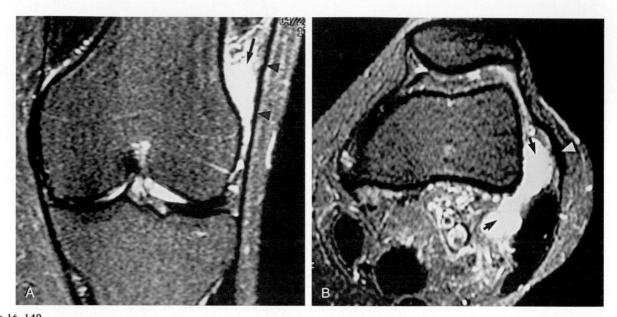

Figure 16–149
Iliotibial tract friction syndrome: MR imaging.

In this 45 year old woman with classic clinical findings of the iliotibial tract friction syndrome, coronal **(A)** and transaxial **(B)** fat-suppressed fast spin echo MR images (TR/TE, 4000/108) show an abnormal collection of fluid (arrows) between the iliotibial tract (arrowheads) and femur. Whether the fluid accumulates in a separate bursa or in a lateral extension of the knee joint in instances of the iliotibial tract friction syndrome is not clear. (Courtesy of A.G. Bergman, M.D., Stanford, California.)

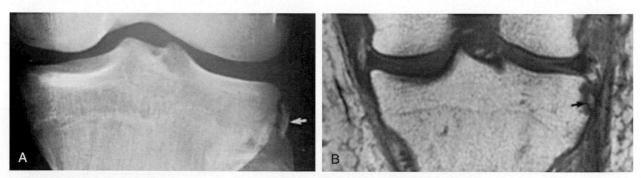

Figure 16–150
Injuries of the lateral capsular ligament (Segond fracture): Routine radiography and MR imaging. This fracture is almost always associated with a tear of the anterior cruciate ligament secondary to the twisting mechanism responsible for both injuries.

A On routine views, the fracture (arrow) is identified as a longitudinal sliver of bone adjacent to the lateral tibial plateau.

B In a coronal T1-weighted spin echo MR image (TR/TE, 500/12), a bone fragment (arrow) is identified at the margin of the lateral tibial plateau. The soft tissues in this region are poorly defined as a result of edema and hemorrhage.

(From Pavlov H, Torg JS: The Running Athlete. Chicago, Year Book, 1987.)

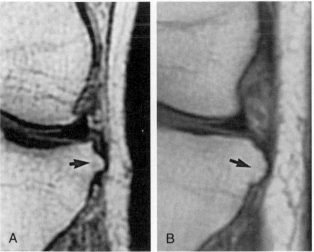

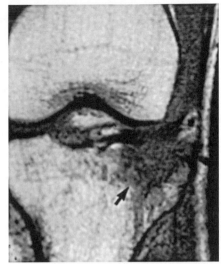

Figure 16–151
Injuries of the lateral capsular ligament (Segond fracture): MR imaging. Examples of the appearance of a healed Segond fracture (arrows) are shown using coronal T1-weighted (**A,** TR/TE, 560/25; **B,** TR/TE, 416/18) spin echo MR images. The anterior cruciate ligament was torn in the patient illustrated in **A** and was intact in the patient illustrated in **B.** (**A,** Courtesy of E. Bosch, M.D., Santiago, Chile; **B,** courtesy of D. Goodwin, M.D., Hanover, New Hampshire.)

Figure 16–153
Injuries of the lateral capsular ligament (Segond fracture): MR imaging. A coronal T1-weighted (TR/TE, 800/25) spin echo MR image shows low signal intensity (arrow) in the lateral aspect of the proximal portion of the tibia, indicating marrow edema. A large joint effusion is evident. The fracture fragment is not well seen. A tear of the anterior cruciate ligament also was present.

16–153). The fracture fragment itself often is not visible, owing to its small size. Associated injuries to the cruciate ligaments and menisci often are visible, and some of these may be accompanied by additional bone injuries with resulting marrow edema.

Plantaris Muscle Injuries

The plantaris muscle is thin and small and lies just deep to the lateral head of the gastrocnemius muscle in the proximal portion of the lower leg. It extends obliquely downward and medially to accompany the Achilles tendon. The muscle may be absent in 7 to 10 per cent of persons.[614] When present, the muscle originates from the distal aspect of the lateral supracondylar line of the femur just superior and medial to the lateral head of the gastrocnemius muscle as well as from the oblique popliteal ligament in the posterior aspect of the knee.[614] The myotendinous junction occurs at the level of the origin of the soleus muscle from the tibia. The long plantaris tendon lies between the medial head of the gastrocnemius muscle and the soleus muscle. Despite its intimate relationship to the Achilles tendon, it often remains intact when the Achilles tendon ruptures.[614]

The proximal aspect of the plantaris tendon may rupture owing to violent contracture of the muscle. This injury is known as "tennis leg," and it causes lower leg pain, especially in athletes.[615, 616] Resulting clinical

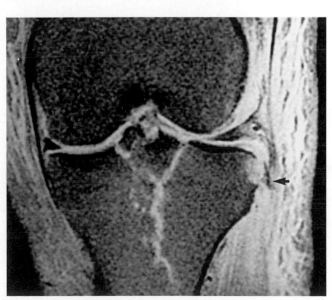

Figure 16–152
Injuries of the lateral capsular ligament (Segond fracture): MR imaging. A coronal fat-suppressed fast spin echo (TR/TE, 1400/20) MR image reveals a Segond fracture (arrow) associated with a tibial plateau fracture and soft tissue edema. (Courtesy of D. Goodwin, M.D., Hanover, New Hampshire.)

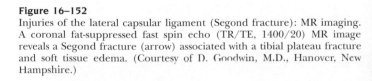

manifestations may resemble those of a rupture of the gastrocnemius muscle. A less severe injury, a muscle strain, also may be encountered. Associated injuries include tears of the anterior cruciate ligament, arcuate ligament, and muscles in the posterolateral corner of the knee, such as the lateral head of the gastrocnemius, soleus, and popliteus muscles.

MR imaging may be helpful in accurate diagnosis.[614] Findings include abnormal signal intensity in the injured muscle or myotendinous junction, fluid collections between the medial head of the gastrocnemius muscle and soleus muscle, and bone contusions (Fig. 16–154).

Abnormalities of the Anterior Supporting Structures

Anatomic Considerations

In the anterior aspect of the knee, ligaments, muscles, aponeuroses, and joint capsule converge to surround the centrally located patella, providing an adequate stabilizing system (Fig. 16–155).[617] These structures, individually or in small groups, lead to forces on the patella that are oriented superiorly (quadriceps muscles), inferiorly (patellar tendon), medially (medial patellar retinaculum and vastus medialis muscle), or laterally (lateral patellar retinaculum, vastus lateralis muscle, and iliotibial tract). Together they stabilize the patella, owing to both passive and active elements.

Passive soft tissue stabilizers are the patellar tendon, medial and lateral patellofemoral ligaments, medial and lateral meniscopatellar ligaments, and portions of the fascia lata. The major passive stabilizer of the patella is the patellar tendon (also referred to as the patellar ligament), extending from the inferior pole of the patella to the tibial tuberosity. This is a broad, flat structure 4 to 6 cm in length and approximately 7 mm in thickness, which diminishes in width from top to bottom. The patellar tendon is approximately 3 cm wide superiorly and 2.5 cm wide inferiorly at its insertion site in the tibial tuberosity.[618] The course of the patellar tendon is almost parallel to the long axis of the lower extremity, although it commonly reveals a slightly oblique lateral orientation from proximal to distal, which contributes to a tendency toward lateral displacement of the patella.[617] Capsular condensations or retinacula link the patella to surrounding structures. Many variations in the anatomy of these capsular condensations exist, however.[619] For example, some authors emphasize those structures that connect the patella to both medial and lateral epicondyles of the femur and to the anterior portions of the medial and lateral menisci. Medially, these condensations include the medial patellofemoral ligament above and the medial meniscopatellar ligament below; laterally, these condensations include the lateral patellofemoral ligament above and the lateral meniscopatellar ligament below.[617] Further lateral reinforcement is provided by the patellar expansion of the fascia lata. Other authors emphasize a superficial

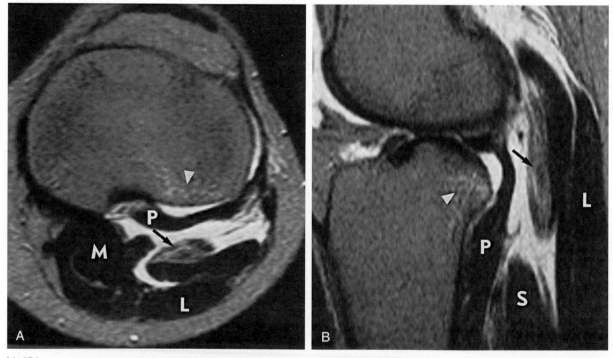

Figure 16–154

Plantaris muscle injuries: MR imaging. A strain of the plantaris muscle occurred in association with a rupture of the anterior cruciate ligament, a sprain of the arcuate ligament, and bone contusions in the lateral compartment of the knee in a 35 year old male skier who had sustained a twisting injury. Transaxial fat-suppressed T2-weighted (TR/TE, 1900/90) (**A**) and sagittal fat-suppressed T2-weighted (TR/TE, 2700/90) (**B**) spin echo MR images show increased signal intensity within the anterior portion of the plantaris muscle (arrows). A posterolateral tibial bone contusion also is evident (arrowheads). L, Lateral head of the gastrocnemius muscle; M, medial head of the gastrocnemius muscle; P, popliteus muscle and tendon; S, soleus muscle. (From Helms CA, et al: Radiology *195*:201, 1995.)

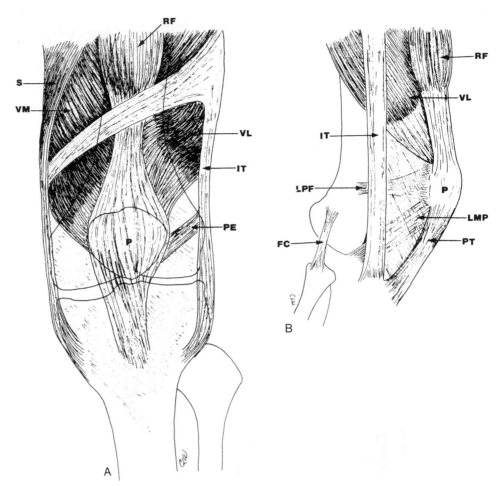

Figure 16–155
Anterior supporting structures: Anatomic considerations.

A Frontal view. Identified structures include the rectus femoris muscle (RF), the vastus medialis (VM) and vastus lateralis (VL) muscles, the sartorius muscle (S), the iliotibial tract (IT) and its patellar extension (PE), and the patella (P).

B Lateral view. Identified structures include the rectus femoris muscle (RF), the vastus lateralis muscle (VL), the iliotibial tract (IT), the patellar tendon (PT), the fibular (lateral) collateral ligament (FC), the patella (P), the lateral meniscopatellar ligament (LMP), and the lateral patellofemoral ligament (LPF).

(From Ficat RP, Hungerford DS: Disorders of the Patello-Femoral Joint. Baltimore, Williams and Wilkins, 1977, pp 16, 17.)

oblique band of the lateral retinaculum that extends from the iliotibial band to the patella,[620, 621] the delicate nature and often absence of the medial and lateral patellofemoral ligaments,[621, 622] the dependence of the width of the lateral patellofemoral ligament on the shape of the patella,[622] the negative correlation between the length of the patellar tendon and the width of the medial patellofemoral ligament,[623] and the presence of medial and lateral patellotibial ligaments (Fig. 16–156).[620, 621] Regardless of these variations, as a group, the lateral soft tissue stabilizers are stronger than the medial soft tissue stabilizers.

The four components of the quadriceps muscle represent the active elements of the soft tissue stabilizers.

Figure 16–156
Anterior supporting structures: Anatomic considerations. Patellofemoral and patellotibial ligaments. These structures act as static stabilizers of the patella. (From Linton RC, Indelicato PA: The knee. *In* JC DeLee, D Drez Jr [Eds]: Orthopaedic Sports Medicine: Principles and Practice. Philadelphia, WB Saunders Co, 1994, p 1168.)

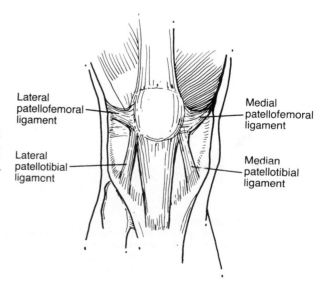

These components are the rectus femoris, vastus lateralis, vastus medialis, and vastus intermedius muscles, which terminate as four tendons that merge several centimeters above the patella, forming the quadriceps tendon, and subsequently attach to the patella. Except for the rectus femoris, all of these muscles take origin from the proximal half of the femur; the rectus femoris originates partly from the pelvis and anterior region of the hip.[619] Three layers of the quadriceps tendon can be identified. The tendon of the rectus femoris muscle is located in the superficial layer. As it descends, its tendinous fibers become deeper in location, situated beneath the fleshy muscle fibers. This tendon attaches to the anterior surface of the patella, with a distal extension that continues on to attach to the superficial part of the patellar tendon. The intermediate or middle layer of the quadriceps tendon results from the fusion of the tendons of the vastus lateralis and vastus medialis muscles. Together, the fused tendons of these two muscles attach to the base of the patella, just posterior to the insertion site of the rectus femoris fibers; individually, they extend over the lateral and medial borders of the patella.[617] They contribute to the medial and lateral retinacula by the continuation of their aponeurosis or investing fascia.[619] The tendon of the vastus intermedius muscle occupies the third, and deepest, layer of the quadriceps tendon, inserting into the base of the patella.

Some authors emphasize a separate distal portion of the vastus medialis muscle, designated the vastus medialis obliquus (Fig. 16–157).[623] The fibers of this muscle arise from the distal medial intermuscular septum and adductor tubercle and insert on the proximal and medial aspect of the patella. These fibers function mainly to balance the normally dominant laterally directed forces on the patella. Similarly, a vastus lateralis obliquus muscle has been described with variable anatomic features.[624] The genu articularis muscle is the final component of the extensor mechanism, arising from the distal portion of the femur and inserting into the suprapatellar pouch.[619, 1139] This muscle retracts the pouch proximally as the knee extends, an action that may not occur properly when a thickened suprapatellar plica is present.

Several bursae exist superficial and deep to these anterior supporting structures. The deep infrapatellar, or pretibial, bursa is situated at the base of the infrapatellar fat body, between the patellar tendon in front and the anterosuperior portion of the tibia behind. Prepatellar bursae exist in front of the patella itself. They may be situated in the subcutaneous tissue, in the aponeurosis, or in the tendinous fibers.

Variations in the shape of the patella, as well as of the patellar surface of the femur, are well recognized,[625–628] and some of these may be causative factors of patellar instability and retropatellar pain. Several classification systems exist for patellar shape (Fig. 16–158), that of Wiberg[625] being cited most often. The Wiberg classification system includes three types of patellar configuration: type 1 patellae have medial and lateral patellar facets, approximately equal in size, both with a concave appearance; type 2 patellae (the most common type) also have concave articular surfaces, with the medial facet being slightly smaller than the lateral facet; and type 3 patellae possess a small medial facet with a convex articular surface. The value of this and other classification systems of patellar (and distal femoral) shape in predicting the likelihood of patellofemoral instability has yet to be proved, and the precision of detecting patellar shape on the basis of axial radiographs of the knee (or transaxial sections provided by CT or MR imaging) requires further study.

The patella has several functions, the most important of which is strengthening the force of knee extension by providing a more anterior fulcrum for this movement. The relationship of the patella and the femur depends on the degree of flexion or extension of the knee. In the fully extended position, the patella lies above the trochlear surface of the femur, and it rests on a layer of subsynovial fat.[625] Its precise position in a mediolateral direction in the extended knee depends on the degree of contraction of the quadriceps mechanism.[617] Furthermore, the "screw home" mechanism of the femorotibial joint that occurs in the final degrees of extension, in which the tibia rotates externally with respect to the femur, lateralizes the tibial tubercle.[617] This external rotation produces a valgus vector between the line of pull of the quadriceps tendon and that of the patellar tendon, designated the Q angle. This vector is resisted by the passive and active medial stabilizers of the knee. As the knee is flexed, the tibia rotates internally, decreasing the Q angle and the lateral vector, and contact of the patella and the trochlea increases, initially involving the lower pole of the patella, and later more

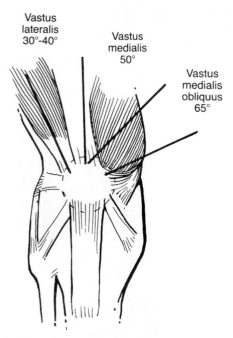

Figure 16–157

Anterior supporting structures: Anatomic considerations. Various muscular elements of the quadriceps. Different portions attach at different angles to the long axis of the thigh, creating various vectors of force. (From Linton RC, Indelicato PA: The knee. *In* JC DeLee, D Drez Jr [Eds]: Orthopaedic Sports Medicine: Principles and Practice. Philadelphia, WB Saunders Co, 1994, p 1166.)

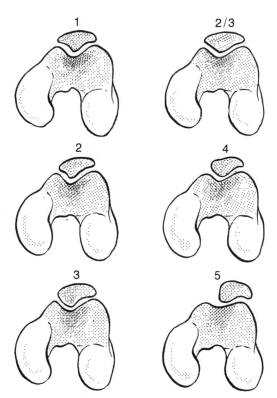

Figure 16–158
Patella: Anatomic variations in shape. Patellar configurations have been delineated by Wiberg, Baumgarten, and other investigators and are summarized in this drawing. For each image, the medial condyle is depicted on the left and the lateral condyle is depicted on the right. Type 1 patellae have equal facets, which are slightly concave. Type 2 patellae are similar, with concave surfaces and a smaller medial facet. Type 3 patellae possess a small medial facet with a convex surface. Type 2/3 patellae have a flat medial facet. Type 4 patellae possess a small or absent medial facet. Type 5 (Jagerhut) patellae demonstrate no medial facet, no central ridge, and lateral subluxation.

and more of the patellar surface. Increasing stability is afforded by the trochlea as it embraces the patella.[617] The point at which the patella becomes centered in the trochlea varies, although at 90 degrees of knee flexion, centering of the patella in the trochlea is an almost universal finding.[629] At this degree of flexion, or with further flexion of the knee beyond 90 degrees, the quadriceps tendon and, eventually, the odd facet of the patella articulate with portions of the femur.[627, 630] The size of the contact area between femur and patella varies according to the position of the knee. In general, the contact area is greater with increasing degrees of knee flexion.[630]

In a departure from conventional descriptions of the functional anatomy and biomechanics of the patellofemoral joint, Ho and Jaureguito[666] highlight 12 basic concepts fundamental to an understanding of these very complex subjects. Their analysis includes the following information.

Concept 1: Variations in the anatomy of the quadriceps mechanism from one person to another are the norm rather than the exception.
Concept 2: Specific characteristics of the quadriceps complex correlate significantly with patellar shape. As in-

dicated earlier, variations in the lateral structures of the quadriceps complex are especially striking,[622] and modifications of the shape of the patella (a sesamoid bone formed within the substance of the quadriceps tendon) reflect a response to the forces acting on it.
Concept 3: The medial patellofemoral ligament is the major restraint to lateral displacement of the patella. In one study, this ligament contributed more than 50 per cent of the restraint to lateral displacement of the patella, whereas the patellomeniscal ligament and associated retinacular fibers of the deep capsular layer of the knee contributed about 20 per cent of this restraint.[667]
Concept 4: Patellar motion occurs in 6 degrees of freedom relative to the femur with flexion and extension of the knee. Thus, the motion arc of the patella is complex, involving both rotation and translation. As the knee is extended, the patella translates anteriorly, medially, and proximally and, simultaneously, it rotates into valgus angulation in the coronal plane, internally in the transaxial plane, and into extension in the sagittal plane.
Concept 5: The relationship between the patella and the tibia also changes in a complex way during flexion and extension of the knee. With extension of the knee, the patella shifts anteriorly with respect to the tibia, the patellar tendon extends about 30 degrees in the sagittal plane, the patella extends about 20 degrees relative to the tibia, and the patella shifts proximally.
Concept 6: Patellar motion is the result of interaction of three bones (femur, tibia, patella), one bone-tendon unit (patella-patellar tendon-tibia), and one muscle complex (quadriceps mechanism).
Concept 7: Patellofemoral contact area changes in both size and location with knee flexion. As the knee flexes from 20 to 90 degrees, the contact area increases by more than one third in size and moves proximally. This increase in the patellofemoral contact area with increasing knee flexion serves to dissipate the greater contact forces that occur in the flexed knee.
Concept 8: Patellofemoral contact force, in the sagittal plane, is maximal between 60 and 110 degrees of knee flexion. Patellofemoral contact force depends on three factors: the quadriceps tendon tensile force, the patellar tendon tensile force, and the angle between them.
Concept 9: Force across the patellofemoral joint also has a laterally directed component in the coronal plane. The angle of the component vector forces commonly is measured as the quadriceps, or Q, angle. The smaller the Q angle, the less is the magnitude of the laterally directed forces.
Concept 10: Patellofemoral contact pressure, which depends on both contact force and area, also is maximal between 60 and 90 degrees of knee flexion.
Concept 11: The tensile force of the patellar tendon is greater than that of the quadriceps tendon with mild knee flexion and less than that of the quadriceps tendon with moderate to severe knee flexion.
Concept 12: The anteroposterior thickness of the patella

provides a mechanical advantage for the quadriceps mechanism in extending the knee.

Pathologic Considerations

Abnormalities of the anterior supporting structures of the knee are related to alterations in the anatomy of the patella and adjacent patellar articular surface of the femur and the constantly changing compressive and tensile forces generated during the complex movement of this joint. The syndromes and disorders related to disuse, overuse, misuse, or injuries of various anterior supporting structures include chondromalacia patellae, patellar tendinitis, disruption of the quadriceps musculature and tendon and of the patellar tendon, osteochondritis dissecans of the patella, osteochondral fractures of the patella and femur, patellar instability with subluxation or dislocation, Osgood-Schlatter disease, and deep infrapatellar and prepatellar bursitis. A review of some of these entities is provided in the following sections of this chapter, but the interested reader also should refer to Chapter 8 dealing with osteochondritis dissecans and osteochondral fractures of the patella. Consideration of chondromalacia patellae also is included in the discussion of the assessment of articular cartilage later in this chapter.

Patellar Tendinitis

Patellar tendinitis appears to represent an overuse syndrome related to sudden and repetitive extension of the knee that may occur in persons, particularly athletes, involved in such activities as kicking, jumping, and running.[631–633] This syndrome, often referred to as jumper's knee, leads to local pain, swelling, and tenderness that ultimately may result in disruption of the patellar tendon. As the major histologic findings associated with patellar tendinitis are not those of inflammation but rather those of fiber failure, mucoid degeneration, and fibrinoid necrosis,[631, 634] the term tendinitis may be inappropriate, as inflammatory changes may represent the response to the injury rather than the primary event.[635] Clinical manifestations include activity-related pain below the patella that initially is intermittent but may become persistent.[632] Men are involved more commonly than women.

It is apparent that similar physical activities lead to age-associated overuse syndromes of the infrapatellar region. In growing children, for example, Osgood-Schlatter disease affecting the tibial tuberosity is seen (Fig. 16–159); in adolescents and young adults, Sinding-Larsen-Johansson disease or insertional tendinopathy in the inferior margin of the patella is encountered; and in the young adult, the patellar tendon itself may be affected.

Routine radiographs usually do not provide diagnostic information in cases of patellar tendinitis. Soft tissue swelling, thickening of the patellar tendon, and obscuration of portions of the infrapatellar fat body may be evident, but these findings are depicted more easily on CT scans and MR images. Bone scintigraphy shows nonspecific accumulation of the radionuclide in the

infrapatellar soft tissues or patella.[636] Ultrasonography reveals an enlarged and hypoechoic tendon, particularly in its proximal portion.[637–639] With CT, the enlarged tendon with central expansion near the inferior pole of the patella and with decreased attenuation values is evident.[638]

MR images in the sagittal plane display the entire length of the patellar tendon (Fig. 16–160).[640, 641] In an analysis of such images in asymptomatic persons, Schweitzer and associates[642] noted that the mean thickness of the patellar tendon was 5.2 mm, being slightly thicker in men. The mean ratio of the thickness of the patellar tendon to the thickness of the quadriceps tendon in this study was 0.72. Focal regions of increased signal intensity within the patellar tendon in T1-weighted spin echo MR images were frequent, particularly proximally, and the signal intensity did not increase in T2-weighted spin echo MR images. Schweitzer and coworkers[642] also observed subtle buckling of the patellar tendon in these asymptomatic persons, a finding that was more prominent in those with joint effusions.

Reiff and associates[643] studied the appearance of the patellar tendon in patients without anterior knee pain using gradient echo MR imaging sequences. They noted some variability in the anteroposterior width, or thickness, of the tendon, particularly superiorly and inferiorly; although widths greater than 7 mm in the proximal aspect of the tendon were encountered both in men and in women, values above 8 mm were very infrequent. Furthermore, these investigators noted increased signal intensity in the superior portion of the tendon in 75 per cent of subjects and in the inferior portion of the tendon in 43 per cent of subjects.

Transaxial MR images in normal persons typically display an ovoid patellar tendon. This imaging plane is ideal for examination of the retinacula.

MR imaging in patients with patellar tendinitis shows an enlarged sagittal diameter of the tendon, with a mean value of 10.9 mm in one series (Fig. 16–161).[635] The proximal portion of the patellar tendon usually is thickened more than its distal portion,[1142] but in severe cases both portions may be involved.[635, 638] An indistinct margin to the posterior aspect of the tendon may be combined with regions of increased intratendinous signal intensity.[634, 635, 1141] The increased signal intensity may be more evident on STIR images or with the use of intravenous administration of a gadolinium compound.[644]

As indicated previously, in certain MR imaging sequences, such as spoiled gradient recalled images in the steady state (spoiled GRASS), foci of increased signal intensity may be seen in tendons that are not enlarged. The cause of these foci is not clear. Regions of cartilage metaplasia or mucoid degeneration may be responsible for these changes. Mucoid degeneration has been documented as a histologic occurrence in patellar tendons, sometimes in association with cystic enlargement (mucoid cysts) of the tendon.[645, 1140]

The application of intravenous gadolinium-enhanced MR imaging sequences to the analysis of disorders of the patellar tendon has indicated a spectrum of abnormalities affecting the entheseal region of the proximal

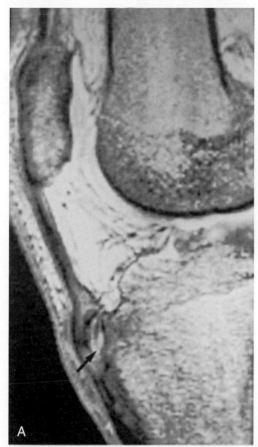

Figure 16–159

Osgood-Schlatter disease: MR imaging.

A A sagittal gradient echo MR image (fast imaging with steady-state precession [FISP]) (TR/TE, 30/10; flip angle, 40 degrees) in a 21 year old man demonstrates a small ossicle separate from the tibial tuberosity (arrow) and a patellar tendon that is of normal size except for mild thickening distally.

B, C In this 35 year old woman, sagittal T1-weighted (TR/TE, 650/20) **(B)** and T2-weighted (TR/TE, 1800/90) **(C)** spin echo MR images reveal a prominent tibial tuberosity, deep infrapatellar bursitis (arrows), and anterior displacement of the patellar tendon. A large separate ossicle (arrowhead) is seen.

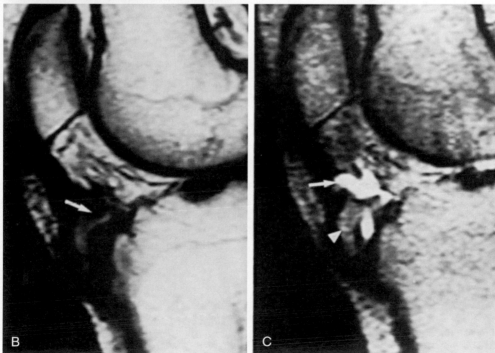

Illustration continued on following page

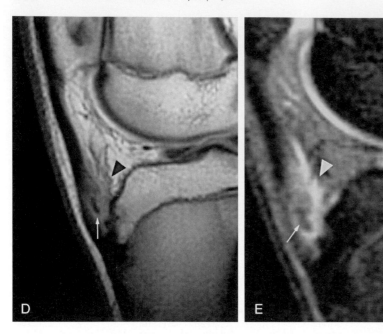

Figure 16–159 *Continued*

D, E In a 14 year old girl, a bone fragment (arrows) and surrounding edema (arrowheads) are evident in sagittal proton density (TR/TE, 2100/20) spin echo **(D)** and MPGR (TR/TE, 700/18; flip angle, 30 degrees) **(E)** MR images. (Courtesy of D. Berthoty, M.D., Las Vegas, Nevada.)

portion of the tendon.[644] The vulnerability of this insertional area is well recognized, and it is subject to a vast array of problems, which include patellar tendinitis, proliferative enthesopathy, avulsion injury, Sinding-Larsen-Johansson disease, patellar sleeve injury, and partial or complete tendon rupture. Different patterns of contrast enhancement of signal intensity would be expected and have been observed,[644] although the precise clinical value of intravenous administration of a gadolinium compound in assessing patellar tendon abnormalities is not yet clear. As in the tendons of other regions of

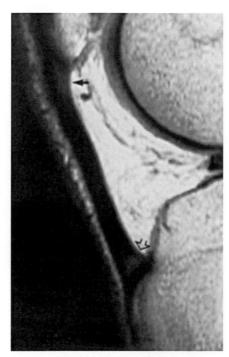

Figure 16–160
Normal patellar tendon: MR imaging. As shown in this sagittal proton density–weighted (TR/TE, 3000/20) spin echo MR image, the patellar tendon typically is of low signal intensity throughout its length, although intermediate signal intensity in the posterior margin of the proximal portion of the tendon (solid arrow) and in a triangular area near its distal insertion (open arrow) may be evident. (Courtesy of J. Yu, M.D., Columbus, Ohio.)

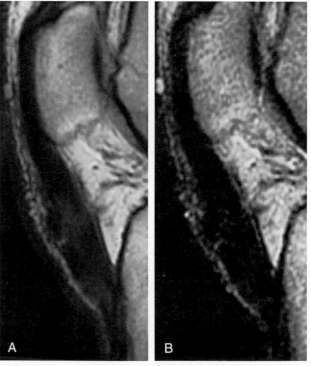

Figure 16–161
Chronic patellar tendinitis: MR imaging. Sagittal proton density–weighted (TR/TE, 2200/30) **(A)** and T2-weighted (TR/TE, 2200/80) **(B)** spin echo MR images show marked thickening of the entire patellar tendon, more pronounced in the middle and distal segments, and indistinctness of the anterior margin of the tendon. No increase in signal intensity within the patellar tendon is seen in **B.** (Courtesy of J. Yu, M.D., Columbus, Ohio.)

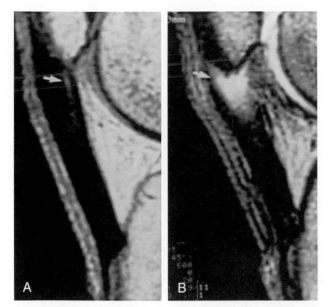

Figure 16–162
Partial tears of the patellar tendon: MR imaging. A sagittal T1-weighted (TR/TE, 850/25) spin echo MR image **(A)** and a sagittal MPGR MR image (TR/TE, 600/20; flip angle, 45 degrees) **(B)** reveal a partial tear (arrows) involving the proximal portion of the patellar tendon and thickening of the entire tendon, indicating chronic patellar tendinitis. The findings of partial patellar tendon rupture are much more pronounced in **B**. (Courtesy of S. Fernandez, M.D., Mexico City, Mexico.)

the body (such as the ankle), a continuum of alterations appears to exist, which range from tendon degeneration or inflammation (i.e., tendinitis) to partial or complete disruption or tearing of the tendon. This underscores the dictum that normal tendons rarely, if ever, rupture.

Quadriceps Tendinitis

Involvement of the quadriceps tendon by a condition similar to patellar tendinitis is rare.[619] More typically, avulsion injuries at the patellar insertion sites of the quadriceps tendon are observed.

Tears of the Patellar and Quadriceps Tendons

Indirect forces applied to the extensor mechanism of the knee can lead to failure of one or more of its components, including the patella, quadriceps tendon, or patellar tendon.[646] Failure of the patella, resulting in fracture, is common, especially in adults (see later discussion). Systemic disorders, such as rheumatoid arthritis, chronic renal disease, and systemic lupus erythematosus, contribute to failure of the quadriceps and patellar tendons, although such failure, particularly of the patellar tendon, may occur in the absence of these causative factors. Patellar tendon ruptures are not uncommon in persons with chronic patellar tendinitis, and they may occur spontaneously or after vigorous physical exercise. Failure of the patellar tendon usually occurs at its junction with the inferior pole of the patella or, less commonly, with the tibial tuberosity, although intrasub-

stance disruption of the patellar tendon also may occur. Complete tears of the patellar tendon are associated with a high position of the patella, designated patella alta. Incomplete tears are unassociated with this change in patellar position. Although CT and ultrasonography can be used to verify complete or incomplete tears of the patellar tendon, MR imaging displays these tears most vividly (Figs. 16–162, 16–163, and 16–164). Typically, the tendon is thickened, and complete or incomplete disruption of its fibers is evident. In recent tears, foci of increased signal intensity are observed in the patellar tendon and adjacent soft tissues on T2-weighted spin echo, certain gradient echo, and STIR images.

Partial or complete tears of the quadriceps tendon may result from an injury involving a direct blow to the tendon or forceful flexion of the knee[647]; or they may occur spontaneously in association with such chronic diseases as systemic lupus erythematosus, rheumatoid arthritis, gout, or renal failure, or after corticosteroid therapy.[648–653] Rarely, spontaneous rupture of the quadriceps tendon occurs in healthy persons.[654, 655] Unilateral or bilateral tendon disruptions have been described. The clinical diagnosis of a complete tear of the quadriceps tendon usually is obvious from the patient's history, his or her inability to extend the knee, a hemarthrosis or soft tissue hematoma, and a palpable or visible gap in the soft tissues above the patella.[635, 656–658] Delays in such diagnosis are encountered, however, which in one report ranged from 14 days to 1 year after the injury.[656]

Routine radiographic findings associated with complete tears of the quadriceps tendon include soft tissue

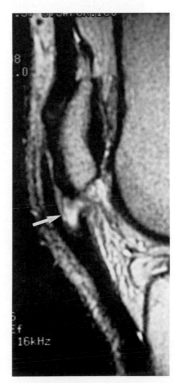

Figure 16–163
Complete tears of the patellar tendon: MR imaging. The sagittal T2-weighted (TR/TE, 4466/90) spin echo MR image vividly displays the site of tendon disruption (arrow).

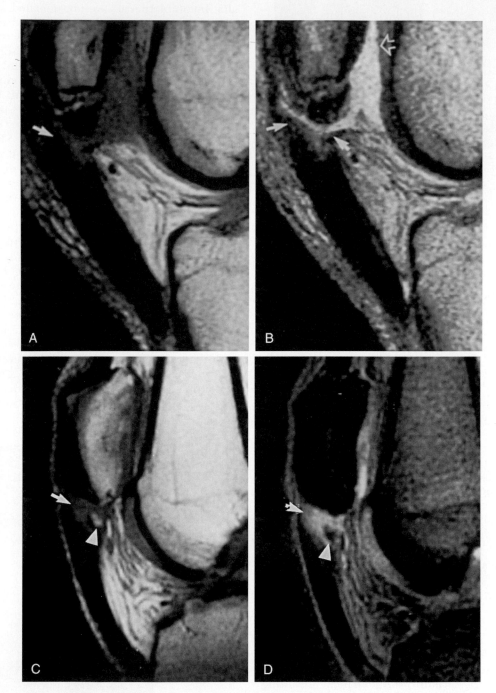

Figure 16–164
Complete tears of the patellar tendon: MR imaging.

   A, B Sagittal proton density–weighted (TR/TE, 2000/20) **(A)** and T2-weighted (TR/TE, 2000/80) **(B)** spin echo MR images reveal complete disruption (solid arrows) of the patellar tendon at its proximal insertion site. The tendon is thickened, fragmentation of the lower pole of the patella is seen, soft tissue edema is present, and a hemarthrosis with a fluid level (open arrow) is evident. (Courtesy of J. Lyons, M.D., San Diego, California.)

   C, D In a second patient, similar findings (arrows) including bone fragmentation (arrowheads) are shown in sagittal proton density–weighted (TR/TE, 1000/20) spin echo **(C)** and MPGR (TR/TE, 550/15; flip angle, 20 degrees) **(D)** MR images. (Courtesy of M. Schweitzer, M.D., Philadelphia, Pennsylvania.)

swelling, distortion of soft tissue planes above the patella, an inferior position of the patella (patella infera or patella baja), calcification or ossification within portions of an avulsed patellar fragment, and an undulating patellar tendon.[651] Similar but less dramatic findings accompany partial tears of the quadriceps tendon. Standard arthrography in cases of partial[659] or complete[660] disruptions of the quadriceps tendon may be diagnostic. Contrast material introduced into the knee joint will extend outside the quadriceps tendon[661] and, in some cases, will extend into the deep infrapatellar or prepatellar bursa. Owing to the superficial location of the quadriceps tendon, ultrasonography also may be used in its assessment.[662, 663]

Sagittal MR images display the quadriceps tendon in exquisite detail (Fig. 16–165). A laminated appearance with two, three, or four layers of tissue characterizes the MR imaging appearance of the normal quadriceps tendon.[664] This laminated structure is more evident in the medial aspect of the tendon, and its lateral portion may appear as a single thick band of low signal intensity. Transaxial MR images confirm that the superficial layer of the quadriceps tendon originates from the rectus femoris muscle, the deep layer originates from the vastus intermedius muscle, and the middle layer (or layers) is composed of fibers derived from the vastus medialis and vastus lateralis muscles.[664] The average thickness (anteroposterior plane) of the quadriceps tendon, defined in MR images, is approximately 8 mm, and its average width (mediolateral plane) is approximately 35 mm.

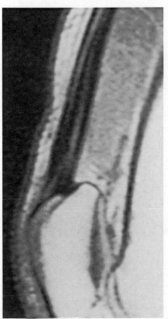

Figure 16–165

Normal quadriceps tendon: MR imaging. A sagittal proton density–weighted (TR/TE, 3000/20) spin echo MR image shows a trilaminar appearance of the quadriceps tendon. The superficial layer relates to the tendon of the rectus femoris muscle, the middle layer relates to the tendons of the vastus medialis and vastus lateralis muscles, and the deep layer relates to the tendon of the vastus intermedius muscle. (Courtesy of J. Yu, M.D., Columbus, Ohio.)

With the knee in full extension, the normal quadriceps tendon appears as a relatively straight band of tissue of low signal intensity in sagittal MR images, and in these images the patellar tendon also is straight and of low signal intensity. Tears of the quadriceps tendon lead to partial or complete interruption of its fibers (Figs. 16–166, 16–167, 16–168, and 16–169), displayed in all three imaging planes.[657, 658, 664] An undulating, corrugated, or wrinkled appearance to the patellar tendon in the sagittal MR images is secondary evidence of disruption of the quadriceps tendon or some other portion of the extensor mechanism (Fig. 16–170),[657] although it is not a specific finding (appearing as a normal finding in a hyperextended knee). In cases of partial tears of the quadriceps tendon, the alterations in its morphology, as depicted by MR imaging, are more subtle, although careful assessment of serial transaxial images usually allows a correct diagnosis.[664] With either partial or complete tears of this tendon, hemorrhage and edema lead to an increase in signal intensity on T2-weighted spin echo and some gradient echo MR images in the acute stage.[640, 641]

Patellofemoral Instability

Patellofemoral instability is a frequent and complex problem that has been studied extensively. The clinical diagnosis of such instability often is difficult, as the resulting symptoms and signs may simulate those of other disorders of the knee. Although observation of the manner in which the patella moves with respect to the femur during flexion and extension of the knee can be accomplished during physical examination, alterations in such movement may be subtle and, further, disagreement exists regarding the precise normal position of the patella during various degrees of flexion and extension of the knee.[629, 665] It is not surprising, therefore, that clinicians have turned to other diagnostic techniques in an effort to provide verification of patellofemoral tracking abnormalities.

Routine radiography, employing standard radiographic projections, has been used to define the position of the patella, particularly in the vertical plane. On the basis of the lateral projection, the position of the patella relative to the joint line can be ascertained. A high-riding patella, or patella alta, has been associated with recurrent lateral patellar subluxations or dislocations, chondromalacia patellae, Sinding-Larsen-Johansson disease, and joint effusions.[617, 667–670, 1144] A low-riding patella, or patella baja, has been identified in neuromuscular disorders, in achondroplasia, and after certain surgical procedures involving transfer of the tibial tuberosity.[617] A number of different methods based on the patellar position in the lateral radiograph have been described to confirm the presence of patella alta or patella baja[1143]; the Insall-Salvati ratio[669] and methods described by Blumensaat,[671] Brattstrom,[672] and Labelle and Laurin[673] are most popular. The advantage of the Insall-Salvati method is its nondependency on the degree of flexion of the knee joint. This technique requires determination of the length of the patellar tendon and that of the patella (Fig. 16–171). The normal

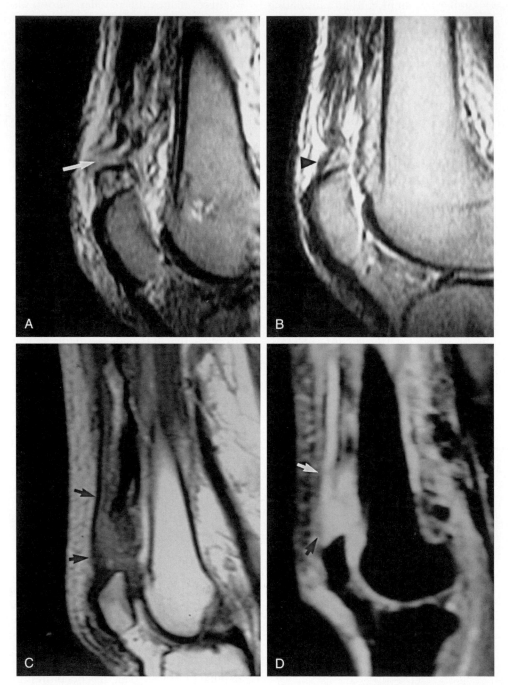

Figure 16–166

Partial and complete tears of the quadriceps tendon: MR imaging.

   A, B This 76 year old man stumbled and then was unable to extend either knee. Sagittal T2-weighted (TR/TE, 2000/80) spin echo MR images reveal a complete tear of the quadriceps tendon (arrow) of the right knee **(A)** and a partial tear of the quadriceps tendon (arrowhead) of the left knee **(B).** The patient had no underlying systemic disorder. Surgery confirmed the MR imaging findings.

   C, D In a 72 year old man, a sagittal T1-weighted (TR/TE, 500/15) spin echo MR image **(C)** and a sagittal STIR MR image (TR/TE, 3675/19; inversion time, 140 msec) **(D)** show disruption of most of the quadriceps tendon, although the tendinous fibers (arrows) of the rectus femoris muscle are intact.

Figure 16–167
Complete tears of the quadriceps tendon: MR imaging. Transaxial proton density–weighted (TR/TE, 2000/30) **(A)** and sagittal T2-weighted (TR/TE, 2500/80) **(B)** spin echo MR images reveal evidence of an acute complete tear (arrows) of the quadriceps tendon. (Courtesy of D. Levey, M.D., Corpus Christi, Texas.)

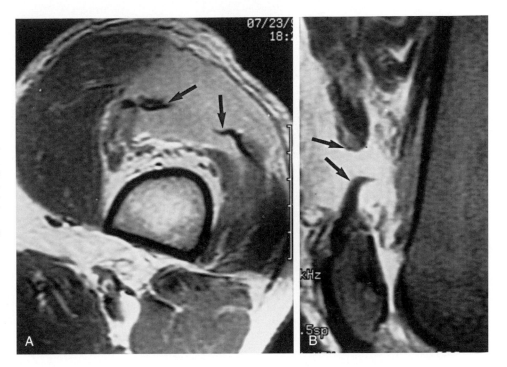

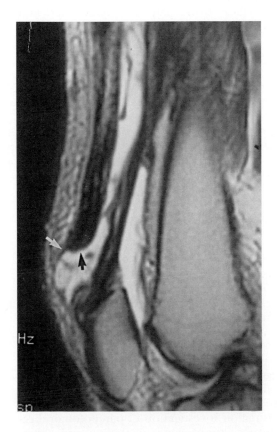

Figure 16–168
Partial tears of the quadriceps tendon: MR imaging. Although some tendinous fibers of the vastus medialis muscle remain attached to the patella, most of the quadriceps tendon is disrupted (arrows), as shown in a sagittal fast spin echo (TR/TE, 3300/102) MR image. (Courtesy of D. Goodwin, M.D., Hanover, New Hampshire.)

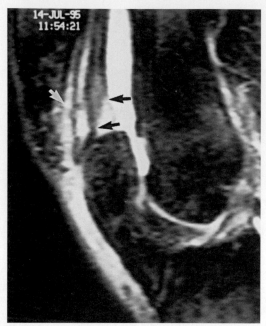

Figure 16–169
Partial tears of the quadriceps tendon: MR imaging. This sagittal STIR MR image (TR/TE, 2755/19; inversion time, 140 msec) shows an acute partial tear (arrows) of the quadriceps tendon that occurred spontaneously in a 74 year old woman.

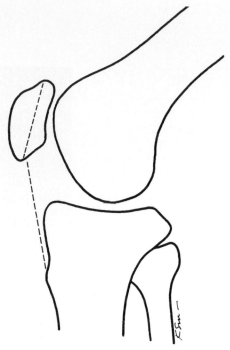

Figure 16–171
Patellar position: Insall-Salvati method. The ratio of patellar tendon length to the greatest diagonal length of the patella may be used to diagnose patella alta.

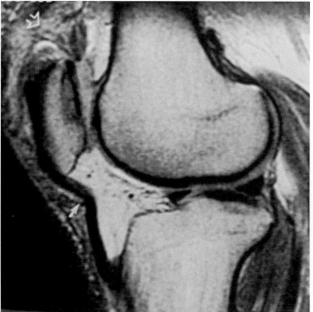

Figure 16–170
Complete tear of the quadriceps tendon: MR imaging. A sagittal proton density–weighted (TR/TE, 2000/20) spin echo MR image demonstrates an abnormal contour of the patellar tendon (solid arrow) related to a complete tear (open arrow) of the quadriceps tendon.

ratio is approximately 1. Drawbacks to this method, including inability to identify precisely the insertion site of the patellar tendon and, more importantly, variations in patellar shape, have led to interest in a modified

Insall-Salvati ratio, in which the length or location of the articular surface of the patella is determined and compared with the position of the joint line or the length of the patellar tendon.[674–676]

Axial radiographic views used to access the configuration of the trochlea, the patellar shape, and the relationship of the patella to the femur also have been employed.[617] A variety of different techniques, noted earlier in this chapter, are available, but all emphasize the inadequacy of the standard "skyline" view in assessing the patellar position. As this view is obtained with knee flexion beyond 90 degrees, it does not allow examination of the patellofemoral relationships in lesser degrees of knee flexion, during which patellar instability is a greater problem. Thus, axial radiographic projections obtained with 20, 30, or 45 degrees of knee flexion have advantages when compared with the skyline view,[617, 677, 678] and may allow detection not only of patellar displacement but also of patellar tilt when a number of lines are constructed and angles measured (Fig. 16–172).

Transaxial images provided by CT and MR imaging (Fig. 16–173) allow assessment of patellar position with the knee extended and with minor degrees of knee flexion (with and without contraction of the quadriceps mechanism).[629, 665, 679–684] As with routine radiographs, a number of lines are constructed on the transaxial CT or MR images and the angles between these lines are measured to document the presence of patellar subluxation, patellar tilt, or both conditions.[683] Both imaging techniques also allow investigation of patellofemoral relationships during various stages of flexion and extension of the knee, usually accomplished by obtaining multiple static images that are viewed in a movie for-

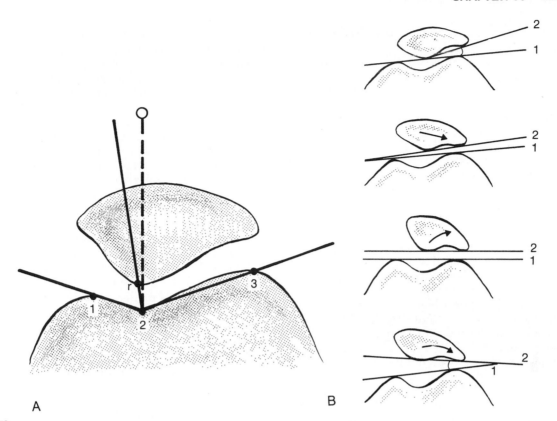

A

B

Figure 16–172

Patellar position: Methods of measurement of lateral patellar displacement and patellar tilt.

A Merchant and coworkers (Merchant AC, et al: J Bone Joint Surg [Am] *56*:1391, 1974) have suggested that on an axial radiograph, the line connecting the median ridge of the patella (r) and trochlear depth (2) should fall medial to or slightly lateral to a line (O) bisecting angle 1-2-3. Here the first line lies medial to line O, a normal finding.

B Laurin and coworkers have indicated other measurements that might be appropriate. The upper two diagrams reveal the normal situation; the lower two diagrams indicate the abnormal situation. On axial radiographs, normally an angle formed between a line connecting the anterior aspect of the femoral condyles (1) and a second line along the lateral facet of the patella (2) opens laterally. In patients with subluxation of the patella, these lines are parallel or the angle of intersection opens medially. In practice, abnormal patellar tilting (as shown in the bottom two diagrams) can occur without patellar subluxation.

(**B,** From Laurin CA, et al: J Bone Joint Surg [Am] *60*:55, 1978.)

mat.[685] Kinematic MR imaging of the patellofemoral joint has been studied extensively by Shellock and colleagues,[686–690] Brossmann and coworkers,[691, 692] and Niitsu and colleagues.[693] Newer modifications of these techniques allow active movement by the patient, loading the knee to better simulate walking or other physical activities, rapid scanning with a variety of gradient re-

called imaging methods, and motion-triggered cine MR imaging. These methods have provided information regarding patterns of lateral subluxation of the patella; the excessive lateral pressure syndrome associated with tilting of the patella (with little or no associated lateral displacement), which increases with flexion of the knee; and medial displacement of the patella, which may oc-

Figure 16–173

Patellofemoral instability: CT scanning. This transaxial CT scan, obtained with the knees flexed 20 degrees, shows lateral subluxation of both patellae.

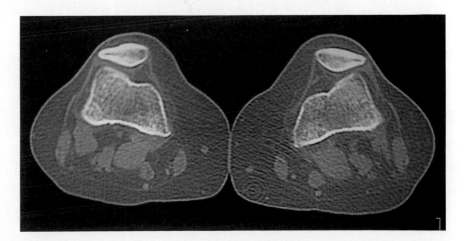

cur as a complication of arthroscopic lateral retinacular release.[687, 694]

Lateral dislocation (or subluxation) of the patella often is a transient phenomenon, with spontaneous reduction.[695] Diagnosis made on the basis of results of physical examination and clinical history may be difficult, and identification of characteristic osteochondral and avulsion fractures on routine radiographs provides important information in many cases (see Chapter 8 and later discussion). Patellar dislocations usually result from a twisting injury with the knee in flexion and the femur rotated internally on a fixed foot. The patella is pulled laterally from the trochlea and across the lateral femoral condyle, leading to osteochondral injuries of the medial patellar facet, lateral femoral condyle, or both structures.[696] The medial retinaculum is injured as a result of distraction, or a small avulsion fracture occurs at the patellar site of attachment of the medial retinaculum. These pathologic findings can be observed directly on MR images of the knee obtained shortly after the injury (Figs. 16–174, 16–175, and 16–176).[696–698] Bone contusions lead to signal intensity changes in the marrow that reflect edema (Fig. 16–177).[699, 700] The location of the marrow edema in the lateral femoral condyle after a patellar dislocation may be more lateral and superior to that seen with anterior cruciate ligament injuries.[696] A sprain of the medial retinaculum is characterized by thickening and increased signal intensity in T2-weighted spin echo MR images, related to edema and hemorrhage; disruption and avulsion of the retinaculum are associated with loss of integrity of its fibers, with similar changes in signal intensity.[696] Defects in the articular cartilage of the patella also may be evident, but their detection with MR imaging often requires specialized sequences (see later discussion). After a lateral patellar dislocation, the patella may assume a more lateral position or may be tilted abnormally, owing to loss of integrity of the medial retinaculum.

Excessive Lateral Pressure Syndrome

Although traditionally axial radiographs of the knee have been used to diagnose lateral subluxation of the patella with respect to the femur, they occasionally demonstrate a normally located patella that is abnormally tilted to the lateral side. This finding led to the concept of an excessive lateral pressure syndrome affecting the articular surface of the lateral facet of the patella and that of the adjacent articular portion of the femur. The clinical manifestations of this syndrome have been well summarized by Ficat and Hungerford.[617] Adults or adolescents are affected, and patellofemoral pain, sometimes precipitated by an injury, is evident. Manual subluxation of the patella while the patient flexes the knee may initiate or aggravate the pain. Loss of articular cartilage in the lateral facet of the patella and adjacent articular portion of the femur, in addition to sclerosis and cyst formation in the subchondral bone of the patella and femur, may be observed. The cartilage loss is believed to be more extensive than and to differ in location from that seen in classic chondromalacia patellae.[617] Causes of the excessive lateral pressure syndrome are not clear, but they may relate to breakdown in one or more of the structures that contribute to medial stability of the patella (e.g., medial retinaculum and vastus medialis muscle) or to alterations in the shape of the lateral trochlea or lateral articular facet of the patella.[617]

Chondromalacia Patellae

Chondromalacia patellae is a term applied to cartilage loss involving one or more portions of the patella that leads to patellofemoral pain. Initially described in 1924 by Aleman[701] as a cause of crepitus and synovitis of the knee, the term has been applied loosely to a host of different disorders causing patellofemoral pain, in which loss of patellar cartilage either is not documented, is not present, or occurs in combination with other morphologic changes. This has led to the designation patellofemoral pain syndrome as a more appropriate description of those diseases associated with retropatellar pain.[617, 627, 702] Such disorders include (but are not limited to) prepatellar bursitis, deep infrapatellar bursi-

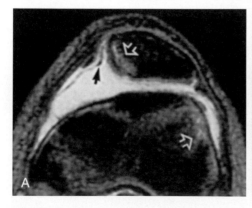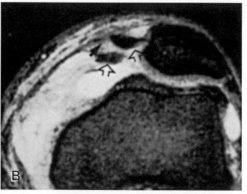

Figure 16–174

Patellofemoral instability: MR imaging.

A A transaxial MPGR MR image (TR/TE, 500/11; flip angle, 15 degrees) shows disruption of the medial patellar retinaculum (solid arrow) and marrow edema with increased signal intensity (open arrows) in the medial aspect of the patella and the lateral femoral condyle. A large joint effusion is present.

B A transaxial MPGR MR image (TR/TE, 500/11; flip angle, 15 degrees) in a second patient shows disruption of the medial patellar retinaculum (solid arrow) and two bone fragments (open arrows) that originated from the medial aspect of the patella. Note the large joint effusion and soft tissue edema. (Courtesy of S.K. Brahme, M.D., La Jolla, California.)

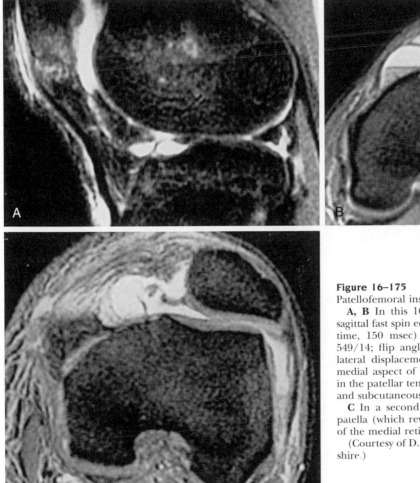
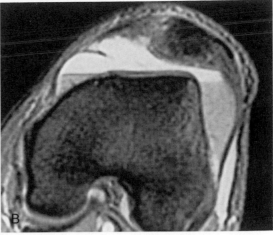

Figure 16–175
Patellofemoral instability: MR imaging.

A, B In this 16 year old girl with an acute injury, sagittal fast spin echo STIR (TR/TE, 3000/28; inversion time, 150 msec) **(A)** and transaxial MPGR (TR/TE, 549/14; flip angle, 15 degrees) **(B)** MR images show lateral displacement of the patella, a fracture of the medial aspect of the patella, abnormal signal intensity in the patellar tendon, a hemarthrosis with a fluid level, and subcutaneous edema.

C In a second patient, note the laterally displaced patella (which reveals cartilage irregularity) and a tear of the medial retinaculum.

(Courtesy of D. Goodwin, M.D., Hanover, New Hampshire.)

tis, pes anserinus bursitis, the plica syndrome, the excessive lateral pressure syndrome, osteoarthritis, and even meniscal tears.

Fundamental to the diagnosis of chondromalacia pa-

tellae is the presence of histologic abnormalities affecting the articular cartilage of the patella. Whether specific histologic findings in the articular cartilage allow separation of chondromalacia from other processes that

Figure 16–176
Patellofemoral instability: MR imaging. A transaxial FLASH (TR/TE, 400/20; flip angle, 10 degrees) MR image shows disruption (arrow) of the tendon of the vastus lateralis muscle in a patient with a previous traumatic medial dislocation of the patella.

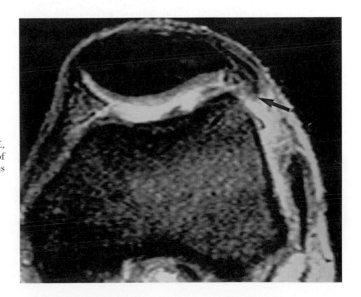

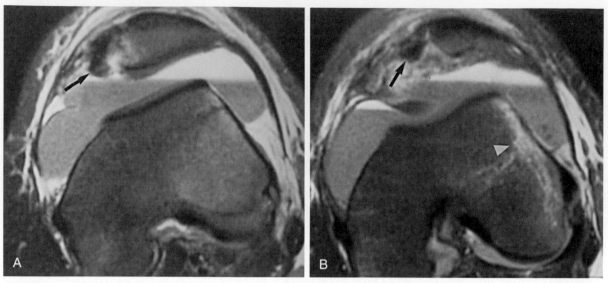

Figure 16–177

Patellofemoral instability: MR imaging. Transaxial fat-suppressed fast spin echo (TR/TE, 3500/85) MR images, with **A** located superior to **B,** reveal evidence of a previous lateral dislocation of the patella. Findings include a hemarthrosis (with fluid levels), disruption of the medial patellar retinaculum, fragmentation of the medial pole of the patella (arrows) and a bone bruise (arrowhead) in the lateral femoral condyle. (Courtesy of D. Witte, M.D., Memphis, Tennessee.)

involve the patellar cartilage is not clear. Goodfellow and colleagues[627] defined two separate processes, basal degeneration and surface degeneration, that affected the patellar cartilage. Basal degeneration was defined as fasciculation of collagen in the middle and deep zones of cartilage (that later might affect the chondral surface) and was believed to occur in the ridge separating the medial and odd facets of the patella in young persons, perhaps related to excessive pressure. Surface degeneration was thought to begin in the young and progress throughout life, perhaps culminating in osteoarthritis of the patellofemoral joint.

Numerous classification systems for chondromalacia patellae have been proposed, generally based on the anatomic extent or the severity of the articular cartilage loss in the patella. As assessment of patellar articular cartilage on the basis of routine and advanced imaging methods is difficult and often inadequate, accurate classification of chondromalacia patellae requires direct observation and even probing of the articular surface of the patella, which can be accomplished arthroscopically. Arthroscopically evident grades of chondromalacia have been described[703]: (1) fibrillation or softening of articular cartilage involving one or more facets of the patella, without involvement of the femur; (2) erosion or fragmentation of the articular surface that is limited to the patella; and (3) changes in the articular cartilage in both the patella and the femur. Another classification system is based on the anatomic distribution of the changes in the patellar articular cartilage[702]: (1) involving the lateral facet, usually just lateral to the median ridge; (2) involving the medial facets, particularly the odd facet; (3) affecting the median ridge and extending into the medial and lateral facets; (4) involving the central portion of the medial and lateral facets with sparing of the median ridge; and (5) affecting the entire articular cartilage (global chondromalacia). In one addi-

tional classification system, the extent and depth of the articular cartilage alterations are emphasized[704]: (1) softening and swelling of the cartilage; (2) fissuring and fragmentation of the cartilage in an area 1 cm or less in diameter; (3) fissuring and fragmentation of the cartilage in an area greater than 1 cm in diameter; and (4) erosion of the entire cartilage coat with exposure of subchondral bone. Classification of cartilage changes in the patella also has been based on MR imaging characteristics (see later discussion).[679]

As there is no universally agreed on definition of chondromalacia patellae, its cause also is not clear. Potential factors include single or recurrent acute episodes of trauma, chronic stress (as in the excessive lateral pressure syndrome), patellofemoral instability, and anatomic or developmental variations in bone morphology.

Assessment of cartilage loss involving the patella using imaging techniques generally is inadequate. Positive findings on routine radiographs require significant and often severe loss of articular cartilage, manifested as joint space narrowing, and secondary changes in the subchondral bone, evident as sclerosis, cyst formation, and osteophytosis. Standard arthrography and arthrography coupled with conventional tomography or CT scanning also are deficient in the diagnosis of early or mild loss of articular cartilage. Imbibition of contrast material in areas of abnormal cartilage may be observed (Fig. 16–178), but this finding is neither sensitive nor specific, as it also may occur when arthrographic images are not obtained immediately after injection of the contrast material. Fissuring and ulceration of articular cartilage are more specific, and the addition of subtracted CT arthrographic images can produce vivid demonstrations of chondromalacia patellae (see Fig. 16–178). Positive results with bone scintigraphy usually indicate more advanced disease with involvement of the subchondral bone. The patellar cartilage is not accessible to investiga-

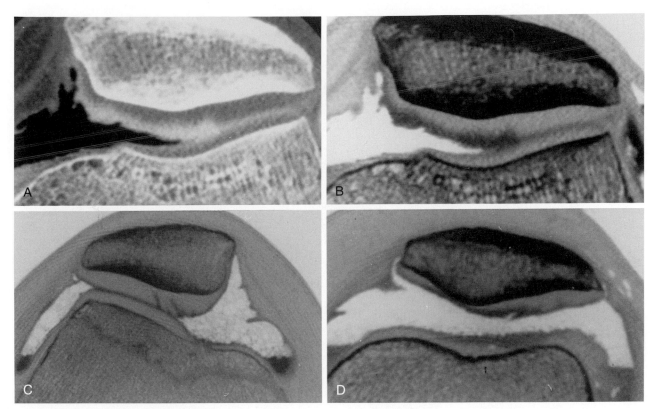

Figure 16–178
Chondromalacia patellae: CT arthrography.
A, B Transaxial CT arthrographic images (using double contrast technique) filmed without (**A**) and with (**B**) subtraction technique show imbibition of radiopaque contrast material and cartilage fibrillation and ulceration.
C, D Two additional subtracted CT arthrographic images in other patients reveal cartilage fissuring and contrast material imbibition.
(Courtesy of A. D'Abreau, M.D., Porto Alegre, Brazil.)

tion with ultrasonography. MR imaging appears to represent the best of an otherwise mediocre group of noninvasive diagnostic techniques for the assessment of patellar cartilage, but it too has many deficiencies. As these deficiencies are not limited to evaluation of the patellar cartilage but apply also to analysis of other articular surfaces in the knee, they are discussed later in this chapter.

Abnormalities of the Central Supporting Structures

Anatomic Considerations

The anterior and posterior cruciate ligaments are intracapsular, extrasynovial structures (Fig. 16–179).[562, 705, 706] These bands of dense tissue connect the femur and tibia and are enveloped by a mesentery-like fold of synovium that originates from the posterior intercondylar region of the knee. In one cadaveric study, the mean length of the anterior cruciate ligament was approximately 3.5 cm, and its central portion had a mean width of approximately 1 cm; the mean length of the posterior cruciate ligament was approximately 3.8 cm, and its central portion had a mean width of approximately 1.3 cm.[707] In another study, the cross-sectional area of the posterior

cruciate ligament was found to be approximately 1.5 times larger than that of the anterior cruciate ligament at the proximal and midsubstance levels but was only 1.2 times larger at the most distal level.[708] Although not all investigators agree that the posterior cruciate ligament is longer than the anterior cruciate ligament, the general consensus is that it is stronger than the anterior cruciate ligament.[709]

The anterior cruciate ligament is attached proximally to a fossa on the posterior aspect of the medial surface of the lateral femoral condyle.[705] Distally, this ligament is attached to a fossa in front of and lateral to the tibial spines. This attachment site fans out like a foot, allowing the anterior cruciate ligament to tuck under the roof of the intercondylar notch.[562] A few fascicles of the anterior cruciate ligament may blend with the anterior attachment of the lateral meniscus, and the anterior cruciate ligament passes beneath the transverse (geniculate) ligament.[705] The tibial attachment of the anterior cruciate ligament is stronger and wider than the femoral attachment.[707, 710] The proximal attachment is oriented primarily in the longitudinal axis of the femur, and the distal attachment is in the anteroposterior axis of the tibia.[562] Because of this anatomic arrangement, a twist of the anterior cruciate ligament fibers occurs when the knee moves from extension to flexion. A twist of the anterior cruciate ligament also is evident in the coronal

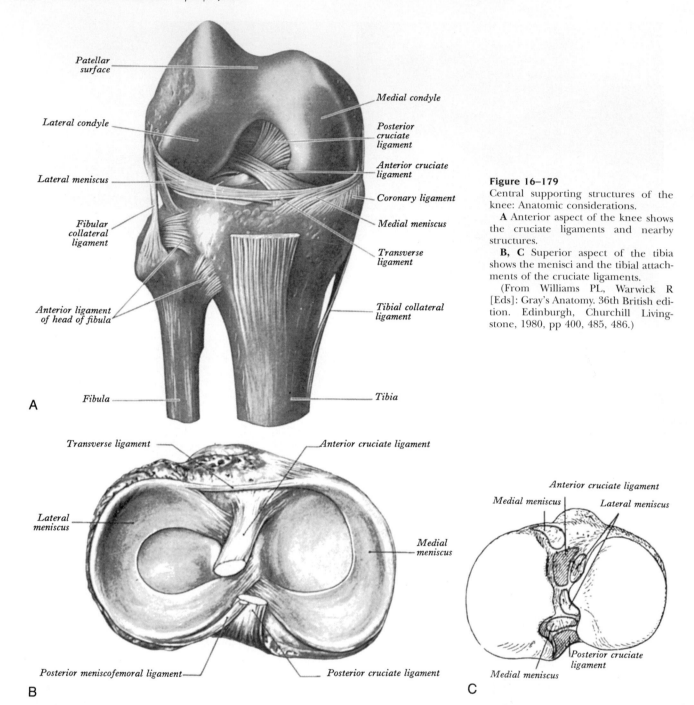

Patellar surface

Medial condyle

Lateral condyle

Posterior cruciate ligament

Anterior cruciate ligament

Lateral meniscus

Coronary ligament

Medial meniscus

Fibular collateral ligament

Transverse ligament

Anterior ligament of head of fibula

Tibial collateral ligament

A

Fibula

Tibia

Transverse ligament

Anterior cruciate ligament

Lateral meniscus

Medial meniscus

Posterior meniscofemoral ligament

Posterior cruciate ligament

B

Anterior cruciate ligament

Medial meniscus

Lateral meniscus

Posterior cruciate ligament

Medial meniscus

C

Figure 16–179
Central supporting structures of the knee: Anatomic considerations.

A Anterior aspect of the knee shows the cruciate ligaments and nearby structures.

B, C Superior aspect of the tibia shows the menisci and the tibial attachments of the cruciate ligaments.

(From Williams PL, Warwick R [Eds]: Gray's Anatomy. 36th British edition. Edinburgh, Churchill Livingstone, 1980, pp 400, 485, 486.)

plane, with external rotation of the fibers by approximately 90 degrees as they approach the tibial surface.[562, 707, 711]

The posterior cruciate ligament attaches inferiorly to the tibia in a depression just posterior to and below its articular surface.[705] This attachment site is intracapsular, however. It is rectangular[562] and quite thin.[705] Some fibers of the posterior cruciate ligament extend laterally, to blend with the attachment site of the posterior horn of the lateral meniscus. The proximal, and functionally more important, attachment site of the posterior cruciate ligament is the posterior aspect of the lateral surface of the medial femoral condyle. The femoral attachment

is shaped like a half-moon[707] and extends into the intercondylar notch. The longitudinal axis of this femoral attachment is described as more horizontal than that of the anterior cruciate ligament[705] or as being in the anteroposterior plane of the femur.[562] The meniscofemoral ligaments of Humphrey and Wrisberg are intimate with the femoral attachment site of the posterior cruciate ligament (see previous discussion). The total cross-sectional area of the meniscofemoral ligaments is about 20 per cent of that of the posterior cruciate ligament.[708]

The spatial orientation of the anterior and posterior cruciate ligaments has been summarized by Arnoczky and Warren.[705] These ligaments cross each other as they extend through the joint. The anterior cruciate ligament courses anteriorly, medially, and distally as it passes from the femur to the tibia, and it turns on itself in a lateral or outward spiral. The posterior cruciate ligament passes posteriorly, laterally, and distally as it extends from the femur to the tibia, and it is narrowest in its midportion. The cruciate ligaments attach to the femur and tibia, not as a single cord, but as a collection of individual fascicles.[705] Although there is some disagreement regarding the presence and number of distinct fascicular bundles,[706] a consensus indicates that two groups of fascicles are evident in both cruciate ligaments. In the anterior cruciate ligament, these two groups are designated the anteromedial bundle or band (arising from the proximal aspect of the femoral attachment and inserting in the anteromedial aspect of the tibial attachment) and the larger posterolateral bundle or bulk (representing the remaining bulk of fascicles that are inserted in the posterolateral aspect of the tibial attachment).[705, 706] As the knee moves from flexion to extension, the anterior cruciate ligament twists on itself, and the functional bundles become manifest. When the knee is extended, the posterolateral bundle is tight, whereas the anteromedial bundle is moderately lax; as the knee is flexed, the anteromedial bundle is tight and the posterolateral bundle is lax.[705] The fascicles in the anteromedial bundle are believed to be longest in flexion, and they may be the primary component that resists anterior displacement of the tibia in flexion; the fascicles in the posterolateral bundle are believed to be longest in extension and may be the primary component that resists hyperextension.[706, 712] In the posterior cruciate ligament, the fascicles are divided into a larger anterior (or anterolateral) portion and a posterior (or posteromedial) portion. The anterior fascicles tighten in flexion of the knee, and the posterior fascicles tighten in extension.[705] Together, portions of the anterior cruciate ligament and the posterior cruciate ligament are taut throughout the range of motion of the knee.

Histologically, the anterior and posterior cruciate ligaments consist mainly of dense fibrous tissue, which, with age, may reveal foci of eosinophilic or mucoid degeneration (or of both types of degeneration).[713] The ligaments are composed of collagen fibrils and, at their site of attachment to bone, in common with all ligaments, transitional zones of fibrocartilage and mineralized cartilage are evident.[714, 715] The cruciate ligaments are covered by a synovial lining that, as indicated earlier, originates at the posterior inlet of the intercondylar notch and extends to the anterior tibial attachment of the anterior cruciate ligament. The predominant source of blood supply to the cruciate ligaments is the middle geniculate artery, which pierces the posterior capsule of the knee joint, although an additional blood supply is derived from the intrapatellar fat pad via the inferior medial and lateral geniculate arteries.[562] The osseous attachments of the cruciate ligaments contribute little to their vascularity. Nerve fibers are derived from terminal branches of the tibial nerve.[716] Such fibers course through the synovial lining of the cruciate ligaments and extend as far anteriorly as the fat pad. Mechanoreceptors are found on the surface of the cruciate liga-

ments amid fibrous and fatty tissue, well beneath the external synovial sheath.[717, 718]

Pathologic Considerations

The anterior cruciate ligament functions as the primary restraint to anterior displacement of the tibia at the knee, but it offers no restraint to posterior displacement of the tibia. Experimental sectioning of the anterior cruciate ligament leads to greater anterior movement of the tibia in 30 degrees of knee flexion than in 90 degrees of flexion.[596] In one study, such sectioning increased anterior tibial displacement from 2.8 mm to 13.0 mm, with a mean value of 6.7 mm.[596] The anterior cruciate ligament also functions as a secondary restraint to tibial rotation, particularly internal rotation of the tibia and with full extension of the knee.[719] Increased tibial rotation is greater when both the anterior cruciate ligament and the medial collateral ligament are sectioned than when either structure is sectioned alone.[567] The anterior cruciate ligament also serves as a minor secondary restraint to varus-valgus angulation at full extension of the knee, although the anterior cruciate ligament appears to offer little additional restraint to such angulation beyond that afforded by the medial collateral ligament and lateral collateral ligament.[596]

The posterior cruciate ligament is the primary restraint to posterior displacement of the tibia at the knee.[596] An increase in such displacement after sectioning of the posterior cruciate ligament is greater at 90 degrees of knee flexion than it is at 30 degrees of knee flexion.[719, 720] The posterior cruciate ligament acts as a major secondary restraint to external tibial rotation, particularly at 90 degrees of flexion, but does not appear to limit internal rotation of the tibia.[596, 719] The posterior cruciate ligament serves as a minor secondary restraint to varus-valgus angulation.[596]

Experimental data provide the following conclusions.[596] Isolated disruption of the anterior cruciate ligament increases anterior movement of the tibia, most evident at 30 degrees of knee flexion, providing the basis for the Lachman test (see later discussion). Isolated disruption of the posterior cruciate ligament increases posterior movement of the tibia, particularly at 75 to 90 degrees of knee flexion, forming the basis for the posterior sag sign (see later discussion). Disruptions of the anterior cruciate ligament, medial collateral ligament, and midportion of the medial aspect of the joint capsule result in large increases in anterior displacement, varus angulation, and internal rotation of the tibia. Disruptions of the anterior cruciate ligament, lateral collateral ligament, and deep posterolateral structures dramatically increase anterior displacement, varus angulation, and external rotation of the tibia. Combined injury of the posterior cruciate ligament, lateral collateral ligament and deep posterolateral structures results in large increases in posterior displacement of the tibia, varus angulation from full extension to 90 degrees of flexion, and external rotation from 30 degrees to 90 degrees of flexion.

Hughston and coworkers[573] divided the instability patterns into two types: straight instabilities (without a rotary component) and rotary instabilities (either simple or combined). By definition, straight instabilities exhibit abnormal motion at the knee without rotation, opening in a manner similar to a book or a door.[575] The common factor exhibited by all straight instability patterns is that, in forced hyperextension, the deficient posterior cruciate ligament is unable to prevent opening of the knee joint and translation of the tibia.[575] Four patterns of straight instability may accompany injuries to the posterior cruciate ligament.[573]

1. Straight medial instability represents instability in hyperextension and is caused by a tear of the posterior cruciate ligament combined with a tear of the medial ligaments of the knee.[573] A positive abduction stress test with the knee in full extension is observed. If the anterior cruciate ligament also is torn, a minimal rotational wobble is evident.[575]

2. Straight lateral instability represents lateral opening of the joint without rotation. It results from tears of the lateral ligaments and the posterior cruciate ligament.[573] It is confirmed by a positive adduction test, accomplished with the knee in full extension. If the anterior cruciate ligament also is torn, a minor rotational wobble again is seen.[575]

3. Straight posterior instability relates to a tear of the posterior cruciate ligament, which may occur as an isolated phenomenon (caused by a force that displaces the tibia posteriorly while the knee is in 90 degrees of flexion) or in combination with injury to the posterior oblique ligament and the arcuate complex of the knee.[573] The large posterior bulk of the posterior cruciate ligament is the site of disruption. This form of instability is manifest by a positive posterior drawer test.

4. Straight anterior instability results from disruption of the posterior cruciate ligament, which may occur in isolation or in combination with tears of the anterior cruciate ligament and the medial and lateral capsular ligaments. It is demonstrated by positive results on several different types of anterior drawer testing, depending on which specific structures are torn. If there is no rotational component, the positive anterior drawer sign persists in internal rotation and external rotation of the knee, as well as in the neutral position.[575]

Three types of simple rotary instabilities exist.[573]

1. Anteromedial rotary instability relates to momentary subluxation of the medial tibial plateau anteriorly and externally on the femur.[575] When mild, this pattern of instability relates to tears of the medial capsule, posterior oblique ligament, and medial collateral ligament; when severe, the anterior cruciate ligament also is injured. Results of an anterior drawer sign with the tibia in external rotation and an abduction stress test with the knee in 30 degrees of flexion are positive.

2. Anterolateral rotary instability is associated with anterior translation and internal rotation of the lateral plateau of the tibia on the femur. Tears of the anterior cruciate ligament and, in some cases, of the lateral capsular ligament and iliotibial tract are present.[573, 575] The results of adduction stress testing are mildly posi-

tive, and jerk and pivot shift testing may be required for diagnosis.[575]

3. Posterolateral rotary instability usually relates to a direct blow that creates varus angulation and hyperextension of the knee, producing posterolateral subluxation of the tibia on the femur. The sites of injury do not include the cruciate ligaments, but rather are the lateral collateral ligament, arcuate ligament, popliteus tendon, and lateral head of the gastrocnemius muscle.[575] A positive posterolateral drawer sign results.

The instability patterns of the knee are complex, do not all fit into this classification system, and may exist in various combinations of these classic types. Proper identification of the type of injury requires careful physical examination, with reliance on the results of many different tests accomplished during application of stress to the injured knee. These tests are described in great detail by Hughston and coworkers.[573] Daniel and Stone[721] have provided a short summary of these tests. Two important tests for anterior cruciate ligament integrity are the Lachman test and pivot shift test. The Lachman test assesses anterior knee laxity and stiffness, accomplished in about 20 degrees of knee flexion. An increase in joint laxity and a decrease in end-point stiffness are signs of injury to the anterior cruciate ligament. A number of different pivot shift tests are described, usually leading to anterior subluxation and subsequent reduction of the tibia, with knee flexion and extension from 10 to 40 degrees as a sequela of anterior cruciate ligament disruption.[721] Two fundamental tests are used to evaluate the integrity of the posterior cruciate ligament.[721] The 90 degree quadriceps active test is performed with the patient in a supine position, with the hip flexed 45 degrees, the knee flexed 90 degrees, and the foot on the table. With contraction of the quadriceps musculature, exaggerated posterior movement of the tibia occurs (positive sag sign). The patient then is asked to slide the foot along the tabletop. Anterior translation of the tibia occurs when the tibia is subluxed posteriorly secondary to disruption of the posterior cruciate ligament.[721] The second test for posterior cruciate ligament integrity is the posterior drawer test, which documents posterior subluxation of the tibia. The test is more useful in acute than in chronic injuries of the posterior cruciate ligament. A posteromedial pivot shift of the knee also has been described, in which positive results relate to injuries not only of the posterior cruciate ligament but also of the medial and posterior collateral ligaments and the posterior oblique ligament.[722]

Physical examination provides important information regarding which ligament or ligaments are torn. In the acute stage, however, difficulty arises owing to pain, muscle spasm, and guarding.[723] The results of carefully performed stress testing may allow precise determination of sites of injury. In some instances, physical examination performed with the patient under general anesthesia is required. Noyes and Grood[724] have outlined four concepts that must be understood for proper diagnosis of injuries of the ligaments of the knee: (1) diagnosis of a ligament injury must be expressed as a specific anatomic defect; (2) physical examination must be interpreted using knowledge of three-dimensional motions of the knee; (3) patterns of rotary instability can be characterized by separate subluxations that occur to the medial and lateral tibial plateaus; and (4) diagnosis of ligament and capsular defects requires the use of selected laxity tests for which the primary and secondary restraints have been determined experimentally. These authors also indicated that terms must be precisely defined. They suggested that the term instability should be used only in a general sense to indicate excessive motion of the knee joint, that the term laxity should be used only in a general sense to indicate slackness or loosening of a ligament, and that the term subluxation represents incomplete or partial displacement at the knee and requires further descriptive terms to indicate precisely which portions of the joint are malaligned.

Anterior Cruciate Ligament Injuries

Injuries to the anterior cruciate ligament are among the most frequent sequelae of knee trauma. In one series, almost 40 per cent of ligamentous injuries of the knee involved the anterior cruciate alone and, in an additional 35 per cent of cases, the anterior cruciate ligament was injured in combination with other ligamentous disruptions, particularly those of the medial collateral ligament.[725] Approximately 60 to 75 per cent of acute traumatic hemarthroses are associated with anterior cruciate ligament injury. The classic mechanism of injury to the anterior cruciate ligament (which frequently is evident in skiers[726] and American football players) is indirect trauma leading to decelerating, hyperextension, or twisting forces, often accompanied by an audible pop and the rapid onset of pain, soft tissue swelling, and disability. The combination of external rotation of the tibia with respect to the femur, knee flexion, and valgus stress may produce an anterior cruciate ligament injury, often combined with additional injuries to the medial collateral ligament and the medial meniscus.[723, 727–730] O'Donoghue's triad of injury consists of a tear of the anterior cruciate ligament, complete disruption of the medial collateral ligament, and a tear of the peripheral portion of the medial meniscus. Even when initial injuries are isolated to the anterior cruciate ligament, chronic instability in the anterior cruciate ligament-deficient knee subsequently can lead to additional injuries, such as meniscal tears. The midsubstance of the anterior cruciate ligament is injured most commonly (approximately 70 per cent of cases), followed in frequency by its proximal portion (approximately 20 per cent of cases), and its distal portion (approximately 10 per cent of cases).

Clinical assessment of the knee in patients with anterior cruciate ligament injuries includes physical examination with stress testing.[731] Instillation of a local anesthetic agent into the joint or, in some cases, the use of general anesthesia may be required, particularly when muscle spasm or patient apprehension precludes adequate evaluation. The correct assessment of the severity of knee instability and its type requires the attention of an experienced orthopedic surgeon, and the results of

stress tests, which may be accomplished with instrumented ligament-testing devices, should be compared with those of the opposite (uninjured) knee. One instrument used for measuring instability of the knee is a KT1000 arthrometer.[732] This instrument allows quantitative analysis of tibial displacement in relation to the femur by tracking the distance between one sensor pad in contact with the tibial tubercle and a second in contact with the patella.[733, 734] The role of arthroscopy in the diagnosis and management of acute knee injuries, including partial and complete tears of the anterior cruciate ligament, is well established. Precise diagnosis requires arthroscopic assessment of the menisci and chondral surfaces as well as the anterior cruciate ligament.[735–737] Arthroscopy also can be used to evaluate knees with chronically deficient anterior cruciate ligaments. In either acute or chronic tears of the anterior cruciate ligament, arthroscopic difficulty may arise if the synovial membrane overlying the torn ligament is intact.

As with any method of analysis, the diagnostic value of the clinical examination in patients with tears of the anterior cruciate ligament depends, foremost, on the skill and diligence of the examiner. When performed carefully, the results of stress testing (with or without the use of arthrometry) often are reliable and sufficient for diagnosis. Data that are used to support the opinion that such clinical testing eliminates the need for imaging studies (particularly MR imaging) can be found,[732, 1118] but these data often do not consider any additional information (beyond the status of the anterior cruciate ligament) that the imaging examination may provide. Furthermore, the clinical diagnosis of partial tears of the anterior cruciate ligament is known to be difficult.[738] With this in mind, most examining physicians use one or more of a number of imaging methods in patients in whom they believe anterior cruciate ligament injury is present.

Routine Radiography. In patients with acute tears of the anterior cruciate ligament, nonspecific soft tissue swelling and a joint effusion may be evident. Although a narrow intercondylar notch (owing to developmental or acquired [e.g., osteophytes] factors) increases the risk for rupture of the anterior cruciate ligament,[1145] the finding lacks specificity. Several fractures of the proximal portion of the tibia and distal portion of the femur, however, are specific for or imply the likelihood of an injury to the anterior cruciate ligament.

1. *Avulsion fracture of the anterior tibial eminence.* These avulsion fractures occur at the site of attachment of the anterior cruciate ligament and are more frequent in children and young adolescents than in older adolescents and adults (in whom injuries of the cruciate ligament itself occur). Avulsion fractures of the anterior tibial eminence, especially in adults, may be associated with additional fractures and other injuries, such as medial ligamentous and meniscal tears. Undisplaced fractures appear as a horizontal fracture line at the base of the anterior portion of the tibial spine; displaced fractures are accompanied by upward movement of the anterior portion of the fragment, which may become

completely detached or even inverted.[739] Avulsion fractures involving the femoral site of attachment of the anterior cruciate ligament are rare.[740]

2. *Lateral tibial rim fracture (Segond fracture).* As indicated earlier, a fracture fragment arising at the site of tibial attachment of the lateral capsular ligament reveals a high association with anterior cruciate ligament instability. The fragment usually is located lateral and just inferior to the joint line on the anteroposterior and tunnel radiographic projections (see Fig. 16–150).

3. *Posterior fracture of the lateral tibial plateau.* A subtle fracture of the posterior part of the lateral tibial plateau, visible on the lateral radiograph of the knee, may relate to an avulsion injury at the insertion site of the posterior portion of the joint capsule.[741] In one study, 11 of 25 patients with tears of the anterior cruciate ligament documented by MR imaging revealed this fracture pattern.[741] These posterior tibial fractures may be associated with fractures of the lateral tibial rim (Segond fracture). Compression fractures of the posterior portion of the lateral tibial plateau or fractures at the site of attachment of the semimembranosus tendon also may be observed in patients with anterior cruciate ligament tears. These fractures lead to an irregular contour of the plateau on lateral radiographs of the knee.[741]

4. *Osteochondral fracture of the lateral femoral condyle.* A constant localized chondral or transchondral lesion occurring in the region of the condylopatellar sulcus of the lateral femoral condyle has been observed at the time of surgical reconstruction of anterior cruciate ligament-deficient knees.[742, 743] During surgery in some patients it was possible to pull the lateral or posterolateral margin of the tibia into the sulcus, suggesting that the lesion was the result of an impaction fracture similar to the Hill-Sachs lesion that accompanies an anterior dislocation of the glenohumeral joint. Retrospectively, the sulcus was shown to be abnormal on the lateral radiograph of the knee in many patients.[744] In one study, only one of 47 patients with clinically intact anterior cruciate ligaments had a condylopatellar sulcus greater than 1 mm deep (as measured on the lateral radiograph), whereas two of 52 patients with acute tears of the anterior cruciate ligament and 13 of 70 patients with chronic tears of the anterior cruciate ligament had a sulcus equal to or greater than 1.5 mm deep.[745] The significance of this finding, which has been designated the lateral notch sign,[745] is supported by (1) histologic data that document the presence of focal areas of degenerated cartilage with localized invagination of cartilage into subchondral bone of the condylopatellar sulcus in patients with chronic anterior cruciate ligament tears,[744] and (2) MR imaging findings in patients with acute tears of the anterior cruciate ligament that include marrow edema (presumably resulting from injury) in the region of the sulcus (see later discussion). The lateral notch sign is considered present when the depth of the sulcus is greater than 1.5 to 2 mm (Figs. 16–180 and 16–181). The sign appears to be a specific indicator of an anterior cruciate ligament-deficient knee, but it is insensitive, probably occurring in fewer than 5 per cent of patients with torn anterior cruciate ligaments.[1146] It is not clear, however, if the deepening of the sulcus represents an osteochondral fracture or a developmental abnormality that predisposes to, rather than results from, the injury mechanism that causes an anterior cruciate ligament tear.

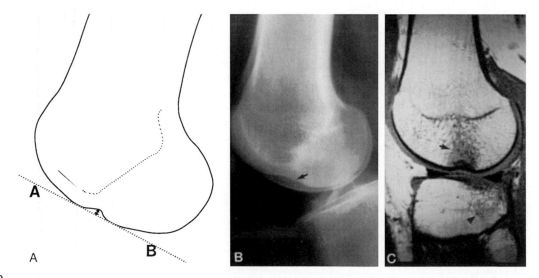

Figure 16–180

Injuries of the anterior cruciate ligament: Routine radiography. Osteochondral fracture of the lateral femoral condyle.

 A Method of measuring the depth of the lateral condylopatellar sulcus. A line (AB) drawn tangentially across the lower articular surface of the lateral femur forms the reference line. The depth of the sulcus is measured perpendicular to this line at the deepest point (arrowheads). (From Cobby MJ, et al: Radiology *184*:855, 1992.)

 B In a patient with a chronic tear of the anterior cruciate ligament, note the prominent condylopatellar sulcus (arrow).

 C In a different patient with a torn anterior cruciate ligament and a deep lateral condylopatellar sulcus, a T1-weighted (TR/TE, 800/30) spin echo MR image shows alterations in marrow signal intensity in the midportion of the lateral femoral condyle (arrow) and in the posterolateral portion of the tibia (arrowhead). These findings are consistent with marrow edema related to impaction fractures. (Courtesy of M. Pathria, M.D., San Diego, California.)

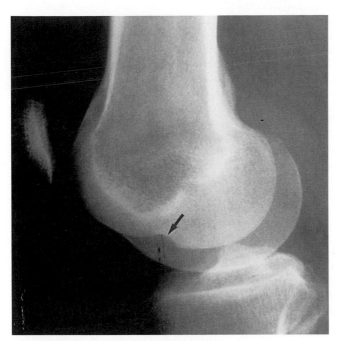

Figure 16–181
Injuries of the anterior cruciate ligament: Routine radiography. Osteochondral fracture of the lateral femoral condyle. Note the very prominent lateral condylopatellar sulcus (arrow).

Arthrography. Several arthrographic techniques have been employed for the evaluation of cruciate ligament injuries, with varying degrees of success. Initial techniques using double contrast arthrography were accurate in fewer than 50 per cent of cases, stimulating investigation with modified methods of examination. Some investigators report success using a lateral view of the knee, which is flexed to 90 degrees over the edge of the table[746] or elevated above the table,[747] or employing single positive contrast examinations.[748] Other investigators indicate approximately 75 to 90 per cent accuracy in diagnosing anterior cruciate ligament tears using conventional tomography.[749] This technique is improved if tomographic exposures are obtained immediately after injection, although this is time-consuming, delaying the meniscal examination.

In a series of articles, Pavlov and collaborators[750–754] emphasized the role of double contrast arthrography in the evaluation of the cruciate ligaments. When accomplished by an experienced arthrographer, the accuracy of the technique surpasses 90 per cent,[752] although similar accuracy has been reported from clinical examination alone.[755] The fundamental arthrographic criterion of a normal anterior cruciate ligament is an anterior synovial surface that is "ruler-straight."[752] This ligament is considered to be lax but intact if the anterior synovial surface is bowed and concave anteriorly. The arthrographic abnormalities associated with disruption of the anterior cruciate ligament are more definite when simultaneous visualization of the posterior cruciate ligament is accomplished (decreasing the likelihood of technical inadequacies) and include nonvisualization, a wavy, lumpy, or acutely angulated anterior surface, irregularity of the inferior attachment of the ligament, pooling of the contrast medium in the usual location of the ligament, and visualization of the plica synovialis infrapatellaris (the infrapatellar synovial fold, which otherwise is easily misinterpreted as evidence of a normal anterior cruciate ligament).[750–753]

An alternative approach to the diagnosis of tears of cruciate ligaments is provided by CT alone or combined with arthrography of the knee. Prior descriptions of the CT technique that is required to evaluate the cruciate ligaments have been conflicting not only with respect to the need for intra-articular contrast material but also with respect to whether the contrast material should be radiopaque material, air, or both. There is no uniform agreement regarding the position of the knee in the CT gantry, the need for angulation of the gantry, or the benefit of reformatted or even three-dimensional images.

Ultrasonography. The diagnostic value of ultrasonography in the detection of rupture of the anterior cruciate ligament is not known. In one study, sonography was performed in 37 patients with a recent traumatic hemarthrosis of the knee who had no bone abnormalities on plain film examination and no history of a previous knee injury.[756] The presence of a hypoechoic collection along the lateral wall of the femoral intercondylar notch was interpreted as a hematoma at the femoral attachment site of the anterior cruciate ligament. Sonography was 91 per cent sensitive and 100 per cent specific in judging the status of the anterior cruciate ligament using MR imaging and arthroscopy as the gold standards.

MR Imaging

Technical Considerations. As with the menisci of the knee, spin echo MR imaging is the most popular method used to assess the anterior cruciate ligament (as well as the posterior cruciate ligament). The best plane for analysis of either cruciate ligament is the sagittal plane, but supplementary data supplied by coronal and transaxial MR images are important.[757] In one study, combined analysis of MR images in all three planes led to an improvement in the sensitivity (98 per cent) and specificity (93 per cent) for determining the status of the anterior cruciate ligament when compared with the sensitivity (94 per cent) and specificity (84 per cent) derived from analysis of the sagittal images alone.[758] The sagittal images commonly are obtained with the leg externally rotated 15 to 30 degrees and therefore represent sagittal oblique images; alternatively, they are obtained by determining the orientation of the anterior cruciate ligament from initial transaxial (or coronal) MR images and using a sagittal oblique imaging plane parallel to this orientation (i.e., a 15 to 30 degree internally rotated imaging plane).[759–762] The use of T1- and T2-weighted spin echo MR images or proton density and T2-weighted spin echo MR images in the sagittal plane is helpful for determining changes in signal intensity in the anterior cruciate ligament that may accompany acute or subacute injuries. T2-weighted images also improve the contrast between the anterior cruciate ligament and a surrounding joint effusion. The sagittal images usually are 3 or 4 mm thick. The use of volumetric (three-dimensional Fourier transform) gradient echo MR images approximately 1 mm thick also may be useful. Gradient echo MR imaging may be coupled with cine technique to provide dynamic, rather than static, data.[763] The leg is extended during the acquisition of the MR images,[762] although the value of slight or moderate flexion of the knee (in an attempt to separate the anterior cruciate ligament from the roof of the intercondylar notch) has not been tested fully.[1197]

Normal Anterior Cruciate Ligament. Identification of the normal anterior cruciate ligament begins with analysis of the sagittal MR images (Fig. 16–182). In choosing a proper sagittal section in which the normal anterior cruciate ligament should be visualized, it often is helpful to find one that displays the intercondylar roof of the femur as a straight line of low signal intensity. Typically, in this section (or sections), the anterior cruciate ligament appears as a straight band of low signal intensity whose course parallels that of the intercondylar line.

The anterior cruciate ligament may not be seen in its entirety in this image (or images), but the course of the visible portion of the ligament still should be parallel to this line of low signal intensity. The anterior cruciate ligament may be seen as a uniform structure of low signal intensity or as one composed of individual fibers of low signal intensity. The individual fibers are identified most frequently at the tibial attachment site of the anterior cruciate ligament. Sometimes two bands (anterior and posterior) of fibers are seen within the anterior cruciate ligament. The posterior band may reveal increased signal intensity in comparison to the anterior band. Indeed, even the anterior band may show regions of increased signal intensity, particularly near its attachment to the tibia, presumably representing regions of fat. With gradient echo MR images, the anterior band is seen regularly, but it may be difficult to see the fibers of the posterior portion of the anterior cruciate ligament. The femoral insertion site of the anterior cruciate ligament may look bulbous, probably related to partial volume artifacts produced by the thickness of the

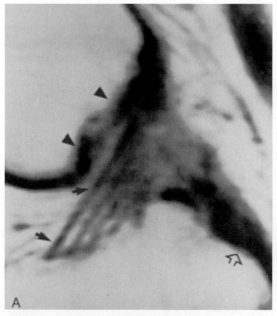
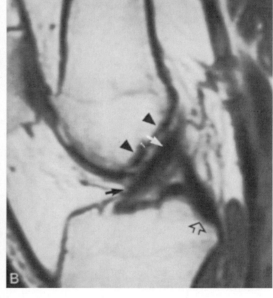
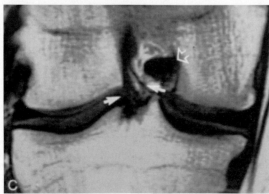

Figure 16–182
Normal anterior cruciate ligament: MR imaging.

A Sagittal proton density–weighted (TR/TE, 2000/20) spin echo MR image. The intercondylar roof (arrowheads) is seen as a straight line of low signal intensity. The anterior cruciate ligament (solid arrows) is seen as individual fibers whose course is straight and parallel to the course of the intercondylar roof. The tibial insertion site of the posterior cruciate ligament (open arrow) also is apparent.

B Sagittal proton density–weighted (TR/TE, 2000/20) spin echo MR image. In this example, the intercondylar roof (arrowheads) again is visualized as a straight line of low signal intensity. Although individual fibers of the anterior cruciate ligament are not seen, the ligament (solid arrows) is of low signal intensity and has a course that is parallel to the course of the intercondylar roof. The tibial insertion site of the posterior cruciate ligament (open arrow) is evident.

C Coronal proton density–weighted (TR/TE, 2000/20) spin echo MR image. Fibers of the anterior cruciate ligament (solid arrows) are seen coursing from the lateral femoral condyle to the anterior portion of the tibia. The femoral insertion site of the posterior cruciate ligament (open arrow) is evident.

sagittal images and resulting in visualization of a portion of the lateral femoral condyle.

In coronal (see Fig. 16–182) and transaxial MR images, the normal anterior cruciate ligament again can be identified. It may not be seen in its entirety in these images, but portions of it are visible and, in the coronal plane, individual fibers may be visualized.

The dominant pattern of signal intensity in the normal anterior cruciate ligament is low, although it is not as low as the signal intensity in the posterior cruciate ligament. The cause of the relative increased signal intensity in the anterior cruciate ligament (Fig. 16–183), particularly in elderly persons, is not clear.[713] Ligament architecture may be a causative factor, leading to increased signal intensity in the anterior cruciate ligament. The obliquely oriented fibers of the anterior cruciate ligament may result in more pronounced volume averaging artifacts during the MR imaging examination. Fat localized between the distal diverging fascicles of the anterior cruciate ligament also represents a potential source for its increased signal intensity. Furthermore, in older persons, regions of mucoid or myxoid changes within the anterior cruciate ligament may be responsible for changes in its signal intensity.[713] Finally, calcium pyrophosphate dihydrate crystal deposition in the cruciate ligaments is not infrequent and also may be responsible for alterations in signal intensity (Fig. 16–184).

Anterior Cruciate Ligament Tears. MR imaging represents a sensitive (90 to 98 per cent), specific (90 to 100 per cent), and accurate (90 to 95 per cent) method for identifying tears of the anterior cruciate ligament.[758, 759, 762, 764] In one study, its sensitivity in the analysis of the anterior cruciate ligament was superior to that provided by clinical tests such as the Lachman test and the anterior drawer sign.[764] MR imaging also appeared to be more specific and, possibly, more sensitive than arthrography in demonstrating tears of the anterior cruciate ligament.[764] The ability of MR imaging to allow differentiation between acute and chronic tears of the anterior cruciate ligament and to permit identification of partial tears of this ligament remains unclear,[765] although reported data indicate decreased accuracy of the examination in these situations (see later discussion).[766–768] The MR imaging diagnosis of injuries to the anterior cruciate ligament relates to the documentation of (1) abnormalities in the anterior cruciate ligament itself; (2) alterations in the appearance of other structures (e.g., posterior cruciate ligament and patellar tendon) related to the abnormal alignment of the tibia and femur that results from an anterior cruciate ligament tear; (3) abnormalities that result from bone impaction forces that occur in the course of the injury itself or from the resultant anterolateral instability that accompanies the injury to the anterior cruciate ligament; and (4) miscellaneous abnormalities (Table 16–1).[769–773, 1147] Of these types of abnormalities, those occurring in the anterior cruciate ligament itself are direct evidence of its injury; those reflecting altered alignment of the tibia and femur are indirect but strong evidence of anterior cruciate ligament injury; and those occurring in the adjacent bone are supportive of the diagnosis of an injury to the anterior cruciate ligament and mandate critical assessment (or reassessment) of the ligament. Furthermore, MR imaging allows confirmation of additional soft tissue damage, such as a tear of the medial meniscus (40 to 80 per cent of cases of acute or chronic tears of the anterior cruciate ligament)[430] or disruption of the medial supporting structures, or both (O'Donoghue's triad[744]), which is known to be associated with anterior cruciate ligament injury.

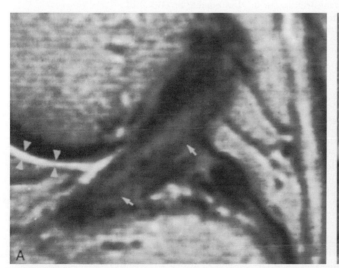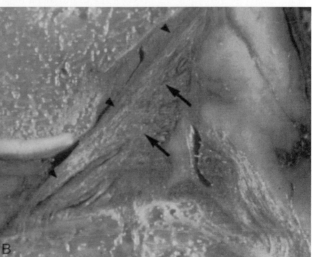

Figure 16–183

Normal anterior cruciate ligament: MR imaging—variations in signal intensity related to eosinophilic degeneration.

A A sagittal T2-weighted (TR/TE, 2000/70) spin echo MR image shows regions of intermediate signal intensity (arrows) in the anterior cruciate ligament. The increased signal intensity is not as great as that of the adjacent joint fluid (arrowheads).

B A corresponding sagittal anatomic section shows that the anterior fibers (arrowheads) of the anterior cruciate ligament are parallel to the imaging plane, whereas the posterior fibers (arrows) of the anterior cruciate ligament have a less steep course and are oriented more obliquely with regard to the sagittal plane. A photomicrograph (not shown) showed extensive eosinophilic degeneration in the anterior cruciate ligament.

(From Hodler J, et al: AJR *159*:357, 1992.)

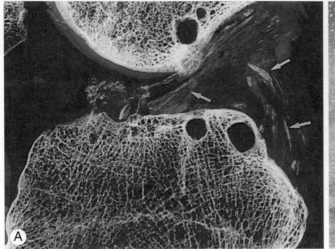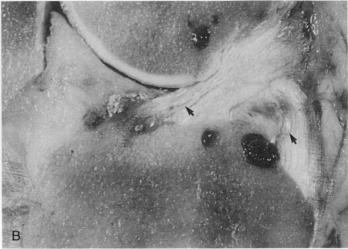

Figure 16–184

Crystal deposition in the anterior and posterior cruciate ligament: Routine radiography. Calcium pyrophosphate dihydrate crystal deposition is evident centrally in the knee, particularly within the cruciate ligaments (arrows), as shown with sagittal section radiography (**A**) and photography (**B**).

1. Abnormalities of the anterior cruciate ligament itself. The two major alterations occurring within the ligament itself are changes in its morphology or course and changes in its signal intensity.[758, 759, 762, 768, 770, 1148] A complete tear of the anterior cruciate ligament is accompanied by disruption of all of its fibers and an irregular or wavy contour. These findings are more evident in sagit- tal than in coronal MR images, although an indistinct anterior cruciate ligament in coronal MR images through the intercondylar notch, referred to as the empty notch sign, is an important finding of a complete tear of the anterior cruciate ligament, having been noted in 92 per cent of such tears in one study.[770] In sagittal MR images, the course of the completely torn

Table 16–1. SOME INDIRECT MR IMAGING FINDINGS ASSOCIATED WITH TEARS OF THE ANTERIOR CRUCIATE LIGAMENT

Finding	Comments
Osseous and Cartilaginous Findings	
Segond fracture	Fracture of the lateral tibial rim or adjacent marrow edema, or both
Bone bruises	Bone bruise in the posterolateral tibial plateau, in the lateral femoral condyle, or in both locations
	Bone bruise in the anterior tibia, in the anterior femoral condyles, or in both locations
Deepened notch in the lateral femoral condyle	Notch depth between 1 and 2 mm is suggestive and over 2 mm is diagnostic of cruciate ligament tear
Focal cartilaginous defect in the lateral femoral condylar notch	Cartilaginous defect may be accompanied by deepened notch or bone bruise, or both
Ligamentous and Tendinous Findings	
Buckling of the posterior cruciate ligament (PCL)	Positive finding when any segment of PCL is concave posteriorly in sagittal images
Posterior PCL line	Positive finding when a line drawn tangent to the posteroinferior portion of the PCL, as seen in sagittal images, fails to intersect the distal medullary cavity of the femur
Coronal PCL sign	Positive finding when entire length of PCL is seen in a single coronal image
Coronal fibular collateral ligament (FCL) sign	Positive finding when entire length of FCL is seen in a single coronal image
Buckling of the patellar tendon	Positive finding when such buckling observed in sagittal images occurs in the absence of quadriceps tendon rupture or hyperextension of knee
Miscellaneous Findings	
Anterior translation of tibia	Positive finding when line drawn from posterior cortex of medial or lateral femoral condyle fails to pass within 5 mm of posterior cortex of tibia in sagittal images
	Positive finding ("uncovered lateral meniscus") when a vertical line drawn tangent to the most posterior cortical margin of the lateral tibial plateau intersects any portion of the posterior horn of the lateral meniscus in sagittal images
	Positive finding (posterior femoral line sign) when a line drawn at a 45 degree angle from the posterosuperior corner of Blumensaat's line fails to intersect the flat portion of the proximal tibial surface in sagittal images
Shearing injury of infrapatellar fat body	Positive finding when a linear region of high signal intensity is seen in the middle of the fat body in sagittal images

Figure 16–185
Injuries of the anterior cruciate ligament: MR imaging. Chronic complete anterior cruciate ligament tears with alterations in ligament morphology and course.

A A sagittal proton density–weighted (TR/TE, 2150/30) spin echo MR image shows a depressed anterior cruciate ligament (arrow) whose course no longer parallels that of the intercondylar roof.

B A sagittal proton density–weighted (TR/TE, 2000/30) spin echo MR image shows a similar finding (arrow) in a second patient with a chronically torn anterior cruciate ligament.

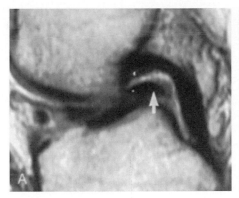
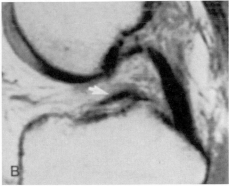

anterior cruciate ligament may appear depressed (Fig. 16–185), with a decreased slope of residual fibers extending almost parallel to the tibial surface rather than at an angle to this surface and parallel to the intercondylar roof (as is characteristic of the normal anterior cruciate ligament). In some chronic complete tears of the anterior cruciate ligament, the development of scar tissue results in an angulated appearance of the ligament (Fig. 16–186) or, in some cases, a continuous band of low signal intensity that simulates the appearance of a normal anterior cruciate ligament (Figs. 16–187 and 16–188).[775] A focal angulation in this band may allow a correct diagnosis of a torn anterior cruciate ligament even in these cases.[765] With acute or chronic tears of some but not all of the fibers of the anterior cruciate ligament, the ligament may appear attenuated, or small, and its course may or may not be altered (see later discussion) (Fig. 16–189). Rarely, developmental hypoplasia of the cruciate ligaments produces a similar appearance (Fig. 16–190).

The presence of increased signal intensity within the anterior cruciate ligament on proton density–weighted and T2-weighted spin echo MR images usually indicates an acute or subacute injury resulting in complete or partial disruption of the ligament (Figs. 16–189 and 16–191). This pattern of increased signal intensity appears to reflect edematous soft tissues, not joint fluid, in the intercondylar notch.[765] A cloudlike or amorphous mass of increased signal intensity, with well-defined margins, may be evident. Although such edema is indicative of a recent tear of the anterior cruciate ligament, its absence does not exclude the presence of a recent

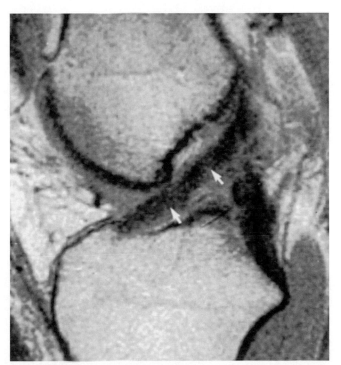

Figure 16–187
Injuries of the anterior cruciate ligament: MR imaging. Chronic complete anterior cruciate ligament tears with scar tissue. A sagittal proton density–weighted (TR/TE, 2000/20) spin echo MR image shows a relatively straight band (arrows) with low signal intensity that bridges the expected origin and insertion of the anterior cruciate ligament. The appearance simulates that of a normal anterior cruciate ligament. At arthroscopy, a chronically torn anterior cruciate ligament that was scarred to the posterior cruciate ligament was found. (From Vahey TN, et al: Radiology *181*:251, 1991.)

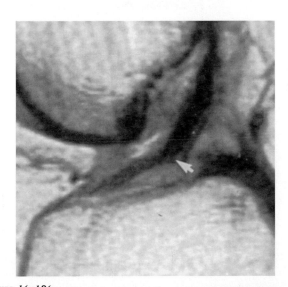

Figure 16–186
Injuries of the anterior cruciate ligament: MR imaging. Chronic complete anterior cruciate ligament tears with scar tissue. A sagittal proton density–weighted (TR/TE, 2000/20) spin echo MR image shows a focally angular (arrow) but intact band with low signal intensity that represents a combination of anterior cruciate ligament fragments and associated bridging fibrous scar. (From Vahey TN, et al: Radiology *181*:251, 1991.)

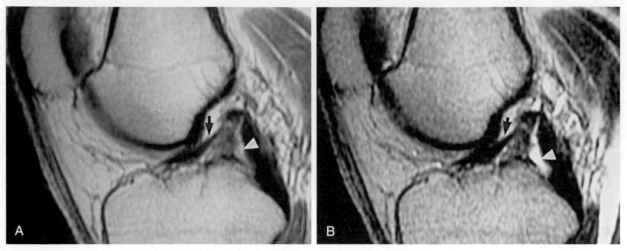

Figure 16–188
Injuries of the anterior cruciate ligament: MR imaging. Chronic complete anterior cruciate ligament tears with scar tissue. As shown on sagittal proton density–weighted (TR/TE, 2200/30) **(A)** and T2-weighted (TR/TE, 2200/80) **(B)** spin echo MR images, the course of the torn anterior cruciate ligament (arrows) is depressed only minimally owing to adhesions between it and the posterior cruciate ligament. A secondary finding of a tear of the anterior cruciate ligament is the presence of fluid (arrowheads) in the triangular space between the two cruciate ligaments, indicative of disruption of the synovial lining that is reflected over the ligaments (see text for details).

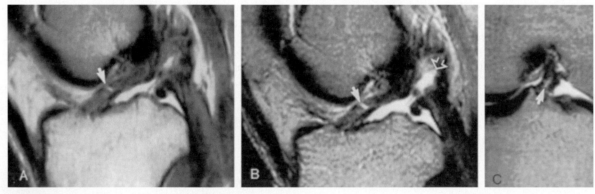

Figure 16–189
Injuries of the anterior cruciate ligament: MR imaging. Acute partial anterior cruciate ligament tears with alterations in ligament morphology and signal intensity. Sagittal proton density–weighted (TR/TE, 4000/21) **(A)** and T2-weighted (TR/TE, 4000/105) **(B)** fast spin echo MR images and a coronal T2-weighted (TR/TE, 3200/108) fast spin echo MR image **(C)** show an attenuated appearance of the anterior cruciate ligament with intraligamentous regions (solid arrows) of high signal intensity. Note the joint fluid that is collecting between the anterior cruciate ligament and posterior cruciate ligament (open arrow), consistent with a tear of the synovial lining that surrounds the cruciate ligaments.

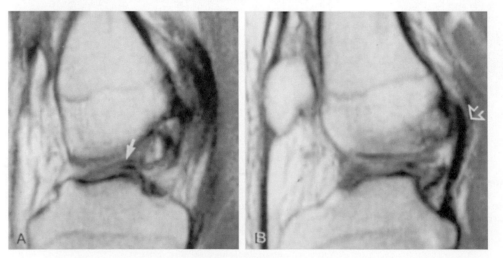

Figure 16–190
Hypoplasia of the cruciate ligaments: MR imaging. In this 19 year old man with hypoplasia of the femur, tibia, and patella, the anterior cruciate ligament (solid arrow) and the posterior cruciate ligament (open arrow) also are hypoplastic, as seen in sagittal proton density–weighted (TR/TE, 2200/15) spin echo MR images **(A, B).** Also note the hypoplastic quadriceps and patellar tendons and anterior translation of the tibia with respect to the femur. (Courtesy of J. Hodler, M.D., Zurich, Switzerland.)

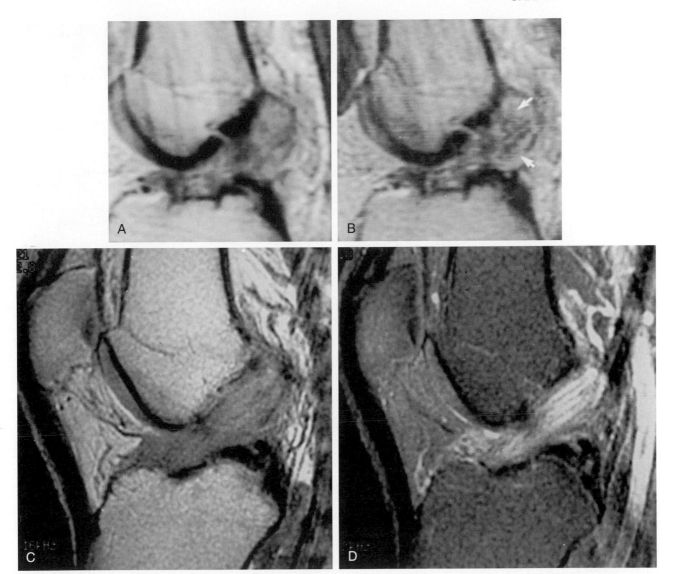

Figure 16–191

Injuries of the anterior cruciate ligament: MR imaging. Acute complete anterior cruciate ligament tears with alterations in intraligamentous signal intensity.

A, B In sagittal proton density–weighted (TR/TE, 2500/20) **(A)** and T2-weighted (TR/TE, 2500/60) **(B)** spin echo MR images, the anterior cruciate ligament is not visualized. In **B,** note a generalized increase in signal intensity (arrows) in an amorphous mass near the femoral site of insertion of the anterior cruciate ligament.

C, D In a second patient, a sagittal proton density–weighted (TR/TE, 1600/30) spin echo MR image **(C)** reveals an amorphous region of intermediate signal intensity about the anterior cruciate ligament. The sagittal fat-suppressed fast spin echo (TR/TE, 2700/36) MR image **(D)** shows diffuse high signal intensity in this region.

tear.[765] With chronic tears of the anterior cruciate ligament, edema usually is not evident. The presence of joint fluid about the chronically torn ligament, however, may simulate the appearance of edema in the MR images.[765] Indeed, alterations in the distribution of joint fluid represent one of the miscellaneous abnormalities associated with disruption of the cruciate ligaments (see later discussion).

Barry and associates[1148] categorized MR imaging abnormalities related directly to the appearance of the anterior cruciate ligament into five patterns, based on an analysis of 91 patients with arthroscopically-proven tears of this ligament: type 1 (diffuse increase in signal intensity within the ligament on T2-weighted spin echo MR images and ligament enlargement—48 per cent of

knees); type 2 (horizontally oriented ligament—21 per cent of knees); type 3 (nonvisualization of ligament—18 per cent of knees); type 4 (discontinuity of ligament—11 per cent of knees); and type 5 (vertically oriented ligament—2 per cent of knees). Although this study did not attempt to differentiate between acute and chronic ligamentous tears, the results indicated that if the anterior cruciate ligament is horizontally oriented, discontinuous, or vertically oriented, it is definitely torn; and that type 1 or 3 abnormalities are associated with a high although not absolute positive predictive value for such tear.

Although, as indicated in the following discussion, additional soft tissue and bone abnormalities seen with MR imaging may serve as clues to the presence of an anterior cruciate ligament tear, the alterations in the ligament itself represent the most important findings of such a tear (particularly a complete tear), allowing correct diagnosis in more than 90 per cent of cases.[770, 1149] False-positive diagnoses may occur, however, owing to the presence of foci of mucinous or myxoid change within the ligament,[729] partial volume averaging of the anterior cruciate ligament with the lateral femoral condyle or with periligamentous fat, and suboptimal selection of the sagittal imaging plane to view the ligament.[770] False-negative diagnoses may result from the formation of scar tissue with adherence of the anterior cruciate ligament to the posterior cruciate ligament (simulating a normal course and signal intensity of the anterior cruciate ligament) or from partial tears in which residual intact fibers lead to an appearance of a normal anterior cruciate ligament (see later discussion).[775] Assessment of all three imaging planes is required to minimize these diagnostic errors. Furthermore, attention should be paid to any additional soft tissue or bone abnormalities that may accompany disruptions of the anterior cruciate ligament.

2. Alterations in other structures related to abnormal alignment of the tibia and femur. Anterior cruciate ligament injuries are associated with anterolateral instability that may be manifested as a forward shift of the tibia with respect to the femur.[776] This shift, if severe, can be recognized easily, owing to the position of the two bones (Fig. 16–192). A line drawn from the posterior cortex of the medial or lateral femoral condyle will fail to pass within 5 mm of the posterior cortex of the tibia on sagittal MR images.[773] If the shift is subtle, its recognition depends on minor alterations in the configuration of

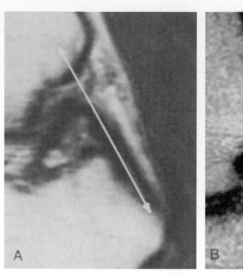

Figure 16–193
Injuries of the anterior cruciate ligament: MR imaging—normal and abnormal configuration of the posterior cruciate ligament.
  A Normal appearance. As shown in this T1-weighted (TR/TE, 600/20) spin echo MR image, a line drawn along the course of the lower portion of the posterior cruciate ligament, when extended superiorly, intersects the femur.
  B Acute complete anterior cruciate ligament tear. As shown in a sagittal T2-weighted (TR/TE, 2000/70) spin echo MR image, the appearance of the posterior cruciate ligament may be altered in association with a complete tear of the anterior cruciate ligament. In this case, acute angulation of the posterior cruciate ligament is evident. A line drawn along the course of the lower portion of the posterior cruciate ligament, when extended superiorly, does not intersect the femur. (Courtesy of S. K. Brahme, M.D., La Jolla, California.)

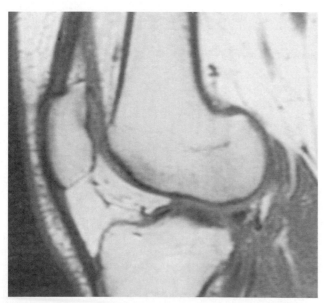

Figure 16–192
Injuries of the anterior cruciate ligament: MR imaging. Chronic complete anterior cruciate ligament tears with anterior translation of the tibia. A sagittal T1-weighted (TR/TE, 600/20) spin echo MR image shows obvious forward movement of the tibia with respect to the lateral femoral condyle. Note uncovering of the posterior horn of the lateral meniscus (see text).

or relationship among other structures in the knee. Examples of these alterations include a relative posterior displacement of the lateral meniscus compared with the posterior margin of the lateral tibial plateau (uncovered lateral meniscus sign), a change in the curvature of the posterior cruciate ligament, and undulation of the patellar tendon.[777]

The uncovered lateral meniscus sign is positive if a vertical line drawn tangent to the posterior-most cortical margin of the lateral tibial plateau on sagittal MR images intersects any part of the posterior horn of the lateral meniscus; this sign is negative if the vertical line does not intersect the lateral meniscus but rather is posterior to the meniscus.[770] In one study, the uncovered lateral meniscus sign was positive in 18 per cent of cases in which an anterior cruciate ligament tear was present and was negative in all cases in which the anterior cruciate ligament was normal.[770]

Changes in the curvature of the posterior cruciate ligament in cases of tears of the anterior cruciate ligament have been emphasized in some reports.[770, 778, 779] A forward shift in the position of the tibia with respect to the femur occurs in patients with anterior cruciate ligament-deficient knees, and this shift may alter the appearance of the smooth curve of the posterior cruciate ligament (Fig. 16–193). In some instances, owing to a more vertical configuration of the middle and distal portions of the posterior cruciate ligament, much of the length of this ligament is seen on a single coronal MR

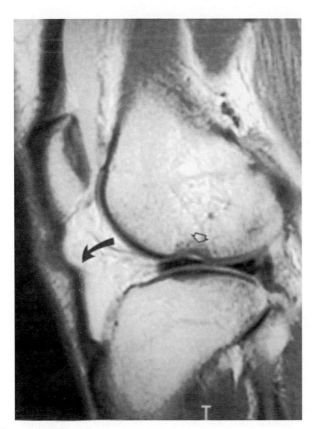

Figure 16–194

Injuries of the anterior cruciate ligament: MR imaging. Acute complete anterior cruciate ligament tears with redundancy of the patellar tendon and osteochondral impaction fractures. A sagittal proton density–weighted (TR/TE, 2000/30) spin echo MR image shows buckling of the patellar tendon (curved solid arrow) and an alteration in signal intensity (open arrow) in the lateral condylopatellar sulcus related to an impaction injury. A large joint effusion is present. (From Cobby MJ, et al: Radiology *184*:855, 1992.)

Undulation and redundancy of the patellar tendon may result from forward movement of the tibia with respect to the femur (Fig. 16–194), but a similar appearance relates to hyperextension of the knee at the time of the MR imaging examination and a tear of the quadriceps tendon. The patellar tendon sign of a tear of the anterior cruciate ligament appears to be both insensitive and nonspecific.[642]

A forward shift of the tibia in patients with a tear of the anterior cruciate ligament also may produce subtle changes in the appearance of other structures about the knee, such as the fibular collateral ligament, which may be visualized in its entirety on a single coronal MR image.[773] This finding, however, in common with the others noted previously, is not sensitive. Indeed, the absence of any or all of the secondary signs associated with femorotibial malalignment on MR imaging examinations does not exclude the diagnosis of a tear of the anterior cruciate ligament.[772] Their presence, however, should stimulate a more critical appraisal of the status of this ligament.[773]

3. Abnormalities related to bone impaction forces. Impaction of portions of the femur and tibia may occur acutely in patients with anterolateral instability of the knee. Subcortical infraction and medullary edema and hemorrhage lead to changes in signal intensity of the affected bone marrow, a finding designated a bone bruise (see Chapter 8). Typically, bone bruises lead to geographic or reticular areas of decreased signal intensity on T1-weighted spin echo MR images and increased signal intensity on T2-weighted spin echo MR images obtained soon after the injury. Their conspicuity is increased in short tau inversion recovery (STIR) MR images and those obtained with fat suppression techniques.[781]

In patients with acute tears of the anterior cruciate ligament, bone bruises have been observed most often in the midportion of the lateral femoral condyle (near the condylopatellar sulcus) and in the posterior portion of the lateral tibial plateau (Figs. 16–195 and 16–196).[744, 782–786] Using MR imaging, Murphy and coworkers[782] detected bone impaction sites involving the posterolateral portion of the tibial plateau in 94 per cent and the lateral femoral condyle in 91 per cent of 32 patients with surgically confirmed acute complete tears of the anterior cruciate ligament. Only one of six patients with a partial tear of the anterior cruciate ligament displayed similar findings. Kaplan and collabo-

image.[773] A line drawn along the inferior portion of the posterior cruciate ligament and extended superiorly on sagittal MR images normally intersects the medullary cavity of the femur; when this line does not intersect the femur but extends parallel to it, a positive posterior cruciate sign is present.[779] Alternatively, the curvature of the posterior cruciate ligament can be quantified on the basis of the sagittal MR images.[770] In common with the uncovered lateral meniscus sign, altered curvature of the posterior cruciate ligament appears to be a specific but insensitive indicator of a tear of the anterior cruciate ligament.[770, 780]

Figure 16–195

Injuries of the anterior cruciate ligament: MR imaging. Acute complete anterior cruciate ligament tears with osteochondral impaction fractures. Sagittal (A) and coronal (B) T2-weighted (TR/TE, 2000/80) spin echo MR images in a patient with an acute tear of the anterior cruciate ligament reveal one typical site of bone injury, appearing as a region of high signal intensity (arrows) in the posterolateral aspect of the proximal portion of the tibia.

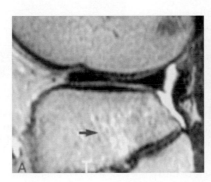
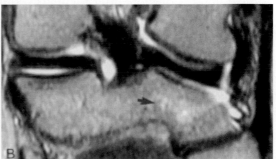

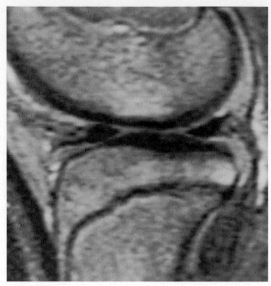

Figure 16–196

Injuries of the anterior cruciate ligament: MR imaging. Acute complete anterior cruciate ligament tears with osteochondral impaction fractures. High signal intensity is identified on the T2-weighted spin echo MR image (TR/TE, 2000/80) in the posterior and middle aspect of the proximal part of the lateral portion of the tibia and the middle to anterior aspects of the lateral femoral condyle. (Courtesy of H. Pavlov, M.D., New York, New York.)

rators[783] detected 89 occult fractures in MR imaging examinations of 56 knees in patients with acute complete tears of the anterior cruciate ligament. The posterior aspect of the lateral tibial plateau was involved in every case, either as an isolated finding or associated with additional lesions, especially in the midportion of the lateral femoral condyle. Tung and associates[770] detected MR imaging findings compatible with a bone bruise in 44 per cent of patients with a complete tear of the anterior cruciate ligament and in 9 per cent of patients who had a normal anterior cruciate ligament at the time of arthroscopy. In patients with a torn anterior cruciate ligament and one or more bone bruises, these bruises were seen in the posterior aspect of the lateral tibial plateau in 32 per cent of cases, in this tibial region and the middle aspect of the lateral femoral condyle in 36 per cent of cases, and in the lateral femoral condyle and medial femoral condyle in 23 per cent of cases. These last investigators emphasized the time-dependent nature of the bone bruises, indicating that they rarely were seen when the MR imaging examination was performed 9 weeks or more after the injury. Results of this study indicated a 73 per cent prevalence of bone bruise in patients with anterior cruciate ligament tear who underwent MR imaging within 9 weeks of injury, and in 91 per cent of cases the lateral compartment of the knee was involved. The authors concluded that the pattern of bone bruise involving the posterior compartment of the lateral tibial plateau, alone or together with that of the middle aspect of the lateral femoral condyle, occurs predominantly but not exclusively in association with acute complete anterior cruciate ligament tear, a conclusion echoed in other studies.[1150] Such bruises usually

are not evident when the patient is examined 9 weeks or more after the knee injury.

The precise location of bone bruises in patients with disruption of the anterior cruciate ligament shows some variability, however, owing in part to the degree of knee flexion at the time of injury. With increased flexion of the knee, the bruise in the lateral femoral condyle may be located more posterior than that occurring with less flexion of the knee.[785] In skiers, for example, in whom ligament injury may be associated with a greater degree of knee flexion than in persons involved in nonskiing-related injuries, a different distribution of bone bruises associated with disruption of the anterior cruciate ligament has been emphasized.[726] Such bruises may involve the posterior portions of both the medial and lateral tibial plateaus and are less frequent in the lateral femoral condyle. Anterior bone bruises involving the tibia and lateral femoral condyle also may accompany certain injuries resulting in disruption of the anterior cruciate ligament.

Other patterns of bone contusion occurring in patients with anterior cruciate ligament tears are those related to avulsion fractures. These occur in the lateral tibial rim (Segond fracture) and posterior margin of the lateral tibial plateau, related to capsular avulsions of the tibia (see Fig. 16–150). Marrow edema is evident on the MR imaging examinations, but the fracture fragments may not be appreciated. Anterior cruciate ligament deficiency also may accompany avulsion fractures at its sites of insertion (Fig. 16–197).

4. Miscellaneous abnormalities. A shearing injury of Hoffa's fat pad has been emphasized as a secondary sign of disruption of the anterior cruciate ligament.[773] A transverse line of high signal intensity in the middle of

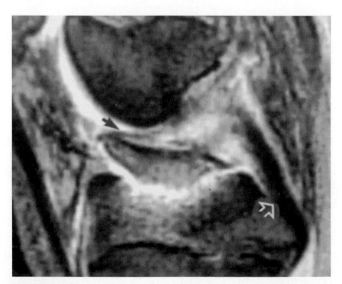

Figure 16–197

Injuries of the anterior cruciate ligament: MR imaging. Acute avulsion of the anterior tibial eminence. A sagittal MPGR MR image (TR/TE, 600/20; flip angle, 45 degrees) shows a displaced avulsion fracture of the tibial eminence. Note the insertion of the anterior cruciate ligament (solid arrow) into the fracture fragment. The site of attachment of the posterior cruciate ligament (open arrow) is not involved. (Courtesy of S. Fernandez, M.D., Mexico City, Mexico.)

the infrapatellar fat body is seen on sagittal T2-weighted spin echo MR images. The sensitivity and specificity of this sign are not clear, however.

In knees in which the cruciate ligaments are intact, integrity of the adjacent synovial lining is expected. In such knees, joint fluid may appear in front of the anterior cruciate ligament and behind the posterior cruciate ligament, but this fluid does not accumulate in a triangular space between the cruciate ligaments that is extrasynovial in location (Figs. 16–198 and 16–199). With disruption of either or both of the cruciate ligaments, the synovial lining about these ligaments may be torn, allowing fluid to enter this triangular space (Fig. 16–200). The absence of fluid in this space, however, does not exclude the presence of a cruciate ligament injury, presumably because the adjacent synovial sheath remains intact.

Incomplete Tears of the Anterior Cruciate Ligament. The term "partial" tear of the anterior cruciate ligament is used inconsistently in the literature, is rarely defined, and sometimes is replaced by such designations as ligament laxity and incompetence. This term implies that some, but not all, of the ligament fibers are torn. The reported frequency of partial, or incomplete, tears is 10 to 28 per cent of all tears of the anterior cruciate ligament.[717] In animals, partial tears of this ligament have shown little potential for healing.[717] In humans, also, sequential clinical assessments in cases of partial tear of the anterior cruciate ligament treated conservatively have shown little change in stability of the joint; patients with normal stability of the knee at the time of initial evaluation generally demonstrate normal stability at follow-up examination and those with pathologic anterior displacement of the tibia at the time of initial assessment reveal similar findings on later examinations.[717]

Partial tears of the anterior cruciate ligament often are associated with symptoms and a hemarthrosis. On physical examination, instability of the knee may be evident,[787] although the degree of instability is less than that associated with complete tears of the ligament, and arthrometric testing may be normal.[717] A definitive diagnosis is provided by arthroscopy in which both torn and intact fibers of the anterior cruciate ligament are identified.

A number of investigations have examined the diagnostic role assumed by MR imaging in patients with incomplete tears of the anterior cruciate ligament.[766–768] Although opinions vary, such diagnosis clearly is more difficult than that of a complete tear of the anterior cruciate ligament (Figs. 16–201 and 16–202). MR imaging findings of abnormal intraligamentous signal intensity, bowing of the ligament, and inability to identify all of the fibers of the ligament are not highly sensitive or specific in the diagnosis of incomplete tears of the anterior cruciate ligament.[766, 767] Secondary findings of cruciate ligament injury, including bone bruises, are less frequent when incomplete (rather than complete) tears are present.[767, 788] In one study, bone bruises were identified in only 12 per cent of 42 patients with partial tears of the anterior cruciate ligament (the diagnosis

of partial tear being confirmed by arthroscopy in 20 patients), compared with a 72 per cent frequency of such bruises in 29 patients with complete tears of the anterior cruciate ligament (all such tears being confirmed at the time of arthroscopy or reconstructive surgery).[788] In another study, posterior displacement of the posterior horn of the lateral meniscus and injury to the popliteus muscle were found to be useful secondary findings on MR imaging examinations in the identification of complete versus partial tears of the anterior cruciate ligament.[767] It is evident that further data are required to better define the diagnostic importance of MR imaging in assessing incomplete tears of this ligament.

Postoperative Anterior Cruciate Ligament

As disruption of the anterior cruciate ligament represents the most frequent of all the ligamentous injuries of the knee, a great deal of thought and study has been directed at its treatment. Left untreated, progressive deterioration of the knee joint, manifested as meniscal tears, further ligamentous damage, and cartilage loss, may occur. Radiographic evidence of osteoarthritis has been reported in approximately one third of patients with anterior cruciate ligament disruption who have been studied serially over a period of years.[789, 790] Many variables, however, enter into the decision regarding the need for surgical intervention and the precise type of procedure required.[791] Whether the anterior cruciate ligament is torn completely or partially and the presence or absence of meniscal and other ligamentous damage influence this decision. Furthermore, lifestyle of the patient also plays a significant role in the decision-making process. Persons who are athletic (i.e., high risk lifestyle) are more likely candidates for surgery than those who are sedentary or who are involved in only modest amounts of physical activity. In patients in whom a conservative therapeutic approach is chosen, functional bracing and modifications in lifestyle may represent a sufficient treatment protocol, particularly in instances of isolated or partial tears of the anterior cruciate ligament.

Principles of Ligament Reconstruction. Operative procedures employed for the treatment of the torn anterior cruciate ligament include primary repair of the ligament, ligament repair plus augmentation using various autogenous grafts, and ligament reconstruction using autogenous materials, allografts (e.g., patellar tendon, Achilles tendon, iliotibial band and fascia lata), or prosthetic devices.[792–794] Of the autogenous intra-articular reconstructions, the bone-patellar tendon-bone graft has become the anterior cruciate ligament substitute to which all others are being compared.[792] The success of this procedure, or other similar ones in which the iliotibial tract, semitendinosus tendon, or gracilis tendon is used as the autogenous graft material, depends on a number of factors, including the structural and material properties of the graft, the intra-articular positioning of the graft, initial tensioning of the graft during implanta-

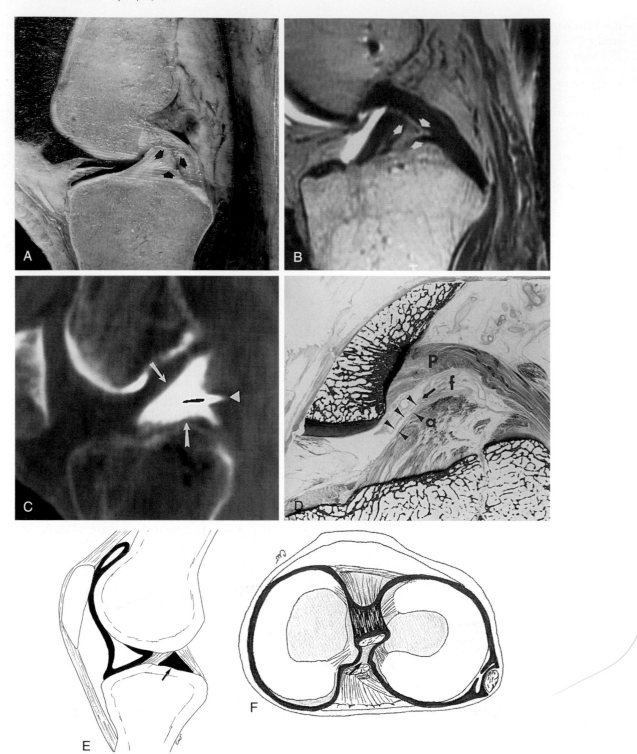

Figure 16–198

Normal anterior and posterior cruciate ligaments: MR imaging. Triangular space of the cruciate ligaments (TSC).

A, B After maximum distention of a cadaveric knee joint with 100 mg of a gadolinium-containing solution, a sagittal section of the knee was obtained. The photograph of the section **(A)** shows that no fluid has entered the TSC (arrows), indicative of an intact pericruciate synovial lining. A sagittal T1-weighted (TR/TE, 800/25) fat-suppressed spin echo MR image **(B)** at the same sagittal level confirms the absence of the gadolinium compound in the TSC (arrows).

C In a second cadaver, iodinated contrast material was injected directly into the TSC. A sagittal CT image confirms that all of the contrast agent remains in the TSC (arrows). An artifact related to the needle is seen (arrowhead).

D A histologic preparation of a midsagittal section shows the anterior (a) and posterior (p) cruciate ligaments. The TSC containing loose connective tissue and fat (f) is seen. The synovial lining (arrowheads) covers the anterior aspect of the anterior cruciate ligament. A small recess is seen (arrow) between the cruciate ligaments.

E, F Schematic drawings of sagittal **(E)** and transverse **(F)** sectional anatomy of the knee show the relationship of the synovial membrane (bold lines) to the cruciate ligaments and the location of the TSC (arrows).

(Courtesy of S. Lee, M.D., Los Angeles, California.)

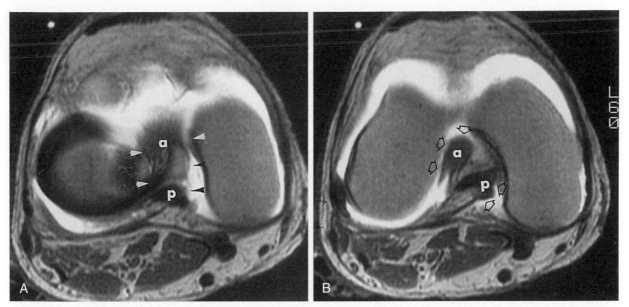

Figure 16–199

Normal anterior and posterior cruciate ligaments: MR imaging. Triangular space of the cruciate ligaments (TSC). After intra-articular injection of a gadolinium-containing solution into a cadaveric knee, transaxial fat-suppressed T1-weighted (TR/TE, 800/25) spin echo MR images, with **A** being 4 mm caudad to **B,** show the fluid surrounding both medial and lateral aspects of the anterior (a) and posterior (p) cruciate ligaments. The synovial membrane attachments (arrowheads in **A,** open arrows in **B**) are seen. (Courtesy of S. Lee, M.D., Los Angeles, California.)

tion, fixation of the graft, and the postoperative rehabilitation regimen.[792]

The choice of the patellar tendon graft has theoretical advantages. In experimental situations, preparations using bone-patellar tendon-bone graft material have been stronger than those using the semitendinosus or gracilis tendon.[795, 796] Furthermore, the bone-to-bone apposition

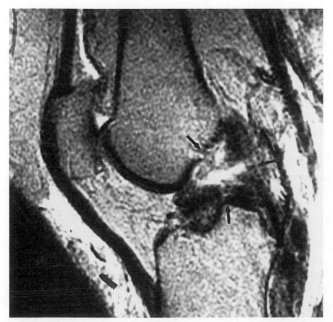

Figure 16–200

Injuries of the anterior cruciate ligament: MR imaging—acute complete anterior cruciate ligament tear with fluid in the TSC. This sagittal T2-weighted (TR/TE, 2000/80) spin echo MR image shows the fluid (arrows) within the TSC, confirming disruption of the pericruciate synovial lining.

used with this graft procedure provides immediate and secure fixation, enabling joint motion soon after surgery. The structural properties of the bone-patellar tendon-bone graft change with time after the surgical procedure. Experimentally, stiffness and ultimate failure of the strength of this preparation decrease over a period of months after surgery, related to increased water content in the graft and, perhaps, to changes in the profile of the collagen fiber and rearrangement of its ultrastructural morphometry.[797] In animals and in humans, the remodeling process occurring in the graft has been documented repeatedly and is believed to be consistent with synovial revascularization.[798]

The middle third of the patellar tendon with its accompanying bone plugs or blocks is used.[799] The femoral insertion site chosen generally is close to or at the normal insertion site of the anterior cruciate ligament. Similarly, the tibial insertion site of the graft usually corresponds closely to that of the anterior cruciate ligament itself. The principle guiding the selection of appropriate femoral and tibial insertion sites is isometry. Isometric points are those regions of ligamentous attachment to the femur and the tibia that allow the graft to undergo minimal (or no) change in its length and associated load during flexion and extension of the knee.[800] Identification of such isometric points is complicated by the fact that the graft has material and geometric properties different from those of the normal anterior cruciate ligament.[792] Furthermore, the anterior cruciate ligament is composed of bands of fibers, each with different morphologic characteristics. As the anteromedial band of the anterior cruciate ligament demonstrates the least amount of change in length during knee movement, autogenous graft procedures probably should reproduce the function of this band of the ligament by assuming its sites of femoral and tibial attach-

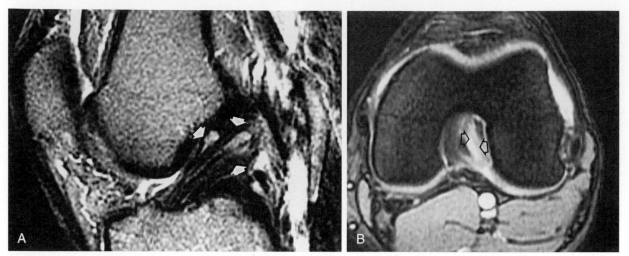

Figure 16–201

Injuries of the anterior cruciate ligament: MR imaging. Acute incomplete (partial) anterior cruciate ligament tear. This 43 year old man had suffered an acute knee injury 3 weeks prior to the MR imaging examination. A clinical examination suggested insufficiency of the anterior cruciate ligament. No arthroscopy was performed. The patient recovered completely with conservative treatment.

A A sagittal T2-weighted (TR/TE, 2000/80) spin echo MR image shows local fluid collections (arrows) within the substance of the anterior cruciate ligament.

B A transaxial MPGR (TR/TE, 500/17; flip angle, 20 degrees) MR image confirms intraligamentous fluid collections (arrows).

ment.[793] In replacements of the anterior cruciate ligament, isometry is less sensitive to the site of tibial attachment of the graft than to the site of femoral attachment. Accurate positioning of the femoral tunnel through which the graft passes appears to be critical.[793] If this tunnel is placed too far anteriorly with respect to the normal anatomic insertion site of the anterior cruciate ligament, high strain along the graft occurs as the knee is flexed; in such cases, knee flexion may be restricted, or over a period of time, the graft may elongate.[792, 793] Graft placement posterior or distal to the normal site of femoral attachment of the anterior cruciate ligament leads to similar problems during knee extension. Although the position of the tibial tunnel (through which the graft passes) is less critical to the success of the surgery, this tunnel should be positioned so that the graft does not impinge against the roof of the intercondylar notch when the knee is fully extended.[792, 801–805] In recent years, anterior notch plasty (roofplasty) has been used as an ancillary procedure in an attempt to decrease the frequency and severity of such impingement.[805]

After proper positioning of the graft is achieved, an appropriate graft tension is chosen based on the desire to restore normal joint kinematics.[792] This choice is difficult, owing to a viscoelastic response that occurs in all grafts that may lead to stress relaxation. Secure fixation of the graft to the host bone also is essential to surgical success. For bone-patellar tendon-bone grafts, large diameter interference-fit screws often are used to fix the bone plugs to the walls of the femoral and tibial tunnels. These screws serve to press the bone plug against the side of the drill hole, and they may be combined with additional screws or staples used to secure the adjacent soft tissue. Finally, rehabilitation of the knee after surgery is essential, but the need for immobilization or early mobilization of the knee is not agreed on, resulting in different rehabilitation protocols.[792]

A variety of prosthetic devices and other means have been used as artificial substitutes for the torn anterior cruciate ligament. Three general types of artificial ligaments exist: prostheses (which are designed to replace the ligament permanently); scaffolds (which produce support for ingrowing tissue by possibly inducing orientated ingrowth of collagen); and stents (which temporarily protect an autogenous graft from excessive strain during the period of its revascularization and collagen maturation).[806] Such artificial ligaments have considerable appeal owing to the theoretical advantage of immediate strength and therefore a rapid return to full function. In practice, however, numerous complications are seen, leading to the current popularity of the bone-patellar tendon-bone graft procedure.

The success of surgical repair of the torn anterior cruciate ligament is influenced by the procedure chosen, the skill of the orthopedic surgeon, and the resolve of the patient during the many months of rehabilitation.[807] Postoperative stiffness of the knee represents a frequent and disabling problem. Failure to regain full extension of the knee after anterior cruciate ligament reconstruction procedures may result from graft impingement (see later discussion), fat pad fibrosis, reflex sympathetic dystrophy, and intra-articular adhesions. The patellar entrapment syndrome (i.e., infrapatellar contracture syndrome) results in a loss of knee extension or knee flexion, with reduced patellar mobility.[808, 1151] It may relate to adherence of the patella to the adjacent infrapatellar fat body, leading to contracture of the patellar tendon, a low-lying patella (patella baja or infera), and loss of patellar cartilage. The cyclops lesion is a fibrous nodule that develops anterior to the tibial insertion site of the graft, within the intercondylar notch, and that may lead to loss of knee extension (see later discussion).[809]

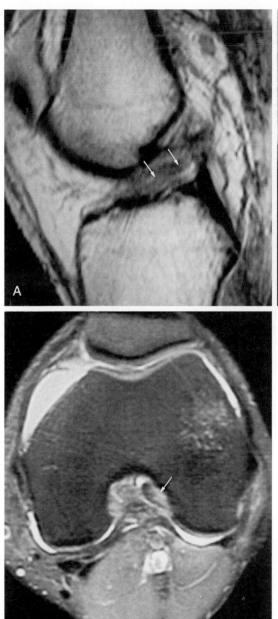

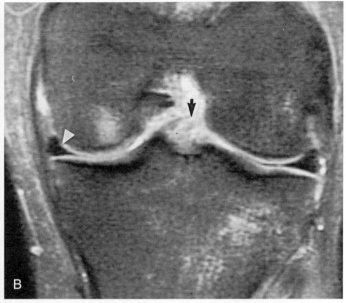

Figure 16–202

Injuries of the anterior cruciate ligament: MR imaging. Acute incomplete (partial) anterior cruciate ligament tear. A 25 year old man had suffered an acute knee injury approximately 2 weeks before the MR imaging examination. Clinical evaluation indicated an insufficient anterior cruciate ligament, and arthroscopy confirmed a tear of the anterior bundle of the anterior cruciate ligament and a medial meniscal tear.

A A sagittal proton density–weighted (TR/TE, 2200/30) spin echo MR image reveals altered morphology of the anterior cruciate ligament (arrows) with slight depression of the course of its fibers.

B A coronal fat-suppressed fast spin echo (TR/TE, 4000/18) MR image shows high signal (arrow) among the fibers of the anterior cruciate ligament, bone bruises of the lateral portion of the tibia and medial femoral condyle, and a tear of the medial meniscus (arrowhead) manifested as a contour abnormality.

C A transaxial fat-suppressed fast spin echo (TR/TE, 3500/17) MR image shows abnormal signal intensity (arrow) near the femoral insertion site of the anterior cruciate ligament and a lateral femoral bone bruise. The MR imaging findings were interpreted as evidence of a complete tear of the anterior cruciate ligament.

Routine Radiography. The normal radiographic appearance of the knee after reconstruction of the anterior cruciate ligament has been summarized by Manaster and coworkers.[810] Both frontal and lateral radiographs provide indirect information regarding the placement of the graft material, based on the position of the tunnels in the femur and the tibia (Fig. 16–203). As indicated previously, these tunnels should exit at the level of the joint in regions close to or at the normal sites of attachment of the anterior cruciate ligament. In the lateral projection, the tibial osseous tunnel begins distally near the tibial tuberosity, courses posteriorly, and exits the tibial articular surface immediately anterior to the anterior tibial spine; in the frontal projection, this tunnel begins in the medial side of the tibia, courses laterally, and exits the tibial articular surface at the intercondylar eminence of the tibial plateau.[810] In the lateral projection, the intra-articular point of entrance of the femoral tunnel is at the intersection of two lines representing the posterior femoral cortex and the intercondylar shelf; in the frontal projection, the femoral osseous tunnel begins laterally, just superior to the lateral femoral condyle, and emerges on the superolateral aspect of the intercondylar notch.[810]

Radiographic findings associated with improper placement of the anterior cruciate ligament graft material (i.e., nonisometric attachment) include the identification of osseous tunnels in the femur and tibia that vary from the normal landmarks noted previously. The construction of a number of lines on lateral radiographs of the maximally extended knee has been used to identify improperly oriented tibial tunnels.[811] The location

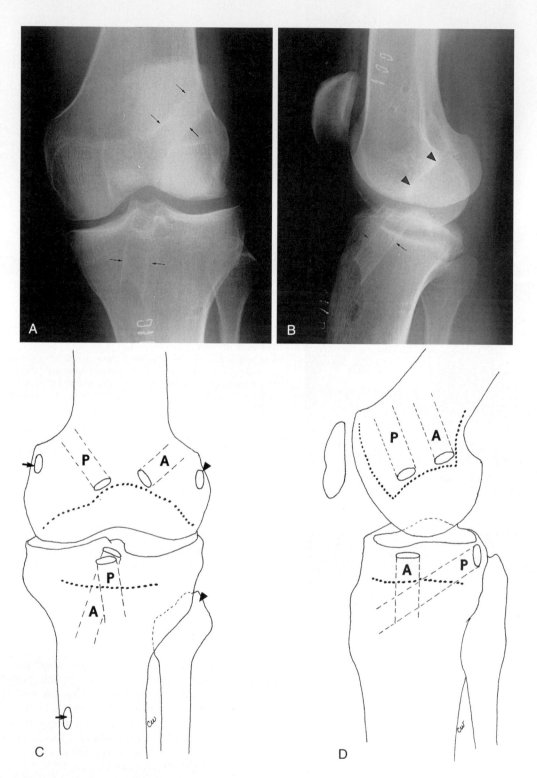

Figure 16–203

Postoperative anterior cruciate ligament: Routine radiography— normal appearance.

A, B The anteroposterior (**A**) and lateral (**B**) radiographs show the location of the tunnels (arrows) in the femur and tibia. In **B,** note that the tibial tunnel is located posterior to the line of the intercondylar roof (arrowheads) of the femur.

C, D Frontal (**C**) and lateral (**D**) diagrams reveal the isometric positions for replacements of the anterior (A) and posterior (P) cruciate ligaments. Isometric positions for the proximal and distal attachments of replacements for the medial (arrows) and lateral (arrowheads) collateral ligaments also are shown. (Redrawn with permission from BJ Manaster, RSNA Categorical Course in Musculoskeletal Radiology, 1993, p 211.)

of a tibial tunnel that is completely anterior to the line of the intercondylar roof (Blumensaat's line), as seen in these radiographs, is consistent with impingement on the anterior portion of the graft by the intercondylar roof (Fig. 16–204).[811] Indeed, ideally, the tibial tunnel should be posterior and parallel to the intercondylar roof.[803, 804] In patients with hyperextension of the knee and a vertically oriented slope to the intercondylar roof, a more posterior position of the tibial tunnel may be required.[804] Additional radiographic abnormalities include breakage of the screws or staples, fracture of the bone plugs, fracture of the patella (related to the donor sites of the bone blocks), heterotopic ossification, osteonecrosis of the femoral condyles, patella baja (related to the patellar entrapment syndrome), and patella alta (related to avulsion or rupture of the patellar tendon) (Fig. 16–204*B*).[808, 810, 812–814, 1152–1154]

MR Imaging. Postoperative impingement of the anterior cruciate ligament graft may occur in the intercondylar notch, blocking full extension of the knee and causing erosion and possible disruption of the graft. Clinically, roof impingement also causes effusions in the knee, anterior knee pain, and recurrent instability.[815] Although routine radiography may provide indirect evidence of such impingement,[811] MR imaging allows direct visualization of the graft itself and potentially is a superior imaging method in establishing the diagnosis of graft impingement, cystic degeneration and rupture (Figs. 16–205 and 16–206).[1155] Despite an initial report that indicated a limited role for MR imaging in the assessment of reconstructed anterior cruciate ligaments,[816] some subsequent investigations of the diagnostic role of MR imaging in this assessment have led to more promising results. Rak and associates[817] empha-

sized a poorly delineated graft and buckling of the posterior cruciate ligament as MR imaging findings consistent with graft inadequacy. The low signal intensity of the normal graft material has been emphasized,[818, 819] and an increase in signal intensity in the graft, particularly in the distal two thirds of its intra-articular portion, has been attributed to impingement of the graft by the intercondylar roof.[811, 820] The results of some studies suggest that persistent low signal intensity in the graft is an indicator of the absence of roof impingement, but the presence of increased signal intensity, although suggesting roof impingement, may occur with or without clinical evidence of knee instability.[820] Further diagnostic difficulty regarding the interpretation and clinical significance of regions of increased signal intensity within the graft relates to the known occurrence of remodeling of the graft (with revascularization and cellular ingrowth) in the early postoperative period.[821] Such remodeling may lead to some variability in the appearance of the graft on MR imaging studies. In one study, only two of 15 autografts (bone-patellar tendon-bone grafts) in clinically stable knees appeared as bands of low signal intensity in the MR images.[822] More recent reports, however, indicate a degree of optimism regarding the value of MR imaging in assessing the precise position of the intraosseous tunnels, the integrity of the graft, and the presence of graft impingement.[823–827, 1156] Oblique sagittal MR imaging along the course of the graft may be valuable. The role of intravenous administration of a gadolinium compound is not clear. MR imaging also reveals time-dependent changes in configuration and signal intensity within the patellar tendon when a portion of it has been used for the anterior cruciate ligament reconstructive procedure.[828]

A localized form of anterior arthrofibrosis, designated

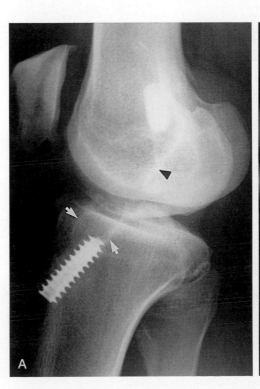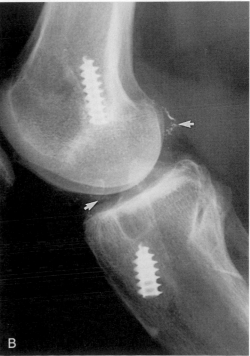

Figure 16–204

Postoperative anterior cruciate ligament: Routine radiography—abnormal appearance.

A Anterior placement of the tibial tunnel. In a fully extended lateral radiograph of the knee, note the abnormal anterior location of the tibial tunnel (arrows) with respect to the line of the intercondylar roof of the femur (arrowhead). Interference screws are seen.

B Metal debris. In this lateral radiograph of a partially flexed knee, intra-articular metal debris (arrows) is evident.

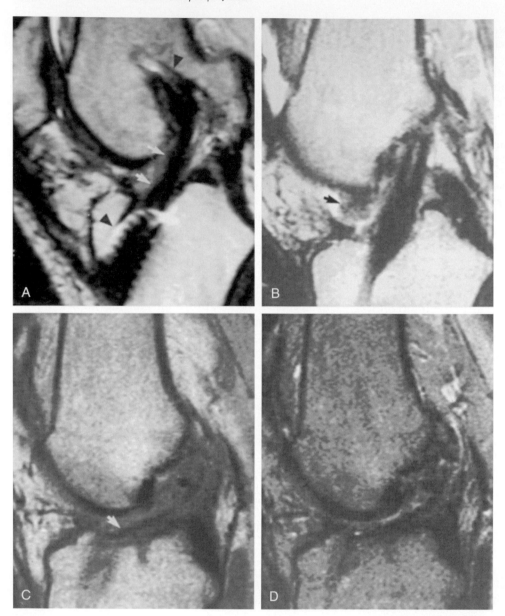

Figure 16–205

Postoperative anterior cruciate ligament: MR imaging.

A Normal appearance. A sagittal T2-weighted (TR/TE, 3800/100) spin echo MR image in an asymptomatic patient with a bone–patellar tendon–bone autograft shows the sites of the intraosseous tunnels (arrowheads) and a graft (arrows) that is straight in contour and of low signal intensity. A slight increase in signal intensity in the distal portion of the patellar tendon is evident.

B Cyclops lesion. A sagittal T2-weighted (TR/TE, 8000/135) spin echo MR image shows a nodular region (arrow) of low signal intensity anterior to the reconstructed anterior cruciate ligament. At surgery, a fibrous nodule, or cyclops lesion, was found.

C, D Autograft rupture. Sagittal proton density–weighted (TR/TE, 2400/20) (**C**) and T2-weighted (TR/TE, 2400/80) (**D**) spin echo MR images reveal only a portion of the autograft (arrow) and, in **D,** adjacent high signal intensity.

(**B–D,** Courtesy of M. Recht, M.D., Cleveland, Ohio.)

Figure 16–206

Postoperative anterior cruciate ligament: MR imaging. Cystic degeneration of the graft (solid arrow) within the tibial tunnel (arrowheads) is associated with an anterior soft tissue mass (open arrow), as shown in a sagittal three-dimensional GRASS (TR/TE, 51/13; flip angle, 20 degrees) MR image. (Courtesy of S. Eilenberg, M.D., San Diego, California.)

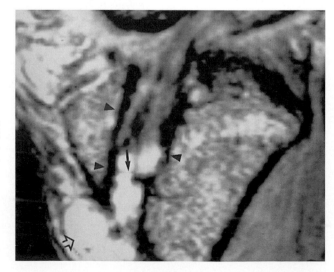

the cyclops lesion, occurs with a frequency of 1 to 10 per cent after reconstruction of the anterior cruciate ligament. The name is derived from the headlike appearance and reddish-blue color of the lesion, observed at arthroscopy, which resemble the features of an eye. The lesion may result from debris related to the drilling and preparation of the tibial tunnel or from exposed and injured ligament fibers due to graft impingement. The dominant signal intensity pattern of the cyclops lesion is low, consistent with fibrous tissue.[829] The lesion is located anterior to the graft (Figs. 16–205*B* and 16–207).

Posterior Cruciate Ligament Injuries

Injuries to the posterior cruciate ligament are less frequent than those to the anterior cruciate ligament, they require greater force, and they initially may be unrecognized, leading to a delay in diagnosis.[830] Injuries to this ligament represent approximately 5 to 20 per cent of all knee injuries. The usual mechanism of injury producing a tear of the posterior cruciate ligament is a force applied to the anterior aspect of the proximal portion of the tibia with the knee flexed. This mechanism occurs from a fall or from striking the knee against the dash-board (i.e., passenger in a car). Posterior cruciate ligament injuries also may result from extreme hyperextension or hyperflexion of the knee or from rotational or valgus forces applied to the knee.[831–833] They may occur as an isolated phenomenon (30 per cent of cases) or in association with other capsular, ligamentous, or meniscal injuries (70 per cent of cases).

DeLee and associates[834] identify four separate mechanisms of injury, the first three of which often lead to an isolated injury of the posterior cruciate ligament:

1. The application of a posteriorly directed force on the anterior aspect of the flexed knee. This mechanism, the most common type, leads to an isolated midsubstance tear of the posterior cruciate ligament.

2. A fall onto the flexed knee with the foot in plantar flexion. If the foot is in dorsiflexion, the force is delivered to the patellofemoral joint, not the posterior cruciate ligament.

3. Hyperflexion alone without the application of a posteriorly directed force. This mechanism may result in proximal avulsion of the posterior cruciate ligament from the femur with the adjacent perichondrium and periosteum, in which case the injury generally can be repaired successfully.

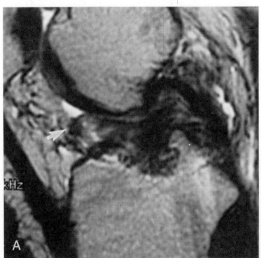

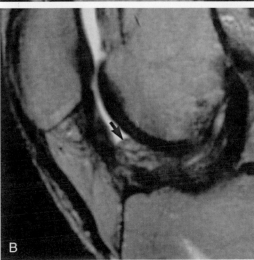

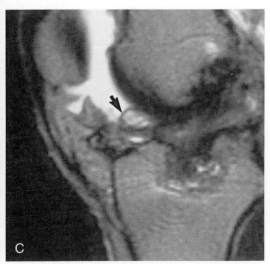

Figure 16–207

Postoperative anterior cruciate ligament: MR imaging—cyclops lesion.

A In a young woman with inability to extend the knee after anterior cruciate ligament repair, an area of low signal intensity (arrow) is seen in a sagittal fast spin echo (TR/TE, 4483/95) MR image. (Courtesy of D. Salonen, M.D., Toronto, Ontario, Canada.)

B, C Two additional examples of a cyclops lesion (arrows) are shown on fat-suppressed fast spin echo MR images (**B,** TR/TE, 3600/119; **C,** TR/TE, 8000/112). (Courtesy of M. Recht, M.D., Cleveland, Ohio.)

4. The application of an anteriorly directed force to a hyperextended knee with the foot fixed on the ground. This mechanism often results in injury to both cruciate ligaments.

Isolated injuries of the posterior cruciate ligament often involve its midsubstance and, in this situation, are difficult to repair. Those involving the proximal attachment site of the ligament, as noted previously, can be repaired, and those involving the distal, or tibial, attachment site are rare and also can be repaired.[834]

Although the reported prevalence of posterior cruciate ligament injuries is low (less than 20 per cent of all ligamentous injuries of the knee), subtle clinical findings in some cases of isolated injury to the posterior cruciate ligament may lead to missed diagnoses. Pain, swelling, and a hemarthrosis[835] may be evident; however, the frequent lack of soft tissue swelling or ecchymosis in these cases may result in a diagnosis of a knee sprain with conservative (and often inadequate) therapy.[836] The posterior drawer test, in which stress is applied to the anterior surface of the tibia in an attempt to produce posterior translation of the tibia with respect to the femur, is positive in 30 to 75 per cent of cases of posterior cruciate ligament tears, and a posterior sag sign represents additional evidence of such a tear.[721] Although arthroscopy can provide direct evidence of a tear of the posterior cruciate ligament, diagnostic problems arise owing to incomplete visualization of this ligament at arthroscopy when the anterior cruciate ligament is intact or misinterpretation of a normal meniscofemoral ligament of Humphrey as an intact posterior cruciate ligament. Arthroscopic findings include direct observation of the ligament tear and indirect evidence of such a tear, including the "sloppy" anterior cruciate ligament sign, in which laxity of the anterior cruciate ligament due to posterior displacement of the tibia is evident.[837] Imaging studies can be used to supplement the clinical assessment.[838]

Routine Radiography. In cases of injury to the posterior cruciate ligament, routine radiographs may reveal avulsion fractures at the tibial site of insertion of the ligament. This may occur in adults or in children. A joint effusion may be present. Owing to the nonspecific nature of a joint effusion and to the infrequent occurrence of an avulsion fracture, however, routine radiography rarely contributes to the diagnosis of a posterior cruciate ligament injury.

MR Imaging

Normal Posterior Cruciate Ligament. The posterior cruciate ligament normally appears as a bandlike structure of low signal intensity on sagittal, coronal, and transaxial MR images (Fig. 16–208).[839] In sagittal MR images, it is arcuate in shape when the knee is in a neutral position or mildly flexed. With increasing flexion, the ligament becomes taut and, with hyperextension, it appears lax.[840] The posterior cruciate ligament is seen in its entirety in a single MR image or possibly two contiguous MR images in the sagittal plane. The meniscofemoral ligament, consisting of the anterior (ligament of Humphrey) and

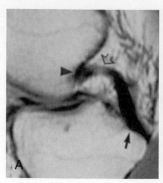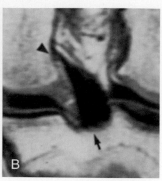

Figure 16–208
Normal posterior cruciate ligament: MR imaging.
A Sagittal proton density–weighted (TR/TE, 2000/20) spin echo MR image. Note the femoral (arrowhead) and tibial (solid arrow) insertion sites of the posterior cruciate ligament. It has an arcuate course and is of low signal intensity except for its proximal portion (open arrow), where intermediate signal intensity may relate to the magic angle phenomenon.
B Coronal proton density–weighted (TR/TE, 2000/20) spin echo MR image. The femoral (arrowhead) and tibial (solid arrow) insertion sites of the posterior cruciate ligament again are identified. The ligament is of low signal intensity and has a smooth contour.

posterior (ligament of Wrisberg) branches, leads to ovoid regions of low signal intensity, either applied to the surface of the posterior cruciate ligament or adjacent to it.[92] In the coronal plane, the posterior cruciate ligament again is identified in a single MR image or perhaps two contiguous MR images. It possesses a gentle curve. Occasionally, in elderly persons, mucoid or eosinophilic degeneration in the posterior cruciate ligament may lead to regions of intermediate signal intensity (Fig. 16–209).

Posterior Cruciate Ligament Tears. Tears of the posterior cruciate ligament usually occur in its midsubstance, or less commonly, at its femoral or tibial insertion site.[840, 841] Disruption of all or a portion of its fibers is evident on the MR imaging examination, especially in sagittal images (Figs. 16–210 and 16–211). Regions of high signal intensity within the ligament may be evident on T2-weighted spin echo MR images in cases of acute or subacute tears of the posterior cruciate ligament (see Fig. 16–210). These regions may relate to hemorrhage or joint fluid collecting within the torn ligament. The diagnosis of avulsion fractures of the tibia at the site of insertion of the posterior cruciate ligament is possible with MR imaging (Fig. 16–212), although correlation with routine radiography is required.

Sonin and associates[842] reported the MR imaging findings in 47 patients with injury to the posterior cruciate ligament, the diagnosis being confirmed arthroscopically in 24 patients. Complete tears (45 per cent), partial tears (47 per cent), and bone avulsions (8 per cent) were seen. Associated ligamentous (38 per cent) or meniscal (47 per cent) injuries were frequent. Regions of altered signal intensity in the bone marrow, compatible with contusions or fractures, also were common (36 per cent). Localization of such regions to the anterior portion of the tibial articular surface is particularly characteristic (Fig. 16–213).

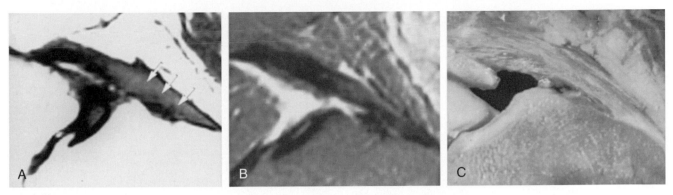

Figure 16–209
Normal posterior cruciate ligament: MR imaging. Variations in signal intensity related to eosinophilic degeneration. Sagittal T1-weighted (TR/TE, 500/20) **(A)** and T2-weighted (TR/TE, 2000/70) **(B)** spin echo MR images show regions of intermediate signal intensity (arrows) that are much more prominent in **A** than in **B**. A corresponding anatomic section **(C)** shows that the posterior cruciate ligament is grossly normal and its fibers are parallel to the sagittal plane. (From Hodler J, et al: AJR *159:*357, 1992.)

Postoperative Posterior Cruciate Ligament

Tears of the posterior cruciate ligament may be treated by primary repair, involving suturing of the ligament, that may be combined with graft augmentation.[843–846] A specific therapeutic strategy, however, often is dictated by the pattern of injury (e.g., acute versus chronic, avulsion fracture versus intrasubstance ligament tear, isolated posterior cruciate ligament tear versus combined tears of multiple ligaments). Acute tears isolated

to the posterior cruciate ligament may be treated nonoperatively, whereas those involving multiple ligaments often require surgical reconstruction. The degree of joint instability often governs the choice of operative or nonoperative treatment of chronic tears of the posterior cruciate ligament. Anatomic reconstruction of the anterolateral component of the posterior cruciate ligament appears to be critical.[1157] At present, the most common technique for reconstruction of the posterior cruciate ligament involves a bone-patellar tendon-bone

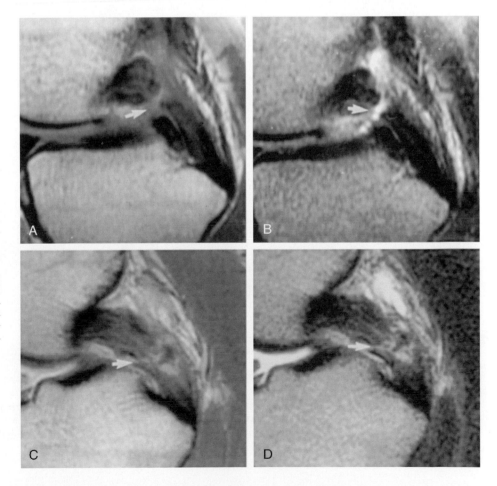

Figure 16–210
Injuries of the posterior cruciate ligament: MR imaging. Acute complete posterior cruciate ligament tears with alterations in ligament morphology and signal intensity.

A, B Sagittal proton density–weighted (TR/TE, 2000/30) **(A)** and T2-weighted (TR/TE, 2000/80) **(B)** spin echo MR images reveal complete disruption (arrows) of the posterior cruciate ligament, with an increase in signal intensity in **B**.

C, D Sagittal proton density–weighted (TR/TE, 2200/20) **(C)** and T2-weighted (TR/TE, 2200/80) **(D)** spin echo MR images in a second patient again show complete disruption (arrows) of the posterior cruciate ligament, with an increase in signal intensity in **D**.

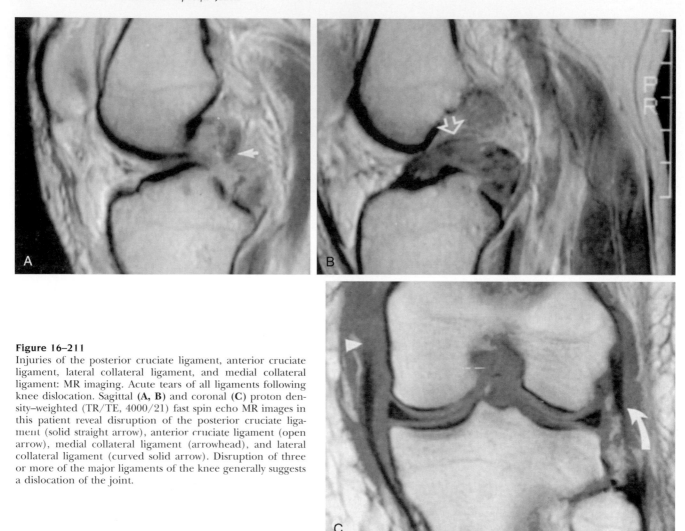

Figure 16–211

Injuries of the posterior cruciate ligament, anterior cruciate ligament, lateral collateral ligament, and medial collateral ligament: MR imaging. Acute tears of all ligaments following knee dislocation. Sagittal **(A, B)** and coronal **(C)** proton density–weighted (TR/TE, 4000/21) fast spin echo MR images in this patient reveal disruption of the posterior cruciate ligament (solid straight arrow), anterior cruciate ligament (open arrow), medial collateral ligament (arrowhead), and lateral collateral ligament (curved solid arrow). Disruption of three or more of the major ligaments of the knee generally suggests a dislocation of the joint.

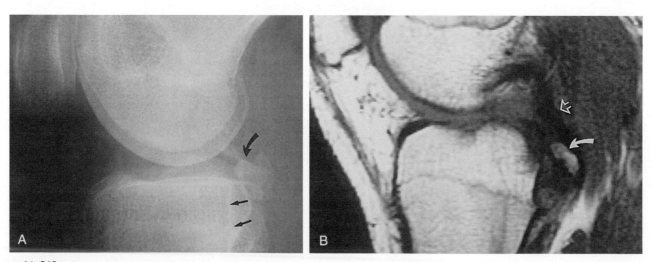

Figure 16–212

Injuries of the posterior cruciate ligament: MR imaging. Acute avulsion of the tibial insertion site of the posterior cruciate ligament. In a 17 year old male patient, a routine radiograph **(A)** shows the avulsed bone fragment (curved arrow) and the parent site in the tibia (straight arrows). A sagittal T1-weighted (TR/TE, 600/15) spin echo MR image **(B)** demonstrates the bone fragment (curved arrow) and attached intact posterior cruciate ligament (open arrow).

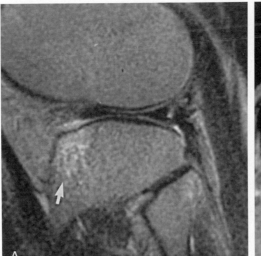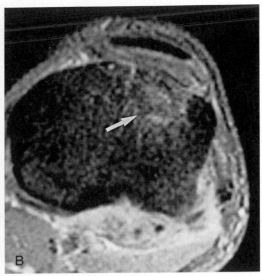

Figure 16–213
Injuries of the posterior cruciate ligament: MR imaging. Anterior tibial bone bruises (arrows) may accompany acute disruption of the posterior cruciate ligament, as shown on sagittal T2-weighted (TR/TE, 2300/85) spin echo (**A**) and transverse MPGR (TR/TE, 533/14; flip angle, 15 degrees) (**B**) MR images. (Courtesy of D. Goodwin, M.D., Hanover, New Hampshire.)

autograft or allograft.[844] An Achilles tendon allograft also may be used. As with procedures used to replace the anterior cruciate ligament, correct placement of femoral and tibial tunnels is critical to the success of grafting procedures used to replace the posterior cruciate ligament. The role of MR imaging in the assessment of the repaired posterior cruciate ligament is not documented.

Fractures and Dislocations

Fractures of the Distal Portion of the Femur

These fractures, which account for about 5 per cent of all femoral fractures, can be classified as supracondylar, intercondylar, or condylar. Most of these injuries result from axial loading combined with varus or valgus stress and rotation. They may occur in association with other injuries, including vascular injuries (e.g., femoral artery), ligamentous disruption of the knee, patellar fractures, fracture-dislocations of the hip, and fractures of the tibial shaft.[847]

The powerful muscles of the thigh lead to characteristic deformities when fractures involve the distal portion of the femur (Fig. 16–214).[848] The muscle pull of the quadriceps and posterior hamstring muscles produces shortening of the femur. As the shaft overrides anteriorly and the gastrocnemius muscles pull posteriorly, the femoral condyles are displaced and angulated posteriorly. When the condyles are separated by the fracture, rotational malalignments are common because of the unrestrained pull of the gastrocnemius muscles and the anterior overriding of the femoral shaft.[848]

Supracondylar fractures (without intra-articular extension) commonly are transverse or slightly oblique in configuration, with varying degrees of displacement and comminution of the fracture fragments.[849, 850] Open or closed fractures are encountered, and injury to the popliteal artery may occur.[851] These supracondylar fractures may be accompanied by a vertical fracture line extending into the knee, leading to *intercondylar fractures*

that possess a T or Y configuration,[852] or a vertical fracture alone may be evident.[853, 854] Incongruity of the surface of the femorotibial or patellofemoral compartment, or of both, is created by displacement at the fracture site. *Condylar fractures,* in which sagittal or coronal fracture lines are isolated to the region of a single condyle,[855] are more difficult to detect on radiographic examination and may require conventional tomography or CT scanning (Fig. 16–215).

Fractures of the Patella

Fractures of the patella result from direct or indirect forces, the latter related to contraction of the quadriceps muscles.[856] Unilateral injuries predominate, although bilateral fractures also are encountered.[857] The three major categories of patellar fractures are trans-

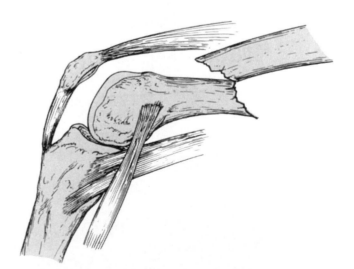

Figure 16–214
Fractures of the distal portion of the femur: Anatomic considerations. A diagram indicates muscle attachments and patterns of bone displacement. See text for details. (From BD Browner, JB Jupiter, AM Levine, et al [Eds]: Skeletal Trauma: Fractures, Dislocations, Ligamentous Injuries. Philadelphia, WB Saunders Co, 1992, p 1643.)

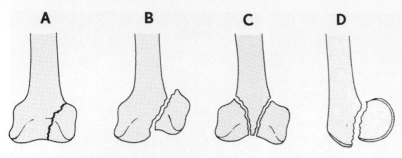

Figure 16–215
Fractures of the distal portion of the femur: Condylar fractures—classification system. Such fractures may be undisplaced (**A**) or displaced (**B–D**), involve one (**A, B**) or both (**C, D**) condyles, and be oriented principally in the sagittal (**A–C**) or coronal (**D**) plane. (From Hohl M, et al: Fractures and dislocations of the knee. *In* CA Rockwood Jr, DP Greene [Eds]: Fractures in Adults. 2nd Ed. Philadelphia, JB Lippincott Co, 1984, p 1444.)

verse, longitudinal (or vertical), and stellate. Transverse fractures are most typical, representing approximately 50 to 80 per cent of all patellar fractures, and generally they are the product of indirect force.[858, 859] They may divide the bone into equal-sized components or involve the superior or, more commonly, the inferior pole. Transverse fractures usually are nondisplaced, are associated with only minimal damage to the articular surfaces of the patella and femur, are unaccompanied by retinacular tears, and are compatible with the patient's still being able to extend the knee (Fig. 16–216). Longitudinal (25 per cent) and stellate or comminuted (20 to 35 per cent) fractures are less frequent and usually result from direct injury, such as striking the dashboard of an automobile (in which case a posterior dislocation of the hip also may be present). Longitudinal patellar fractures also may be avulsive injuries. Osteochondral fractures occur in combination with patellar dislocation (see later discussion). Displacement of the osseous fragments, particularly in instances of comminuted fractures, can be

considerable. Ischemic necrosis is a complication of patellar fractures, involving the proximal fragment and appearing 1 to 3 months after the injury.[860]

Fragmentation and separation of the lower pole of the patella is referred to as Sinding-Larsen-Johansson disease (Fig. 16–217), representing a stress-related phenomenon, although the mechanism of injury is debated.[861] A patellar sleeve fracture also involves the lower pole of the patella.[862, 863] Seen in children and adolescents, this fracture generally relates to an avulsion injury produced by hyperextension of the knee and is characterized by an avulsed fragment containing bone and a substantial sleeve of cartilage. Inability to extend the knee fully and, in some cases, a palpable defect about the inferior pole of the patella may be evident. The size of the patellar fragment and, indeed, the severity of the injury may not be apparent on routine radiographs owing to the invisible nature of cartilage. Thus, MR imaging represents a useful ancillary method for the assessment of this injury. The size of the cartilage com-

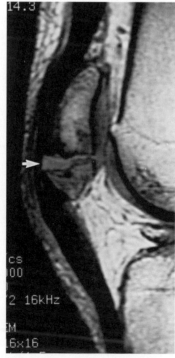

Figure 16–216
Patellar fractures. A sagittal proton density–weighted (TR/TE, 2000/20) spin echo MR image reveals a slightly displaced transverse patellar fracture (arrow) with adjacent marrow edema and an intact extensor mechanism. (Courtesy of D. Witte, M.D., Memphis, Tennessee.)

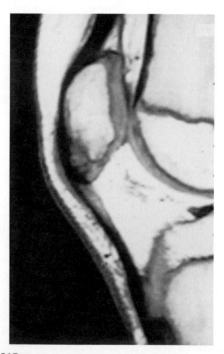

Figure 16–217
Sinding-Larsen-Johansson disease: MR imaging. In a 12 year old child, a sagittal T1-weighted (TR/TE, 650/15) spin echo MR image reveals bone irregularity in the lower pole of the patella. (Courtesy of D. Levey, M.D., Corpus Christi, Texas.)

ponent of the avulsed fragment and the extra-articular or intra-articular pattern of the fracture line can be ascertained with MR imaging, dictating in part the manner in which the injury is treated.[862]

Of related interest, fracture and dislocation of another sesamoid bone about the knee, the fabella, are reported.[864, 865]

Fractures of the Proximal Portion of the Tibia

These fractures (Fig. 16–218), which may be extra-articular or intra-articular, may be overlooked entirely on routine radiography. CT scanning frequently is required for accurate assessment of these injuries, and the tomographic techniques allow further analysis of the extent of displacement and depression of the articular segment.[866-870] MR imaging represents an additional method for diagnosis of occult fractures of the tibial plateau.[871] The relative benefits of CT scanning (including spiral CT techniques and image reconstruction)[872] versus MR imaging[873] (Fig. 16–219) in the assessment of fractures of the tibial plateau are not clear, although the latter technique allows the detection of associated ligamentous and meniscal injuries.[873]

Tibial plateau fractures result from a variety of mechanisms, which include vertical compression, varus or valgus forces, and twisting,[850] and they may be accompanied by injuries to the cruciate or collateral ligaments of the knee. Although they may occur in young persons, including those involved in athletics,[874] tibial plateau fractures predominate in middle-aged and elderly persons. Isolated lateral plateau fractures (75 to 80 per cent of all fractures of the tibial plateaus) and combined lateral and medial plateau fractures (10 to 15 per cent of all such fractures) are more frequent than isolated medial plateau fractures (5 to 10 per cent of all plateau fractures).[875] Available classification systems emphasize the location and configuration of the fracture lines.[876-880]

Important imaging considerations with respect to tibial fractures include the detection of lipohemarthrosis, avulsion fractures and sites of ligamentous detachment (femoral condyles, fibular head, and intercondylar eminence), meniscal injuries, abnormal widening of the joint space during the application of stress, and disruption of the articular surface. As an approximate guideline, surgical reduction generally is advised for fractures of the tibial plateau that are depressed or displaced by more than 1 cm.[880] Recognized complications of these injuries include peroneal nerve involvement, ruptures of the popliteal artery, residual varus or valgus angulation, and osteoarthritis.[881, 882]

Fractures of the tibial spine or intercondylar eminence result from violent twisting, abduction-adduction injuries, or direct contact with the adjacent femoral condyle and are indicative of possible damage to the cruciate ligaments of the knee.[850] Varying degrees of osseous displacement are seen.[883] Either the anterior

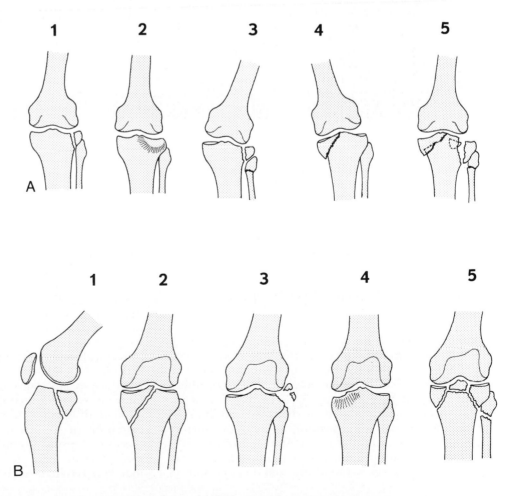

Figure 16–218
Fractures of the proximal portion of the tibia: Classification systems.

A Fractures of the tibial plateau. 1, Minimally displaced. 2, Local compression. 3, Split compression. 4, Total condylar depression. 5, Bicondylar.

B Fracture-dislocations of the knee. 1, Split fracture. 2, Entire plateau fracture. 3, Rim avulsion. 4, Rim compression. 5, Four-part fracture.

(**A,** From Hohl M: J Bone Joint Surg [Am] *49*:1456, 1967; **B,** from Hohl M, Moore TM: Articular fractures of the proximal tibia. *In* CM Evarts [Ed]: Surgery of the Musculoskeletal System. New York, Churchill Livingstone, 1983. Used by permission.)

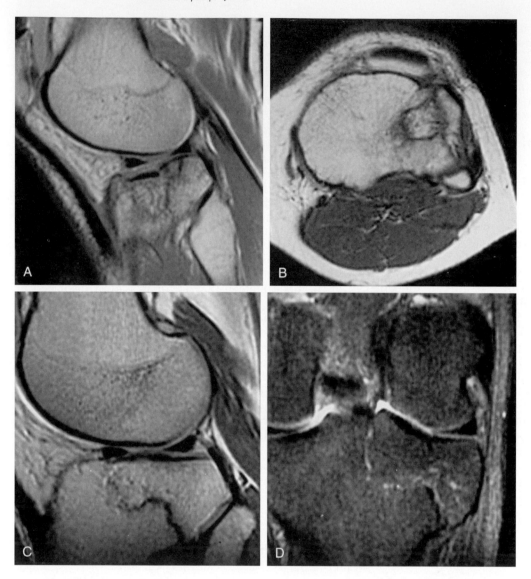

Figure 16–219

Fractures of the proximal portion of the tibia: MR imaging.

A, B A depressed and comminuted fracture of the lateral tibial plateau is seen on a sagittal proton density–weighted (TR/TE, 1800/20) spin echo MR image **(A)** and on a transaxial T1-weighted (TR/TE, 420/15) spin echo MR image **(B)**.

C, D A nondepressed subacute linear fracture of the lateral tibial plateau is demonstrated on a sagittal proton density–weighted (TR/TE, 2700/32) spin echo MR image **(C)** and on a coronal fat-suppressed fast spin echo (TR/TE, 4000/18) MR image **(D)**. (Courtesy of D. Goodwin, M.D., Hanover, New Hampshire.)

tibial spine or, less commonly, the posterior tibial spine is affected, and rarely both are involved. Avulsion injuries of the anterior tibial spine occur more commonly in children and in adolescents than in adults and, in children, often result from a fall while bicycling.[884] Such fractures in adults typically are accompanied by ligamentous and meniscal injury, whereas in children they may appear as an isolated phenomenon.[885]

Fractures of the Proximal Portion of the Fibula

Isolated fractures of the head or neck of the fibula are distinctly uncommon; the detection of a fracture in these regions should prompt a search for a ligamentous injury or fracture of the knee or ankle.[875] The combination of an adduction stress to the knee, rupture of the lateral capsular and ligamentous structures, an injury of the peroneal nerve, and, possibly, an avulsion fracture of the fibula is termed the ligamentous peroneal nerve syndrome.[850, 886] Additional complications of fractures of the proximal portion of the fibula include contusion or

traction of the biceps tendon, injury to the anterior tibial artery, and avulsion of the fibular head with possible intra-articular entrapment.[850]

Knee Dislocation

Knee dislocation is a rare but serious injury due to the neurovascular insult that may result from popliteal artery and peroneal nerve damage.[887–891] Dislocations of the knee require major force; typical causes include high-energy trauma resulting from motor vehicle accidents, industrial injury, or falls from a considerable height. Less commonly, these dislocations occur in collisions with a blow to the knee during sporting activities.[892, 893] Anterior, posterior, lateral, medial, and rotary types of dislocation are recognized. Anterior dislocation is the most common type (30 to 50 per cent of all knee dislocations), apparently resulting from hyperextension of the knee with sequential tearing of the posterior capsule, posterior cruciate ligament, and anterior cruciate ligament. The adjacent popliteal artery may be stretched, leading to thrombosis or laceration.

Posterior dislocations are next in frequency, although in some reported series they have been more common than anterior dislocations.[893] They may result from crushing blows to the leg with force applied to the anterior surface of the proximal tibia, one example being the dashboard injury. The extensor mechanism of the knee may be injured at the same time. Medial, lateral, and rotary (posterolateral) dislocations of the knee are uncommon, but they invariably are associated with damage to the collateral ligaments. Although the precise number of ligaments that are torn, stretched, or avulsed during a knee dislocation varies and depends on the magnitude of the force and the type of dislocation, injury to both cruciate ligaments is common (although not invariable[894]), as is injury to one or both collateral ligaments. As a general rule, the detection of disruption of four major ligaments of the knee (cruciate ligaments and collateral ligaments) implies that a dislocation of the joint has occurred. Rotary, or posterolateral, dislocation of the knee may be irreducible owing to intra-articular invagination of the medial capsule and medial collateral ligament.[893]

Arteriography should be employed to delineate the status of the popliteal artery in patients in whom operative intervention is being contemplated as a result of vascular symptoms and signs.[895] Popliteal artery injury occurs in 25 to 50 per cent of knee dislocations, may accompany posterior or anterior knee dislocations, and is encountered in both low- and high-energy injuries.[896, 897] The popliteal vein and tibial and peroneal nerves also may be injured during knee dislocations.

MR imaging (Figs. 16–220 and 16–221) can be employed to study soft tissue injuries associated with knee dislocations.[1158] In one investigation of 17 patients, all had complete tears of the anterior cruciate ligament, 15 had complete tears of the posterior cruciate ligament, and 12 had tears of the fibular collateral ligament with or without involvement of the tendon of the biceps femoris muscle.[898] Popliteal tendon tears occurred in eight patients and were either complete or incomplete, and such tears were associated with injuries of the peroneal nerve.

Patellar Dislocation

Traumatic dislocation of the patella can be produced by a direct blow or an exaggerated contraction of the quadriceps mechanism. Abnormalities predisposing to displacement may include an abnormally high patella (patella alta), deficient height of the lateral femoral condyle, shallowness of the patellofemoral groove, genu valgum or genu recurvatum, lateral insertion of the patellar tendon, muscular weakness, and excessive tibial torsion.[899, 900] Lateral dislocation predominates, although rare patterns of displacement include vertical (superior) dislocations or rotational dislocations, along either the vertical or the horizontal axis of the bone, the last pattern associated with intercondylar or intra-articular displacement of the patella.[901–909] Medial dislocation of the patella may follow surgical release of the lateral patellar retinaculum.[910] With regard to lateral dislocations of the patella, osteochondral fractures of the me-

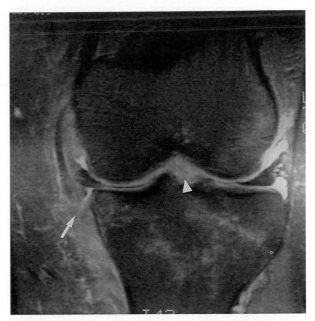

Figure 16–220

Knee dislocation: MR imaging. In a 34 year old man, soft tissue injuries accompanying a knee dislocation included tears of the anterior and posterior cruciate ligaments, medial collateral ligament, and anterior horn of the lateral meniscus. A coronal fat-suppressed fast spin echo MR image (TR/TE, 3983/18) shows disruption of the medial collateral ligament (arrow), a tear of the anterior and posterior cruciate ligaments manifest as an empty intercondylar appearance (arrowhead), and bone bruises in the lateral femoral condyle and proximal portion of the tibia.

dial patellar facet and lateral femoral condyle are common.[911–920]

Proximal Tibiofibular Joint Dislocation

The proximal tibiofibular joint exists between the lateral condyle of the tibia and the head of the fibula, and it communicates with the knee joint in approximately 10 per cent of adults.[921–924] Apposing bony facets are covered with articular cartilage, and the bones are connected by a fibrous capsule and anterior and posterior ligaments. The fibrous capsule, which is attached to the margins of the tibial and fibular articular facets, is much thicker anteriorly than posteriorly. The anterior ligament passes obliquely upward from the front of the fibular head to the front of the lateral condyle of the tibia; the posterior ligament passes obliquely upward from the back of the fibular head to the back of the lateral condyle of the tibia. The posterior ligament is covered by the popliteus tendon. Superior support is provided by the fibular collateral ligament, extending from the lateral aspect of the fibular head to the lateral femoral epicondyle.

Although rare, proximal tibiofibular joint dislocation may be seen in parachuting, hang-gliding, sky-diving, and horseback riding injuries. Anterior or, less frequently, posterior dislocation of the fibular head can be noted.[925–930] Peroneal nerve injury can appear after a posterior dislocation of this joint. Rarely, a superior dislocation can be seen, which is associated with injury

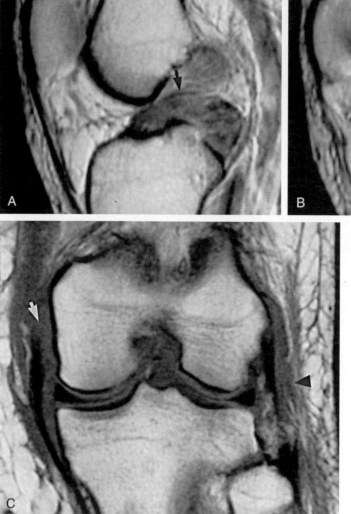

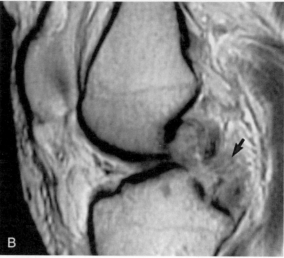

Figure 16–221

Knee dislocation: MR imaging. In a 33 year old woman, soft tissue injuries accompanying a knee dislocation included tears of both cruciate ligaments, a tear of the medial collateral ligament, and a sprain of the lateral collateral ligament.

A, B Sagittal fast spin echo MR images (TR/TE, 4000/21) show tears of the anterior cruciate (arrow, **A**) and posterior cruciate (arrow, **B**) ligaments.

C A coronal T1-weighted (TR/TE, 750/20) spin echo MR image reveals disruption of the medial collateral ligament (arrow) and edema (arrowhead) about the lateral collateral ligament.

to the interosseous membrane and superior dislocation of the lateral malleolus.

Subluxation of the proximal tibiofibular joint refers to excessive and symptomatic movement without frank dislocation.[931–934] This is a self-limited condition of youth with decreasing symptoms as the patient approaches skeletal maturity, although persistent symptoms and signs may require surgical intervention. Although radiographs may be normal, MR imaging may reveal bone bruises (Fig. 16–222).

Cartilage Abnormalities

Anatomic Considerations

Articular hyaline cartilage is a complex structure whose integrity is fundamental to proper joint function. Covering the articulating ends of bones in synovial joints, articular cartilage has unique structural characteristics that provide an extremely smooth and resilient surface that can withstand the high pressure and rapid velocity

generated during normal articular movement. Articular cartilage is composed primarily of collagen and proteoglycans.

Macroscopic and microscopic analysis of articular cartilage indicates a structure whose composition changes throughout its substance (Figs. 16–223 and 16–224). Its superficial (or tangential) zone, representing approximately 5 to 10 per cent of its total thickness, is composed of flattened and elongated cells oriented parallel to the surface of the joint. The collagen fibers are horizontally disposed and are independent of fibers in other zones,[935] and the matrix contains less proteoglycan than that present in other zones. The second zone, located deep to the superficial zone and designated the transitional or intermediate stratum, contains chondrocytes that are larger and occur singly or in groups. The third zone, designated the radiate stratum, contains columns of large cells that are oriented perpendicular to the surface, after the pattern of collagen deposition. This is the largest layer of articular cartilage, representing 70 to 80 per cent of its total thickness. The fourth and deepest zone, designated the calcified stratum, is com-

Figure 16–222
Proximal tibiofibular joint: Subluxation (MR imaging). Although the precise mechanism of injury was not clear in this 39 year old man, the "kissing" bone bruises (arrows) about the proximal tibiofibular joint, as shown on coronal fat-suppressed fast spin echo (TR/TE, 4000/20) **(A)** and sagittal fast spin echo STIR (TR/TE, 3000/28; inversion time, 150 msec) **(B)** MR images, are consistent with a previous subluxation of the joint (or direct injury). Note fluid in the proximal tibiofibular joint. (Courtesy of D. Goodwin, M.D., Hanover, New Hampshire.)

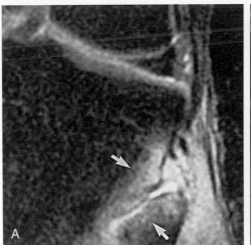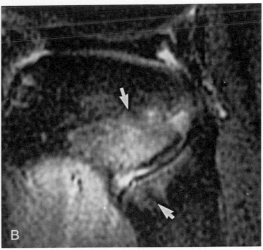

posed of nonviable cells and heavily calcified matrix. The inferior surface of the calcified zone of cartilage is irregular or undulating, with tongues of tissue that extend into and interdigitate with the subchondral bone. The tidemark represents a basophilic line, recognized on histologic analysis, that marks the junction between the calcified and noncalcified cartilage. The subchondral bone contains a thin plate that overlies the cancellous trabeculae that surround the marrow elements.

Nourishment of articular cartilage is derived from three sources: the synovial fluid, through a process of intrusion and extrusion of fluid that occurs with normal movement; the vessels of the synovial membrane; and the vessels of the underlying marrow cavity, which may penetrate or extend completely through the calcified layer of cartilage.

Pathologic Considerations

Healing of articular cartilage after an acute injury or a chronic insult is marginal at best, owing to its relative avascularity and its sparse cellularity. Healing of a cartilage defect that does not involve the subchondral bone plate relies entirely on chondrocyte proliferation at the margins of the injured area. Although chondrocytes can proliferate, the response generally is inadequate to lead to complete healing of the lesion. With cartilage injuries that extend to the subchondral bone plate, a healing response characterized by granulation tissue and fibroblastic proliferation is evident.[936, 937] The resulting fibrocartilaginous scar tissue differs morphologically from normal hyaline cartilage.

The overall cellularity, fluid content, and collagen

Figure 16–223
Cartilage abnormalities: Anatomic considerations. A schematic representation of the orientation of the collagen fibers in articular cartilage is provided. (Adapted from Mow VC, Fithian DC, Kelly MA: Fundamentals of articular cartilage. *In* JW Ewing [Ed]: Articular Cartilage and Knee Joint Function: Basic Science and Arthroscopy. New York, Raven Press, 1990, p 1.)

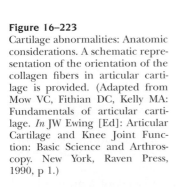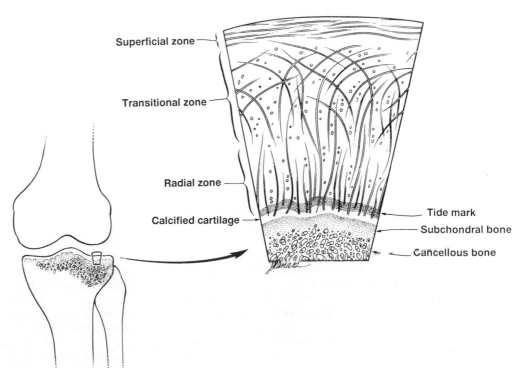

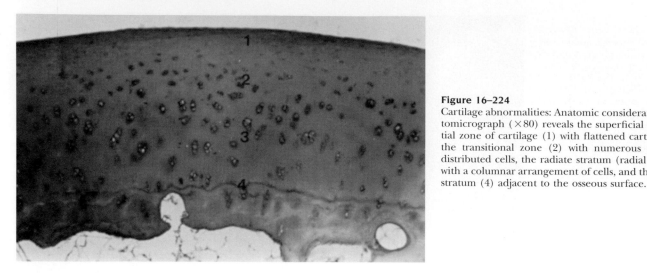

Figure 16–224

Cartilage abnormalities: Anatomic considerations. Photomicrograph (×80) reveals the superficial or tangential zone of cartilage (1) with flattened cartilage cells, the transitional zone (2) with numerous irregularly distributed cells, the radiate stratum (radial zone) (3) with a columnar arrangement of cells, and the calcified stratum (4) adjacent to the osseous surface.

and glycosaminoglycan composition of articular cartilage does not change significantly with age.[938] Although aging articular cartilage appears yellow, no evidence has been found to suggest that this pigment has any functional significance.[938] Cartilage fibrillation, however, is an age-dependent process, occurring initially at the periphery of the joint surfaces and in the superficial layers.[939, 940] Splitting, fraying, and pitting of the articular surface characterize this fibrillation, which on chemical analysis is associated with depletion of glycosaminoglycans and with normal collagen concentration.[938] Such cartilage fibrillation is not regarded as synonymous with osteoarthritis, although it may progress to involve the deeper layers of cartilage. The initial stages of osteoarthritis are characterized by softening of the articular cartilage, with disruption occurring along the planes of the collagen fibrils. This process may extend vertically, involving deeper layers of the cartilage, progressing to reach the tidemark and, with abrasion of the abnormal cartilage, exposing the subchondral bone. The changes of osteoarthritis resemble those of aging but, in loaded (i.e., weight-bearing) portions of a joint, are more extensive. The morphologic changes of osteoarthritis, however, certainly resemble those of aging, differing primarily in extent. The relationships of those changes in articular cartilage that relate to aging, those that relate to osteoarthritis, and those that are designated as chondromalacia are not clear.

Cartilage Degeneration

Owing to the difficulty in distinguishing among the cartilage alterations of aging and those occurring in chondromalacia and osteoarthritis, all of the findings are considered together here. In a subsequent section of this chapter, imaging findings associated with advanced stages of osteoarthritis are considered.

From an imaging standpoint, many of the standard methods (e.g., conventional radiography, magnification radiography, arthrographic and tomoarthrographic techniques, and ultrasonography) used to evaluate cartilage degeneration also estimate chondral loss.[941–943] None of these is ideal. Some, such as standard radiography, require the use of films obtained during weight-bearing or application of stress, and others, such as arthrographic methods, require the injection of contrast material. Ultrasonography is applicable only when the articular surfaces can be positioned in such a manner as to allow their assessment with probes placed on the skin surface. Scintigraphy generally requires the presence of changes in the subchondral bone. MR imaging, however, appears unique in its ability to demonstrate not only cartilage loss but also internal chondral derangement.

Arthrography. The role of arthrography in the diagnosis of chondromalacia of the patella has been the subject of debate. Most observers regard its role as minor or nonexistent,[944, 945] although others are more optimistic.[946, 947] The posterior surface of the patella is V-shaped, with medial and lateral facets separated by an osseous ridge. Routine lateral projections during arthrography demonstrate only a small amount of the patellar cartilaginous surface, that near the apex of the ridge. Axial projections increase the cartilaginous area that can be visualized, and oblique projections tangential to the medial and lateral facets may further improve this visualization.[948] If overhead and fluoroscopic filming is supplemented with conventional tomography or CT scanning, the diagnosis of chondromalacia indeed may be substantiated by arthrography in some patients.[949–952] On arthrography, chondromalacia produces absorption or inhibition of contrast material by the patellar cartilage (see Fig. 16–178). Nodular elevation, fissuring, or diminution of the cartilaginous surface may be apparent.

Ultrasonography. The role of ultrasonography in the assessment of the articular cartilage is limited by the need to position the joint in such a manner as to provide proximity to the articular surface for a probe placed on the skin.[1159] Although acute flexion of the knee allows sonographic analysis of portions of the articular cartilage in the femoral condyles, the cartilage in the proximal portion of the tibia and the posterior surface of the patella is not evaluated. Information derived from this procedure, therefore, is incomplete.

Scintigraphy. In general, bone scintigraphy is regarded as a technique that is able to detect subchondral bone abnormalities occurring in moderate to advanced stages of osteoarthritis. In some studies, however, abnormal accumulation of bone-seeking radionuclides in subchondral bone was found to be a reliable predictor of subsequent loss of joint space.[953, 954] In these investigations, a negative bone scan proved to be a powerful negative predictor with regard to the development of joint space loss over the ensuing 5 years.

MR Imaging

Normal Articular Cartilage. The application of MR imaging to the assessment of articular cartilage, particularly that of the knee, has been the subject of numerous investigations. Owing to its excellent contrast resolution, its ever-increasing spatial resolution, and the ability to obtain images in any plane, the superiority of MR imaging to other imaging methods in this assessment seems guaranteed. In practice, however, the usefulness of MR imaging in providing clinically important information on the integrity of the articular cartilage is not certain. Although severe chondral abnormalities, including full-thickness defects and denudation of the articular surface, are delineated with MR imaging, the detection of more superficial cartilage lesions with this imaging method is far more challenging. Despite the application of modified sequences and newer methods of MR imaging, the results of prior investigations have been inconsistent and often have not withstood critical analysis. A multitude of MR pulse sequences have been advocated, including T1-weighted,[955–957] proton density–weighted,[958] and T2-weighted[958–960] standard spin echo sequences; fast spin echo sequences[961]; T1-weighted inversion recovery sequences[962]; magnetization transfer contrast sequences[159, 963]; fat-suppressed sequences[964, 965]; and both two- and three-dimensional gradient recalled echo sequences.[966–970] The reported sensitivity and specificity for detecting cartilage lesions with these sequences have ranged from a low of 31 per cent[967] (sensitivity) and 50 per cent[959] (specificity) to a high of 100 per cent[959, 969] for each. Another technique, MR arthrography enhanced with intra-articular administration of gadolinium compounds, has been shown to be effective in the detection of cartilage abnormalities,[971, 972] but this method is time-consuming and invasive.

In addition to the uncertainty regarding the efficacy of these sequences in allowing the depiction of cartilage lesions, the appearance of normal cartilage with the various sequences also is unclear. The majority of descriptions of cartilage in spin echo and gradient echo images has indicated a homogeneous signal intensity or a subtle bilaminar appearance (Fig. 16–225).[955, 967, 968] A study using high-resolution spin echo imaging found a trilaminar appearance of normal cartilage.[973] The cause of the different signal intensities in the three layers is uncertain, but it was postulated that the different layers corresponded to the different histologic zones of cartilage.[973] The thin surface layer was believed to represent the histologically superficial zone, with the middle layer representing the transitional zone and the deep layer representing a combination of the deep radiate zone, the calcified cartilage zone, and the subchondral bone.

Recht and collaborators,[974] in a study of cadaveric knees in which multiple MR imaging methods were employed, found that a bilaminar or trilaminar appearance of articular cartilage occasionally was present with spin echo and certain gradient echo sequences, but this was not a consistent finding. The reason for this was uncertain. With fat-suppressed spoiled gradient recalled acquisition in the steady state (SPGR) sequences, cartilage appeared to have a trilaminar appearance, consisting of a superficial region of high signal intensity, an intermediate region of low signal intensity, and a deep region of high signal intensity (Fig. 16–226). Determination of the cause of the different signal intensities in the three layers and their histologic correlation was not possible in this study. The superficial location of the outer region of high intensity suggested the possibility that this region corresponded to the histologically apparent superficial zone of cartilage.

Rubenstein and collaborators,[975] using spin echo MR imaging sequences in the analysis of bovine articular cartilage, also detected a trilaminar appearance of normal cartilage, with signal intensity characteristics corresponding closely to those reported by Recht and coworkers.[974] Results of polarized light microscopy of histologic specimens confirmed the existence of three zones, and transmission electron microscopy showed different collagen arrangements in the zones. With rotation of the specimens with respect to the main magnetic field, an isotropic effect on signal intensity was noted, especially in the hypointense second lamina. Because of the preferential alignment of water molecules associated with collagen, angular rotation of the cartilage in the direction of minimum dipolar coupling (55 degrees to the magnetic field, i.e., the magic angle) caused the cartilage to have a homogeneous appearance. Rubenstein and colleagues[975] concluded that the MR imaging appearance of the three layers of articular cartilage is strongly influenced by an isotropic arrangement of the collagen and by the alignment of the specimen relative to the magnetic field, and that similar principles can be expected to apply to MR imaging characteristics of normal human articular cartilage.

The results of available studies underscore the complexity of the issue of MR imaging of articular cartilage. As the MR imaging appearance of normal articular cartilage is not agreed on and certainly is influenced by the precise imaging method or sequence employed, disagreement regarding the value of MR imaging in assessing abnormal cartilage is to be expected (see later discussion). Normal MR phenomena (e.g., magic angle) and artifacts (e.g., truncation artifact) clearly can influence the manner in which normal (and abnormal) cartilage is displayed on MR images.[1198] This display also is modified when compression is applied to the chondral surface.[1160] Ultimately, the role of MR imaging in this regard may relate not to the analysis of the morphology of articular cartilage but to its physiology. Specifically, the integrity of articular cartilage depends on proper nutrition, in which nutrients and waste products are moved into and out of the cartilage matrix, mainly as a

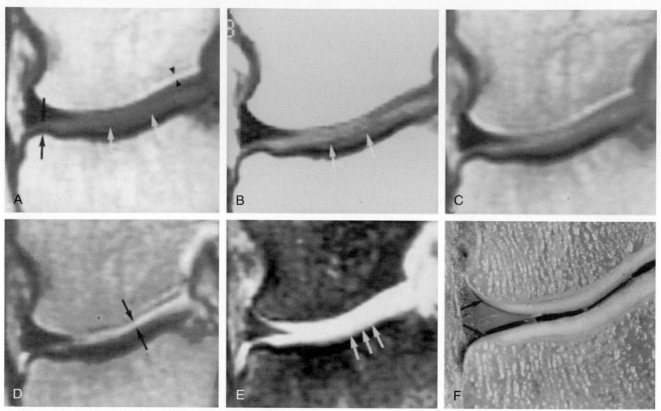

Figure 16-225

Normal articular cartilage: MR imaging. Femoral and tibial articular cartilage (lateral compartment) without macroscopically visible focal defects examined with spin echo and gradient echo sequences.

A Coronal T1-weighted (TR/TE, 600/20) spin echo MR image. Cartilage is represented by a superficial layer of intermediate signal intensity and a deep layer of low signal intensity (black arrows). The presence of a chemical shift artifact is suggested, which may explain the difference in thickness of the deep hypointense layer between the tibial and femoral sides. A hyperintense line at the periphery of the femoral fat marrow is consistent with this suggestion (arrowheads). The normal articular cartilage shows slight irregularity (white arrows).

B Coronal T1-weighted (TR/TE, 600/20) spin echo MR image photographed with meniscal windowing. Slight cartilage irregularity is more pronounced (arrows).

C Coronal proton density–weighted (TR/TE, 2000/20) spin echo MR image. There is reduced contrast. The cartilage appears to be more homogeneous.

D Coronal T2-weighted (TR/TE, 2000/70) spin echo MR image. The superficial layer of cartilage is narrower. The differentiation between the cartilage surface and the joint fluid is difficult (arrows).

E Coronal MPGR MR image (TR/TE, 450/15; flip angle, 15 degrees). The superficial layer of cartilage demonstrates high signal intensity. Differentiation between the fluid and the surface of the articular cartilage is difficult. Cartilage irregularities potentially simulate fluid-filled ulcerations (arrows).

F Corresponding anatomic section. The cartilage is grossly normal. Note that its thickness is significantly less at the periphery of the joint.

(From Hodler J, et al: J Comput Assist Tomogr *16*:597, 1992.)

result of diffusion of synovial fluid.[976–978] Although the most widely used technique for the in vitro evaluation of diffusive transport in cartilaginous tissues is the radioactive tracer method[979, 980] (in which measurements are made of the intrachondral flux of a radioisotope contained in a bath to which the cartilage is exposed), MR imaging also may be employed for this purpose.[981]

Abnormal Articular Cartilage. The use of MR imaging in the study of abnormal cartilage has been investigated extensively. Although MR imaging sequences and techniques have varied, analysis of the knee, particularly the patellofemoral joint, has received the most attention. The choice of the patellofemoral joint is a wise one, owing to the thickness of the normal articular cartilage of the patella, the frequent occurrence of chondromalacia patellae and osteoarthritis of the patellofemoral

compartment, and the adequate display of this compartment provided by transaxial MR images. Numerous MR imaging sequences have been employed in the study of the patellar articular cartilage, some more successfully than others. As a general rule, any MR imaging sequence that is insensitive to the detection of abnormal patellar cartilage will be even less sensitive to cartilage changes in other locations, such as the femorotibial compartments, glenohumeral joint, ankle, and hip, owing to more complex regional anatomy. In fact, in any site, angular or curved articular surfaces can lead to diagnostic difficulty during MR imaging, owing to partial volume artifacts that lead to superimposition of subchondral bone and articular cartilage. Thin section imaging displays that can be accomplished with the use of volumetric gradient echo MR sequences may diminish these artifacts but not eliminate them.

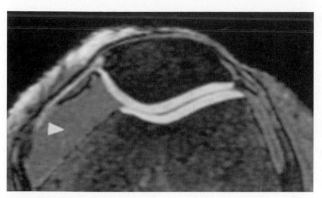

Figure 16–226
Normal articular cartilage: MR imaging. Patellofemoral articular cartilage. Transaxial 3DFT SPGR MR image (TR/TE, 52/10; flip angle, 60 degrees) obtained with chemical presaturation of fat (ChemSat). The articular cartilage is of high signal intensity, and the bone and synovial fluid (arrowhead) are of low signal intensity. The articular cartilage possesses a trilaminar appearance, best appreciated in the lateral patellar facet and the lateral femoral condyle; the superficial portion of articular cartilage is of high signal intensity, a thin intermediate region shows low signal intensity, and the deep portion of the articular cartilage is of high signal intensity.

The choice of a standard by which the results of MR imaging of articular cartilage can be assessed creates added difficulty. Although gross morphologic and histologic analysis can be used as a standard in cadaveric studies, arthroscopy generally is chosen as the standard in patient studies. Differences in examiner expertise, terminology, sites of analysis, and techniques of measurement (landmarks may be better defined on cross-sectional images than during arthroscopy) are encountered that make arthroscopy a less than ideal standard by which to judge the sensitivity and specificity of MR imaging abnormalities.

With MR imaging, two fundamental findings of abnormal articular cartilage are sought: altered thickness and modified signal intensity. With regard to the first, detection of decreased thickness of articular cartilage as the sine qua non for cartilage abnormality is an oversimplification. Diminution in cartilage thickness is a well-known manifestation of moderate to advanced osteoarthritis; however, thickening of cartilage may occur after its injury, a finding documented repeatedly in animal models in which the knee has been rendered unstable with surgical techniques.[982–984] Cartilage, like other connective tissues, swells when injured, a finding that is well documented during arthroscopic assessment of chondromalacia. The cause of posttraumatic cartilage thickening is not clear; an increase in proteoglycan content, of water, or of both, may be important in the pathogenesis of cartilage thickening.[984, 985] Thus, the increase in thickness may represent hypertrophy secondary to repair or edema due to recurrent injury in the experimentally produced unstable knee.[986] Long-term studies in such knees have indicated that cartilage breakdown and loss may follow the stage of cartilage thickening.[987] Similarly, thickening of articular cartilage may represent an early manifestation of osteoarthritis in humans, and progressive loss of articular cartilage may indicate more advanced disease.

The accurate determination of increased or decreased cartilage thickness with MR imaging requires identification of its most superficial and deepest layers on sequential images in any plane. An ideal MR imaging sequence used to assess articular cartilage is one that, among other attributes, allows precise definition of the interfaces between the surface of the cartilage and the joint space and between the deepest layer of cartilage and the subchondral bone. The interface between the deepest layer of cartilage and the subchondral bone is anatomically complex, however, consisting of a layer of calcified cartilage, a subchondral bone plate, and the adjacent spongy trabeculae and marrow of the subchondral bone. Furthermore, the interface between the superficial layer of cartilage and the joint space changes according to the congruency of the apposing articular surfaces, the presence of any gap or tissue void between these surfaces, and the presence, amount, and composition of joint fluid. Thus, identification of a specific MR imaging sequence that provides good delineation of these two interfaces in one particular clinical situation and in one anatomic location does not necessarily indicate that this same sequence is useful in other situations and in different anatomic sites. The presence of a joint effusion generally is regarded as an advantage in delineation with MR imaging of superficial changes in the articular cartilage, so long as an imaging sequence is chosen that accentuates the differences in signal intensity of the fluid and the articular cartilage. This principle forms the basis for the use of MR arthrography (with intra-articular instillation of saline solution or gadolinium compounds) in the assessment of articular cartilage, especially in patients in whom native joint fluid is either absent or minimal (see later discussion). With spin echo MR imaging, T2-weighted sequences lead to an arthrogram-like effect in patients with joint effusions, with synovial fluid hyperintense relative to hyaline cartilage. Multislice gradient echo MR sequences (employing a longer echo time and low flip angle) also lead to this arthrogram-like effect (Fig. 16–227).[988] Alternatively, if a single slice or volumetric positive contrast technique is desired, a minimal repetition time (TR), minimal

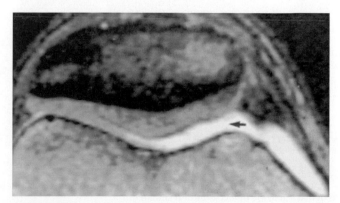

Figure 16–227
Normal articular cartilage: MR imaging. Patellofemoral articular cartilage. Transaxial MPGR MR image (TR/TE, 450/20; flip angle, 15 degrees). The presence of joint fluid (arrow) of high signal intensity allows improved visualization of the surface of the articular cartilage.

echo time (TE), intermediate flip angle GRASS sequence may be used.[988] Evaluation of intrinsic cartilage lesions is facilitated by optimizing contrast-to-noise ratios between synovial fluid and hyaline cartilage. A multiplanar sequence for this purpose would have a minimal TE and a large flip angle, leading to a T1-weighted appearance with synovial fluid hypointense relative to hyaline cartilage.[988] If a single scan or three-dimensional technique is desired, a GRASS sequence at minimal TR and TE and intermediate flip angle may be used.

The second fundamental finding of cartilage abnormality is altered signal intensity. The clinical significance of this finding, however, in the absence of alterations in cartilage thickness or surface irregularities of cartilage is not entirely clear, as correlative histologic and histochemical data generally are lacking. Some previous MR imaging studies of patellofemoral cartilage have employed grading systems in which the lowest grade has consisted of intrachondral alterations of signal intensity (hypointensity or hyperintensity) occurring in the absence of chondral surface irregularities or alterations of cartilage thickness,[679, 974] but the reported data do not allow assessment of the clinical significance of this grade of abnormality.

Complicating the MR imaging analysis of abnormal articular cartilage are technical and anatomic pitfalls. The chemical shift artifact is the spatial misrepresentation of predominantly water-containing tissue versus fat-containing tissue that occurs along the frequency-encoding axis.[989] The articular cartilage whose surface is perpendicular to this axis appears thicker or thinner than it actually is, leading to diagnostic error. Rotation of the frequency-encoding and phase-encoding gradients allows more accurate appraisal of the true thickness of this articular cartilage. Ringing artifacts (i.e., Gibbs or truncation artifacts) also can lead to errors in the assessment of articular cartilage with MR imaging.[1198] These artifacts, which result in concentric curvilinear lines of

low signal intensity displayed throughout the image, may relate to data interpolation when a smaller acquisition matrix is interpolated into a larger display matrix and become problematic along linear tissue interfaces where there are abrupt transitions in signal intensity. Ringing artifacts occur in both the frequency-encoded and phase-encoded directions (they are more likely in the latter direction), and their spacing (although not their amplitude) can be diminished with greater sampling of the higher frequencies in k-space (e.g., 256 phase-encoded steps). Finally, as indicated previously, partial volume averaging artifacts also can lead to improper analysis of cartilage integrity.

A description of the most frequently employed MR imaging techniques for cartilage assessment follows.

1. Standard spin echo sequences. Standard T1-weighted and T2-weighted spin echo images have been used to analyze hyaline cartilage (Figs. 16–228 and 16–229). The T1-weighted spin echo MR images provide good anatomic detail and high contrast between cartilage and subchondral bone, but they are associated with poor contrast between cartilage and joint fluid. The advantages of T2-weighted spin echo MR images include an arthrogram-like effect when a joint effusion is present and the ability to delineate signal intensity changes within the articular cartilage; their disadvantages include poor contrast between articular cartilage and subchondral bone and insufficient resolution to allow detection of contour abnormalities in the absence of a joint effusion. Hayes and collaborators,[955] in a cadaveric study of the patellar cartilage, found T1-weighted spin echo MR images to be satisfactory for defining cartilage morphology, allowing detection of focal cartilage lesions (as small as 3 or 4 mm in diameter) and diffuse chondral thinning. With these images, contrast between joint fluid and cartilage was found to be less than that provided by T2-weighted spin echo MR images, but adequate to permit visualization of more advanced cartilage

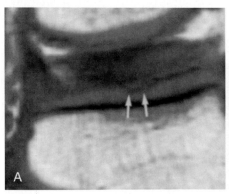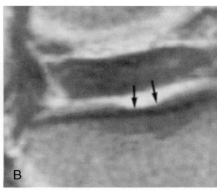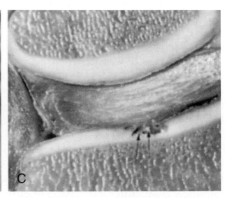

Figure 16–228

Articular cartilage abnormalities: MR imaging. Femorotibial articular cartilage (lateral compartment). Standard spin echo MR images. Focal defect in the tibial articular cartilage.

  A Coronal oblique T1-weighted (TR/TE, 600/20) spin echo MR image. The tibial cartilage is focally thinned (arrows). The depth of the articular cartilage defect is underestimated.

  B Coronal oblique T2-weighted (TR/TE, 2000/70) spin echo MR image. The defect is filled with hyperintense joint fluid that depicts the extent of the defect more exactly but not its precise form (arrows).

  C Corresponding anatomic section. A deep focal defect nearly extends to the subchondral bone. Fibrillation within the defect may explain part of the fact that the T1-weighted MR images led to an underestimation of the size of the defect (arrows).

  (From Hodler J, et al: J Comput Assist Tomogr *16*:597, 1992.)

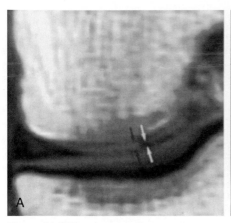
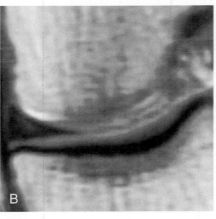
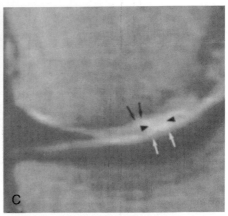
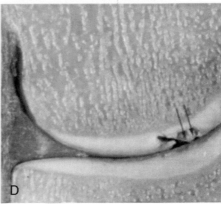

Figure 16–229

Articular cartilage abnormalities: Standard spin echo MR imaging—femorotibial articular cartilage (medial compartment), focal defect in the femoral articular cartilage.

A Coronal T1-weighted (TR/TE, 600/20) spin echo MR image. The lateral (more central) part of the defect is hypointense (white arrows). Medially (more peripherally), minimally increased signal intensity is seen within the deep hypointense cartilage layer (black arrows).

B Coronal proton density–weighted (TR/TE, 2000/20) spin echo MR image. The lateral part of the defect is less obvious, while hyperintensity is more marked than on the T1-weighted spin echo MR image in the medial part of the defect.

C Coronal T2-weighted (TR/TE, 2000/70) spin echo MR image. The medial part of the defect is well demarcated (black arrows), while differentiation between the lateral part of the lesion and the joint fluid is difficult (arrowheads). The presence of joint fluid simulates cartilage irregularity on the tibial surface (white arrows).

D Corresponding anatomic section. A gross cartilage defect with some tissue within the lateral (central) part (arrows) is evident.

(From Hodler J, et al: J Comput Assist Tomogr *16*:597, 1992.)

lesions. These investigators indicated that T2-weighted spin echo MR images were less useful because of decreased spatial resolution, poor contrast between subchondral bone and cartilage, and poor delineation of changes in signal intensity within the cartilage. Speer and coworkers[967] noted the value of an arthrogram-like effect on T2-weighted spin echo MR images provided by a joint effusion in the detection of partial-thickness and full-thickness cartilage lesions of the knee. DeSmet and colleagues[990] noted distinctive defects or fissures of high signal intensity in the patellar articular cartilage on sagittal T2-weighted spin echo MR images that corresponded to arthroscopically proved sites of chondromalacia. McCauley and associates[958] also emphasized the importance of T2-weighted, as well as proton density–weighted, spin echo MR images in the diagnosis of cartilage lesions, using arthroscopy as the gold standard and noting the complementary nature of findings derived from each of these sequences. The posterior surface of the patella was evaluated. In their study of chondromalacia patellae, focal cartilage abnormalities in signal intensity or contour on one or both of these sequences yielded the highest correlation with the arthroscopic diagnosis of chondromalacia. In a commentary on this investigation, Hodler and Resnick[957] indicated that they had confirmed several of these findings, mainly (1) the importance of focal changes in signal intensity in the diagnosis of localized cartilage defects; (2) the infrequency of direct depiction of chondral contour abnormalities; (3) the relative insensitivity of proton density–weighted images alone; and (4) the value of the combined analysis of different MR imaging

sequences. These last investigators also indicated that MR imaging is better suited for visualization of cartilaginous defects that do not contain any tissue, rather than those containing residual fibrillated cartilage or granulation tissue. Hodler and collaborators[991] subsequently reported an MR imaging investigation of femorotibial articular cartilage in cadavers in which they concluded that the value of those MR imaging sequences (i.e., T1-weighted, proton density–weighted, and T2-weighted spin echo sequences, as well as multiplanar gradient recalled sequences) used routinely in the analysis of internal derangements of the knee in the detection of focal defects of the hyaline cartilage is limited. Brown and Quinn,[992] using proton density–weighted and T2-weighted spin echo MR images, concluded that such images were valuable only in the diagnosis of advanced lesions of chondromalacia patellae. Colin and associates,[993] employing standard spin echo MR sequences in 37 patients, found that such sequences had an accuracy of 73 per cent, a sensitivity of 47 per cent, and a specificity of 96 per cent in the detection of femorotibial cartilage lesions when arthroscopy was used as the gold standard. Van Leersum and collaborators,[994] in an investigation of the reliability of various spin echo MR imaging sequences (as well as gradient echo and fat suppressed fast spin echo sequences) in the analysis of the thickness of patellar cartilage in cadaveric specimens, determined that the T1-weighted spin echo MR images were most accurate.

2. Standard spin echo sequences combined with fat-suppression techniques. Although many fat-suppression techniques are available, most are based on four methods or their modifications[995]: Dixon and chopper methods, the hybrid method, frequency-selection presaturation (ChemSat), and short tau inversion recovery (STIR). The Dixon and chopper methods are based on the production of separate water-based and fat-based MR images, and the hybrid method in the spin echo mode of data acquisition uses a single two-excitation MR imaging sequence.[995] The ChemSat technique initially involves the selective excitation of fat (as compared to water) with a narrow-band pulse in the absence of any gradients, and it subsequently dephases the signal of fat with added gradients and then immediately continues with the choice of a specific imaging sequence.[995] The ChemSat technique is most effective when high field strength magnets are used. Inhomogeneities in the magnetic field lead to inconsistent fat suppression in some cases, an artifact that can be minimized through the use of a smaller field of view.

The assessment of articular cartilage using fat-suppression methods combined with standard spin echo technique has received limited attention (Fig. 16–230). In one study, Chandnani and coworkers[964] used both standard and hybrid suppression methods with and without the intra-articular injection of saline solution and gadopentetate dimeglumine in the analysis of femorotibial cartilage in cadaveric knees. These investigators found the hybrid fat suppression technique combined with T1-weighted spin echo MR imaging sequences with or without saline injection to be superior to standard spin echo MR images alone in the visualization of the articular cartilage. With this method, intra-articular fluid is of low signal intensity compared with the high signal intensity of the articular cartilage. Thus, the interfaces between the chondral surface (of high signal intensity) and the joint fluid (of low signal intensity), and between the chondral surface (of high signal intensity) and the subchondral bone (of low signal intensity), are well seen. Koskinen and collaborators,[996] in a study of cadaveric patellae with a low field strength magnet, arrived at similar conclusions. König and associates[966] also found chemical shift (and gradient refocused) images to be more useful than standard spin echo MR sequences in the detection of early osteoarthritis, although they indicated that the presence of a joint effusion led to some diagnostic difficulty in the assessment of articular cartilage. Rose and associates[997] investigated 71 patients with anterior knee pain and suspected chondromalacia patellae in whom arthroscopy of the knee had been performed using a variety of MR imaging sequences, including transaxial standard spin echo (and fast spin echo) sequences with fat suppression. Early and advanced stages of chondromalacia patellae were detected reliably on analysis of the MR images, with high specificity and positive predictive value. The results of most of these investigations reinforce the concept that fat-suppression imaging methods combined with standard spin echo MR imaging, by changing the dynamic range of the images, afford excellent contrast between articular cartilage and surrounding structures in both the presence and absence of a joint effusion, but its effectiveness in delineating intrachondral abnormalities is not proved.

3. STIR sequences. Although STIR sequences are used extensively for the analysis of infections, tumors, and traumatic disorders of bone and soft tissue, their application to the assessment of articular cartilage lesions has received little attention. STIR imaging sequences are effective in depressing the signal intensity in the bone marrow and, therefore, may allow clear separation between the articular cartilage and subchondral bone. The interface between cartilage and joint fluid generally is poorly delineated with such sequences, however, as both fluid and cartilage reveal high (fluid) or moderately high (cartilage) signal intensity. STIR imaging is extremely sensitive in the detection of joint fluid, subchondral cystic lesions containing such fluid, and marrow alterations in regions of subchondral bone sclerosis.[998]

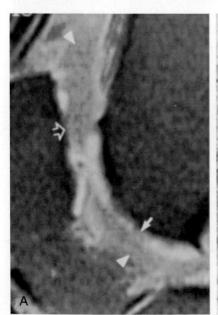
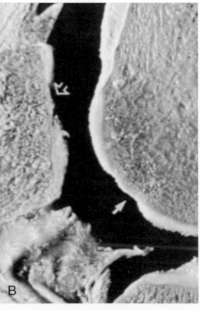

Figure 16–230

Articular cartilage abnormalities: MR imaging. Patellofemoral articular cartilage. T1-weighted spin echo MR images with hybrid method of fat suppression. Cartilage fibrillation and erosion. A sagittal T1-weighted (TR/TE, 500/20) spin echo MR image after the intra-articular injection of saline solution **(A)** shows cartilage thinning in the femoral condyle (solid arrow) and erosion of cartilage (open arrow) in the patella. Note the low signal intensity of the saline solution (arrowheads). The cartilage findings (solid and open arrows) are corroborated in the corresponding anatomic section **(B).** (From Chandnani V, et al: Radiology *178*:557, 1991.)

4. Fast spin echo sequences. Fast spin echo MR imaging sequences are used increasingly to provide images with the desired type of contrast in a shorter acquisition time. For example, heavily T2-weighted images can be obtained far more rapidly with fast spin echo than with standard spin echo techniques. The disadvantages of the fast spin echo method include a loss of spatial resolution along the phase-encoded axis that is exaggerated on images obtained with short echo times and that leads to image blurring and to a decrease in the number of images that can be obtained at any given repetition time (when compared with standard spin echo methods). Furthermore, as fat reveals a relatively high signal intensity even in heavily T2-weighted fast spin echo images, the combination of fast spin echo imaging and fat-suppression techniques has become popular.

The application of fast spin echo MR imaging sequences to cartilage analysis has not been studied extensively. In common with T2-weighted standard spin echo methods, an arthrogram-like effect provided by joint fluid on fast spin echo images obtained with long repetition times may prove useful in delineating the chondral surface. Such was the case in one study by Broderick and coworkers,[961] who used a dual fast spin echo pulse sequence combined with fat suppression to evaluate the knees in patients with osteoarthritis and in normal persons. These investigators indicated that cartilage and adjacent fluid could be differentiated easily in short TE and long TR images. In almost all cases, contrast resolution allowed detection of inhomogeneity of signal intensity in diseased cartilage, and correlation of MR imaging findings and those at arthroscopy was high. A tendency of cartilage abnormalities to be underestimated with this fast spin echo technique also was noted, however.

Fast spin echo MR imaging sequences often are combined with fat suppression in the analysis of musculoskeletal disorders. As one example, this combination method has been used to assess traumatic abnormalities of the marrow (e.g., bone bruises) and the collateral ligaments, and, in some institutions, it is a routine sequence in the imaging protocol for the knee. When fluid is present in the joint, fat-suppressed fast spin echo MR imaging sequences allow detection of chondral degeneration and injury (Fig. 16–231).

The role of fast spin echo STIR MR imaging sequences in the assessment of cartilage is not year clear, although the advantages and disadvantages of this technique are similar to those of conventional STIR sequences.

5. Gradient recalled echo sequences. Both two- and three-dimensional gradient recalled echo (GRE) sequences have been used to study articular cartilage.[966–970, 974, 988, 999–1003, 1161–1163] Many of these sequences provide high contrast between articular cartilage, synovial fluid, and subchondral bone; some allow the acquisition of radial sections that are perpendicular to the articular surface (Fig. 16–232), and those using volumetric acquisition allow thin contiguous scans and reformatting of image data in any plane that is desired (see Fig. 16–232). Disagreement exists regarding the selection of specific GRE scanning parameters that are optimal for analysis of articular cartilage, however. As examples, fast imaging with steady precession (FISP) with a flip angle of 70 degrees and a short TR has been advocated for the assessment of degenerative changes in hyaline cartilage[1004]; and short TR fast low-angle shot (FLASH) sequences with a flip angle of 12 degrees have been considered appropriate for the general evaluation of articular cartilage.[966] In a detailed analysis of various GRE techniques that were used to assess the patellofemoral joint in normal volunteers, Yao and coworkers[988] arrived at the following conclusions:

a. For optimal contrast-to-noise ratios (synovial fluid-cartilage), the best multiplanar sequence (for TE less than 23 msec) is with a short TE and a large flip angle (e.g., TR/TE, 400/9; flip angle, 73 degrees).

b. If a single scan or three-dimensional technique providing optimal contrast-to-noise ratios is desired, a GRASS sequence at minimal TR and TE and intermediate flip angle (e.g., TR/TE, 18/9; flip angle, 32 degrees) is best.

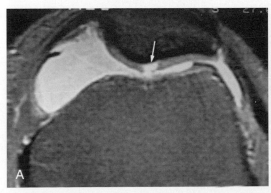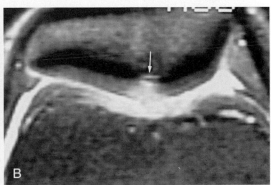

Figure 16–231

Articular cartilage abnormalities: MR imaging. Fast spin echo MR images with fat suppression.

A In a transaxial fat-suppressed fast spin echo (TR/TE, 3500/17; echo train, 8) MR image, note the focal defect (arrow) in the patellar articular cartilage. Fluid within the defect, as in this case, is more likely to occur when a large joint effusion is present.

B In a second patient, a transaxial fat-suppressed fast spin echo (TR/TE, 4400/17; echo train, 8) MR image shows a similar patellar lesion (arrow). At the time of arthroscopy, a flap of cartilaginous tissue was evident at this site. With probing, this flap moved in and out of the chondral defect.

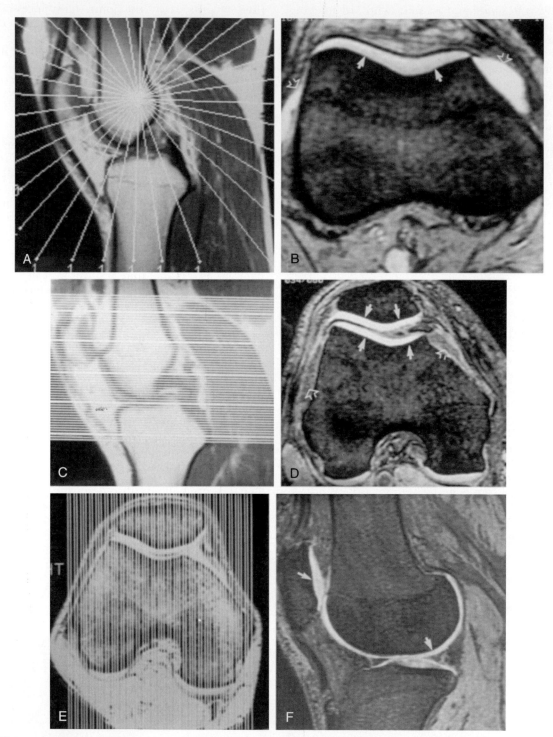

Figure 16–232

Normal articular cartilage: MR imaging—femoral, tibial, and patellar articular cartilage, gradient recalled echo sequences.

A, B MPGR MR images with radial sections to assess femoral cartilage. From a sagittal T1-weighted (TR/TE, 450/20) spin echo MR localizer image **(A)**, radial sections can be programmed such that the plane of individual images is perpendicular to the articular surface of the distal portion of the femur. One such MPGR MR image (TR/TE, 450/15; flip angle, 20 degrees) is shown **(B).** Note the high signal intensity of articular cartilage (solid arrows) with a trilaminar appearance and the high signal intensity of joint fluid (open arrows).

C, D 3DFT SPGR acquisition in the steady state with assessment of patellar and femoral cartilage. From a similar sagittal T1-weighted (TR/TE, 450/20) spin echo MR localizer image **(C)**, transaxial SPGR MR images (TR/TE, 52/10; flip angle, 60 degrees) obtained with chemical presaturation of fat (ChemSat) **(D)** can be obtained. Note the high signal intensity of articular cartilage (solid arrows) and the low signal intensity of joint fluid (open arrows).

E, F 3DFT SPGR acquisition in the steady state with assessment of femoral and tibial cartilage. From a transaxial MPGR MR image (TR/TE, 450/15; flip angle, 20 degrees) **(E)**, sagittal SPGR MR images (TR/TE, 52/10; flip angle, 60 degrees) obtained with chemical presaturation of fat (ChemSat) **(F)** can be obtained. Note the high signal intensity and trilaminar appearance of the articular cartilage (solid arrows).

c. For optimal signal-to-noise ratios (for both synovial fluid and hyaline cartilage), the best multiplanar sequence employs a short TE and an intermediate flip angle (e.g., TR/TE, 400/9; flip angle, 30 degrees).

d. If a short TR, high signal-to-noise technique is desired, GRASS (e.g., TR/TE, 18/9; flip angle, 13 degrees) is superior to FLASH.

Recht and colleagues[974] assessed the patellofemoral articular cartilage in cadavers using the intra-articular administration of saline solution and a number of GRE sequences and standard spin echo sequences, including the following: two fat-suppressed three-dimensional spoiled GRASS (SPGR) sequences; a nonfat-suppressed three-dimensional SPGR sequence; a three-dimensional GRASS sequence; and T1-weighted, proton density–weighted, and T2-weighted spin echo sequences (Fig. 16–233). Using grading systems for the severity of the cartilage as seen in the various MR images, and for the confidence level of the observer, and employing close MR imaging-pathologic correlation, these investigators found that the fat-suppressed three-dimensional SPGR sequences provided the most accurate results, with a

sensitivity of 96 per cent, a specificity of 95 per cent, and an accuracy of 95 per cent. The two SPGR sequences (TR/TE, 52/5; flip angle, 30 degrees; and TR/TE, 52/10; flip angle, 60 degrees) revealed a trilaminar appearance in regions of normal articular cartilage. With these sequences, regions of abnormal cartilage were characterized by loss of the surface layer and sometimes of the deeper layers of cartilage (Fig. 16–234). Abnormal low signal intensity frequently was seen in the articular cartilage adjacent to the area of cartilage loss. No statistically significant difference was identified between the two fat-suppressed SPGR sequences in the detection of lesions. The sequence with flip angle of 60 degrees and echo time of 10 msec was slightly superior for allowing correct staging of the cartilage lesions; in this sequence, 24 of 25 lesions were graded within one grade of the corresponding macroscopic grade. Although these results are promising, the SPGR sequences are time-consuming, and their effectiveness in displaying cartilage abnormalities in regions other than the patellofemoral joint (Fig. 16–235) is not proved.[1162] Furthermore, the optimal flip angle for demonstrating articular cartilage is not agreed on.[1002]

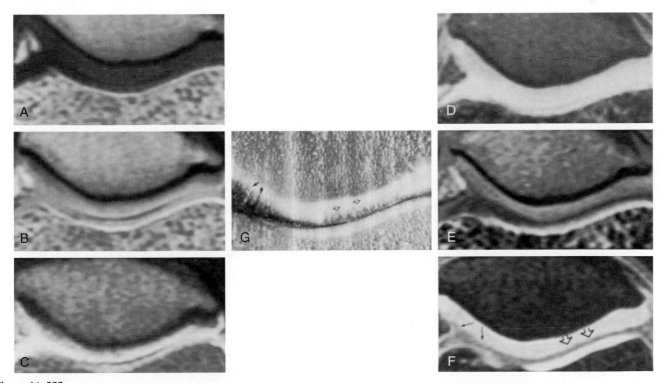

Figure 16–233
Articular cartilage abnormalities: MR imaging—patellar articular cartilage, spin echo and gradient recalled echo sequences. A variety of transaxial MR imaging sequences are used to analyze a grade 2 cartilage lesion (minor surface fibrillation or loss of less than 50 per cent of the cartilage thickness) of the lateral patellar facet and a grade 3 cartilage lesion (severe surface fibrillation or loss of more than 50 per cent of the cartilage thickness but without exposure of subchondral bone) of the medial patellar facet.
A T1-weighted (TR/TE, 500/14) spin echo MR image.
B Proton density–weighted (TR/TE, 2000/20) spin echo MR image.
C T2-weighted (TR/TE, 2000/70) spin echo MR image.
D Three-dimensional Fourier transform (3DFT) GRASS MR image (TR/TE, 40/10; flip angle, 30 degrees).
E 3DFT spoiled GRASS MR image (TR/TE, 40/5; flip angle, 30 degrees).
F 3DFT fat-suppressed (ChemSat) spoiled GRASS MR image (TR/TE, 52/10; flip angle, 60 degrees).
The medial (solid arrows) and lateral (open arrows) patellar facet lesions are indicated in the corresponding transverse anatomic section (**G**).
The patellar cartilage abnormalities are seen best in **F** (solid arrows and open arrows). The absence of cartilage in the medial femoral condyle is secondary to the plane of sectioning and is not a true cartilage lesion.
(From Recht MT, et al: Radiology *187*:473, 1993.)

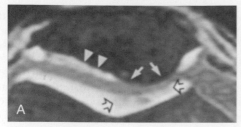

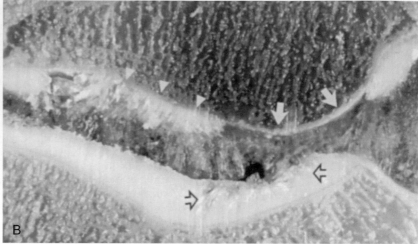

Figure 16–234

Articular cartilage abnormalities: MR imaging—patellar and femoral articular cartilage. A transaxial 3DFT SPGR acquisition in the steady state MR image (TR/TE, 60/10; flip angle, 60 degrees) obtained with chemical presaturation of fat (ChemSat) (**A**) and a corresponding transverse anatomic section (**B**) are shown. In **A,** the articular cartilage of the patella is focally absent (solid arrows) or severely thinned (arrowheads), and that of the femur reveals surface irregularity and altered signal intensity (between open arrows). The corresponding cartilage regions are indicated (closed and open arrows and arrowheads) in **B.** (From Recht MT, et al: Radiology *187:*473, 1993.)

One modification of the three-dimensional gradient echo technique that has been found useful in improving contrast between cartilage and joint fluid (without fat suppression) relates to combining the signals from the first and second gradient echoes, which form immediately after and immediately before each radiofrequency pulse.[1163] Such a technique, designated dual energy in the steady state (DESS), was optimized using the following parameters: bandwidth of 98 Hz per pixel, TR of 30 msec, TE of 7.1 msec, and flip angle of 60 degrees.[1163] The clinical usefulness of the DESS sequence is not yet proved, however.

With the application of three-dimensional gradient echo MR imaging sequences to cartilage analysis, three-dimensional image displays of articular cartilage and quantitative assessment of cartilage volume are possible.[1005–1007, 1164–1166] Specialized computer workstations often are required to minimize errors related to calculations of cartilage thickness and, ultimately, cartilage volume.

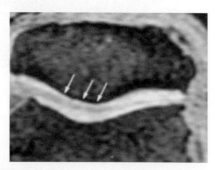

Figure 16–235

Articular cartilage abnormalities: MR imaging—patellar articular cartilage. A transaxial 3DFT SPGR acquisition in the steady state MR image (TR/TE, 58/10; flip angle, 60 degrees) obtained with chemical presaturation of fat (ChemSat) shows diffuse cartilage thinning (arrows) involving mainly the medial portion of the patella. Fluid of low signal intensity is seen between the femoral and patellar cartilage.

6. MR arthrography. MR arthrography has been used in the evaluation of many joints, including the knee. The rationale for its application to the assessment of articular cartilage is the improved visualization of the chondral surface that results when joint fluid is present. MR arthrography can be accomplished with the intra-articular injection of saline solution or gadolinium compounds; the advantages of gadolinium contrast agent administration include its high signal intensity on T1-weighted spin echo MR images, which allows for high spatial resolution and shorter examination time (Fig. 16–236). As MR arthrography can be coupled with other MR imaging techniques, including various gradient re-called sequences, injection of saline solution also may be employed. In one study in which focal defects were created in the articular cartilage in cadaveric knees, MR arthrography using gadolinium compounds, as compared with saline solution, allowed detection of smaller chondral lesions.[971] In another study of chondromalacia patellae in 27 patients, MR arthrography using gadolinium compounds was more sensitive than CT arthrography in the detection of chondral abnormalities.[1001]

Some disadvantages exist to the use of MR arthrography. As with standard arthrography, a needle puncture and proper localization of the needle in the joint are required, lengthening examination time. An underestimation of cartilage thickness, particularly with gradient echo imaging, may occur. In part, this may result from a delay in examination time, allowing imbibition of the gadolinium compound (or saline solution) into the superficial layers of cartilage. Overestimation of cartilage thickness, particularly with T1-weighted spin echo imaging, also may be encountered. Furthermore, the long-term effects of gadolinium compounds on the articular cartilage and synovial membrane are not known.

An alternative (and indirect) method of MR arthrography employs intravenous administration of a gadolinium compound with delayed imaging. The rationale of the technique relates to intra-articular movement, or

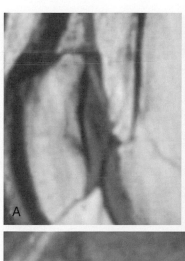
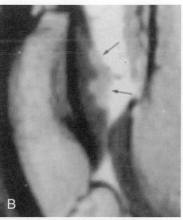
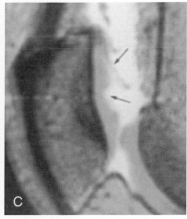

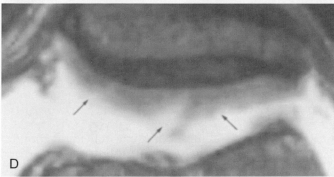

Figure 16–236

Articular cartilage abnormalities: MR arthrography—patellar articular cartilage.

A A sagittal T1-weighted (TR/TE, 700/15) spin echo MR image shows subtle alterations in signal intensity in the patellar articular cartilage.

B In the same patient, a sagittal T1-weighted (TR/TE, 700/15) spin echo MR image obtained following the intra-articular injection of a gadolinium compound shows surface irregularity of the patellar articular cartilage (arrows) with imbibition of fluid.

C In the same patient, a sagittal three-dimensional MR image using fast imaging with steady-state precession (FISP) (TR/TE, 30/10; flip angle, 35 degrees) obtained after the intra-articular administration of a gadolinium compound better defines the surface irregularity of the patellar articular cartilage (arrows).

D In the same patient, a transaxial three-dimensional MR image using FISP (TR/TE, 30/10; flip angle, 35 degrees) obtained after the intra-articular administration of a gadolinium compound dramatically displays the extent of articular cartilage abnormalities in the patella (arrows).

(Courtesy of J. Kramer, M.D., Vienna, Austria.)

seepage, of the contrast agent from the synovial membrane over a period of time that can be shortened if the joint is exercised. The success of such indirect MR arthrography generally relies on the presence of a native effusion in the joint to be examined. Few centers currently are using this method to assess articular cartilage, however.

7. Magnetization transfer contrast. Magnetization transfer contrast (MTC), or saturation transfer imaging, is a newer MR imaging method that improves contrast in gradient recalled sequences and that is sensitive to the interaction between water and macromolecules.[1008] With MTC, low-power radiofrequency irradiation is applied off resonance to selectively saturate ^1H nuclei with a short T2, as part of a conventional gradient recalled echo MR imaging sequence. The saturation of the short T2 component then is transferred to the bulk water protons via a magnetization exchange process, which is highly selective for water protons.[1008, 1009] MTC, therefore, provides unique information regarding the interaction between water and macromolecules.[1009] Compared with standard gradient recalled echo MR images, MTC images demonstrate increased contrast between many tissue pairs.[1009] When applied to the analysis of the knee, MTC has been shown to improve contrast in standard single-section gradient recalled echo images with regard to fat-muscle, muscle-flowing blood, and cartilage-synovial fluid interfaces (Figs. 16–237 and 16–238).[1010] The improvement of contrast between the articular cartilage and synovial fluid also is apparent on three-dimensional images,[1008] images that otherwise are associated with decreased contrast. Although contrast generation with MTC is complex, MTC images and T2-weighted images generally reveal increased signal intensity in similar regions.[1008] Thus, synovial fluid is of high signal intensity on MTC images. The sharp contrast generated between the cartilage and the synovial fluid with MTC suggests that the cartilage contains macromolecules that strongly interact with water protons.[1010] With MTC, hypertrophic synovial tissue also reveals increased signal intensity, underscoring the potential of saturation transfer imaging to allow discrimination among cartilage, joint fluid, and pannus.[159]

Results of recent studies using MTC and MTC subtraction techniques have been promising. The dependence of MTC on collagen concentration appears likely, and alterations in collagen structure theoretically should be detectable with these imaging methods.[1011] MTC also may be sensitive to alterations in glycosaminoglycans and other components of cartilage matrix.[1012] The most powerful use of MTC imaging ultimately may relate to its combination with other MR imaging measurements that are sensitive in detecting cartilage degeneration,

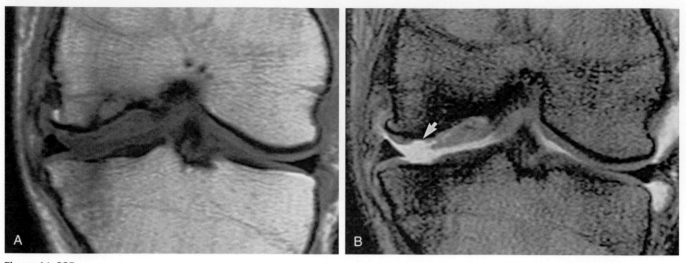

Figure 16–237

Articular cartilage abnormalities: MR imaging with magnetization transfer contrast (MTC). Compared with a coronal T1-weighted (TR/TE, 650/20) spin echo MR image **(A)**, a MPGR (TR/TE, 683/15; flip angle, 40 degrees) MR image obtained with MTC **(B)** allows far better delineation of the lesion (arrow) in the femoral articular cartilage. Osteochondritis dissecans of the medial femoral condyle is seen. (Courtesy of S. Eilenberg, M.D., San Diego, California.)

such as those resulting from diffusion and sodium MR imaging.[1012–1014]

8. Ultrashort echo time projection reconstruction MR imaging. Proton reconstruction MR imaging with echo times (TE) as short as 50 μsec has been used to obtain signal from structures (such as tendons) with very short T2 relaxation times.[1167] Similar imaging has been applied to the assessment of articular cartilage.[1168] Preliminary data have indicated superior delineation of patellar cartilage (in cadavers) when compared to three-dimensional fat-suppressed SPGR images and MTC techniques[1168] (see Fig. 16–238).

Osteoarthritis

The abnormalities of osteoarthritis are not confined to articular cartilage. The subchondral bone also is involved either prior or subsequent to the appearance of chondral alterations. The early subchondral bone abnormalities may be detected with bone scintigraphy (see previous discussion) or MR imaging (see later discussion), and later abnormalities consisting of bone sclerosis, subchondral cysts, and osteophytes are readily apparent on routine radiographs.[1015–1027]

As MR imaging is a tomographic technique, gauging the extent of cartilage and subchondral bone based on findings on MR images appears to be more sensitive and accurate than routine radiographic images. Focal cartilage lesions and chondral abnormalities in the less involved femorotibial compartment are assessed far better with MR imaging than with conventional radiography (Fig. 16–239). The subchondral changes delineated with MR imaging in patients with osteoarthritis of the knee vary in their morphology and signal intensity, and the precise histologic causes of these changes often are not clear. As examples of this, regions of high signal intensity on T2-weighted spin echo, certain gradient echo, and STIR MR imaging sequences, when localized

to subchondral bone, may reflect subchondral cysts containing fluid or granulation tissue, marrow edema, or both; and regions of low signal intensity in the subchondral bone as seen with these imaging sequences may reflect the presence of fibrous tissue, trabecular thickening, or a combination of the two.[1028, 1169] The appearance of osteophytes on MR images varies according to their location (e.g., central versus marginal) and the amount of marrow within them (Figs. 16–240 and 16–241). Additional findings of osteoarthritis of the knee, including joint effusions, stress fractures, and intra-articular bodies (see later discussion) also can be evident on the MR imaging examination. Furthermore, the possibility exists that qualitative assessment of the various MR imaging findings of osteoarthritis of the knee, coupled with quantitative assessment of relaxation times of pathologic tissue, provides useful information regarding the progression of the disease and its response to therapeutic intervention.[1029]

Chondral and Osteochondral Injury

Two types of fractures involve articular cartilage: shearing fractures that produce chondral or osteochondral lesions confined to the superficial surfaces of the joint; and fractures in periarticular bone that also pass through the articular cartilage of the joint.[1030] These latter fractures often extend perpendicularly through the cartilage as a direct extension of the fracture line within the bone. Resulting incongruity of the joint surface often is underestimated with routine radiography and is assessed more actively with imaging methods that allow indirect (e.g., arthrography) or direct (e.g., MR imaging) visualization of the chondral surface.

Chondral and osteochondral lesions, as well as osteochondritis dissecans, are discussed in detail in Chapter 8. As many of these lesions involve the articular surfaces of the knee (e.g., femoral condyles, patella), a few additional comments are appropriate here. Rotary or shear-

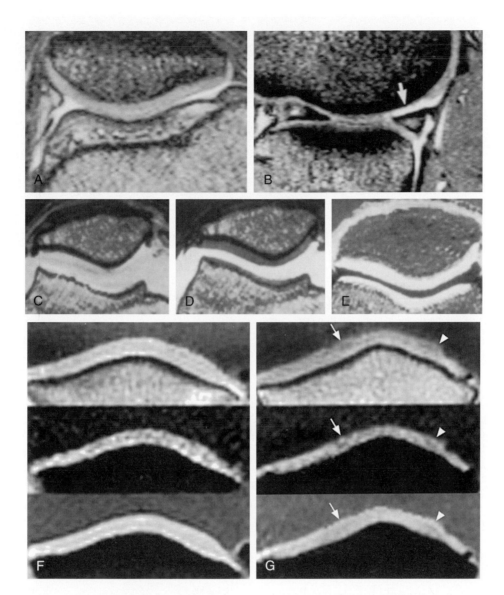

Figure 16–238

Normal and abnormal articular cartilage: MR imaging with magnetization transfer contrast (MTC), saturation transfer (ST) imaging, or ultrashort echo time projection reconstruction MR imaging—patellar and femoral articular cartilage.

A Normal patellar articular cartilage. A transaxial single section gradient recalled echo MR image (TR/TE, 650/15; flip angle, 40 degrees) obtained with MTC reveals the smooth patellar articular cartilage, which is of low signal intensity when compared with the joint fluid.

B Abnormal femoral articular cartilage. In a sagittal single section gradient recalled echo MR image obtained with MTC, a chondral defect (arrow) of the lateral femoral condyle is apparent. Note fluid of high signal intensity within the cartilage defect.

C–E Normal patellar and femoral articular cartilage. Transaxial images in an unfrozen cadaveric knee after the intra-articular injection of 55 ml of saline solution to simulate a joint effusion. Conventional 3DFT GRASS MR image (TR/TE, 60/7; flip angle, 20 degrees) **(C)**; addition of on-resonance pulsed ST to the sequence in **C (D)**; and ST subtraction image, obtained by subtracting image **D** from image **C (E)**. Note the decreased signal intensity of articular cartilage in **D** compared to **C**. This leads to an improvement in contrast between cartilage and fluid, but it decreases the contrast at the cartilage-bone interface. In **E,** ST subtraction provides high contrast at both the cartilage-fluid and cartilage-bone interfaces.

(**A, B** Courtesy of M. Solomon, M.D., San Jose, California; **C-E,** courtesy of C. Peterfy, M.D., and H. Genant, M.D., San Francisco, California.)

F, G Normal **(F)** and abnormal **(G)** patellar cartilage. Comparison of ultrashort echo time projection reconstruction (PR) MR imaging (TR/TE, 400/0.15) (top images in **F** and **G**), MTC (TR/TE, 400/6) MR imaging (middle images in **F** and **G**), and fat-suppressed three-dimensional SPGR (TR/TE, 50/10; flip angle, 60 degrees) MR imaging (bottom images in **F** and **G**).

In **F**, note the trilaminar appearance and high signal intensity of articular cartilage with PR MR imaging, the high signal intensity and nonlaminar appearance of articular cartilage with MTC MR imaging, and the high signal intensity and trilaminar appearance of articular cartilage with SPGR MR imaging.

In **G**, PR MR imaging shows two lesions. The lesion on the left (arrow) is characterized by decreased signal intensity in the middle layer of cartilage and preservation of the surface layer; the lesion on the right (arrowhead) is characterized by hypertrophy of articular cartilage and decreased signal intensity in the superficial and middle layers of cartilage. MTC MR imaging reveals only minor changes of signal intensity at the sites (arrow, arrowhead) of cartilage abnormality. With SPGR MR imaging, the lesion on the left (arrow) is not apparent; the lesion on the right (arrowhead) is associated with cartilage hypertrophy and a normal appearance of the superficial layer of cartilage. When the MR imaging findings were correlated to histologic findings in these cadaveric patellae, PR MR imaging was found to be most accurate.

(Courtesy of J. Brossmann, M.D., and L.R. Frank, Ph.D., San Diego, California.)

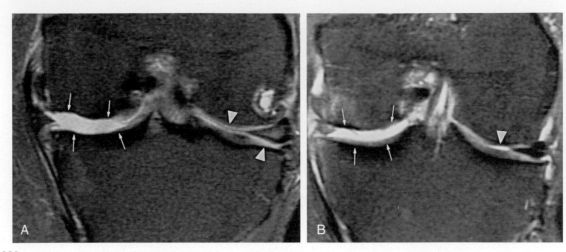

Figure 16–239
Osteoarthritis: MR imaging.

A In this patient with medial joint space loss and chondrocalcinosis evident on routine radiographs (not shown), a coronal fat-suppressed fast spin echo (TR/TE, 3000/18) MR image shows denudation of femoral and tibial articular cartilage (arrows) in the medial femorotibial compartment, mild to moderate loss of femoral and tibial articular cartilage (arrowheads) in the lateral femorotibial compartment, medial meniscal degeneration, and a lateral femoral subchondral cyst.

B In a second patient, severe cartilage loss in the medial femorotibial compartment (arrows), moderate cartilage loss in the lateral femorotibial compartment (arrowhead), and medial meniscal degeneration are evident in a coronal fat-suppressed fast spin echo (TR/TE, 3950/18) MR image. Note marrow edema in the medial femoral condyle.

ing forces generated by acute trauma or impaction forces occurring during a joint dislocation can lead to injury of the articular surface in which a portion of the surface is avulsed. The injuries may be purely chondral, may include a tiny or large fragment of bone and the entire overlying cartilage, or rarely, may involve bone alone if the overlying cartilage has already been eroded by an unrelated joint process.[1030] The resulting fragment may remain in situ or it may be partially or completely detached. If completely detached, it may become a free body in the joint, sometimes lodging and becoming embedded in a distant portion of the synovial membrane.

The pathologic characteristics of chondral and osteochondral fractures have been described in detail by Milgram.[1030–1033] The cartilage injury often is more complex than a simple fracture line, consisting of comminution and crushing of cartilage tissue. Beneath the dis-

rupted chondral fragment, the remaining cartilage may appear relatively normal or may demonstrate a blister-like effect. Acutely, any bone that has been separated along with the overlying cartilage appears normal histologically and, at its base, local hemorrhage and crushing of exposed trabeculae may be observed. In more chronic cases, the osteochondral fragment may be attached by a soft tissue pedicle to its site of origin. The composition of this pedicle varies: it may be secure or loose, cartilaginous or fibrous, long or short, and avascu-

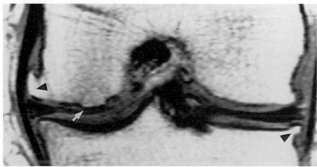

Figure 16–240
Osteoarthritis: MR imaging. A coronal T1-weighted (TR/TE, 800/20) spin echo image reveals a central osteophyte (arrow) in the medial femoral condyle and marginal osteophytes (arrowheads). (Courtesy of A. Motta, M.D., Cleveland, Ohio.)

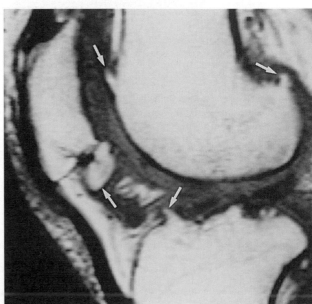

Figure 16–241
Osteoarthritis: MR imaging. A sagittal T1-weighted (TR/TE, 600/15) spin echo MR image shows multiple osteophytes containing fatty marrow (arrows).

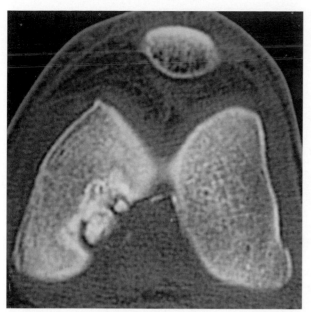

Figure 16–242
Osteochondritis dissecans: CT scanning. A transaxial CT scan shows a classic lesion in the inner aspect of the medial femoral condyle. Note the presence of multiple fragments of bone.

lar or vascular.[1030] In the knee, osteochondral fractures of the femoral condyles commonly result in a mobile lesion containing considerable portions of overlying, intact cartilage and fibrous and cartilaginous pedicles. At any site, repair at the base of an osteochondral lesion is associated with fibrocartilaginous proliferative tissue

derived from subchondral bone. Even empty craters may contain such tissue.

The detection of an osteochondral fragment containing a sizeable piece of bone that is located in its original osseous bed, is free in the joint cavity, or is embedded in the synovial membrane can be accomplished reasonably well with routine radiography, conventional tomography, or CT scanning (Fig. 16–242). The detection of an osteochondral fragment containing a small piece of bone or a purely chondral fragment located in any of these sites frequently requires additional imaging methods, such as standard arthrography, conventional arthrotomography, computed arthrotomography, or MR imaging, that provide indirect or direct evidence that such a fragment is present.

Evaluation of chondral and osteochondral fractures and osteochondritis dissecans with MR imaging has received considerable attention.[1034–1042] Such evaluation includes analysis of the site and size of the lesion, the integrity of the overlying cartilage, and, in the case of osteochondritis dissecans, the stability of the lesion. When a lesion is associated with intact cartilage and is not ballotable at the time of arthroscopy (or open surgery), it is regarded as stable. A lesion that is loose in situ is ballotable, although the overlying cartilage is normal.[1038] Grossly loose lesions are associated with a disrupted chondral surface and partial or complete separation of the fragment. The MR imaging criteria used to judge stability generally are based on the appearance of the junctional zone between the fragment and the parent bone (Figs. 16–243 and 16–244). The absence of high signal intensity in this zone on T2-weighted spin echo and certain gradient echo sequences usually indi-

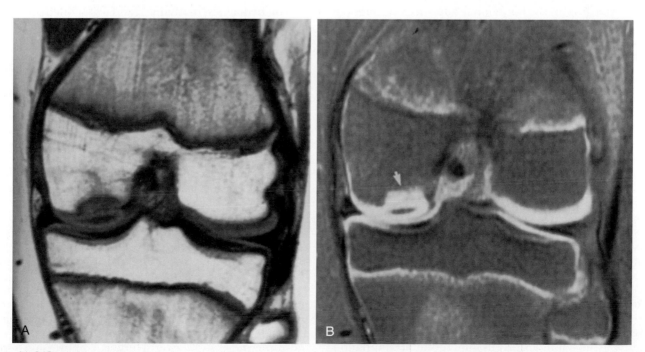

Figure 16–243
Osteochondritis dissecans: MR imaging. Coronal T1-weighted (TR/TE, 600/20) **(A)** and T1-weighted (TR/TE, 800/20) **(B)** spin echo MR images, the latter image obtained with fat suppression, show the typical location of osteochondritis dissecans in the inner aspect of the medial femoral condyle. In **B,** note the high signal intensity at the base of the lesion (arrow), a poor prognostic sign. (From Bosch E, et al: Physician Sportsmed *21*:116, 1993.)

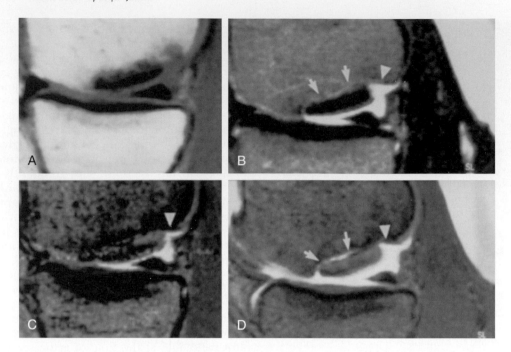

Figure 16–244

Osteochondritis dissecans: MR imaging and MR arthrography.

A, B Sagittal T1-weighted (TR/TE, 700/15) **(A)** and T2-weighted (TR/TE, 2500/90) **(B)** spin echo MR images show a large osteochondral lesion in the medial femoral condyle. In **B,** note a slight increase in signal intensity at the base of the lesion (arrows), which represents either fluid or granulation tissue. Also in **B,** because of the high signal intensity of the joint fluid, a posterior defect in the articular cartilage is apparent (arrowhead). Note the large synovial cyst.

C In the same patient, a sagittal three-dimensional MR image using FISP shows the posterior disruption of the articular cartilage (arrowhead) but fails to reveal increased signal intensity at the base of the lesion.

D In the same patient, a sagittal three-dimensional FISP MR image obtained after the intra-articular administration of a gadolinium compound reveals definite fluid (arrows) at the base of the lesion, indicating a poor prognosis. The posterior cartilaginous defect again is seen (arrowhead).

(Courtesy of J. Kramer, M.D., Vienna, Austria.)

cates a stable lesion.[1037, 1038] The presence of such high signal intensity in the junctional zone is a strong (although not infallible) indicator of an unstable lesion. High signal intensity may result from granulation tissue at the base of the lesion or it may relate to fluid that extends from the joint cavity through cartilage defects. Although the presence of joint fluid in the base of the lesion clearly indicates cartilage violation, differentiation between this fluid and granulation tissue with MR imaging is difficult in some cases. MR arthrography, in which gadolinium compounds injected intra-articularly can be detected at the interface of the fragment and parent bone, can confirm disruption of the articular cartilage. MR imaging after the intravenous administration of gadolinium compounds, in which accentuation of signal intensity occurs in the junctional zone, provides strong evidence that granulation tissue is present. These supplementary methods improve the accuracy of MR imaging in defining stability in cases of osteochondritis dissecans, although large lesions (equal to or greater than 0.8 cm²) and those with thick (equal to or greater than 3 mm) sclerotic margins as defined by routine radiography generally are unstable.[1038] Furthermore, bone scintigraphy can be used to judge lesion stability, as unstable lesions usually reveal accumulation of the radionuclide in flow, blood pool, and delayed phases of the examination.[1038] Thus, the relative value of MR imaging in the analysis of lesion stability is not clear.

The role of MR imaging in allowing direct assessment of the cartilage surface in cases of osteochondritis dissec-

ans or chondral or osteochondral fractures is limited by the inadequacies of many standard sequences in the accurate delineation of articular cartilage (see previous discussion) (Fig. 16–245). The role of MR imaging in determining the presence of necrosis in fragments containing considerable quantities of bone also is not clear. Finally, the relative value of MR imaging, in comparison to other imaging methods, in the detection of free bodies within the joint or those embedded in the synovial membrane is questionable (see later discussion). MR imaging, however, is sensitive in the diagnosis of occult subcortical femoral and tibial fractures that, with time, may progress to osteochondral sequelae.[1039]

Surgical methods applied to the treatment of osteochondritis dissecans (and osteochondral fractures or lesions) in the knee and elsewhere include excision of the chondral or osteochondral fragment, débriding the crater (at the parent site of the fragment), and various types of fixation and grafting. With regard to fixation techniques, bone pegs typically derived from the tibia may be inserted into drill holes in the osteochondral fragment and subjacent bone to fix the fragment in place.[1043, 1044] Pins may be used instead of bone plugs, although a subsequent arthrotomy is necessary to remove the pins.[1045, 1046] Even Herbert compression screws have been used to fix the fragment.[1047] Osteochondral grafting procedures, usually employing an allograft, represent a departure from these fixation techniques.[1048, 1049] Such grafts, which have been used for other purposes, such as in the treatment of tibial plateau fractures,[1050]

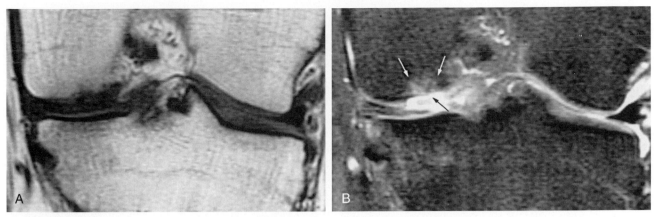

Figure 16–245
Osteochondral fracture: MR imaging. An acute osteochondral lesion of the medial femoral condyle is not well evaluated on a coronal T1-weighted (TR/TE, 433/12) spin echo MR image **(A)** but is well shown (arrows) on a coronal fat-suppressed fast spin echo (TR/TE, 4000/18) MR image **(B).** The medial meniscus also is torn, as was the anterior cruciate ligament.

are fixed in place with Kirschner wires, screws, or resorbable synthetic or autogenous material.[1051] Although the reported data are preliminary, MR imaging may prove useful in monitoring the incorporation of the allograft (Fig. 16–246).[1052]

Intra-Articular Bodies

Although intra-articular bodies composed of cartilage alone or cartilage and bone together may be evident in virtually any joint, those of the knee are encountered

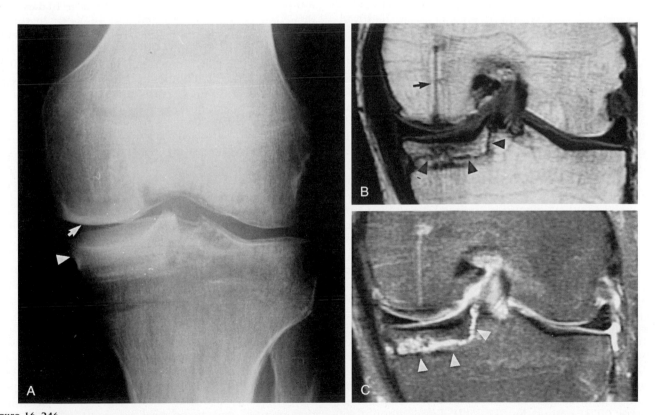

Figure 16–246
Osteochondral allograft: MR imaging.
   A Routine radiograph reveals osteochondral allografts used to replace the femoral (arrow) and tibial (arrowhead) articular surfaces in the medial femorotibial compartment. The femoral allograft appears to be completely incorporated. On the tibial side, a thin radiolucent line is seen between the allograft and parent bone.
   B On a coronal T1-weighted (TR/TE, 900/12) spin echo MR image, a line of low signal intensity (arrowheads) at the base and side of the tibial allograft is seen. The femoral allograft appears to be fully incorporated. The vertical line of low signal intensity (arrow) marks the site of insertion of resorbable synthetic material used to hold the graft in place.
   C On a coronal fat-suppressed fast spin echo (TR/TE, 4000/18) MR image, note the zone of high signal intensity (arrowheads) at the base and side of the tibial graft, compatible with the presence of granulation tissue. In both **B** and **C,** the signal intensity of the marrow in the allografts is identical to that of normal fatty marrow, and the articular cartilage of the allografts appears grossly normal.

most frequently. Any process that leads to acute disruption or chronic disintegration of the articular surface can give rise to one or more free or synovium-embedded intra-articular bodies. Examples of such processes include chondral and osteochondral fractures, osteochondritis dissecans, osteoarthritis, neuropathic osteoarthropathy, rheumatoid arthritis, gout, calcium pyrophosphate dihydrate crystal deposition disease, calcium hydroxyapatite crystal deposition disease, osteonecrosis, and rheumatoid arthritis. Furthermore, primary synovial (osteo)chondromatosis, a rare disorder of unknown cause, leads to metaplasia of the synovial lining with the formation of cartilage nodules that may calcify or ossify and become free within the joint cavity.

Regardless of their source of origin, intra-articular bodies all demonstrate similar histopathologic alterations once they are free in the joint space.[1030] They receive their nutrition from the synovial fluid and may contain any or all of the principal cells of bone tissue (i.e., osteoblasts, osteocytes, chondroblasts, chondrocytes, fibroblasts, osteoclasts, and their precursor cells). The osteoblasts and osteoclasts can differentiate and perform their functions without the presence of any blood supply.[1030] The origin of these cells may be the nidi of the free bodies themselves or, more likely, the synovial membrane. The surface cells of free bodies form more cartilaginous layers than osseous layers; as these layers are formed, the deeper cells are deprived of their nutrition, die, and calcify.[1030]

Calcified free or embedded intra-articular bodies that are large usually are identified easily with routine radiography. Classically, they appear layered, without recognizable trabeculae. Occasionally, irregular radiodense nodules at the periphery of the bodies create a mulberry-like appearance.[1053] Smaller bodies, unless heavily calcified, are more difficult to detect with routine radiography or, sometimes, even with conventional tomography or CT scanning. With any of these imaging methods, the search for intra-articular bodies is more rewarding if normal recesses and dependent portions of the knee (or other joint) are analyzed carefully. Common locations for intra-articular bodies in the knee are the suprapatellar recess (particularly when a suprapatellar plica is present), popliteus tunnel, recesses beneath the menisci, and the intercondylar notch.[1054] Free bodies within the knee may pass into an adjacent synovial cyst. Multiple intra-articular bodies in the knee are present in approximately 30 per cent of cases.[1054] A calcified area localized to the region of the posterior horn of the medial meniscus may represent a meniscal ossicle rather than an intra-articular body (see previous discussion).

The detection of small calcified or noncalcified bodies in the knee may require arthrography or the combination of arthrography and either conventional tomography or CT scanning (Fig. 16–247). Large amounts of air with or without a small amount of radiopaque contrast material are injected in the joint. Transaxial CT scanning may be employed with the patient supine or prone, depending on the suspected location of the fragment. Care must be exercised so that the tibial spines are not misinterpreted as evidence of intra-articular osseous bodies.

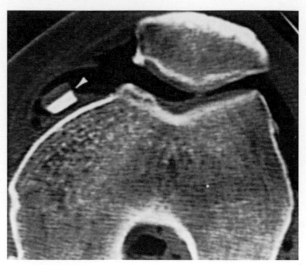

Figure 16–247

Intra-articular bodies: CT arthrography. After the introduction of air into the knee joint, a transaxial CT scan reveals the fragment (arrowhead), consisting of cartilage and bone in the medial aspect of the joint.

Small calcified or noncalcified bodies in the knee may escape detection with MR imaging, especially if a joint effusion is not present. A joint effusion makes their detection easier (Figs. 16–248 and 16–249). In the absence of a knee effusion, MR arthrography may represent an effective technique for demonstrating such bodies (see Fig. 16–248). In general, however, the diagnosis of free or embedded bodies in the knee is better accomplished with computed arthrotomography than with MR imaging.

Abnormalities of Subchondral Bone

Occult Injuries

The detection of occult injuries in the distal portion of the femur and the proximal portion of the tibia with MR imaging has been emphasized repeatedly[759, 770, 782, 783, 1039, 1055–1058, 1170] and is discussed in Chapter 8. Many of these injuries result from forces that lead to impaction of one articular surface against another, and they frequently are accompanied by additional insults to the menisci and to intra-articular (i.e., cruciate) and periarticular ligaments. Experimentally, transarticular loading has led to fractures through the zone of calcified cartilage and subchondral bone, frequently with step-off displacement and little or no change in the gross appearance of the articular cartilage; MR imaging has documented soft tissue swelling, joint effusions, and alterations of signal intensity in the bone marrow as transient accompanying phenomena.[1059] Such alterations in signal intensity within subchondral marrow after injury to the knee (or to other joints) have led to the introduction of the term "bone bruise."[1057] The precise histologic correlates of a bone bruise are not clear, although microfractures of trabeculae and hyper-

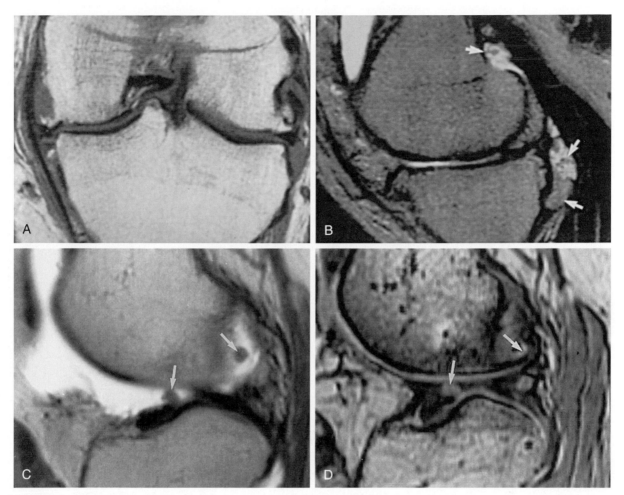

Figure 16–248

Intra-articular bodies: MR imaging.

A, B In this patient with severe osteoarthritis of the knee, a coronal T1-weighted (TR/TE, 800/25) spin echo MR image **(A)** shows loss of the medial femorotibial joint space and osteophytes in the marginal regions of the femur and tibia. A sagittal T2-weighted (TR/TE, 2000/80) spin echo MR image **(B)** reveals multiple intra-articular bodies (arrows) appearing as foci of low signal intensity surrounded by joint fluid of high signal intensity.

C, D After the placement of two cartilaginous bodies (3 mm in size) in a cadaveric knee joint, a T1-weighted (TR/TE, 500/20) spin echo MR arthrographic (i.e., gadolinium compound) image obtained with fat suppression in the sagittal plane **(C)** shows these bodies exquisitely (arrows). A sagittal spoiled GRASS (SPGR) MR image (TR/TE, 52/10; flip angle, 60 degrees) **(D)** shows these bodies as regions of high signal intensity (arrows). (Courtesy of J. Brossmann, M.D., San Diego, California.)

emia, edema, and hemorrhage in adjacent marrow probably contribute to the changes in signal intensity. Reticulated regions of low signal intensity are apparent in T1-weighted spin echo MR images, and similar regions of inhomogeneous high signal intensity are observed in T2-weighted spin echo MR images (Fig. 16–250). STIR and certain fat suppression imaging sequences display these lesions dramatically as areas of high signal intensity within involved marrow (see Fig. 16–250). The MR imaging characteristics of bone bruises are similar to those noted in cases of transient painful bone marrow edema.

Additional occult cartilage and bone injuries about the knee include stress fractures (insufficiency and fatigue fractures) (Fig. 16–251), osteochondral fractures (Fig. 16–252), and acute fractures of the femoral condyles and tibial plateaus (Fig. 16–253) that generally extend into the chondral surfaces.[1057] Although differentiation among these injuries generally is possible on the basis of MR imaging findings coupled with information derived from the patient's history, clinical examination, and results of other imaging studies, this is not always possible. A constant component of all types of occult injury is a poorly defined area of decreased signal intensity in T1-weighted spin echo MR images and of increased signal intensity in T2-weighted spin echo MR images within the bone marrow, presumably related to edema, hemorrhage, hyperemia, or even osteonecrosis, or combinations of these findings.[1057] This may be the only component of a bone bruise, whereas with osteochondral fractures, stress fractures, and acute fractures, additional MR imaging features may be evident (see Chapter 8). These occult injuries may occur together or in isolation, and one type of injury, such as a bone bruise, later may develop into another type.[1039] The sensitivity of the MR imaging examination in detection of any of these occult injuries is equal to and probably better than bone scintigraphy, even single photon emis-

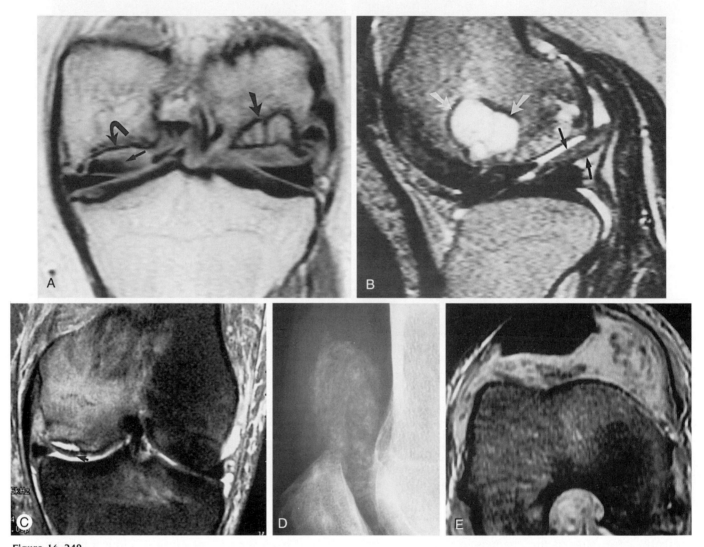

Figure 16–249
Intra-articular bodies: MR imaging.

A, B Osteochondritis dissecans. In a 25 year old woman with involvement of both femoral condyles, coronal proton density–weighted (TR/TE, 2100/20) **(A)** and sagittal T2-weighted (TR/TE, 2700/90) **(B)** spin echo MR images show extensive contour irregularity and cyst formation in subchondral bone (large arrows) and multiple intra-articular osteochondral fragments (small arrows).

C Steroid-induced osteonecrosis. In this 87 year old man, osteonecrosis of the medial femoral condyle is associated with a small, partially displaced osteochondral fragment (arrow), marrow edema in the femur and tibia, and a degenerative medial meniscus, as seen on a coronal fat-suppressed fast spin echo (TR/TE, 5000/48) MR image. Subcutaneous edema also is present.

D, E Calcium pyrophosphate dihydrate (CPPD) crystal deposition disease. This disorder may be associated with widespread intra-articular deposition of CPPD crystals, as shown in a routine radiograph **(D)** and transaxial MPGR MR image (TR/TE, 450/15; flip angle, 60 degrees) **(E)**. In this case, both CPPD and hydroxyapatite crystals were recovered from the joint.

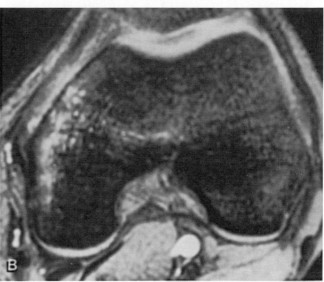

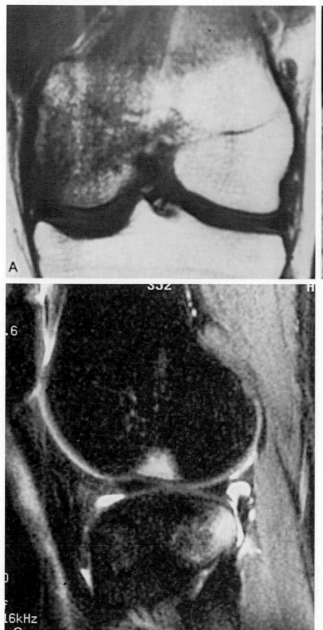

Figure 16–250

Bone bruises: MR imaging.

A In a T1-weighted spin echo MR image (TR/TE, 500/12), a geographic area of decreased signal intensity within the medial femoral condyle is identified in the coronal plane.

B In the transaxial multiplanar gradient recalled (MPGR) sequence (TR/TE, 350/18; flip angle, 30 degrees), high signal intensity is seen along the medial femoral condylar margin, indicative of hemorrhage, edema, and associated microfracture.

C A sagittal STIR MR image (TR/TE, 4950/19; inversion time, 160 msec) shows bone bruises of high signal intensity in the lateral femoral condyle and lateral tibial plateau, characteristic of an injury to the anterior cruciate ligament.

(**A, B,** Courtesy of H. Pavlov, M.D., New York, New York; **C,** courtesy of D. Berthoty, M.D., Las Vegas, Nevada.)

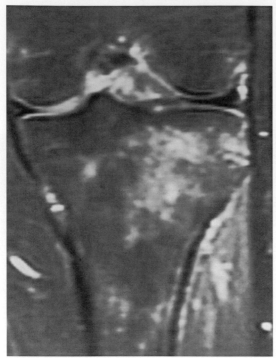

Figure 16–251
Stress fractures: MR imaging. In this patient who developed knee pain after starting a new jogging program, a coronal T1-weighted (TR/TE, 750/20) spin echo MR image obtained with chemical presaturation of fat (ChemSat) and after the intravenous injection of a gadolinium compound reveals areas of increased signal intensity in the lateral tibial plateau. (From Bosch E, et al: *Physician Sportsmed 21*:116, 1993.)

sion computed tomography (SPECT). The specificity of the MR imaging examination surely is superior to bone scintigraphy and, by modifying and shortening the MR imaging examination, its cost may not differ significantly from that of bone scintigraphy. In all cases, when an occult injury to cartilage and subchondral bone is detected with MR imaging, attention must be directed to other structures, such as the menisci and the collateral and cruciate ligaments, that also may be injured.

Hematopoietic Hyperplasia

A report in 1989 by Deutsch and coworkers[1060] was the first to emphasize the occurrence of islands of hypercel-lular but otherwise normal-appearing hematopoietic marrow in the metaphysis of the distal end of the femur in asymptomatic persons, particularly obese premeno-pausal women who also are cigarette smokers. These islands demonstrated low signal intensity on both T1-weighted and T2-weighted spin echo images, prompting initial concern about the possibility of occult myelopro-liferative neoplasms. A similar alteration of marrow signal intensity about the knee in an obese woman subse-quently was reported by Schuck and Czarnecki,[1061] and in this patient, marrow alterations were noted not only in the distal portion of the femur but also in the proxi-mal portion of the tibia, proximal aspect of the femora, and iliac crest. Shellock and collaborators[1062] observed a high prevalence (43 per cent) of hematopoietic bone marrow hyperplasia in the distal femoral metaphysis of marathon runners when compared with healthy volun-teers (3 per cent) and with patients with symptoms of knee disorders (15 per cent). The femoral epiphysis and the proximal portion of the tibia were not affected. These authors postulated that the frequency of such marrow hyperplasia in marathon runners may indicate a response to the anemia encountered in highly condi-tioned aerobically trained athletes. Other investigators also have confirmed the presence of hematopoietic bone marrow about the knee, emphasizing its localiza-tion to the femoral metaphysis, some variability in the pattern of decreased marrow signal intensity, and accen-tuated changes in signal intensity when opposed-phase gradient echo MR sequences are employed.[1063, 1065]

The major differential diagnostic considerations of MR imaging findings are lymphoma or other myelopro-liferative disorders (Fig. 16–254), myelofibrosis (Fig. 16–255), and sickle cell anemia or other hemoglobinopa-thies. Although benign hematopoietic hyperplasia may not be confined to the distal femoral metaphysis in all cases, this distribution provides the most important clue to correct diagnosis. Furthermore, the absence of in-creased signal intensity on T2-weighted spin echo MR images favors a diagnosis of benign hematopoietic hy-perplasia over that of most primary and secondary bone tumors and osteomyelitis.

Osteonecrosis

Ischemic necrosis involving the bones about the knee is second in frequency only to that of the femoral head.

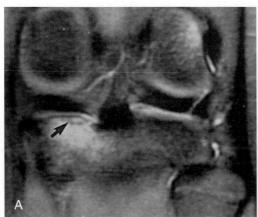
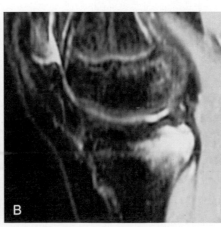

Figure 16–252
Osteochondral fractures: MR imaging.
A A small osteochondral fracture (arrow) of the posterior aspect of the medial tibial plateau is surrounded by marrow edema, as shown on a coronal fat-suppressed fast spin echo (TR/TE, 3950/18) MR image.
B The sagittal STIR MR image (TR/TE, 3667/17; inversion time, 150 msec) shows dramatic edema, although the fracture itself is not identified.

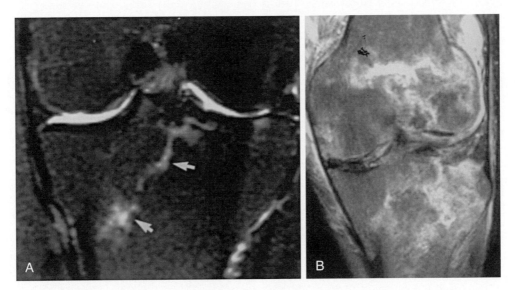

Figure 16–253
Occult acute fractures: MR imaging.

A Although routine radiographs were normal in this patient who had sustained an injury to the knee, a coronal T2-weighted (TR/TE, 4000/102) fast spin echo MR image obtained with chemical presaturation of fat (ChemSat) reveals the fracture line (arrows) in the tibial plateau.

B A coronal fat-suppressed fast spin echo MR image (TR/TE, 3500/76) in a 72 year old man with a remote injury of the knee and acute trauma shows acute fractures of the distal portion of the femur and tibial plateaus manifested as regions of high signal intensity. (Courtesy of D. Berthoty, M.D., Las Vegas, Nevada.)

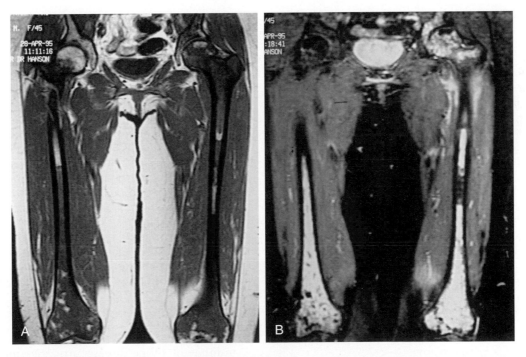

Figure 16–254
Non-Hodgkin's lymphoma: Disseminated disease—MR imaging.

A A coronal T1-weighted (TR/TE, 600/17) spin echo MR image reveals tumor of low signal intensity diffusely distributed in the marrow of the femora and left innominate bone.

B With STIR imaging (TR/TE, 4000/19; inversion time, 140 msec), the involved regions are of high signal intensity.
(Courtesy of D. Wilcox, M.D., Kansas City, Missouri.)

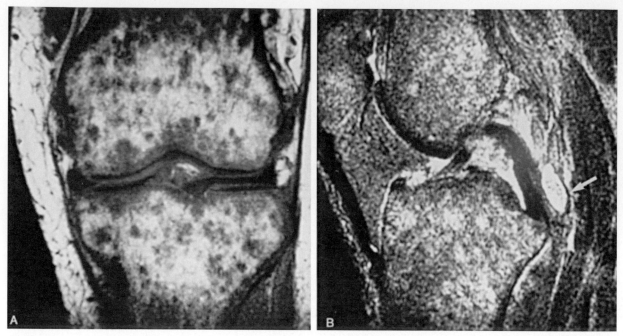

Figure 16–255

Myelofibrosis: MR imaging. This 71 year old woman had myelofibrosis and hepatosplenomegaly. Routine radiographs of the femora showed periostitis. The coronal T1-weighted (TR/TE, 800/20) spin echo MR image **(A)** shows inhomogeneous signal intensity in the bone marrow of the distal end of the femur and proximal end of the tibia. The sagittal T2-weighted (TR/TE, 2000/80) spin echo MR image **(B)** again reveals inhomogeneous signal intensity in the bone marrow. The findings are consistent with hyperplastic red marrow, granulation tissue, and fibrosis. An incidental finding is a probable ganglion (arrow) arising near the posterior cruciate ligament. (Courtesy of G. Greenway, M.D., Dallas, Texas.)

Typical sites of involvement are the femoral condyles and proximal portion of the tibia, although involvement of the diaphyseal and metaphyseal regions of the femur and tibia is encountered. Ischemic necrosis of the patella is rare and usually is associated with a patellar fracture, previous surgery, or the administration of corticosteroid medications. Osteonecrosis of the fibula is extremely rare.

The causes of osteonecrosis are diverse (Figs. 16–256 and 16–257), and, in some cases, no causative factors can be identified, a situation designated primary (or spontaneous) osteonecrosis. Primary osteonecrosis about the knee is a condition of middle-aged and elderly men and women who develop the spontaneous onset of knee pain (Figs. 16–258, 16–259, and 16–260). The weight-bearing portion of the medial femoral condyle is affected most frequently, although involvement of the lateral femoral condyle or the medial or lateral regions of the proximal portion of the tibia, or combinations of these sites, is encountered. One or both knees may be affected, and an association of this condition with meniscal tears and, later, with osteoarthritis is recognized. The major alternative diagnostic consideration is osteochondritis dissecans (Table 16–2).

A variety of imaging methods may be used to diagnose osteonecrosis about the knee, of which bone scintigraphy and MR imaging are most sensitive, and to define its distribution and extent. The classic feature of bone necrosis as displayed by bone scintigraphy is the increased accumulation of the radiopharmaceutical agent at or near the site of involvement, although decreased accumulation or no accumulation (i.e., cold lesion) of

the radionuclide may be found in the acute stages of the process. The MR imaging features of osteonecrosis are more variable, influenced by the stage of the process. Decreased signal intensity in the involved bone marrow in T1-weighted spin echo MR images and increased signal intensity in this region in T2-weighted spin echo MR images usually are evident (Figs. 16–261 and 16–262), even in early stages of osteonecrosis. Later findings in cases of osteonecrosis involving the femoral condyles or subchondral bone of the tibia include flattening of the articular surface and areas of persistent low signal intensity that reflect the presence of bone sclerosis (Fig. 16–263). Similar findings are displayed by more conventional techniques, such as routine radiography and conventional tomography.

Widespread infarcts in the diaphyseal and metaphyseal regions of the femur and tibia lead to serpentine areas about the lesions whose signal intensity characteristics relate to the presence of sclerotic bone and granulation tissue.

Other Disorders

A number of other disease processes may involve the bones about the knee. These include osteomyelitis and septic arthritis (Figs. 16–264 and 16–265), Blount's disease (Fig. 16–266), multiple epiphyseal dysplasias (Fig. 16–267), and Paget's disease (Fig. 16–268).

Of the many bone tumors and tumor-like lesions that are found about the knee (Table 16–3), several deserve emphasis. *Osteochondromas* are most frequently observed in this location. They may be solitary or multiple (Fig.

Text continued on page 745

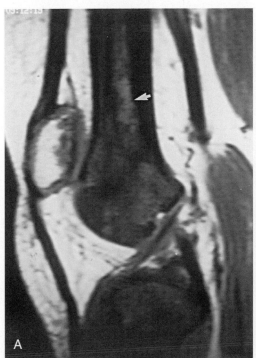

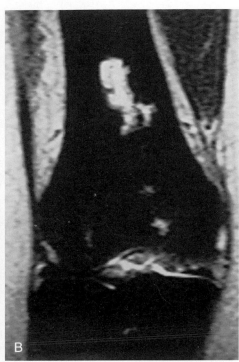

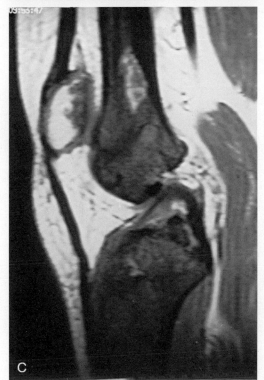

Figure 16–256

Sickle cell anemia: Marrow ischemia—MR imaging.

A Findings on this sagittal T1-weighted (TR/TE, 886/15) spin echo MR image include cortical thickening (especially in the femoral shaft) and markedly decreased signal intensity of the marrow in the femur, tibia, and posterior portion of the patella. A focus of intermediate signal intensity (arrow) is seen in the distal aspect of the femur.

B A coronal T2-weighted (TR/TE, 1950/90) spin echo MR image shows high signal intensity in this femoral region displayed on marrow of markedly decreased signal intensity.

C After the intravenous administration of a gadolinium compound, enhancement of signal intensity in the femoral lesion is evident, when compared to findings in **A.** These findings, combined with clinical data, are consistent with the presence of acute infarction.

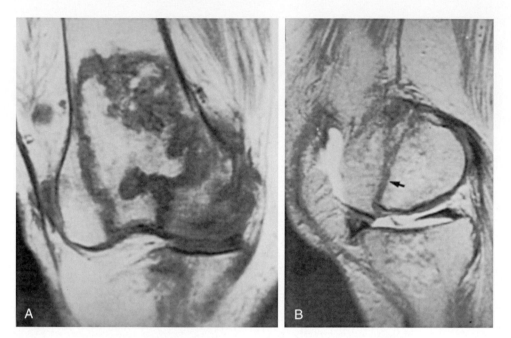

Figure 16–257
Osteonecrosis: MR imaging. This patient developed knee pain after a fall.

A A coronal T1-weighted (TR/TE, 600/20) spin echo MR image shows classic features of osteonecrosis involving the distal portion of the femur. Observe the serpentine margin of the lesion with low signal intensity.

B A sagittal T2-weighted (TR/TE, 2000/70) spin echo MR image shows a fracture (arrow) through the area of osteonecrosis in the medial femoral condyle. Osteonecrosis also involves the adjacent tibial plateau, and a joint effusion is seen.

  (Courtesy of S.K. Brahme, M.D., San Diego, California.)

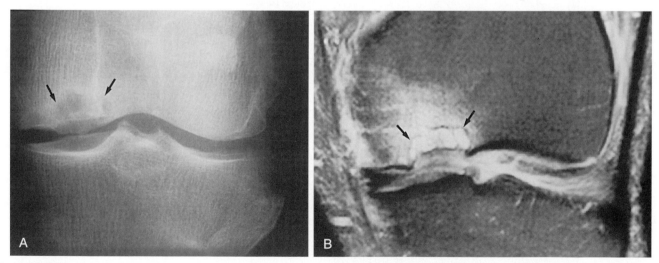

Figure 16–258
Primary (spontaneous) osteonecrosis about the knee: Routine radiography and MR imaging. In this 58 year old man, a routine radiograph **(A)** shows flattening of the medial femoral condyle and large subchondral cysts (arrows). After the intravenous injection of a gadolinium compound, a coronal fat-suppressed T1-weighted (TR/TE, 700/20) spin echo MR image **(B)** shows marked enhancement of signal intensity of the lesion (arrows) and adjacent marrow edema.

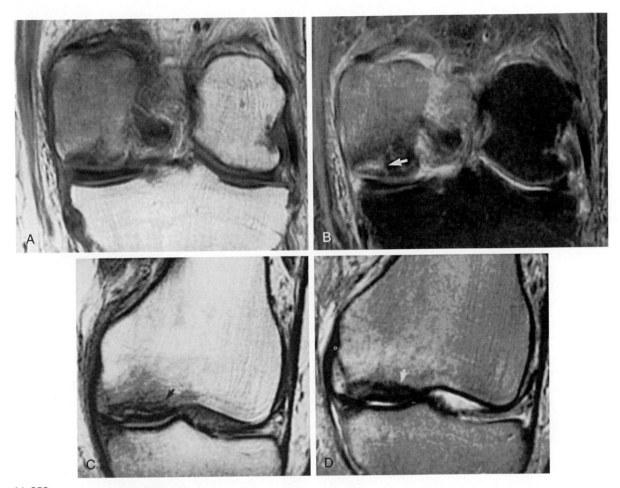

Figure 16–259

Primary (spontaneous) osteonecrosis about the knee: MR imaging.

A, B In this 81 year old man, a coronal T1-weighted (TR/TE, 800/16) spin echo MR image **(A)** shows flattening of the medial femoral condyle, a subchondral band of low signal intensity, and patchy regions of low signal intensity throughout the medial condyle. On a coronal fat-suppressed fast spin echo (TR/TE, 3000/21) MR image **(B),** the necrotic region is seen (arrow), diffuse condylar edema is evident, and subcutaneous edema also is apparent.

C, D In this 67 year old woman with the abrupt onset of knee pain, a coronal proton density (TR/TE, 1000/20) spin echo MR image **(C)** reveals flattening of the medial femoral condyle, with a subchondral zone of low signal intensity (arrow). Broader areas of low signal intensity involve the medial femoral condyle and medial tibial plateau. On a coronal T2-weighted (TR/TE, 3000/76) spin echo image **(D),** the area of necrosis again is evident (arrow). Note the bone marrow edema, with high signal intensity, in the medial femoral condyle and medial tibial plateau. Additional findings include a joint effusion, a torn medial meniscus (not well shown), and subcutaneous edema. (Courtesy of M. Schweitzer, M.D., Philadelphia, Pennsylvania.)

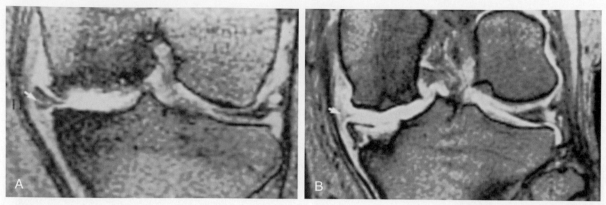

Figure 16–260

Spontaneous osteonecrosis about the knee: MR imaging.

A Medial femoral condyle. A coronal multiplanar gradient recalled (MPGR) MR image (TR/TE, 600/20; flip angle, 45 degrees) shows cartilage loss in both the medial femoral condyle and medial tibial plateau, a subchondral zone of osteonecrosis in the medial femoral condyle, diminished signal intensity in the adjacent tibial plateau consistent with bone sclerosis, a joint effusion, and a tear (arrow) of the medial meniscus. The findings are those of spontaneous osteonecrosis of the medial femoral condyle with secondary osteoarthritis.

B Medial tibial plateau. A similar coronal MPGR image (TR/TE, 600/20; flip angle, 45 degrees) reveals osteonecrosis in the medial tibial plateau with depression and fracture of the articular surface, loss of articular cartilage, sclerosis with low signal intensity in the medial femoral condyle, a joint effusion, and a torn medial meniscus (arrow).

(Courtesy of S. Fernandez, M.D., Mexico City, Mexico.)

Table 16–2. SPONTANEOUS OSTEONECROSIS VERSUS OSTEOCHONDRITIS DISSECANS (ABOUT THE KNEE)

	Spontaneous Osteonecrosis	**Osteochondritis Dissecans**
Age of onset	Middle-aged and elderly	Adolescent
Symptoms	Pain, tenderness, swelling, restricted motion	Variable; may be lacking
Typical location	Weight-bearing surface of medial femoral condyle	Non–weight-bearing surface of medial femoral condyle
Probable pathogenesis	Trauma, perhaps related to meniscal tear; or vascular insult	Trauma
Sequelae	Degenerative joint disease; intra-articular osteocartilaginous bodies	Intra-articular osteocartilaginous bodies

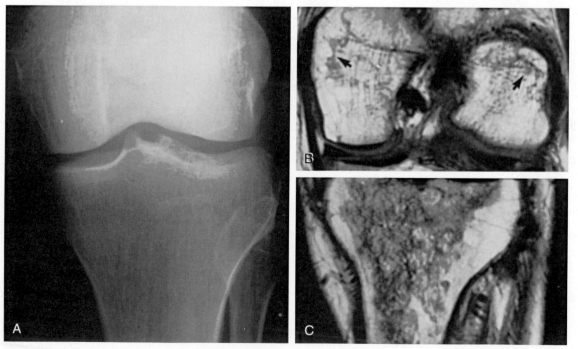

Figure 16–261

Osteonecrosis: MR imaging.

A The routine radiograph is normal.

B, C Two coronal T1-weighted (TR/TE, 750/20) spin echo MR images show characteristic findings of osteonecrosis involving both femoral condyles (arrows) and tibia.

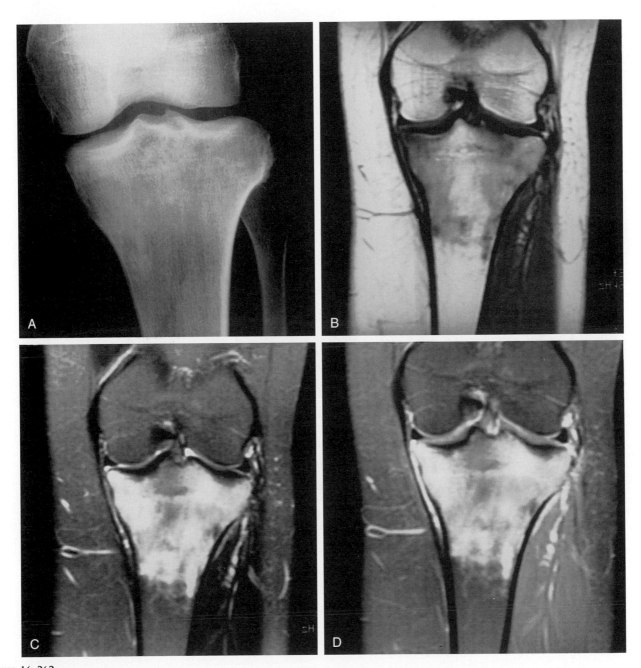

Figure 16–262
Osteonecrosis: MR imaging.
  A The routine radiograph shows patchy osteosclerosis in the tibia. The findings are not specific for osteonecrosis.
  B Inhomogeneous regions of low signal intensity are evident on a coronal T1-weighted (TR/TE, 733/17) spin echo MR image.
  C, D Coronal fat-suppressed fast spin echo (TR/TE, 3600/85) **(C)** and fat-suppressed T1-weighted (TR/TE, 700/17) spin echo **(D)** MR images, the latter obtained after intravenous gadolinium contrast agent administration, show similar findings. Note inhomogeneous but mainly high signal intensity in the tibia. The findings, again, are not specific.

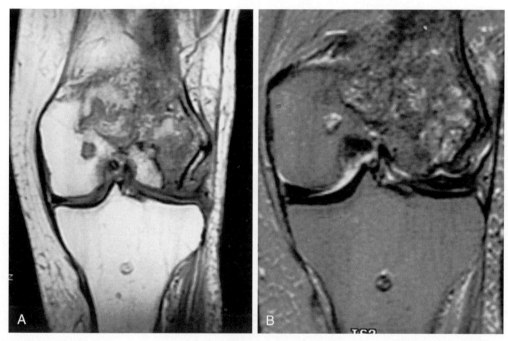

Figure 16–263
Primary (spontaneous) osteonecrosis about the knee: MR imaging. In this 73 year old woman, coronal T1-weighted (TR/TE, 600/22) **(A)** and T2-weighted (TR/TE, 2400/90) **(B)** spin echo MR images show widespread osteonecrosis in the lateral femoral condyle and femoral metaphysis, with small foci of osteonecrosis in the tibia and a tear of the lateral meniscus. No underlying cause for the changes could be identified. (Courtesy of D. Artenian, M.D., Fresno, California.)

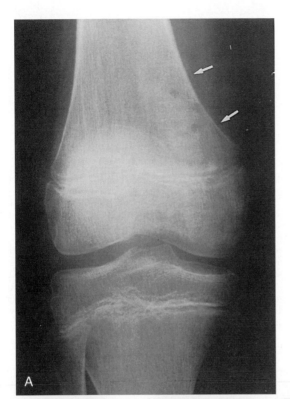

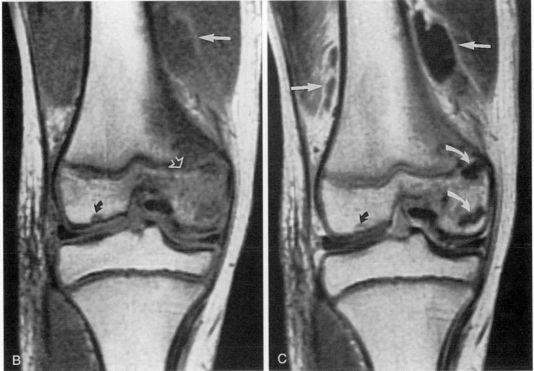

Figure 16–264

Osteomyelitis and septic arthritis: Routine radiography and MR imaging. In a 12 year old boy, a routine radiograph **(A)** reveals subtle periostitis (arrows). A T1-weighted (TR/TE, 500/20) spin echo MR image in the coronal plane **(B)** shows abnormal marrow signal intensity (open arrow), a subchondral bone erosion (curved arrow), and a soft tissue abscess (straight arrow). After intravenous administration of a gadolinium compound, a coronal T1-weighted (TR/TE, 500/20) spin echo MR image **(C)** confirms enhancement of signal intensity in the area of the subchondral bone erosion (curved black arrow) and the presence of bone (curved white arrows) and soft tissue (straight white arrows) abscesses.

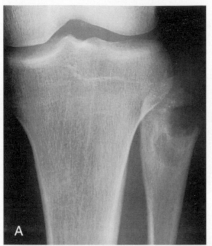

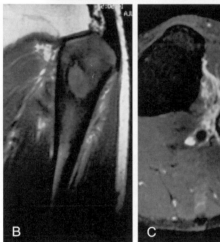

Figure 16–265
Brodie's abscess: MR imaging.

A In a 20 year old man with a 1 month history of pain, a routine radiograph shows an irregular osteolytic lesion in the proximal portion of the fibula. It has a sclerotic margin and is associated with bone expansion. The findings are characteristic of a Brodie's abscess.

B A coronal T1-weighted (TR/TE, 578/15) spin echo MR image reveals the lesion and surrounding marrow edema.

C On a transverse fat-suppressed T1-weighted (TR/TE, 770/15) spin echo MR image after intravenous administration of a gadolinium contrast agent, note the low signal intensity (arrow) within the center of the abscess and high signal intensity in the periphery of the abscess, nearby bone marrow, and adjacent soft tissues.

Figure 16–266
Blount's disease: Infantile tibia vara. MR imaging.

A In this young girl, a coronal T1-weighted (TR/TE, 550/15) spin echo MR image shows defective ossification of the medial portion of the tibial epiphysis (arrow) with a slanted bone contour. The unossified epiphyseal cartilage is visible as a region of intermediate signal intensity (arrowhead).

B A coronal gradient echo MR image (FISP) (TR/TE, 30/17; flip angle, 20 degrees) with volumetric acquisition (2.5 mm thick section) reveals the abnormal bone contour (arrow) and the unossified cartilage, appearing as a region of high signal intensity (arrowhead).

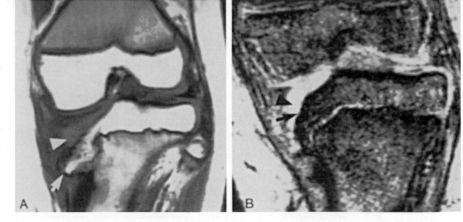

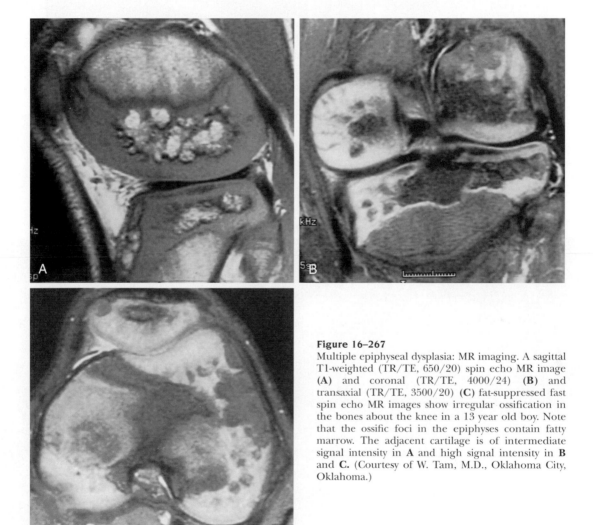

Figure 16–267
Multiple epiphyseal dysplasia: MR imaging. A sagittal T1-weighted (TR/TE, 650/20) spin echo MR image **(A)** and coronal (TR/TE, 4000/24) **(B)** and transaxial (TR/TE, 3500/20) **(C)** fat-suppressed fast spin echo MR images show irregular ossification in the bones about the knee in a 13 year old boy. Note that the ossific foci in the epiphyses contain fatty marrow. The adjacent cartilage is of intermediate signal intensity in **A** and high signal intensity in **B** and **C.** (Courtesy of W. Tam, M.D., Oklahoma City, Oklahoma.)

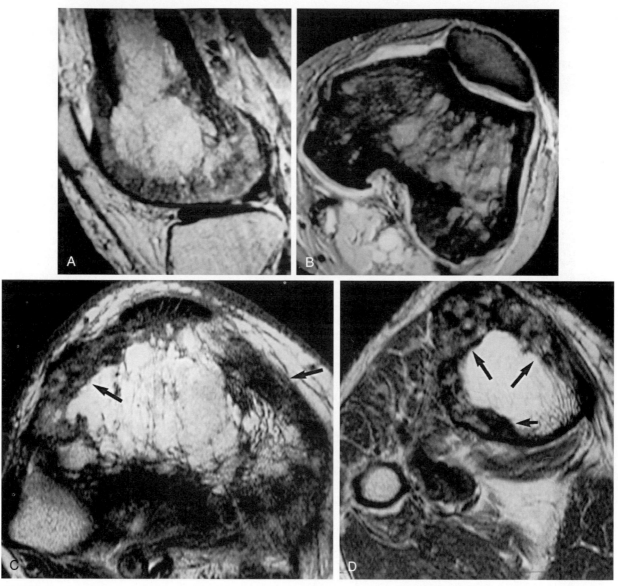

Figure 16–268
Paget's disease: MR imaging.
   A, B The classic coarsened trabecular pattern of Paget's disease is seen in the distal portion of the femur on sagittal T2-weighted (TR/TE, 2200/80) spin echo **(A)** and transaxial MPGR (TR/TE, 600/15; flip angle, 20 degrees) **(B)** MR images. (Courtesy of T. Broderick, M.D., Orange, California.)
   C, D In a second patient, transverse T1-weighted (TR/TE, 450/20) spin echo MR images, with **C** located above **B,** show marked thickening of the tibial cortex (arrows) with normal signal intensity in the adjacent bone marrow. (Courtesy of S. Siegel, M.D., New York, New York.)

Table 16–3. TUMORS AND TUMOR-LIKE LESIONS OF BONE: FREQUENCY OF INVOLVEMENT OF BONES ABOUT THE KNEE

Lesion	Frequency, %*
Enostosis	20
Osteoid osteoma	20
Osteoblastoma	15
Osteosarcoma	65
Enchondroma	15
Periosteal chondroma	25
Chondroblastoma	40
Chondromyxoid fibroma	48
Osteochondroma	37
Chondrosarcoma	16
Nonossifying fibroma	70
Desmoplastic fibroma	18
Fibrosarcoma	60
Giant cell tumor	58
Malignant fibrous histiocytoma	50
Lipoma	28
Hemangioma	5
Hemangiopericytoma	9
Hemangioendothelioma	45
Neurofibroma/neurilemoma	8
Simple bone cyst	10
Aneurysmal bone cyst	17
Adamantinoma†	85
Ewing's sarcoma	30

*Approximate figure based on analysis of major reports containing the greatest number of cases.

†Lesions affecting any part of the tibia are included in the analysis.

16–269) and, although classically metaphyseal in origin, may involve the epiphysis (Fig. 16–270). Complications of osteochondromas include their fracture (Fig. 16–271), adjacent bursitis (Fig. 16–272), compression of nearby nerves or vessels, and malignant degeneration (Figs. 16–273 and 16–274). *Giant cell tumors* also are very common in the bones about the knee (Fig. 16–275). *Enchondromas* (Fig. 16–276) and *chondroblastomas* (Fig. 16–277) frequently localize in these same sites. Epiphyseal involvement is characteristic of both giant cell tumors and chondroblastomas, whereas enchondromas are encountered more often in the metaphysis and diaphysis. Although not located invariably in the cortex, *osteoid osteomas* in this location have characteristic imaging features (Fig. 16–278). Other tumors or tumor-like lesions found about the knee include fibrous cortical defects (nonossifying fibromas) (Fig. 16–279) and both conventional (Fig. 16–280) and parosteal (Fig. 16–281) osteosarcomas.

Cystic and proliferative changes in the posteromedial aspect of the cortex of the distal portion of the femur occur at the sites of attachment of tendinous fibers of the adductor magnus muscle and those of the medial head of the gastrocnemius muscle. Terms applied to these changes include periosteal (or cortical) desmoids and avulsive cortical irregularities. The latter term is preferred, owing to the nature of the alterations, which appear to represent a traction enthesopathy. Although resulting radiographic abnormalities generally are diagnostic, the findings occasionally may be misinterpreted as evidence of a malignant neoplasm. CT scanning or MR imaging is effective in providing a correct diagnosis

in such cases (Fig. 16–282).[1171, 1172] With MR imaging, high signal intensity about the cystic or proliferative cortical region in T2-weighted images should not be considered inconsistent with the diagnosis of this non-neoplastic process.

Developmental Abnormalities

Congenital Subluxation and Hyperextension of the Knee

Congenital subluxation and hyperextension of the knee is a rare congenital deformity.[1066–1072] A definite female preponderance is seen. Hereditary factors appear to be important in some cases,[1073–1076] although other factors may be important in the causation of this condition.[1077–1080] The severity of the deformity varies.[1081, 1082] Radiographs confirm the anterior position of the proximal portion of the tibia with respect to the distal end of the femur and, possibly, lateral subluxation and valgus deformity of the knee. Anterior tibial bowing and patellar hypoplasia also may be seen. Arthrography or MR imaging (Fig. 16–283) can delineate flattening of the chondral surface in the posterior tibial epiphysis and obliteration of the suprapatellar pouch secondary to local fibrous adherence to the quadriceps muscle. Surgical observations confirm the presence of ablation of the suprapatellar pouch and also reveal quadriceps fibrosis, anterior dislocation of the hamstring tendons, dysplasia of the articular surfaces of the femur and tibia, and elongation and attenuation of the anterior cruciate ligament.[1071]

Bipartite Patella and Dorsal Defect of the Patella

The occurrence of multiple ossification centers in a sesamoid bone, of which the bipartite patella is the best example, has long been regarded as a normal variation with little or no clinical significance. Ogden and collaborators[1083] and others[1084–1086] have challenged this concept, emphasizing that local pain may accompany this patellar variation and, further, that histologic analysis suggests the presence of a chronic chondro-osseous tensile failure of the bone in skeletally immature persons, similar to that occurring in Osgood-Schlatter and Sinding-Larsen-Johansson lesions. The bipartite patella usually, but not invariably, is bilateral. The predilection for the superolateral aspect of the bone (Figs. 16–284 and 16–285), with rare exceptions, remains the radiographic hallmark of the finding, usually allowing differentiation from acute fractures and anomalies[1087] of the patella. Rarely, other forms of partition of the patella, either in the sagittal[1088] or coronal[1089] plane, are encountered.

The dorsal defect of the patella initially was believed to be a variation in normal ossification of the bone,[1090, 1091] perhaps related to bipartite patella, and occurring in 0.3 to 1 per cent of persons,[1092, 1093] either unilaterally or bilaterally.[1094–1096] More recently, a trau-

Text continued on page 757

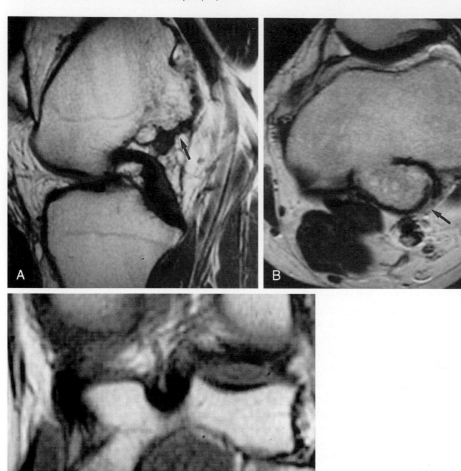

Figure 16–269
Solitary osteochondroma: MR imaging.

A, B Sagittal proton density–weighted (TR/TE, 1800/18) spin echo **(A)** and transaxial fast spin echo (TR/TE, 2500/40) **(B)** MR images show a typical broad-based osteochondroma (arrows) arising from the posterior surface of the distal portion of the femur. Continuity of cortical and medullary bone in the outgrowth with that of the parent bone is obvious. The popliteal vessels are displaced. (Courtesy of S. Eilenberg, M.D., San Diego, California.)

C A coronal T1-weighted (TR/TE, 600/15) spin echo MR image shows an osteochondroma (arrows) arising from the posterior surface of the tibia. Continuity of the cortical and medullary bone of the osteochondroma with that of the tibia is evident. (Courtesy of V. Chandani, M.D., San Antonio, Texas.)

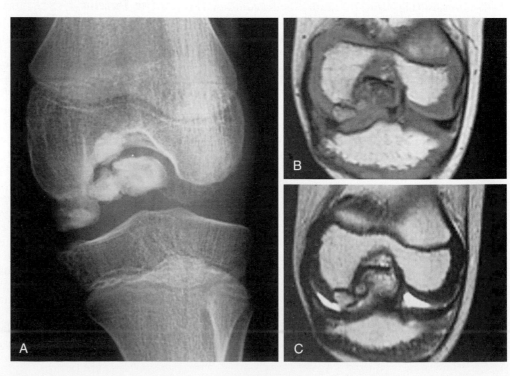

Figure 16–270
Dysplasia epiphysealis hemimelica (Trevor's disease): MR imaging. In a 5 year old boy, routine radiography **(A)** shows ossific foci about the medial aspect of the knee, characteristic of this condition. Coronal T1-weighted (TR/TE, 670/25) spin echo **(B)** and fast spin echo (TR/TE, 6445/130) **(C)** MR images show fatty marrow within these foci, which extend into the intercondylar region of the joint. Note subtle erosion of bone, leading to an irregular and widened condylar tunnel. (Courtesy of T. Hughes, M.D., Christchurch, New Zealand.)

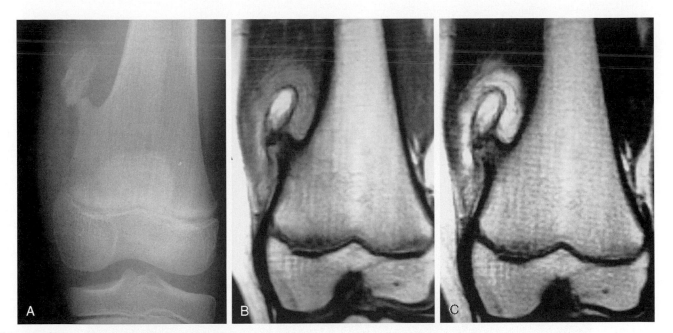

Figure 16–271
Solitary osteochondroma: Fracture. MR imaging.
   A The routine radiograph shows a fracture through the base of an osteochondroma of the femur.
   B, C Coronal proton density–weighted (TR/TE, 2000/22) **(B)** and T2-weighted (TR/TE, 2000/90) **(C)** spin echo MR images show the fracture as well as altered signal intensity in the marrow of the osteochondroma and in the soft tissues around it. Without routine radiography, accurate interpretation of the MR images would be difficult.
   (Courtesy of B. Flannigan, M.D., Los Angeles, California.)

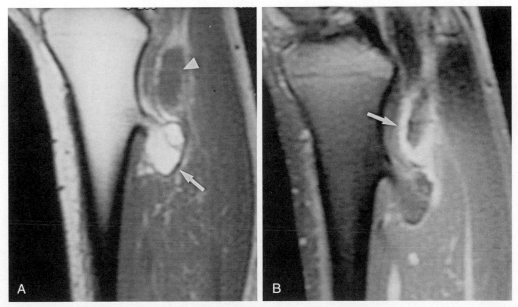

Figure 16–272
Osteochondroma: Bursitis, MR imaging. In a 36 year old man, a sagittal T1-weighted (TR/TE, 633/11) spin echo MR image **(A)** shows an osteochondroma (arrow) arising from the posterior aspect of the proximal portion of the tibia. A collection of fluid (arrowhead) is seen above the osteochondroma. After the intravenous administration of a gadolinium compound, a sagittal fat-suppressed T1-weighted (TR/TE, 633/11) spin echo MR image **(B)** shows enhancement of signal intensity in the wall of the inflamed bursa (arrow). (Courtesy of L. White, M.D., Toronto, Ontario, Canada.)

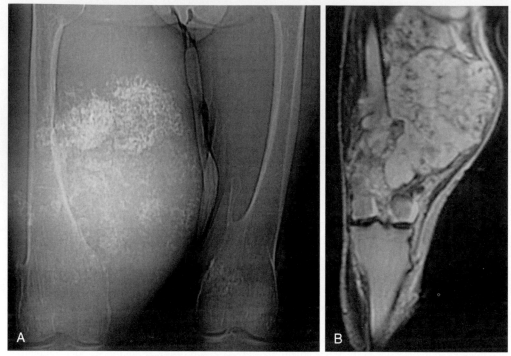

Figure 16–273
Hereditary multiple exostoses: Malignant transformation, MR imaging. In this patient with an enlarging mass about the right femur, the scout film **(A)** from a CT examination shows an irregular calcified mass adjacent to the right femur, multiple osteochondromas about the knees, and modeling deformities of the femoral necks. The mass has caused erosion of the adjacent regions of the femur. On a T2-weighted coronal spin echo MR image **(B)**, the mass is lobulated, is nonhomogeneous but mainly of high signal intensity, and extends into the femur. Osteochondromas involve the ipsilateral tibia. The mass proved to be a chondrosarcoma. (Courtesy of D. Goodwin, M.D., Hanover, New Hampshire.)

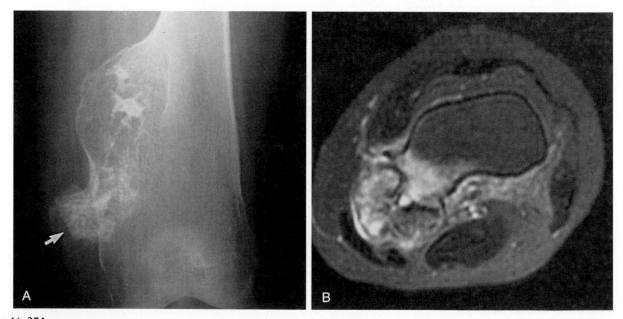

Figure 16–274
Osteochondroma: Malignant degeneration, MR imaging. In this patient with multiple hereditary exostoses, a routine radiograph **(A)** reveals multiple osteochondromas, one of which (arrow) is irregular in outline. A transaxial fat-suppressed fast spin echo (TR/TE, 4166/104) MR image **(B)** shows high signal intensity within and about the osteochondroma and in the adjacent marrow of the femur. A chondrosarcoma was the cause of these findings. (Courtesy of L. White, M.D., Toronto, Ontario, Canada.)

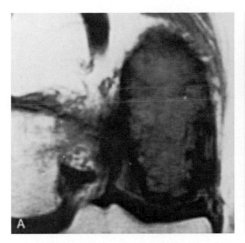

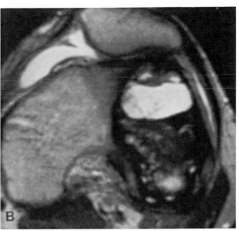

Figure 16–275
Giant cell tumor: MR imaging—femur. In a 26 year old man, a coronal T1-weighted (TR/TE, 775/20) spin echo MR image **(A)** reveals the tumor of low signal intensity involving the lateral femoral condyle. In a transaxial T2-weighted (TR/TE, 2000/70) spin echo MR image **(B)** the tumor is of inhomogeneous signal intensity; there is high signal intensity anteriorly and mainly low signal intensity posteriorly. A joint effusion is present. (Courtesy of M. Mitchell, M.D., Halifax, Nova Scotia, Canada.)

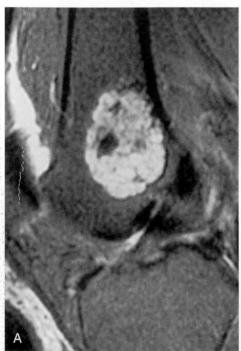

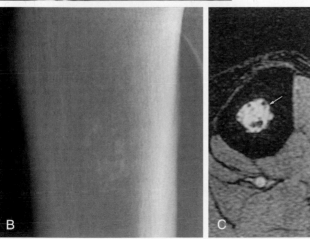

Figure 16–276
Enchondroma: MR imaging.

   A A sagittal STIR MR image (TR/TE, 3500/28; inversion time, 160 msec) shows a typical enchondroma of the distal portion of the femur. It is well-defined and lobulated and is composed of lobules of high signal intensity. Foci of calcification appear as regions of low signal intensity. (Courtesy of D. Goodwin, M.D., Hanover, New Hampshire.)

   B, C A lateral radiograph shows distinctive small focal calcific collections in the medullary cavity of the tibia **(B)**. A transaxial three-dimensional spoiled gradient recalled acquisition in the steady state (SPGR) MR image (TR/TE, 50/10; flip angle, 60 degrees) obtained with chemical presaturation of fat (ChemSat) **(C)** reveals the lesion of high signal intensity (arrow) in the tibia. Note foci of low signal intensity representing calcification and mild endosteal erosion. A biopsy was not performed.

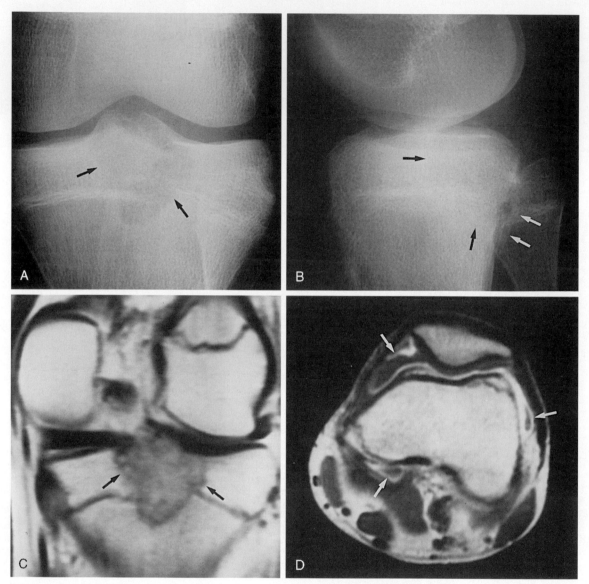

Figure 16–277
Chondroblastoma: MR imaging.

A, B Frontal **(A)** and lateral **(B)** radiographs reveal the lesion (black arrows) in the tibial epiphysis and metaphysis and adjacent periostitis (white arrows).

C After intravenous administration of a gadolinium contrast agent, a coronal T1-weighted (TR/TE, 500/30) spin echo MR image reveals slight enhancement of signal intensity in the tumor (arrows).

D On a transverse T1-weighted (TR/TE, 800/30) spin echo MR image at the level of the patella, gadolinium enhancement of signal intensity in an inflamed synovial membrane (arrows) is evident.

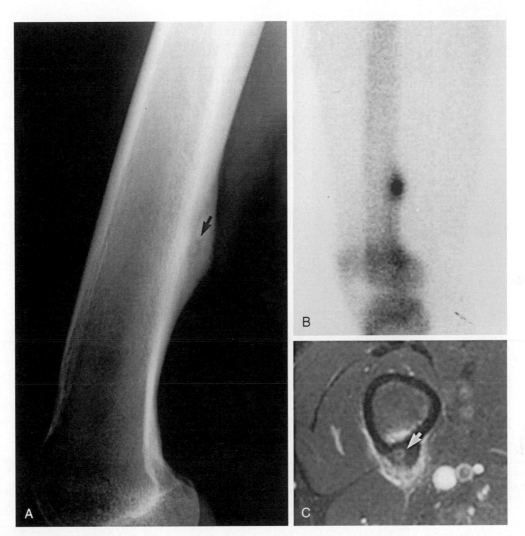

Figure 16–278

Osteoid osteoma: MR imaging.

A Observe the partially calcified nidus (arrow) in the posterior cortex of the femur, with associated mature periosteal reaction leading to cortical thickening.

B During bone scintigraphy, a lateral view of the femur shows intense uptake of the radionuclide at the site of the cortical lesion.

C A fat-saturated transaxial T1-weighted (TR/TE, 600/29) spin echo MR image obtained after intravenous administration of a gadolinium compound shows the partially calcified nidus (arrow) with enhancement of signal intensity in the adjacent marrow and soft tissues.

(Courtesy of D. Goodwin, M.D., Hanover, New Hampshire.)

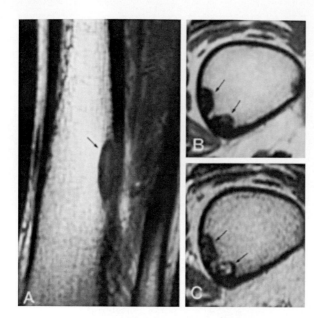

Figure 16–279
Nonossifying fibroma (fibrous cortical defect): MR imaging.

A Tibia. A coronal T1-weighted (TR/TE, 600/25) spin echo MR image in this 18 year old boy documents an elongated eccentric lesion (arrow) in the lateral aspect of the tibia. It is sharply defined and of low signal intensity. It remained of low signal intensity in T2-weighted spin echo MR images. (Courtesy of A. Peck, M.D., Portland, Oregon.)

B, C Femur. Multiple eccentric lesions (arrows) in the distal femoral metaphysis are well delineated in transaxial T1-weighted (TR/TE, 400/20) **(B)** and T2-weighted (TR/TE, 2000/80) **(C)** spin echo MR images in this 14 year old boy. One of the lesions shows an increase in signal intensity in **C.** (Courtesy of P. VanderStoep, M.D., St. Cloud, Minnesota.)

Figure 16–280
Conventional osteosarcoma: MR imaging. This 17 year old man had a 2 month history of knee pain.

A A routine radiograph reveals an osteolytic lesion involving the medial aspect of the metaphysis of the femur. A Codman's triangle (arrow) is seen.

B A coronal T1-weighted (TR/TE, 700/20) spin echo MR image shows the intraosseous and extraosseous extent of the tumor.

C A coronal T2-weighted (TR/TE, 2500/80) spin echo MR image obtained with chemical presaturation of fat (ChemSat) shows high signal intensity in the tumor, as well as a joint effusion. A total knee arthroplasty was performed.

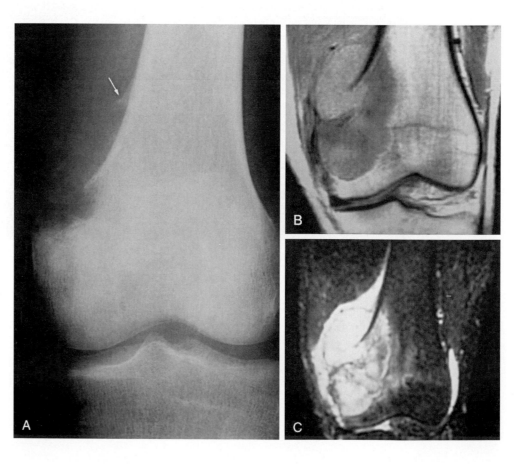

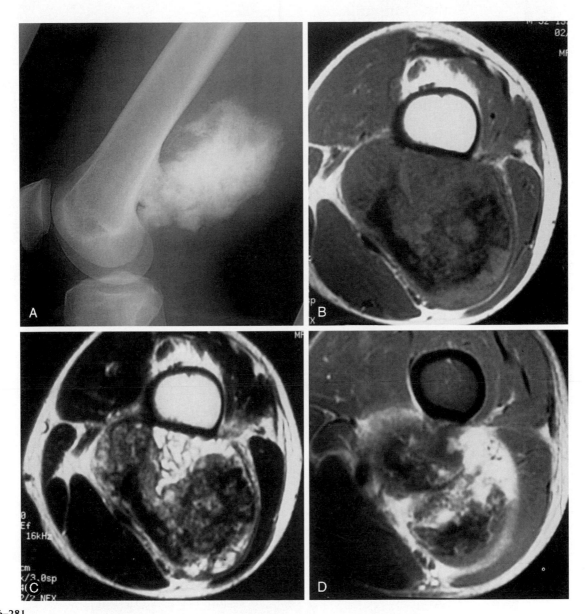

Figure 16–281

Parosteal osteosarcoma: MR imaging.

  A A lateral radiograph demonstrates an ossifying lesion, irregular in outline, posterior to the distal portion of the femur. A more mature-appearing stalk appears to connect the lesion to the femur.

  B A transaxial T1-weighted (TR/TE, 500/17) spin echo MR image shows the large lesion, inhomogeneous in signal intensity. The marrow of the femur appears normal.

  C A transaxial T2-weighted (TR/TE, 2300/90) spin echo MR image documents the inhomogeneous signal intensity in the mass. Portions of it remain of low signal intensity; other areas show high signal intensity. Adjacent musculature is displaced.

  D A transaxial fat-suppressed T1-weighted (TR/TE, 600/17) spin echo MR image obtained after intravenous gadolinium contrast agent administration reveals irregular enhancement of signal intensity in the tumor.

  (Courtesy of C. Chen, M.D., Kaoshiung, Taiwan, and G.S. Huang, M.D., Taipei, Taiwan.)

Illustration continued on following page

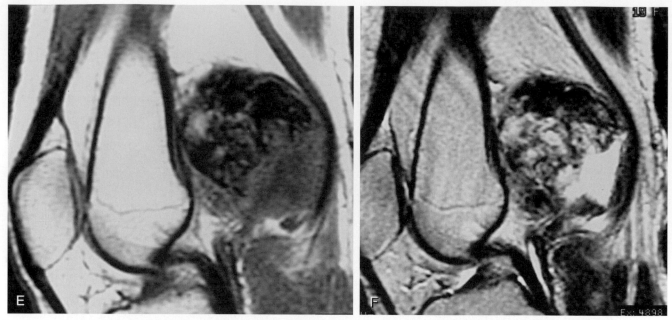

Figure 16–281 *Continued*

E, F In a second patient, a large parosteal osteosarcoma is displayed in sagittal T1-weighted (TR/TE, 600/13) **(E)** and T2-weighted (TR/TE, 4000/87) **(F)** spin echo MR images. The popliteal vessels are displaced, and the femur is not involved. (Courtesy of S. Fernandez, M.D., Mexico City, Mexico.)

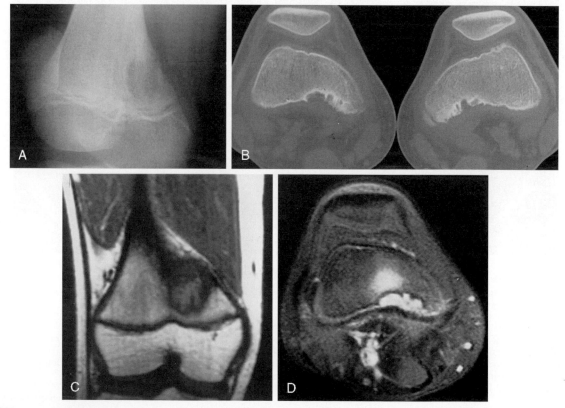

Figure 16–282

Periosteal (juxtacortical) desmoid: MR imaging. This 11 year old female gymnast developed right knee pain over a 6 month period.

A An oblique radiograph shows an osteolytic lesion involving the posteromedial surface of the femur.

B A transaxial CT scan confirms the presence of lesions in both femora. Note irregular erosion of the posterior surface of both bones.

C A coronal T1-weighted (TR/TE, 578/15) spin echo MR image of the right femur shows low signal intensity in the lesion.

D A transaxial fat-suppressed T1-weighted (TR/TE, 625/15) spin echo MR image of the right femur, obtained after intravenous administration of a gadolinium compound, reveals enhancement of signal intensity in the lesion and in the adjacent marrow (presumably indicative of edema).

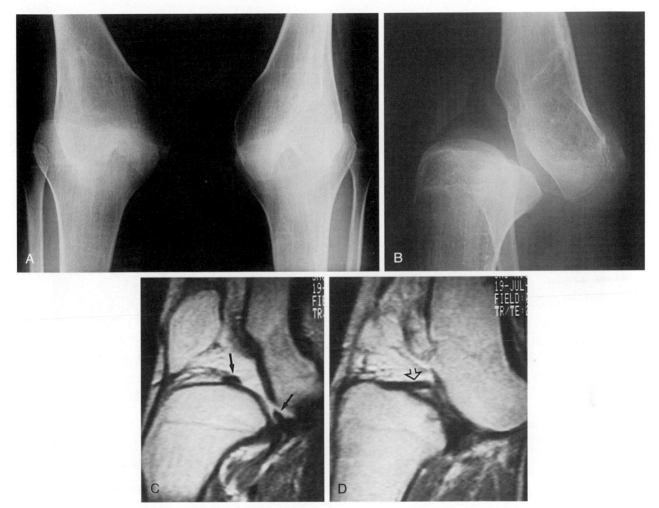

Figure 16–283
Congenital dislocation of the knee: Routine radiography and MR imaging. In a 22 year old man, frontal radiographs (**A**) of both knees reveal bilateral, symmetric anterior dislocations of the knees. A lateral radiograph of the left knee (**B**) shows the anterior dislocation of the tibia and fibula with respect to the femur. Note flattening of the distal anterior femoral surface. Two sagittal proton density–weighted (TR/TE, 2500/40) spin echo MR images (**C, D**) reveal posterior displacement of the anterior and posterior horns of the medial meniscus (arrows, **C**) and stretching of the anterior cruciate ligament (arrow, **D**).

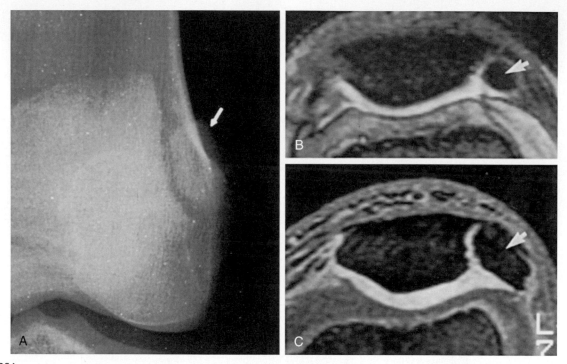

Figure 16–284

Bipartite patella: Routine radiography and MR imaging.

A Localization to the superolateral aspect of the patella (arrow) is the most characteristic radiographic finding.

B In a transaxial gradient echo (MPGR) MR image (TR/TE, 500/17; flip angle, 20 degrees) obtained with chemical presaturation of fat (ChemSat), the separate ossification center (arrow) in the superolateral aspect of the patella is evident. Cartilage with high signal intensity is seen between the ossicle and remaining portion of the patella and on the posterior articular surface of the bone.

C In a different patient, a transaxial gradient echo (SPGR) MR image (TR/TE, 58/10; flip angle, 60 degrees) obtained with volumetric acquisition and chemical presaturation of fat (ChemSat), resulting in a section thickness of 1.5 mm, shows a larger ossicle (arrow) in the superolateral portion of the patella. The cartilage again reveals high signal intensity. The accompanying joint effusion is of low signal intensity. (Courtesy of M. Recht, M.D., Cleveland, Ohio.)

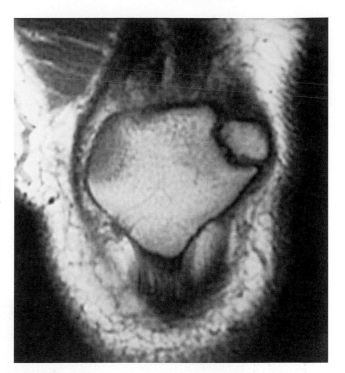

Figure 16–285
Bipartite patella: MR imaging. As shown in a coronal T1-weighted (TR/TE, 983/16) spin echo MR image, localization to the superolateral aspect of the bone is characteristic of this accessory ossification center of the patella.

matic pathogenesis related to traction occurring in the insertion site of the vastus lateralis muscle has been emphasized.[1093] In common with a bipartite patella, the dorsal defect occurs in the superolateral aspect of the bone and the two conditions may coexist in the same person.[1093] Histologically, the dorsal defect is characterized by the presence of nonspecific fibrous components with or without areas of bone necrosis. Although patients with this finding generally are asymptomatic, local pain and tenderness may be present.[1097]

The radiographic characteristics of the dorsal defect of the patella include a well-circumscribed lesion in the superolateral portion of the bone, adjacent to the articular cartilage. CT confirms the typical location of the defect and may demonstrate fissuring of the adjacent superficial, or external, surface of the bone. MR imaging (Fig. 16–286) reveals some variability in the signal intensity characteristics of the dorsal patellar defect: On T1-weighted spin echo MR images, the lesion may be inhomogeneous, with signal that is isointense or slightly hyperintense to that of articular cartilage, or, in some areas, that is hypointense to that of articular cartilage; on gradient echo images, the signal intensity of the lesion generally is equal to or greater than that of the cartilage.[1098] Although, in general, the articular cartilage adjacent to the dorsal defect is intact, this is not uniformly the case.[1099] Healing of the dorsal defect of the patella may occur spontaneously or after surgical intervention. New bone initially develops at the margins of the lesion and proceeds centrally.[1093] Dorsal defects rarely are observed after the third decade of life.

Vascular Abnormalities

Aneurysms

Aneurysms not infrequently involve the popliteal artery and produce a mass in the popliteal space that superfi-

cially simulates joint disease or a soft tissue tumor. Clinical examination almost always reveals intrinsic pulsation, however, and the aneurysm will not expand the suprapatellar bursa, as would a knee joint effusion. Popliteal aneurysms rarely rupture but are prone to thrombose or produce downstream embolization. Although diagnosis is readily confirmed with ultrasonography or MR imaging, arteriography of the aneurysm and adjacent vessels is indicated in planning surgery (Figs. 16–287 and 16–288).

Several authors report the development of arterial aneurysms in association with osteochondromas about the knee joint. The usual proximity of the popliteal

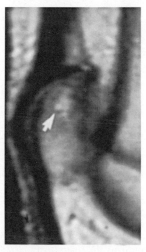

Figure 16–286
Dorsal defect of the patella: MR imaging. A sagittal T2-weighted (TR/TE, 2000/60) spin echo MR image shows a subchondral lesion (arrow) with high signal intensity in the superior portion of the patella. The lesion was of low signal intensity on T1-weighted images (not shown).

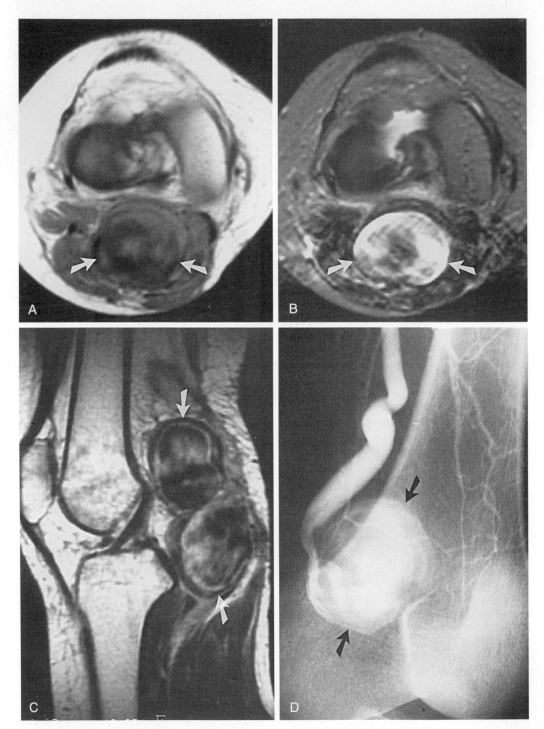

Figure 16–287

Popliteal artery aneurysm: MR imaging and arteriography. This 19 year old male patient had undergone surgical resection of aggressive fibromatosis that had required use of a saphenous vein graft to replace involved portions of the popliteal artery. Transaxial T1-weighted (TR/TE, 600/20) **(A)** and T2-weighted (TR/TE, 3000/100) **(B)** spin echo MR images and a sagittal T1-weighted (TR/TE, 400/20) spin echo MR image obtained after intravenous administration of a gadolinium compound **(C)** show the aneurysm (arrows) at the vascular graft site. Arteriography **(D)** confirms the diagnosis (arrows).

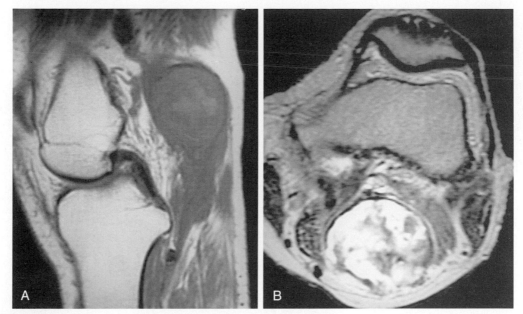

Figure 16–288
Popliteal artery aneurysm: MR imaging. A partially thrombosed popliteal artery aneurysm is shown with sagittal T1-weighted (TR/TE, 800/11) spin echo (**A**) and transaxial T2-weighted (TR/TE, 2766/80) spin echo (**B**) MR images. Note the inhomogeneous signal intensity of the aneurysm in both images.

artery to the rough aspect of the osteochondroma and the mechanical trauma secondary to motion of the knee joint combine to produce chronic arterial injury and eventual aneurysm (Fig. 16–289).

Cystic Mucinous Degeneration

Cystic mucinous degeneration may involve the popliteal artery (Fig. 16–290). The usual manifestations are ischemic, often of abrupt onset in young men, secondary to arterial obstruction by the cyst; rarely the mass is palpable, simulating a primary articular lesion. Hemorrhage into the cyst may occur, producing an intramural hematoma. The cause is unknown; a congenital origin is postulated by some investigators because the condition may affect relatively young patients.[1100, 1101]

Popliteal Artery Entrapment Syndrome

The popliteal artery entrapment syndrome is produced by compression of the popliteal artery by the medial head of the gastrocnemius muscle. It generally is manifested as intermittent claudication in a young, otherwise normal patient. The compression usually is due to either (1) abnormal position of the popliteal artery medial to the medial head of the gastrocnemius muscle, or (2) compression of a normally situated popliteal artery by an anomalous laterally inserting slip from the medial head of the gastrocnemius.[1102, 1103] A variety of other muscle anomalies may produce this syndrome, however.[1104] Furthermore, a functional type of popliteal entrapment syndrome may relate only to hypertrophy of the gastrocnemius muscle.

The diagnosis of this condition can be established by arteriography, ultrasonography, CT scanning, or MR imaging.[1105–1109] With regard to MR imaging, the method

may be more sensitive if accomplished both at rest and during active plantar flexion against resistance.[1108]

Venous Disease

The swelling and tenderness of thrombophlebitis sometimes may simulate joint disease clinically. Venography is the most definitive diagnostic procedure. In the presence of thrombosis of lower extremity veins, intraluminal defects due to thrombi are almost always visualized. Fresh thrombi largely fill the obstructed venous lumen, and commonly they demonstrate convex proximal and distal margins. A thin rim of contrast medium may be insinuated between the thrombus and the venous wall.

Vascular injection or MR imaging also allows diagnosis of a variety of other venous abnormalities, including varicosities, venous aneurysms, and arteriovenous fistula (Fig. 16–291). Of interest, intraosseous lesions of the tibia may accompany some of these abnormalities (Fig. 16–292).

Soft Tissue Abnormalities

Virtually any infectious or neoplastic process may involve the soft tissues about the knee. Of the soft tissue tumors, lipomas (Fig. 16–293), liposarcomas (Fig. 16–294), malignant fibrous histiocytomas, synovial sarcomas (Fig. 16–295), and neurogenic tumors (Figs. 16–296 to 16–300) are encountered most commonly. The importance of MR imaging in displaying the extent of the tumor and its relationship to surrounding vessels and nerves is not disputed, although the method often does not allow a specific diagnosis in most cases. Similarly, MR imaging can be used to delineate the extent of soft tissue infections. Abscesses can be diagnosed reliably (Fig. 16–301).

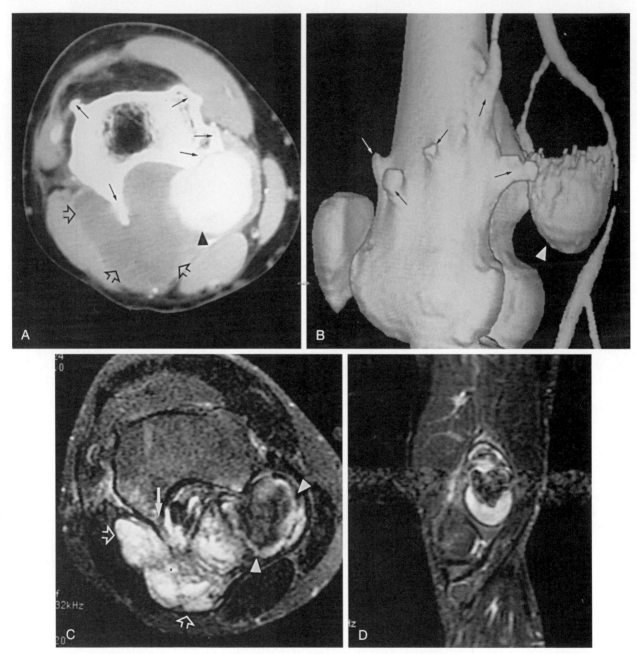

Figure 16–289

Hereditary multiple exostoses: Pseudoaneurysm of popliteal artery. This 15 year old boy with known hereditary multiple exostoses developed an enlarging mass behind the knee, which was believed to represent malignant transformation of an osteochondroma.

A A transverse CT scan obtained after intravenous administration of an iodinated contrast agent shows several osteochondromas (solid arrows), a contrast-opacified aneurysm (arrowhead), and a more lateral portion of the mass (open arrows) with inhomogeneous appearance, which represented an organized hematoma.

B A three-dimensional display of the CT data shows the aneurysm (arrowhead) and osteochondromas (solid arrows).

C A transaxial fat-suppressed fast spin echo MR image (TR/TE 4000/91), at about the same level as **A,** shows the aneurysm (arrowheads), organized hematoma (open arrows), and causative osteochondroma (solid arrow).

D A sagittal STIR (TR/TE, 4000/65; inversion time, 150 msec) MR image shows the aneurysm with prominent flow artifacts.

(Courtesy of L. White, M.D., Toronto, Ontario, Canada.)

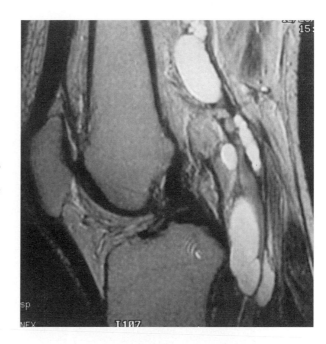

Figure 16–290
Cystic mucinous degeneration of the popliteal artery: MR imaging. In a 63 year old man with claudication, a sagittal fast spin echo (TR/TE, 3000/102) MR image shows cystic areas of high signal intensity along the course of the popliteal artery. (Courtesy of D. Witte, M.D., Memphis, Tennessee.)

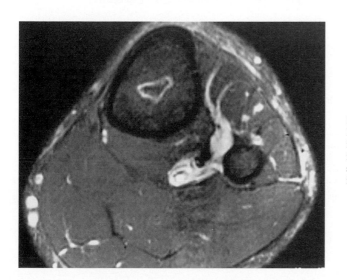

Figure 16–291
Klippel-Trenaunay syndrome: MR imaging. Note the presence of abnormalities of both superficial and deep veins as well as a focus of osteonecrosis in the tibia on this transaxial fat-suppressed T1-weighted (TR/TE, 847/22) spin echo MR image obtained after the intravenous injection of a gadolinium compound.

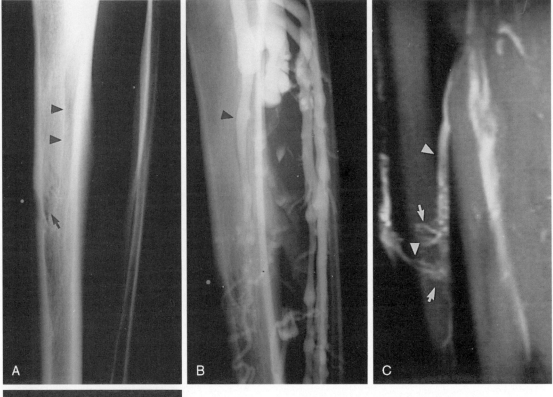

Figure 16–292

Venous malformation: MR imaging.

A In a 46 year old man with prominent varicose veins, a lateral radiograph shows a serpentine lesion of the tibia (arrow) and an enlarged vascular channel (arrowheads).

B A venogram reveals irregular and tortuous intraosseous veins, with one vein (arrowhead) occupying the vascular channel.

C This sagittal fat-suppressed fast spin echo MR image (TR/TE, 4000/13) shows tortuous intraosseous veins (arrows) with large major venous channels extending through the anterior and posterior cortices (arrowheads) of the tibia.

D The transaxial fat-suppressed fast spin echo MR image (TR/TE, 4550/126) confirms the presence of venous varicosities outside and within (arrow) the bone.

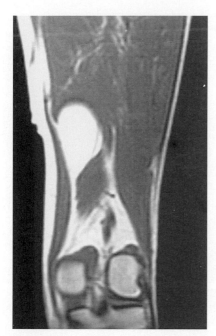

Figure 16–293
Lipoma: MR imaging. An intermuscular lipoma, with homogeneous high signal intensity, is displayed in a coronal T1-weighted (TR/TE, 966/10) spin echo MR image.

Muscle Abnormalities

MR imaging is well suited to the analysis of a variety of muscle disorders, including anomalous muscles (e.g., the tensor fasciae suralis originating from the semitendinosus muscle and contributing to the Achilles tendon[1173]) and dermatomyositis and polymyositis. Kaufman and associates[1174] provided one of the early descriptions of the role of MR imaging in this regard. They examined five patients with polymyositis and eight with dermatomyositis; eight of these 13 patients had clinically active disease. Using standard spin echo techniques, these investigators observed muscle atrophy, fatty replacement of muscles, and intramuscular regions of decreased signal intensity that correlated in extent with the activity of the disease processes. Keim and coworkers[1175] and Hernandez and collaborators[1176] studied patients with juvenile dermatomyositis using both T1- and T2-weighted spin echo imaging. At the outset of the disease, a significant increase in signal intensity on the T2-weighted MR images occurred in the involved muscle groups. With clinical improvement, this signal intensity returned to normal and, with the recurrence of clinically evident disease activity, an increase in signal intensity at sites of muscle involvement again was noted on the T2-weighted images. The authors postulated that shifts in the distribution of water due to muscle inflammation and infarction were responsible for the imaging abnormalities. They also indicated that similar alterations in signal intensity could occur in muscles affected by infection, infarction, trauma, and rhabdomyolysis. The investigators discounted the effect of steroid-induced myopathy in the production of the MR imaging abnormalities.

Other studies generally have confirmed the usefulness of this imaging method in the assessment of the degree, activity, and distribution of muscle involvement in dermatomyositis and polymyositis. Differences have been found in the patterns of muscle abnormalities in these inflammatory disorders when compared with congenital myopathies and muscular dystrophies,[1177] although in all disease categories, certain muscles appear to be less affected than others, perhaps related to specific anatomic and functional characteristics.[1177] In some investigations, predominant involvement of the vastus lateralis muscle and, to a lesser extent, the vastus intermedius and vastus medialis muscles, with relative sparing of the rectus femoris and biceps femoris muscles, has been noted in patients with dermatomyositis.[1178] T1 and T2 values in affected muscles have been higher than those in normal controls.[25] P-31 spectra of the diseased muscles have shown decreased concentrations of adenosine triphosphate and phosphocreatine, and these metabolic data have correlated with clinical assessment.[1178] Preliminary evidence also has suggested that a correlation exists between histopathologic findings and the degree of abnormality revealed by MR spectroscopy.[1174, 1179]

Although most of the reported investigations of the value of MR imaging in the assessment of inflammatory muscle disease have stressed standard spin echo sequences, some of the more recent ones have employed modified imaging parameters. One of these, fat suppression, has shown promise in this regard.[1180] As an example, Fraser and colleagues[1181] compared quantitative and qualitative indices of signal intensity in muscle in patients with myositis to two measures of disease activity: a subjective global impression of disease activity and a quantitative measure of such activity based on level of muscle enzymes and strength. Seventeen patients had

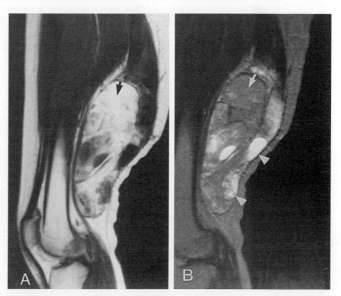

Figure 16–294
Liposarcoma: MR imaging. Sagittal T1-weighted (TR/TE, 500/16) **(A)** and T2-weighted (TR/TE, 2500/80) **(B)** spin echo MR images of a myxoid liposarcoma located behind the femur show inhomogeneity of signal intensity. Observe regions (arrows) of signal intensity identical to that of fat and others (arrowheads) with high signal intensity in **B**. (Courtesy of P. Ellenbogen, M.D., Dallas, Texas.)

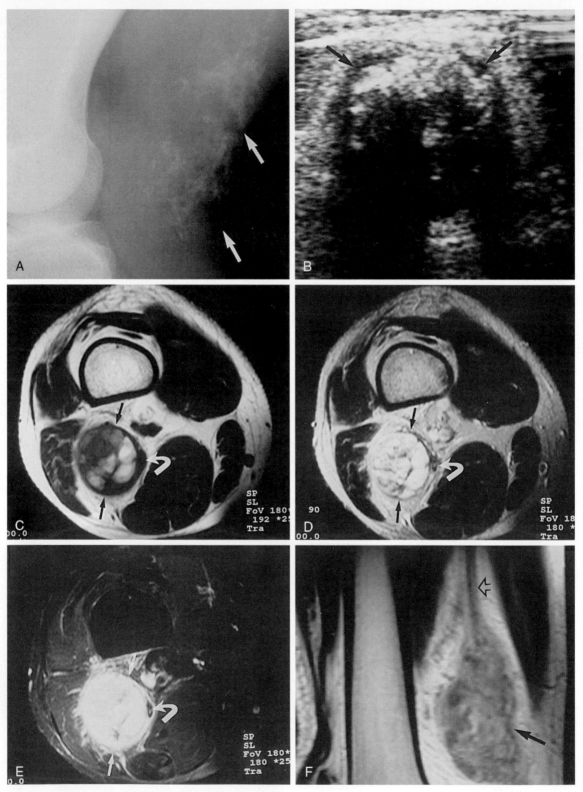

Figure 16–295

Synovial sarcoma: MR imaging.

A Routine radiography reveals an irregularly calcified mass (arrows) behind the knee in a 24 year old man.

B Ultrasonography documents an echogenic mass (arrows) with acoustic shadowing.

C, D Transaxial T1-weighted (TR/TE, 600/15) **(C)** and T2-weighted (TR/TE, 2700/90) **(D)** spin echo MR images reveal a mass (straight arrows) with heterogeneous signal intensity that is displacing the tibial nerve (curved arrows).

E A transaxial fat-suppressed T1-weighted (TR/TE, 650/15) spin echo MR image obtained after the intravenous administration of a gadolinium contrast agent shows enhanced signal intensity in the mass (straight arrows) and the displaced tibial nerve (curved arrow).

F A sagittal T1-weighted (TR/TE, 420/15) spin echo MR image obtained after gadolinium injection documents the enhanced signal intensity in the mass (solid arrow) and its relationship to the tibial nerve (open arrow).

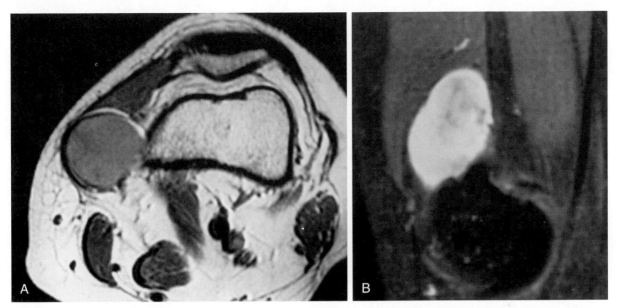

Figure 16–296

Neurofibroma: MR imaging. A solitary neurofibroma adjacent to the medial aspect of the distal portion of the femur is of intermediate signal intensity in a transaxial proton density (TR/TE, 1808/22) spin echo MR image **(A)** and of high signal intensity in a sagittal fat-suppressed T1-weighted (TR/TE, 775/15) spin echo MR image obtained after the intravenous administration of a gadolinium contrast agent **(B).** The appearance is not specific.

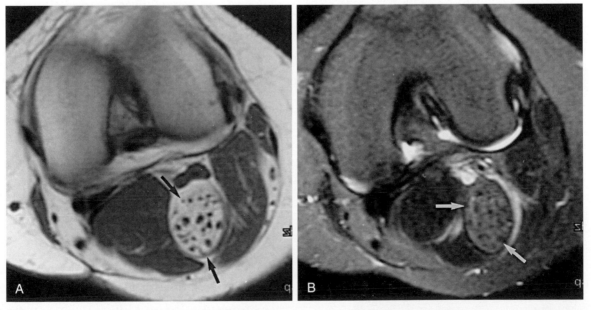

Figure 16–297

Fibrolipomatous hamartoma of the tibial nerve: MR imaging. Transaxial T1-weighted (TR/TE, 600/12) spin echo **(A)** and fat-suppressed fast spin echo (TR/TE, 3300/84) **(B)** MR images show the characteristic features of this lesion (arrows). Note that the hamartoma contains abundant fat mixed with longitudinally oriented or tubular structures of low signal intensity. Fibrolipomatous hamartomas are encountered more often about the median nerve in the carpal tunnel of the wrist. (Courtesy of D. Witte, M.D., Memphis, Tennessee.)

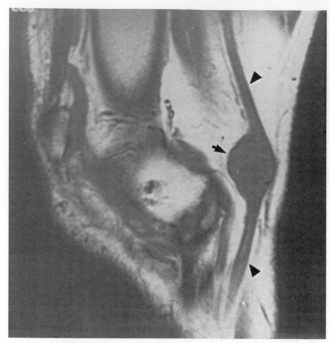

Figure 16–298
Neurilemoma: MR imaging. Note the fusiform soft tissue mass (arrow) of low signal intensity on a sagittal T1-weighted (TR/TE, 600/20) spin echo MR image. The adjacent portions of the tibial nerve (arrowheads) are apparent. (Courtesy of R. Stiles, M.D., Atlanta, Georgia.)

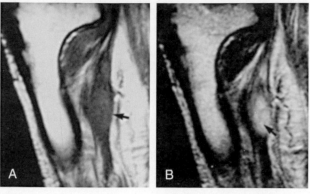

Figure 16–300
Stump neuroma: MR imaging. In a 20 year old man with a previous amputation of the leg below the level of the knee, sagittal T1-weighted (TR/TE, 700/20) **(A)** and T2-weighted (TR/TE, 2000/70) **(B)** spin echo MR images show a neuroma (arrows) of the tibial nerve with homogeneous, low signal intensity in **A** and inhomogeneous high signal intensity in **B**. (Courtesy of C. Sebrechts, M.D., San Diego, California.)

polymyositis, 10 had dermatomyositis, and 13 had inclusion body myositis (see later discussion). These investigators used T1- and T2-weighted spin echo sequences and a short tau (inversion time) inversion recovery (STIR) sequence. The last, characterized by a 180 degree inversion pulse prior to a standard spin echo technique, can be designed to suppress the signal of fat. T2-weighted images were found useful in identifying abnormally high signal intensity in muscle, particularly in patients with acute or newly diagnosed disease; however, in those with chronic disease, differentiation of areas of myositis and of fatty infiltration was difficult. STIR imaging improved diagnostic accuracy, with areas of muscle inflammation displaying high signal intensity on a background of depressed signal of fat. Both transaxial and coronal images provided useful information, and the signal intensity of affected muscles on the STIR sequences was higher in patients with clinically active disease than in those with inactive disease. Of interest, differences in the distribution patterns of disease were seen with MR imaging in dermatomyositis and polymyositis versus inclusion body myositis. In polymyositis, involvement was greater in the anterior than in the posterior compartment in the leg, and a more focal pattern of increased signal intensity was seen.

Hernandez and coworkers[1182] confirmed the value of fat suppressed MR imaging in the evaluation of muscle disease in a small group of children with dermatomyositis or similar disorders. In their study, a hybrid fat suppression technique was employed.[1183] This hybrid method uses two distinct techniques to suppress the signal from fat. In the first, a 180 degree refocusing radiofrequency pulse is shifted temporarily to render the water and fat components of the signal in and out of phase on alternate acquisitions. Subtraction of these echoes during signal averaging ideally yields only the desired water signal.[1182] In the second technique, a frequency-selected binomial pulse precedes the spin echo segment of the sequences to saturate the fat signal selectively with little effect on the water signal.[1182] In a direct comparison of conventional T2-weighted spin echo images and T2-weighted fat suppressed images, Hernandez and coworkers found that the latter method improved the detection of muscle abnormalities owing to the greater contrast provided by the suppression of the fat

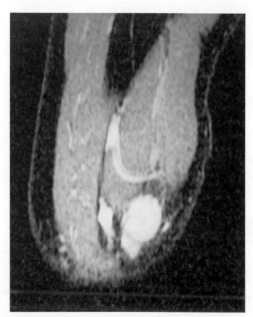

Figure 16–299
Stump neuroma: MR imaging. These neuromas typically are of high signal intensity on STIR MR images, as shown in this sagittal image (TR/TE, 3666/17; inversion time, 150 msec) in a 30 year old man with an amputation below the knee.

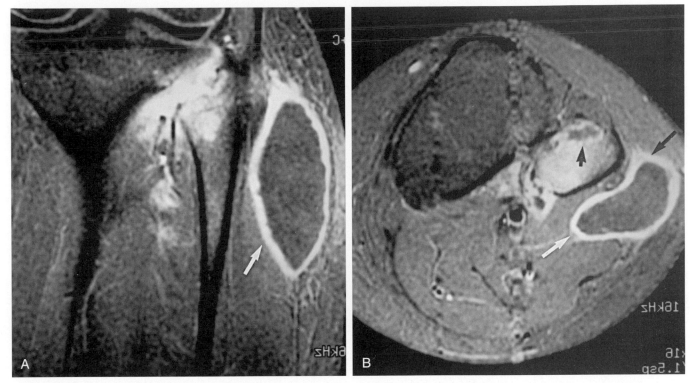

Figure 16–301

Soft tissue abscess and osteomyelitis: MR imaging—tuberculosis. Coronal **(A)** and transverse **(B)** fat-suppressed T1-weighted (TR/TE, 600/15) spin echo MR images obtained after the intravenous administration of a gadolinium compound show tuberculous abscesses (arrows) in the soft tissue and fibula, manifest as ringlike enhancement of signal intensity, and osteomyelitis (of the fibula). (Courtesy of Y. Lee, M.D., Seoul, Korea.)

signal (Fig. 16–302). The signal intensity in unaffected muscles was decreased to a greater extent than that in involved muscles, presumably related to a greater concentration of fat in normal musculature. Abnormal muscles demonstrated higher signal intensity owing to prolongation of the T2 relaxation time, which likely is due to accumulation of extracellular water.

These fat suppression methods have been employed increasingly in the analysis of disorders of the musculoskeletal system. Basically, by reducing the masking effect of fat, these techniques accentuate the visibility of alterations in tissue water.[1182] The resulting regions of high signal intensity are not diagnostic of any particular pathologic condition (i.e., tumor, infection, edema), but

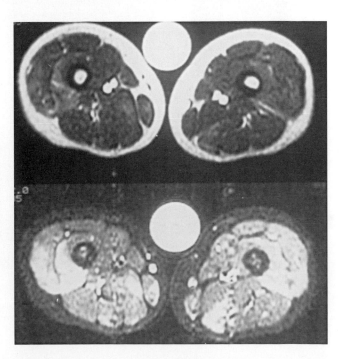

Figure 16–302

Dermatomyositis and polymyositis: MR imaging. This 7 year old girl had clinical and serologic evidence of dermatomyositis. In the top image, a T2-weighted (TR/TE, 2500/80) spin echo MR image of the thighs, in the transverse plane, reveals subtle abnormalities in signal intensity of the vastus lateralis muscle on the right side. In the bottom image, a fat-suppressed T2-weighted (TR/TE, 2500/80) spin echo MR image delineates more extensive muscle abnormalities in both thighs. (Reproduced with permission from Hernandez RJ, et al: Radiology *182*:217, 1992.)

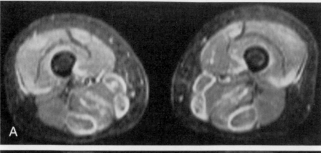

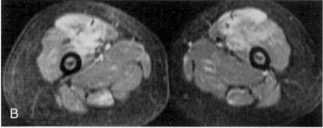

Figure 16–303

Polymyositis: MR imaging.

A Transaxial STIR MR image (TR/TE, 1500/30; inversion time, 100 msec) shows ringlike hyperintensity around the muscles in the thighs, indicative of myofascial edema.

B Identical transaxial STIR MR image obtained more proximally reveals typical patchy areas of hyperintensity within the muscles.

(Reproduced with permission from Adams EM, et al: Radiographics *15*:563, 1995.)

ratio, a limited number of available sections, and suppression that is not specific for fat.[1185-1187] Furthermore, enhancement techniques using intravenous administration of gadolinium compounds are not compatible with STIR imaging. Hybrid methods of chemical shift imaging produce fat suppression while maintaining images with high contrast and a good signal to noise ratio.

In one study, MR imaging was found to be cost-effective in analysis of patients with polymyositis owing to its displaying areas in the muscle most suitable for biopsy.[1188] When biopsies are obtained in regions with extensive muscle edema and little muscle atrophy, the number of false negative results may be reduced.

On analysis of reported experience with MR imaging in patients with polymyositis and dermatomyositis, it becomes evident that this method shows great promise in several respects: it reveals signal intensity alterations in muscle that correlate with disease activity; changes in signal patterns can be used to monitor response to therapy; muscle sites suitable for biopsy can be ascertained; additional findings related to abnormalities in subcutaneous and myofascial tissue may be seen (Figs. 16–303 and 16–304); and specific findings on MR imaging studies may allow differentiation of these muscle diseases and others. Furthermore, signal intensity of involved muscles appears to correlate with muscle strength, although abnormal MR imaging findings and serum levels of muscle enzymes may have different sensitivities.[1180]

Inclusion body myositis represents a separate category of muscle disease that can be distinguished from dermatomyositis and polymyositis. It was Chou's report in 1967[1189] that initially called attention to an inflammatory process of muscle characterized by the presence of intranuclear and cytoplasmic inclusions within cells derived

in the clinical setting of myositis, edematous tissue clearly can be distinguished from fat when such techniques are used. An advantage of the STIR method is that contrast for T1 and T2 effects is additive, making it extremely sensitive in the detection of changes in water content[1184]; disadvantages include a poor signal to noise

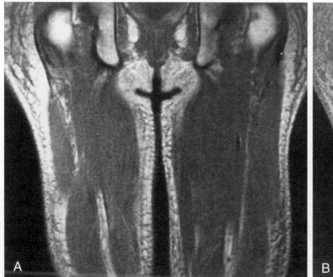

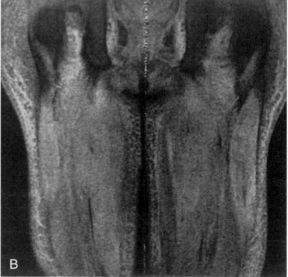

Figure 16–304

Polymyositis: MR imaging.

A Coronal T1-weighted spin echo MR image shows marked reticulation of the subcutaneous fat.

B Coronal STIR MR image (TR/TE, 1500/30; inversion time, 100 msec) confirms inflammation and edema in the subcutaneous fat, appearing as regions of high signal intensity.

(Reproduced with permission from Adams EM, et al: Radiographics *15*:563, 1995.)

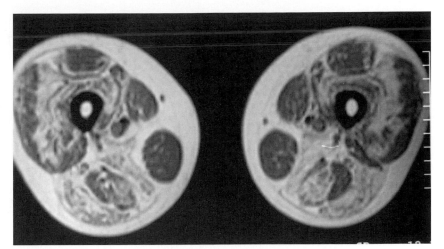

Figure 16–305
Inclusion body myositis: MR imaging. The predominant abnormality in this patient, as displayed in a transverse T1-weighted (TR/TE, 700/15) spin echo MR image of both thighs, is symmetrical fatty replacement of multiple muscles.
(Courtesy of J. Kramer, M.D., Vienna, Austria.)

from muscle biopsy. Other reports subsequently appeared of cases of myositis in which similar histopathologic findings were evident.[1190, 1191] Inclusion body myositis is a rare disease occurring predominantly in men. The age of onset is variable, with the disease appearing from the second through the eighth decades of life.[1192–1194] Clinical findings resemble those of polymyositis. In contrast to polymyositis, however, there is little or no association with malignancy or connective tissue disease, and patients with inclusion body myositis show resistance to high-dose corticosteroid therapy.[1192] Also, as outlined earlier, MR imaging (Fig. 16–305) may reveal distinctive changes in this disease.[1181]

SUMMARY

As in other anatomic regions, the knee is affected by a large number of diverse disorders. Of particular importance are traumatic abnormalities of the menisci and the medial, lateral, anterior, and central supporting structures. Furthermore, many diseases of the synovial membrane, some unique to the knee, may be encountered. Traumatic and degenerative processes of articular cartilage in the knee are of great clinical importance. Although many imaging methods may be used for the assessment of internal derangements and related disorders of the knee, MR imaging currently appears to be optimal.

REFERENCES

1. Walmsley R: Joints. *In* GJ Romanes (Ed): Cunningham's Textbook of Anatomy. 11th Ed. London, Oxford University Press, 1972.
2. Resnick D, Newell JD, Guerra J Jr, et al: Proximal tibiofibular joint: Anatomic-pathologic-radiographic correlation. AJR *131*:133, 1978.
3. Weston WJ: The deep infrapatellar bursa. Australas Radiol *17*:212, 1973.
4. Warwick R, William PL: Gray's Anatomy. 35th British Ed. Philadelphia, WB Saunders Co, 1973.
5. Leffers D: Dislocations and soft tissue injuries of the knee. *In* BD Browner, JB Jupiter, AM Levine, et al (Eds): Skeletal Trauma: Fractures, Dislocations, Ligamentous Injuries. Philadelphia, WB Saunders Co, 1992, p. 1717.
6. Eisenberg RL, Hedgcock MW, Williams EA, et al: Optimum radiographic examination for consideration of compensation awards. III. Knee, hand, and foot. AJR *135*:1075, 1980.
7. Cockshott WP, Racoveanu NT, Burrows DA, et al: Use of radiographic projections of knee. Skel Radiol *13*:131, 1985.
8. Camp JD, Coventry MB: Use of special views in roentgenography of the knee joint. US Naval Med Bull *42*:56, 1944.
9. Singer AM, Naimark A, Felson D, et al: Comparison of overhead and cross-table lateral views for detection of knee-joint effusion. AJR *144*:973, 1985.
10. Bradley WG, Ominsky SH: Mountain view of the patella. AJR *136*:53, 1981.
11. Hughston JC: Subluxation of the patella. J Bone Joint Surg [Am] *50*:1003, 1968.
12. Wiberg G: Roentgenographic and anatomic studies on the femoropatellar joint. Acta Orthop Scand *12*:319, 1941.
13. Furmaier A, Breit A: Über die Roentgenologie des Femoropatellargelenks. Arch Orthop Unfallchir *45*:126, 1952.
14. Merchant AC, Mercer RL, Jacobsen RH, et al: Roentgenographic analysis of patellofemoral congruence. J Bone Joint Surg [Am] *56*:1391, 1974.
15. Ficat P, Phillips J, Bizour H: Le défilé fémoro-patellaire. Rev Méd Toulouse *6*:241, 1970.
16. Ficat RP, Hungerford DS: Disorders of the Patello-Femoral Joint. Baltimore, Williams & Wilkins Co, 1977, p. 40.
17. Laurin CA, Dussault R, Levesque HP: The tangential x-ray investigation of the patellofemoral joint: X-ray technique, diagnostic criteria and their interpretation. Clin Orthop *144*:16, 1979.
18. Leach RE, Gregg T, Ferris JS: Weight-bearing radiography in osteoarthritis of the knee. Radiology *97*:265, 1970.
19. Arlbäck S: Osteoarthrosis of the knee: A radiographic investigation. Acta Radiol Suppl *277*:7, 1968.
20. Leonard LM: The importance of weight-bearing x-rays in knee problems. J Maine Med Assoc *62*:101, 1971.
21. Hagstedt B, Norman O, Olsson TH, et al: Technical accuracy in high tibial osteotomy for gonarthrosis. Acta Orthop Scand *51*:963, 1980.
22. Jacobsen K: Radiologic technique for measuring instability in the knee joint. Acta Radiol (Diagn) *18*:113, 1977.
23. Rijke AM, Tegtmeyer CJ, Weiland DJ, et al: Stress examination of the cruciate ligaments: A radiologic Lachman test. Radiology *165*:867, 1987.
24. Harrison RB, Wood MB, Keats TE: The grooves of the distal articular surface of the femur—a normal variant. AJR *126*:751, 1976.
25. Jacobsen K: Landmarks of the knee joint on the lateral radiograph during rotation. ROFO *125*:399, 1976.
26. Ravelli A: Zum Roetgenbild des menschlichen Kniegelenkes. ROFO *71*:614, 1949.
27. Danzig LA, Newell JD, Guerra J Jr, et al: Osseous landmarks of the normal knee. Clin Orthop *156*:201, 1981.
28. Blumensaat C: Die Lageabweichugen und Verrenkungen der Kniescheibe. Ergebn Chir Orthop *31*:149, 1938.
29. Jacobsen K, Bertheussen K, Gjerloff CC: Characteristics of the line of Blumensaat. Acta Orthop Scand *45*:764, 1974.
30. Hall FM: Radiographic diagnosis and accuracy in knee joint effusions. Radiology *115*:49, 1975.
31. Butt WP, Lederman H, Chuang S: Radiology of the suprapatellar region. Clin Radiol *34*:511, 1983.
32. Engelstad BL, Friedman EM, Murphy WA: Diagnosis of joint effusion on lateral and axial projections of the knee. Invest Radiol *3*:188, 1981.
33. Lewis RW: Roentgenographic study of soft tissue pathology in and about the knee joint. AJR *65*:200, 1951.
34. Bachman AL: Roentgen diagnosis of knee-joint effusion. Radiology *46*:462, 1946.
35. Harris RD, Hecht HL: Suprapatellar effusions: A new diagnostic sign. Radiology *97*:1, 1970.
36. Friedman AC, Naidich TP: The fabella sign: Fabella displacement in synovial effusion and popliteal fossa masses. Radiology *127*:113, 1978.
37. Weston WJ: The extrasynovial and capsular fat pads on the posterior aspect of the knee joint. Skel Radiol *2*:87, 1977.

38. Dalinka MK, Cohen GS, Wershba M: Knee arthrography. CRC Crit Rev Radiol Sci *4*:1, 1973.
39. Kaye JJ: Knee arthrography today. Radiology *157*:265, 1985.
40. Freiberger RH, Pavlov H: Knee arthrography. Radiology *166*:489, 1988.
41. Langer JE, Meyer SJF, Dalinka MK: Imaging of the knee. Radiol Clin North Am *28*:975, 1990.
42. Keats TE, Staatz DS, Bailey RW: Pneumoarthrography of the knee. Surg Gynecol Obstet *94*:361, 1952.
43. Lindblom K: The arthrographic appearance of the ligaments of the knee joint. Acta Radiol *19*:582, 1938.
44. Lindblom K: Arthrography of the knee, a roentgenographic and anatomical study. Acta Radiol (Suppl) *74*:7, 1948.
45. Andrén L, Wehlin L: Double contrast arthrography of the knee with horizontal roentgen ray beam. Acta Orthop Scand *29*:307, 1960.
46. Tegtmeyer CJ, McCue FC III, Higgins SM, et al: Arthrography of the knee: A comparative study of the accuracy of single and double contrast techniques. Radiology *132*:37, 1979.
47. Freiberger RH, Killoran PJ, Cardona G: Arthrography of the knee by double contrast method. AJR *97*:736, 1966.
48. Gerber AM, Resnick D: Knee joint puncture after patellectomy. Clin Orthop *154*:337, 1981.
49. Butt WP, McIntyre JL: Double contrast arthrography of the knee. Radiology *92*:487, 1969.
50. Angell FL: Fluoroscopic technique of double contrast arthrography of the knee. Radiol Clin North Am *9*:85, 1971.
51. Mink JH, Dickerson R: Air or CO_2 for knee arthrography? AJR *134*:991, 1980.
52. Angell FL: A restraint device for arthrography of the knee. Radiology *98*:186, 1971.
53. Gelmon MI, Riding LJ: Arthrography of the knee. Appl Radiol *4*:19, 1975.
54. Gilula LA: A simplified stress device for knee arthrography. Radiology *122*:828, 1977.
55. Levinsohn EM: A new simple restraining device for fluoroscopically monitored knee arthrography. Radiology *122*:827, 1977.
56. Nicks AJ, Mihalko M: A simple device to open the knee joint space during double contrast arthrography. Radiology *122*:827, 1977.
57. Lee KR, Sanders WF: A practical stress device for knee arthrography. Radiology *127*:542, 1978.
58. Rosenthal DI, Murray WT, Jauernek RR, et al: Stressing the knee joint for arthrography. Radiology *134*:250, 1980.
59. Bowen AD III: Have you tried this knee arthrography stress device? AJR *134*:197, 1980.
60. Martin IR, Stoner P: An efficient apparatus for liver arthrography. Br J Radiol *58*:483, 1985.
61. Salazar JE, Sebes JI, Scott RL: The supine view in double-contrast knee arthrography. AJR *141*:585, 1983.
62. Hammond DI, Liver JA: Prone and supine views in double-contrast knee arthrography. J Can Assoc Radiol *35*:262, 1984.
63. Weaver JW: Stereoscopic spot filming in arthrography. AJR *138*:172, 1982.
64. de Carvalho A, Jurik AG: Joint fluid after aspiration: A disturbing factor in knee arthrography. Acta Radiol Diagn *26*:715, 1985.
65. Sedgwick WG, Gilula LA, Lesker PA, et al: Wear particles: Their value in knee arthrography. Radiology *136*:11, 1980.
66. Hotchkiss RN, Tew WP, Hungerford DS: Cartilaginous debris in the injured human knee: Correlation with arthroscopic findings. Clin Orthop *168*:144, 1982.
67. Evans CH, Mears DC, Stanitski CL: Ferrographic analysis of wear in human joints: Evaluation by comparison with arthroscopic examination of symptomatic knees. J Bone Joint Surg [Br] *4*:572, 1982.
68. Kean DM, Worthington BS, Preston BJ, et al: Nuclear magnetic resonance imaging of the knee: Examples of normal anatomy and pathology. Br J Radiol *56*:355, 1983.
69. Moon KL Jr, Genant HK, Helms CA, et al: Musculoskeletal applications of nuclear magnetic resonance. Radiology *147*:161, 1983.
70. Li KC, Henkelman RM, Poon PY, et al: MR imaging of the normal knee. J Comput Assist Tomogr *8*:1147, 1984.
71. Reicher MA, Rauschning W, Gold RH, et al: High-resolution magnetic resonance imaging of the knee joint: Normal anatomy. AJR *145*:895, 1985.
72. Reicher MA, Bassett LW, Gold RH: High-resolution magnetic resonance imaging of the knee joint: Pathologic correlations. AJR *145*:903, 1985.
73. Burk DL Jr, Kanal E, Brunberg JA, et al: 1.5-T surface-coil MRI of the knee. AJR *147*:293, 1986.
74. Soudry M, Lanir A, Angel D, et al: Anatomy of the normal knee as seen by magnetic resonance imaging. J Bone Joint Surg [Br] *68*:117, 1986.
75. Turner DA, Prodromos CC: Magnetic resonance imaging of knee injuries. Semin Ultrasound CT MR *7*:339, 1986.
76. Gallimore GW Jr, Harms SE: Knee injuries: High-resolution MR images. Radiology *160*:457, 1986.
77. Harms SE, Muschler G: Three-dimensional MR imaging of the knee using surface coils. J Comput Assist Tomogr *10*:773, 1986.
78. Beltran J, Noto AM, Mosure JC, et al: The knee: Surface-coil MR imaging at 1.5 T. Radiology *159*:747, 1986.
79. Mandelbaum BR, Finerman GAM, Reicher MA, et al: Magnetic resonance imaging as a tool for evaluation of traumatic knee injuries: Anatomical and pathoanatomical correlations. Am J Sports Med *14*:361, 1986.

80. Reicher MA, Hartzman S, Duckwiler GR, et al: Meniscal injuries: Detection using MR imaging. Radiology *159*:753, 1986.
81. Reicher MA, Hartzman S, Bassett LW, et al: MR imaging of the knee. I. Traumatic disorders. Radiology *162*:547, 1987.
82. Cruess JV III, Mink J, Levy TL, et al: Meniscal tears of the knee: Accuracy of MR imaging. Radiology *164*:445, 1987.
83. Stoller DW, Martin C, Crues JV III, et al: Meniscal tears: Pathologic correlation with MR imaging. Radiology *163*:731, 1987.
84. Bellon EM, Keith MW, Coleman PE, et al: Magnetic resonance imaging of internal derangements of the knee. Radiographics *8*:95, 1988.
85. Mesgarzadeh M, Schneck CD, Bonakdarpour A: Magnetic resonance imaging of the knee and correlation with normal anatomy. Radiographics *8*:707, 1988.
86. Tyrrell RL, Gluckert K, Pathria M, et al: Fast three-dimensional MR imaging of the knee: Comparison with arthroscopy. Radiology *166*:865, 1988.
87. Herman LJ, Beltran J: Pitfalls in MR imaging of the knee. Radiology *167*:775, 1988.
88. Haggar AM, Froelich JW, Hearshen DO, et al: Meniscal abnormalities of the knee: 3DFT fast-scan GRASS MR imaging. AJR *150*:1341, 1988.
89. Spritzer CE, Vogler JB, Martinez S, et al: MR imaging of the knee: Preliminary results with a 3DFT GRASS pulse sequence. AJR *150*:597, 1988.
90. Silva I Jr, Silver DM: Tears of the meniscus as revealed by magnetic resonance imaging. J Bone Joint Surg [Am] *70*:199, 1988.
91. Van Heuzen EP, Golding RP, Van Zanten TEG, et al: Magnetic resonance imaging of meniscal lesions of the knee. Clin Radiol *39*:658, 1988.
92. Watanabe AT, Carter BC, Teitelbaum GP, et al: Normal variations in MR imaging of the knee: Appearance and frequency. AJR *153*:341, 1989.
93. Mink JH, Deutsch AL: Magnetic resonance imaging of the knee. Clin Orthop *244*:29, 1989.
94. Bassett LW, Grover JS, Seeger LL: Magnetic resonance imaging of knee trauma. Skel Radiol *19*:401, 1990.
95. Rothschild PA, Domesek JM, Kaufman L, et al: MR imaging of the knee with a 0.064-T permanent magnet. Radiology *175*:775, 1990.
96. Manaster BJ: Magnetic resonance imaging of the knee. Semin Ultrasound CT MR *11*:307, 1990.
97. Kursunoglu-Brahme S, Resnick D: Magnetic resonance imaging of the knee. Orthop Clin North Am *21*:561, 1990.
98. Reeder JD, Matz SO, Becker L, et al: MR imaging of the knee in the sagittal projection: Comparison of three-dimensional gradient-echo and spin-echo sequences. AJR *153*:537, 1989.
99. Solomon SL, Totty WG, Lee JKT: MR imaging of the knee: Comparison of three-dimensional FISP and two-dimensional spin-echo pulse sequences. Radiology *173*:739, 1989.
100. Gay SB, Chen NC, Burch JJ, et al: Multiplanar reconstruction in magnetic resonance evaluation of the knee: Comparison with film magnetic resonance interpretation. Invest Radiol *28*:142, 1993.
101. Harms SE, Flamig DP, Fisher CF, et al: New method for fast MR imaging of the knee. Radiology *173*:743, 1989.
102. Hajek PC, Baker LL, Sartoris DJ, et al: MR arthrography: Anatomic-pathologic investigation. Radiology *163*:141, 1987.
103. Hajek PC, Sartoris DJ, Neumann C, et al: Potential contrast agents for MR arthrography: In vitro evaluation and practical observations. AJR *149*:97, 1987.
104. Engel A: Magnetic resonance knee arthrography: Enhanced contrast by gadolinium complex in the rabbit and in humans. Acta Orthop Scand (Suppl 240) *61*:3, 1990.
105. Boden SD, Labropoulos PA, Vailas JC: MR scanning of the acutely injured knee: Sensitive, but is it cost effective? Arthroscopy *6*:306, 1990.
106. Ruwe PA, Wright J, Randall RL, et al: Can MR imaging effectively replace diagnostic arthroscopy? Radiology *183*:335, 1992.
107. Spiers ASD, Meagher T, Ostlere SJ, et al: Can MRI of the knee affect arthroscopic practice? A prospective study of 58 patients. J Bone Joint Surg [Br] *75*:49, 1993.
108. Noble J: Unnecessary arthroscopy. J Bone Joint Surg [Br] *74*:797, 1992.
109. Senghas RE: Indications for magnetic resonance imaging. J Bone Joint Surg [Am] *73*:1, 1991.
110. Boden SD, Davis DO, Dina TS, et al: A prospective and blinded investigation of magnetic resonance imaging of the knee: Abnormal findings in asymptomatic subjects. Clin Orthop *282*:177, 1992.
111. Hodler J, Yu JS, Steinert HC, et al: MR imaging versus alternative imaging techniques. MRI Clin North Am *3*:591, 1995.
112. Haramati N, Staron RB, Cushin S, et al: Value of the coronal plane in MRI of internal derangement of the knee. Skel Radiol *23*:211, 1994.
113. Munk PL, Helms CA, Genant HK, et al: Magnetic resonance imaging of the knee: Current status, new directions. Skel Radiol *18*:569, 1989.
114. Buckwalter KA, Braunstein EM, Janizek DB, et al: MR imaging of meniscal windows: Narrow versus conventional window width photography. Radiology *187*:827, 1993.
115. Vahlensieck M, Lang P, Seelos K, et al: Musculoskeletal MR imaging: Turbo (fast) spin-echo versus conventional spin-echo and gradient-echo imaging at 0.5 tesla. Skel Radiol *23*:607, 1994.
116. Fellner C, Geissler A, Held P, et al: Signal, contrast, and resolution in optimized PD- and T2-weighted turbo SE images of the knee. J Comput Assist Tomogr *19*:96, 1995.

117. Rubin DA, Kneeland JB, Listerud J, et al: MR diagnosis of meniscal tears of the knee: Value of fast spin echo vs conventional spin-echo pulse sequences. AJR 162:1131, 1994.

118. Peterfy CG: Answer. AJR 165:734, 1995.

119. Hilfiker P, Zanetti M, Debatin JF, et al: Fast spin-echo inversion-recovery imaging versus fast T2-weighted spin-echo imaging in bone marrow abnormalities. Invest Radiol 30:110, 1995.

120. Weinberger E, Shaw DWW, White KS, et al: Nontraumatic pediatric musculoskeletal MR imaging: Comparison of conventional and fast-spin-echo short inversion time inversion-recovery technique. Radiology 194:721, 1995.

121. Quinn SF, Brown TR, Szumowski JKT: Menisci of the knee: Radial MR imaging correlated with arthroscopy in 259 patients. Radiology 185:577, 1992.

122. Heron CW, Calvert PT: Three-dimensional gradient-echo MR imaging of the knee: Comparison with arthroscopy in 100 patients. Radiology 183:839, 1992.

123. Araki Y, Ootani F, Tsukaguchi I, et al: MR diagnosis of meniscal tears of the knee: Value of axial three-dimensional Fourier transformation GRASS images. AJR 158:587, 1992.

124. Aubel S, Heyd RL, Thaete FL, et al: MR knee imaging: Axial 3DFT GRASS pulse sequence versus spin-echo imaging for detecting meniscal tears. Magn Reson Imaging 10:531, 1992.

125. Hopkins KL, Li KCP, Bergman G: Gadolinium-DTPA-enhanced magnetic resonance imaging of musculoskeletal infectious processes. Skel Radiol 24:325, 1995.

126. Schoenberg NY, Beltran J: Contrast enhancement in musculoskeletal imaging: Current status. Radiol Clin North Am 32:337, 1994.

127. Harris ED Jr: Biology of the joint. In WN Kelley, ED Harris Jr, S Ruddy, et al (Eds): Textbook of Rheumatology. 2nd Ed. Philadelphia, WB Saunders Co, 1985, p. 254.

128. Pedowitz RA, Gershuni DH, Crenshaw AG, et al: Intraarticular pressure during continuous passive motion of the human knee. J Orthop Res 7:530, 1989.

129. Knight AD, Levick JR: Physiological compartmentation of fluid within the synovial cavity of the rabbit knee. J Physiol 331:1, 1982.

130. Schweitzer ME, Falk A, Berthoty D, et al: Knee effusion: Normal distribution of fluid. AJR 159:361, 1992.

131. Kaneko K, De Mony EH, Robinson AE: Distribution of joint effusion in patients with traumatic knee joint disorders: MRI assessment. Clin Imaging 17:176, 1993.

132. Schweitzer ME, Falk A, Pathria M, et al: MR imaging of the knee: Can changes in the intracapsular fat pads be used as a sign of synovial proliferation in the presence of an effusion? AJR 160:823, 1993.

133. Gillquist J, Hagberg G, Oretorp N: Arthroscopy in acute injuries of the knee joint. Acta Orthop Scand 48:190, 1977.

134. Noyes FR, Basset RW, Grood ES, et al: Arthroscopy in acute traumatic hemarthrosis of the knee. J Bone Joint Surg [Am] 62:687, 1980.

135. Maffulli N, Binfield PM, King JB, et al: Acute haemarthrosis of the knee in athletes: A prospective study of 106 cases. J Bone Joint Surg [Br] 75:945, 1993.

136. Davie B: The significance and treatment of haemarthrosis of the knee following trauma. Med J Aust 1:1355, 1969.

137. Wilkinson A: Traumatic haemarthrosis of the knee. Lancet 2:13, 1965.

138. Weinberger A, Schumacher HR: Experimental joint trauma: Synovial response to blunt trauma and inflammatory reaction to intraarticular injections of fat. J Rheumatol 8:380, 1981.

139. Baer AN, Wright EP: Lipid laden macrophages in synovial fluid: A late finding in traumatic arthritis. J Rheumatol 14:848, 1987.

140. Lawrence C, Seife B: Bone marrow in joint fluid: A clue to fracture. Ann Intern Med 74:740, 1971.

141. Berk RN: Liquid fat in the knee joint after trauma. N Engl J Med 277:1411, 1967.

142. Kling DH: Fat in traumatic effusions of the knee joint. Am J Surg 6:71, 1929.

143. Gregg JR, Nixon JE, DiStefano V: Neutral fat globules in traumatized knees. Clin Orthop 132:219, 1978.

144. Graham J, Goldman JA: Fat droplets and synovial fluid leukocytes in traumatic arthritis. Arthritis Rheum 21:76, 1978.

145. Rabinowitz JL, Gregg JR, Nixon JE: Lipid composition of the tissues of human knee joints. II. Synovial fluid in trauma. Clin Orthop 190:292, 1984.

146. Pierce CB, Eaglesham DC: Traumatic lipohemarthrosis of the knee. Radiology 39:655, 1942.

147. Saxton HM: Lipohaemarthrosis. Br J Radiol 35:122, 1962.

148. Arger PH, Oberkircher PE, Miller WT: Lipohemarthrosis. AJR 121:97, 1974.

149. Train JS, Hermann G: Lipohemarthrosis: Its occurrence with occult cortical fracture of the knee. Orthopedics 3:416, 1980.

150. Sacks BA, Rosenthal DI, Hall FM: Capsular visualization in lipohemarthrosis of the knee. Radiology 122:31, 1977.

151. Bianchi S, Zwass A, Abdelwahab IF, et al: Sonographic evaluation of lipohemarthrosis: Clinical and in vitro study. J Ultrasound Med 14:279, 1985.

152. Egund N, Nilsson LT, Wingstrand H, et al: CT scans and lipohaemarthrosis in hip fractures. J Bone Joint Surg [Br] 72:379, 1990.

153. Kier R, McCarthy SM: Lipohemarthrosis of the knee: MR imaging. J Comput Assist Tomogr 14:395, 1990.

154. Kursunoglu-Brahme S, Riccio T, Weisman MH, et al: Rheumatoid knee: Role of gadopentetate-enhanced MR imaging. Radiology 176:831, 1990.

155. Singson RD, Zalduondo FM: Value of unenhanced spin-echo MR imaging in distinguishing between synovitis and effusion of the knee. AJR 159:569, 1992.

156. Ostergaard M, Lorenzen I, Henriksen O: Dynamic gadolinium-enhanced MR imaging in active and inactive immunoinflammatory gonarthritis. Acta Radiol 35:275, 1994.

157. Drapé J-L, Thelen P, Gay-Depassier P: Intra-articular diffusion of Gd-DOTA after intravenous injection in the knee: MR imaging evaluation. Radiology 188:227, 1993.

158. Winalski CS, Aliabadi P, Wright RJ, et al: Enhancement of joint fluid with intravenously administered gadopentetate dimeglumine: Technique, rationale, and implications. Radiology 187:179, 1993.

159. Peterfy CG, Majumdar S, Lang P, et al: MR imaging of the arthritic knee: Improved discrimination of cartilage, synovium, and effusion with pulsed saturation transfer and fat-suppressed T1-weighted sequences. Radiology 191:413, 1994.

160. Pipkin G: Knee injuries: The role of the suprapatellar plica and suprapatellar bursa in simulating internal derangements. Clin Orthop 74:161, 1971.

161. Harty M, Joyce JJ III: Synovial folds in the knee joint. Orthop Rev 7:91, 1977.

162. Deutsch AL, Resnick D, Dalinka MK, et al: Synovial plicae of the knee. Radiology 141:627, 1981.

163. Apple JS, Martinez S, Hardaker WT, et al: Synovial plicae of the knee. Skel Radiol 7:251, 1982.

164. Jackson RW: The sneaky plicae. J Rheumatol 7:251, 1982.

165. Jouanin T, Dupont JY, Halimi P, et al: The synovial folds of the knee joint: Anatomical study based on the dissection of 200 knee joints. Anat Clin 4:47, 1982.

166. Kinnard P, Levesque RY: The plica syndrome: A syndrome of controversy. Clin Orthop 183:141, 1984.

167. Dorfmann H, Orengo PH, Amarenco G: Pathology of the synovial folds in the knee: The value of arthroscopy. Rev Rhum Mal Osteoartic 50:324, 1983.

168. Harrewyn JM, Algnan M, Renoux M, et al: Pathological synovial folds in the knee joint (synovial plica): Arthroscopic treatment. Rev Rhum Mal Osteoartic 49:3, 1982.

169. Gray DJ, Gardner E: Prenatal development of the human knee and superior tibiofibular joints. Am J Anat 86:235, 1950.

170. Pipkin G: Lesions of the suprapatellar plica. J Bone Joint Surg [Am] 32:363, 1950.

171. Patel D: Plica as a cause of anterior knee pain. Orthop Clin North Am 17:273, 1986.

172. Aprin H, Shapiro J, Gershwind M: Arthrography (plica views): A noninvasive method for diagnosis and prognosis of plica syndrome. Clin Orthop 183:90, 1984.

173. Frija G, Halimi PH, Dupont JY, et al: Expression radiologique des plicae du genou. Ann Radiol 25:375, 1982.

174. Schäfer H: Synovialfalten des kniegelenkes: Die Plica parapatellaris medialis. ROFO 147:640, 1987.

175. Boven F, De Boeck M, Potvliege R: Synovial plicae of the knee on computed tomography. Radiology 147:805, 1983.

176. Hodge JC, Ghelman B, O'Brien SJ, et al: Synovial plicae and chondromalacia patellae: Correlation of results of CT arthrography with results of arthroscopy. Radiology 186:827, 1993.

177. Richmond JC, McGinty JB: Segmental arthroscopic resection of the hypertrophic mediopatellar plica. Clin Orthop 178:185, 1983.

178. Nottage WM, Sprague NF III, Auerbach BJ, et al: The medial patellar plica syndrome. Am J Sports Med 11:211, 1983.

179. Vaughan-Lane T, Dandy DJ: The synovial shelf syndrome. J Bone Joint Surg [Br] 64:475, 1982.

180. Jackson RW, Marshall DJ, Fujisawa Y: The pathologic medial shelf. Orthop Clin North Am 13:307, 1982.

181. Flanagan JP, Trakru S, Meyer M, et al: Arthroscopic excision of symptomatic medial plica: A study of 118 knees with 1–4 year follow-up. Acta Orthop Scand 65:408, 1994.

182. Dory MA: Arthrographic recognition of the mediopatellar plica of the knee. Radiology 150:608, 1984.

183. Thijn CJP, Hillen B: Arthrography and the medial compartment of the patello-femoral joint. Skel Radiol 11:183, 1984.

184. Hardaker WT Jr, Whipple TL, Bassett FM III: Diagnosis and treatment of the plica syndrome of the knee. J Bone Joint Surg [Am] 62:221, 1980.

185. Dalinka MK, Garofola J: The infrapatellar synovial fold: A cause for confusion in the evaluation of the anterior cruciate ligament. AJR 127:589, 1976.

186. Johnson DP, Eastwood DM, Witherow PJ: Symptomatic synovial plicae of the knee. J Bone Joint Surg [Am] 75:1485, 1993.

187. Klein W: The medial shelf of the knee: A follow up study. Arch Orthop Traum Surg 102:67, 1983.

188. Schulitz KP, Hille E, Kochs W: The importance of the mediopatellar synovial plica for chondromalacia patellae. Arch Orthop Traum Surg 102:37, 1983.

189. Moller H: Incarcerating mediopatellar synovial plica syndrome. Acta Orthop Scand *52:*357, 1981.

190. Reid GD, Glasgow M, Gordon DA, et al: Pathological plicae of the knee mistaken for arthritis. J Rheumatol *7:*573, 1980.

191. Cooke TD, Wyllie J: Anatomic separation of the suprapatellar pouch spares its involvement by rheumatoid synovitis in the knee. Rheumatol Int *1.*99, 1981.

192. Amatuzzi MM, Fazzi A, Varella MH: Pathologic synovial plica of the knee: Results of conservative management. Am J Sports Med *18:*466, 1990.

193. San Dretto MA, Wartinbee DR, Carrerra GF, et al: Suprapatellar plica synovialis: A common arthrographic finding. J Can Assoc Radiol *33:*163, 1982.

194. Zeiss J, Booth RL Jr, Woldenberg LS, et al: Post-traumatic synovitis presenting as a mass in the suprapatellar bursa of the knee: MRI appearance. Clin Imaging *17:*81, 1993.

195. Katz DS, Levinsohn EM: Pigmented villonodular synovitis of the sequestered suprapatellar bursa. Clin Orthop *306:*204, 1994.

196. Reider B, Marshall JL, Warren RF: Persistent vertical septum in the human knee joint. J Bone Joint Surg [Am] *63:*1185, 1981.

197. Darlington D, Hawkins CF: Nail-patella syndrome with iliac horns and hereditary nephropathy: Necropsy report and anatomical dissection. J Bone Joint Surg [Br] *49:*164, 1967.

198. Wilson PD, Eyre-Brook AL, Francis JD: A clinical and anatomical study of the semimembranosus bursa in relation to popliteal cyst. J Bone Joint Surg *20:*963, 1938.

199. Lindgren PG, Willén R: Gastrocnemio-semimembranosus bursa and its relation to the knee joint. Acta Radiol *18:*497, 1977.

200. Doppman JL: Baker's cyst and the normal gastrocnemiosemimembranosus bursa. AJR *94:*646, 1965.

201. Burleson RJ, Bickel WH, Dahlin DC: Popliteal cyst: Clinico-pathologic survey. J Bone Joint Surg [Am] *38:*1265, 1956.

202. Rauschning W: Anatomy and function of the communication between knee joint and popliteal bursae. Ann Rheum Dis *39:*354, 1980.

203. Rauschning W, Fredriksson BA, Wilander E: Histomorphology of idiopathic and symptomatic popliteal cysts. Clin Orthop *164:*306, 1982.

204. Lindgren PG, Willen R: Gastrocnemio-semimembranosus bursa and its relation to the knee joint. I. Anatomy and histology. Acta Radiol Diagn *18:*497, 1977.

205. Baker WM: Formation of synovial cysts in leg in connection with disease of knee joint. St. Bartholomew's Hosp Rep *13:*245, 1877.

206. Wigley RD: Popliteal cysts: Variations on a theme of Baker. Semin Arthritis Rheum *12:*1, 1982.

207. Gristina AG, Wilson PD: Popliteal cysts in adults and children: Review of 90 cases. Arch Surg *88:*357, 1964.

208. Hoffman BK: Cystic lesions of popliteal space. Surg Gynecol Obstet *116:*551, 1963.

209. Jayson MIV, Dixon AS: Intra-articular pressure in rheumatoid arthritis of the knee. III. Pressure changes during joint use. Ann Rheum Dis *29:*401, 1970.

210. Taylor AR, Rana NA: A valve: An explanation of the formation of popliteal cysts. Ann Rheum Dis *32:*419, 1973.

211. Lindgren PG, Rauschning W: Clinical and arthrographic studies on the valve mechanism in communicating popliteal cysts. Arch Orthop Traum Surg *95:*245, 1979.

212. Palmer DG: Anteromedial synovial cysts at the knee joint in rheumatoid disease. Australas Radiol *16:*79, 1972.

213. Seidl G, Scherak O, Hofner W: Antefemoral dissecting cysts in rheumatoid arthritis. Radiology *133:*343, 1979.

214. Shepherd JR, Helms CA: Atypical popliteal cyst due to lateral synovial herniation. Radiology *140:*66, 1981.

215. O'Dell JR, Andersen PA, Hollister JR, et al: Anterior tibial mass: An unusual complication of popliteal cysts. Arthritis Rheum *27:*113, 1984.

216. Corbetti F, Schiavon F, Fiocco U, et al: Unusual antefemoral dissecting cyst. Br J Radiol *58:*675, 1985.

217. Thevenon A, Hardouin P, Duquesnoy B: Popliteal cyst presenting as an anterior tibial mass. Arthritis Rheum *28:*477, 1985.

218. Podgorski M, Edmonds J: Bidirectional knee joint rupture. J Rheumatol *12:*1180, 1985.

219. Eyanson S, Macfarlane JD, Brandt KD: Popliteal cyst mimicking thrombophlebitis as the first indication of knee disease. Clin Orthop *144:*215, 1979.

220. Schmidt MC, Workman JB, Barth WF: Dissection or rupture of a popliteal cyst: A syndrome mimicking thrombophlebitis in rheumatic diseases. Arch Intern Med *134:*694, 1974.

221. Swett HA, Jaffe RB, McIff EB: Popliteal cysts: Presentation as thrombophlebitis. Radiology *115:*613, 1975.

222. Solomon L, Berman L: Synovial rupture of knee joint. J Bone Joint Surg [Br] *54:*460, 1972.

223. Gordon GV, Edell S, Brogadir SP, et al: Baker's cysts and true thrombophlebitis: Report of two cases and review of the literature. Arch Intern Med *139:*40, 1979.

224. Patrone NA, Ramsdell GM: Baker's cyst and venous thrombosis. South Med J *74:*768, 1981.

225. Iacano V, Gauvin G, Zimbler S: Giant synovial cyst of the calf and thigh in a patient with granulomatous synovitis. Clin Orthop *115:*220, 1976.

226. Pallardy G, Fabre P, Ledoux-Lebard G, et al: L'arthrographie du genou dans l'étude des bursites et des kystes synoviaux. J Radiol Electrol Med Nucl *50:*481, 1969.

227. Shapiro RF, Resnick D, Castles JJ, et al: Fistulization of rheumatoid joints: Spectrum of identifiable syndromes. Ann Rheum Dis *34:*489, 1975.

228. Perri JA, Rodnan GP, Mankin HJ: Giant synovial cysts of the calf in patients with rheumatoid arthritis. J Bone Joint Surg [Am] *50:*709, 1968.

229. Fedullo LM, Bonakdarpour A, Moyer RA, et al: Giant synovial cysts. Skel Radiol *12:*90, 1984.

230. Hertzanu Y, Mendelsohn DB, Firer P: Calcified bodies in a giant Baker's cyst. S Afr Med J *65:*973, 1984.

231. Rosenthal DI, Schwartz AN, Schiller AL: Case report 179. Skel Radiol *7:*142, 1981.

232. Kattapuram SV: Case report 181. Skel Radiol *7:*279, 1982.

233. McLeod BC, Charters JR, Straus AK, et al: Gas-like radiolucencies in a popliteal cyst. Rheumatol Int *3:*143, 1983.

234. Wilson AJ, Ford LT, Gilula LA: Migrating mouse: A sign of dissecting popliteal cyst. AJR *150:*867, 1988.

235. Molpus WM, Shah HR, Nicholas RW, et al: Case report 731. Skel Radiol *21:*266, 1992.

236. Lapayowker MS, Cliff MM, Tourtelotte CD: Arthrography in the diagnosis of calf pain. Radiology *95:*319, 1970.

237. Pastershank SP, Mitchell DM: Knee joint bursal abnormalities in rheumatoid arthritis. J Can Assoc Radiol *28:*199, 1977.

238. Wolfe RD, Colloff B: Popliteal cysts: An arthrographic study and review of the literature. J Bone Joint Surg [Am] *54:*1057, 1972.

239. Bryan RS, DiMichele JD, Ford GL Jr: Popliteal cysts: Arthrography as an aid to diagnosis and treatment. Clin Orthop *50:*203, 1967.

240. Grepl J: Beitrag zur positiven Arthrographie bei pathologischen Veränderungen der Bursae popliteae. ROFO *119:*84, 1973.

241. Clark JM: Arthrography diagnosis of synovial cysts of the knee. Radiology *115:*480, 1975.

242. Cooperberg PL, Tsang I, Truelove L, et al: Grey scale ultrasound in the evaluation of rheumatoid arthritis of the knee. Radiology *126:*759, 1978.

243. Ambanelli U, Manganelli P, Nervetti A, et al: Demonstration of articular effusions and popliteal cysts with ultrasound. J Rheumatol *3:*134, 1976.

244. Carpenter JR, Hattery RR, Hunder GG, et al: Ultrasound evaluation of the popliteal space: Comparison with arthrography and physical examination. Mayo Clin Proc *51:*498, 1976.

245. Rudikoff JC, Lynch JJ, Philipps E, et al: Ultrasound diagnosis of Baker cyst. JAMA *235:*1054, 1976.

246. Moore CP, Sarti DA, Lovie JS: Ultrasonographic demonstration of popliteal cysts in rheumatoid arthritis: A noninvasive technique. Arthritis Rheum *18:*577, 1975.

247. Meire HB, Lindsay DJ, Swinson DR, et al: Comparison of ultrasound and positive contrast arthrography in the diagnosis of popliteal and calf swellings. Ann Rheum Dis *33:*221, 1974.

248. Szer IS, Klein-Gitelman M, DeNardo BA, et al: Ultrasonography in the study of prevalence and clinical evolution of popliteal cysts in children with knee effusions. J Rheumatol *19:*458, 1992.

249. Pathria MN, Zlatkin M, Sartoris DJ, et al: Ultrasonography of the popliteal fossa and lower extremities. Radiol Clin North Am *26:*77, 1988.

250. Fam AG, Wilson SR, Holmberg S: Ultrasound evaluation of popliteal cysts in osteoarthritis of the knee. J Rheumatol *9:*428, 1982.

251. Lukes PJ, Herberts P, Zachrisson BE: Ultrasound in the diagnosis of popliteal cysts. Acta Radiol Diagn *21:*663, 1980.

252. Gompels BM, Darlington LG: Evaluation of popliteal cysts and painful calves with ultrasonography: Comparison with arthrography. Ann Rheum Dis *41:*355, 1982.

253. Harper J, Schubert F, Benson MD, Hayes P: Ultrasound and arthrography in the detection of ruptured Baker's cysts. Australas Radiol *26:*281, 1982.

254. Hermann G, Yeh H-C, Lehr-Janus C, Berson BL: Diagnosis of popliteal cyst: Double-contrast arthrography and sonography. AJR *137:*369, 1981.

255. Levin MH, Nordyke RA, Ball JJ: Demonstration of dissecting popliteal cysts by joint scans after intra-articular isotope injections. Arthritis Rheum *14:*591, 1971.

256. Abdel-Dayem HM, Barodawala YK, Papademetriou T: Scintigraphic arthrography: Comparison with contrast arthrography and future applications. Clin Nucl Med *7:*516, 1982.

257. Lamki L: Baker's cyst: Radionuclide arthrographic findings. Clin Nucl Med *10:*147, 1985.

258. Wallner RJ, Dadparvar S, Croll MN, Brady LW: Demonstration of an infected popliteal (Baker's) cyst with three-phase skeletal scintigraphy. Clin Nucl Med *10:*153, 1985.

259. Cooper RA: Computerized tomography (body scan) of Baker's cyst. J Rheumatol *5:*184, 1978.

260. Schwimmer M, Edelstein G, Heiken JP, Gilula LA: Synovial cysts of the knee: CT evaluation. Radiology *154:*175, 1985.

261. Lee KR, Tines SC, Price HI, De Smet AA, Neff JR: The computed tomographic findings of popliteal cysts. Skel Radiol *10:*26, 1983.

262. Lee KR, Tines SC, Yoon JW: CT findings of suprapatellar synovial cysts. J Comput Assist Tomogr *8:*296, 1984.

263. Grepl J: Wert der positiven Arthrographie zur Diagnostik und Pathogenese retrofemoraler Bakerzysten. Z Orthop *120:*1, 1982.

264. Dixon AS, Grast C: Acute synovial rupture in rheumatoid arthritis: Clinical and experimental observations. Lancet *1:*742, 1964.

265. Tait GBW, Bach F, Dixon AS: Acute synovial rupture: Further observations. Ann Rheum Dis *23*:273, 1965.

266. Hull RG, Rennie JAN, Eastmond CJ, et al: Nuclear magnetic resonance (NMR) tomographic imaging for popliteal cysts in rheumatoid arthritis. Ann Rheum Dis *43*:56, 1984.

267. Lieberman JM, Yulish BS, Bryan PJ, et al: Magnetic resonance imaging of ruptured Baker's cyst. Can Assoc Radiol J *39*:295, 1988.

268. Cardinal E, Dussault RG, Kaplan PA: Imaging and differential diagnosis of masses within a joint. Can Assoc Radiol J *45*:363, 1994.

269. Treadwell EL: Synovial cysts and ganglia: The value of magnetic resonance imaging. Semin Arthritis Rheum *24*:61, 1994.

270. Janzen DL, Peterfy CG, Forbes JR, et al: Cystic lesions around the knee joint: MR imaging findings. AJR *163*:155, 1994.

271. Fielding JR, Franklin PD, Kustan J: Popliteal cysts: A reassessment using magnetic resonance imaging. Skel Radiol *20*:433, 1991.

272. Dungan DH, Seeger LL, Grant EG: Case report 707. Skel Radiol *21*:52, 1992.

273. Barbaric ZL, Young LW: Synovial cyst in juvenile rheumatoid arthritis. AJR *116*:655, 1972.

274. Toyama WM: Familial popliteal cysts in children. Am J Dis Child *124*:586, 1972.

275. Rauschning W, Lindgren PG: Popliteal cysts (Baker's cysts) in adults. I. Clinical and roentgenological results of operative excision. Acta Orthop Scand *50*:583, 1979.

276. DeSmet AA, Neff JR: Knee arthrography for the preoperative evaluation of juxta-articular masses. Radiology *143*:633, 1982.

277. Griffiths HT, Elston CW, Colton CL, et al: Popliteal masses masquerading as popliteal cysts. Ann Rheum Dis *43*:60, 1984.

278. Bogumill GP, Bruno PD, Barrick EF: Malignant lesions masquerading as popliteal cysts: A report of three cases. J Bone Joint Surg [Am] *63*:474, 1981.

279. Littlejohn GO, Brand CA, Ada A, et al: Popliteal cysts and deep venous thrombosis: Tc-99m red blood cell venography. Radiology *155*:237, 1985.

280. Giyanani VL, Grozinger KT, Gerlock AJ Jr, et al: Calf hematoma mimicking thrombophlebitis: Sonographic and computed tomographic appearance. Radiology *154*:779, 1985.

281. Robb D: Obstruction of the popliteal artery by synovial cyst. Br J Surg *48*:221, 1960.

282. Haid SP, Conn J, Bergan JJ: Cystic adventitial disease of the popliteal artery. Arch Surg *101*:765, 1970.

283. Shute K, Rothnie NG: The aetiology of cystic arterial disease. Br J Surg *60*:397, 1973.

284. Firooznia H, Golimbu C, Rafii M, et al: Computerized tomography in diagnosis of compression of the common peroneal nerve by ganglion cysts. Comput Radiol *7*:343, 1983.

285. Gambari PI, Giuliani G, Poppi M, et al: Ganglionic cysts of the peroneal nerve at the knee: CT and surgical correlation. J Comput Assist Tomogr *14*:801, 1990.

286. Muckart RD: Compression of the common peroneal nerve by intramuscular ganglion from the superior tibio-fibular joint. J Bone Joint Surg [Br] *58*:241, 1976.

287. Barrie HJ, Barrington TW, Colwill JC, et al: Ganglion migrans of the proximal tibiofibular joint causing lesions in the subcutaneous tissue, muscle, bone, or peroneal nerve: Report of three cases and review of the literature. Clin Orthop *149*:211, 1980.

288. Bianchi S, Abdelwahab IF, Kenan S, et al: Intramuscular ganglia arising from the superior tibiofibular joint: CT and MR evaluation. Skel Radiol *24*:253, 1995.

289. Ward WG, Eckardt JJ: Ganglion cyst of the proximal tibiofibular joint causing anterior compartment syndrome: A case report and anatomical study. J Bone Joint Surg [Am] *76*:1561, 1994.

290. Burk DL Jr, Dalinka MK, Kanal E, et al: Meniscal and ganglion cysts of the knee: MR evaluation. AJR *150*:331, 1988.

291. Present DA, Hudson TM, Enneking WF: Computed tomography of extraosseous ganglia. Clin Orthop *202*:249, 1986.

292. Matsumoto K, Hukuda S, Ogata M: Juxta-articular bone cysts at the insertion of the pes anserinus: Report of two cases. J Bone Joint Surg [Am] *72*:286, 1990.

293. Zeiss J, Coombs RJ, Booth RL Jr, et al: Chronic bursitis presenting as a mass in the pes anserinus bursa: MR diagnosis. J Comput Assist Tomogr *17*:137, 1993.

294. Forbes JR, Helms CA, Janzen DL: Acute pes anserine bursitis: MR imaging. Radiology *194*:525, 1995.

295. Abdelwahab IF, Kenan S, Hermann G, et al: Periosteal ganglia: CT and MR imaging features. Radiology *188*:245, 1993.

296. Muckle DS, Monahan P: Intra-articular ganglion of the knee: Report of two cases. J Bone Joint Surg [Br] *54*:520, 1972.

297. Caan P: Zystenbildung (Ganglion) im Ligamentum cruciatum anti genus. Deutsche Zeitschrift Chir *186*:403, 1924.

298. Sjovall H: Ein Fall von Ganglion in einem rupturierten Ligamentum cruciatum genus post. Acta Chir Scand *87*:331, 1942.

299. Levine J: A ganglion of the anterior cruciate ligament. Surgery *24*:836, 1948.

300. Chang W, Rose DJ: Ganglion cysts of the anterior cruciate ligament: A case report. Bull Hosp Joint Dis *48*:182, 1988.

301. Yasuda K, Majima T: Intra-articular ganglion blocking extension of the knee: Brief report. J Bone Joint Surg [Br] *70*:837, 1988.

302. Kaempffe F, D'Amato C: An unusual intra-articular ganglion of the knee with intraosseous extension: A case report. J Bone Joint Surg [Am] *71*:773, 1989.

303. Brown MF, Dandy DJ: Intra-articular ganglia in the knee. J Arthrosc Rel Res *6*:322, 1990.

304. Liu SH, Osti L, Mirzayan R: Ganglion cysts of the anterior cruciate ligament: A case report and review of the literature. J Arthrosc Rel Surg *10*:110, 1994.

305. Garcia A, Hodler J, Vaughn L, et al: Case report 677. Skel Radiol *20*:373, 1991.

306. Nokes SR, Koonce TW, Montanez J: Ganglion cysts of the cruciate ligaments of the knee: Recognition on MR images and CT-guided aspiration. AJR *162*:1503, 1994.

307. Savage L, Garth WP Jr: Intra-articular synovial cyst of the knee originating from a chondral fracture of the medial femoral condyle: A case report. J Bone Joint Surg [Am] *76*:1394, 1994.

308. McLaren DB, Buckwalter KA, Vahey TN: The prevalence and significance of cyst-like changes at the cruciate ligament attachments in the knee. Skel Radiol *21*:365, 1992.

309. Myllymäki T, Tikkakoski T, Typpö T, et al: Carpet-layer's knee. An ultrasonographic study. Acta Radiol Diagn *34*:496, 1993.

310. Hoffa A: Influence of adipose tissue with regard to the pathology of the knee joint. JAMA *43*:795, 1904.

311. Smilie IS: Lesions of the infrapatellar fat pad and synovial fringes: Hoffa's disease. Acta Orthop Scand *33*:371, 1963.

312. Magi M, Barca A, Bucca C, et al: Hoffa disease. Ital J Orthop Traumatol *17*:211, 1991.

313. Metheny JA, Mayor MB: Hoffa's disease: Chronic impingement of the infra-patellar fat pad. Am J Knee Surg *1*:134, 1988.

314. Ogilvie-Harris DJ, Giddens J: Hoffa's disease: Arthroscopic resection of the infrapatellar fat pad. Arthroscopy *10*:184, 1994.

315. Kohn D, Deiler S, Rudert M: Arterial blood supply of the infrapatellar fat pad: Anatomy and clinical consequences. Acta Orthop Trauma Surg *114*:72, 1995.

316. Wolfe RD, Giuliano VJ: Double-contrast arthrography in the diagnosis of pigmented villonodular synovitis of the knee. AJR *110*:793, 1970.

317. Greenfield MM, Wallace KM: Pigmented villonodular synovitis. Radiology *54*:350, 1950.

318. Sanderud A: Pigmented villonodular synovitis. Acta Orthop Scand *24*:155, 1955.

319. Hughes TH, Sartoris DJ, Schweitzer ME, et al: Pigmented villonodular synovitis: MRI characteristics. Skel Radiol *24*:7, 1995.

320. Frot B, Palazzo E, Zietoun F, et al: Villonodular synovitis of the knee: Contribution of magnetic resonance imaging. Rev Rhum Mal Osteoartic [Engl Ed] *61*:157, 1994.

321. Palumbo RC, Matthews LS, Reuben JM: Localized pigmented villonodular synovitis of the patellar fat pad: A report of two cases. Arthroscopy *10*:400, 1994.

322. Van Meter CD, Rowdon GA: Localized pigmented villonodular synovitis presenting as a locked lateral meniscal bucket handle tear: A case report and review of the literature. Arthroscopy *10*:309, 1994.

323. Crittenden JJ, Jones DM, Santarelli AG: Knee arthrogram in synovial chondromatosis. Radiology *94*:133, 1970.

324. Prager RJ, Mall JC: Arthrographic diagnosis of synovial chondromatosis. AJR *127*:344, 1976.

325. Kramer J, Recht M, Deely DM, et al: MR appearance of idiopathic synovial osteochondromatosis. J Comput Assist Tomogr *17*:772, 1993.

326. Resnick D, Oliphant M: Hemophilia-like arthropathy of the knee associated with cutaneous and synovial hemangiomas: Report of 3 cases and review of the literature. Radiology *114*:323, 1975.

327. Forrest J, Staple TW: Synovial hemangioma of the knee: Demonstration by arthrography and arteriography. AJR *112*:512, 1971.

328. Cotten A, Flipo R-M, Herbaux B, et al: Synovial hemangioma of the knee: A frequently misdiagnosed lesion. Skel Radiol *24*:257, 1995.

329. Weitzman G: Lipoma arborescens of the knee: Report of a case. J Bone Joint Surg [Am] *47*:1030, 1965.

330. Burgan DW: Lipoma arborescens of the knee: Another cause of filling defects on a knee arthrogram. Radiology *101*:583, 1971.

331. Hermann G, Hochberg F: Lipoma arborescens: Arthrographic findings. Orthopedics *3*:19, 1980.

332. Armstrong SJ, Watt I: Lipoma arborescens of the knee. Br J Radiol *62*:178, 1989.

333. Martinez D, Millner PA, Coral A, et al: Case report 745. Skel Radiol *21*:393, 1992.

334. Feller JF, Rishi M, Hughes EC: Lipoma arborescens of the knee: MR demonstration. AJR *163*:162, 1994.

335. Grieten M, Buckwalter KA, Cardinal E, et al: Case report 873. Skel Radiol *23*:652, 1994.

336. Blais RE, LaPrade RF, Chaljub G, et al: The arthroscopic appearance of lipoma arborescens of the knee. Arthroscopy *11*:623, 1995.

337. Pudlowski RM, Gilula LA, Kyriakos M: Intra-articular lipoma with osseous metaplasia: Radiographic-pathologic correlation. AJR *132*:471, 1979.

338. Fischer B, Munaretto F, Fritschy D, et al: An unusual arthroscopic discovery: An intraarticular schwannoma of the knee. Arthroscopy *10*:113, 1994.

339. Renström P, Johnson RJ: Anatomy and biomechanics of the menisci. Clin Sports Med *9*:523, 1990.

340. Arnoczky SP: Gross and vascular anatomy of the meniscus and its role in meniscal healing, regeneration, and remodeling. *In* VC Mow, SP Arnoczky, DW Jackson (Eds): Knee Meniscus: Basic and Clinical Foundations. New York, Raven Press, 1992, p. 1.

341. Sintzoff SA Jr, Gevenois PA, Andrianne Y, et al: Transverse geniculate ligament of the knee: Appearance at plain radiography. Radiology *180*:259, 1991.

342. Kohn D, Moreno B: Meniscus insertion anatomy as a basis for meniscus replacement: A morphological cadaveric study. Arthroscopy *11*:96, 1995.

343. Heller L, Langman J: The meniscofemoral ligaments of the human knee. J Bone Joint Surg [Br] *46*:307, 1964.

344. Kaplan EB: The lateral meniscofemoral ligaments of the knee joint. Bull Hosp Joint Dis *17*:1765, 1956.

345. Hassine D, Feron JM, Henry-Feugeas MC, et al: The meniscofemoral ligaments: Magnetic resonance imaging and anatomic correlations. Surg Radiol Anat *14*:59, 1992.

346. Ingman AM, Ghosh P, Taylor TKF: Variation of collagenous and non-collagenous proteins of human knee joint menisci with age and degeneration. Gerontologia *20*:212, 1974.

347. Adams ME, Hukins DWL: The extracellular matrix of the meniscus. *In* VC Mow, SP Arnoczky, DW Jackson (Eds): Knee Meniscus: Basic and Clinical Foundations. New York, Raven Press, 1992, p. 15.

348. Bullough PG, Munuera L, Murphy J, et al: The strength of the menisci of the knee as it relates to their fine structure. J Bone Joint Surg [Am] *52*:564, 1970.

349. Peters TJ, Smillie IS: Studies on the chemical composition of the menisci of the knee joint with special reference to the horizontal cleavage lesion. Clin Orthop *86*:245, 1972.

350. Petersen W, Tillmann B: Age-related blood and lymph supply of the knee menisci: A cadaver study. Acta Orthop Scand *66*:308, 1995.

351. Bylski-Austrow DJ, Malumed J, Meade T, et al: Knee joint contact pressure decreases after chronic meniscectomy relative to the acutely meniscectomized joint: A mechanical study in the goat. J Orthop Res *11*:796, 1993.

352. Radin EL, Paul IL: Does cartilage compliance reduce skeletal impact loads? Arthritis Rheum *13*:139, 1970.

353. Voloshin AS, Wosk J: Shock absorption of meniscectomized and painful knees: A comparative in-vivo study. J Biomed Eng *5*:157, 1983.

354. Kurosawa H, Fukuboyashi T, Nakajima H: Load-bearing mode of the knee: Physical behavior of the knee joint with or without menisci. Clin Orthop *149*:283, 1980.

355. Krause WE, Pope MD, Johnson RJ, et al: Mechanical changes in the knee after meniscectomy. J Bone Joint Surg [Am] *58*:599, 1976.

356. Fu FH, Baratz M: Meniscal injuries. *In* JC DeLee, D Drez Jr (Eds): Orthopaedic Sports Medicine: Principles and Practice. Philadelphia, WB Saunders Co, 1994, p. 1146.

357. Di Carlo EF: Pathology of the meniscus. *In* SP Arnoczky, DW Jackson (Eds): Knee Meniscus: Basic and Clinical Foundations. New York, Raven Press, 1992, p. 117.

358. Hough AJ, Webber RJ: Pathology of the meniscus. Clin Orthop *252*:32, 1990.

359. Fahmy NRM, William EA, Noble J: Meniscal pathology and osteoarthritis of the knee. J Bone Joint Surg [Br] *65*:24, 1983.

360. Sokoloff L, Varma AA: Chondrocalcinosis in surgically resected joints. Arthritis Rheum *31*:750, 1988.

361. Noble J, Hamblen DL: The pathology of the degenerative meniscus lesion. J Bone Joint Surg [Br] *57*:180, 1975.

362. Adams ME, Billingham MEJ, Muir H: The glycosaminoglycans in menisci in experimental and natural osteoarthritis. Arthritis Rheum *26*:69, 1983.

363. Ricklin P, Ruttimann A, Del Buono MS: Meniscus Lesions: Diagnosis, Differential Diagnosis, and Therapy. 2nd Ed. New York, Grune & Stratton, 1983.

364. Shogry MEC, Pope TL Jr: Vacuum phenomenon simulating meniscal or cartilaginous injury of the knee at MR imaging. Radiology *180*:513, 1991.

365. Hodler J, Haghighi P, Pathria MN, et al: Meniscal changes in the elderly: Correlation of MR imaging and histologic findings. Radiology *184*:221, 1992.

366. Day B, Mackenzie WG, Shim SS, et al: The vascular and nerve supply of the human meniscus. Arthroscopy *1*:58, 1985.

367. Ferrer-Roca O, Vilalta C: Lesions of the meniscus. I. Macroscopic and histologic findings. Clin Orthop *146*:289, 1980.

368. Crues JV III, Stoller DW: The menisci. *In* JH Mink, MA Reicher, JV Crues III (Eds): Magnetic Resonance Imaging of the Knee. New York, Raven Press, 1987, p. 55.

369. Vangsness CT Jr, Ghaderi B, Hohl M, et al: Arthroscopy of meniscal injuries with tibial plateau fractures. J Bone Joint Surg [Br] *76*:488, 1994.

370. Grenier R, du Tremblay P: Clinical judgement versus arthrography for diagnosing knee lesions. Can J Surg *23*:186, 1980.

371. Selby B, Richardson ML, Nelson BD, et al: Sonography in the detection of meniscal injuries of the knee: Evaluation in cadavers. AJR *149*:549, 1987.

372. McDonnell CH III, Jeffrey RB Jr, Bjorkengren AG, et al: Intraarticular sonography for imaging the knee menisci: Evaluation in cadaveric specimens. AJR *159*:573, 1992.

373. Selby B, Richardson ML, Montana MA, et al: High resolution sonography of the menisci of the knee. Invest Radiol *21*:332, 1986.

374. Marymont JV, Lynch MA, Henning CE: Evaluation of meniscus tears of the knee by radionuclide imaging. Am J Sports Med *11*:432, 1983.

375. Collier BD, Johnson RP, Carrera GF, et al: Chronic knee pain assessed by SPECT: Comparison with other modalities. Radiology *157*:795, 1985.

376. Passariello R, Trecco F, de Paulis F, et al: Meniscal lesions of the knee joint: CT diagnosis. Radiology *157*:29, 1985.

377. Steinbach LS, Helms CA, Sims RE, et al: High resolution computed tomography of knee menisci. Skel Radiol *16*:11, 1987.

378. Manco LG, Lozman J, Coleman ND, et al: Noninvasive evaluation of knee meniscal tears: Preliminary comparison of MR imaging and CT. Radiology *163*:727, 1987.

379. Manco LG, Kavanaugh JH, Lozman J, et al: Diagnosis of meniscal tears using high-resolution computed tomography: Correlation with arthroscopy. J Bone Joint Surg [Am] *69*:498, 1987.

380. Manco LG, Berlow ME, Czajka J, et al: Bucket-handle tears of the meniscus: Appearance at CT. Radiology *168*:709, 1988.

381. Manco LG, Berlow ME: Meniscal tears—comparison of arthrography, CT, and MRI. CRC Crit Rev Diagn Imaging *29*:151, 1989.

382. Lindblom K: Arthrography of the knee, a roentgenographic and anatomical study. Acta Radiol (Suppl) *74*:7, 1948.

383. Montgomery CE: Synovial recesses in knee arthrography. AJR *121*:86, 1974.

384. Russell E, Hamm R, LePage JR, et al: Some normal variations of knee arthrograms and their anatomical significance. J Bone Joint Surg [Am] *60*:66, 1978.

385. Nicholas JA, Freiberger RH, Killoran PJ: Double contrast arthrography of the knee: Its value in the management of 225 knee derangements. J Bone Joint Surg [Am] *52*:203, 1970.

386. Heiser S, LaBriola JH, Meyers MH: Arthrography of the knee. Radiology *79*:822, 1962.

387. McIntyre JL: Arthrography of the lateral meniscus. Radiology *105*:531, 1972.

388. Jelaso DV: The fascicles of the lateral meniscus: An anatomic-arthrographic correlation. Radiology *114*:335, 1975.

389. Wickstrom KT, Spitzer RM, Olsson HE: Roentgen anatomy of the posterior horn of the lateral meniscus. Radiology *116*:617, 1975.

390. Fetto JF, Marshall JL, Ghelman B: An anomalous attachment of the popliteus tendon to the lateral meniscus: Case report. J Bone Joint Surg [Am] *59*:548, 1977.

391. Pavlov H, Goldman AB: The popliteus bursa: An indicator of subtle pathology. AJR *134*:313, 1980.

392. Freiberger RH, Killoran PJ, Cardona G: Arthrography of the knee by double contrast method. AJR *97*:736, 1966.

393. Butt WP, McIntyre JL: Double contrast arthrography of the knee. Radiology *92*:487, 1969.

394. Ringertz HG: Arthrography of the knee. I. Localization of lesions. Acta Radiol Diagn *14*:138, 1973.

395. Ringertz HG: Arthrography of the knee. II. Isolated and combined lesions. Acta Radiol Diagn *17*:235, 1976.

396. Hall FM: Buckled meniscus. Radiology *126*:89, 1978.

397. Bramson RT, Staple TW: Double contrast knee arthrography in children. AJR *123*:838, 1975.

398. Stenström R: Diagnostic arthrography of traumatic lesions of the knee joint in children. Ann Radiol *18*:391, 1975.

399. Saddawi ND, Hoffman BK: Tear of the attachment of a normal medial meniscus of the knee in a four year old child. J Bone Joint Surg [Am] *52*:809, 1970.

400. Shakespeare DT, Rigby HS: The bucket-handle tear of the meniscus: A clinical and arthrographic study. J Bone Joint Surg [Br] *65*:383, 1983.

401. Fitzgerald SW: Magnetic resonance imaging of the meniscus: Advanced concepts. MRI Clin North Am *2*:349, 1994.

402. Anderson MW, Raghavan N, Seidenwurm DJ, et al: Evaluation of meniscal tears: Fast spin-echo versus conventional spin-echo magnetic resonance imaging. Acad Radiol *2*:209, 1995.

403. Stone KR, Stoller DW, Irving SG, et al: 3D MRI volume sizing of the knee meniscus cartilage. Arthroscopy *10*:641, 1994.

404. Kaplan PA, Dussault RG: Magnetic resonance imaging of the knee: Menisci, ligaments, tendons. Top Magn Reson Imaging *5*:228, 1993.

405. Vahey TN, Bennett HT, Arrington LE, et al: MR imaging of the knee: Pseudotear of the lateral meniscus caused by the meniscofemoral ligament. AJR *154*:1237, 1990.

406. Mesgarzadeh M, Moyer R, Leder DS, et al: MR imaging of the knee: Expanded classification and pitfalls to interpretation of meniscal tears. RadioGraphics *13*:489, 1993.

407. Carpenter WA: Meniscofemoral ligament simulating tear of the lateral meniscus: MR features. J Comput Assist Tomogr *14*:1033, 1990.

408. Brantigan OC, Voshell AF: The tibial collateral ligament: Its function, its bursae, and its relation to the medial meniscus. J Bone Joint Surg *25*:121, 1943.

409. Lee JK, Yao L: Tibial collateral ligament bursa: MR imaging. Radiology *178*:855, 1991.

410. Chew FS: Medial meniscal flounce: Demonstration on MR imaging of the knee. AJR *155*:199, 1990.

411. Davis SJ, Teresi LM, Bradley WG, et al: The "notch" sign: Meniscal contour deformities as indicators of tear in MR imaging of the knee. J Comput Assist Tomogr *14*:975, 1990.

412. Turner DA, Rapoport ML, Erwin WD, et al: Truncation artifact: A potential pitfall in MR imaging of the menisci of the knee. Radiology *179*:629, 1991.

413. Peterfy CG, Janzen DL, Tirman PFJ, et al: "Magic-angle" phenomenon: A cause of increased signal in the normal lateral meniscus on short-TE MR images of the knee. AJR *163*:149, 1994.

414. Negendank WG, Fernandez-Madrid FR, Heilbrun LK, et al: Magnetic resonance imaging of meniscal degeneration in asymptomatic knees. J Orthop Res *8*:311, 1990.

415. Kaplan PA, Nelson NL, Garvin KL, et al: MR of the knee: The significance of high signal in the meniscus that does not clearly extend to the surface. AJR *156*:333, 1991.

416. De Smet AA, Norris MA, Yandow DR, et al: MR diagnosis of meniscal tears of the knee: Importance of high signal in the meniscus that extends to the surface. AJR *161*:101, 1993.

417. Dillon EH, Pope CF, Jokl P, et al: Follow-up of grade 2 meniscal abnormalities in the stable knee. Radiology *181*:849, 1991.

418. Kursunoglu-Brahme S, Schwaighofer B, Gundry C, et al: Jogging causes acute changes in the knee joint: An MR study in normal volunteers. AJR *154*:1233, 1990.

419. Shellock FG, Deutsch AL, Mink JH, et al: Do asymptomatic marathon runners have an increased prevalence of meniscal abnormalities? An MR study of the knee in 23 volunteers. AJR *157*:1239, 1991.

420. Shellock F, Mink JH: Knees of trained long-distance runners: MR imaging before and after competition. Radiology *179*:635, 1991.

421. Brunner MC, Flower SP, Evancho AM, et al: MRI of the athletic knee: Findings in asymptomatic professional basketball and collegiate football players. Invest Radiol *24*:72, 1989.

422. Reinig JW, McDevitt ER, Ove PN: Progression of meniscal degenerative changes in college football players: Evaluation with MR imaging. Radiology *181*:255, 1991.

423. Glashow JL, Katz R, Schneider M, et al: Double-blind assessment of the value of magnetic resonance imaging in the diagnosis of anterior cruciate and meniscal lesions. J Bone Joint Surg [Am] *71*:113, 1989.

424. Boeree NR, Watkinson AF, Ackroyd CE, et al: Magnetic resonance imaging of meniscal and cruciate injuries of the knee. J Bone Joint Surg [Br] *73*:452, 1991.

425. Zobel MS, Borrello JA, Siegel MJ, et al: Pediatric knee MR imaging: Pattern of injuries in the immature skeleton. Radiology *190*:397, 1994.

426. De Smet AA, Norris MA, Yandow DR, et al: Diagnosis of meniscal tears of the knee with MR imaging: Effect of observer variation and sample size on sensitivity and specificity. AJR *160*:555, 1993.

427. Quinn SF, Brown TF: Meniscal tears diagnosed with MR imaging versus arthroscopy: How reliable a standard is arthroscopy? Radiology *181*:843, 1991.

428. Justice WW, Quinn SF: Error patterns in the MR imaging evaluation of menisci of the knee. Radiology *196*:617, 1995.

429. De Smet AA, Tuite MJ, Norris MA, et al: MR diagnosis of meniscal tears: Analysis of causes of errors. AJR *163*:1419, 1994.

430. DeSmet AA, Graf BK: Meniscal tears missed on MR imaging: Relationship to meniscal tear patterns and anterior cruciate ligament tears. AJR *162*:905, 1994.

431. Firooznia H, Golimbu C, Rafii M: MR imaging of the menisci. Fundamentals of anatomy and pathology. MRI Clin North Am *2*:325, 1994.

432. Tuckman GA, Miller WJ, Remo JW, et al: Radial tears of the menisci: MR findings. AJR *163*:395, 1994.

433. Wright DH, DeSmet AA, Norris M: Bucket-handle tears of the medial and lateral menisci of the knee: Value of MR imaging in detecting displaced fragments. AJR *165*:621, 1995.

434. Singson RD, Feldman F, Staron R, et al: MR imaging of displaced bucket-handle tear of the medial meniscus. AJR *156*:121, 1991.

435. Weiss KL, Morehouse HT, Levy IM: Sagittal MR images of the knee: A low-signal band parallel to the posterior cruciate ligament caused by a displaced bucket-handle tear. AJR *156*:117, 1991.

436. Haramati N, Staron RB, Rubin S, et al: The flipped meniscus sign. Skel Radiol *22*:273, 1993.

437. Vande Berg B, Malghem J: Arthrographic pseudotear of the anterior horn of the lateral meniscus caused by a displaced meniscal fragment. Skel Radiol *22*:600, 1993.

438. Woods GW, Chapman DR: Reparable posterior meniscocapsular disruption in anterior cruciate ligament injuries. Am J Sports Med *12*:381, 1984.

439. El-Khoury GY, Usta HY, Berger RA: Meniscotibial (coronary) ligament tears. Skel Radiol *11*:191, 1984.

440. Tyson LL, Daughters TC Jr, Ryu RKN, et al: MRI appearance of meniscal cysts. Skel Radiol *24*:421, 1995.

441. Becton JL, Young HH: Cysts of the semilunar cartilage of the knee. Arch Surg *90*:708, 1985.

442. Lantz B, Singer KM: Meniscal cysts. Clin Sports Med *9*:707, 1990.

443. Parisien JS: Arthroscopic treatment of cysts of the menisci: A preliminary report. Clin Orthop *257*:154, 1990.

444. Passler JM, Hofer HP, Peicha G, et al: Arthroscopic treatment of meniscal cysts. J Bone Joint Surg [Br] *75*:303, 1993.

445. Glasgow MMS, Allen PW, Blakeway C: Arthroscopic treatment of cysts of the lateral meniscus. J Bone Joint Surg [Br] *75*:299, 1993.

446. Hernandez FJ: Cysts of the semilunar cartilage of the knee: A light and electron microscopic study. Acta Orthop Scand *47*:436, 1976.

447. Burgan DW: Arthrographic findings in meniscal cysts. Radiology *101*:579, 1971.

448. Wroblewski M: Trauma and the cystic meniscus: Review of 500 cases. Injury *4*:319, 1971.

449. Raine GET, Gonet LCL: Cysts of the menisci of the knee. Postgrad Med J *48*:49, 1972.

450. Spence KF Jr, Robertson RJ: Medial meniscal cysts. Orthopedics *9*:1093, 1986.

451. Mills CA, Henderson IJP: Cysts of the medial meniscus: Arthroscopic diagnosis and management. J Bone Joint Surg [Br] *75*:293, 1993.

452. Ferrer-Roca O, Vilalta C: Lesions of the meniscus. II. Horizontal cleavages and lateral cysts. Clin Orthop *146*:301, 1980.

453. Barrie HJ: The pathogenesis and significance of meniscal cysts. J Bone Joint Surg [Br] *61*:184, 1979.

454. Coral A, van Holsbeeck M, Adler RS: Imaging of meniscal cyst of the knee in three cases. Skel Radiol *18*:451, 1989.

455. Edwards MSD, Hirigoyen M, Burge PD: Compression of the common peroneal nerve by a cyst of the lateral meniscus: A case report. Clin Orthop *316*:131, 1995.

456. Enis JE, Ghandur-Mnaymneh L: Cyst of the lateral meniscus causing erosion of the tibial plateau: A case report. J Bone Joint Surg [Am] *61*:441, 1979.

457. Kay SP, Gold RH, Bassett LW: Meniscal pneumatocele: A case report of spontaneous, persistent intra-articular and juxta-articular gas. J Bone Joint Surg [Am] *67*:1117, 1985.

458. Mason RJ, Friedman SJ, Frassica SJ: Medial meniscal cyst of the knee simulating a solitary bone lesion: A case report and review of the literature. Clin Orthop *304*:190, 1994.

459. Hasegawa Y, Ishimura M, Tamai S, et al: Chondromatosis within a meniscal cyst of the knee. Arthroscopy *11*:115, 1995.

460. Chen W-C, Wu J-J, Chang C-Y, et al: Computed tomography of a meniscal cyst. Orthopedics *10*:1569, 1987.

461. De Flaviis L, Scaglione P, Nessi P, et al: Ultrasound in degenerative cystic meniscal disease of the knee. Skel Radiol *19*:441, 1990.

462. Buckwalter JA, Dryer RF, Mickelson MR: Arthrography in juxtaarticular cysts of the knee: Two cases diagnosed by delayed roentgenograms. J Bone Joint Surg [Am] *61*:465, 1979.

463. Schafer H: Das Meniskusganglion: Früherkennung durch Ausmessung standardisierter Arthrogramme. ROFO *136*:505, 1982.

464. Hall FM: Arthrography of the discoid lateral meniscus. AJR *128*:993, 1977.

465. Haveson SB, Rein BI: Lateral discoid meniscus of the knee: Arthrographic diagnosis. AJR *109*:581, 1970.

466. Smillie IS: The congenital discoid meniscus. J Bone Joint Surg [Br] *30*:671, 1948.

467. Kaplan EB: Discoid lateral meniscus of the knee joint: Nature, mechanism and operative treatment. J Bone Joint Surg [Am] *39*:77, 1957.

468. Fisher AGT: The disk-shaped external semilunar cartilage. Br Med J *1*:688, 1936.

469. Cave EF, Staples OS: Congenital discoid meniscus: A cause of internal derangement of the knee. Am J Surg *54*:371, 1941.

470. Jeannopoulos CL: Observations on discoid menisci. J Bone Joint Surg [Am] *32*:649, 1950.

471. Dickhaut SC, DeLee JC: The discoid lateral-meniscus syndrome. J Bone Joint Surg [Am] *64*:1068, 1982.

472. Murdoch G: Congenital discoid medial semilunar cartilage. J Bone Joint Surg [Br] *38*:564, 1956.

473. Riachi E, Phares A: An unusual deformity of the medial semilunar cartilage. J Bone Joint Surg [Br] *45*:146, 1963.

474. Richmond DA: Two cases of discoid medial cartilage. J Bone Joint Surg [Br] *40*:268, 1958.

475. Ross JA, Tough ICK, English TA: Congenital discoid cartilage: Report of a case of discoid medial cartilage with an embryological note. J Bone Joint Surg [Br] *40*:262, 1958.

476. Weiner B, Rosenberg N: Discoid medial meniscus: Association with bone changes in the tibia. A case report. J Bone Joint Surg [Am] *56*:171, 1974.

477. Resnick D, Goergen TG, Kaye JJ, et al: Discoid medial meniscus. Radiology *121*:575, 1976.

478. Dickason JM, Del Pizzo W, Blazina ME, et al: A series of ten discoid medial menisci. Clin Orthop *168*:75, 1982.

479. Johnson RG, Simmons EH: Discoid medial meniscus. Clin Orthop *167*:176, 1982.

480. Hermann G, Berson BL: Discoid medial meniscus: Two cases of tears presenting as locked knee due to athletic trauma. Am J Sports Med *12*:74, 1984.

481. Comba D, Quaglia F, Magliano GE: Massive discoid medial meniscus: A case report. Acta Orthop Scand *56*:340, 1985.

482. Philippon J: Étude des malformations congénitales méniscales par arthropneumographie. J Radiol Electrol Med Nucl *40*:1, 1959.

483. Moes CAF, Munn JD: The value of knee arthrography in children. J Can Assoc Radiol *16*:226, 1965.

484. Nathan PA, Cole SC: Discoid meniscus—a clinical and pathological study. Clin Orthop *64*:107, 1969.

485. Schonholtz GJ, Koenig TM, Prince A: Bilateral discoid medial menisci: A case report and literature review. J Arthrosc *9*:315, 1993.

486. Dashefsky JH: Discoid lateral meniscus in three members of a family. J Bone Joint Surg [Am] *53*:1208, 1971.

487. Busch MT: Meniscal injuries in children and adolescents. Clin Sports Med 9:661, 1990.
488. Woods GW, Whelan JM: Discoid meniscus. Clin Sports Med 9:695, 1990.
489. Kulowski J, Rickett HW: The relation of discoid meniscus to cyst formation and joint mechanics. J Bone Joint Surg 29:900, 1947.
490. Washington ER III, Root L, Liener VC: Discoid lateral meniscus in children: Long-term follow-up after excision. J Bone Joint Surg [Am] 77:1357, 1995.
491. Engber WD, Mickelson MR: Cupping of the lateral tibial plateau associated with a discoid meniscus. Orthopedics 4:904, 1981.
492. Weiner B, Rosenberg N: Discoid medial meniscus: Association with bone changes in the tibia: A case report. J Bone Joint Surg [Am] 56:171, 1974.
493. Aichroth PM, Patel DV, Marx CL: Congenital discoid lateral meniscus in children: A follow-up study and evolution of management. J Bone Joint Surg [Br] 73:932, 1991.
494. Berson BL, Hermann G: Torn discoid menisci of the knee in adults: Four case reports. J Bone Joint Surg [Am] 61:303, 1979.
495. Howe MA, Buckwalter KA, Braunstein EM, et al: Case report 483. Skel Radiol 17:293, 1988.
496. Silverman JM, Mink JH, Deutsch AL: Discoid menisci of the knee: MR imaging appearance. Radiology 173:351, 1989.
497. Blacksin MF, Greene B, Botelho G: Bilateral diskoid medial menisci diagnosed by magnetic resonance imaging: A case report. Clin Orthop 285:214, 1992.
498. Hamada M, Shino K, Kawano K, et al: Usefulness of magnetic resonance imaging for detecting intrasubstance tear and/or degeneration of lateral discoid meniscus. Arthroscopy 10:645, 1994.
499. Stark JE, Siegel MJ, Weinberger E, et al: Discoid menisci in children: MR features. J Comp Assist Tomogr 19:608, 1995.
500. Neuschwander DC, Drez D Jr, Finney TP: Lateral meniscal variant with absence of the posterior coronary ligament. J Bone Joint Surg [Am] 74:1186, 1992.
501. Symeonides PP, Ioannides G: Ossicles in the knee menisci: Report of three cases. J Bone Joint Surg [Am] 54:1288, 1972.
502. Weaver JB: Calcification and ossification of the menisci. J Bone Joint Surg 42:873, 1942.
503. Rosen IE: Unusual intrameniscal lunulae: Three case reports. J Bone Joint Surg [Am] 40:925, 1958.
504. Glass RS, Barnes WM, Kells DU, et al: Ossicles of knee menisci: Report of seven cases. Clin Orthop 111:163, 1975.
505. Bernstein RM, Olsson HE, Spitzer RM, et al: Ossicle of the meniscus. AJR 127:785, 1976.
506. Mariani PP, Puddo G: Meniscal ossicle: A case report. Am J Sports Med 9:392, 1981.
507. Pederson HE: The ossicles of the semilunar cartilages of rodents. Anat Rec 105:1, 1949.
508. Ganey TM, Ogden JA, Abou-Madi N, et al: Meniscal ossification. II. The normal pattern in the tiger knee. Skel Radiol 23:173, 1994.
509. Mitrovic DR: Ossification of human menisci. Arthritis Rheum 34:638, 1991.
510. Ogden JA, Ganey TM, Arrington JA, et al: Meniscal ossification. I. Human. Skel Radiol 23:167, 1994.
511. Richmond JC, Sarno RC: Arthroscopic treatment of medial meniscal avulsion fractures. Arthroscopy 4:117, 1988.
512. Richmond JC, Sarno RC: Posttraumatic intracapsular bone fragments: Association with meniscal tears. AJR 150:159, 1988.
513. Tuite MJ, DeSmet AA, Swan JS, et al: MR imaging of a meniscal ossicle. Skel Radiol 24:543, 1995.
514. Liu SH, Osti L, Raskin A, et al: Meniscal ossicles: Two case reports and a review of the literature. Arthroscopy 10:296, 1994.
515. Yu JS, Resnick D: Meniscal ossicle: MR imaging appearance in three patients. Skel Radiol 23:637, 1994.
516. Schnarkowski P, Tirman PFJ, Fuchigama KD, et al: Meniscal ossicle: Radiographic and MR imaging findings. Radiology 196:47, 1995.
517. Yao J, Yao L: Magnetic resonance imaging of a symptomatic meniscal ossicle. Clin Orthop 293:225, 1993.
518. Radin EL, de Lamotte F, Maquet P: Role of the menisci in the distribution of stress in the knee. Clin Orthop 185:290, 1984.
519. Kurosawa H, Fukubayashi T, Nakajima H: Load-bearing mode of the knee joint: Physical behavior of the knee joint with or without menisci. Clin Orthop 149:283, 1980.
520. Korkala O, Karaharju E, Gronblad M, et al: Articular cartilage after meniscectomy: Rabbit knees studied with the scanning electron microscope. Acta Orthop Scand 55:273, 1984.
521. Jackson JP: Degenerative changes in the knee after meniscectomy. Br Med J 2:525, 1968.
522. Appel H: Late results after meniscectomy in the knee joint: A clinical and roentgenologic follow-up investigation. Acta Orthop Scand (Suppl) 133:6, 1970.
523. Tapper EM, Hoover NW: Late results after meniscectomy. J Bone Joint Surg [Am] 51:517, 1969.
524. Noble J, Erat K: In defense of the meniscus: A prospective study of 200 meniscectomy patients. J Bone Joint Surg [Br] 62:7, 1980.
525. Shapiro F, Glimcher MJ: Induction of osteoarthrosis in the rabbit knee joint: Histologic changes following meniscectomy and meniscal lesions. Clin Orthop 147:287, 1980.
526. Rangger C, Klestil T, Gloetzer W, et al: Osteoarthritis after arthroscopic partial meniscectomy. Am J Sports Med 23:240, 1995.
527. Arnoczky SP, Warren RF: The microvasculature of the meniscus and its response to injury—an experimental study in the dog. Am J Sports Med 11:131, 1983.
528. Arnoczky SP, Cooper TG, Stadelmaier DM, et al: Magnetic resonance signals in healing menisci: An experimental study in dogs. Arthroscopy 10:552, 1994.
529. De Haven KE: Peripheral meniscal repair: An alternative to meniscectomy. J Bone Joint Surg [Br] 63:463, 1981.
530. Hamberg P, Gillquist J, Lysholm J: Suture of new and old peripheral meniscal tears. J Bone Joint Surg [Am] 65:193, 1983.
531. Gershuni DH, Skyhar MJ, Danzig LA, et al: Experimental models to promote healing of tears in the avascular segment of canine knee menisci. J Bone Joint Surg [Am] 71:1363, 1989.
532. DeHaven KE, Arnoczky SP: Meniscal repair. I. Basic science indications for repair, and open repair. J Bone Joint Surg [Am] 76:140, 1994.
533. De Young DJ, Flo GL, Tvedten H: Experimental medial meniscectomy in dogs undergoing cruciate ligament repair. J Am Anim Hosp Assoc 16:639, 1980.
534. Kim JM, Moon MS: Effects of synovectomy upon regeneration of meniscus in rabbits. Clin Orthop 141:287, 1979.
535. Burr DB, Radin EL: Meniscal function and the importance of meniscal regeneration in preventing late medial compartment osteoarthrosis. Clin Orthop 171:121, 1982.
536. Arnoczky SP, Warren RN, Kaplan N: Meniscal remodeling following partial meniscectomy: An experimental study in the dog. Arthroscopy 1:248, 1985.
537. van Arkel ERA, DeBoer H: Human meniscal transplantation: Preliminary results at 2 to 5 year follow-up. J Bone Joint Surg [Br] 77:589, 1995.
538. Johnson DL: Meniscal reconstruction: Present and future. Oper Techniques Orthop 5:276, 1995.
539. Patten RM, Rolfe BA: MRI of meniscal allografts. J Comput Assist Tomogr 19:243, 1995.
540. Siegel MC, Roberts CS: Meniscal allografts. Clin Sports Med 12:59, 1993.
541. Northmore-Ball MD, Dandy DJ, Jackson RW: Arthroscopic, open partial, and total meniscectomy. J Bone Joint Surg [Br] 65:400, 1983.
542. Tregonning RJA: Closed partial meniscectomy: Early results for single tears with meniscal symptoms. J Bone Joint Surg [Br] 65:378, 1983.
543. Goodfellow JW: Closed meniscectomy. J Bone Joint Surg [Br] 65:373, 1983.
544. Heatley FW: The meniscus—can it be repaired? J Bone Joint Surg [Br] 62:397, 1980.
545. Cabaud HE, Rodkey WG, Fitzwater JE: Medial meniscus repairs: An experimental and morphologic study. Am J Sports Med 9:129, 1981.
546. Danzig L, Resnick D, Gonsalves M, et al: Blood supply to the normal and abnormal menisci of the human knee. Clin Orthop 172:271, 1983.
547. Doyle JR, Eisenberg JH, Orth MW: Regeneration of knee menisci: A preliminary report. J Trauma 6:50, 1966.
548. Smillie IS: Observations on the regeneration of the semilunar cartilages in man. Br J Surg 31:398, 1944.
549. Goldenberg RR: Refracture of a regenerated internal semilunar cartilage. J Bone Joint Surg 17:1054, 1935.
550. Massare C, Bard M, Tristant H: Intérêt de l'arthrographie du genou dans les gonalgies après meniscectomie: Revue de 200 dossiers personnels. J Radiol Electrol Med Nucl 55:401, 1974.
551. Debnam JW, Staple TW: Arthrography of the knee after meniscectomy. Radiology 113:67, 1974.
552. Laasonen EM, Wilppula E: Why a meniscectomy fails. Acta Orthop Scand 47:672, 1976.
553. Dandy DJ, Jackson RW: The diagnosis of problems after meniscectomy. J Bone Joint Surg [Br] 57:349, 1975.
554. Hall FM: MR diagnosis of recurrent meniscal tears: How soon we forget. AJR 162:1502, 1994.
555. Yu JS, Resnick D: Imaging of the knee. Curr Opin Orthop 4:56, 1993.
556. Smith DK, Totty WG: The knee after partial meniscectomy: MR imaging features. Radiology 176:141, 1990.
557. Kent RH, Pope CF, Lynch JK, et al: Magnetic resonance imaging of the surgically repaired meniscus: Six month follow-up. Magn Res Imaging 9:335, 1991.
558. Deutsch AL, Mink JH, Fox JM, et al: Peripheral meniscal tears: MR findings after conservative treatment or arthroscopic repair. Radiology 176:485, 1990.
559. Farley TE, Howell SM, Love KF, et al: Meniscal tears: MR and arthrographic findings after arthroscopic repair. Radiology 180:517, 1991.
560. Applegate GR, Flannigan BD, Tolin BS, et al: MR diagnosis of recurrent tears in the knee: Value of intraarticular contrast material. AJR 161:821, 1993.
561. Odgaard A, Pedersen CM, Bentzen SM, et al: Density changes at the proximal tibia after medial meniscectomy. J Orthop Res 7:744, 1989.
562. Burks RT: Gross anatomy. In D Daniel, W Akeson, J O'Connor (Eds): Knee Ligaments: Structure, Function, Injury, and Repair. New York, Raven Press, 1990, p. 59.
563. Warren LF, Marshall JL, Girgis F: The prime static stabilizers of the medial side of the joint. J Bone Joint Surg [Am] 56:665, 1974.

564. Hennigan SP, Schneck CD, Mesgardazeh M, et al: The semimembranosus-tibial collateral ligament bursa: Anatomical study and magnetic resonance imaging. J Bone Joint Surg [Am] 76:1322, 1994.

565. Hughston JC, Eilers AF: The role of the posterior oblique ligament in repairs of acute medial (collateral) ligament tears of the knee. J Bone Joint Surg [Am] 55:923, 1973.

566. Hughston JC: The importance of the posterior oblique ligament in repairs of acute tears of the medial ligaments in knees with and without an associated rupture of the anterior cruciate ligament: Results of long-term follow-up. J Bone Joint Surg [Am] 76:1328, 1994.

567. Brantigan OC, Voshell AF: The mechanics of the ligaments and menisci of the knee joint. J Bone Joint Surg 23:44, 1941.

568. Linton RC, Indelicato PA: Medial ligament injuries. In JC DeLee, D Drez Jr (Eds): Orthopaedic Sports Medicine: Principles and Practice. Philadelphia, WB Saunders Co, 1994, p. 1261.

569. Grood ES, Noyes FR, Butler DL, et al: Ligamentous and capsular restraints preventing medial and lateral laxity in intact human cadaver knees. J Bone Joint Surg [Am] 63:1257, 1981.

570. Markolf KL, Mensch JS, Amstutz HC: Stiffness and laxity of the knee—the contributions of the supporting structures: A quantitative in vitro study. J Bone Joint Surg [Am] 58:583, 1976.

571. Seering WP, Piziali RL, Nagel DA, et al: The function of the primary ligaments of the knee in varus-valgus and axial rotation. J Biomech 13:785, 1980.

572. Shoemaker SC, Markolf KL: Effects of joint load on the stiffness and laxity of ligament-deficient knees: An in vitro study of the anterior cruciate and medial collateral ligaments. J Bone Joint Surg [Am] 67:136, 1985.

573. Hughston JC, Andrews JR, Cross MJ, et al: Classification of knee ligament instabilities. I. The medial compartment and cruciate ligaments. J Bone Joint Surg [Am] 58:159, 1976.

574. Hughston JC, Andrews JR, Cross MJ, et al: Classification of knee ligament instabilities. II. The lateral compartment. J Bone Joint Surg [Am] 58:173, 1976.

575. Andrews JR, Axe MJ: The classification of knee ligament instability. Orthop Clin North Am 16:69, 1985.

576. Indelicato PA: Injury to the medial capsuloligamentous complex. In JA Feagin (Ed): The Crucial Ligaments: Diagnosis and Treatment of Ligamentous Injuries About the Knee. New York, Churchill Livingstone, 1988, p. 197.

577. O'Donoghue DH: Surgical treatment of fresh injuries to major ligaments of the knee. J Bone Joint Surg [Am] 32:791, 1950.

578. Engle CP, Noguchi M, Ohland KJ, et al: Healing of the rabbit medial collateral ligament following an O'Donoghue triad injury: Effects of anterior cruciate ligament reconstruction. J Orthop Res 12:357, 1994.

579. Frank CB, Bray R, Chimich D, et al: Abnormality of the contralateral ligament after injuries of the medial collateral ligament: An experimental study in rabbits. J Bone Joint Surg [Am] 76:403, 1994.

580. Turner DA, Prodromos CC, Petasnick JP, et al: Acute injury of the ligaments of the knee: Magnetic resonance evaluation. Radiology 154:717, 1985.

581. Tehranzadeh J, Kerr R, Amster J: Magnetic resonance imaging of tendon and ligament abnormalities. II. Pelvis and lower extremities. Skel Radiol 21:79, 1992.

582. Garvin GJ, Munk PL, Vellet AD: Tears of the medial collateral ligament: Magnetic resonance imaging findings and associated injuries. J Can Assoc Radiol 44:199, 1993.

583. Schweitzer ME, Tran D, Deely DM, et al: Medial collateral ligament injuries: Evaluation of multiple signs, prevalence and location of associated bone bruises, and assessment with MR imaging. Radiology 194:825, 1995.

584. Yao L, Dungan D, Seeger LL: MR imaging of tibial collateral ligament injury: Comparison with clinical examination. Skel Radiol 23:521, 1994.

585. Mirowitz SA, Shu HH: MR imaging evaluation of knee collateral ligaments and related injuries: Comparison of T1-weighted, T2-weighted, and fat-saturated T2-weighted sequences—correlation with clinical findings. J Magn Res Imaging 4:725, 1994.

586. Yao L, Lee JK: Avulsion of the posteromedial tibial plateau by the semimembranosus tendon: Diagnosis with MR imaging. Radiology 172:513, 1989.

587. Vanek J: Posteromedial fracture of the tibial plateau is not an avulsion injury: A case report and experimental study. J Bone Joint Surg [Br] 76:290, 1994.

588. Seebacher JR, Inglis AE, Marshall JL, et al: The structure of the posterolateral aspect of the knee. J Bone Joint Surg [Am] 64:536, 1982.

589. Reider B, Marshall JL, Koslin RT, et al: The anterior aspect of the knee joint. J Bone Joint Surg [Am] 63:351, 1981.

590. Terry GC, Hughston JD, Norwood LA: The anatomy of the iliopatellar band and iliotibial tract. Am J Sports Med 14:39, 1986.

591. Jakob RP, Warner JP: Lateral and posterolateral rotatory instability of the knee. In JC DeLee, D Drez Jr (Eds): Orthopaedic Sports Medicine: Principles and Practice. Philadelphia, WB Saunders Co, 1994, p. 1275.

592. Last RJ: The popliteus muscle and the lateral meniscus. J Bone Joint Surg [Br] 32:93, 1950.

593. Cohn AK, Mains DB: Popliteal hiatus of the lateral meniscus. Am J Sports Med 7:221, 1979.

594. Veltri DM, Warren RF: Posterolateral instability of the knee. J Bone Joint Surg [Am] 76:460, 1994.

595. De Lee JC, Riley MB, Rockwood CA Jr: Acute posterolateral rotary instability of the knee. Am J Sports Med 11:199, 1983.

596. Shoemaker SC, Daniel DM: The limits of knee motion: In vitro studies. In D Daniel, W Akeson, J O'Connor (Eds): Knee Ligaments: Structure, Function, Injury, and Repair. New York, Raven Press, 1990, p. 153.

597. Ruiz ME, Erickson SJ: Medial and lateral supporting structures of the knee: Normal MR imaging anatomy and pathologic findings. MRI Clin North Am 2:381, 1994.

598. Sebastianelli WJ, Hanks GA, Kalenak A: Isolated avulsion of the biceps femoris insertion: A case report. Clin Orthop 259:200, 1990.

599. Rose DJ, Parisien JS: Popliteus tendon rupture: Case report and review of the literature. Clin Orthop 226:113, 1988.

600. Tria AJ, Johnson CD, Zawadsky JP: The popliteus tendon. J Bone Joint Surg [Am] 71:714, 1989.

601. Geissler WB, Corso SR, Caspari RB: Isolated rupture of the popliteus with posterior tibial nerve palsy. J Bone Joint Surg [Br] 74:811, 1992.

602. Naver L, Aalberg JR: Avulsion of the popliteus tendon: A rare cause of chondral fracture and hemarthrosis. Am J Sports Med 13:423, 1985.

603. Nakhostine M, Perko M, Cross M: Isolated avulsion of the popliteus tendon. J Bone Joint Surg [Br] 77:242, 1995.

604. Brown TR, Quinn SF, Wensel JP, et al: Diagnosis of popliteus injuries with MR imaging. Skel Radiol 24:511, 1995.

605. Orava S: Iliotibial tract friction syndrome in athletes: An uncommon exertion syndrome on the lateral side of the knee. Br J Sports Med 12:69, 1978.

606. Martens M, Libbrecht P, Burssens A: Surgical treatment of the iliotibial band friction syndrome. Am J Sports Med 17:651, 1989.

607. Noble CA: Iliotibial band friction syndrome in runners. Am J Sports Med 8:232, 1980.

608. Murphy BJ, Hechtman KS, Uribe JW, et al: Iliotibial band friction syndrome: MR imaging findings. Radiology 185:569, 1992.

609. Segond P: Recherches cliniques et experimentales sur les epanchements sanguins du genou par entorse. Prog Med 7:297, 1879.

610. Bock GW, Bosch E, Mishra DK, et al: The healed Segond fracture: A characteristic residual bone excrescence. Skel Radiol 23:555, 1994.

611. Johnson LL: Lateral capsular ligament complex: Anatomical and surgical considerations. Am J Sports Med 7:156, 1979.

612. Hess T, Rupp S, Hopf T, et al: Lateral tibial avulsion fractures and disruptions to the anterior cruciate ligament: A clinical study of their incidence and correlation. Clin Orthop 303:193, 1994.

613. Weber WN, Neumann CH, Barakos JA, et al: Lateral tibial rim (Segond) fractures: MR imaging characteristics. Radiology 180:731, 1991.

614. Helms CA, Fritz RC, Garvin GJ: Plantaris muscle injury: Evaluation with MR imaging. Radiology 195:201, 1995.

615. Froimson AE: Tennis leg. JAMA 209:415, 1969.

616. Anouchi YS, Parker RD, Seitz WH: Posterior compartment syndrome of the calf resulting from misdiagnosis of a rupture of the medial head of the gastrocnemius. J Trauma 27:678, 1987.

617. Ficat RP, Hungerford DS: Disorders of the Patello-femoral Joint. Baltimore, Williams & Wilkins, 1977.

618. Reider B, Marshall JL, Koslin B, et al: The anterior aspect of the knee joint: An anatomic study. J Bone Joint Surg [Am] 63:351, 1981.

619. Walsh WM: Patellofemoral joint. In JC DeLee, D Drez Jr (Eds): Orthopaedic Sports Medicine: Principles and Practice. Philadelphia, WB Saunders Co, 1994, p. 1163.

620. Fulkerson JP, Gossling HR: Anatomy of the knee joint lateral retinaculum. Clin Orthop 153:183, 1980.

621. Terry GC: The anatomy of the extensor mechanism. Clin Sports Med 8:163, 1989.

622. Reider B, Marshall JL, Koslin B, et al: The anterior aspect of the knee joint: An anatomical study. J Bone Joint Surg [Am] 63:351, 1981.

623. Lieb FF, Perry J: Quadriceps function: An anatomical and mechanical study using amputated limbs. J Bone Joint Surg [Am] 50:1535, 1968.

624. Hallisey MJ, Doherty N, Bennett WF: Anatomy of the junction of the vastus lateralis tendon and the patella. J Bone Joint Surg [Am] 69:545, 1987.

625. Wiberg G: Roentgenographic and anatomic studies of the femoropatellar joint, with special reference to chondromalacia patellae. Acta Orthop Scand 12:319, 1941.

626. Goodfellow JW, Hungerford DS, Zindel M: Patellofemoral mechanics and pathology. I. Functional anatomy of the patellofemoral joint. J Bone Joint Surg [Br] 58:287, 1976.

627. Goodfellow JW, Hungerford DS, Woods C: Patellofemoral joint mechanics and pathology. II. Chondromalacia patellae. J Bone Joint Surg [Br] 58:291, 1976.

628. Outerbridge RE: Further studies on the etiology of chondromalacia patellae. J Bone Joint Surg [Br] 46:179, 1964.

629. Delgado-Martins H: A study of the position of the patella using computerized tomography. J Bone Joint Surg [Br] 61:443, 1976.

630. Hungerford DS, Barry M: Biomechanics of the patellofemoral joint. Clin Orthop 144:9, 1979.

631. Martens M, Wouters P, Burssens A, et al: Patellar tendinitis: Pathology and results of treatment. Acta Orthop Scand 53:445, 1982.

632. Blazina ME, Kerlan RK, Jobe FW, et al: Jumper's knee. Orthop Clin North Am 4:665, 1973.

633. Roels J, Martens M, Mulier JC, et al: Patellar tendinitis (jumper's knee). Am J Sports Med 6:362, 1978.
634. Bodne D, Quinn SF, Murray WT, et al: Magnetic resonance images of chronic patellar tendinitis. Skel Radiol 17:24, 1988.
635. El-Khoury GY, Wira RL, Berbaum KS, et al: MR imaging of patellar tendinitis. Radiology 184:849, 1992.
636. Kahn D, Wilson MA: Bone scintigraphic findings in patellar tendinitis. J Nucl Med 28:1768, 1987.
637. Mourad K, King J, Guggiana P: Computed tomography and ultrasound imaging of jumper's knee—patellar tendinitis. Clin Radiol 39:162, 1988.
638. Davies SG, Baudouin CJ, King JB, et al: Ultrasound, computed tomography and magnetic resonance imaging in patellar tendinitis. Clin Radiol 43:52, 1991.
639. O'Keefe D: Ultrasound in clinical orthopaedics. J Bone Joint Surg [Br] 74:488, 1992.
640. Sonin AH: Magnetic resonance imaging of the extensor mechanism. MRI Clin North Am 2:401, 1994.
641. Sonin AH, Fitzgerald SW, Bresler ME, et al: MR imaging appearance of the extensor mechanism of the knee: Functional anatomy and injury patterns. Radiographics 15:367, 1995.
642. Schweitzer ME, Mitchell DG, Ehrlich SM: The patellar tendon: Thickening, internal signal, buckling, and other MR variants. Skel Radiol 22:411, 1993.
643. Reiff DB, Heenan SD, Heron CW: MRI appearance of the asymptomatic patellar tendon on gradient echo imaging. Skel Radiol 24:123, 1995.
644. McLoughlin RF, Raber EL, Vellet AD, et al: Patellar tendinitis: MR imaging features, with suggested pathogenesis and proposed classification. Radiology 197:843, 1995.
645. Scranton PE Jr, Farrar EL: Mucoid degeneration of the patellar ligament in athletes. J Bone Joint Surg [Am] 74:435, 1992.
646. Siwek CW, Rao JP: Ruptures of the extensor mechanism of the knee joint. J Bone Joint Surg [Am] 63:932, 1981.
647. Scuderi C: Quadriceps tendon rupture. Am J Surg 95:626, 1958.
648. Levy M, Seelefreund M, Maor P, et al: Bilateral spontaneous and simultaneous rupture of the quadriceps tendon in gout. J Bone Joint Surg [Br] 53:510, 1971.
649. Potasman I, Bassan HN: Multiple tendon ruptures in systemic lupus erythematosus: Case report and review of the literature. Ann Rheum Dis 43:347, 1984.
650. Lotem N, Robson MD, Rosenfield JB: Spontaneous rupture of the quadriceps tendon in patients on chronic hemodialysis. Ann Rheum Dis 33:428, 1974.
651. Newburg A, Wales L: Radiographic diagnosis of quadriceps tendon rupture. Radiology 125:367, 1977.
652. David HG, Green JT, Grant AJ, et al: Simultaneous bilateral quadriceps rupture: A complication of anabolic steroid abuse. J Bone Joint Surg [Br] 77:159, 1994.
653. Lombardi LJ, Cleri DJ, Epstein E: Bilateral spontaneous quadriceps tendon rupture in a patient with renal failure. Orthopedics 18:187, 1995.
654. Walker LG, Glick H: Bilateral spontaneous quadriceps tendon ruptures: A case report and review of the literature. Orthop Rev 8:867, 1989.
655. Nabors ED, Kremchek TE: Bilateral rupture of the extensor mechanism of the knee in healthy adults. Orthopedics 18:477, 1995.
656. Ramsey RH, Mueller GE: Quadriceps tendon rupture: A diagnostic trap. Clin Orthop 70:161, 1970.
657. Berlin RC, Levinsohn EM, Chrisman H: The wrinkled patellar tendon: An indication of abnormality in the extensor mechanism of the knee. Skel Radiol 20:181, 1991.
658. Kuivila TE, Brems JJ: Diagnosis of acute rupture of the quadriceps tendon by magnetic resonance imaging: A case report. Clin Orthop 262:236, 1991.
659. Smason JB: Post-traumatic fistula connecting prepatellar bursa with knee joint: Report of a case. J Bone Joint Surg [Am] 54:1553, 1972.
660. Jelaso DV, Morris GA: Rupture of the quadriceps tendon: Diagnosis by arthrography. Radiology 116:621, 1975.
661. Aprin H, Broukhim B: Early diagnosis of acute rupture of the quadriceps tendon by arthrography. Clin Orthop 185:185, 1985.
662. Laine H, Harjula A, Peltokaillio P: Ultrasound in the evaluation of the knee and patellar regions. J Ultras Med 6:33, 1987.
663. Bianchi S, Zwass A, Abdelwahab IF, et al: Diagnosis of tears of the quadriceps tendon of the knee: Value of sonography. AJR 162:1137, 1994.
664. Zeiss J, Saddemi SR, Ebraheim NA: MR imaging of the quadriceps tendon: Normal layered configuration and its importance in cases of tendon rupture. AJR 159:1031, 1992.
665. Schutzer SF, Ramsby GR, Fulkerson JP: The evaluation of patellofemoral pain using computerised tomography: A preliminary report. Clin Orthop 204:286, 1986.
666. Ho SSW, Jaureguito JW: Functional anatomy and biomechanics of the patellofemoral joint. Oper Tech Sports Med 2:238, 1994.
667. Conlan T, Garth WP, Lemons TE: Evaluation of the medial soft tissue restraints of the extensor mechanism of the knee. J Bone Joint Surg [Am] 75:682, 1993.
668. Insall JN, Falvo KA, Wise DN: Chondromalacia patellae. J Bone Joint Surg [Am] 58:1, 1976.
669. Insall JN, Salvati E: Patella position in the normal knee joint. Radiology 101:101, 1971.
670. Insall J, Goldberg V, Salvati E: Recurrent dislocation and the high-riding patella. Clin Orthop 88:67, 1972.
671. Blumensaat C: Die Lageabweichungen und Verrenkungen der Kniescheibe. Ergeb Chir Orthop 31:149, 1938.
672. Brattstrom H: Patella alta in non-dislocating knee joints. Acta Orthop Scand 41:578, 1970.
673. Labelle H, Laurin CA: Radiological investigation of normal and abnormal patellae. J Bone Joint Surg [Br] 57:530, 1975.
674. Blackburne JS, Peel TE: A new method of measuring patellar height. J Bone Joint Surg [Br] 59:241, 1977.
675. de Carvalho A, Andersen AH, Toop S, et al: A method for assessing the height of the patella. Int Orthop 9:195, 1985.
676. Gresalmer RP, Meadows S: The modified Insall-Salvati ratio for assessment of patellar height. Clin Orthop 282:170, 1992.
677. Merchant AC, Mercer RL, Jacobsen RM, et al: Roentgenographic analysis of patellofemoral congruence. J Bone Joint Surg [Am] 56:1391, 1974.
678. Laurin CA, Dussault R, Levesque HP: The tangential x-ray investigation of the patellofemoral joint: X-ray technique, diagnostic criteria, and interpretation. Clin Orthop 144:16, 1979.
679. Conway WF, Hayes CW, Loughran T, et al: Cross-sectional imaging of the patellofemoral joint and surrounding structures. RadioGraphics 11:195, 1991.
680. Inoue M, Shino K, Hirose H, et al: Subluxation of the patella: Computed tomography of patellofemoral congruence. J Bone Joint Surg [Am] 70:1331, 1988.
681. Martinez S, Korokken M, Fondren FB, et al: Diagnosis of patellofemoral malalignment by computed tomography. J Comput Assist Tomogr 7:1050, 1983.
682. Koskinen SK, Taimela S, Nelimarkka O, et al: Magnetic resonance imaging of patellofemoral relationships. Skel Radiol 22:403, 1993.
683. Shea KP: Radiographic evaluation of the patellofemoral joint. Oper Tech Sports Med 2:256, 1994.
684. Jones RB, Bartlett EC, Vainright JR, et al: CT determination of tibial tubercle lateralization in patients with anterior knee pain. Skel Radiol 24:505, 1995.
685. Stanford W, Phelan J, Kathol MH, et al: Patellofemoral joint motion: Evaluation by ultrafast computed tomography. Skel Radiol 17:487, 1988.
686. Shellock FG, Mink JH, Fox JM: Patellofemoral joint: Kinematic MR imaging to assess tracking abnormalities. Radiology 168:551, 1988.
687. Shellock FG, Mink JH, Deutsch AL, et al: Patellar tracking abnormalities: Clinical experience with kinematic MR imaging in 130 patients. Radiology 172:799, 1989.
688. Shellock FG, Foo TKF, Deutsch AL, et al: Patellofemoral joint: Evaluation during active flexion and ultrafast spoiled GRASS MR imaging. Radiology 180:581, 1991.
689. Shellock FG, Mink JH, Deutsch AL, et al: Kinematic MR imaging of the patellofemoral joint: Comparison of passive positioning and active movement techniques. Radiology 184:574, 1992.
690. Shellock FG, Mink JH, Deutsch AL, et al: Patellofemoral joint: Identification of abnormalities with active-movement, "unloaded" versus "loaded" kinematic MR imaging techniques. Radiology 188:575, 1993.
691. Brossmann J, Muhle C, Schröder C, et al: Patellar tracking patterns during active and passive knee extension: Evaluation with motion-triggered cine MR imaging. Radiology 187:205, 1993.
692. Brossmann J, Muhle C, Büll CC, et al: Evaluation of patellar tracking in patients with suspected patellar malalignment: Cine MR imaging vs arthroscopy. AJR 162:361, 1994.
693. Niitsu M, Akisada M, Anno I, et al: Moving knee joint: Technique for kinematic MR imaging. Radiology 174:569, 1990.
694. Hughston JC, Deese M: Medial subluxation of the patella as a complication of lateral release. Am J Sports Med 16:383, 1988.
695. Hughston JC: Patellar subluxation: A recent history. Clin Sports Med 8:153, 1989.
696. Kirsch MD, Fitzgerald SW, Friedman H, et al: Transient lateral patellar dislocation: Diagnosis with MR imaging. AJR 161:109, 1993.
697. Gilbert TJ, Johnson E, Detlie T, et al: Patellar dislocation: Medial retinacular tears, avulsion fractures, and osteochondral fragments. Orthopedics 16:732, 1993.
698. Kreitner K-F, Grebe P, Runkel M, et al: Stellenwert der MR-Tomographie bei traumatischen Patellaluxation. ROFO 163:32, 1995.
699. Virolainen H, Visuri T, Kuusela T: Acute dislocation of the patella: MR findings. Radiology 189:243, 1993.
700. Lance E, Deutsch AL, Mink JH: Prior lateral patellar dislocation: MR imaging findings. Radiology 189:905, 1993.
701. Aleman O: Chondromalacia post-traumatica patellae. Acta Chir Scand 63:149, 1928.
702. Ficat RP, Phillippe J, Hungerford DS: Chondromalacia patellae: A system of classification. Clin Orthop 144:55, 1979.
703. Jackson RW: Etiology of chondromalacia patellae. Instr Course Lect 25:36, 1976.
704. Outerbridge RE: The etiology of chondromalacia patellae. J Bone Joint Surg [Br] 43:752, 1961.
705. Arnoczky SP, Warren RF: Anatomy of the cruciate ligaments. In JA Feagin Jr (Ed): The Crucial Ligaments. New York, Churchill Livingstone, 1988, p. 179.

706. Dye SF, Cannon WD Jr: Anatomy and biomechanics of the anterior cruciate ligament. Clin Sports Med 7:715, 1988.

707. Girgis FG, Marshall JL, Monajem ARS: The cruciate ligaments of the knee joint: Anatomical, functional, and experimental analysis. Clin Orthop 106:216, 1975.

708. Harner CD, Livesay GA, Kashiwaguchi S, et al: Comparative study of the size and shape of human anterior and posterior cruciate ligaments. J Orthop Res 13:429, 1995.

709. Kennedy JC, Hawkins RJ, Willis RB, et al: Tension studies of human knee ligaments: Yield point, ultimate failure, and disruption of the cruciate and tibial collateral ligaments. J Bone Joint Surg [Am] 58:350, 1976.

710. Arnoczky SP: Anatomy of the anterior cruciate ligament. Clin Orthop 172:19, 1983.

711. Odensten M, Gillquist J: Functional anatomy of the anterior cruciate ligament and a rationale for reconstruction. J Bone Joint Surg [Am] 67:257, 1985.

712. Cabaud HE: Biomechanics of the anterior cruciate ligaments. Clin Orthop 172:26, 1983.

713. Hodler J, Haghighi P, Trudell D, et al: The cruciate ligaments of the knee: Correlation between MR appearance and gross and histologic findings in cadaveric specimens. AJR 159:357, 1992.

714. Danylchuk KD, Finlay JB, Kreck JP: Microstructural organization of human and bovine cruciate ligaments. Clin Orthop 131:294, 1978.

715. Cooper RR, Misol S: Tendon and ligament insertion: A light and electron microscopic study. J Bone Joint Surg [Am] 52:1, 1970.

716. Kennedy JC, Weinberg HW, Wilson AS: The anatomy and function of the anterior cruciate ligament. J Bone Joint Surg [Am] 56:223, 1974.

717. Daniel DM, Fritschy D: Anterior cruciate ligament injuries. *In* JC DeLee, D Drez Jr (Eds): Orthopaedic Sports Medicine: Principles and Practice. Philadelphia, WB Saunders Co, 1994, p. 1313.

718. Jennings AG: A proprioceptive role for the anterior cruciate ligament: A review of the literature. J Orthop Rheumatol 7:3, 1994.

719. Markolf KL, Mensch JS, Amstutz HC: Stiffness and laxity of the knee—contributions of the supporting structures: A quantitative in vitro study. J Bone Joint Surg [Am] 58:583, 1976.

720. Grood ES, Stowers SF, Noyes FR: Limits of motion in the human knee: Effect of sectioning the posterior cruciate ligament and posterolateral structures. J Bone Joint Surg [Am] 70:88, 1988.

721. Daniel DM, Stone ML: Diagnosis of knee ligament injury: Tests and measurements of joint laxity. *In* JA Feagin Jr (Ed): The Crucial Ligaments. New York, Churchill Livingstone, 1988, p. 287.

722. Owens TC: Posteromedial pivot shift of the knee: A new test for rupture of the posterior cruciate ligament. A demonstration in six patients and a study of anatomical specimens. J Bone Joint Surg [Am] 76:532, 1994.

723. Noyes FR, Mooar PA, Matthews DS, et al: The symptomatic anterior cruciate deficient knee. I. The long-term functional disability in athletically active individuals. J Bone Joint Surg [Am] 65:154, 1983.

724. Noyes FR, Grood ES: Diagnosis of knee ligament injuries: Clinical concepts. *In* JA Feagin Jr (Ed): The Crucial Ligaments. New York, Churchill Livingstone, 1988, p. 261.

725. Balkfors B: The course of knee-ligament injuries. Acta Orthop Scand 198:1, 1982.

726. Speer KP, Warren RF, Wickiewicz TL, et al: Observations on the injury mechanism of anterior cruciate ligament tears in skiers. Am J Sports Med 23:77, 1995.

727. Fetto JF, Marshall JL: The natural history and diagnosis of anterior cruciate ligament insufficiency. Clin Orthop 147:29, 1980.

728. Feagin JA, Curl WW: Isolated tear of the anterior cruciate ligament: 5-year follow-up study. Am J Sports Med 4:95, 1976.

729. Feagin JA: The syndrome of the torn anterior cruciate ligament. Orthop Clin North Am 10:81, 1979.

730. Arnold JA, Coker TP, Heaton LM, et al: Natural history of anterior cruciate tears. Am J Sports Med 7:305, 1979.

731. Kim S-J, Kim H-K: Reliability of the anterior drawer test, the pivot test, and the Lachman test. Clin Orthop 317:237, 1995.

732. Liu SH, Osti L, Henry M, et al: The diagnosis of acute complete tears of the anterior cruciate ligament: Comparison of MRI, arthrometry, and clinical examination. J Bone Joint Surg [Br] 77:586, 1995.

733. Malcolm LL, Daniel DM, Stone ML, et al: The measurement of anterior knee laxity after ACL reconstructive surgery. Clin Orthop 196:35, 1985.

734. Daniel DM, Malcolm LL, Losse G, et al: Instrumented measurement of anterior laxity of the joint. J Bone Joint Surg [Am] 67:720, 1985.

735. Noyes FR, Bassett RW, Grood ES, et al: Arthroscopy in acute traumatic hemarthrosis of the knee. J Bone Joint Surg [Am] 62:687, 1980.

736. Gillquist J, Hagberg G, Oretorp N: Arthroscopy in acute injuries of the knee joint. Acta Orthop Scand 48:190, 1977.

737. De Haven KE: Diagnosis of acute knee injuries with hemarthrosis. Am J Sports Med 8:9, 1980.

738. Lintner DM, Kamaric E, Moseley JB, et al: Partial tears of the anterior cruciate ligament: Are they clinically detectable? Am J Sports Med 23:111, 1995.

739. Meyers MH, McKeever FM: Fracture of the intercondylar eminence. J Bone Joint Surg [Am] 41:209, 1959.

740. Eady JL, Cardenas CD, Sopa D: Avulsion of the femoral attachment of the anterior cruciate ligament in a seven-year-old child. J Bone Joint Surg [Am] 64:1376, 1982.

741. Stallenberg B, Gevenois PA, Sintzoff SA Jr, et al: Fracture of the posterior aspect of the lateral tibial plateau: Radiographic sign of anterior cruciate ligament tear. Radiology 187:821, 1993.

742. Losee RE, Johnson TR, Southwick WO: Anterior subluxation of the lateral tibial plateau. J Bone Joint Surg [Am] 60:1015, 1978.

743. Galway HR, MacIntosh DL: The lateral pivot shift: A symptom and sign of anterior cruciate ligament insufficiency. Clin Orthop 147:45, 1980.

744. Cobby MJ, Schweitzer ME, Resnick D: The deep lateral femoral notch: An indirect sign of a torn anterior cruciate ligament. Radiology 184:855, 1992.

745. Warren RF, Kaplan N, Bach BR: The lateral notch sign of anterior cruciate ligament insufficiency. Am J Knee Surg 1:119, 1988.

746. Mittler S, Freiberger RH, Harrison-Stubbs M: A method of improving cruciate ligament visualization in double contrast arthrography. Radiology 102:441, 1972.

747. Arcomano JP, Anetrella LJ: Visualizing the anterior cruciate ligament. AJR 138:1189, 1982.

748. Reider B, Clancy W, Langer LO: Diagnosis of cruciate ligament injury using single contrast arthrography. Am J Sports Med 12:451, 1984.

749. Dalinka MK, Gohel VK, Rancier L: Tomography in the evaluation of the anterior cruciate ligament. Radiology 108:31, 1973.

750. Pavlov H, Torg JS: Double contrast arthrographic evaluation of the anterior cruciate ligament. Radiology 126:661, 1978.

751. Pavlov H, Freiberger RH: An easy method to demonstrate the cruciate ligaments by double contrast arthrography. Radiology 126:817, 1978.

752. Pavlov H, Warren RF, Sherman MF, et al: The accuracy of double-contrast arthrographic evaluation of the anterior cruciate ligament: A retrospective review of one hundred and sixty-three knees with surgical confirmation. J Bone Joint Surg [Am] 65:175, 1983.

753. Pavlov H: The radiographic diagnosis of the anterior cruciate ligament deficient knee. Clin Orthop 172:57, 1983.

754. Brody GA, Pavlov H, Warren RF, et al: Plica synovialis infra-patellaris: Arthrographic sign of anterior cruciate ligament disruption. AJR 140:767, 1983.

755. Braunstein EM: Anterior cruciate ligament injuries: A comparison of arthrographic and physical diagnosis. AJR 138:423, 1982.

756. Ptasznik R, Feller J, Bartlett J, et al: The value of sonography in the diagnosis of traumatic rupture of the anterior cruciate ligament of the knee. AJR 164:1461, 1995.

757. Lerman JE, Gray DS, Schweitzer ME, et al: MR evaluation of the anterior cruciate ligament: Value of axial images. J Comput Assist Tomogr 19:604, 1995.

758. Fitzgerald SW, Remer EM, Friedman H, et al: MR evaluation of the anterior cruciate ligament: Value of supplementing sagittal images with coronal and axial images. AJR 160:1233, 1993.

759. Remer EM, Fitzgerald SW, Friedman H, et al: Anterior cruciate ligament injury: MR imaging diagnosis and patterns of injury. RadioGraphics 12:901, 1992.

760. Buckwalter KA, Pennes DR: Anterior cruciate ligament: Oblique sagittal MR imaging. Radiology 175:276, 1990.

761. Vellet AD, Fowler P, Marks P, et al: Accuracy of non-orthogonal MR imaging in acute disruption of the anterior cruciate ligament. Radiology 173(P):233, 1989.

762. Mink JH, Levy T, Crues JV III: Tears of the anterior cruciate ligament and menisci of the knee: MR imaging evaluation. Radiology 167:769, 1988.

763. Niitsu M, Anno I, Fukubayashi T, et al: Tears of the cruciate ligaments and menisci: Evaluation with cine MR imaging. Radiology 178:859, 1991.

764. Lee JK, Yao L, Phelps CT, et al: Anterior cruciate ligament tears: MR imaging compared with arthroscopy and clinical tests. Radiology 166:861, 1988.

765. Vahey TN, Broome DR, Kaye KJ, et al: Acute and chronic tears of the anterior cruciate ligament: Differential features at MR imaging. Radiology 181:251, 1991.

766. Umans H, Wimpfheimer O, Haramati N, et al: Diagnosis of partial tears of the anterior cruciate ligament of the knee: Value of MR imaging. AJR 165:893, 1995.

767. Yao L, Gentili A, Petrus L, et al: Partial ACL rupture: An MR diagnosis? Skel Radiol 24:247, 1995.

768. Vahey T, Meyer SF, Shelbourne KD, et al: MR imaging of anterior cruciate ligament injuries. MRI Clin North Am 2:365, 1994.

769. Kaye JJ: Ligament and tendon tears: Secondary signs. Radiology 188:616, 1993.

770. Tung GA, Davis LM, Wiggens ME, et al: Tears of the anterior cruciate ligament: Primary and secondary signs at MR imaging. Radiology 188:661, 1993.

771. Liu SH, Osti Dorey F, et al: Anterior cruciate ligament tear: A new diagnostic index on magnetic resonance imaging. Clin Orthop 302:147, 1994.

772. Gentili A, Seeger LL, Yao L, et al: Anterior cruciate ligament tear: Indirect signs at MR imaging. Radiology 193:835, 1994.

773. Robertson PL, Schweitzer ME, Bartolozzi AR, et al: Anterior cruciate ligament tears: Evaluation of multiple signs with MR imaging. Radiology 193:829, 1994.

774. Staron RB, Haramati N, Feldman F, et al: O'Donoghue's triad: magnetic resonance imaging evidence. Skel Radiol 23:633, 1994.

775. Leach WJ, King JB: Posterior reattachment of the torn anterior cruciate ligament. J Bone Joint Surg [Br] 76:159, 1994.

776. Chan WP, Peterfy C, Fritz RC, et al: MR diagnosis of complete tears of the anterior cruciate ligament of the knee: Importance of anterior subluxation of the tibia. AJR 162:355, 1994.

777. McCauley TR, Moses M, Kier R, et al: MR diagnosis of tears of anterior cruciate ligament of the knee: Importance of ancillary findings. AJR 162:115, 1994.

778. Boeree NR, Ackroyd CE: Magnetic resonance imaging of anterior cruciate ligament rupture: A new diagnostic sign. J Bone Joint Surg [Br] 74:614, 1992.

779. Schweitzer ME, Cervilla V, Kursunoglu-Brahme S, et al: The PCL line: An indirect sign of anterior cruciate ligament injury. Clin Imaging 16:43, 1992.

780. Vahey TN, Hunt JE, Shelbourne KD: Anterior translocation of the tibia at MR imaging: A secondary sign of anterior cruciate ligament tear. Radiology 187:817, 1993.

781. Kapelov SR, Teresi LM, Bradley WG, et al: Bone contusions of the knee: Increased lesion detection with fast spin-echo MR imaging with spectroscopic fat saturation. Radiology 189:901, 1993.

782. Murphy BJ, Smith RL, Uribe JW, et al: Bone signal abnormalities in the posterolateral tibia and lateral femoral condyle in complete tears of the anterior cruciate ligament: A specific sign? Radiology 182:221, 1992.

783. Kaplan PA, Walker CW, Kilcoyne RF, et al: Occult fracture patterns of the knee associated with anterior cruciate ligament tears: Assessment with MR imaging. Radiology 183:835, 1992.

784. Kaneko K, Demouy EH, Brunet ME: Correlation between occult bone lesions and meniscoligamentous injuries in patients with traumatic knee joint disease. Clin Imaging 17:253, 1993.

785. Stein LN, Fischer DA, Fritts HM, et al: Occult osseous lesions associated with anterior cruciate ligament tears. Clin Orthop 313:187, 1995.

786. Fowler PJ: Bone injuries associated with anterior cruciate ligament disruption. Arthroscopy 10:453, 1994.

787. Buckley SC, Barrack RL, Alexander AH: The natural history of conservatively treated partial anterior cruciate ligament tears. Am J Sports Med 17:221, 1989.

788. Zeiss J, Paley K, Murray K, et al: Comparison of bone contusion seen by MRI in partial and complete tears of the anterior cruciate ligament. J Comput Assist Tomogr 19:773, 1995.

789. McDaniel WJ, Dameron TB: Untreated ruptures of the anterior cruciate ligament: A follow-up. J Bone Joint Surg [Am] 62:696, 1980.

790. McDaniel WJ, Dameron TB: The untreated anterior cruciate ligament rupture. Clin Orthop 172:158, 1983.

791. Daniel DM, Fithian DC: Indications for ACL surgery. Arthroscopy 10:434, 1994.

792. Beynnon BD, Johnson RJ, Fleming BC: The mechanics of anterior cruciate ligament reconstruction. In DW Jackson (Ed): The Anterior Cruciate Ligament: Current and Future Concepts. New York, Raven Press, 1993, p. 259.

793. Johnson RJ, Beynnon BD, Nichols CE, et al: Current concepts review: The treatment of injuries to the anterior cruciate ligament. J Bone Joint Surg [Am] 74:140, 1992.

794. Swenson TM, Fu FH: Graft selection for anterior cruciate ligament reconstruction. Oper Tech Orthop 5:261, 1995.

795. Noyes FR, Butler D, Grood E, et al: Biomechanical analysis of human ligament grafts used in knee ligament repairs and reconstruction. J Bone Joint Surg [Am] 66:344, 1984.

796. Noyes FR, Butler D, Paulos LE, et al: Intra-articular cruciate reconstruction. 1. Perspectives on graft strength, vascularization, and immediate motion after replacement. Clin Orthop 172:71, 1983.

797. McFarland EG, Morrey BF, An KN, et al: The relationship of vascularity and water content to tensile strength in a patellar tendon replacement of the anterior cruciate in dogs. Am J Sports Med 14:436, 1986.

798. Yasuda K, Tomiyama Y, Ohkoshi Y, et al: Arthroscopic observations of autogenetic quadriceps and patellar tendon grafts after anterior cruciate ligament reconstruction of the knee. Clin Orthop 246:217, 1989.

799. Clancy WG, Ray M, Zoltan J: Nonoperative or operative treatment of acute anterior cruciate ligament tears. J Bone Joint Surg [Am] 70:1483, 1988.

800. Grood ES, Hefzy MS, Butler DL, et al: On the placement and the initial tension of anterior cruciate ligament substitutes. Trans Orthop Res Soc 8:92, 1983.

801. Burns GS, Howell SM: The effect of tibial hole placement and roofplasty on impingement of anterior cruciate ligament reconstructions. Trans Orthop Res 17:656, 1992.

802. Hefzy MS, Grood ES: Sensitivity of insertion locations on length patterns of anterior cruciate ligament fibers. J Biomech Eng 108:73, 1986.

803. Jackson DW, Gasser SI: Tibial tunnel placement in ACL reconstruction. Arthroscopy 10:124, 1994.

804. Howell SM, Barad SJ: Knee extension and its relationship to the slope of the intercondylar roof: Implications for positioning the tibial tunnel in anterior cruciate ligament reconstructions. Am J Sports Med 23:288, 1995.

805. Muneta T, Yamamoto H, Ishibashi T, et al: The effects of tibial tunnel placement and roofplasty on reconstructed anterior cruciate ligament knees. Arthroscopy 11:57, 1995.

806. Moyen B, Lerat J-L: Artificial ligaments for anterior cruciate replacement: A new generation of problems. J Bone Joint Surg [Br] 76:173, 1994.

807. Vergis A, Gillquist J: Graft failure in intra-articular anterior cruciate ligament reconstructions: A review of the literature. Arthroscopy 11:312, 1995.

808. Paulos LE, Rosenberg TD, Drawbert J, et al: Infrapatellar contracture syndrome: An unrecognized cause of knee stiffness with patella entrapment and patella infera. Am J Sports Med 15:331, 1987.

809. Jackson DW, Schaefer RK: Cyclops syndrome: Loss of extension following intra-articular ACL reconstruction. Arthroscopy 6:171, 1990.

810. Manaster BJ, Remley K, Newman AP, et al: Knee ligament reconstruction: Plain film analysis. AJR 150:337, 1988.

811. Howell SM, Clark JA: Tibial tunnel placement in anterior cruciate ligament reconstructions and graft impingement. Clin Orthop 283:187, 1992.

812. Christen B, Jakob RP: Fractures associated with patellar ligament grafts in cruciate ligament surgery. J Bone Joint Surg [Br] 74:617, 1992.

813. Bonamo JJ, Krinick RM, Sporn AA: Rupture of the patellar ligament after use of its central third for anterior cruciate ligament reconstruction: A report of two cases. J Bone Joint Surg [Am] 66:1294, 1984.

814. McCarroll JR: Fracture of the patella during a golf swing following reconstruction of the anterior cruciate ligament: A case report. Am J Sports Med 11:26, 1983.

815. Watanabe BM, Howell SM: Arthroscopic findings associated with roof impingement of an anterior cruciate ligament graft. Am J Sports Med 23:616, 1995.

816. Moeser P, Bechtold RE, Clark T, et al: MR imaging of anterior cruciate ligament repair. J Comput Assist Tomogr 13:105, 1989.

817. Rak KM, Gillogly SD, Schaefer RA, et al: Anterior cruciate ligament reconstruction: Evaluation with MR imaging. Radiology 178:553, 1991.

818. Allgayer B, Gradinger R, Lehner K, et al: Die Kernspintomographie zur Beurteilung des vorderen Kreuzbandersatzes mit Sehnentransplantaten. ROFO 155:294, 1991.

819. Autz G, Goodwin C, Singson RD: Magnetic resonance evaluation of anterior cruciate ligament repair using the patellar tendon double bone block technique. Skel Radiol 20:585, 1991.

820. Howell SM, Berns GS, Farley TE: Unimpinged and impinged anterior cruciate ligament grafts: MR signal intensity measurements. Radiology 179:639, 1991.

821. Howell SM, Clark JA, Blasier RD: Serial magnetic resonance imaging of hamstring anterior cruciate ligament autografts during the first year of implantation: A preliminary study. Am J Sports Med 19:42, 1991.

822. Yamato M, Yamagishi T: MRI of patellar tendon anterior cruciate ligament autografts. J Comput Assist Tomogr 16:604, 1992.

823. Howell SM, Clark JA, Farley TE: Serial magnetic resonance study assessing the effects of impingement on the MR image of the patellar tendon graft. Arthroscopy 8:350, 1992.

824. Cheung Y, Magee TH, Rosenberg ZS, et al: MRI of anterior cruciate ligament reconstruction. J Comput Assist Tomogr 16:134, 1992.

825. Maywood RM, Murphy BJ, Uribe JW, et al: Evaluation of arthroscopic anterior cruciate ligament reconstruction using magnetic resonance imaging. Am J Sports Med 21:523, 1993.

826. Wacker F, Schilling A, Dihlmann SW, et al: Die Kernspintomographie bei autologer Plastik des vorderen Kreuzbandes: Vergleich zweier Operationsmethoden. ROFO 162:51, 1995.

827. Sanchis-Alfonso V, Martinez-Sanjuan V, Gastaldi-Orquin E: The value of MRI in the evaluation of the ACL deficient knee and in the post-operative evaluation after ACL reconstruction. Eur J Radiol 16:126, 1993.

828. Coupens SD, Yates CK, Sheldon C, et al: Magnetic resonance imaging evaluation of the patellar tendon after use of its central one-third for anterior cruciate ligament reconstruction. Am J Sports Med 20:332, 1992.

829. Recht MP, Piraino DW, Cohen MAH, et al: Localized anterior arthrofibrosis (cyclops lesion) after reconstruction of the anterior cruciate ligament: MR imaging findings. AJR 165:383, 1995.

830. Covey DC, Sapega AA: Injuries of the posterior cruciate ligament. J Bone Joint Surg [Am] 75:1376, 1993.

831. Fowler PJ, Messieh SS: Isolated PCL injuries in athletes. Am J Sports Med 15:553, 1987.

832. Bianchi M: Acute tears of the PCL: Clinical study and results of operative treatment in 27 cases. Am J Sports Med 11:308, 1983.

833. Cross MJ, Powell JF: Long-term followup of PCL rupture: A study of 116 cases. Am J Sports Med 12:292, 1984.

834. DeLee JC, Bergfeld JA, Drez D Jr, et al: The posterior cruciate ligament. In JC DeLee, D Drez Jr (Eds): Orthopaedic Sports Medicine: Principles and Practice. Philadelphia, WB Saunders Co, 1994, p. 1374.

835. Fanelli GC: Posterior cruciate ligament injuries in trauma patients. J Arthrosc Rel Surg 9:291, 1993.

836. Barton TM, Torg JS, Das M: PCL insufficiency: A review of the literature. Sports Med 1:419, 1984.

837. Fanelli GC, Giannotti BF, Edson CJ: The posterior cruciate ligament arthroscopic evaluation and treatment. Arthroscopy 10:637, 1994.

838. Rubinstein RA Jr, Shelbourne D, McCarroll JR, et al: The accuracy of the clinical examination in the setting of posterior cruciate ligament injuries. Am J Sports Med 22:550, 1994.

839. Sonin AH, Fitzgerald SW, Hoff FL, et al: MR imaging of the posterior cruciate ligament: Normal, abnormal, and associated injury patterns. Radiographics 15:551, 1995.

840. Grover JS, Bassett LW, Gross ML, et al: Posterior cruciate ligament: MR imaging. Radiology *174*:527, 1990.
841. Hunter JC, Chapman JR: Isolated avulsion of the posterior cruciate ligament: An uncommon dashboard injury. AJR *164*:1190, 1995.
842. Sonin AH, Fitzgerald SW, Friedman II, et al: Posterior cruciate ligament injury: MR imaging diagnosis and patterns of injury. Radiology *190*:455, 1994.
843. Fu FH, Harner CD, Johnson DL, et al: Biomechanics of knee ligaments: Basic concepts and clinical application. J Bone Joint Surg [Am] *75*:1716, 1993.
844. Anderson JK, Noyes FR: Principles of posterior cruciate ligament reconstruction. Orthopedics *18*:493, 1995.
845. Malek MM: Arthroscopic allograft: Posterior cruciate ligament reconstruction. Oper Tech Sports Med *3*:157, 1995.
846. Schulte KR, Harner CD: Management of isolated posterior cruciate ligament injuries. Oper Tech Orthop *5*:270, 1995.
847. Siliski JM, Mahring M, Hofer HP: Supracondylar-intercondylar fractures of the femur: Treatment by internal fixation. J Bone Joint Surg [Am] *71*:95, 1989.
848. Helfet DL: Fractures of the distal femur. *In* BD Browner, JB Jupiter, AM Levine, et al (Eds): Skeletal Trauma: Fractures, Dislocations, Ligamentous Injuries. Philadelphia, WB Saunders Co, 1992, p. 1643.
849. Seinsheimer F III: Fractures of the distal femur. Clin Orthop *153*:169, 1980.
850. Hohl M, Larson RL, Jones DC: Fractures and dislocations of the knee. *In* CA Rockwood Jr, DP Green (Eds): Fractures in Adults. 2nd Ed. Philadelphia, JB Lippincott Co, 1984, p. 1429.
851. Klingensmith W, Oles P, Martinez H: Arterial injuries associated with dislocation of the knee or fracture of the lower femur. Surg Gynecol Obstet *120*:961, 1965.
852. Neer CS, Grantham SA, Shelton ML: Supracondylar fracture of the adult femur. J Bone Joint Surg *49*:591, 1967.
853. Pogrund H, Husseini N, Bloom R, Finsterbush A: The cleavage intercondylar fracture of the femur. Clin Orthop *160*:74, 1981.
854. Giles JB, DeLee JC, Heckman JD, Keever JE: Supracondylar-intercondylar fractures of the femur treated with a supracondylar plate and lag screw. J Bone Joint Surg [Am] *64*:864, 1982.
855. Lewis SL, Pozo JL, Muirhead-Allwood WFG: Coronal fractures of the lateral femoral condyle. J Bone Joint Surg [Br] *71*:118, 1989.
856. Carpenter JE, Kasman R, Matthews LS: Fractures of the patella. J Bone Joint Surg [Am] *75*:1550, 1993.
857. Hensal F, Nelson T, Pavlov H, Torg JS: Bilateral patellar fractures from indirect trauma: A case report. Clin Orthop *178*:207, 1983.
858. Lotke PA, Ecker ML: Transverse fractures of the patella. Clin Orthop *158*:180, 1981.
859. Bostrom A: Fracture of the patella: A study of 422 patellar fractures. Acta Orthop Scand (Suppl) *143*:5, 1972.
860. Scapinelli R: Blood supply of the human patella: Its relation to ischaemic necrosis after fracture. J Bone Joint Surg [Br] *49*:563, 1967.
861. Heckman JD, Alkire CC: Distal patellar pole fractures: A proposed common mechanism of injury. Am J Sports Med *12*:424, 1984.
862. Bates DG, Hresko MT, Jaramillo D: Patellar sleeve fracture: Demonstration with MR imaging. Radiology *193*:825, 1994.
863. Shands PA, McQueen DA: Demonstration of avulsion fracture of the inferior pole of the patella by magnetic resonance imaging: A case report. Radiology *193*:825, 1994.
864. Dashefsky JH: Fracture of the fabella: A case report. J Bone Joint Surg [Am] *59*:698, 1977.
865. Frey C, Bjorkengren A, Sartoris D, et al: Knee dysfunction secondary to dislocation of the fabella. Clin Orthop *222*:223, 1987.
866. Rafii M, Lamont JG, Firooznia H: Tibial plateau fractures: CT evaluation and classification. CRC Crit Rev Diagn Imaging *27*:91, 1987.
867. Elstrom J, Pankovich AM, Sassoon H, Rodriguez J: The use of tomography in the assessment of fractures of the tibial plateau. J Bone Joint Surg [Am] *58*:551, 1976.
868. Rafii M, Firooznia H, Golimbu C, Bonamo J: Computed tomography of tibial plateau fractures. AJR *142*:1181, 1984.
869. Newberg AH, Greenstein R: Radiographic evaluation of tibial plateau fractures. Radiology *126*:319, 1978.
870. Dias JJ, Stirling AJ, Finlay DBL, Gregg PJ: Computerised axial tomography for tibial plateau fractures. J Bone Joint Surg [Br] *69*:84, 1987.
871. Barrow BA, Fajman WA, Parker LM, et al: Tibial plateau fractures: Evaluation with MR imaging. Radiographics *14*:553, 1994.
872. McEnery KW, Wilson AJ, Pilgram TK, et al: Fractures of the tibial plateau: Value of spiral CT coronal plane reconstructions for detecting displacement in vitro. AJR *163*:1177, 1994.
873. Kode L, Lieberman JM, Motta AO, et al: Evaluation of tibial plateau fractures: Efficacy of MR imaging compared with CT. AJR *163*:141, 1994.
874. McConkey JP, Meeuwisse W: Tibial plateau fractures in alpine skiing. Am J Sports Med *16*:159, 1988.
875. Rogers LF: Radiology of Skeletal Trauma. 2nd Ed. New York, Churchill Livingstone, 1992.
876. Anglen JO, Healy WL: Tibial plateau fractures. Orthopedics *11*:1527, 1988.
877. Honkonen SE, Järvinen MJ: Classification of fractures of the tibial condyles. J Bone Joint Surg [Br] *74*:840, 1992.
878. Hohl M: Tibial condylar fractures. J Bone Joint Surg [Am] *49*:1455, 1967.
879. Moore TM: Fracture-dislocation of the knee. Clin Orthop *156*:128, 1981.
880. Waddell JP, Johnston DWC, Neidre A: Fractures of the tibial plateau: A review of ninety-five patients and comparison of treatment methods. J Trauma *21*:376, 1981.
881. Ottolenghi CE: Vascular complications in injuries about the knee joint. Clin Orthop *165*:148, 1982.
882. Jensen DB, Bjerg-Nielsen A, Laursen N: Conventional radiographic examination in the evaluation of sequelae after tibial plateau fractures. Skel Radiol *17*:330, 1988.
883. Meyers MH, McKeever FM: Fracture of the intercondylar eminence of the tibia. J Bone Joint Surg [Am] *41*:209, 1959.
884. Nichols JN, Tehranzadeh J: A review of tibial spine fractures in bicycle injury. Am J Sports Med *15*:172, 1987.
885. Kendall NS, Hsu SY, Chan K-M: Fracture of the tibial spine in adults and children: A review of 31 cases. J Bone Joint Surg [Br] *74*:848, 1992.
886. Platt H: On the peripheral nerve complications of certain fractures. J Bone Joint Surg *10*:403, 1928.
887. Hill JA, Rana NA: Complications of posterolateral dislocation of the knee: Case report and literature review. Clin Orthop *154*:212, 1981.
888. Kennedy JC: Complete dislocation of the knee joint. J Bone Joint Surg [Am] *45*:889, 1963.
889. Reckling FW, Peltier LF: Acute knee dislocations and their complications. J Trauma *9*:181, 1969.
890. Meyers MH, Harvey JR Jr: Traumatic dislocation of the knee joint: A study of eighteen cases. J Bone Joint Surg [Am] *53*:16, 1971.
891. Taylor AR, Arden GP, Rainey HA: Traumatic dislocation of the knee: A report of forty-three cases with special reference to conservative treatment. J Bone Joint Surg [Br] *54*:96, 1972.
892. Frassica FJ, Sim FH, Staeheli JW, et al: Dislocation of the knee. Clin Orthop *263*:200, 1991.
893. Roman PD, Hopson CN, Zenni EJ Jr: Traumatic dislocation of the knee: A report of 30 cases and literature review. Orthop Rev *16*:917, 1987.
894. Cooper DE, Speer KP, Wickiewicz TL, et al: Complete knee dislocation without posterior cruciate ligament disruption. Clin Orthop *284*:228, 1992.
895. Kaufman SL, Martin LG: Arterial injuries associated with complete dislocation of the knee. Radiology *184*:153, 1992.
896. Bloom MH: Traumatic knee dislocation and popliteal artery occlusion. Phys Sports Med *15*:143, 1987.
897. McCoy GF, Hannon DG, Barr RJ, et al: Vascular injury associated with low-velocity dislocations of the knee. J Bone Joint Surg [Br] *69*:285, 1987.
898. Yu JS, Goodwin D, Salonen D, et al: Complete dislocation of the knee: Spectrum of associated soft-tissue injuries depicted by MR imaging. AJR *164*:135, 1995.
899. Brattstrom H: Shape of the intercondylar groove normally and in recurrent dislocation of the patella. Acta Orthop Scand (Suppl) *68*:5, 1964.
900. Brattstrom H: Patella alta in non-dislocating knee joints. Acta Orthop Scand *41*:578, 1970.
901. Frangakis EK: Intra-articular dislocation of the patella: A case report. J Bone Joint Surg [Am] *56*:423, 1974.
902. Allen FJ: Intercondylar dislocation of the patella. S Afr Med J *18*:66, 1944.
903. Deaderick C: Case of rupture of quadriceps femoris tendon with dislocation of the patella beneath the intercondyloid groove of the femur. Ann Surg *11*:102, 1890.
904. Feneley RCL: Inter-articular dislocation of the patella: Report of a case. J Bone Joint Surg [Br] *50*:653, 1968.
905. Murakami Y: Intra-articular dislocation of the patella: A case report. Clin Orthop *171*:137, 1982.
906. Moed BR, Morawa LG: Acute traumatic lateral dislocation of the patella: An unusual case presentation. J Trauma *22*:516, 1982.
907. Hanspal RS: Superior dislocation of the patella. Injury *16*:487, 1985.
908. van den Brock TAA, Moll PJ: Horizontal rotation of the patella. Acta Orthop Scand *56*:436, 1985.
909. Corso SJ, Thal R, Forman D: Locked patellar dislocation with vertical axis rotation: A case report. Clin Orthop *279*:190, 1992.
910. Miller PR, Klein RM, Teitge RA: Medial dislocation of the patella. Skel Radiol *20*:429, 1991.
911. Milgram JE: Tangential osteochondral fracture of the patella. J Bone Joint Surg *25*:271, 1943.
912. Morscher E: Cartilage-bone lesions of the knee joint following injury. Reconstr Surg Traumatol *12*:2, 1971.
913. Ahstrom JP: Osteochondral fracture in the knee joint associated with hypermobility and dislocation of the patella. J Bone Joint Surg [Am] *47*:1491, 1965.
914. Frandsen PA, Kristensen H: Osteochondral fracture associated with dislocation of the patella: Another mechanism of injury. J Trauma *19*:195, 1979.
915. McDougall A, Brown JD: Radiological sign of recurrent dislocation of the patella. J Bone Joint Surg [Br] *50*:841, 1968.
916. Freiberger RH, Kotzen LM: Fracture of the medial margin of the patella, a finding diagnostic of lateral dislocation. Radiology *88*:902, 1967.
917. Rorabeck CH, Bobechko WP: Acute dislocation of the patella with osteochondral fracture: A review of eighteen cases. J Bone Joint Surg [Br] *58*:237, 1976.

918. Jacobsen K, Metz P: Occult traumatic dislocation of the patella. J Trauma 16:829, 1976.

919. Vainionpää S, Laasonen E, Pätiälä H, Rusanen M, Rokkannen P: Acute dislocation of the patella. Acta Orthop Scand 57:331, 1986.

920. Nietosvaara Y, Aalto K, Kallio PE: Acute patellar dislocation in children: Incidence and associated osteochondral fractures. J Pediatr Orthop 14:513, 1994.

921. Resnick D, Newell JD, Guerra J Jr, et al: Proximal tibiofibular joint: Anatomic-pathologic-radiographic correlation. AJR 131:133, 1978.

922. Ogden JA: The anatomy and function of the proximal tibiofibular joint. Clin Orthop 101:186, 1974.

923. Jacobsen K: Landmarks of the knee joint on the lateral radiograph during rotation. ROFO 125:399, 1976.

924. Veth RPH, Kingma LM, Nielsen HKL: The abnormal proximal tibiofibular joint. Arch Orthop Trauma Surg 102:167, 1984.

925. Ogden JA: Dislocation of the proximal fibula. Radiology 105:547, 1972.

926. Parkes JC II, Zelko RR: Isolated acute dislocation of the proximal tibiofibular joint: Case report. J Bone Joint Surg [Am] 55:177, 1973.

927. Conforty B, Tal E, Margulies Y: Anterior dislocation of the head of the fibula. J Trauma 20:902, 1980.

928. Falkenberg P, Nygaard H: Isolated anterior dislocation of the proximal tibiofibular joint. J Bone Joint Surg [Br] 65:310, 1983.

929. Weinert CR Jr, Raczka R: Recurrent dislocation of the superior tibiofibular joint: Surgical stabilization by ligament reconstruction. J Bone Joint Surg [Am] 68:126, 1986.

930. Gianchino AA: Recurrent dislocations of the proximal tibiofibular joint. J Bone Joint Surg [Am] 68:1104, 1986.

931. Ogden JA: Subluxation and dislocation of the proximal tibiofibular joint. J Bone Joint Surg [Br] 56:145, 1974.

932. Baciu CC, Tudor A, Olaru I: Recurrent luxation of the superior tibiofibular joint in the adult. Acta Orthop Scand 45:772, 1974.

933. Sijbrandij S: Instability of the proximal tibio-fibular joint. Acta Orthop Scand 49:621, 1978.

934. Sharma P, Daffner RH: Case report 389. Skel Radiol 15:505, 1986.

935. Teshima R, Otsuka T, Takasu N, et al: Structure of the most superficial layer of articular cartilage. J Bone Joint Surg [Br] 77:460, 1995.

936. Campbell CJ: The healing of cartilage defects. Clin Orthop 64:45, 1969.

937. Landells JW: The reactions of injured human articular cartilage. J Bone Joint Surg [Br] 39:548, 1957.

938. Harris ED Jr: Biology of the joint. In WN Kelley, ED Harris Jr, S Ruddy, et al (Eds): Textbook of Rheumatology. Philadelphia, WB Saunders Co, 1985, p. 254.

939. Meachim G: Light microscopy of Indian ink preparations of fibrillated cartilage. Ann Rheum Dis 31:457, 1972.

940. Byers PD, Contepomi CA, Farker TA: A postmortem study of the hip joint. Ann Rheum Dis 29:15, 1970.

941. Buckland-Wright JC, MacFarlane DG, Jasani K, et al: Quantitative microfocal radiographic assessment of osteoarthritis of the knee from weight bearing tunnel and semiflexed standing views. J Rheumatol 21:1734, 1994.

942. Buckland-Wright JC, MacFarlane DG, Lynch JA, et al: Quantitative microfocal radiography detects changes in osteoarthritis knee joint space width in patients in placebo controlled trial of NSAID therapy. J Rheumatol 22:937, 1995.

943. Anderson PW, Maslin P: Tomography applied to knee arthrography. Radiology 110:271, 1974.

944. Thomas RH, Resnick D, Alazraki NP, et al: Compartmental evaluation of osteoarthritis of the knee: A comparative study of available diagnostic modalities. Radiology 116:585, 1975.

945. Kaufmann J, Langlotz M: Ist die idiopathische Chondropathia patellae mit radiologischen methoden Diagnostizierbar? ROFO 141:422, 1984.

946. Horns JW: The diagnosis of chondromalacia by double contrast arthrography of the knee. J Bone Joint Surg [Am] 59:119, 1977.

947. Thijn CJP: Double contrast arthrography in meniscal lesions and patellar chondropathy. Radiol Clin Biol 45:345, 1976.

948. Rau WS, Kauffmann G: Röntgendiagnostik des Knorpelschadens am Kniegelenk. Radiologe 18:451, 1978.

949. Reichelt A, Hehne HJ, Rau WS, et al: Die doppel Kontrast-arthrographie bei der Chondropathia patellae—klinische und experimentelle Studie zur Pathogenese und Diagnostik. Z Orthop 117:746, 1979.

950. Reiser M, Karpf P-M, Bernett P: Diagnosis of chondromalacia patellae using CT arthrography. Eur J Radiol 2:181, 1982.

951. Boven F, Bellemans M-A, Geurts J, et al: A comparative study of the patello-femoral joint on axial roentgenogram, axial arthrogram, and computed tomography following arthrography. Skel Radiol 8:179, 1982.

952. Boven F, Bellemans M-A, Geurts J, et al: The value of computed tomography scanning in chondromalacia patellae. Skel Radiol 8:183, 1982.

953. McCrae F, Shouls J, Dieppe P, et al: Scintigraphic assessment of osteoarthritis of the knee joint. Ann Rheum Dis 51:938, 1992.

954. Dieppe P, Cushnaghan J, Young P, et al: Prediction of the progression of joint space narrowing in osteoarthritis of the knee by bone scintigraphy. Ann Rheum Dis 52:557, 1993.

955. Hayes CW, Sawyer RW, Conway WF: Patellar cartilage lesions: In vitro detection and staging with MR imaging and pathologic correlation. Radiology 176:479, 1990.

956. Yulish BS, Montanez J, Goodfellow DB, et al: Chondromalacia patellae: Assessment with MR imaging. Radiology 164:763, 1987.

957. Hodler J, Resnick D: Chondromalacia patellae. AJR 158:101, 1992.

958. McCauley TR, Kier R, Lynch KJ, et al: Chondromalacia patellae: Diagnosis with MR imaging. AJR 158:101, 1992.

959. Handelberg F, Shahabpour M, Casteleyn P: Chondral lesions of the patella evaluated with computed tomography, magnetic resonance imaging, and arthroscopy. Arthroscopy 6:24, 1990.

960. Wojtys E, Wilson M, Buckwalter K, et al: Magnetic resonance imaging of knee hyaline cartilage and intraarticular pathology. Am J Sports Med 15:455, 1987.

961. Broderick LS, Turner DA, Renfrew DL, et al: Severity of articular cartilage abnormality in patients with osteoarthritis: Evaluation with fast spin-echo MR vs arthroscopy. AJR 162:99, 1994.

962. Lehner KB, Rechl HP, Gmeinwieser JK, et al: Structure, function and degeneration of bovine hyaline cartilage: Assessment with MR imaging in vitro. Radiology 170:495, 1989.

963. Wolff SD, Chesnick S, Frank JA, et al: Magnetization transfer contrast imaging of the knee. Radiology 179:623, 1991.

964. Chandnani VP, Ho C, Chu P, et al: Knee hyaline cartilage evaluated with MR imaging: A cadaveric study involving multiple imaging sequences and intraarticular injection of gadolinium and saline solution. Radiology 178:557, 1991.

965. Totterman S, Weiss SL, Szumowski J, et al: MR fat suppression technique in the evaluation of normal structure of the knee. J Comput Assist Tomogr 13:473, 1989.

966. König H, Sauter R, Deimling M, et al: Cartilage disorders: Comparison of spin-echo, CHESS, and FLASH sequence MR images. Radiology 164:753, 1987.

967. Speer KP, Spritzer CE, Goldner JL, et al: Magnetic resonance imaging of traumatic knee articular cartilage injuries. Am J Sports Med 19:396, 1991.

968. Tyrrell RL, Gluckert K, Pathria M, et al: Fast three-dimensional MR imaging of the knee: Comparison with arthroscopy. Radiology 166:865, 1988.

969. Heron CW, Calvert PT: Three-dimensional gradient-echo MR imaging of the knee: Comparison with arthroscopy in 100 patients. Radiology 183:839, 1992.

970. Reiser MF, Bongartz G, Erlemann R, et al: Magnetic resonance in cartilaginous lesions of the knee joint with three-dimensional gradient-echo imaging. Skel Radiol 17:465, 1988.

971. Gylys-Morin VM, Hajek PC, Sartoris DJ, et al: Articular cartilage defects: Detectability in cadaver knees with MR. AJR 148:1153, 1987.

972. Kramer J, Stiglbauer R, Engel A, et al: MR contrast arthrography (MRA) in osteochondrosis dissecans. J Comput Assist Tomogr 16:254, 1992.

973. Modl JM, Sether LA, Haughton VM, et al: Articular cartilage: Correlation of histologic zones with signal intensity at MR imaging. Radiology 181:853, 1991.

974. Recht MP, Kramer J, Marcelis S, et al: Abnormalities of articular cartilage in the knee: Analysis of available MR techniques. Radiology 187:473, 1993.

975. Rubenstein JD, Kim JK, Morava-Protzner I, et al: Effects of collagen orientation on MR imaging characteristics of bovine articular cartilage. Radiology 188:219, 1993.

976. Maroudas A: Physicochemical properties of articular cartilage. In MAR Freeman (Ed): Adult Articular Cartilage. London, Pitman Medical, 1979, p. 215.

977. Maroudas A, Weinberg PD, Parker KH: The distributions and diffusivities of small ions in chondroitin sulphate, hyaluronate and some proteoglycan solutions. Biophys Chem 32:257, 1988.

978. Maroudas A, Schneiderman R, Popper O: The role of water, proteoglycan, and collagen in solute transport in cartilage. In KE Kuettner, R Schleyerbach, JG Peyron, et al (Eds): Articular Cartilage and Osteoarthritis. New York, Raven Press, 1992, p. 355.

979. Maroudas A: Distribution and diffusion of solutes in articular cartilage. Biophys J 10:365, 1970.

980. Torzilli PA, Adams TC, Mis RJ: Transient solute diffusion in articular cartilage. J Biomech 2:203, 1987.

981. Burstein D, Gray ML, Hartman AL, et al: Diffusion of small solutes in cartilage as measured by nuclear magnetic resonance (NMR) spectroscopy and imaging. J Orthop Res 11:465, 1993.

982. Brandt KD, Adams ME: Exuberant repair of articular cartilage damage: Effect of anterior cruciate ligament transection in the dog. Trans Orthop Res Soc 14:584, 1989.

983. Vignon E, Arlot M, Hartman D, et al: Hypertrophic repair of articular cartilage in experimental osteoarthrosis. Ann Rheum Dis 42:82, 1983.

984. Braunstein EM, Brandt KD, Albrecht M: MRI demonstration of hypertrophic articular cartilage repair in osteoarthritis. Skel Radiol 19:335, 1990.

985. Adams ME, Brandt KD: Hypertrophic repair of canine articular cartilage in osteoarthritis after anterior cruciate ligament transection. J Rheumatol 18:428, 1991.

986. Pritzker KPH: Posttraumatic cartilage hypertrophy: Edema or repair? J Rheumatol 18:314, 1991.

987. Brandt KD, Braunstein EM, Visco DM, et al: Anterior (cranial) cruciate ligament transection in the dog: A bona fide model of osteoarthritis, not merely of cartilage injury and repair. J Rheumatol 18:436, 1991.

988. Yao L, Sinha S, Seeger LL: MR imaging of joints: Analytic optimization of GRE techniques at 1.5 T. AJR 158:339, 1992.

989. Hayes CW, Conway WF: Evaluation of articular cartilage: Radiographic and cross-sectional imaging techniques. RadioGraphics 12:409, 1992.

990. De Smet AA, Monu JUV, Fisher DR, et al: Signs of patellar chondromalacia on sagittal T2-weighted magnetic resonance imaging. Skel Radiol 21:103, 1992.

991. Hodler J, Berthiaume M-J, Schweitzer ME, et al: Knee joint hyaline cartilage defects: A comparative study of MR and anatomic sections. J Comput Assist Tomogr 16:597, 1992.

992. Brown TR, Quinn SF: Evaluation of chondromalacia of the patellofemoral compartment with axial magnetic resonance imaging. Skel Radiol 22:325, 1993.

993. Colin T, Provost N, Begin J, et al: Contribution of magnetic resonance imaging to the evaluation of femorotibial cartilage lesions. Rev Rhum Mal Osteoartic [Engl Ed] 61:297, 1994.

994. van Leersum MD, Schweitzer ME, Gannon F, et al: Thickness of patellofemoral articular cartilage as measured on MR imaging: sequence comparison of accuracy, reproducibility, and interobserver variation. Skel Radiol 24:431, 1995.

995. Tien RD: Fat-suppression MR imaging in neuroradiology: Techniques and clinical application. AJR 158:369, 1992.

996. Koskinen SK, Komu M, Aho HJ, et al: MR imaging of patellar cartilage degeneration at 0.02T: Study of 23 cadaveric patellae. Acta Radiol 32:514, 1991.

997. Rose PM, Demlow TA, Szumowski J, et al: Chondromalacia patellae: Fat-suppressed MR imaging. Radiology 193:437, 1994.

998. McAlindon TEM, Watt I, McCrae F, et al: Magnetic resonance imaging in osteoarthritis of the knee: Correlation with radiographic and scintigraphic findings. Ann Rheum Dis 50:14, 1991.

999. Nakanishi K, Inoue M, Harada K, et al: Subluxation of the patella: Evaluation of patellar articular cartilage with MR imaging. Br J Radiol 65:662, 1992.

1000. Chan WP, Lang P, Stevens MP, et al: Osteoarthritis of the knee: Comparison of radiography, CT, and MR imaging to assess extent and severity. AJR 157:799, 1991.

1001. Gagliardi JA, Chung EM, Chandnani VP, et al: Detection and staging of chondromalacia patellae: Relative efficacies of conventional MR imaging, MR arthrography, and CT arthrography. AJR 163:629, 1994.

1002. Disler DG, Peters TL, Muscoreil SJ, et al: Fat-suppressed spoiled GRASS imaging of knee hyaline cartilage: Technique optimization and comparison with conventional MR imaging. AJR 163:887, 1994.

1003. Adam G, Prescher A, Nolte-Ernsting C, et al: MRT des hyalinen Kniegelenkknorpels: Tierexperimentelle und klinische Untersuchungen. ROFO 160:143, 1994.

1004. Bongartz G, Bock E, Horbach T, et al: Degenerative cartilage lesions of the hip: magnetic resonance evaluation. Magn Res Imaging 7:179, 1989.

1005. Pilch L, Stewart C, Gordan D, et al: Assessment of cartilage volume in the femorotibial joint with magnetic resonance imaging and 3D computer reconstruction. J Rheumatol 21:2307, 1994.

1006. Eckstein F, Sittek H, Milz S, et al: The morphology of articular cartilage assessed by magnetic resonance imaging (MRI). Reproducibility and anatomic correlation. Surg Radiol Anat 16:429, 1994.

1007. Eckstein F, Sittek H, Gavazzeni A, et al: Der Kniegelenksknorpel in der Magnetresonanztomographie: MR-Chondrovolumetrie (MR-CVM) mittels fettunterdruckter FLASH-3D-Sequenz. Radiologe 35:87, 1995.

1008. Wolff SD, Balaban RS: Magnetization transfer contrast (MTC) and tissue water proton relaxation in vivo. Magn Reson Med 10:135, 1989.

1009. Wolff SD, Eng J, Balaban RS: Magnetization transfer contrast: Method for improving contrast in gradient-recalled-echo images. Radiology 179:133, 1991.

1010. Wolff SD, Chesnick S, Frank JA, et al: Magnetization transfer contrast: MR imaging of the knee. Radiology 179:623, 1991.

1011. Vahlensieck M, Dombrowski F, Leutner C, et al: Magnetization transfer contrast (MTC) and MTC-subtraction: Enhancement of cartilage lesions and intracartilaginous degeneration in vitro. Skel Radiol 23:535, 1994.

1012. Gray ML, Burnstein D, Lesperance LM, et al: Magnetization transfer in cartilage and its constituent macromolecules. Mag Reson Med 34:319, 1995.

1013. Jelicks LA, Paul PK, O'Byrne E, et al: Hydrogen-1, sodium-23, and carbon 13 MR spectroscopy of cartilage degeneration in vitro. J Magn Reson Imaging 3:565, 1993.

1014. Burnstein D, Gray ML, Hartman AL, et al: Diffusion of small solutes in cartilage as measured by nuclear magnetic resonance (NMR) spectroscopy and imaging. J Orthop Res 11:465, 1993.

1015. Parker F Jr, Keefer CS, Myers WK, et al: Histologic changes in the knee joint with advancing age: Relation to degenerative arthritis. Arch Pathol 17:516, 1934.

1016. Casscells SW: Gross pathological changes in the knee joint of the aged individual: A study of 300 cases. Clin Orthop 132:225, 1978.

1017. Wiley AM: Pathological and clinical aspects of degenerative disease of the knee. Can J Surg 11:14, 1968.

1018. Ostlere SJ, Seeger LL, Eckardt JJ: Subchondral cysts of the tibia secondary to osteoarthritis of the knee. Skel Radiol 19:287, 1990.

1019. Pottenger LA, Phillips FM, Draganich LF: The effect of marginal osteophytes on reduction of varus-valgus instability in osteoarthritic knees. Arthritis Rheum 33:853, 1990.

1020. Kindynis P, Haller J, Kang HS, et al: Osteophytes of the knee: Anatomic, radiologic, and pathologic investigation. Radiology 174:841, 1990.

1021. Hernborg J, Nilsson BE: Age and sex incidence of osteophytes in the knee joint. Acta Orthop Scand 44:66, 1973.

1022. Hernborg J, Nilsson BE: The relationship between osteophytes in the knee joint, osteoarthritis and aging. Acta Orthop Scand 44:69, 1973.

1023. Martin LM, Bourne RB, Rorabeck CH: Stress fractures associated with osteoarthritis of the knee: A report of three cases. J Bone Joint Surg [Am] 70:771, 1988.

1024. Lepoutre C: Sésamoid douloureux (sésamoide dujumeau externe): Guérison par l'extirpation. Rev Orthop 16:234, 1929.

1025. Mangieri JV: Peroneal-nerve injury from an enlarged fabella: A case report. J Bone Joint Surg [Am] 55:395, 1973.

1026. Weiner D, Macnab I, Turner M: The fabella syndrome. Clin Orthop 126:213, 1977.

1027. Bergenudd H, Johnell O, Redlund-Johnell I, et al: The articular cartilage after osteotomy for medial gonarthrosis: Biopsies after 2 years in 19 cases. Acta Orthop Scand 63:413, 1992.

1028. Bergman AG, Willen HK, Lindstrand AL, et al: Osteoarthritis of the knee: Correlation of subchondral MR signal abnormalities with histopathologic and radiographic features. Skel Radiol 23:445, 1994.

1029. Gahunia HK, LeMaire C, Babyn PS, et al: Osteoarthritis in Rhesus Macaque knee joint: Quantitative magnetic resonance imaging tissue characterization of articular cartilage. J Rheumatol 22:1747, 1995.

1030. Milgram JW: Radiologic and Histologic Pathology of Nontumorous Diseases of Bones and Joints. Northbrook, IL, Northbrook Publishing Company, 1990, pp 265, 281.

1031. Milgram JW: The classification of loose bodies in human joints. Clin Orthop 124:282, 1977.

1032. Milgram JW: The development of loose bodies in human joints. Clin Orthop 124:292, 1977.

1033. Milgram JW: Radiological and pathological manifestations of osteochondritis dissecans of the distal femur. Radiology 126:305, 1978.

1034. Nelson DW, DiPaola J, Colville M, et al: Osteochondritis dissecans of the talus and knee: Prospective comparison of MR and arthroscopic classifications. J Comput Assist Tomogr 14:804, 1990.

1035. Adam G, Bühne M, Prescher A, et al: Stability of osteochondral fragments of the femoral condyle: Magnetic resonance imaging with histopathologic correlation in an animal model. Skel Radiol 20:601, 1991.

1036. Lehner K, Heuck A, Rodammer G, et al: MRI bei der Osteochondrosis dissecans. ROFO 147:191, 1987.

1037. De Smet AA, Fisher DR, Graf BK, et al: Osteochondritis dissecans of the knee: Value of MR imaging in determining lesion stability and the presence of articular cartilage defects. AJR 155:549, 1990.

1038. Mesgarzadeh M, Sapega AA, Bonakdarpour A, et al: Osteochondritis dissecans: Analysis of mechanical stability with radiography, scintigraphy, and MR imaging. Radiology 165:775, 1987.

1039. Vellet AD, Marks PH, Fowler PJ, et al: Occult posttraumatic osteochondral lesions of the knee: Prevalence, classification, and short-term sequelae evaluated with MR imaging. Radiology 178:271, 1991.

1040. Munk PL, Vellet AD: Lesions of cartilage and bone around the knee. Top Magn Res Imaging 5:249, 1993.

1041. Ochi M, Sumen Y, Kanda T, et al: The diagnostic value and limitation of magnetic resonance imaging on chondral lesions in the knee joint. Arthroscopy 10:176, 1994.

1042. Kramer J, Scheurecker A, Mohr A: Osteochondrale Lasionen. Radiologe 35:109, 1995.

1043. Gillespie HS, Day B: Bone peg fixation in the treatment of osteochondritis dissecans of the knee. Clin Orthop 143:125, 1979.

1044. Johnson EW, McLeod TL: Osteochondral fragments of the distal end of the femur fixed with bone pegs. J Bone Joint Surg [Am] 59:677, 1977.

1045. Smillie IS: Treatment of osteochondritis dissecans. J Bone Joint Surg [Br] 39:248, 1957.

1046. Lipscomb PR Jr, Lipscomb PR Sr, Bryan RS: Osteochondritis dissecans of the knee with loose fragments. J Bone Joint Surg [Am] 60:235, 1978.

1047. Thomson NL: Osteochondritis dissecans and osteochondral fragments managed by Herbert compression screw fixation. Clin Orthop 224:71, 1987.

1048. Garrett JC: Osteochondritis dissecans. Clin Sports Med 10:569, 1991.

1049. Garrett JC, Kress KH, Mudano M: Osteochondritis dissecans of the femoral condyle in the adult. Arthroscopy 8:474, 1992.

1050. Locht RC, Gross AE, Langer F: Late osteochondral allograft resurfacing for tibial plateau fractures. J Bone Joint Surg [Am] 66:328, 1984.

1051. Meyers MH, Akeson W, Convery FR: Resurfacing of the knee with fresh osteochondral allograft. J Bone Joint Surg [Am] 71:704, 1989.

1052. Smith DS, Sharp DC, Resendes M: MRI of healing osteochondritis dissecans fragment with absorbable pins. J Comput Assist Tomogr 18:832, 1994.

1053. Freund E: Chondromatosis of the joints. Arch Surg 34:670, 1937.

1054. Dandy DJ, O'Carroll PF: The removal of loose bodies from the knee under arthroscopic control. J Bone Joint Surg [Br] 64:473, 1982.

1055. Yao L, Lee JK: Occult intraosseous fracture: Detection with MR imaging. Radiology 167:749, 1988.

1056. Lynch TCP, Crues JV III, Morgan FW, et al: Bone abnormalities of the knee: Prevalence and significance at MR imaging. Radiology 171:761, 1989.

1057. Mink JH, Deutsch AL: Occult cartilage and bone injuries of the knee: Detection, classification, and assessment with MR imaging. Radiology 170:823, 1989.

1058. Capps GW, Hayes CW: Easily missed injuries around the knee. Radio-Graphics 14:1191, 1994.

1059. Thompson RC Jr, Vener MJ, Griffiths HJ, et al: Scanning electron-microscopic and magnetic resonance-imaging studies of injuries to the patellofemoral joint after acute transarticular loading. J Bone Joint Surg [Am] 75:704, 1993.

1060. Deutsch AL, Mink JH, Rosenfelt FP, et al: Incidental detection of hematopoietic hyperplasia on routine knee MR imaging. AJR 152:333, 1989.

1061. Schuck JE, Czarnecki DJ: MR detection of probable hematopoietic hyperplasia involving the knees, proximal femurs, and pelvis. AJR 153:655, 1989.

1062. Shellock FG, Morris E, Deutsch AL, et al: Hematopoietic bone marrow hyperplasia: High prevalence on MR images of the knee in asymptomatic marathon runners. AJR 158:335, 1992.

1063. Lang PL, Fritz R, Vahlensieck M, et al: Residuales und rekonvertiertes hämatopoetisches Knochenmark im distalen Femur. ROFO 156:89, 1992.

1064. Lang PL, Fritz R, Majumdar S, et al: Hematopoietic bone marrow in the adult knee: Spin-echo and opposed-phase gradient-echo MR imaging. Skel Radiol 22:95, 1993.

1065. Poulton TB, Murphy WD, Duerk JL, et al: Bone marrow reconversion in adults who are smokers: MR imaging findings. AJR 161:1217, 1993.

1066. Niebauer JJ, King DE: Congenital dislocation of the knee. J Bone Joint Surg [Am] 42:207, 1960.

1067. Carlson DH, O'Connor J: Congenital dislocation of the knee. AJR 127:465, 1976.

1068. Laurence M: Genu recurvatum congenitum. J Bone Joint Surg [Br] 49:121, 1967.

1069. Curtis BH, Fisher RL: Congenital hyperextension with anterior subluxation of the knee. J Bone Joint Surg [Am] 51:255, 1969.

1070. Bell MJ, Atkins RM, Sharrard WJW: Irreducible congenital dislocation of the knee: Aetiology and management. J Bone Joint Surg [Br] 69:403, 1987.

1071. Johnson E, Audell R, Oppenheim WL: Congenital dislocation of the knee. J Pediatr Orthop 7:194, 1987.

1072. Bensahel H, Dal Monte A, Hjelmstedt A, et al: Congenital dislocation of the knee. J Pediatr Orthop 9:174, 1989.

1073. McFarlane AL: A report on four cases of congenital genu recurvatum occurring in one family. Br J Surg 34:388, 1947.

1074. Provenzano RW: Congenital dislocation of the knee: Report of a case. N Engl J Med 236:360, 1947.

1075. Dungy C, Leupp M: Congenital hyperextension of the knees in twins. Clin Pediatr 23:169, 1984.

1076. Katz MP, Grogono BJS, Soper KC: The etiology and treatment of congenital dislocation of the knee. J Bone Joint Surg [Br] 49:112, 1967.

1077. Shattock SG: Genu recurvatum in a foetus at term. Trans Pathol Soc Lond 42:280, 1891.

1078. Jacobsen K, Vopalecky F: Congenital dislocation of the knee. Acta Orthop Scand 56:1, 1985.

1079. Middleton DS: The pathology of congenital genu recurvatum. Br J Surg 22:696, 1935.

1080. Ferris B, Aichroth P: The treatment of congenital knee dislocation: A review of nineteen knees. Clin Orthop 216:135, 1987.

1081. Ahmadi B, Shahriaree H, Silver CM: Severe congenital genu recurvatum: Case report. J Bone Joint Surg [Am] 61:622, 1979.

1082. Ferris BD, Jackson AM: Congenital snapping knee: Habitual anterior subluxation of the tibia in extension. J Bone Joint Surg [Br] 72:453, 1990.

1083. Ogden JA, McCarthy SM, Jokl P: The painful bipartite patella. J Pediatr Orthop 2:263, 1982.

1084. Green WT Jr: Painful bipartite patellae: A report of three cases. Clin Orthop 110:197, 1975.

1085. Lawson JP: Symptomatic radiographic variants in extremities. Radiology 157:625, 1985.

1086. Ogata K: Painful bipartite patella: A new approach to operative treatment. J Bone Joint Surg [Am] 76:573, 1994.

1087. Weinberg S: Case report 177. Skel Radiol 7:223, 1981.

1088. Hägglund G, Pettersson H: A case of bilateral duplication of the patella. Acta Orthop Scand 60:725, 1989.

1089. Gasco J, Del Pino JM, Gomar-Sancho F: Double patella: A case of duplication in the coronal plane. J Bone Joint Surg [Br] 69:602, 1987.

1090. Goergen TG, Resnick D, Greenway G, et al: Dorsal defect of the patella: A characteristic radiographic lesion. Radiology 130:333, 1979.

1091. Haswell DM, Berne AS, Graham CB: The dorsal defect of the patella. Pediatr Radiol 4:238, 1976.

1092. Johnson JF, Brogden BG: Dorsal defect of the patella: Incidence and distribution. AJR 139:339, 1982.

1093. van Holsbeeck M, Vandamme B, Marchal G, et al: Dorsal defect of the patella: Concept of its origin and relationship with bipartite and multipartite patella. Skel Radiol 16:304, 1987.

1094. Owsley DW, Mann RW: Bilateral dorsal defect of the patella. AJR 154:1347, 1990.

1095. Hunter LY, Hensinger RN: Dorsal defect of the patella with cartilaginous involvement: A case report. Clin Orthop 143:131, 1979.

1096. Denham RH: Dorsal defect of the patella. J Bone Joint Surg [Am] 66:116, 1984.

1097. Safran MR, McDonough P, Seeger L, et al: Dorsal defect of the patella. J Pediatr Orthop 14:603, 1994.

1098. Ho VB, Kransdorf MJ, Jelinek JS, et al: Dorsal defect of the patella: MR features. J Comput Assist Tomogr 15:474, 1991.

1099. Sueyoshi Y, Shimozaki E, Matsumoto T, et al: Two cases of dorsal defect of the patella with arthroscopically visible cartilage surface perforations. Arthroscopy 9:164, 1993.

1100. DeLaurentis DA, Wolferth CC, Wolf FM, et al: Mucinous adventitial cysts of the popliteal artery in an 11 year old girl. Surgery 74:456, 1973.

1101. Schlesinger A, Gottesman L: Cystic degeneration of the popliteal artery. AJR 127:1043, 1976.

1102. Inada K, Hirose M, Iwashima Y, et al: Popliteal artery entrapment syndrome: A case report. Br J Surg 65:613, 1978.

1103. Insua JA, Young JR, Humphries AW: Popliteal artery entrapment syndrome. Arch Surg 101:771, 1970.

1104. Rosset E, Hartung O, Brunet C, et al: Popliteal artery entrapment syndrome. Surg Radiol Anat 17:161, 1995.

1105. Mailis A, Lossing A, Ashby P, et al: Intermittent claudication of tibial vessels as a result of calf muscle hypertrophy: Case report. J Vasc Surg 16:116, 1992.

1106. Rizzo RJ, Flinn WR, Iao RS, et al: Computed tomography for the evaluation of arterial disease in the popliteal fossa. J Vasc Surg 11:112, 1990.

1107. Di Marzo L, Cavallaro A, Sciacca V, et al: Diagnosis of popliteal artery entrapment syndrome: The role of duplex scanning. J Vasc Surg 13:434, 1991.

1108. Di Cesare E, Marsili L, Marino G, et al: Stress MR imaging for evaluation of popliteal artery entrapment. J Magn Res Imaging 4:617, 1994.

1109. McGuinness G, Durham JD, Rutherford RB, et al: Popliteal artery entrapment: Findings at MR imaging. J Vasc Intervent Radiol 2:241, 1991.

1110. Terry GC, Tagert BE, Young MJ: Reliability of the clinical assessment in predicting the cause of internal derangements of the knee. Arthroscopy 11:568, 1995.

1111. MacKenzie R, Dixon AK, Keene GS, et al: Magnetic resonance imaging of the knee: Assessment of effectiveness. Clin Radiol 51:245, 1996.

1112. Vahlensieck M, Peterfy CG, Wischer T, et al: Indirect MR arthrography: Optimization and clinical applications. Radiology 200:249, 1996.

1113. Matellic TM, Aronsson DD, Boyd DW Jr, et al: Acute hemarthrosis of the knee in children. Am J Sports Med 23:668, 1995.

1114. Lugo-Olivieri CH, Scott WW Jr, Zerhouni EA: Fluid-fluid levels in injured knees: Do they always represent lipohemarthroses? Radiology 198:499, 1996.

1115. Kim S-J, Choe W-S: Pathologic infrapatellar plica: A report of two cases and literature review. Arthroscopy 12:236, 1996.

1116. Otsuka Y, Mizuta H, Nakamura E, et al: Tenosynovial giant-cell tumor arising from the anterior cruciate ligament of the knee. Arthroscopy 12:496, 1996.

1117. Donahue F, Turkel D, Mnaymneh W, et al: Hemorrhagic prepatellar bursitis. Skeletal Radiol 25:298, 1996.

1118. Rose NE, Gold SM: A comparison of accuracy between clinical examination and magnetic resonance imaging in the diagnosis of meniscal and anterior cruciate ligament tears. Arthroscopy 12:398, 1996.

1119. Dixon AK: Magnetic resonance imaging of meniscal tears of the knee. J Bone Joint Surg [Br] 78:174, 1996.

1120. Rothstein CP, Laorr A, Helms CA, et al: Semimembranosus–tibial collateral ligament bursitis: MR imaging findings. AJR 166:875, 1996.

1121. MacKenzie R, Palmer CR, Lomas DJ, et al: Magnetic resonance imaging of the knee: Diagnostic performance statistics. Clin Radiol 51:251, 1996.

1122. Miller GK: A prospective study comparing the accuracy of the clinical diagnosis of meniscal tear with magnetic resonance imaging and its effect on clinical outcome. Arthroscopy 12:406, 1996.

1123. Pedowitz RA, Feagin JA, Rajagopalan S: A surgical algorithm for treatment of cystic degeneration of the meniscus. Arthroscopy 12:209, 1996.

1124. Barber FA: Editorial overview. Arthroscopy 12:216, 1996.

1125. Kim S-J, Choi C-H: Bilateral complete discoid medial menisci combined with anomalous insertion and cyst formation. Arthroscopy 12:112, 1996.

1126. Shea KG, Westin C, West J: Anomalous insertion of the medial meniscus of the knee. A case report. J Bone Joint Surg [Am] 77:1894, 1995.

1127. Kim S-J, Jeon C-H, Koh C-H: A ring-shaped lateral meniscus. Case report. Arthroscopy 11:738, 1995.

1128. Ohana N, Plotquin D, Atar D: Bilateral hypoplastic lateral meniscus. Case report. Arthroscopy 11:740, 1995.

1129. Pollard ME, Kang Q, Berg EE: Radiographic sizing for meniscal transplantation. Arthroscopy 11:684, 1995.

1130. Potter HG, Rodeo SA, Wickiewicz TL, et al: MR imaging of meniscal allografts: Correlation with clinical and arthroscopic outcomes. Radiology 198:509, 1996.

1131. Tuite MJ, DeSmet AA: MR of the postoperative knee. Topics Magn Res Imag 8:2, 1996.

1132. Santori N, Condello V, Adriani E, et al: Osteonecrosis after arthroscopic medial meniscectomy. Case report. Arthroscopy 11:220, 1996.

1133. Muscolo DL, Costa-Paz M, Makino A, et al: Osteonecrosis of the knee following arthroscopic meniscectomy in patients over 50 years old. Arthroscopy 12:273, 1996.

1134. Rozbruch SR, Wickiewicz TL, DiCarlo EF, et al: Osteonecrosis of the knee following arthroscopic laser meniscectomy. Arthroscopy 12:245, 1996.

1135. Maynard MJ, Deng X, Wickiewicz TL, et al: The popliteofibular ligament. Rediscovery of a key element in posterolateral stability. Am J Sports Med 24:311, 1996.

1136. Yu JS, Salonen DC, Hodler J, et al: Posterolateral aspect of the knee: Improved MR imaging with a coronal oblique technique. Radiology *198*:199, 1996.

1137. Jones CDS, Keene GCR, Christie AD: The popliteus as a retractor of the lateral meniscus of the knee. Arthroscopy *11*:270, 1995.

1138. Westrich GH, Hannafin JA, Potter HG: Isolated rupture and repair of the popliteus tendon. Case report. Arthroscopy *11*:628, 1995.

1139. Puig S, Dupuy DE, Sarmiento A, et al: Articular muscle of the knee: A muscle seldom recognized on MR imaging. AJR *166*:1057, 1996.

1140. Khan KM, Bonar F, Desmond PM, et al: Patellar tendinosis (jumper's knee): Findings at histopathologic examination, US, and MR imaging. Radiology *200*:821, 1996.

1141. Yu JS, Popp JE, Kaeding CC, et al: Correlation of MR imaging and pathologic findings in athletes undergoing surgery for patellar tendinitis. AJR *165*:115, 1995.

1142. Johnson DP, Wakeley CJ, Watt I: Magnetic resonance imaging of patellar tendonitis. J Bone Joint Surg [Br] *78*:452, 1996.

1143. Berg EE, Mason SL, Lucas MJ: Patellar height ratios. A comparison of four measurement methods. Am J Sports Med *24*:218, 1996.

1144. Brossmann J, Koch S, Schwarzenberg H, et al: Effect of intraarticular pressure on patellar position. Computed tomography study in cadaveric specimens. Invest Radiol *31*:67, 1996.

1145. Lund-Hanssen H, Gannon J, Engebretsen L, et al: Intercondylar notch width and the risk for anterior cruciate ligament rupture. A case-control study in 46 female handball players. Acta Orthop Scand *65*:529, 1994.

1146. Yu JS, Bosch E, Pathria MN, et al: Deep lateral femoral sulcus: Study of 124 patients with anterior cruciate ligament tear. Emerg Radiol *2*:129, 1995.

1147. Brandser EA, Riley MA, Berbaum KS, et al: MR imaging of anterior cruciate ligament injury: Independent value of primary and secondary signs. AJR *167*:121, 1996.

1148. Barry KP, Mesgarzadeh M, Triolo J, et al: Accuracy of MRI patterns in evaluating anterior cruciate ligament tears. Skeletal Radiol *25*:365, 1996.

1149. Falchook FS, Tigges S, Carpenter WA, et al: Accuracy of direct signs of tears of the anterior cruciate ligament. J Canad Assoc Radiol *47*:114, 1996.

1150. Snearly WN, Kaplan PA, Dussault RG: Lateral-compartment bone contusions in adolescents with intact anterior cruciate ligaments. Radiology *198*:205, 1996.

1151. Paulos LE, Wnorowski DC, Greenwald AE: Infrapatellar contracture syndrome. Diagnosis, treatment, and long-term followup. Am J Sports Med *22*:440, 1994.

1152. Ogilvie-Harris DJ, Sekyi-Otu A: Periarticular heterotopic ossification: A complication of arthroscopic anterior cruciate ligament reconstruction using a two-incision technique. Arthroscopy *11*:677, 1995.

1153. Athanasian EA, Wickiewicz TL, Warren RF: Osteonecrosis of the femoral condyle after arthroscopic reconstruction of a cruciate ligament. Report of two cases. J Bone Joint Surg [Am] *77*:1418, 1995.

1154. Recht MP, Piraino DW, Applegate G, et al: Complications after anterior cruciate ligament reconstruction: Radiographic and MR findings. AJR *167*:705, 1996.

1155. Victoroff BN, Paulos L, Beck C, et al: Subcutaneous pretibial cyst formation associated with anterior cruciate ligament allografts: A report of four cases and literature review. Arthroscopy *11*:486, 1995.

1156. Grøntvedt T, Engebretsen L, Rossvoil I, et al: Comparison between magnetic resonance imaging findings and knee stability: Measurements after anterior cruciate ligament repair with and without augmentation. A five-to seven-year followup of 52 patients. Am J Sports Med *23*:729, 1995.

1157. Harner CD, Xerogeanes JW, Livesay GA, et al: The human posterior ligament complex: An interdisciplinary study. Ligament morphology and biomechanical evaluation. Am J Sports Med *23*:736, 1995.

1158. Twaddle BC, Hunter JC, Chapman JR, et al: MRI in acute knee dislocation. A prospective study of clinical, MRI, and surgical findings. J Bone Joint Surg [Br] *78*:573, 1996.

1159. Castriota-Scanderbeg A, De Micheli V, Scarale MG, et al: Precision of sonographic measurement of articular cartilage: inter- and intraobserver analysis. Skeletal Radiol *25*:545, 1996.

1160. Andresen R, Radmer S, König H, et al: MR diagnosis of retropatellar chondral lesions under compression. A comparison with histological findings. Acta Radiol *37*:91, 1996.

1161. Recht MP, Piraino DW, Paletta GA, et al: Accuracy of fat-suppressed three-dimensional spoiled gradient-echo FLASH MR imaging in the detection of patellofemoral articular cartilage abnormalities. Radiology *198*:209, 1996.

1162. Disler DG, McCauley TR, Kelman CG, et al: Fat-suppressed three-dimensional spoiled gradient-echo MR imaging of hyaline cartilage defects in the knee: Comparison with standard MR imaging and arthroscopy. AJR *167*:127, 1996.

1163. Hardy PA, Recht MP, Piraino D, et al: Optimization of a dual echo in the steady state (DESS) free-precession sequence for imaging cartilage. JMRI *6*:329, 1996.

1164. Piplani MA, Disler DG, McCauley TR, et al: Articular cartilage volume in the knee: Semiautomated determination from three-dimensional reformations of MR images. Radiology *198*:855, 1996.

1165. Marshall KW, Mikulis DJ, Guthrie BM: Quantification of articular cartilage using magnetic resonance imaging and three-dimensional reconstruction. J Orthop Res *13*:814, 1995.

1166. Sittek H, Eckstein F, Gavazzeni A, et al: Assessment of normal patellar cartilage volume and thickness using MRI: An analysis of currently available pulse sequences. Skeletal Radiol *25*:55, 1996.

1167. Koblik PD, Freeman DM: Short echo time magnetic resonance imaging of tendon. Invest Radiol *12*:1095, 1993.

1168. Brossmann J, Frank LR, Pauly JM, et al: Ultrashort echo time projection reconstruction MR imaging of cartilage with histopathologic correlation: Comparison with fat-suppressed spoiled GRASS and magnetization transfer contrast MR imaging. Radiology, in press.

1169. Nolte-Ernsting CCA, Adam G, Bühne M, et al: MRI of degenerative bone marrow lesions in experimental osteoarthritis of canine knee joints. Skeletal Radiol *25*:413, 1996.

1170. Delzell PB, Schils JP, Recht MP: Subtle fractures about the knee: Innocuous-appearing yet indicative of significant internal derangement. AJR *167*:699, 1996.

1171. Hyman AA, Heiser WJ, Kim SE, et al: An excavation of the distal femoral metaphysis: a magnetic resonance imaging study. A case report. J Bone Joint Surg [Am] *12*:1897, 1995.

1172. Yamazaki T, Maruoka S, Takahashi S, et al: MR findings of avulsive cortical irregularity of the distal femur. Skeletal Radiol *24*:43, 1995.

1173. Chason DP, Schultz SM, Fleckenstein JL: Tensor fasciae suralis: Depiction on MR images. AJR *165*:1220, 1995.

1174. Kaufman LD, Gruber BL, Gersten DP, et al: Preliminary observations on the role of magnetic resonance imaging for polymyositis and dermatomyositis. Ann Rheum Dis *46*:569, 1987.

1175. Keim DR, Hernandez RJ, Sullivan DB: Serial magnetic resonance imaging in juvenile dermatomyositis. Arthritis Rheum *34*:1580, 1991.

1176. Hernandez RJ, Keim DR, Sullivan DB, et al: Magnetic resonance imaging appearance of the muscles in childhood dermatomyositis. J Pediatr *117*:546, 1990.

1177. Lamminen AE: Magnetic resonance imaging of primary skeletal muscle disease: Patterns of distribution and severity of involvement. Br J Radiol *63*:946, 1990.

1178. Park JH, Vansant JP, Kumar NG, et al: Dermatomyositis: Correlative MR imaging and P-31 MR spectroscopy for quantitative characterization of inflammatory disease. Radiology *177*:473, 1990.

1179. Borghi L, Savoldi F, Scelsi R, et al: Nuclear magnetic resonance response of protons in normal and pathological human muscles. Exp Neurol *81*:89, 1983.

1180. Hernandez RJ, Sullivan DB, Chenevert TL, et al: MR imaging in children with dermatomyositis: Musculoskeletal findings and correlation with clinical and laboratory findings. AJR *161*:359, 1993.

1181. Fraser DD, Frank JA, Dalakas M, et al: Magnetic resonance imaging in the idiopathic inflammatory myopathies. J Rheumatol *18*:1693, 1991.

1182. Hernandez RJ, Keim DR, Chenevert TL, et al: Fat-suppressed MR imaging of myositis. Radiology *182*:217, 1992.

1183. Szumowski J, Eisen JK, Vinitski S, et al: Hybrid methods of chemical-shift imaging. Magn Reson Med *9*:379, 1989.

1184. Adams EM, Chow CK, Premkumar A, et al: The idiopathic inflammatory myopathies: Spectrum of MR imaging findings. Radiographics *15*:563, 1995.

1185. Dousset M, Weissleder R, Hendrick RE, et al: Short T1 inversion-recovery imaging of the liver: Pulse-sequence optimization and comparison with spin-echo imaging. Radiology *171*:327, 1989.

1186. Bydder GM, Young IR: MR imaging: Clinical use of the inversion recovery sequence. J Comput Assist Tomogr *9*:659, 1985.

1187. Shuman WP, Baron RL, Peters MJ, et al: Comparison of STIR and spin-echo MR imaging at 1.5 T in 90 lesions of the chest, liver, and pelvis. AJR *152*:852, 1989.

1188. Schweitzer ME, Fort J: Cost-effectiveness of MR imaging in evaluating polymyositis. AJR *165*:1469, 1995.

1189. Chou SM: Myxovirus-like structure in a case of human polymyositis. Science *158*:1453, 1967.

1190. Yunis EJ, Samaha FJ: Inclusion body myositis. Lab Invest *25*:240, 1971.

1191. Carpenter S, Karpati G, Heller I, et al: Inclusion body myositis: A distinct variety of inflammatory myopathy. Neurology *28*:8, 1978.

1192. Calabrese LH, Mitsumoto H, Chou SM: Inclusion body myositis presenting as treatment-resistant polymyositis. Arthritis Rheum *30*:397, 1987.

1193. Sayers ME, Chou SM, Calabrese LH: Inclusion body myositis: Analysis of 32 cases. J Rheumatol *19*:1385, 1992.

1194. Wortmann RL: The dilemma of treating patients with inclusion body myositis. J Rheumatol *19*:1327, 1992.

1195. Trieshmann HW Jr, Mosure JC: The impact of magnetic resonance imaging of the knee on surgical decision making. Arthroscopy *12*:550, 1996.

1196. Nemeth WC, Sanders BL: The lateral synovial recess of the knee: Anatomy and role in chronic iliotibial band friction syndrome. Arthroscopy *12*:574, 1996.

1197. Niitsu M, Ikeda K, Fukubayashi T, et al: Knee extension and flexion: MR delineation of normal and torn anterior cruciate ligaments. J Comp Assist Tomogr *20*:322, 1996.

1198. Erickson SJ, Waldschmidt JG, Czervionke LF, et al: Hyaline cartilage: Truncation artifact as a cause of trilaminar appearance with fat-suppressed three-dimensional spoiled gradient-recalled sequences. Radiology *201*:260, 1996.

In common with other musculoskeletal sites, the ankle and foot are affected by a variety of disease processes, which include developmental, articular, inflammatory, and neoplastic disorders. Joints, bones, tendons, ligaments, muscles, other soft tissues, or combinations of these structures are involved. Although routine radiography remains fundamental to analysis and diagnosis of these disorders, other imaging methods, especially MR imaging, have become increasingly important in such assessment in recent years. These methods require considerable knowledge of regional anatomy if the resulting images are to be interpreted correctly, anatomy that is made complex owing, in part, to angular osseous surfaces and tendons whose orientation changes dramatically as they pass from the lower leg into the foot. This chapter emphasizes important anatomic features of the ankle and foot and the application of newer imaging techniques to the evaluation of some of the disease processes that affect these regions of the body.

ANATOMY

A brief description of the anatomy of the foot and ankle is included here. More complete discussions of this

anatomy are contained in appropriate sections of this chapter.

Osseous Anatomy

The distal end of the tibia contains the medial malleolus and articular surface (Fig. 17–1). The medial malleolus is formed by two colliculi separated by a groove (i.e., intercollicular groove). The anterior colliculus extends more inferiorly than the posterior colliculus. The superficial portion of the medial (tibial collateral or deltoid) collateral ligament inserts in the anterior border and medial surface of the anterior colliculus; the tibiotalar component of the deep portion of the medial collateral ligament inserts in the posterior border of the anterior colliculus, the intercollicular groove, and the anterior portion of the posterior colliculus.[1] The broad malleolus has an articular facet on its lateral surface, which is comma-shaped in configuration. On the posterior surface of the distal tibia is a groove, just lateral to the medial malleolus, related to the tendon of the tibialis posterior muscle. The inferior surface of the tibia repre-

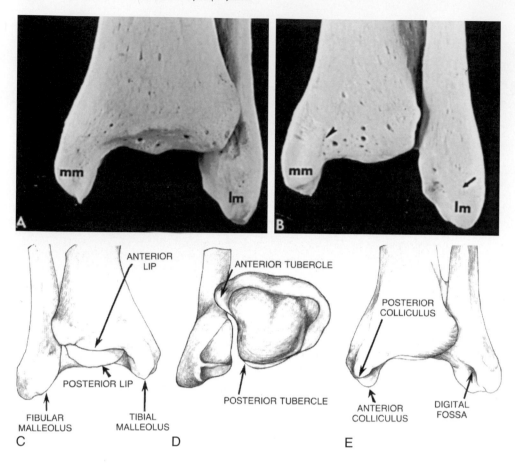

Figure 17–1
Distal ends of the tibia and fibula: Osseous anatomy.

A, B Anterior (**A**) and posterior (**B**) aspects. Observe the medial malleolus (mm), lateral malleolus (lm), groove for the tendon of the tibialis posterior muscle (arrowhead), and groove for the peroneal tendons (arrow).

C–E Frontal (**C**), inferior (**D**), and posterior (**E**) aspects of distal portions of tibia and fibula. (Reproduced with permission from Kelikian H, Kelikian AS: Disorders of the Ankle. Philadelphia, WB Saunders Co, 1985, p. 8.)

sents the articular area for the talus. It is smooth, wider anteriorly than posteriorly, concave anteriorly to posteriorly, and minimally convex medially to laterally. The posterior margin of the articular surface is lower than the anterior margin, and the direct attachment of the transverse portion of the posterior tibiofibular ligament on the lateral half of this margin forms a labrum.[1] The articular surface on the inferior tibia is continuous with that on the medial malleolus. The triangular fibular notch is on the lateral side of the tibia. This notch represents the site of attachment of various ligaments that connect the distal tibia and fibula.

The distal end of the fibula contains the lateral malleolus (see Fig. 17–1). This structure projects more inferiorly than the medial malleolus and contains a triangular facet on its medial surface for articulation with the talus, and an irregular surface above this facet for the interosseous ligament. Posterior to the convex articular facet is a depression, the malleolar fossa. The posterior surface of the lateral malleolus contains a sulcus, often shallow, in which the tendon of the peroneus brevis muscle resides; the tendon of the peroneus longus muscle lies more superficially.

The dorsal surface of the talus contains the trochlear articular surface (Fig. 17–2). This surface is convex anteriorly to posteriorly and concave from side to side. The medial surface of the talar body possesses a facet that articulates with the medial malleolus. The lateral surface of the body contains a triangular articular facet that is intimate with the lateral malleolus.

Assessment of alignment of the ankle on radiographs is important in the evaluation of this joint after trauma. Small degrees of lateral displacement of the talus on the tibia may result in the rapid development of secondary degenerative arthritis. It has been shown that even 1 mm of lateral displacement of the talus reduces the tibiotalar contact areas by 42 per cent.[2] Incomplete ligament tears may result in relatively small amounts of displacement, which may be difficult to detect radiographically. This has stimulated investigators to propose radiographic criteria for assessment of tibiotalar alignment.[3]

A short, concave cortical line representing the posteromedial surface of the talus was used by some investigators to determine tibiotalar displacement.[4] This line actually delineates the insertion of the deep deltoid fibers, however, and does not represent the true medial articular surface. In addition, this line cannot be identified precisely with moderate internal or external rotation of the talus, precluding accurate measurements on rotation radiographs. The main pitfalls of previously reported measurement techniques include (1) inability to accurately identify the posteromedial border of the talus with extreme degrees of rotation, (2) lack of an identifiable posterolateral talar landmark, and (3) variations in the weight-bearing line of the tibia with rotation, because this bone is not a true cylinder even above the metaphysis.

In the adult, the coronal plane of the ankle is oriented in about 15 to 20 degrees of external rotation

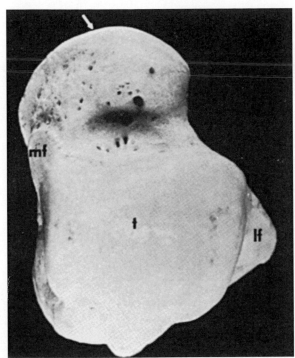

Figure 17–2

Talus: Osseous anatomy. Dorsal aspect. Structures include the trochlear surface (t), medial facet (mf) for articulation with the medial malleolus, and lateral facet (lf) for articulation with the lateral malleolus. The distal surface (arrow) of the talus articulates with the tarsal navicular surface.

with reference to the coronal plane of the knee[5] and therefore the lateral malleolus is slightly posterior to the medial malleolus. To obtain a true anteroposterior radiograph of the tibiotalar joint, the ankle must be positioned with the medial and lateral malleoli parallel to the tabletop; that is, in about 15 to 20 degrees of internal rotation, or the mortise view.[6] This positioning places the medial articular surface tangent to the x-ray beam, and the short concave line representing the posteromedial surface of the talus falls slightly lateral to the medial articular surface. With this view, the radiographic medial clear space represents the actual width of the medial joint space. In adults, the normal interosseous space is about 2.5 to 3.5 mm.[7]

Articular Anatomy

Talocrural (Ankle) Joint

The articular surfaces are cartilage-covered and the bones are connected by a fibrous capsule and by the deltoid, anterior and posterior talofibular, and calcaneofibular ligaments (Fig. 17–3).[8] The fibrous capsule is attached superiorly to the medial and lateral malleoli and tibia and inferiorly to the talus. The talar attachment of the capsule is close to the margins of the trochlear surface except anteriorly, where the attachment to the neck of the talus is located at some distance from the articular margin. The capsule is weak both anteriorly and posteriorly, but it is reinforced medially

and laterally by various ligaments. A synovial membrane lines the inner aspect of the capsule and extends for a short vertical distance between the tibia and fibula. In this latter area, cartilage may be found on the osseous surfaces, continuous with that in the ankle joint.

The surrounding ligaments include the following[8]:

1. Deltoid (medial, or tibial, collateral) ligament. This medial ligament is triangular and is attached above to the apex and the posterior and anterior borders of the medial malleolus. It contains superficial, middle, and deep fibers, although classification of the fibers of this ligament is not uniform (see later discussion). Superficial fibers run anteriorly to the tuberosity of the tarsal navicular bone and blend with the plantar calcaneonavicular ligament. Middle fibers attach to the sustentaculum tali of the calcaneus, and deep and posterior fibers pass to the medial talar surface, including its tubercle.

2. Anterior talofibular ligament. This ligament extends from the anterior margin of the lateral malleolus to the lateral articular facet on the neck of the talus.

3. Posterior talofibular ligament. This ligament attaches to the lateral malleolar fossa and extends horizontally to the lateral tubercle of the talus and medial malleolus.

4. Calcaneofibular ligament. This structure extends from the lateral malleolus to the lateral surface of the calcaneus. It is crossed by the peroneus longus and peroneus brevis tendons. These last three ligaments (i.e., anterior talofibular, posterior talofibular, calcaneofibular) constitute the lateral ligamentous complex of the ankle.

The soft tissue anatomy of the talocrural joint governs the radiographic manifestations of an articular effusion. On lateral radiographs, an ankle effusion produces a teardrop-shaped dense shadow anterior to the joint, extending along the neck of the talus,[9] a finding that is accentuated when the ankle is dorsiflexed.[10] A similar radiodense area in the posterior aspect of the joint or a lobulated mass (indicative of articular communication with the posterior subtalar joint) in this region is an additional, although less reliable, sign of an ankle effusion.

Distal Tibiofibular Joint

This fibrous joint consists of a strong interosseous ligament that unites the convex surface of the medial distal fibula and the concave surface of the adjacent fibular notch of the tibia (see later discussion). Additionally, the anterior and posterior tibiofibular ligaments reinforce this joint. Below this ligamentous joint, an upward prolongation of the synovial membrane of the ankle (talocrural joint) can extend 3 to 5 mm. This synovial recess may be associated with cartilaginous surfaces on the tibia and fibula.

Talocalcaneal Joints[11, 12]
(Figs. 17–4, 17–5, and 17–6)

The talocalcaneal joints are two in number: the subtalar (posterior talocalcaneal or posterior subtalar) joint and

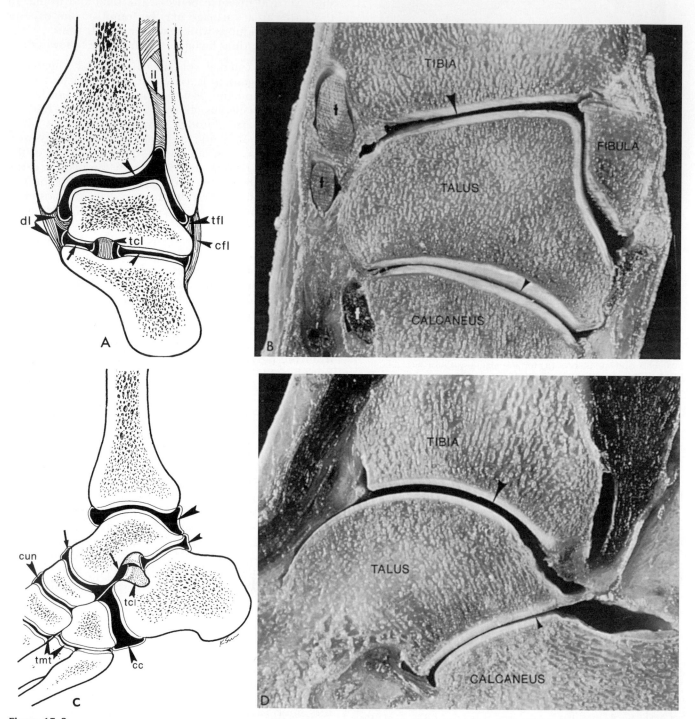

Figure 17–3

Talocrural (ankle) joint: Articular anatomy.

A, B A drawing and photograph of a coronal section through the distal ends of the tibia, fibula, and talus, outlines the ankle joint (large arrowheads), interosseous ligament (il) of tibiofibular syndesmosis, interosseous talocalcaneal ligament (tcl), portions of the deltoid ligament (dl), posterior talofibular ligament (tfl), calcaneofibular ligament (cfl), surrounding tendons (t), subtalar joint (small arrowheads), and talocalcaneonavicular joint (arrow).

C, D Some of the same structures as in **A** and **B** can be identified in a drawing and photograph of a sagittal section of the ankle. Additional joints that can be seen are the calcaneocuboid (cc), cuneonavicular (cun), and tarsometatarsal (tmt) joints.

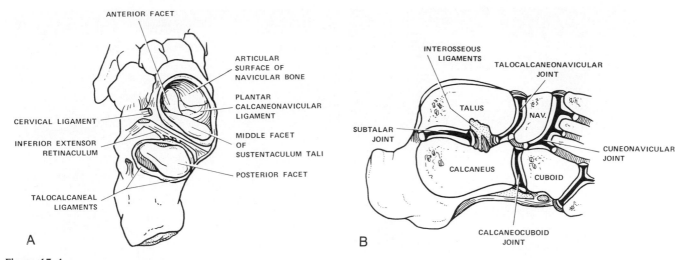

Figure 17–4

Talocalcaneal joints: Articular anatomy.

A Superior surface of calcaneus. Note the broad convex posterior talar facet separated from the anterior and middle talar facets by the tarsal canal and its ligamentous structures. Two completely independent synovium-lined joints are formed.

B Oblique section of the foot. The interosseous ligaments between the talus and calcaneus are well shown, and the two separate talocalcaneal articulations are indicated. Note the independent calcaneocuboid and cuneonavicular joint cavities.

(From Resnick D: Radiology *111*:581, 1974.)

Figure 17–5

Talocalcaneal joints: Sagittal cross-sectional anatomy.

A A lateral sagittal section through the fibula (F) and ankle (A) demonstrates the subtalar articulation (open arrow) between the posterior facets of the talus and calcaneus. The tarsal sinus (1) and posterior talofibular ligament (black dot) are indicated. A separate calcaneocuboid joint (2) is evident.

B A more medial sagittal section outlines the talocalcaneonavicular (curved arrows) and subtalar (open arrow) joint cavities completely separated by the contents of the tarsal sinus (1). The calcaneocuboid articulation (2) again is indicated.

(From Resnick D: Radiology *111*:581, 1974.)

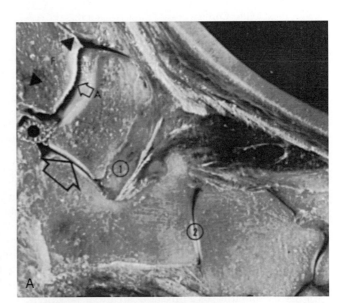

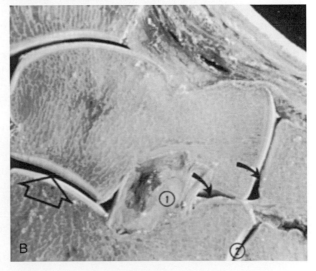

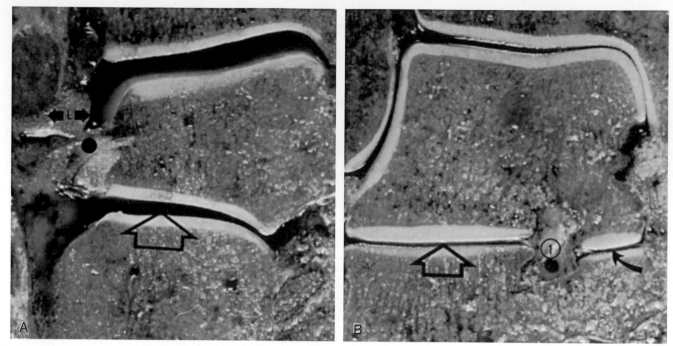

Figure 17–6

Talocalcaneal joints: Coronal cross-sectional anatomy.

A A section through the subtalar articulation (open arrow) is shown. The lateral (L) malleolus and posterior talofibular ligament (black dot) are indicated.

B A more anterior section outlines separate subtalar (open arrow) and talocalcaneonavicular (curved arrow) joints. The interosseous ligaments (1) are labeled.

(From Resnick D: Radiology *111*:581, 1974.)

the talocalcaneonavicular (anterior subtalar) joint. These joints are separated by the tarsal canal and sinus and their contents.

The subtalar joint exists between the posterior talar facet of the calcaneus and the posterior calcaneal facet of the talus. The talar facet is oval and concave and extends distally and laterally at an angle of approximately 45 degrees with the sagittal plane. The posterior calcaneal facet is oval and convex anteroposteriorly. This synovium-lined joint, which may communicate with the talocrural or ankle joint in approximately 10 to 20 per cent of persons,[11–14] contains a capsule that contributes to the interosseous talocalcaneal ligament, the major bond between talus and calcaneus. Additional structures binding talus and calcaneus are the anterior talocalcaneal ligament (extending from the lateral talar tubercle to the proximal medial calcaneus), the medial talocalcaneal ligament (extending from the medial talar tubercle to the sustentaculum tali), and the lateral talocalcaneal ligament (extending from the lateral surface of the talus to that of the calcaneus).

The talocalcaneonavicular joint also is a synovium-lined joint, which exists between the head of the talus, the posterior surface of the navicular bone, the anterior articular surface of the calcaneus, and the proximal surface of the plantar calcaneonavicular ligament, or ''spring'' ligament. The distal surface of the head of the talus is oval and convex, directed inferiorly and medially to articulate with the oval, concave proximal surface of the navicular bone. The plantar surface of the talar head has three articular areas separated by indistinct

osseous ridges: the posterior area is large and oval, is convex in shape, and articulates with the sustentaculum tali of the calcaneus; the second area, anterolateral to the posterior area, is flattened, articulating with the superior surface of the calcaneus; and the navicular area, directed distally, is oval and convex, articulating with the tarsal navicular bone. The anterior articular surface of the talus also contacts the plantar calcaneonavicular ligament. This ligament has a central area that consists of fibrocartilage and bridges the triangular space between the anterior and middle talar facets of the calcaneus and navicular bone. The posterior surface of the joint capsule contributes to the interosseous ligament. On its medial side, this joint is enlarged or deepened by a portion of the deltoid ligament, which is attached to the plantar calcaneonavicular ligament. Movements are coordinated between the talocalcaneonavicular and subtalar joints and include inversion and eversion of the foot.

Calcaneocuboid Joint (Fig. 17–7)

This joint is formed between apposing quadrilateral facets on the calcaneus and cuboid bones, and its capsule is reinforced by surrounding ligaments, including the long plantar ligament (extending from the plantar surface of the calcaneus to the cuboid and third through fifth metatarsals) and the plantar calcaneocuboid ligament (extending from calcaneus to cuboid). The calcaneocuboid and talocalcaneonavicular joints often are referred to collectively as the transverse tarsal joint.

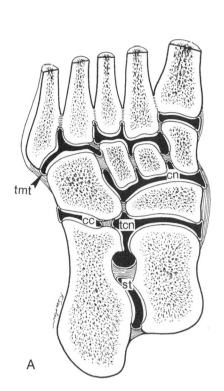
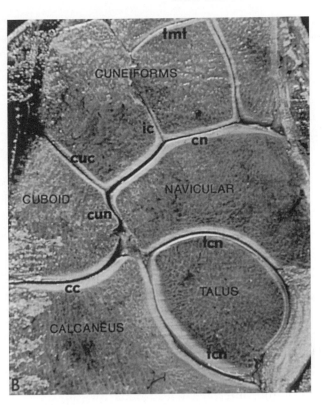

Figure 17–7
Joints of the midfoot: Articular anatomy.
   A, B Drawing and photograph of an oblique transverse section through the midfoot outlines the following joints: subtalar (st), talocalcaneonavicular (tcn), cuneonavicular (cn), calcaneocuboid (cc), cuboideonavicular (cun), cuneocuboid (cuc), intercuneiform (ic), and tarsometatarsal (tmt) joints.

Movements at the calcaneocuboid joint are limited to gliding and rotation.

Cuneonavicular, Intercuneiform, Cuneocuboid, and Cuboideonavicular Joints
(see Fig. 17–7)

The cuneonavicular joint is formed between the concave articular surfaces of the posterior portion of the three cuneiform bones and the convex distal surface of the navicular bone. The articular capsule of this joint is continuous with two intercuneiform joints (small joint cavities between the proximal portions of the cuneiform bones), cuneocuboid joint (articulation between apposing facets on the cuboid bone and lateral cuneiform), and cuboideonavicular joint (inconstant cavity between cuboid and navicular bones). Movements at all of these joints occur simultaneously and include slight amounts of gliding and rotation of one bone on another.

Tarsometatarsal and Intermetarsal Joints

The medial cuneiform and first metatarsal bones possess an independent medial tarsometatarsal joint (see Fig. 17–7). The intermediate tarsometatarsal joint is located between the second and third metatarsal bones and the intermediate and lateral cuneiform bones. This joint may communicate with the intercuneiform and cuneonavicular joints. The lateral tarsometatarsal joint exists between the distal aspect of the cuboid and the base of the fourth and fifth metatarsal bones. A limited amount of gliding motion may occur between tarsals and metatarsal bones, the motion being accentuated at the medial tarsometatarsal joint. The tarsometatarsal joints extend distally between the metatarsal bases as intermetatarsal joints. Slight gliding motion can occur at these latter joints.[15]

Metatarsophalangeal Joints

The metatarsophalangeal joints, which are synovial joints, exist where the rounded heads of the metatarsal bones approximate the cupped surfaces of the proximal phalanges (Fig. 17–8). The articular portions of the metatarsal heads include the distal and plantar aspects of the bone but do not include the dorsal surface. The plantar aspect of the first metatarsal bone is unique, containing two longitudinal grooves separated by a ridge. Each groove may articulate with a sesamoid bone.[15–18] Fibrous capsules surround these joints. The thin dorsal portion of these capsules frequently is intimate with small bursae that separate the capsule from the extensor tendons. Ligaments about these joints include the plantar ligaments, the deep transverse metatarsal ligaments (which connect the plantar ligaments of adjacent metatarsophalangeal joints), and the collateral ligaments (which are located at each side of the joint and extend from the dorsal tubercle of the metatarsal head to the phalangeal base). Active movements at the metatarsophalangeal joints include extension, flexion,

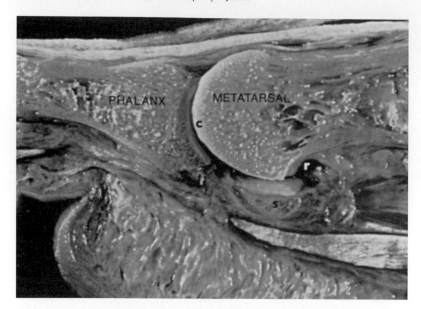

Figure 17–8
Metatarsophalangeal joints: Articular anatomy. A sagittal section through the first metatarsophalangeal joint reveals articular cartilage (c), proximal recesses (r), and a plantar sesamoid (s) bone.

abduction, and adduction. Accessory movements are gliding and rotation of the phalanges.

Interphalangeal Joints

In each foot, the nine interphalangeal joints (two in each of the four lateral digits and one interphalangeal joint of the great toe) separate phalanges and are surrounded by a capsule and two collateral ligaments. The plantar ligament represents a fibrous plate on the plantar surface of the capsule. Active movements at the interphalangeal joints are flexion and extension. Accessory movements are rotation, abduction, and adduction.

Tendon Sheath and Bursal Anatomy

Tendons with accompanying tendon sheaths are intimate with the ankle joint (Fig. 17–9).[19–22] Anteriorly,

sheaths are present about the tendons of the tibialis anterior, extensor hallucis longus, extensor digitorum longus, and peroneus tertius muscles. Medially, sheaths are present about the tendons of the tibialis posterior, flexor digitorum longus, and flexor hallucis longus muscles. Laterally, the common sheath of the tendons of the peroneus longus and peroneus brevis muscles may be appreciated.[23]

Important tendons, aponeuroses, and bursae are located about the calcaneus. The plantar aponeurosis contains strong fibers that adhere to the posteroinferior surface of the bone. The Achilles tendon, which is the thickest and strongest human tendon, attaches to the posterior surface of the calcaneus approximately 2 cm below the upper surface of the bone. The retrocalcaneal bursa exists between the Achilles tendon and the posterosuperior surface of the calcaneus (Fig. 17–10).[24, 25] This bursal space is lined with synovium, which extends

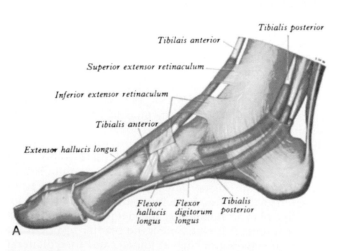
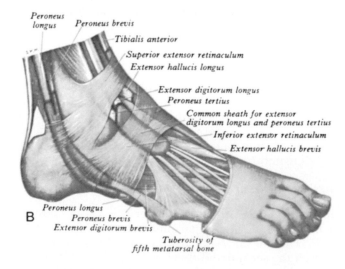

Figure 17–9
Tendon sheaths about the ankle: Normal anatomy.
  A Medial aspect of the ankle.
  B Lateral aspect of the ankle.
  (From Williams PL, Warwick R [Eds]: Gray's Anatomy. 36th British edition. Edinburgh, Churchill Livingstone, 1980, pp. 611, 612.)

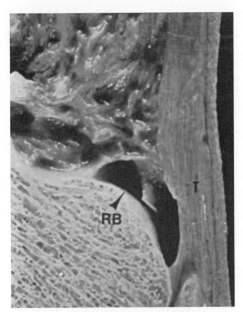

Figure 17–10
Retrocalcaneal bursa: Normal anatomy. In this sagittal section, observe the retrocalcaneal bursa (RB), which is located between the Achilles tendon (T) and upper border of the calcaneus. Above the bursa, the preachilles fat pad can be identified. (From Resnick D, et al: Radiology *125*:355, 1977.)

over both the Achilles tendon and the inferior limit of the preachilles fat pad. The posterior surface of the calcaneus is covered with cartilage.

A triangular radiolucent area, the posterior triangle or preachilles fat pad, is normally observed on lateral radiographs of the ankle. The posterior margin of the triangle is the Achilles tendon and the anterior border is the flexor hallucis longus muscle.[26] Obscuration of portions of the preachilles fat pad occurs in instances of tendinous rupture,[27] but similar findings may indicate accessory or anomalous muscles of the lower calf.

Soft Tissue Anatomy

Crural Interosseous Membrane

The crural interosseous membrane is tightly stretched between the interosseous borders of tibia and fibula.[28] Its upper limit is just inferior to the proximal tibiofibular joint, and its lower limit contains fibers that blend with those about the distal tibiofibular joint. The oblique fibers in the crural interosseous membrane extend inferiorly and laterally from tibia to fibula. A large oval opening in the superior aspect of the membrane allows passage of the anterior tibial vessels; a smaller distal opening allows passage of the perforating branch of the peroneal artery.

Retinacula and Aponeurosis

Owing to the change in orientation of the tendons from a vertical attitude in the lower leg to a horizontal attitude in the foot, five retinacula act to maintain close approximation of the tendons to the bones about the

ankle and thereby prevent bowstringing of these tendons (see Fig. 17–9)[29, 30]:

1. Superior extensor retinaculum. The superior extensor retinaculum is attached to the anterior surface of the lateral malleolus and to the anterior surface of the medial portion of the tibia, and it is continuous with the deep fascia of the lower leg. This structure serves to reinforce the crural fascia and to contain the tendons of the tibialis anterior, extensor hallucis longus, extensor digitorum longus, and peroneus tertius muscles on the dorsal surface of the ankle.

2. Inferior extensor retinaculum. The inferior extensor retinaculum is a Y-shaped structure whose base is attached laterally to the calcaneus. Two limbs or bands are evident medially: An upper limb is located at the level of the ankle and attaches to the medial malleolus; a lower limb attaches to the plantar aponeurosis. This retinaculum serves to prevent bowstringing of the dorsal tendons.

3. Flexor retinaculum. The flexor retinaculum is located medially, enclosing the tarsal tunnel. It extends between the medial malleolus and the calcaneus. Three septa divide the tarsal tunnel into four compartments: The first compartment encloses the tendon of the tibialis posterior muscle; the second compartment encloses the tendon of the flexor digitorum longus muscle; the third compartment encloses the neurovascular bundle (i.e., posterior tibial vessels and the tibial nerve); and the fourth compartment encloses the tendon of the flexor hallucis longus muscle.

4 and 5. Superior and inferior peroneal retinacula. The two peroneal retinacula are laterally located fascial thickenings that extend from the lateral malleolus to the calcaneus. These retinacula serve to hold the tendons of the peroneus longus and brevis muscles firmly in place behind the fibula.

The plantar aponeurosis is a longitudinally oriented, strong fibrous structure located in the plantar aspect of the foot.[30] The central portion is the thickest part of this aponeurosis; this portion arises on the calcaneal tuberosity, initially broadens, and subsequently thins distally before dividing into five separate structures that each extend to one of the toes. The medial and lateral portions of the plantar aponeurosis are thinner and smaller than the central portion. Two vertical intermuscular septa arise from the junction of the central portion of the plantar aponeurosis with the medial and lateral portions, dividing the plantar muscles into medial, lateral, and intermediate groups.[30]

Muscles and Tendons

The anatomy of the musculature of the lower portion of the leg and the foot has been detailed by Jaffe and coworkers.[30] A summary of this anatomy is provided by Schweitzer and Resnick.[29] The musculature of the lower portion of the leg is divided into three compartments: posterior, lateral, and anterior (Fig. 17–11).

1. Posterior compartment. The muscles of the posterior compartment are separated into a superficial layer (consisting of the gastrocnemius, soleus, and plantaris

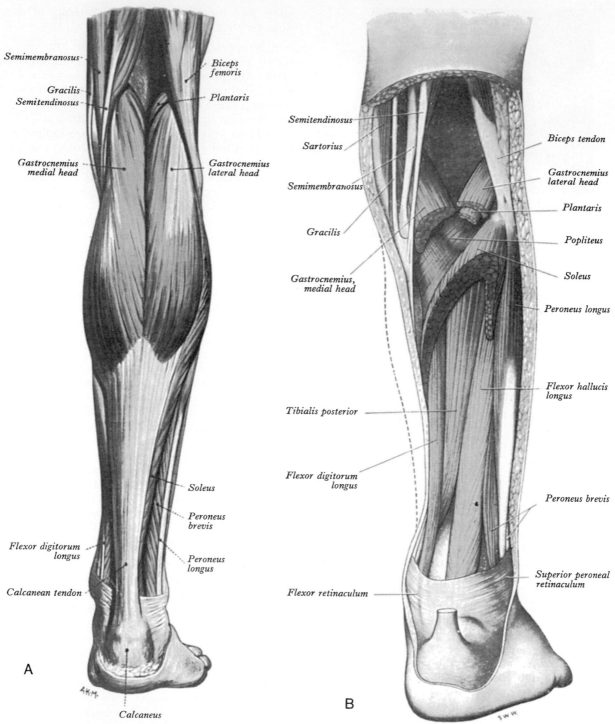

Figure 17–11
Musculature of the lower portion of the leg: Normal anatomy.
  A Posterior aspect, superficial layer of muscles.
  B Posterior aspect, deep layer of muscles.

muscles) and a deep layer (consisting of the popliteus, tibialis posterior, flexor hallucis longus, and flexor digitorum longus muscles). The two heads of the gastrocnemius muscle arise from the medial (medial head) and lateral (lateral head) femoral condyles. These two heads combine in the midcalf to form a single muscle belly that ends in a large, flat tendon, the Achilles tendon.

Deep to the gastrocnemius muscle lies the soleus muscle. This muscle originates as two heads: one head originates from the superior portion of the fibula and the other originates from the posterior and medial aspects of the tibia and the popliteal line. The usual insertion site of the soleus muscle is in the midportion of the Achilles tendon. The small plantaris muscle originates

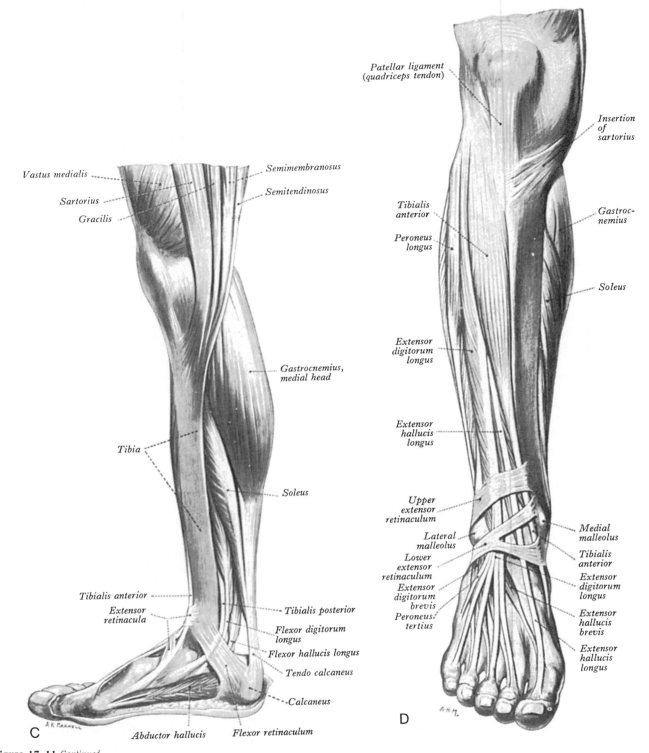

Figure 17–11 *Continued*
C Medial aspect.
D Anterior aspect.
(From Williams PL, Warwick R [Eds]: Gray's Anatomy. 36th British edition, Edinburgh, Churchill Livingstone, 1980, pp. 606–609.)

from the lateral femoral condyle. It forms a tendon in the proximal portion of the leg, and it extends distally to insert in the Achilles tendon.

The most lateral structure in the deep posterior compartment is the flexor hallucis longus muscle. This muscle originates in the posterior aspect of the middle

portion of the fibula, and it extends distally to insert in the distal phalanx of the great toe. The flexor digitorum longus muscle originates from the posterior aspect of the tibia and inserts distally in the form of four slips that pass to the distal phalanges of the second, third, fourth, and fifth toes. The tibialis posterior muscle arises from the posterior aspects of the tibia and fibula and the interosseous membrane. This muscle represents the deepest and most central structure of the posterior compartment. Its distal insertion is in the navicular, cuneiform bones, calcaneus, and metatarsals of the second, third, and fourth toes.

The tendons of the flexor hallucis longus, flexor digitorum longus, and tibialis posterior muscles are intimately related at the level of the medial malleolus. In this region, the tendons lie in a groove, the tendon of the tibialis posterior muscle being most anterior, the tendon of the flexor digitorum longus muscle being in the intermediate position, and the tendon of the flexor hallucis longus muscle being located posteriorly. A mnemonic device ("Tom, Dick, and Harry") can be used to help recall the anterior to posterior relationships of these three tendons: "T" for the tibialis posterior tendon, "D" for the flexor digitorum longus tendon, and "H" for the flexor hallucis longus tendon. The location of the posterior tibial neurovascular bundle (i.e., artery, vein, and nerve) between the tendons of the flexor digitorum longus and flexor hallucis longus muscles can be remembered by expanding the mnemonic device as follows: "Tom, Dick, and *A Very Nervous* Harry."

2. Lateral compartment. The peroneus longus and peroneus brevis muscles lie in the lateral compartment of the lower leg. Both originate from the lateral aspect of the fibula, the origin of the peroneus longus muscle being more superior than that of the peroneus brevis muscle. The myotendinous junction of the peroneus longus occurs above the ankle, at the level of the soleal insertion in the Achilles tendon. The myotendinous junction of the peroneus brevis is located slightly more distally. Both tendons pass lateral to the ankle; the peroneus longus tendon extends medially across the foot to insert in the first metatarsal bone and medial cuneiform; the tendon of the peroneus brevis muscle inserts in the base of the fifth metatarsal bone.

The peroneus brevis and peroneus longus tendons are intimately related at the level of the lateral malleolus. In this location, the peroneus longus tendon is located posterior to the tendon of the peroneus brevis muscle. Above this level, the muscle belly of the peroneus brevis is located posterior to the tendon of the peroneus longus muscle. Below and anterior to the level of the lateral malleolus, the peroneus longus tendon is located inferior and posterior to the peroneus brevis tendon.

3. Anterior compartment. The muscles of the anterior compartment are the extensor digitorum longus, peroneus tertius, extensor hallucis longus, and tibialis anterior.

The extensor digitorum longus is the most lateral muscle in this compartment. It originates from the upper aspect of the tibia and the fibula and the intervening interosseous membrane. Distally, it divides into four slips, which run forward on the dorsum of the foot and extend into the second, third, fourth, and fifth toes. The tendon of the extensor digitorum longus muscle begins at the approximate level of the lateral malleolus.

The peroneus tertius muscle is intimately related to the extensor digitorum longus muscle. It arises from the lower third of the medial surface of the fibula, the adjoining anterior surface of the interosseous membrane, and the anterior crural intermuscular septum. The tendon of the peroneus tertius muscle inserts in the base of the fifth metatarsal bone.

The extensor hallucis longus muscle arises from the middle and distal portions of the fibula and the anterior surface of the interosseous membrane. Its distal attachment is to the dorsal aspect of the base of the distal phalanx of the great toe. The tibialis anterior muscle originates from the lateral aspect of the tibia, from the anterior surface of the interosseous membrane, and from the deep surface of the fascia cruris. The insertion of the tibialis anterior muscle is to the medial and inferior surfaces of the medial cuneiform bone and the adjacent portion of the base of the first metatarsal bone.

The tendons of the tibialis anterior, extensor hallucis longus, and extensor digitorum longus muscles lie alongside each other in the anterior portion of the lower leg. The most medial of these structures is the tibialis anterior tendon and the most lateral is the extensor digitorum longus tendon, with the tendon of the extensor hallucis longus muscle lying in an intermediate position. Another mnemonic device, "Tom, Harry, and Dick," can be used to define the medial to lateral relationships of these three tendons (i.e., "T" for the tibialis anterior, "H" for the extensor hallucis longus, and "D" for the extensor digitorum longus).

The muscles of the foot commonly are described according to layers rather than compartments (Fig. 17–12). The plantar muscles are arranged in four different layers. The muscles in the superficial layer include the abductor hallucis, flexor digitorum brevis, and abductor digiti minimi. These three muscles extend from the tuberosity of the calcaneus to the toes. The abductor hallucis muscle is located medially, arising from the medial aspect of the calcaneal tuberosity, the plantar aponeurosis, and the flexor retinaculum. The fibers of this muscle terminate as a tendon that inserts in the proximal phalanx of the great toe. The medial and lateral plantar vessels and nerve pass deep to the proximal portion of the abductor hallucis muscle.

The flexor digitorum brevis muscle arises by a narrow tendon from the medial aspect of the calcaneal tuberosity and from the plantar aponeurosis. It inserts distally in the middle phalanges of the second, third, fourth, and fifth toes. The abductor digiti minimi muscle is located laterally. It arises in large part from the lateral portion of the calcaneal tuberosity. Distally, its tendon extends over a groove in the plantar surface of the fifth metatarsal bone and attaches to the lateral side of the proximal phalanx of the fifth digit.

The second layer of plantar muscles consists of the quadratus plantae and lumbrical muscles as well as the tendons of the flexor hallucis longus and flexor digitorum longus muscles. The quadratus plantae muscle also is known as the flexor digitorum accessorius muscle. It arises from the medial and lateral portions of the calcaneal tuberosity, and it terminates in tendinous slips

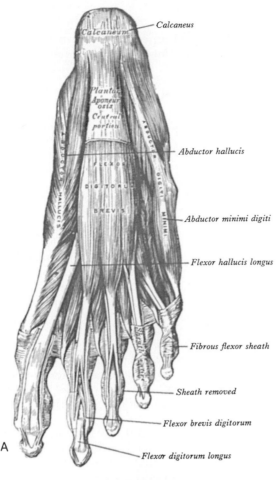

Calcaneus

Plantar
Aponeurosis
Central
portion

Abductor hallucis

Abductor minimi digiti

Flexor hallucis longus

Fibrous flexor sheath

Sheath removed

Flexor brevis digitorum

Flexor digitorum longus

A

Figure 17–12
Musculature of the foot: Normal anatomy.
  A Superficial muscles.
  B Intermediate muscles.
  C Deep muscles.
  (From Williams PL, Warwick R [Eds]: Gray's Anatomy. 36th British edition. Edinburgh, Churchill Livingstone, 1980, pp. 614, 616.)

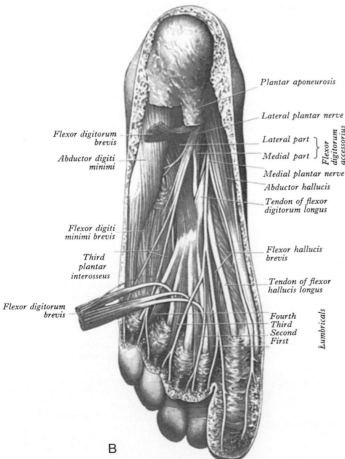

Plantar aponeurosis

Lateral plantar nerve

Lateral part
Medial part } Flexor digitorum accessorius

Medial plantar nerve

Abductor hallucis

Tendon of flexor digitorum longus

Flexor hallucis brevis

Tendon of flexor hallucis longus

Fourth
Third
Second
First

Lumbricals

Flexor digitorum brevis

Abductor digiti minimi

Flexor digiti minimi brevis

Third plantar interosseus

Flexor digitorum brevis

B

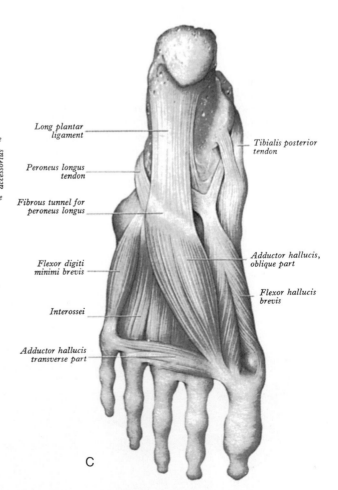

Long plantar ligament

Peroneus longus tendon

Fibrous tunnel for peroneus longus

Flexor digiti minimi brevis

Interossei

Adductor hallucis transverse part

Tibialis posterior tendon

Adductor hallucis, oblique part

Flexor hallucis brevis

C

that join the long flexor tendons to the second, third, and fourth toes. The lumbrical muscles consist of four small muscles extending in a medial to lateral direction. These muscles arise from the tendons of the flexor digitorum longus muscle, and they insert in the dorsal digital expansions in the proximal phalanges.

The third layer of plantar muscles consists of the flexor hallucis brevis, adductor hallucis, and flexor digiti minimi brevis muscles. The flexor hallucis brevis muscle is located medially, originating from the cuboid and lateral cuneiform bones. Distally, this muscle divides into medial and lateral parts, each terminating as a tendon that inserts in the base of the proximal phalanx of the great toe. Each tendon contains a sesamoid bone beneath the first metatarsophalangeal joint. The adductor hallucis muscle arises as two heads. The oblique head originates from the second, third, and fourth metatarsal bases and the long plantar ligament. The transverse head arises from the capsules of the third, fourth, and fifth metatarsophalangeal joints and the deep transverse ligament. The two heads of this muscle join and insert in the lateral sesamoid bone of the great toe and the base of the first phalanx of the hallux. The flexor digiti minimi brevis muscle originates from the medial aspect of the plantar surface of the base of the fifth metatarsal bone, from the cuboid bone, and from the sheath of the peroneus longus tendon. The tendon of the flexor digiti minimi brevis muscle inserts in the base of the proximal phalanx of the fifth toe.

The fourth layer of plantar muscles is the deepest, and it consists of the seven interosseous muscles. These muscles, which originate from the metatarsal bases, are further divided into four dorsal and three plantar muscles. The dorsal interosseous muscles insert laterally in the proximal phalanges; the plantar interosseous muscles insert medially.

The extensor digitorum brevis muscle represents the only intrinsic muscle in the dorsal aspect of the foot. It arises from the superolateral portion of the calcaneus, anterior to the groove for the peroneus brevis tendon, from the interosseous talocalcaneal ligament, and from the inferior extensor retinaculum. This muscle inserts in the lateral aspect of the proximal phalanges of the first, second, third, and fourth toes.

FUNCTION

The functional anatomy of the ankle and foot has been reviewed in great detail by Sarrafian[1] and Mann,[31] many of whose observations are included here. The ankle and subtalar joint complex, although anatomically independent, function as a unit, and their function, in turn, is linked to that of adjacent joints, such as the transverse tarsal joint (i.e., calcaneocuboid joint and talonavicular portion of the talocalcaneonavicular joint) and metatarsophalangeal joints. When functioning normally, these series of joints provide the stable platform of the body in stance and help absorb the impact of ground contact during walking, running, or jumping.[31] Abnormalities in any one of these joints may lead to adaptive changes in another, one example of which is the rounding of the talar dome at the ankle that may accompany subtalar coalition. Forces far greater than body weight accompany a variety of physical activities, particularly those occurring in such sports as American football, basketball, and track, and such forces applied to the ankle and foot are demanding not only of joints but also of surrounding ligaments.

Both the ankle and subtalar joints are highly mobile. At the ankle, movement occurs primarily in the sagittal plane (i.e., dorsiflexion and plantar flexion of the foot) (Fig. 17–13) indicative of the restrictions in movement in the coronal plane resulting from the medial and lateral malleoli and collateral ligaments. Minor components of ankle motion occur about the longitudinal and vertical axes.[1] The precise amounts of plantar flexion and dorsiflexion of the foot that occur normally at the ankle will vary from one person to another, although values of 50 degrees of plantar flexion and 20 degrees of dorsiflexion are useful guidelines.[31] From positions of dorsiflexion to plantar flexion at the ankle joint, the talus and the malleoli remain in contact. Owing to the conical shape of the superior surface of the talus (a

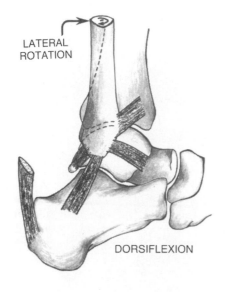

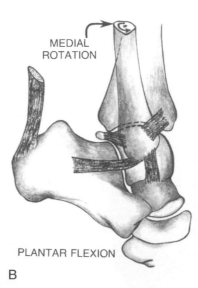

Figure 17–13
Ankle movement: Dorsiflexion and plantar flexion. In dorsiflexion, the fibula rotates on its long axis laterally, creating an anterior gap in the inferior tibiofibular syndesmosis. In plantar flexion, the fibula is pulled forward and medial, and the anterior gap of the syndesmosis is closed. (From Kelikian H, Kelikian AS: Disorders of the Ankle. Philadelphia, WB Saunders Co, 1985, p. 45.)

A

B

surface that is larger anteriorly than posteriorly), plantar flexion of the talus induces a functional varus alignment or supination (Fig. 17–14).[1, 32] The subtalar joint is less constrained than the ankle, being stabilized only by joint configuration and the interosseous ligament.[31] Inversion and eversion occur in this joint; the average range of motion is 25 to 30 degrees of inversion and 5 to 10 degrees of eversion.[1] Inversion and eversion are complex movements, however, and have been regarded as rotary movement of the foot around its own longitudinal axis. They represent triplane movements, which occur in two patterns: pronation-abduction-extension and supination-adduction-flexion.[1] At the time of initial ground contact during walking, the subtalar joint undergoes rapid eversion, a movement that is more prominent in persons with pes planus deformity; subsequently, the subtalar joint undergoes progressive inversion, which reaches a maximum at toe-off, when eversion once again begins.[31] The plantar aponeurosis also serves an important function during these stages of walking. Dorsiflexion of the metatarsophalangeal joints activates the plantar aponeurosis mechanism, which leads to depression of the metatarsal heads, elevation of the longi-

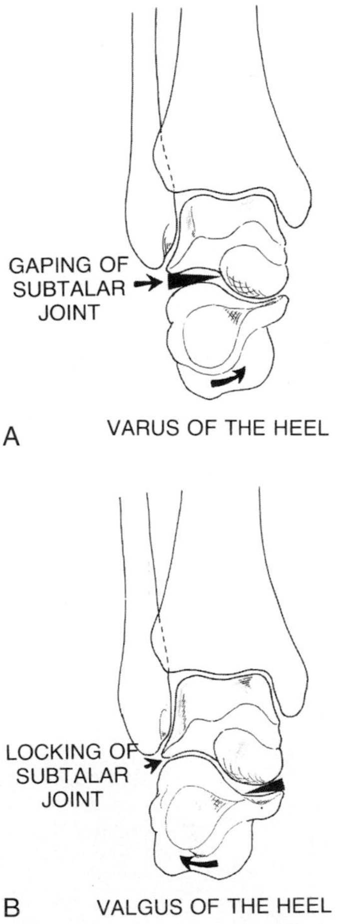

Figure 17–14
Ankle movement: Dorsiflexion and plantar flexion.
A Varus of the heel accompanies plantar flexion.
B Valgus of the heel accompanies dorsiflexion.
(From Kelikian H, Kelikian AS: Disorders of the Ankle. Philadelphia, WB Saunders Co, 1985, p 42.)

tudinal arch of the foot, inversion of the calcaneus, and external rotation of the tibia.[31]

The transverse tarsal joint gains its support from ligamentous structures, and its stability is derived from subtalar joint inversion.[31] The motion at this joint is adduction (normally about 20 degrees) and abduction (normally about 10 degrees). During normal walking, the forefoot is flexible at heel strike to absorb the impact, flexibility being related to eversion of the calcaneus and subtalar joint with unlocking of the transverse tarsal joint; at toe-off, the forefoot is rigid, owing to inversion of the calcaneus and subtalar joint with locking of the transverse tarsal joint.

These observations underscore the close functional linkage of the ankle, subtalar, and transverse tarsal joints and plantar aponeurosis that is essential for walking (as well as running and jumping). Pathologic changes at one or more of these locations will lead to changes at the others, owing to the increased stress placed on them. Initially, these other sites may compensate for dysfunction of one of the components of this linkage, as exemplified by exaggerated motion of the subtalar and transverse tarsal joints that may follow impingement syndromes (with decreased mobility) of the ankle; ultimately, these sites also may fail.[31]

The ankle joint is required to absorb considerable force during the daily activities of life. The load-bearing surface of the ankle joint in normal adults is about 11 cm² to 13 cm², although the area of contact at this joint varies according to the precise position of the talus.[1] Furthermore, a portion of the static load of the leg (approximately 16 or 17 percent) is transmitted by the fibula at the tibiofibular joint.[33] Indeed, the precise position of the fibula at the level of the ankle varies according to the degree of dorsiflexion or plantar flexion of the foot. During dorsiflexion, the intermalleolar distance increases approximately 1.5 mm and lateral rotation of the fibula in the horizontal plane, relative to the tibia, of about 2 or 3 degrees is noted.[34] With weight-bearing, the fibula descends about 2 or 3 mm, perhaps related to the downward pull exerted by the flexors of the foot.[1, 35, 36]

As will be addressed later in this chapter, the stability of the ankle joint depends on both passive and dynamic factors.[1] Passive factors include the contour of the articular surfaces and the integrity of the collateral and distal tibiofibular ligaments, the retinaculae, and the tendon tunnels. Dynamic factors include gravity, muscle action, and the reaction between the foot and ground. The dorsiflexed position of the ankle is the most stable.

IMAGING TECHNIQUES

Although most abnormalities of the ankle and foot are evaluated initially with routine radiography, in some situations conventional radiographs appear unremarkable or do not display the full extent of the process. Other imaging methods, therefore, often are fundamental to analysis of a variety of processes in these locations. These methods are discussed in detail throughout this chapter and include bone scintigraphy and additional radionuclide techniques (as in the assessment of neoplastic and infectious disorders), ultrasonography (for the detection of foreign bodies, joint effusions, ligament and tendon abnormalities, and superficial soft tissue masses), arthrography (as in the evaluation of articular abnormalities and ligament disruptions), CT scanning (which may be applied to the analysis of complex fractures and dislocations), CT arthrography (for the assessment of intra-articular bodies), and MR imaging and MR arthrography (which have many established applications). The technical aspects of each of these methods vary according to the specific clinical situation (see later discussion). General comments related to two of these methods (arthrography and MR imaging) are included here.

Arthrography

Arthrography of the ankle is accomplished under fluoroscopic control with the patient in the recumbent position.[37, 38] A 20 gauge, 1.5 inch needle is introduced into the ankle, and 6 to 10 ml of radiopaque contrast material is injected.

Under normal circumstances, ankle arthrography results in opacification of the articular cavity without evidence of extra-articular leak except for filling of the tendon sheath of the flexor hallucis longus or the flexor digitorum longus, or both, in approximately 20 per cent of patients (Fig. 17–15).[37, 38] The posterior subtalar joint will be opacified in approximately 10 to 20 per cent of patients. All other patterns of contrast medium extravasation are regarded as abnormal.

The normal ankle arthrogram reveals three recesses. In the region of the syndesmosis between distal portions of the tibia and fibula, a small vertical recess, best delineated on oblique radiographs, 1 to 2.5 cm high and approximately 4 mm wide can be observed.[39] Additional anterior and posterior recesses are best visualized on lateral radiographs.

Arthrographic evaluation of either or both talocalcaneal joints has been employed to investigate congenital, traumatic, and articular disorders.[40, 41] The normal arthrogram of the talocalcaneonavicular joint demonstrates a smooth synovial cavity extending in a gradual curve, which is concave posteriorly, about the anterior aspect of the talus (Fig. 17–16). The cavity extends dorsally to the talar neck and ventrally along the plantar aspect of the talus. It covers the sustentaculum tali. There is no communication with the calcaneocuboid, posterior subtalar, or cuneonavicular joints. The contrast-filled posterior subtalar joint appears as a linear dense area between the posterior halves of talus and calcaneus along the lateral aspect of the foot (see Fig. 17–16). A recess appears as a sausage-shaped collection of contrast material at the posterior margin of the joint. Medial and lateral recesses also are evident. No contrast material flows into the region of the sinus tarsi.[41] In 10 to 20 per cent of arthrograms, communication is present between the posterior subtalar joint and the ankle.

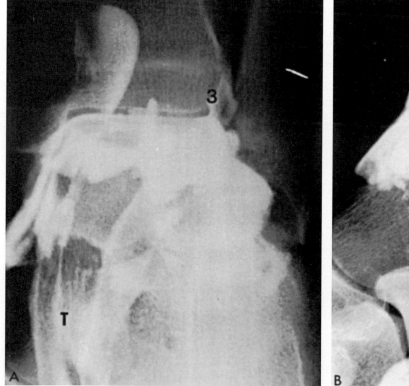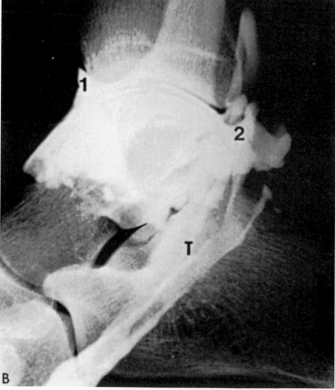

Figure 17–15

Ankle arthrography: Normal arthrogram. Anteroposterior (**A**) and lateral (**B**) views. The tibiotalar joint has been opacified. Note the normal recesses: anterior recess (1), posterior recess (2), and syndesmotic recess (3). Filling of the medial tendon sheaths (T) and posterior subtalar joint (arrowhead) is a normal finding.

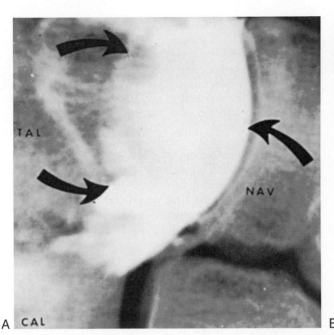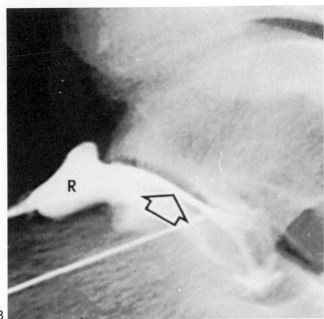

Figure 17–16

Arthrography of the talocalcaneonavicular and posterior subtalar joints: Normal appearance.

A An oblique projection during arthrography of the talocalcaneonavicular joint. Note the partially filled articular cavity (arrows) between the talus (TAL), navicular (NAV), and calcaneus (CAL).

B A lateral projection during arthrography of the posterior subtalar joint reveals filling of the articular cavity (arrow) with visualization of a normal posterior recess (R). The talocalcaneonavicular joint does not opacify.

(From Resnick D: *Radiology 111*:581, 1974.)

Rarely is communication observed between the posterior subtalar joint and talocalcaneonavicular cavity.

Magnetic Resonance Imaging

MR imaging of the foot and ankle poses unique challenges owing, in part, to the small size of the structures of interest (requiring high spatial resolution), the non-orthogonal orientation of many of these structures (necessitating careful selection of imaging planes), the numerous ways in which the patient may be positioned for the examination (supine or prone and, if supine, with the knees flexed or straightened), and the curved external surface of the foot and ankle (which may create technical difficulties, as with fat suppression methods).[42, 43] Although the most successful MR imaging examinations of the ankle and foot are tailored according to the indications for each individual patient, a simplified approach divides this anatomic area into three examination zones[44]: the ankle and hindfoot, the midfoot, and the forefoot. As the midfoot is displayed adequately whether the examination is tailored for the ankle and hindfoot or for the forefoot, further simplification is possible in which only two examination zones are considered. The major indications for examination of the ankle and hindfoot (including the midfoot) are assessment of tendons, ligaments, and osteochondritis dissecans of the talus; the major indication for examination of the forefoot (including the midfoot) is assessment of infection, particularly that of the diabetic foot. For the examination of the ankle, hindfoot, and midfoot, the patient may be placed supine, the foot and ankle are positioned such that the medial malleolus is in the center of the coil, and the foot is allowed to lie in a relaxed position (usually about 10 to 20 degrees of plantar flexion and 10 to 30 degrees of external rotation).[44] For the examination of forefoot and midfoot, the patient can lie supine with the knees flexed or prone with the feet plantar flexed, and the toes are centered in the coil.

In general, examination of only the affected side is superior, allowing a smaller field of view (FOV). In practice, however, having the other (unaffected) side for comparison purposes has distinct advantages, particularly in the assessment of tendons and ligaments. Such comparison usually is not required when the examination is being performed for evaluation of infection or tumor. Furthermore, when necessary, images of both sides can be confined to a single plane, usually the transverse (or transaxial) plane when the ankle and hindfoot are being examined. The choice of a surface coil depends on whether one foot or both feet are included in the images; a send-receive extremity coil is adequate for examination of a single foot and ankle, whereas a head coil may be employed to assess both feet and ankles. A FOV of 12 to 14 cm can be used to examine a single extremity; a larger FOV obviously is required to examine both extremities. Although the larger FOV results in decreased in-plane spatial resolution, such resolution can be improved by decreasing the matrix size of the images. For example, the resolution of an image obtained with a 25 cm FOV and a 256 × 256 matrix is equal to that of a 12 cm FOV and 128 matrix.[42] Slice thickness depends on the precise imaging sequence that is chosen. For spin echo sequences, a slice thickness of 3 or 4 mm is typical.

The three conventional imaging planes used to study the ankle and foot are sagittal, coronal, and transverse (or transaxial) (Plates 14–1 through 14–12). With regard to the foot, the transverse plane is parallel to the plantar surface (i.e., the plantar plane). In almost all instances, at least two and often three imaging planes are employed. Of the three planes, the transaxial plane usually provides the most anatomic information and should be used as part of every examination. Tendons are best displayed in transaxial and sagittal images, and ligaments are best displayed in transaxial and coronal images. Adequate visualization of ankle ligaments may require plantar flexion or dorsiflexion of the foot, or both, however (see later discussion). Adequate visualization of tendons may require use of nonorthogonal planes that are parallel and at right angles to the longitudinal contour of specific tendons. Such planes also are useful in delineating a variety of other soft tissue and bony structures of the ankle and foot.[497]

Little agreement exists regarding the specific imaging sequences required when performing MR imaging examinations of the ankle and foot. Typically, conventional or fast spin echo sequences form at least a portion of the examination, and both T1-weighted and T2-weighted images are obtained. Some form of gradient echo imaging, such as a multiplanar gradient recalled (MPGR) sequence, can be employed with a shallow flip angle to delineate regions of abnormal signal intensity, as in cases of tenosynovitis and tendon tears. Three-dimensional Fourier transform (3DFT) gradient echo imaging sequences are useful in certain situations, owing to the ability to obtain very thin sections and, when the data set is nearly isotropic, to allow reformatted images to be obtained in nonorthogonal planes. One such application relates to the assessment of ligament injuries. MR angiography employing two-dimensional (2D) or 3D time-of-flight (TOF) techniques has found use in the assessment of patients with peripheral vascular disease in the foot and ankle, obviating the need for angiography.[45]

Fat suppression methods often are applied to MR imaging of various anatomic sites, including the ankle and foot. Their benefit is most apparent in the analysis of infections and neoplasms, although these techniques also can be used to detect regions of bone marrow edema accompanying acute injuries or chronic stress reactions. Two types of fat suppression imaging are most popular: short tau (inversion time) inversion recovery (STIR) and chemically selective inversion pulses (spectral presaturation with inversion recovery [SPIR]) or chemically selective saturation pulses (ChemSat).[42] The first of these, STIR, accomplishes apparent fat suppression by employing a short inversion time. It is extremely sensitive to the presence of marrow abnormalities, which typically appear as regions of high signal intensity, and, because of this, represent an important screening method. SPIR or ChemSat imaging sequences also are sensitive to marrow abnormalities and represent true fat suppression methods. Suppression of fat about the foot and ankle may not be uniform with these methods, however, unless ancillary techniques are employed (Fig. 17–17). True fat suppression methods decrease the signal intensity of the predominantly fatty bone marrow and, when coupled with imaging sequences (such as certain fast spin echo sequences) that lead to increased signal intensity at sites of abnormal marrow, can be quite effective. These methods also can be combined with the intravenous administration of a gadolinium contrast agent to accentuate the abnormalities associated with marrow processes. In general, the appearance of such processes on MR images combining fat suppression and intravenous gadolinium contrast agent is similar to that displayed on STIR MR images, although the latter images may lead to an overestimation of the extent of abnormality. Fat suppression methods also can be combined with the intra-articular administration of a gadolinium compound (i.e., MR arthrography), al-

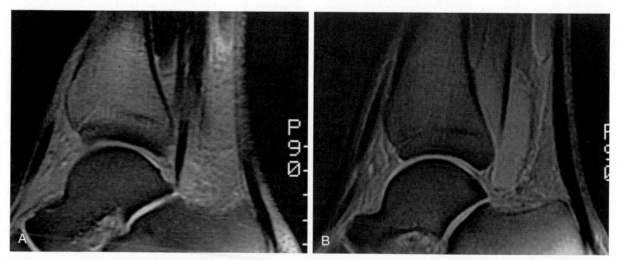

Figure 17–17

MR imaging of the ankle and foot: Fat suppression techniques. When compared to a standard sagittal T1-weighted (TR/TE, 850/12) spin echo MR image obtained with fat suppression (ChemSat) **(A)**, an identical sagittal T1-weighted (TR/TE, 850/12) fat-suppressed MR image in which a bag containing Kaopectate Plus was placed about the ankle **(B)** shows more homogeneous suppression of fat.

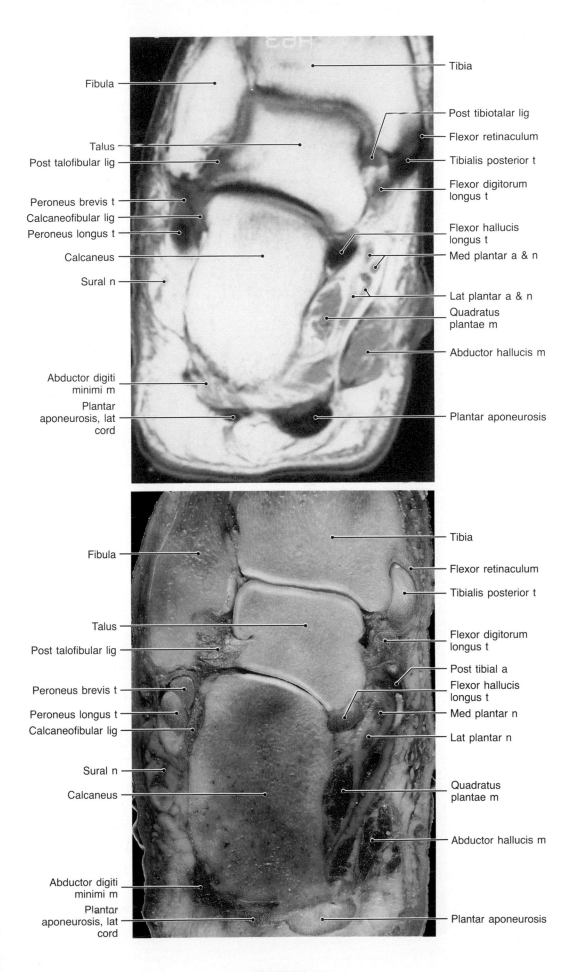

Fibula

Tibia

Talus

Post talofibular lig

Post tibiotalar lig

Flexor retinaculum

Tibialis posterior t

Peroneus brevis t

Calcaneofibular lig

Peroneus longus t

Calcaneus

Sural n

Flexor digitorum
longus t

Flexor hallucis
longus t

Med plantar a & n

Lat plantar a & n

Quadratus
plantae m

Abductor hallucis m

Abductor digiti
minimi m

Plantar
aponeurosis, lat
cord

Plantar aponeurosis

Fibula

Tibia

Flexor retinaculum

Tibialis posterior t

Talus

Post talofibular lig

Flexor digitorum
longus t

Post tibial a

Peroneus brevis t

Peroneus longus t

Calcaneofibular lig

Flexor hallucis
longus t

Med plantar n

Lat plantar n

Sural n

Calcaneus

Quadratus
plantae m

Abductor hallucis m

Abductor digiti
minimi m

Plantar
aponeurosis, lat
cord

Plantar aponeurosis

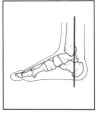

PLATE 17–1

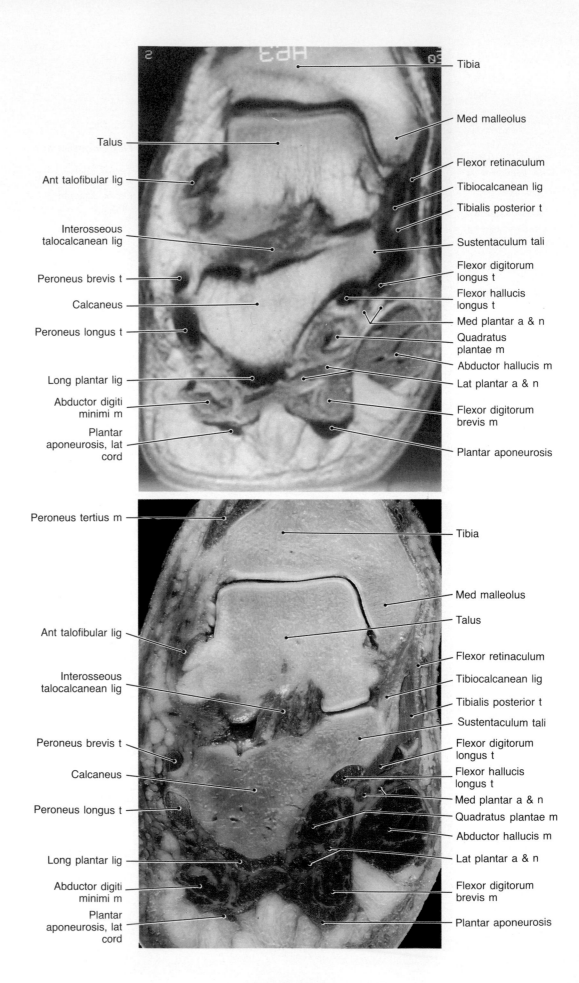

Tibia

Med malleolus

Talus

Ant talofibular lig

Flexor retinaculum

Tibiocalcanean lig

Tibialis posterior t

Interosseous talocalcanean lig

Sustentaculum tali

Flexor digitorum longus t

Peroneus brevis t

Flexor hallucis longus t

Calcaneus

Med plantar a & n

Peroneus longus t

Quadratus plantae m

Abductor hallucis m

Lat plantar a & n

Long plantar lig

Flexor digitorum brevis m

Abductor digiti minimi m

Plantar aponeurosis, lat cord

Plantar aponeurosis

Peroneus tertius m

Tibia

Ant talofibular lig

Med malleolus

Talus

Flexor retinaculum

Interosseous talocalcanean lig

Tibiocalcanean lig

Tibialis posterior t

Sustentaculum tali

Peroneus brevis t

Flexor digitorum longus t

Calcaneus

Flexor hallucis longus t

Peroneus longus t

Med plantar a & n

Quadratus plantae m

Abductor hallucis m

Long plantar lig

Lat plantar a & n

Abductor digiti minimi m

Flexor digitorum brevis m

Plantar aponeurosis, lat cord

Plantar aponeurosis

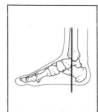

PLATE 17–2

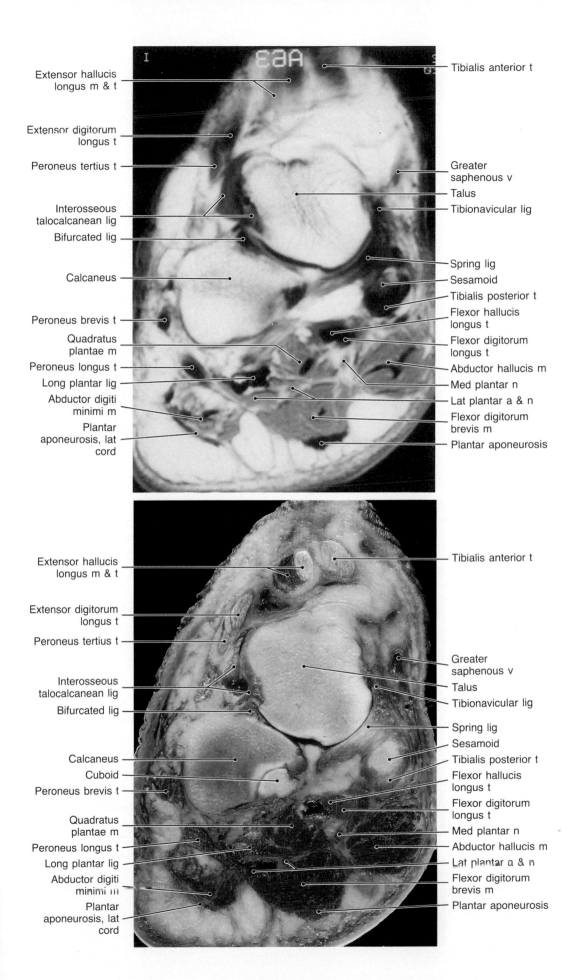

Upper image labels:

Extensor hallucis longus m & t

Extensor digitorum longus t

Peroneus tertius t

Interosseous talocalcanean lig

Bifurcated lig

Calcaneus

Peroneus brevis t

Quadratus plantae m

Peroneus longus t

Long plantar lig

Abductor digiti minimi m

Plantar aponeurosis, lat cord

Tibialis anterior t

Greater saphenous v

Talus

Tibionavicular lig

Spring lig

Sesamoid

Tibialis posterior t

Flexor hallucis longus t

Flexor digitorum longus t

Abductor hallucis m

Med plantar n

Lat plantar a & n

Flexor digitorum brevis m

Plantar aponeurosis

Lower image labels:

Extensor hallucis longus m & t

Extensor digitorum longus t

Peroneus tertius t

Interosseous talocalcanean lig

Bifurcated lig

Calcaneus

Cuboid

Peroneus brevis t

Quadratus plantae m

Peroneus longus t

Long plantar lig

Abductor digiti minimi m

Plantar aponeurosis, lat cord

Tibialis anterior t

Greater saphenous v

Talus

Tibionavicular lig

Spring lig

Sesamoid

Tibialis posterior t

Flexor hallucis longus t

Flexor digitorum longus t

Med plantar n

Abductor hallucis m

Lat plantar a & n

Flexor digitorum brevis m

Plantar aponeurosis

PLATE 17–3

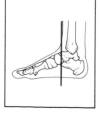

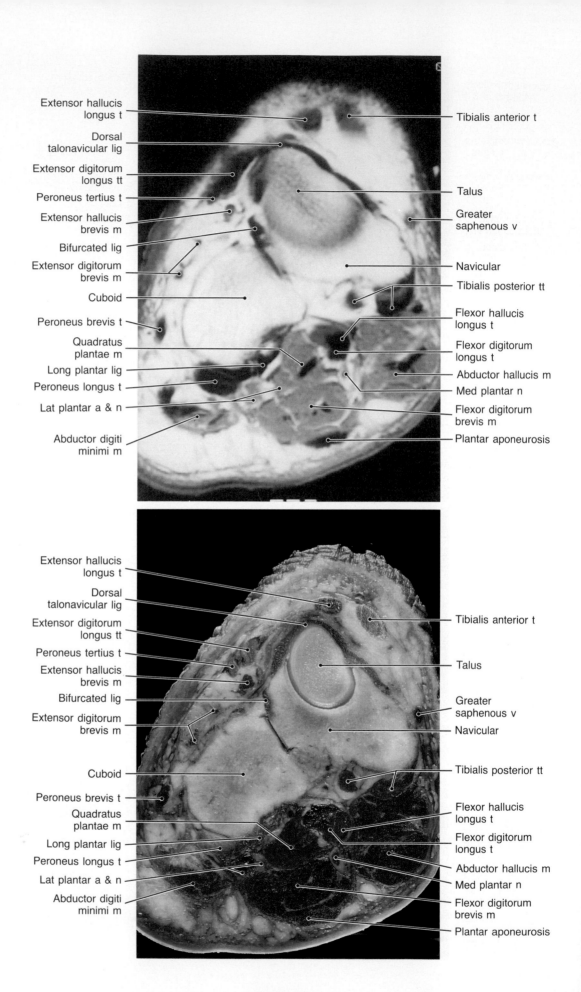

Extensor hallucis longus t

Dorsal talonavicular lig

Extensor digitorum longus tt

Peroneus tertius t

Extensor hallucis brevis m

Bifurcated lig

Extensor digitorum brevis m

Cuboid

Peroneus brevis t

Quadratus plantae m

Long plantar lig

Peroneus longus t

Lat plantar a & n

Abductor digiti minimi m

Tibialis anterior t

Talus

Greater saphenous v

Navicular

Tibialis posterior tt

Flexor hallucis longus t

Flexor digitorum longus t

Abductor hallucis m

Med plantar n

Flexor digitorum brevis m

Plantar aponeurosis

Extensor hallucis longus t

Dorsal talonavicular lig

Extensor digitorum longus tt

Peroneus tertius t

Extensor hallucis brevis m

Bifurcated lig

Extensor digitorum brevis m

Cuboid

Peroneus brevis t

Quadratus plantae m

Long plantar lig

Peroneus longus t

Lat plantar a & n

Abductor digiti minimi m

Tibialis anterior t

Talus

Greater saphenous v

Navicular

Tibialis posterior tt

Flexor hallucis longus t

Flexor digitorum longus t

Abductor hallucis m

Med plantar n

Flexor digitorum brevis m

Plantar aponeurosis

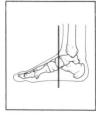

PLATE 17–4

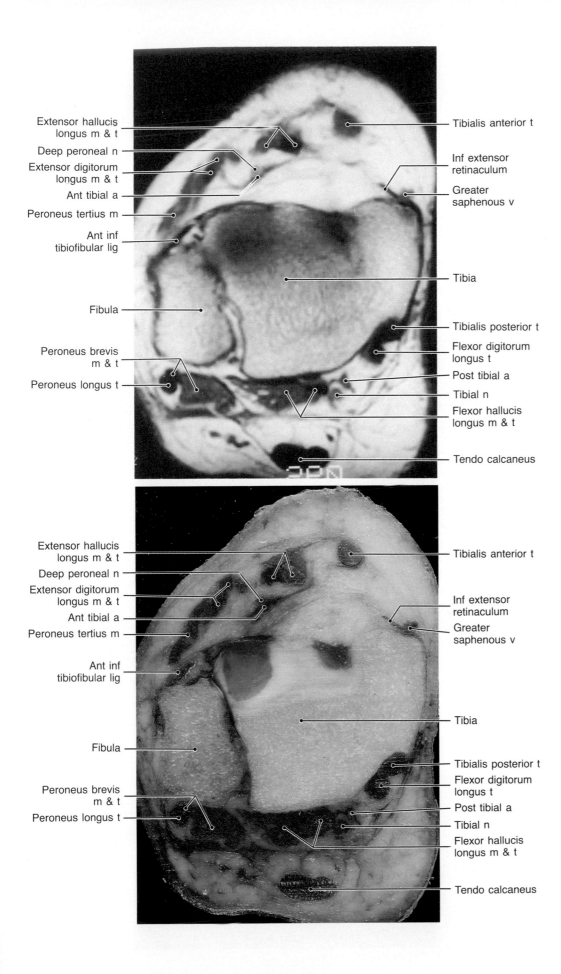

Extensor hallucis longus m & t

Deep peroneal n

Extensor digitorum longus m & t

Ant tibial a

Peroneus tertius m

Ant inf tibiofibular lig

Fibula

Peroneus brevis m & t

Peroneus longus t

Tibialis anterior t

Inf extensor retinaculum

Greater saphenous v

Tibia

Tibialis posterior t

Flexor digitorum longus t

Post tibial a

Tibial n

Flexor hallucis longus m & t

Tendo calcaneus

Extensor hallucis longus m & t

Deep peroneal n

Extensor digitorum longus m & t

Ant tibial a

Peroneus tertius m

Ant inf tibiofibular lig

Fibula

Peroneus brevis m & t

Peroneus longus t

Tibialis anterior t

Inf extensor retinaculum

Greater saphenous v

Tibia

Tibialis posterior t

Flexor digitorum longus t

Post tibial a

Tibial n

Flexor hallucis longus m & t

Tendo calcaneus

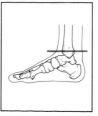

PLATE 17–5

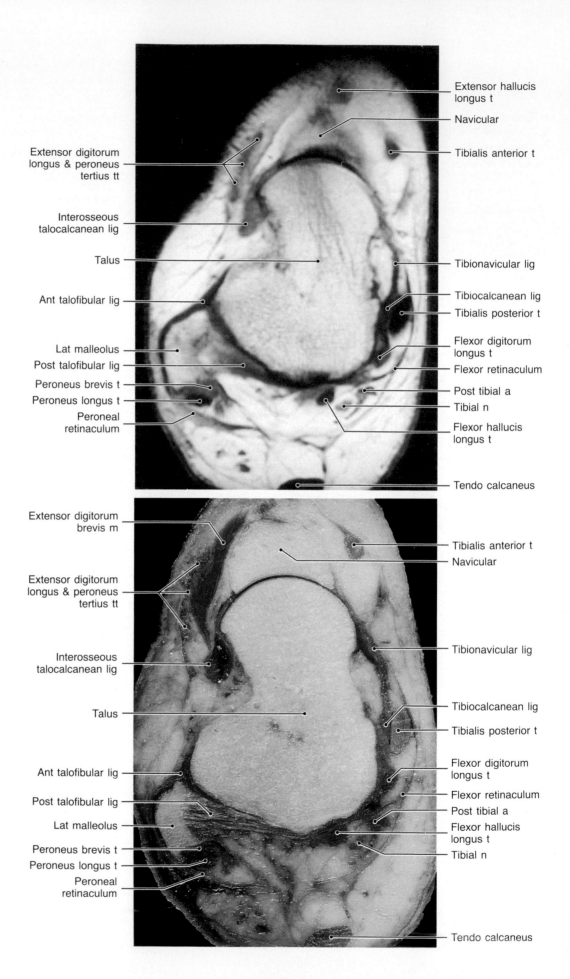

Extensor hallucis longus t

Navicular

Tibialis anterior t

Extensor digitorum longus & peroneus tertius tt

Interosseous talocalcanean lig

Talus

Tibionavicular lig

Ant talofibular lig

Tibiocalcanean lig

Tibialis posterior t

Lat malleolus

Flexor digitorum longus t

Post talofibular lig

Flexor retinaculum

Peroneus brevis t

Post tibial a

Peroneus longus t

Tibial n

Peroneal retinaculum

Flexor hallucis longus t

Tendo calcaneus

Extensor digitorum brevis m

Tibialis anterior t

Navicular

Extensor digitorum longus & peroneus tertius tt

Interosseous talocalcanean lig

Talus

Tibionavicular lig

Tibiocalcanean lig

Tibialis posterior t

Ant talofibular lig

Flexor digitorum longus t

Post talofibular lig

Flexor retinaculum

Lat malleolus

Post tibial a

Peroneus brevis t

Flexor hallucis longus t

Peroneus longus t

Tibial n

Peroneal retinaculum

Tendo calcaneus

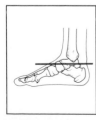

PLATE 17-6

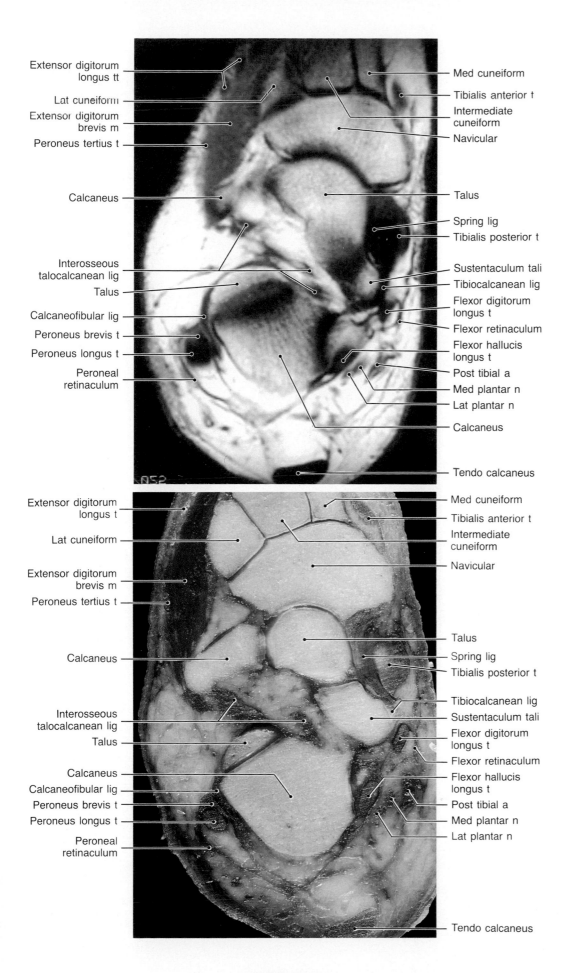

Extensor digitorum longus tt

Lat cuneiform

Extensor digitorum brevis m

Peroneus tertius t

Calcaneus

Interosseous talocalcanean lig

Talus

Calcaneofibular lig

Peroneus brevis t

Peroneus longus t

Peroneal retinaculum

Med cuneiform

Tibialis anterior t

Intermediate cuneiform

Navicular

Talus

Spring lig

Tibialis posterior t

Sustentaculum tali

Tibiocalcanean lig

Flexor digitorum longus t

Flexor retinaculum

Flexor hallucis longus t

Post tibial a

Med plantar n

Lat plantar n

Calcaneus

Tendo calcaneus

Extensor digitorum longus t

Lat cuneiform

Extensor digitorum brevis m

Peroneus tertius t

Calcaneus

Interosseous talocalcanean lig

Talus

Calcaneus

Calcaneofibular lig

Peroneus brevis t

Peroneus longus t

Peroneal retinaculum

Med cuneiform

Tibialis anterior t

Intermediate cuneiform

Navicular

Talus

Spring lig

Tibialis posterior t

Tibiocalcanean lig

Sustentaculum tali

Flexor digitorum longus t

Flexor retinaculum

Flexor hallucis longus t

Post tibial a

Med plantar n

Lat plantar n

Tendo calcaneus

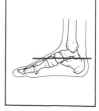

PLATE 17–7

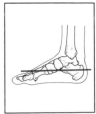

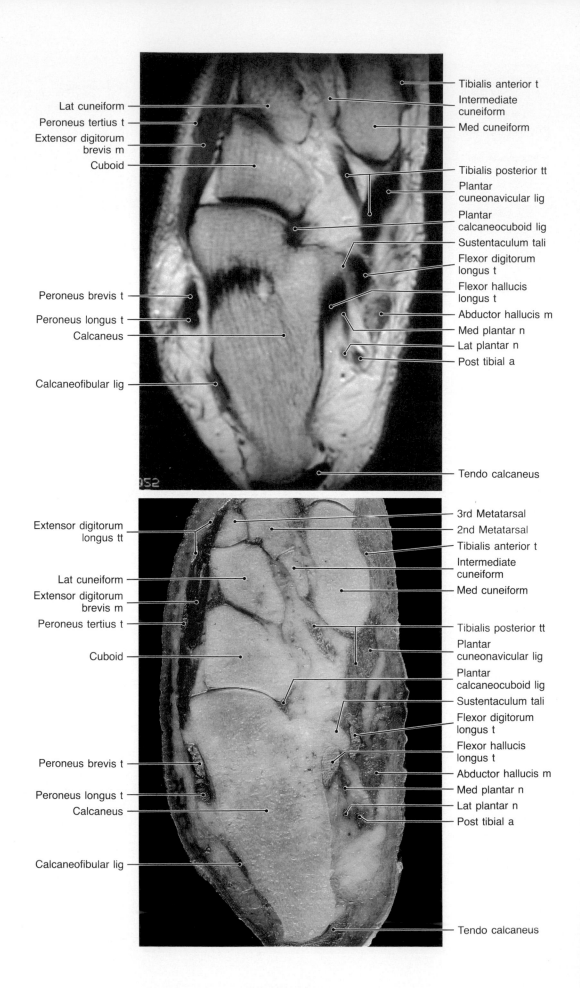

Lat cuneiform

Peroneus tertius t

Extensor digitorum
brevis m

Cuboid

Peroneus brevis t

Peroneus longus t

Calcaneus

Calcaneofibular lig

Tibialis anterior t

Intermediate
cuneiform

Med cuneiform

Tibialis posterior tt

Plantar
cuneonavicular lig

Plantar
calcaneocuboid lig

Sustentaculum tali

Flexor digitorum
longus t

Flexor hallucis
longus t

Abductor hallucis m

Med plantar n

Lat plantar n

Post tibial a

Tendo calcaneus

Extensor digitorum
longus tt

Lat cuneiform

Extensor digitorum
brevis m

Peroneus tertius t

Cuboid

Peroneus brevis t

Peroneus longus t

Calcaneus

Calcaneofibular lig

3rd Metatarsal

2nd Metatarsal

Tibialis anterior t

Intermediate
cuneiform

Med cuneiform

Tibialis posterior tt

Plantar
cuneonavicular lig

Plantar
calcaneocuboid lig

Sustentaculum tali

Flexor digitorum
longus t

Flexor hallucis
longus t

Abductor hallucis m

Med plantar n

Lat plantar n

Post tibial a

Tendo calcaneus

PLATE 17–8

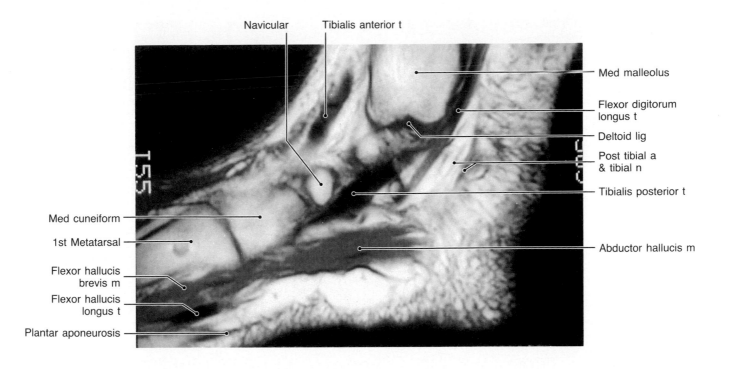

Navicular — Tibialis anterior t

Med malleolus

Flexor digitorum longus t

Deltoid lig

Post tibial a & tibial n

Tibialis posterior t

Med cuneiform

1st Metatarsal

Flexor hallucis brevis m

Flexor hallucis longus t

Plantar aponeurosis

Abductor hallucis m

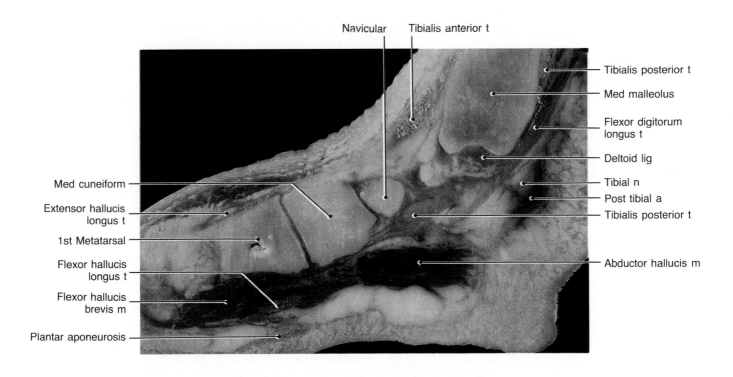

Navicular — Tibialis anterior t

Tibialis posterior t

Med malleolus

Flexor digitorum longus t

Deltoid lig

Tibial n

Post tibial a

Tibialis posterior t

Med cuneiform

Extensor hallucis longus t

1st Metatarsal

Flexor hallucis longus t

Flexor hallucis brevis m

Plantar aponeurosis

Abductor hallucis m

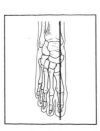

PLATE 17-9

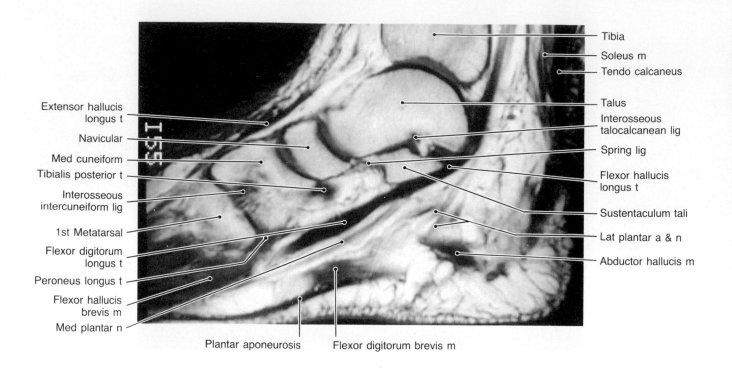

Extensor hallucis longus t

Navicular

Med cuneiform

Tibialis posterior t

Interosseous intercuneiform lig

1st Metatarsal

Flexor digitorum longus t

Peroneus longus t

Flexor hallucis brevis m

Med plantar n

Tibia

Soleus m

Tendo calcaneus

Talus

Interosseous talocalcanean lig

Spring lig

Flexor hallucis longus t

Sustentaculum tali

Lat plantar a & n

Abductor hallucis m

Plantar aponeurosis   Flexor digitorum brevis m

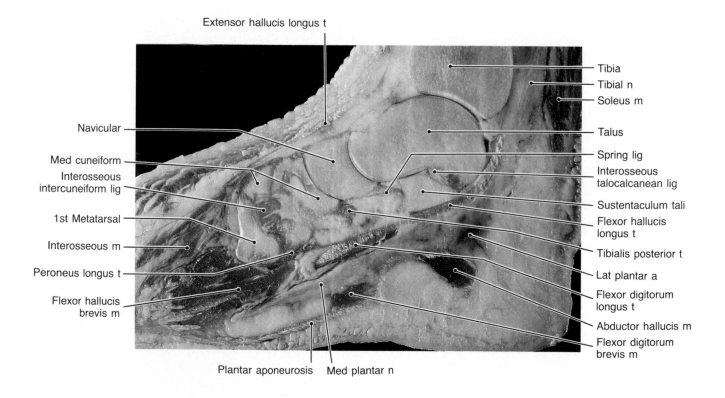

Extensor hallucis longus t

Navicular

Med cuneiform

Interosseous intercuneiform lig

1st Metatarsal

Interosseous m

Peroneus longus t

Flexor hallucis brevis m

Tibia

Tibial n

Soleus m

Talus

Spring lig

Interosseous talocalcanean lig

Sustentaculum tali

Flexor hallucis longus t

Tibialis posterior t

Lat plantar a

Flexor digitorum longus t

Abductor hallucis m

Flexor digitorum brevis m

Plantar aponeurosis   Med plantar n

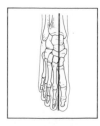

PLATE 17–10

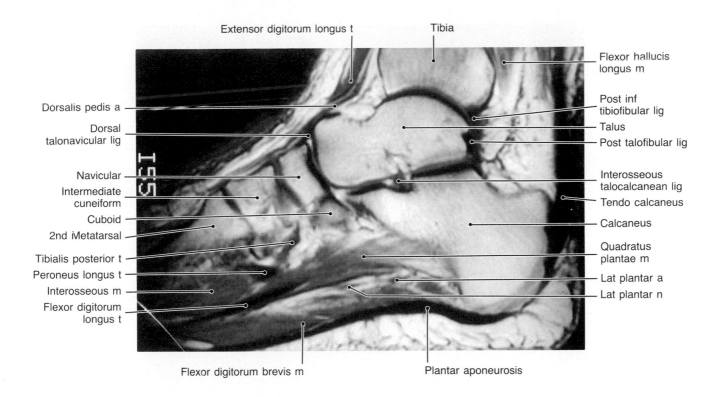

Extensor digitorum longus t   Tibia

Dorsalis pedis a

Dorsal talonavicular lig

Navicular

Intermediate cuneiform

Cuboid

2nd Metatarsal

Tibialis posterior t

Peroneus longus t

Interosseous m

Flexor digitorum longus t

Flexor hallucis longus m

Post inf tibiofibular lig

Talus

Post talofibular lig

Interosseous talocalcanean lig

Tendo calcaneus

Calcaneus

Quadratus plantae m

Lat plantar a

Lat plantar n

Flexor digitorum brevis m   Plantar aponeurosis

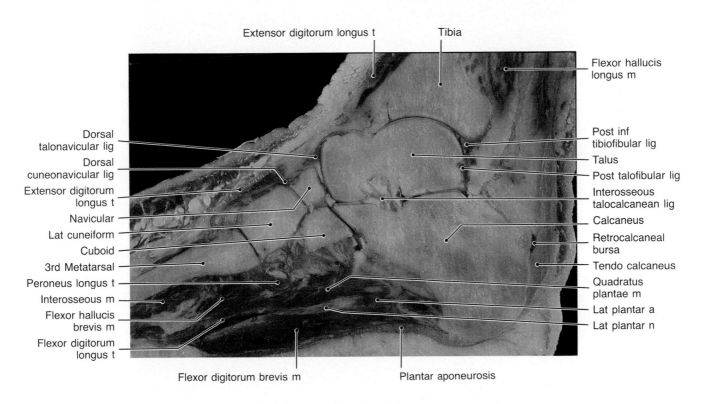

Extensor digitorum longus t   Tibia

Dorsal talonavicular lig

Dorsal cuneonavicular lig

Extensor digitorum longus t

Navicular

Lat cuneiform

Cuboid

3rd Metatarsal

Peroneus longus t

Interosseous m

Flexor hallucis brevis m

Flexor digitorum longus t

Flexor hallucis longus m

Post inf tibiofibular lig

Talus

Post talofibular lig

Interosseous talocalcanean lig

Calcaneus

Retrocalcaneal bursa

Tendo calcaneus

Quadratus plantae m

Lat plantar a

Lat plantar n

Flexor digitorum brevis m   Plantar aponeurosis

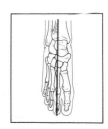

PLATE 17–11

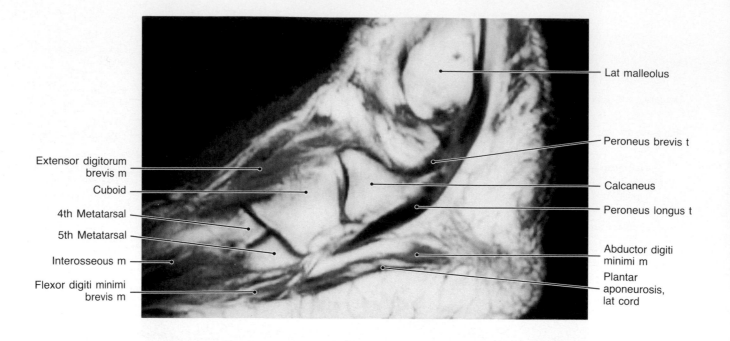

Extensor digitorum brevis m

Cuboid

4th Metatarsal

5th Metatarsal

Interosseous m

Flexor digiti minimi brevis m

Lat malleolus

Peroneus brevis t

Calcaneus

Peroneus longus t

Abductor digiti minimi m

Plantar aponeurosis, lat cord

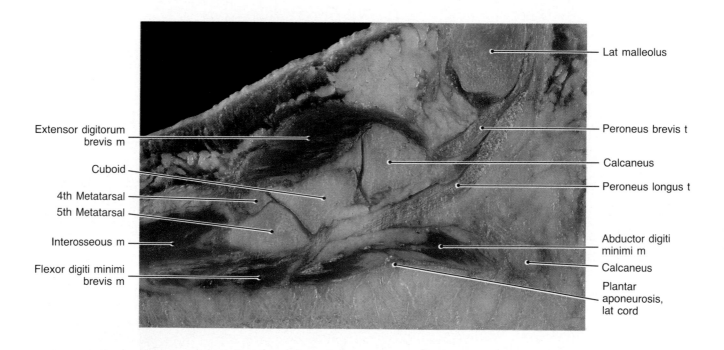

Extensor digitorum brevis m

Cuboid

4th Metatarsal

5th Metatarsal

Interosseous m

Flexor digiti minimi brevis m

Lat malleolus

Peroneus brevis t

Calcaneus

Peroneus longus t

Abductor digiti minimi m

Calcaneus

Plantar aponeurosis, lat cord

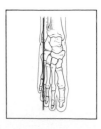

PLATE 17–12

though the indications for this procedure are limited (see later discussion).

Dynamic MR imaging can be accomplished by combining methods of rapid image acquisition with movement of a body part. Although this type of imaging has proved useful in the evaluation of disorders of the temporomandibular, patellofemoral, and radiocarpal joints, data regarding its application to abnormalities of the ankle and foot are incomplete. One potential application of dynamic MR imaging to assessment of abnormalities in these last anatomic sites relates to tendon subluxation or dislocation, particularly of the peroneal tendons (see later discussion), which may be evident only in certain positions of the foot.

SPECIFIC ABNORMALITIES

Fractures and Dislocations

Fractures of the Tibial and Fibular Diaphyses

Of all the long tubular bones, the tibia is fractured most commonly. Direct or indirect forces applied to the tibia can result in fracture (Table 17-1). Indirect forces lead to spiral or oblique fractures of the tibia (as opposed to the transverse or comminuted fractures associated with direct injury), and the fibula may be left intact. Isolated fractures of the shaft of the fibula are uncommon, resulting from a direct blow. More typically, such an apparently isolated fibular fracture in reality is one component of a more complicated injury involving also the ankle (see later discussion).[46] CT may be required in the evaluation of some tibial fractures to assess the relationship of the fracture fragments and the extent of soft tissue injury. In instances of spiral fractures of the tibia, CT provides accurate information regarding the extent of separation of the fragments.[47] Although MR imaging is of great benefit for the detection of stress

fractures and other occult injuries of the lower leg (and foot), its role in the assessment of acute fractures of the shafts of the tibia and fibula is not established.

The frequency and rate of union of tibial fractures have varied in reported series, although Sarmiento and colleagues,[48, 49] using closed reduction and prefabricated bracing of tibial shaft fractures, reported a union rate of 97.5 per cent. The average rate of healing of such fractures in adults is about 16 to 18 weeks in closed injuries and about 4 weeks longer in open injuries. Tibial shaft fractures in children generally heal more quickly. A delayed union of these tibial fractures should be considered present when the fracture line still is readily visible 5 to 6 months after the injury, and a nonunion should be suspected when the fracture line remains apparent more than 6 months after injury.[46] The role of scintigraphy and other imaging methods in the assessment of fracture healing is discussed in Chapter 8.

Additional complications of tibial (and fibular) shaft fractures include malunion, infection, neurovascular injury, and compartment syndromes. Although vascular injury in cases of tibial shaft fracture is uncommon, fractures involving the proximal portion of the diaphysis may be accompanied by occlusion or laceration of the anterior tibial artery. This artery also may be injured when fractures involving the lower portion of the tibia are displaced posteriorly. Posterior tibial artery involvement is rare in cases of tibial shaft fracture, although such involvement may be apparent when a posterior compartment syndrome is present. The common peroneal nerve is the most commonly injured nerve in patients with a fracture of the diaphysis of the tibia or fibula, although such injury is not frequent. Compartment syndromes, as indicated in Chapter 10, may complicate a variety of musculoskeletal injuries, including fractures of the tibial and fibular shafts. The anterior compartment of the lower leg is involved most commonly in these fractures, particularly in closed but also in open fractures. Its frequency is decreased in fractures that are comminuted or are associated with disruption

Table 17-1. FRACTURES OF THE TIBIAL AND FIBULAR SHAFTS

Site	Characteristics	Complications
Tibia	Direct or indirect trauma	Delayed union (no osseous union at 20 weeks) in 5 to 15 per cent of cases
	Associated fractures of the fibula, especially in direct and severe trauma	Nonunion (no osseous union at 6 months to 1 year) is most common in the distal third of tibia
	Transverse or comminuted fracture in direct trauma; oblique or spiral fracture in indirect trauma; sometimes segmental fractures	Infection with or without nonunion
		Vascular injury (to anterior tibial artery or, less commonly, posterior tibial artery)
	Middle and distal thirds > proximal third	Compartment syndrome (anterior > posterior or lateral compartment)
	Minor, moderate, or major categories of injury, the last associated with comminuted and open fractures	Nerve injury (uncommon, peroneal and posterior tibial nerves)
	Prognosis related to amount of displacement, degree of comminution, open or closed fracture, and infection	Refracture (especially in athletes)
	Childhood fractures:	Leg shortening
	Toddler fracture—spiral fracture, undisplaced	Osteoarthritis (if fracture extends into joint)
	Proximal metaphyseal fracture—associated with genu valgum deformity	Reflex sympathetic dystrophy syndrome
		Fat embolism
Fibula	Isolated fractures are rare, related to direct injury	Related to those of the associated tibial or ankle injury
	Associated fractures of the tibia and ankle injuries	

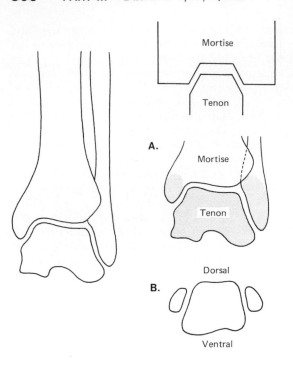

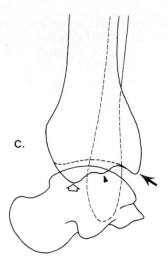

Figure 17–18

Ankle: Normal anatomy.

A Anteroposterior views show the "mortise and tenon" relationship of the tibia, fibula, and talus.

B This diagram illustrates the cross-sectional appearance of the talar side of the ankle joint. Note that the dorsal narrowing of the talus serves to wedge this bone into the mortise, particularly during weight-bearing and dorsiflexion.

C In this lateral view, the long posterior process of the tibia stabilizes the joint dorsally (solid arrow). The anterior (open arrow) and posterior (arrowhead) colliculi of the medial malleolus also are indicated.

of the interosseous membrane (or that are open), as spontaneous decompression of the compartment results. Involvement of the posterior or lateral compartment of the lower leg is less frequent.

In children, distinctive fractures of the tibial shaft include a spiral fracture in the first 3 years of life, designated a toddler's fracture, and a fracture involving the proximal metaphysis of the bone.[50–53] Valgus displacement in these latter fractures may relate to hyperemia with selective stimulation of the medial portion of the tibial physis or to interposition of the periosteum or a portion of the pes anserinus tissues within the fracture site.[54]

Fractures About the Ankle

Fractures about the ankle are among the most common traumatic abnormalities affecting the skeleton. The treatment of ankle injuries is directed toward restoration of anatomic alignment and reestablishment of normal function (Fig. 17–18); in recent years, a general trend toward operative intervention in the treatment of more severe injuries of the ankle has become apparent.[55] It is important to diagnose both fractures and ligamentous injuries to optimize these therapeutic efforts. Stability of the ankle joint depends on the integrity of a ring formed by the tibia, fibula, and talus, united by sur-

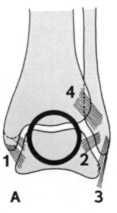
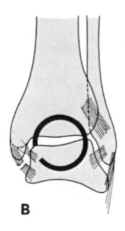
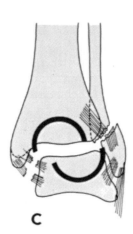

Figure 17–19

Ankle: Stable and unstable characteristics.

A The stability of the ankle joint is determined by the status of a ring comprising the mortise and surrounding ligaments. The latter include the deep and superficial deltoid ligaments (1), the anterior (2) and posterior (not shown) talofibular ligaments, the calcaneofibular ligament (3), the anterior (4) and posterior (not shown) tibiofibular ligaments, the inferior transverse ligament (not shown), and the interosseous membrane and ligament (not shown).

B A single break in this ring will not allow displacement.

C Two or more breaks in the ring allow displacement of the mortise.

rounding ligaments (Fig. 17–19).[56] A single break in the ring does not allow subluxation of the talus in the mortise, whereas two or more breaks in the ring, whether fractures or a fracture in combination with a ruptured ligament, will allow abnormal talar motion. Displacement of the talus in the ankle joint may be evident on routine radiographs including the mortise view. Such displacement, which becomes evident owing to widening of the medial portion of the joint space, generally has been attributed to a lateral shift of the talus, although the primary pattern of instability, in reality, appears to be external rotation of the talus.[55] The application of stress to the ankle during the radiograpic examination can be of considerable diagnostic impor-

tance in the detection of instability and of specific sites of ligamentous disruption (Fig. 17–20).[57–59]

Although ankle fractures may be described using anatomic terminology (e.g., medial or lateral malleolar, bimalleolar, or trimalleolar), such a description fails to consider the mechanism of injury and the associated ligamentous disruptions. A comprehensive classification of ankle fractures based on mechanism of injury was first proposed in 1922.[60] Subsequently, Lauge-Hansen derived a more unified and complete classification system that considered both the mechanism of injury and the associated ligamentous abnormalities.[61, 62] Although it is more complex than other classification systems, the Lauge-Hansen method becomes quite simple to remem-

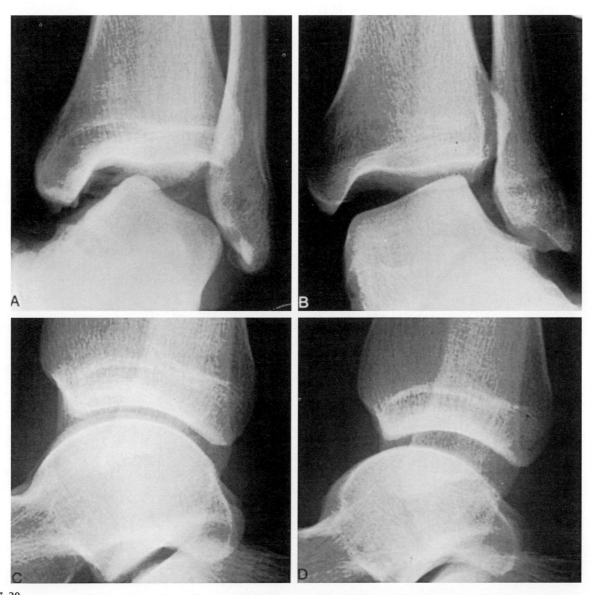

Figure 17–20
Ankle instability: Stress radiography.
  A An anteroposterior varus (inversion) stress view (with the foot in neutral position) shows obvious widening of the lateral portion of the joint, indicating some degree of ligamentous disruption. The tibiotalar angle measured 34 degrees. Small fracture fragments are evident.
  B An anteroposterior valgus (eversion) stress view reveals widening of the medial "clear" space indicative of a rupture of the deltoid ligaments.
  C, D Lateral radiographs were obtained without (**C**) and with (**D**) the application of anterior stress (anterior drawer sign). In **D**, note anterior movement of the talus on the tibia.

ber and apply once the basic terminology and the association between mechanism and radiographic appearance are understood. This method, however, is not ideal; it is based on the position of the foot relative to the body when, in fact, the foot commonly is fixed to the ground with the body in one of several different positions during a fall. Furthermore, interobserver (and even intraobserver) variation in the application of the Lauge-Hansen classification system appears to be large.[63, 64] Still, this system commonly is employed in the description of ankle injuries. Other classification methods do exist, however, including that of Weber (as a modification of the system of Danis), which is based on the position of fibular fracture with respect to the joint line.[46, 55, 65] Although the Weber system is simple to employ, its lack of descriptive detail and the general absence of reference to injury on the medial side of the ankle may limit its clinical usefulness.[66] In the Weber classification system, three patterns of injury are identified, two of which can also be assigned a Lauge-Hansen classification category[65]: Type A injuries (Fig. 17–21) are accompanied by a horizontal fracture of the lateral malleolus below or at the level of the joint space with an oblique fracture of the medial malleolus, corresponding to Lauge-Hansen supination-adduction injuries; type B injuries (Fig. 17–22) are accompanied by a spiral fracture of the lateral malleolus in association with partial disruption of the anterior tibiofibular ligament and a transverse fracture of the medial malleolus or disruption of the deltoid ligament, and they do not correspond precisely to a specific type of injury in the Lauge-Hansen classification system; and type C injuries (Fig. 17–23) are accompanied by a high fibular fracture with

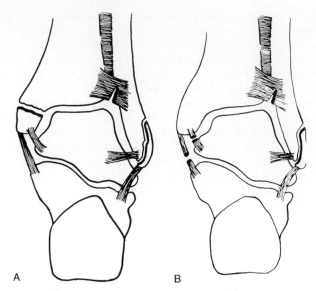

Figure 17–22
Weber type B ankle injury.
  A The typical injury produces spiral fractures of the distal end of the fibula, horizontal fractures of the medial malleolus, and partial disruption of the distal tibiofibular ligaments.
  B Variation of **A**, showing similar lateral changes with rupture of the deltoid ligament and an intact medial malleolus.
  (From Daffner RH: Radiol Clin North Am *28*:395, 1990.)

subsequent disruption of the anterior and posterior tibiofibular ligaments and interosseous membrane and a transverse fracture of the medial malleolus corresponding to Lauge-Hansen pronation–external rotation injuries.
  On the basis of experimental results in cadavers,

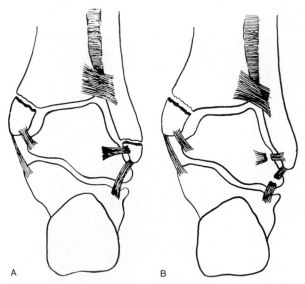

Figure 17–21
Weber type A ankle injuries.
  A The typical injury produces a transverse fracture of the distal fibula at or below the joint space in association with an oblique fracture of the medial malleolus.
  B Variation of **A**, in which there is an intact fibula with rupture of the lateral collateral ligaments and an oblique medial malleolar fracture.
  (From Daffner RH: Radiol Clin North Am *28*:395, 1990.)

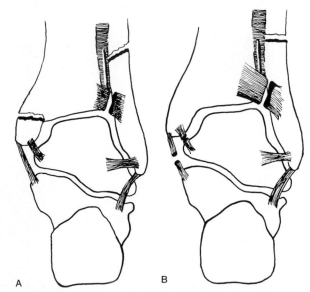

Figure 17–23
Weber type C injury.
  A This injury produces a high fibular fracture with disruption of the interosseous membrane and distal tibiofibular ligaments as well as a horizontal fracture of the medial malleolus.
  B Variant that has the same lateral findings but with an intact medial malleolus and rupture of the deltoid ligament.
  (From Daffner RH: Radiol Clin North Am *28*:395, 1990.)

Lauge-Hansen defined five major predictable fracture complexes.[61, 62, 67] Within each grouping are stages of injury, designated by Roman numerals; the higher the number, the greater the applied force and resultant damage. Each of the groups is designated by two characteristic terms. The first term is either *pronation* or *supination* and refers to the position of the foot at the time of injury (Fig. 17–24). Pronation or supination of the foot tightens various ligamentous and capsular structures of the tibiotalar joint, decreasing flexibility and increasing transmission of forces across the joint to the distal portions of the tibia and fibula. The foot is pronated when there is outward rotation and eversion of the forefoot with abduction of the hindfoot. Supination represents inward rotation and inversion of the forefoot with adduction of the hindfoot.

The second term reflects the direction that the talus is displaced or rotated relative to the mortise formed by the distal regions of the tibia and fibula. Talar displacement can occur in five possible directions: external rotation, in which the talus is displaced externally or laterally; internal rotation, in which the talus is displaced internally or medially; abduction, in which the talus is displaced laterally without significant rotation; adduction, in which the talus is displaced medially without significant rotation; and dorsiflexion, in which the talus is dorsiflexed on the tibia. Thus, with the foot in either pronation or supination, the talus may be subjected to one of five vectors of force—external rotation, internal rotation, abduction, adduction, or dorsiflexion. It also

should be realized that, for example, external rotation of the talus on the tibia and fibula will occur either when the foot is rotated laterally relative to the fixed tibia and fibula or when the body undergoes internal rotation while the foot is fixed. Although these fracture groups result from application of forces with the position and direction of the foot designated, the end result is classified by the radiographic appearance—specifically, in the first four types, by the configuration of the fibular fracture and not by the mechanism of injury deduced from available clinical information. Indeed, an accurate description of the injury rarely is provided by the patient.

1. Supination-external rotation fracture (SER stages I, II, III, and IV). The SER category constitutes almost 60 per cent of all ankle fractures (Fig. 17–25).[67] The fracture complex is caused by external rotation of the supinated foot. In this position, the deltoid ligament is relaxed. External rotation of the foot forces the talus against the fibula, commonly resulting in rupture of the anterior tibiofibular ligament (stage I), although, alternatively, an avulsion fracture arising from the anterior surface of the fibula or tibia (fracture of Tillaux) may be present.[68] Small avulsion fractures usually are not apparent radiographically; furthermore, as most stage I lesions are ligamentous, they too are rarely detected on radiographs. As the mechanism of injury continues, a short oblique fracture of the distal portion of the fibula will occur (stage II). This fracture extends

Figure 17–24
Supination and pronation: Compound motion of the ankle.

A–C, Supination. Supination is a compound motion consisting of adduction and inversion of the forefoot (**A**) combined with inversion of the heel (**B**) as well as plantar flexion of the foot about the ankle joint (**C**). Arrows indicate direction of motion.

D–F, Pronation. Pronation is a compound motion in which there is abduction and eversion of the forefoot (**D**) combined with eversion of the heel (**E**) as well as dorsiflexion of the foot at the ankle joint (**F**). Arrows indicate direction of motion.

(From Daffner RH: Radiol Clin North Am *28*:395, 1990.)

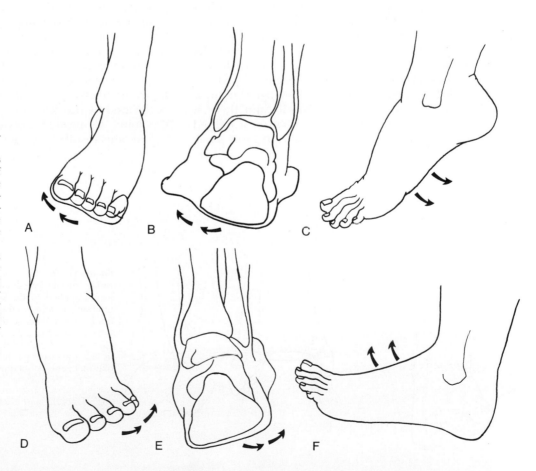

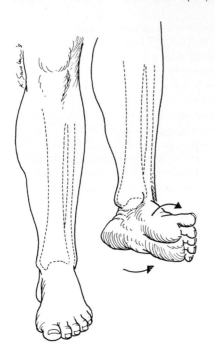

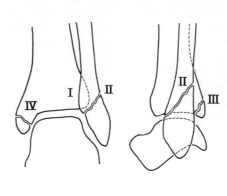

Figure 17–25

Ankle injuries: Supination—external rotation fracture. External rotation forces applied to the supinated foot result initially in a rupture of the anterior tibiofibular ligament (stage I). As the forces continue, a short oblique fracture of the distal portion of the fibula occurs (stage II). The next stage of the injury is a fracture of the posterior aspect of the tibia (stage III). The final stage of the injury is a fracture of the medial malleolus (stage IV).

from the anteromedial aspect of the fibula in a dorsal and proximal direction. It usually is evident within 1.5 cm of the tibiotalar joint and rarely is more than 2.5 cm proximal to this joint. The next stage of injury is a fracture of the posterior aspect of the tibia of varying size (stage III). The majority of SER stage III posterior tibial fractures are small and, in some cases, the injury may advance to stage IV without a posterior tibial fracture. The final stage (stage IV) is characterized by a fracture of the medial malleolus or a rupture of the deltoid ligament. Medial malleolar fractures and deltoid ligament ruptures occur with approximately equal frequency in SER injuries.[67] If a typical SER stage II oblique fibular fracture is noted radiographically and there is no evidence of a medial malleolar fracture, a deltoid injury should be suspected when medial soft tissue swell-

ing or widening of the medial aspect of the tibiotalar joint is apparent.

2. Supination-adduction fracture (SAD stages I and II). The SAD category constitutes about 20 per cent of all ankle fractures (Fig. 17–26).[67] These injuries are produced by a medially directed force acting on the supinated foot. Supination causes tension on the lateral ligaments and, with adduction, either a lateral ligament rupture or transverse (traction or avulsion) fracture of the distal portion of the fibula occurs (SAD stage I). The characteristic transverse fibular fracture usually arises just distal to the tibiotalar joint but, rarely, may be located at the level of or immediately proximal to the joint. Continued pressure from the medially directed talus results in a fracture of the medial malleolus

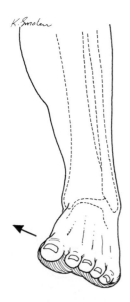

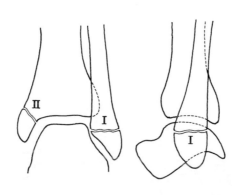

Figure 17–26

Ankle injuries: Supination-adduction fracture. Adduction forces applied to the supinated foot initially result in a traction or avulsion fracture of the distal portion of the fibula or rupture of the lateral ligaments (stage I). As forces continue, a fracture of the medial malleolus or a rupture of the deltoid ligament occurs (stage II). The fibular fracture typically is transverse and that of the medial malleolus is oblique or nearly vertical.

or a rupture of the deltoid ligament (SAD stage II). The malleolar fracture often is oblique or nearly vertical (as is typical of injuries related to compressive forces), but it also may be transverse, a fracture configuration usually attributed to avulsion or traction forces. Thus, the medial malleolar fracture configuration is not significantly distinctive to allow deduction of the mechanism of injury.

The injury to the lateral ligaments, particularly the anterior talofibular ligament, that characterizes the first stage of the SAD complex may represent an avulsion fracture. The fracture fragment often is small and located just distal to the fibular tip, and its identification commonly requires use of a bright light. As a general rule, any small ossicle in this location should be considered evidence of a recent (or remote) injury and not a normal variation of growth.[69]

3 and 4. Pronation–external rotation fracture (PER stages I, II, III, and IV); pronation-abduction fracture (PAB stages I, II, and III).

The PER (Figs. 17–27 and 17–28) and PAB (Fig. 17–29) fractures constitute about 20 per cent of all fractures occurring about the ankle.[67] The two groups commonly are considered together, as fractures of the PER stages I and II, and PAB stages I and II cannot be distinguished radiographically. When the foot is pronated, the deltoid ligament is tense. Forceful external rotation or abduction of the talus results in either deltoid ligament rupture (60 per cent) or fracture of the medial malleolus (40 per cent) (PER or PAB stage I). In a PER or PAB stage II lesion, a rupture of the distal tibiofibular syndesmosis also occurs. This latter injury may be purely ligamentous or may be an avulsion fracture arising from either the anterior or the posterior tubercle or from both. PAB stage III fractures include the injuries of the first two stages combined with a transverse supramalleolar fibular fracture. PER stage III

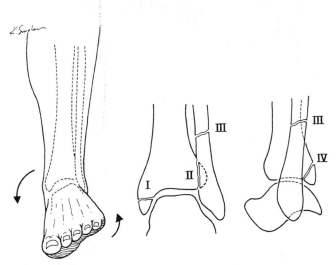

Figure 17–27

Ankle injuries: Pronation—external rotation fracture. Forces of external rotation applied to the pronated foot result initially in rupture of the deltoid ligament or a fracture of the medial malleolus (stage I). As forces continue, there is rupture of the anterior tibiofibular ligament (stage II). A high fibular fracture (stage III) and a fracture of the posterior tibial margin (stage IV) are the final stages in this mechanism of injury.

injuries include the abnormalities in the first two stages and a short spiral fracture of the fibula more than 2.5 cm above the tibiotalar joint. The last-mentioned fibular fracture usually is 6 to 8 cm above the ankle and may even be more proximal in location. Associated rupture of the syndesmosis ligaments and interosseous membrane occurs. PER stage IV fractures include the first three stages in combination with a fracture of the posterior tibial margin. Radiographic detection of the characteristic fibular fracture of either the PAB or PER stage III injury in the absence of a medial malleolar fracture must be associated with a rupture of the deltoid ligament.

Certain diagnostic points regarding these injuries deserve emphasis. A fibular fracture occurring above the joint line and proximal to the distal tibiofibular synostosis may be an important manifestation of an ankle injury. The Dupuytren fracture is one type, occurring in this position and involving the lower portion of the fibular shaft. When it results from a PER injury, the fracture extends from the anterior edge of the fibula in a posteroinferior direction; in a PAB injury the fracture is oblique and extends from the lateral surface of the bone in an inferomedial direction; and in a SER injury, the fibular fracture is oblique, located approximately 4 cm from the distal tip of the fibula, and extends from the anterior edge of the bone in a posterosuperior direction.[46] The Maisonneuve fracture is a second type, involving the proximal portion of the fibular shaft. Although the precise mechanism of this fracture is not agreed on, it is associated with disruption of the distal tibiofibular syndesmosis and a medial malleolar fracture or tear of the deltoid ligament.[70] It may be overlooked on the basis of clinical findings. Alternatively, when discovered, an evaluation of the ankle is required.[71] In one study using MR imaging to evaluate the ankle in five patients with acute Maisonneuve fractures, the anterior tibiofibular ligament was disrupted in all cases, the posterior tibiofibular ligament was disrupted in two patients, and the calcaneofibular (two patients), anterior talofibular (five patients), superficial deltoid (five patients), and deep deltoid (four patients) ligaments also were injured.[498]

Second, in these pronation injuries, the tibiofibular syndesmosis and interosseous membrane always are disrupted to the level of the most inferior portion of a fibular fracture that involves the distal portion of the diaphysis; with Maisonneuve fractures of the proximal fibula such disruption may or may not be present.[46] Measurement of the syndesmotic region, or lateral clear space, of the ankle therefore becomes important. A width greater than 5.5 mm always is abnormal, indicating syndesmotic rupture. A width of 2 to 5.5 mm is suggestive of such injury and may be an indication for stress radiography of the ankle.

5. Pronation-dorsiflexion fracture (PDF stages I, II, III, and IV).

The PDF category of ankle fractures was added to the first four categories to provide an explanation for a group of fractures produced by axial loading (Fig. 17–30).[72] These injuries also are designated pilon (pestle) fractures, as the talus is driven into the tibial

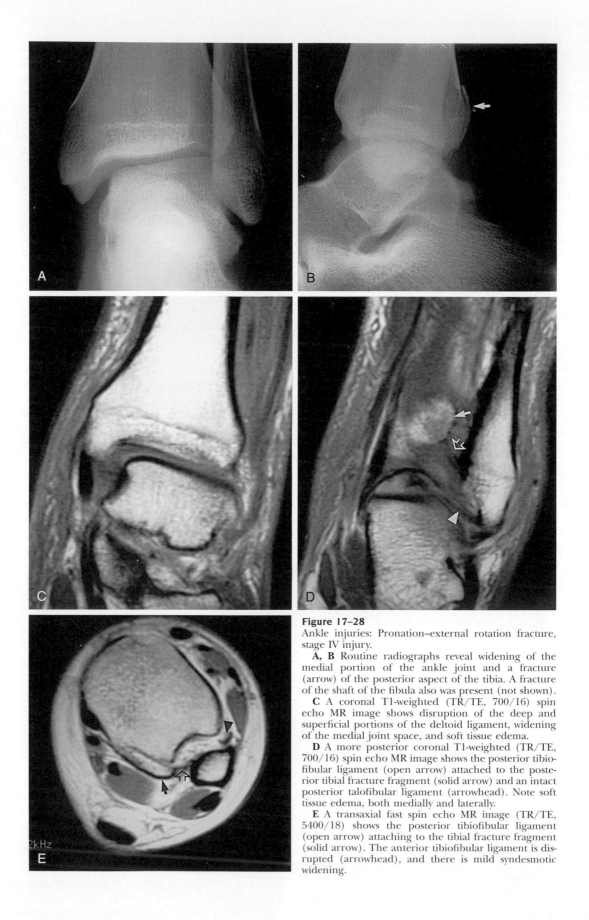

Figure 17–28

Ankle injuries: Pronation–external rotation fracture, stage IV injury.

A, B Routine radiographs reveal widening of the medial portion of the ankle joint and a fracture (arrow) of the posterior aspect of the tibia. A fracture of the shaft of the fibula also was present (not shown).

C A coronal T1-weighted (TR/TE, 700/16) spin echo MR image shows disruption of the deep and superficial portions of the deltoid ligament, widening of the medial joint space, and soft tissue edema.

D A more posterior coronal T1-weighted (TR/TE, 700/16) spin echo MR image shows the posterior tibiofibular ligament (open arrow) attached to the posterior tibial fracture fragment (solid arrow) and an intact posterior talofibular ligament (arrowhead). Note soft tissue edema, both medially and laterally.

E A transaxial fast spin echo MR image (TR/TE, 5400/18) shows the posterior tibiofibular ligament (open arrow) attaching to the tibial fracture fragment (solid arrow). The anterior tibiofibular ligament is disrupted (arrowhead), and there is mild syndesmotic widening.

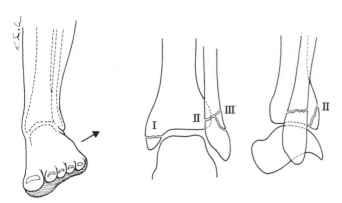

Figure 17–29

Ankle injuries: Pronation-abduction fracture. The first two stages of this injury are identical to those of the pronation–external rotation fracture complex. Stage III is a transverse supramalleolar fibular fracture that may be comminuted laterally.

plafond like a pestle in a mortar.[65, 73–77] Pilon fractures of the tibia constitute less than 0.5 per cent of all ankle fractures.[78] Their mechanism is forced dorsiflexion of the pronated foot, often occurring in a fall from a height, which forces the talus into the ankle mortise. Pilon fractures commonly are associated with additional injuries of the spine, pelvis, and calcaneus, and they may be considered to evolve through several stages. In stage I, a fracture of the medial malleolus is seen. In stage II, a second fracture occurs, arising from the ante-

rior tibial margin. A supramalleolar fracture of the fibula characterizes stage III, and in stage IV it is accompanied by a relatively transverse fracture of the posterior aspect of the tibia, which connects with the anterior tibial fracture. The important radiographic features of PDF fractures are the intra-articular anterior lip fracture of the stage II injury and the comminution of the tibia of the stage IV injury. These features as well as preservation of the normal tibiofibular distance and, in some cases, talar fractures serve to distinguish the pilon injury, which is related to axial compression, from trimalleolar fractures resulting from rotational forces.[77]

Other Fractures. An isolated fracture of the posterior tibial margin is a rare lesion that does not fit precisely into the Lauge-Hansen classification system. The mechanism of injury is compression by the talar dome, a situation that might result from kicking an object with the ankle in a neutral position or in plantar flexion. Fractures of the posterior tibial region occur as an isolated lesion or in combination with other injuries. They may be overlooked on the true lateral view of the ankle; their detection is facilitated by the use of an off-lateral projection achieved by slight external rotation of the patient's foot or by MR imaging (Fig. 17–31).[79] An isolated fracture of the anterior margin of the distal portion of the tibia is an uncommon lesion.

In all varieties of ankle fracture, routine radiography represents the primary means of diagnosis and assess-

Figure 17–30

Ankle injuries: Pronation-dorsiflexion fracture.

A Initially, a fracture of the medial malleolus occurs (stage I). Subsequent injuries include a fracture of the anterior tibial margin (stage II), a supramalleolar fracture of the fibula (stage III), and a transverse fracture of the posterior aspect of the tibia, which connects with the anterior tibial fracture (stage IV).

B, C Stage IV injury. Routine radiography (**B**) and a sagittal T1-weighted (TR/TE, 500/12) spin echo MR image (**C**) show the characteristics of the distal tibial fracture (arrows).

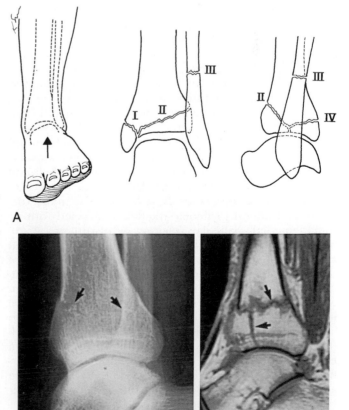

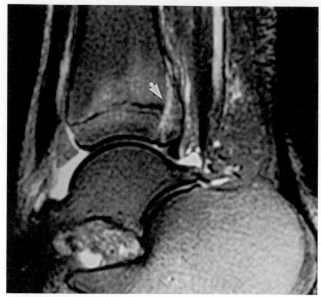

Figure 17–31

Ankle injuries: Occult fracture of the posterior tibial margin. A sagittal fat-suppressed fast spin echo MR image (TR/TE, 3600/108) shows the fracture (arrow), surrounding marrow and soft tissue edema, and an ankle effusion.

ment, although it does not diminish the importance of a thorough physical examination.[80] CT remains important in the assessment of complex injuries,[77, 81] and arthrography occasionally is employed in the evaluation of acute ligamentous injuries (see later discussion). Bone scintigraphy[82] has limited applications in the analysis of ankle injuries. The role of MR imaging in patients with acute ankle trauma or chronic ankle instability is addressed later in this chapter.

The principles guiding therapeutic decisions in patients with ankle injuries have been well summarized by Michelson.[55] Experimental data have indicated that injuries isolated to the lateral side of the ankle do not lead to abnormal mechanics of the ankle joint and that the amount of displacement of the fibula does not determine talar displacement when the ankle is axially loaded. Because of these data and the results of clinical studies, fractures isolated to the lateral malleolus generally are treated conservatively. A bimalleolar injury (defined as a lateral malleolar fracture combined with either a medial malleolar fracture or disruption of the deltoid ligament) can lead to a shift of the talus and alteration in ankle kinematics. Anatomic reduction of the injury, generally accomplished with operative treatment, is the key factor in determining a successful outcome. With regard to syndesmotic injuries, data have indicated that, in the absence of a medial injury, no amount of disruption of the syndesmosis alters the loading characteristics of the ankle. In the presence of a medial injury, the extent of syndesmotic injury determines whether or not the loading characteristics of the ankle are altered. These factors influence the manner (operative versus nonoperative) in which the injuries are treated. Trimalleolar injuries (defined as a bimalleolar injury that is combined with a fracture of the

posterior lip of the tibial plafond) may lead to ankle instability, especially when the fracture fragment is large (i.e., involves more than 30 per cent of the posterior aspect of the tibia). In such cases, reduction and fixation of the fibular fracture frequently reduces the fracture of the posterior malleolus. If not, open reduction and fixation of the posterior malleolar fragment can be accomplished.

Ankle Dislocations

Subluxations and dislocations of the ankle, particularly those in a medial or lateral direction, commonly are associated with fracture of the adjacent malleolar surfaces. Displacements due to extensive ligamentous and capsular injury without fracture can occur. Medial dislocation of the talus appears to be the most common type,[46] although lateral, posterior, anterior, posteromedial, superior, and rotary dislocations also are encountered,[83–85] and any type may be associated with a fracture of the tibial surface. A significant number of these injuries are open. The diagnosis of the specific type of fracture-dislocation usually is accomplished easily by routine radiography; asymmetry of the ankle joint is best delineated on mortise views obtained in 10 degrees of internal rotation.[6] Such assessment is important, as even minor degrees of displacement of the talus with respect to the tibia can result in secondary degenerative joint disease. Arthrography can be used to demonstrate the presence and site of ligamentous injury, although the examination must be accomplished shortly after the traumatic insult (see later discussion).

A peculiar type of ankle injury resulting from severe external rotation of the foot may lead to posterior displacement of the fibula, which becomes locked behind the tibia.[86, 87] This injury, which sometimes is referred to as a Bosworth fracture-dislocation of the ankle,[88] is rare, may be associated with a spiral fracture of the distal fibula, and is easily misdiagnosed on radiographic examination. An anterior variant of this injury also has been described.[89]

Fractures and Dislocations of the Talus

Of the tarsal bones, injuries of the talus deserve some degree of emphasis, as this bone has functional importance in transmitting the body's weight and allowing motion between the lower leg and foot; it also has unique anatomic characteristics that include a tenuous blood supply, which increases its susceptibility to posttraumatic ischemic necrosis, and lack of muscular attachments, which increases the likelihood of dislocation.[90] It is second only to the calcaneus as a site of fracture in the tarsal bones.[91] Avulsion fractures predominate, occurring in the superior surface of the talar neck and the lateral, medial, and posterior aspects of the body[90]; major injuries of the talus also are seen, and these may involve the head, neck, or body, sometimes in association with dislocation of the bone.[92]

Most avulsion fractures are produced by a twisting or rotational force combined with flexion or extension stresses. A longitudinal compression force in combination with acute plantar flexion presumably accounts for the avulsion fracture of the anterosuperior surface of the talar neck; eversion stress may lead to osseous avulsion at the site of attachment of the deep fibers of the deltoid ligament to the body of the talus (Fig. 17–32); the posterior process may be fractured during severe plantar flexion of the foot, owing to its compression between the posterior surface of the tibia and the calcaneus; and disruption of the talar body where the bone projects beneath the tip of the lateral malleolus may result from severe dorsiflexion and external rotation.[93] Those fractures involving the posterior process of the talus may be difficult to differentiate from the os trigonum (see later discussion).

Fractures of the head of the talus are rare.[94] Those of the talar neck are second in frequency to avulsion injuries of the bone (Fig. 17–33). Dorsiflexion related to a force from below or, more rarely, a direct blow to the talus produces this fracture. The extent of the injury varies.[95–97] Complications of talar neck fractures include delayed union or nonunion, infection, osteoarthritis of adjacent joints, and ischemic necrosis.[95, 96, 98, 99] It is the proximal portion of the bone that is affected in ischemic necrosis, with reportable exceptions.[100] Stress fractures of the talar neck also are encountered (see Fig. 17–33). Fractures of the body of the talus are infrequent (Fig. 17–34); they may involve the posterior or lateral process, the articular surface, or all regions, especially in instances of fracture comminution.[101, 102]

Transchondral fractures of the talus (osteochondritis dissecans) are discussed in Chapter 8 and later in this chapter. Acute osteochondral fractures may accompany tangential or impaction forces and often are associated with additional injuries about the ankle (Figs. 17–35 and 17–36).

Subluxations or dislocations of the talus generally are accompanied by fractures of the bone, although they may occur as an isolated phenomenon. They usually are classified as subtalar (peritalar) dislocations and total

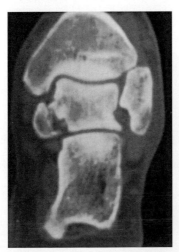

Figure 17–32
Talar injuries: Avulsion fracture of talar body. Fractures of the medial portion of the talus may result from avulsion owing to the attachment site of the deep fibers of the deltoid ligament. (Courtesy of G. Greenway, M.D., Dallas, Texas.)

talar dislocations. The first pattern indicates simultaneous disruption of the talocalcaneal and talonavicular joints.[103–110] Total dislocation of the talus is an extremely infrequent and serious injury in which the talus generally becomes located medially or laterally.[111] Ischemic necrosis of the talus and infection are two important complications.[112]

Fractures of the Calcaneus

The calcaneus is the most common site of tarsal fracture. Although accurate diagnosis commonly is provided by routine and specialized radiographs, the complexity of calcaneal anatomy has prompted considerable interest in CT as a technique that ideally displays the extent of injury.[113–121] Fractures of the calcaneus can be classified broadly into intra-articular (approximately 75 per cent) and extra-articular (approximately 25 per cent of cases); the former are associated with a poorer prognosis owing to displacement of fragments and to disruption of the subtalar joints.[122–125]

Intra-articular fractures generally occur as a result of a vertical fall in which the talus is driven into the cancellous bone of the calcaneus[126]; this mechanism of injury explains the frequency (10 per cent) of bilateral calcaneal fractures as well as the simultaneous occurrence of spinal injuries.[126, 127] CT is a useful technique for the delineation of complex intra-articular fractures. Extra-articular calcaneal fractures result from several different mechanisms, of which twisting forces are most important.[127, 128] Fractures of the anterior process of the calcaneus,[129, 130] related to attachment sites of the ligamentum bifurcatum, may escape detection unless careful analysis of the radiographs is undertaken; acute calcaneal fractures in children, although rare,[131] and stress fractures may be especially difficult to delineate[132] (see later discussion and Chapter 8).

The diagnostic problems encountered in intra-articular fractures are of another sort. Fracture comminution and displacement are common, creating many irregular pieces of bone that are difficult to identify.[133, 134] It is here that conventional tomography[135] or CT scanning[114, 115] is most useful in defining not only the characteristics of the acute injury but also its sequelae, including osteoarthritis of the subtalar joints, malunion, and peroneal tendon dislocation or entrapment between the calcaneus and the fibula. Arthrography, often accomplished by injecting contrast media, corticosteroid medication, and anesthetic agents, can be used to delineate joint abnormalities and sources of articular pain in patients with previous calcaneal fractures.[499, 500]

Fractures of Other Tarsal Bones

Fractures elsewhere in the tarsus are infrequent. Typical sites of injury in the tarsal navicular bone are its dorsal surface near the talonavicular space and the tuberosity and body of the bone.[90] Stress fractures and neuropathic fractures (in diabetes mellitus) of the navicular bone also are encountered (Figs. 17–37 and 17–38). Fractures of the navicular tuberosity may be combined with injuries of the calcaneus and cuboid, whereas isolated

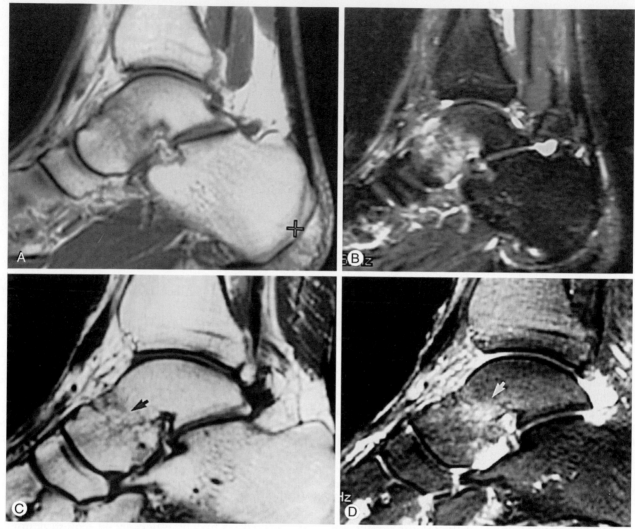

Figure 17–33
Talar injuries: Fractures of the talar neck.

A, B In a 33 year old man, sagittal T1-weighted (TR/TE, 600/20) spin echo **(A)** and fast spin echo STIR (TR/TE, 4000/64; inversion time, 150 msec) **(B)** MR images show a fracture of the talar neck with surrounding marrow edema, the latter appearing as regions of high signal intensity in **B.** (Courtesy of D. Goodwin, M.D., Hanover, New Hampshire.)

C, D Stress fractures of the fatigue or insufficiency type also can affect the talar neck (arrows), as shown in sagittal T1-weighted (TR/TE, 616/15) spin echo **(C)** and fat-suppressed fast spin echo (TR/TE, 2900/85) **(D)** MR images. (Courtesy of M. Starok, M.D., Toronto, Ontario, Canada.)

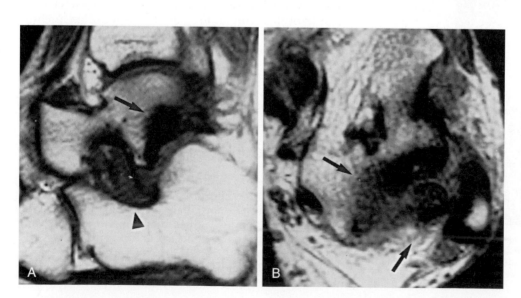

Figure 17–34
Talar injuries: Fractures of the lateral process. Sagittal T1-weighted (TR/TE, 580/15) **(A)** and transaxial proton density–weighted (TR/TE, 1800/22) **(B)** spin echo MR images show a remote fracture (arrows) of the lateral process in a 26 year old man. Note obliteration of the contents of the sinus tarsi (arrowhead, **A**), indicative of the sinus tarsi syndrome.

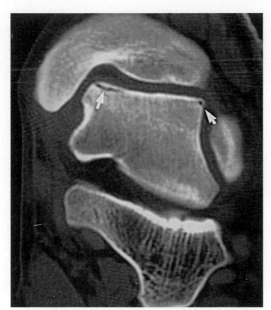

Figure 17–35

Ankle injuries: Osteochondral fracture. A coronal CT scan shows a fracture line (arrows) extending horizontally beneath the bone plate of the talus. (Courtesy of D. Goodwin, M.D., Hanover, New Hampshire.)

fractures of the cuboid and the cuneiform bones are rare. In all instances, differentiation between a fracture and the common accessory bones must be accomplished, and the latter bones themselves may fracture.[136, 137] Fracture of the os peroneum is rare but may be associated with wide separation of the bone fragments, related to the action of the peroneus longus muscle. It may result from direct trauma or indirect stress that results from violent dorsiflexion of the foot. The latter mechanism of injury also may produce a rupture of the peroneus longus tendon.[138, 501] Such rup-

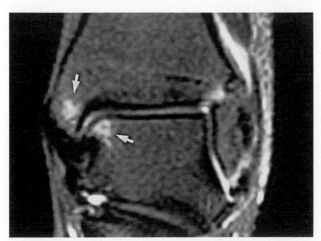

Figure 17 36

Ankle injuries: Subchondral trabecular microfractures. In a female basketball player who sustained a supination injury, a coronal fat-suppressed fast spin echo MR image (TR/TE, 4000/70) shows abnormal high signal intensity in apposing portions of the talus and medial malleolus (arrows) and lateral soft tissue edema. (Courtesy of D. Goodwin, M.D., Hanover, New Hampshire.)

ture leads to displacement of the os peroneum from its normal position adjacent to the lower border of the cuboid bone or the calcaneocuboid joint.

Tarsal Dislocations

Subluxation, dislocation, and fracture-dislocation are common injuries in the midfoot and hindfoot.[139–142] Of particular interest is the Lisfranc's fracture-dislocation of the tarsometatarsal joints (Fig. 17–39).[143–147] Normally, the heads of the metatarsal bones are joined by transverse ligaments.[145] Similarly, the bases of the metatarsal bones reveal ligamentous connections,[148] except between the base of the first and that of the second metatarsal bone. An oblique ligament extends between the medial cuneiform and the second metatarsal base, anchoring the base of this metatarsal bone, which also is stabilized because of its recessed position between the cuneiforms.

Injuries of the tarsometatarsal joints can result from direct or, more commonly, indirect trauma. In the latter situation, violent abduction of the forefoot can lead to lateral displacement of the four lateral metatarsal bones with or without a fracture at the base of the second metatarsal bone and the cuboid bone. Dislocations occurring without fractures, however, are rare. Accompanying dorsal displacement is more frequent than plantar displacement, a predilection that is explained, at least in part, by the relatively wide configuration of the dorsal surface of the base of the second metatarsal bone. The first metatarsal bone may dislocate in the same direction (convergent or ipsilateral dislocation) or in the opposite direction (divergent dislocation) of the other metatarsal bones, depending on the precise vectors of the force.[149, 150]

Radiographic examination usually identifies the dislocation and accompanying fractures, although the findings may be subtle and other techniques, including the application of stress,[147] weight-bearing radiography,[151] and CT,[152] have been emphasized (Fig. 17–40). Tomographic displays are advantageous in demonstrating the relationships among the metatarsal bases and adjacent tarsal bones, and the soft tissue resolution provided by MR imaging also may allow the identification of torn ligaments (Figs. 17–41, 17–42, and 17–43). As anatomic reduction is the key to successful treatment of tarsometatarsal dislocations, this technique also may prove useful in defining the success of the reduction attempts.

Other varieties of tarsal subluxation and dislocation have been described, although most are rare.[153–159]

Metatarsophalangeal and Interphalangeal Joint Dislocations

Dislocations at the metatarsophalangeal joints can occur in any direction, related to the mechanism of injury. The first metatarsophalangeal joint may be affected.[160] Similarly, patterns of dislocation of interphalangeal joints in the foot vary. Sesamoid bone dislocations with or without intra-articular entrapment are rare and usually confined to the first ray.[161–164] Such entrapment, as well as that related to the volar plate,[165] leads to persis-

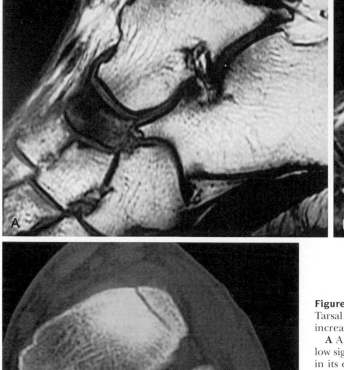

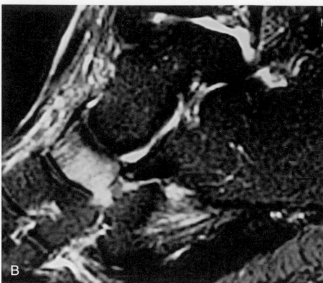

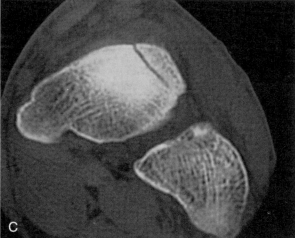

Figure 17–37

Tarsal navicular injuries: Stress fractures. This 60 year old man developed increasing pain in the dorsum of the foot.

A A sagittal T1-weighted (TR/TE, 300/20) spin echo MR image shows low signal intensity throughout the tarsal navicular bone, most prominent in its dorsal and proximal portions.

B On a sagittal fat-suppressed fast spin echo MR image (TR/TE, 4000/92), high signal intensity is evident in the navicular bone.

C The coronal CT scan is far more specific, documenting the navicular stress fracture.

(Courtesy of P. Kindynis, M.D., Geneva, Switzerland.)

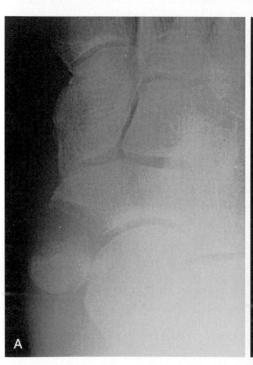

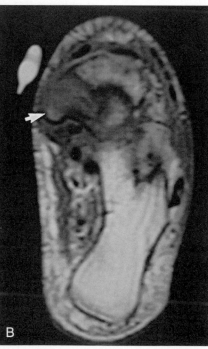

Figure 17–38

Tarsal navicular injuries: Neuropathic fractures. In a 62 year old diabetic man, pain developed spontaneously in the medial aspect of the foot.

A Routine radiograph shows an avulsion fracture of the navicular tuberosity.

B The transverse T1-weighted (TR/TE, 650/11) spin echo MR image shows the avulsed fragment (arrow) and marrow edema.

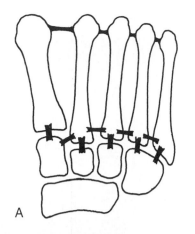
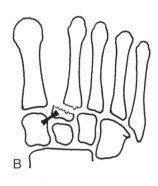

Figure 17–39

Lisfranc's fracture-dislocation of tarsometatarsal joints.

A Normal ligamentous anatomy (see text).

B Lateral dislocation of the second through fifth metatarsal bones may be associated with fractures of the base of the second metatarsal bone and cuboid.

(From Wiley JJ: J Bone Joint Surg [Br] *53*:474, 1971.)

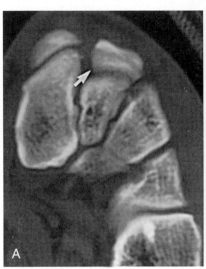
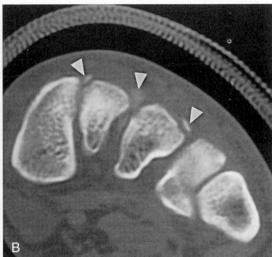

Figure 17–40

Injuries of the tarsometatarsal joints: CT scanning. As demonstrated on transverse (**A**) and coronal (**B**) CT scans, this method can be used to assess tarsometatarsal joint subluxation (arrow) and fractures of the cuneiform and metatarsal bones (arrowheads).

Figure 17–41

Injuries of the tarsometatarsal joints: MR imaging. As the ligament extending between the medial cuneiform bone and the base of the second metatarsal bone (**A,** arrow) is key to the stability of the tarsometatarsal joints, MR imaging may be valuable in demonstrating either an intact (**B,** arrow) or disrupted (**C,** arrow) ligament.

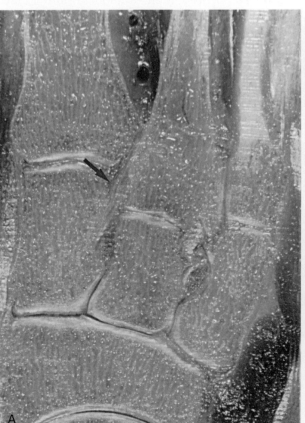
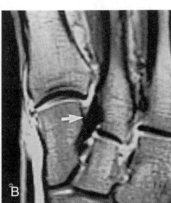
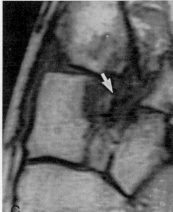

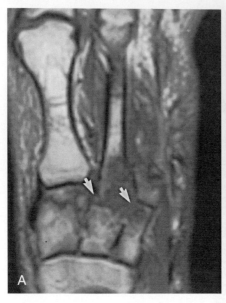 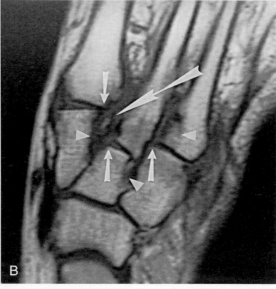

Figure 17–42
Injuries of the tarsometatarsal joints: MR imaging.

A On a transverse T1-weighted (TR/TE, 800/20) spin echo MR image, note subluxation at the tarsometatarsal joints (arrows), with adjacent fractures and bone marrow edema. (Courtesy of D. Goodwin, M.D., Hanover, New Hampshire.)

B In a second patient, an identical T1-weighted spin echo MR image shows subluxation of the first, second, and third tarsometatarsal joints (small arrows), disruption of the Lisfranc ligament (large arrow), and multiple fractures (arrowheads).

tent widening of the joint after attempts at reduction of the dislocation.

Hyperextension of the first metatarsophalangeal joint occurring in American football, soccer, and basketball players may lead to disruption of the plantar aspect of the joint capsule, which tears away from the metatarsal head, an injury designated *turf-toe*, owing to its occurrence on playing fields made of artificial turf.[166–169] Plantar flexion or valgus stress applied to this joint is a less common mechanism of injury. Rarely, hyperextension of the first metatarsophalangeal joint leads to extensive disruption of the plantar plate with lateral dislocation or proximal or distal migration of the sesamoid bones or sesamoid fracture without joint dislocation (Fig. 17–44).[170, 171] Sequelae of any of these hyperextension injuries include chondromalacia of the head of the first metatarsal bone, hallux rigidus or valgus, dorsal osteophytes, and periarticular calcification.[166]

An understanding of this injury requires knowledge of regional anatomy.[169] The medial and lateral sesamoids at the first metatarsophalangeal joint are contained within the tendons of the flexor hallucis brevis muscle and articulate on their dorsal surface with the medial and lateral facets on the plantar surface of the first metatarsal head (Fig. 17–45). Distally, the sesamoids are attached to the base of the proximal phalanx by the plantar plate. A fibrous sheath contains the tendon of the flexor hallucis longus muscle beneath the plantar surface of the two sesamoids. Also contributing to the plantar stability of this joint are the tendons of the abductor and adductor hallucis muscles. Collateral ligaments are located on the medial and lateral aspect of the joint, and these ligaments interdigitate with the

Figure 17–43
Injuries of the tarsometatarsal joints: MR imaging. A coronal fat-suppressed fast spin echo MR image (TR/TE, 5000/48) shows plantar dislocation of the fourth and fifth metatarsal bones (arrows), with abnormal intraosseous high signal intensity. Compare with the opposite normal side.

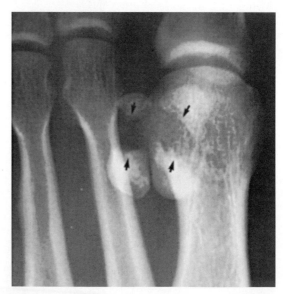

Figure 17–44
Disruption of the plantar capsule of the first metatarsophalangeal joint with displaced sesamoid fractures (turf-toe). Note the diastasis between the fracture fragments (arrows). (Courtesy of B. Howard, M.D., Charlotte, North Carolina.)

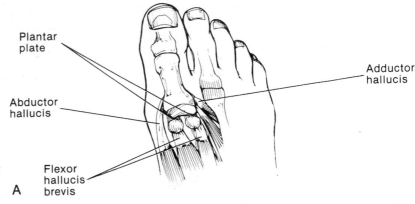

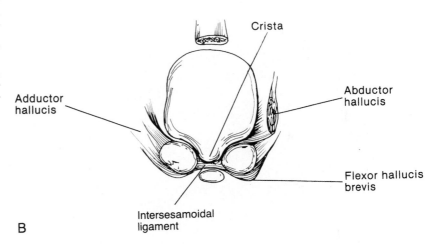

Figure 17–45

Sesamoid bones of the first metatarsophalangeal joint: Normal anatomy.

A The sesamoids are contained in the tendons of the flexor hallucis brevis muscle. The abductor hallucis muscle inserts onto the medial aspect of the medial sesamoid as well as the plantar medial base of the proximal phalanx, and the adductor hallucis muscle inserts onto the lateral aspect of the lateral sesamoid as well as the plantar lateral base of the proximal phalanx.

B The sesamoids articulate with facets on the plantar aspect of the first metatarsal head.

(From Coughlin MJ: Conditions of the forefoot. In JC DeLee, D Drez Jr [Eds]: Orthopaedic Sports Medicine: Principles and Practice. Philadelphia, WB Saunders Co, 1994, p. 1860.)

sesamoid ligaments (Fig. 17–46). Dorsally, the tendons of the extensor hallucis longus and brevis muscles and the hood ligaments of the extensor expansion are found, although dorsal stabilization is much weaker than plantar stabilization.[169]

The normal amount of active extension of the first metatarsophalangeal joint is about 80 degrees, and an additional 25 degrees of extension can be accomplished passively.[172] Beyond this normal range of motion (which differs in men and women and decreases with advancing age), forced hyperextension leads to axial compressive forces on the articular surfaces of the metatarsal head and proximal phalanx of the great toe, resulting in cartilage and bone injury, and to varying degrees of capsular disruption.[169] Rigid soles may limit the degree of extension of the first metatarsophalangeal joint,

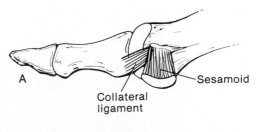

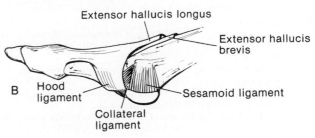

Figure 17–46

Sesamoid bones of the first metatarsophalangeal joint: Normal anatomy.

A The sesamoid and collateral ligaments stabilize the medial and lateral aspects of the first metatarsophalangeal joint.

B The hood ligament of the extensor expansion reinforces the dorsal aspect of the first metatarsophalangeal joint.

(From Coughlin MJ: Conditions of the forefoot. In JC DeLee and D Drez Jr [eds]: Orthopaedic Sports Medicine: Principles and Practice. Philadelphia, WB Saunders Co, 1994, p. 1861.)

whereas flexible soles afford little protection against hyperextension of this joint.

Although routine radiography occasionally reveals osseous and soft tissue abnormalities in patients with turf toe, interest has developed in the diagnostic role of MR imaging in assessing this injury (and other injuries of the plantar surface of the foot) (Fig. 17–47).[173, 174, 502] On T1-weighted spin echo MR images, the normal plantar plate appears as a continuous structure of low signal intensity abutting on the plantar aspect of the metatarsal head and attaching to the base of the proximal phalanx, although it is difficult to distinguish from the thicker, overlying flexor tendons.[173] With gradient echo imaging, the normal plantar plate is slightly hyperintense when

compared to the signal intensity of the flexor tendons and, distally, regions of higher signal intensity in the plantar plate normally may be evident.[173] Signs of rupture of the plantar plate include discontinuity and more widespread areas of increased signal intensity.[174] The site of disruption of the plate may be at the level of the joint or beneath the metatarsal head, and fluid also may be evident in the joint or flexor tendon sheath.

Arthrography with opacification of the first metatarsophalangeal joint also has been used to diagnose disruption of the plantar plate.[173] Positive arthrographic findings include opacification of the flexor tendon sheath. Collateral ligament rupture is accompanied by medial or lateral extravasation of contrast material beyond the

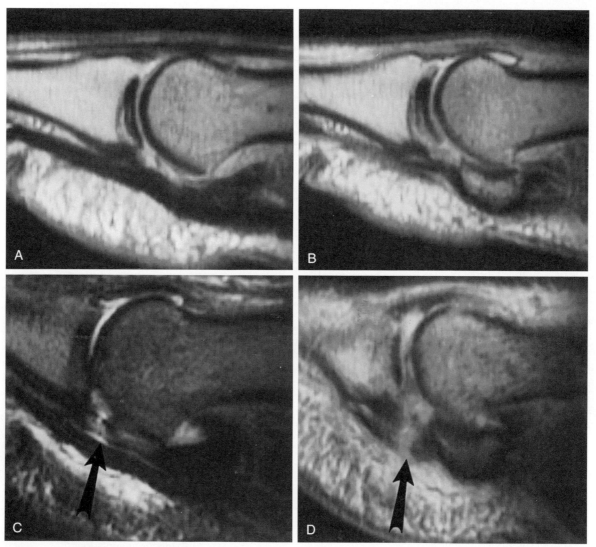

Figure 17–47
Turf toe: MR imaging—sagittal views of the first metatarsophalangeal joint.

A Normal situation. Proton density–weighted spin echo MR image shows the flexor hallucis longus tendon as a plantar structure of low signal intensity.

B Normal situation. In a proton density–weighted spin echo MR image medial to **A,** the plantar capsule extends from the proximal phalanx to the sesamoid bone.

C Turf toe. A T2-weighted spin echo MR image shows a tear (arrow) of the plantar plate and an intact flexor hallucis longus tendon. Note edema and hemorrhage in the plantar soft tissues.

D Turf toe. A proton density–weighted spin echo MR image shows disruption of the plantar plate (arrow).

(From Tewes DP, et al: Clin Orthop *304*:200, 1994.)

confines of the joint and, in some cases, by opacification of intermetatarsal bursae.

Fractures of the Metatarsal Bones and Phalanges

Metatarsal fractures may result from direct or indirect forces or as a response to chronic stress (see Chapter 8) or neuropathic osteoarthropathy.

Fractures of the base of the fifth metatarsal bone have received a great deal of attention in the medical literature.[175–178] Two major types exist: an avulsion fracture of the tuberosity and a transverse fracture of the proximal portion of the diaphysis (Jones fracture).[179] Avulsion of a portion of the tuberosity of the fifth metatarsal bone results from an indirect injury associated with sudden inversion of the foot. Its further pathogenesis is debated, with alternative theories implicating the peroneus brevis tendon or the lateral cord of the plantar aponeurosis in the production of the injury.[178] A fracture in the proximal diaphyseal region of the fifth metatarsal bone, the true Jones fracture, results from either direct or indirect forces and is associated with delayed union or nonunion and refracture.

Fractures of the phalanges of the toes are common and create few diagnostic problems.[180] Of particular importance are displaced intra-articular fractures (which may require surgical reduction) and, in children, physeal injuries of the distal phalanx (the stubbed great toe, which may be open and accompanied by osteomyelitis).[181] Sesamoid fractures, especially in the first ray, also are encountered.

Ligament Abnormalities

Anatomic Considerations

The primary function of the ankle joint is to provide stability during locomotion. Such stability relates not only to the configuration of the three principal bones that form the ankle (tibia, fibula, and talus) but also to the surrounding soft tissue structures, particularly the ligaments, that bind the bones together and the muscles and tendons that regulate ankle movement. Spanning the ankle joint are more than 10 ligaments as well as four retinacula and numerous tendons (some with sheaths), but no muscles save for the occasional fibers of the peroneus tertius muscle.[182] A thick fibrous membrane holds the shafts of the tibia and fibula together, four syndesmotic ligaments bind the lower ends of the bones, and two sets of collateral ligaments connect the malleoli to the talus, calcaneus, and tarsal navicular bone.[183] Despite this extensive arrangement of bones, ligaments, retinacula, tendons, and a fibrous membrane, acute or chronic ankle instability is one of the most important and common problems encountered in clinical practice. Indirect or direct violence can disrupt one or more of these structures, as well as nearby vessels and nerves. Although many types of fractures about the ankle represent direct evidence of this violence (see previous discussion), injury to nearby ligaments ultimately may be responsible for chronic disability.

Anatomically, the ligaments of the ankle are grouped according to their location into three complexes: the tibiofibular complex, the medial complex, and the lateral complex. The ligaments in the lateral complex are injured most commonly, usually related to an inversion stress; the ligaments in the medial complex are injured less frequently, generally as a result of an eversion stress and often in association with a fibular fracture; and the ligaments of the tibiofibular complex may be injured owing to external rotation at the ankle or forced dorsiflexion of the foot, often in combination with a fracture of the fibula.

Tibiofibular Complex. The interlacing fibers of the crural interosseous membrane pass obliquely downward from the interosseous ridge of the tibia to that of the fibula. Descent of the fibula, which occurs during the push-off phase of gait, leads to more acute angulation of these fibers. Just above the inferior tibiofibular syndesmosis, the lower of two apertures in the crural interosseous membrane provides a passageway for the perforating branch of the peroneal artery. In instances of total tibiofibular diastasis in which the syndesmotic ligaments and the distal fibers of the crural interosseous membrane are torn, this artery may be injured.[183]

Four ligaments, collectively designated the syndesmotic ligaments, bind together the apposing portions of the tibia and fibula (Fig. 17–48). From above downward, they are the interosseous ligament, the anterior tibiofibular ligament, the posterior tibiofibular ligament, and

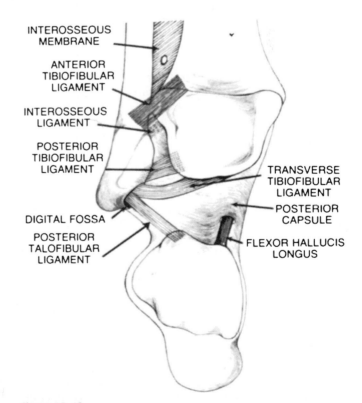

Figure 17–48
Syndesmotic ligaments and related structures: Normal anatomy. See text for details. (From Kelikian H, Kelikian AS: Disorders of the Ankle. Philadelphia, WB Saunders Co, 1985, p. 5.)

the transverse tibiofibular ligament. The anatomy of these ligaments has been well defined by Kelikian and Kelikian.[183] The interosseous ligament represents the lowermost portion of the crural interosseous membrane and consists of short, thick fibers that join the concave surface of the peroneal groove of the tibia to the convex surface of the fibula. It is triangular, with a broad base distally and a pointed apex proximally. In combination with injuries of the crural interosseous membrane, disruption of the interosseous ligament occurs when forces lead to diastasis of the distal portions of the tibia and fibula. In injuries that involve external rotation of the talus with lateral displacement and external rotation of the fibula, an open-book type of disruption of the interosseous ligament occurs in combination with disruption of the anterior tibiofibular ligament.[183]

The anterior tibiofibular ligament extends between the anterolateral surface of the tibia (including the anterior tubercle) to the adjacent anterior surface of the fibula. As the fibers pass from the tibia to the fibula, they are directed downward and laterally. Furthermore, the fibers increase in length from above downward, the lower fibers being longer, sometimes reaching 25 mm.[1] This ligament consists of two or more fascicles, between which branches of the anterior peroneal arteries may pass. The most inferior fibers cover the tibiofibular corner of the joint, passing over a segment of the talus.[1]

This ligament is the weakest of the four syndesmotic ligaments and the first to yield in injuries that produce external rotation of the fibula. In association with oblique fractures of the lateral malleolus, occurring with supination and external rotation at the ankle, an avulsion fracture of the anterior tubercle of the tibia at the site of insertion of the anterior tibiofibular ligament, rather than disruption of the ligament itself, may occur.[183]

The posterior tibiofibular ligament is the posterior counterpart of the anterior tibiofibular ligament, extending from the posterolateral surface of the tibia (including the posterior tubercle) to the adjacent posterior surface of the fibula. The fibers of this ligament pass upward and medially, and some extend more medially, reaching the lateral border of the groove containing the tibialis posterior tendon.[1] External rotation and posterior displacement of the fibula lead to disruption of this ligament or an avulsion fracture of the posterior tibial tubercle.

The transverse tibiofibular ligament represents the lowermost portion of the posterior tibiofibular ligament (and, sometimes is designated the deep component of the posterior tibiofibular ligament), although often it is considered to be a distinct structure.[183] In common with the remaining portions of the posterior tibiofibular ligament, the transverse tibiofibular ligament inserts into the posterior surface of the tibia. Laterally, however, the transverse tibiofibular ligament inserts into the upper part of the lateral malleolar fossa in the posteroinferior portion of the fibula. This ligament extends below the posterior surface of the tibia, contacting the posterior aspect of the talus. The fibers of this ligament are directed upward, medially, and posteriorly, although at the posterior border of the tibial articular surface the fibers become more horizontal or transverse.[1] The ligament contains a proportion of yellow elastic fibers, accounting for its yellowish color, and its internal surface is covered by a synovial membrane.

Medial Complex. The medial or tibial collateral ligament of the ankle is the strong, triangular or fan-shaped deltoid ligament. The deltoid ligament often is divided into superficial and deep portions (Fig. 17–49). The superficial portion of the ligament originates mainly from the anterior colliculus of the tibial malleolus. This portion of the deltoid ligament is divided further into three sets of fibers which, in an anterior to posterior direction, are the tibionavicular, tibiocalcaneal, and posterior tibiotalar fibers. The anterior or tibionavicular part of the superficial portion of the deltoid ligament consists of fibers that pass from their tibial attachment site to the tuberosity of the navicular bone and the medial margin of the plantar calcaneonavicular ligament. The middle or tibiocalcaneal part (the strongest superficial component of the ligament) consists of fibers that descend almost in a perpendicular direction from the medial malleolus to the whole length of the sustentaculum tali of the calcaneus. The posterior tibiotalar part of the superficial portion of the deltoid ligament has fibers that pass laterally and backward to attach to the medial side of the talus and to its medial tubercle. This part is located more deeply than the anterior and middle parts and sometimes is considered together with the deep portion of the deltoid ligament. The deep portion of the deltoid ligament extends from the tip of the medial malleolus to the entire nonarticular medial surface of the body of the talus. The tendons of the tibialis posterior and flexor digitorum longus muscles are located superficial to the deltoid ligament.

Sarrafian[1] has emphasized several anatomic considerations regarding the deltoid ligament:

1. The entire medial ligamentous complex, except the very anterior part, is invested by the deep crural fascia in continuity with the flexor retinaculum.
2. The anterior border of the ligament is covered by the tibialis anterior tendon and, laterally, is continuous with the thin anterior portion of the joint capsule.
3. The middle and posterior segments of the ligament are covered by the obliquely oriented tibialis posterior and flexor digitorum longus tendons.
4. Posteriorly, the ligament is in continuity with the posterior portion of the joint capsule and the posterior talofibular ligament.
5. Except for its deep tibiotalar component, the medial ligament is a continuous fibrous sheet, division of which into various segments is artificial and based only on the specific insertion sites.

The fibers of the deep portion of the deltoid ligament prevent the talus from being displaced laterally. If the deep portion remains intact, displacement of a fractured distal portion of the fibula or tibiofibular diastasis does not occur.[183] The tibionavicular component of the superficial portion of the deltoid ligament suspends the inferior calcaneonavicular or spring ligament which, in turn, supports the head of the talus; the tibiocalcaneal

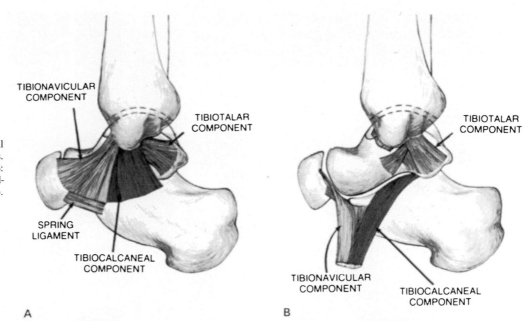

Figure 17–49
Tibial collateral ligament: Normal anatomy. See text for details. (From Kelikian H, Kelikian AS: Disorders of the Ankle. Philadelphia, WB Saunders Co, 1985, p. 20.)

portion of the superficial portion of the deltoid ligament prevents the calcaneus from assuming a valgus alignment.[183]

Lateral Complex. The lateral ligamentous complex of the ankle is referred to as the fibular collateral ligament, consisting of three components, or fasciculi, all of which attach to the lateral (fibular) malleolus (Figs. 17–50 and 17–51). One component connects the lateral malleolus to the calcaneus and is designated the calcaneofibular ligament. Two components connect the lateral malleolus to the anterolateral and posterolateral surfaces of the talus and are designated the anterior talofibular and posterior talofibular ligaments, respectively. These two ligaments fuse with the capsule of the ankle joint,

whereas the calcaneofibular ligament does not.[183] Owing to their location in an anteroposterior plane, these three components of the lateral ligamentous complex of the ankle sometimes are referred to as the anterior (anterior talofibular), middle (calcaneofibular), and posterior (posterior talofibular) segments, or bands.

The anterior talofibular ligament passes from the anterior margin of the fibular malleolus in a forward and medial direction to attach to the lateral articular facet and lateral aspect of the neck of the talus. This ligament sometimes is composed of two bands; a larger upper band may reach the origin of the anterior tibiofibular ligament, and a smaller lower band may reach the origin of the calcaneofibular ligament.[1] The anterior talofibular ligament is horizontal with the talus in neutral posi-

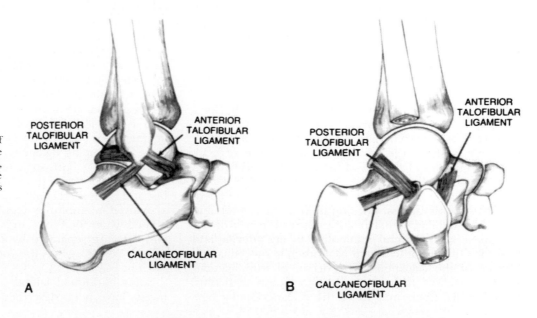

Figure 17–50
Lateral ligamentous complex of the ankle: Normal anatomy. See text for details. (From Kelikian H, Kelikian AS: Disorders of the Ankle. Philadelphia, WB Saunders Co, 1985, p. 20.)

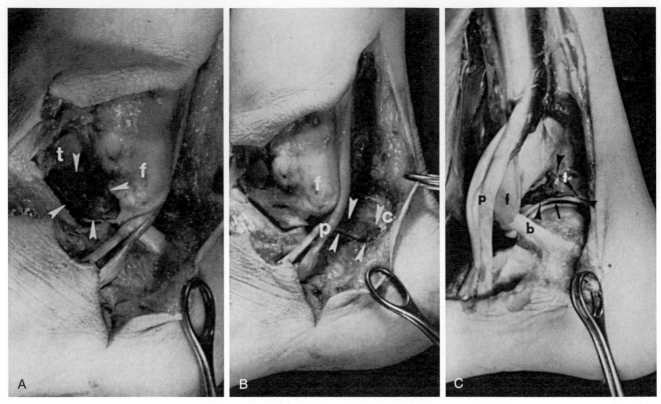

Figure 17–51
Lateral ligamentous complex of the ankle: Normal anatomy—dissection identifying the major lateral ligaments of the ankle (ligaments are painted with tantalum). The anterior talofibular ligament **(A)** (arrowheads) extends from the distal end of the fibula (f) to the talus (t). The calcaneofibular ligament **(B)** (arrowheads) originates from the posterior aspect of the distal part of the fibula (f) and inserts on the superior aspect of the calcaneus (c). It is intimate with the tendons of the peroneal muscles (p). The posterior talofibular ligament **(C)** (arrowheads) extends from the fibula (f) to the talus (t). Note its relationship to the calcaneofibular ligament (b), peroneal tendons (p), and posterior subtalar joint (arrow). (Courtesy of J. Kaye, M.D., New York, New York.)

tion, is directed slightly upward as it passes medially with the talus in dorsiflexion, and is directed downward as it passes medially with the talus in plantar flexion.[1] This component of the lateral ligamentous complex is the weakest and is injured most often. When intact, the anterior talofibular ligament prevents forward displacement of the talus. This ligament passes over a ridge related to the anterior border of the lateral articular facet of the talar body, a part of the ligament that is vulnerable to injury. The intimacy of the anterior talofibular ligament with the joint capsule explains the inevitable occurrence of capsular disruption in cases of anterior talofibular ligament disruption, and the location of the perforating branch of the peroneal artery close to the superficial margin of the anterior talofibular ligament explains the occasional occurrence of traumatic aneurysms of this vessel in cases of anterior talofibular ligament disruption.[183]

The calcaneofibular ligament is long and rounded, and it extends across two joints (the talocrural and posterior subtalar joints) from a depression in front of the apex of the lateral malleolus, in an inferior and posterior direction, to attach to a tubercle on the lateral surface of the calcaneus. The origin of this ligament does not reach the very tip of the lateral malleolus. Occasionally, fibers may unite the calcaneofibular liga-

ment and the inferior band of the anterior talofibular ligament. The tendons of the peroneus longus and peroneus brevis muscles and their sheath cross over this ligament. The calcaneofibular ligament is lax in the standing position and is taut during inversion of the calcaneus. This ligament serves to stabilize the posterior subtalar joint.

The posterior talofibular ligament is a strong, horizontally oriented structure that passes from the lower part of the fossa of the lateral malleolus to the lateral tubercle of the posterior process of the talus. One slip of this ligament, designated the tibial slip or posterior intermalleolar ligament, passes obliquely upward, to attach to the medial malleolus.[505] The posterior talofibular ligament has some features in common with the transverse tibiofibular ligament of the inferior tibiofibular syndesmosis[183]; both structures are located in the coronal plane, both arise from the fossa of the lateral malleolus, and both are deeply seated and partially invested by a synovial membrane. These structures are intimately related when the foot is in a position of plantar flexion, and they are separated by a space (through which the talus is visible) when the foot is in a position of dorsiflexion.

Some additional lateral or posterolateral ankle ligaments have been described that are not present consistently and that are referred to with inconsistent terminology, including such designations as the fibulotalocalcaneal ligament, posterior fibulocalcaneal ligament, and the peroneotalocalcaneal ligament.[1]

Pathologic Considerations

Injuries to the ligaments about the ankle are one of the most frequently encountered consequences of trauma. They typically are seen in young adults, particularly those involved in sports such as basketball and soccer.[184] The lateral ligamentous complex is injured more commonly than the medial or tibiofibular complex. Of the lateral ligaments, the anterior talofibular ligament is affected most frequently, either alone or in combination with an injury of the calcaneofibular ligament.[185–188] Indeed, a predictable sequence of injury may be observed, beginning in the anterior talofibular ligament and followed by involvement of the calcaneofibular and finally the posterior talofibular ligaments. As acute injuries to the ligaments of the ankle may be complicated by chronic dysfunction of the joint, accurate and early diagnosis is important. Clinical assessment employs local palpation of the ligaments, often combined with stress testing, to determine which individual ligaments are injured. Diffuse swelling leads to diagnostic problems in some cases, and severe pain in the acute stage may limit the usefulness of stress maneuvers designed to identify patterns of talar displacement unless the patient is examined under general anesthesia.

Ligamentous injuries are classified on the basis of the specific site or sites of involvement and their severity. The severity of the injury may be categorized as grade I, II, or III. Grade I injuries are the least severe, apparently representing failure of some of the ligamentous fibers, and grade III injuries are the most severe, associated with complete ligamentous disruption and instability of the ankle joint; grade II injuries are intermediate in severity. Instability of the ankle implies abnormal joint motion during the application of varus or valgus stress or positive results during an anterior drawer test (in which the talus moves in a forward direction when anterior stress is placed on the calcaneus).[189] These stress tests (see later discussion) require meticulous technique such that each of the ligaments about the ankle is tested individually. Furthermore, the results of stress testing may be unreliable in the acute stage of injury.[190]

With regard to the lateral ligamentous complex of the ankle, some disagreement exists regarding the functional importance of its various components.[187] The primary function of the anterior and posterior talofibular ligaments is to restrain anterior and posterior displacement, respectively, of the talus in relation to the fibula and tibia; the primary function of the calcaneofibular ligament is to restrain inversion of the calcaneus with respect to the fibula. The anterior talofibular ligament appears to be the primary lateral stabilizer of the ankle joint in all positions of plantar flexion of the foot.[187] Because the majority of ankle sprains occur during plantar flexion, adduction, and inversion, the anterior talofibular ligament is the initial site of disruption, followed next by disruption of the calcaneofibular

ligament and then by disruption of the posterior talofibular ligament. If the ankle is in neutral position at the time of injury, the initial site of abnormality may be the calcaneofibular ligament, although the other two lateral ligaments also may be involved. If the ankle is in dorsiflexion when injured, a syndesmotic rupture is most likely.[187] Isolated, complete rupture of the anterior talofibular ligament occurs in 60 to 70 per cent of ankle sprains. In approximately 40 per cent of cases in which this ligament is disrupted, an associated tear of the calcaneofibular ligament is evident.[183] Isolated tears of the calcaneofibular ligament (i.e., without an associated tear of the anterior talofibular ligament) are very rare, as such tears usually represent the second stage of disruption of the lateral ligamentous complex. When the calcaneofibular ligament is disrupted, associated abnormalities may include avulsion of the base of the fifth metatarsal bone and tears of the medial layer of the common peroneal tendon sheath.[183] Furthermore, as the pattern of injury to the lateral side of the ankle continues, the capsule of the posterior subtalar joint and the lateral talocalcaneal ligament also are torn. The usual mechanism of injury to the lateral ligamentous complex of the ankle is plantar flexion of the foot and inversion at the ankle. Such injuries predominate in young men and in women who wear high-heeled shoes. The posterior talofibular ligament rarely is torn; one mechanism of injury relates to a dislocation of the talus that is not accompanied by a fracture of the distal portion of the fibula.[183] Complete ruptures of the lateral ligaments of the ankle usually are midsubstance tears. Less frequently, insertional disruptions are evident. Partial tears also tend to be midsubstance tears.[187]

Stress testing, often combined with radiography (see Fig. 17–20), applied to assessment of the lateral ligaments of the ankle employs inversion forces with the foot in a neutral position, in a position of plantar flexion, or in both positions. The angle of talar tilt is increased relative to the uninjured side. An anterior drawer sign also can be used, in which a positive response is characterized by forward movement of the talus with respect to the tibia. The value of these tests, however, often is questioned.[519] In general, positive results during stress testing of the lateral ligaments are reliable evidence of abnormality, although falsely negative results may be encountered when stress radiography is employed.[187] With regard to the anterior drawer sign, the importance of performing the examination not only with the ankle in neutral position but also with it in plantar flexion has been emphasized in the diagnosis of anterior talofibular ligament abnormalities[191]; if forward talar translation is more than 6 mm in neutral position and 8 mm in plantar flexion, such abnormalities usually are present.[187] The methods of measurement of such translation on radiographs are variable, however (Fig. 17–52). Furthermore, comparison with the opposite, uninjured side often is required when this test is performed; in general, a difference in the amount of anterior talar translation of greater than 2 or 3 mm is considered evidence of a tear of the anterior talofibular ligament.[187]

With regard to the talar tilt stress test, the position of

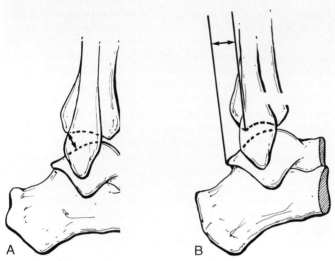

Figure 17-52
The anterior drawer stress radiograph.

A Anterior talar displacement (in millimeters) is recorded by measuring the shortest distance from the most posterior articular surface of the tibia to the talar dome.

B Another, more uncommon method of measuring the anterior displacement of the talus. The perpendicular distance between vertical lines drawn through the posterior lip of the tibia and the posterolateral tubercle of the talus is measured.

(From Renstrom PAFH, Kannus P: Injuries of the foot and ankle. *In* JC DeLee, D Drez Jr [Eds]: Orthopaedic Sports Medicine: Principles and Practice. Philadelphia, WB Saunders Co, 1994, p. 1711.)

the ankle at the time of testing again influences the results of the examination. With the ankle in neutral position, an inversion load places high strain on the calcaneofibular ligament; with progressive plantar flexion of the ankle, increasing strain is placed on the anterior talofibular ligament with an inversion load, while the calcaneofibular ligament becomes more relaxed.[187] When coupled with routine radiography, various methods of measurement of the degree of talar tilting have been described (Fig. 17-53). The extent of abnormal tilting of the talus is influenced by such factors as the method of ankle loading, the amount of the load, the precise position of the ankle during testing, and the number of lateral ligaments that are disrupted. Combined tears of the anterior talofibular and calcaneofibular ligaments allow more tilting of the talus than tears of the anterior talofibular ligament alone. As guidelines, if the talar tilt is between 10 and 20 degrees, the injury to the lateral ligaments is moderate, related to a tear of the anterior talofibular ligament and, possibly, to a tear of the calcaneofibular ligament as well; if the talar tilt is greater than 20 degrees, the rupture generally involves both ligaments; and if the talar tilt is more than 10 degrees greater than on the uninjured side, a combined ligamentous disruption also is likely.[187] Increased diagnostic accuracy is expected when both types of stress tests (anterior drawer and talar tilt) are employed, when they are done carefully, and when both ankles are studied.

Injuries to the medial side of the ankle include avulsion fractures of the medial malleolus or disruption of the deltoid ligament. Widening of the ankle mortise is

encountered more commonly when the deltoid ligament is torn, as fractures of the malleoli are characterized by normal ligamentous connections between the malleoli and the talus.[183] Thus, rupture of the deltoid ligament implies more severe injury, and it may be accompanied not only by widening of the mortise of the talocrural joint but also by significant injuries to the lateral ligaments of the ankle and entrapment of the tendon of the tibialis posterior muscle. Partial tears of the deltoid ligament, with involvement only of its superficial (and anterior) portion, are seen occasionally, although complete tears involving both the superficial and the deep portions of the ligament are encountered more frequently. These complete tears commonly are accompanied by fractures of the lateral malleolus and by lateral or posterolateral displacement of the talus. Indeed, complete tears of the deltoid ligament without additional injuries to the ankle are rare. Tears of the ligament may be interstitial or represent avulsion injuries at its sites of attachment.

With routine radiography, the altered position of the talus may be evident, or the bone may appear to be tilted medially. Occasionally, however, at the time of routine radiography, the displaced talus may have assumed a more normal relationship with the tibia. This has led to such designations as "invisible injury to the deltoid ligament" or "silent displacement of the talus."[183, 192, 193] When displacement of the talus is evident, a widened clear space (the distance between the talar body and the medial malleolus) of the ankle is seen radiographically. Disruption of the deltoid ligament is suggested when this clear space measures 3 mm or more.[183] A stress test employing eversion loading of the ankle can be used to evaluate the deltoid ligament.

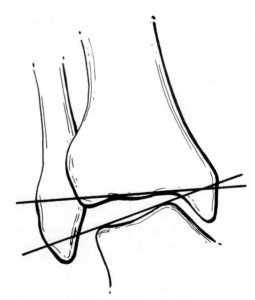

Figure 17-53
The talar tilt (inversion) stress radiograph. The talar tilt angle refers to the angle between two lines drawn to the tibial plafond and the talar dome. During stress, the ankle is in neutral position but is internally rotated 10 to 20 degrees. (From Renstrom PAFH, Kannus P: Injuries of the foot and ankle. *In* JC DeLee, D Drez Jr [Eds]: Orthopedic Sports Medicine: Principles and Practice. Philadelphia, WB Saunders Co, 1994, p. 1713.)

More than 10 degrees of tilting of the talus generally is considered abnormal.[187]

Unusual patterns of posttraumatic deficiency of the deltoid ligament are described. A rupture of the deep portion of the ligament may be accompanied by an avulsion fracture of the medial malleolus at the site of attachment of its superficial portion.[194, 195] Partial tears of the anterior part of the superficial portion of the deltoid ligament (i.e., tibionavicular part) also may occur.

Diastasis of the distal portions of the tibia and fibula relates to injury of the ligaments of the inferior tibiofibular syndesmosis and the adjacent fibers of the crural interosseous membrane. Such diastasis occurs with partial or complete rupture of the syndesmosis ligament complex. Complete ruptures of the syndesmotic ligaments rarely occur without associated fractures and other ligament injuries. Such injuries generally include rupture of the medial ligamentous complex and malleolar fractures; the lateral ligaments of the ankle usually are not injured in cases of syndesmotic ligamentous injuries.[187] The pattern of fibular fracture provides evidence regarding the likelihood of injury to the syndesmosis ligaments. In the Weber classification system, types B and C fibular fractures are associated with syndesmosis injuries in 50 per cent or more of cases, whereas such injuries rarely are associated with type A fibular fractures; in the Lauge-Hansen classification system, the injury mechanisms of syndesmotic ruptures parallel those of deltoid ligament ruptures and include supination-external rotation, pronation-abduction, and pronation-external rotation injuries.[187] Isolated injuries to the syndesmosis have been described in slalom skiers who, during a race, straddle one of the slalom gates, the mechanism of injury related to sudden external rotation of the ankle, contact of the talus and fibula, and diastasis of the syndesmosis.[196]

Diastasis may occur in an anterior to posterior direction (open book injury) or in a posterior to anterior direction. Kelikian and Kelikian[183] have defined three types of tibiofibular diastasis: intercalary diastasis, the least common type, involves disruption of the lowermost fibers of the crural interosseous membrane with intact ligaments of the tibiofibular syndesmosis; anterior tibiofibular diastasis, the most common type, represents the open book injury, in which the anterior ligaments of the tibiofibular syndesmosis are disrupted; and total tibiofibular diastasis, intermediate in frequency, leads to complete disruption of all four syndesmotic ligaments and tearing of the crural interosseous membrane to the level of the associated fracture of the fibula. Intercalary diastasis is an injury of children, occurring prior to closure of the physis in the distal portion of the tibia. Associated physeal injuries of the tibia are seen. Anterior tibiofibular diastasis, leading to disruption of the anterior portion of the syndesmotic ligaments, is associated with external rotation of the talus, disruption of some of the fibers of the interosseous ligament, capsular injury, and in some cases, spiral fractures of the fibula at any level (e.g., Maisonneuve fracture of the proximal portion of the fibula). The diagnosis is facilitated by the presence of associated fractures, not only of the fibula but also of the anterior tubercle of the tibia, of the posterior margin of the distal portion of the tibia, and of the medial malleolus.[183] Total tibiofibular diastasis, which is caused by excessive abduction or external rotation at the ankle, is accompanied almost universally by suprasyndesmotic fractures of the fibula and, in some cases, by an avulsion fracture of the medial malleolus or disruption of the deltoid ligament.

Clinical and radiographic examinations are fundamental to diagnosis of syndesmosis injuries. Clinical findings may be subtle, requiring careful physical examination supplemented with provocative stress tests (e.g., squeeze test, Cotton test).[187] Routine radiographs also may be supplemented with stress testing, and proper analysis includes construction of a number of lines and careful measurements (Table 17-2 and Fig. 17-54).[197-200]

Partial or complete ossification of the syndesmosis has been observed after injury.[187, 201] This complication is encountered most often in athletes, especially American football players, with histories of chronic and recurrent ankle sprains. Operative intervention with removal of the abnormal bone may be required.

Imaging Considerations

Initial assessment of injuries to the medial, lateral, and syndesmotic ligaments about the ankle requires routine radiography, which allows detection of any accompanying fractures, and radiography performed during the application of stress. Complementary imaging methods involve predominantly arthrography, ultrasonography, and MR imaging.

Arthrography. Arthrographic abnormalities associated with ligamentous injuries have been well described (Fig. 17-55).[37, 39, 202-213] With tears of the anterior talofibular ligament, contrast material will be seen both inferior and lateral to the distal fibula on frontal radiographs and anterior to the distal fibula on lateral radiographs. Occasionally, on anteroposterior views, the contrast material will overlie the syndesmosis. With tears of the calcaneofibular ligament, contrast material fills the peroneal tendon sheaths as the inner aspect of the sheaths also is torn.[214-218] Tears of the calcaneofibular ligament are associated with tears of the anterior talofibular ligament, so that the arthrographic findings of both ligament injuries are apparent. The posterior talofibular ligament also may be injured in these instances.

Contrast opacification of the peroneal tendon sheaths, although always an abnormal finding on ankle arthrograms,[215] is not specific for calcaneofibular ligament disruption.[214] Isolated filling of these sheaths is most compatible with a new or old injury to this ligament, whereas such filling combined with leakage of contrast material distal and lateral to the lateral malleolus suggests combined ruptures of the anterior talofibular and calcaneofibular ligaments or an anterior talofibular ligament rupture associated with disruption of the peroneal tendon sheaths. Opacification of the sheaths may be prevented by blood or fibrin clot so that false-negative arthrograms are encountered.[214, 218] With injury to the anterior tibiofibular ligament, extravasation of

Table 17–2. RADIOLOGIC CRITERIA FOR DELTOID LIGAMENT AND SYNDESMOSIS DISRUPTION

Talocrural Angle

This angle is the superior medial angle of a line drawn perpendicular to the distal tibial articular surface and a line joining the tips of both malleoli on the mortise view. The adult talocrucal angle is 83 ± 4 degrees and normally is less than 2 degrees different from the opposite side. Any difference over 5 degrees is abnormal.

Medial Clear Space

This is the distance from the lateral border of the medial malleolus to the medial border of the talus at the level of talar dome on the mortise radiograph. A space over 4 mm is abnormal.

Valgus Talar Tilt

This represents any difference in the width of the joint space proximal to the medial and lateral talar ridges on the mortise radiograph. Two millimeters difference is considered the upper limit of normal.

Syndesmosis A

This measures the tibiofibular clear space from the lateral border of the posterior tibial malleolus (point A) to the medial border of the fibula (point B) on the AP radiograph. This space is normally less than 5 mm and represents a syndesmosis disruption if it is more.

Syndesmosis B

This measures the tibiofibular overlap from the medial border of the fibula (point B) to the lateral border of the anterior tibial prominence (point C) on the AP radiograph. This space is abnormal if it is less than 10 mm.

Talar Subluxation

This is a subjective assessment of congruity of the tibial articular surface and talar dome on the AP radiograph. Any incongruity indicates an abnormality.

All measurements refer to Figure 17–54.

Modified with permission of the publisher from Stiehl JB: Complex ankle fracture dislocations with syndesmotic diastasis. Orthop Rev *14*:499, 1990. Copyright 1990 by Excerpta Medica Inc.

contrast material occurs between distal ends of the tibia and fibula, beyond the syndesmotic recess. Its arthrographic appearance may simulate that of capsular rupture.[219] The arthrographic appearance of injuries to the deltoid ligament is characterized by extravasation of contrast material beyond the medial confines of the joint. Syndesmotic tears are associated with such extravasation between the tibia and the fibula.

The amount of extravasation of contrast material after any of these ligament tears depends on many factors, including the volume of contrast material injected, the degree of surrounding soft tissue injury, the presence of scar tissue from previous injuries, and the length of time from injury to arthrography.[37, 39] Arthrography performed after considerable delay may not reveal the presence of ligamentous injury; arthrography performed after appropriate conservative or operative therapy may not demonstrate previously evident abnormalities.[202]

Ankle arthrography is a reliable method of delineating these ligamentous injuries. Its reported accuracy is 75 to 90 per cent.[204, 205] Some observers report less success, particularly in diagnosing double injuries of the lateral ligaments.[203] In these cases, massive extravasation related to one injury may obscure extravasation related

to a second injury. The combination of ankle arthrography and peroneal tenography may improve diagnostic accuracy in patients with combined lesions of both the anterior talofibular and the calcaneofibular ligaments.[213]

Ultrasonography. As the medial and lateral ligaments of the ankle are located superficially, application of ultrasonography to their assessment is possible.[220, 221] As in other regions of the body, successful ultrasonography of ankle ligaments depends on meticulous technique. Normal ligaments appear as hyperechoic bands of tissue, whereas sonographic findings of ligament injuries include disruption or thickening of the involved structures. Ultrasonography is more feasible for the assessment of the anterior talofibular and calcaneofibular ligaments than for evaluation of other ankle ligaments.

MR Imaging. MR imaging has been used to evaluate ligamentous injuries about the ankle.[222-231, 503, 504] Although standard spin echo MR sequences[223] have been employed, 3DFT gradient recalled MR sequences may provide superior information, owing to the ability to obtain thin contiguous sections.[222, 232] Furthermore, earlier investigations employing MR imaging usually studied the ankle in a neutral position, with no regard to placing the ligaments paraxial to the imaging plane. The value of plantar flexion of the foot as a means to allow better delineation of some of these ligaments with MR imaging was emphasized in one report.[223] In 1992, Schneck and coworkers[224, 225] provided the most detailed description of MR imaging techniques that allowed optimal visualization of the ankle ligaments. Based on a cadaveric study,[224] these investigators analyzed the ap-

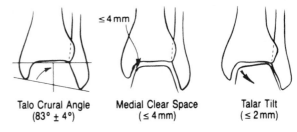

Talo Crural Angle
(83° ± 4°)   Medial Clear Space
(≤ 4 mm)   Talar Tilt
(≤ 2 mm)

Anterior Posterior View

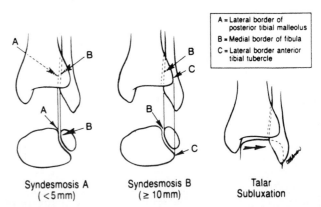

A = Lateral border of posterior tibial malleolus
B = Medial border of fibula
C = Lateral border anterior tibial tubercle

Syndesmosis A
(<5 mm)   Syndesmosis B
(≥ 10 mm)   Talar Subluxation

Figure 17–54

Syndesmotic radiographic criteria. (Reprinted with permission of the publisher from Stiehl JB: Complex ankle fracture dislocations with syndesmotic diastasis. Orthop Rev *14*:499, 1990. Copyright 1990 by Excerpta Medica Inc.)

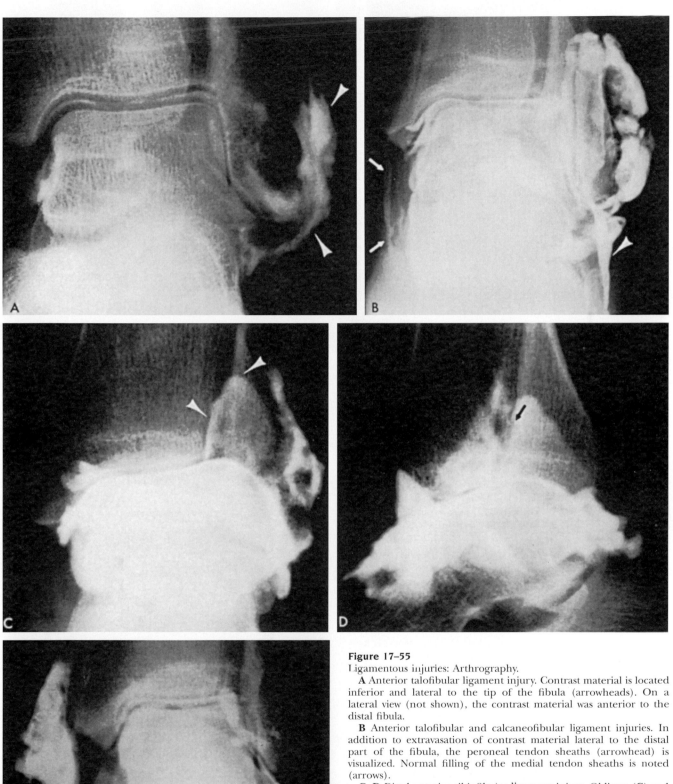

Figure 17–55

Ligamentous injuries: Arthrography.

A Anterior talofibular ligament injury. Contrast material is located inferior and lateral to the tip of the fibula (arrowheads). On a lateral view (not shown), the contrast material was anterior to the distal fibula.

B Anterior talofibular and calcaneofibular ligament injuries. In addition to extravasation of contrast material lateral to the distal part of the fibula, the peroneal tendon sheaths (arrowhead) is visualized. Normal filling of the medial tendon sheaths is noted (arrows).

C, D Distal anterior tibiofibular ligament injury. Oblique (**C**) and lateral (**D**) views reveal extravasation between the distal ends of the tibia and fibula (arrowheads). The normal clear zone anterior to the distal portion of the fibula has been obliterated (arrow).

E Deltoid ligament injury. Contrast material has extravasated beneath and medial to the medial malleolus (arrowhead).

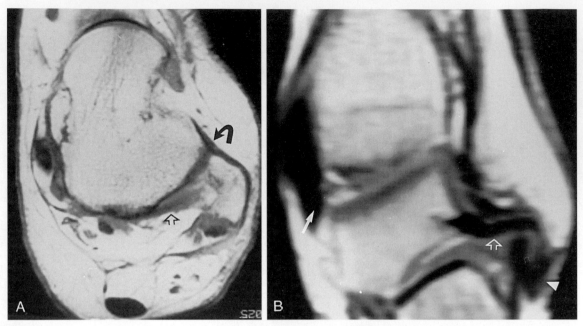

Figure 17–56

Normal ligaments of the ankle: MR imaging—anterior and posterior talofibular ligaments and calcaneofibular ligament. A transaxial T1-weighted (TR/TE, 600/20) spin echo MR image **(A)** and a coronal T1-weighted (TR/TE, 600/20) spin echo MR image **(B)** show the anterior talofibular ligament (curved arrow), posterior talofibular ligament (open arrows), calcaneofibular ligament (arrowhead), and tibiotalar ligament (and tibialis posterior tendon) (straight solid arrow).

pearance of the normal ligaments, employing spin echo MR images and various positions of the foot. They concluded that (1) transaxial images with the foot taped into dorsiflexion of 10 to 20 degrees provided optimized visualization of the anterior, posterior, and inferior tibiofibular ligaments and of the anterior and posterior talofibular ligaments and also provided an overview of the deltoid ligaments; (2) coronal MR images provided full-length views of various parts of the deltoid ligament; (3) transaxial images with the foot taped into plantar flexion of 40 to 50 degrees provided optimized visualization of the calcaneofibular ligament and of some parts of the deltoid ligament; and (4) sagittal images provided the best full-length views of the calcaneonavicular (spring) ligament.

Whether the ankle ligaments are evaluated with the foot in a neutral position, plantar flexed, dorsiflexed, or in combinations of these positions, three MR imaging planes are required to evaluate all of the ligaments of the ankle fully, although the sagittal plane is least valuable. The normal ligaments are thin and of low signal intensity. The anterior talofibular ligament is the easiest to identify, particularly in transaxial MR images (Fig. 17–56). Similarly, the posterior talofibular ligament is identified most readily in the transaxial plane (although it also is seen in coronal images), and its posterior aspect is intimately related to the peroneal longus tendon and its sheath (see Fig. 17–56). A parallel arrangement of individual fibers separated by fibrofatty tissue may be evident, and the tibial slip, or posterior intermalleolar ligament, sometimes can be identified (Fig. 17–57). In the sagittal plane, the posterior talofibular ligament produces one or more foci of low signal intensity adjacent to the posterior surface of the talus, an appearance that

simulates that of an intra-articular body. The calcaneofibular ligament is best evaluated in transaxial and coronal MR images (see Fig. 17–56), although it is not seen in approximately 20 per cent of normal ankles. The peroneus longus and peroneus brevis tendons are located just superficial to the calcaneofibular ligament,

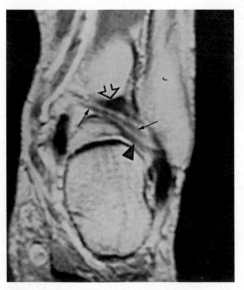

Figure 17–57

Normal ligaments of the ankle: MR imaging. Tibial slip (i.e., posterior intermalleolar ligament) of posterior talofibular ligament and transverse tibiofibular ligament. A coronal proton density–weighted (TR/TE, 4000/20) spin echo MR image shows the following normal ligaments: posterior talofibular ligament (arrowhead), posterior intermalleolar ligament (solid arrows), and transverse tibiofibular ligament (open arrow). (Courtesy of Z.S. Rosenberg, M.D., New York, New York.)

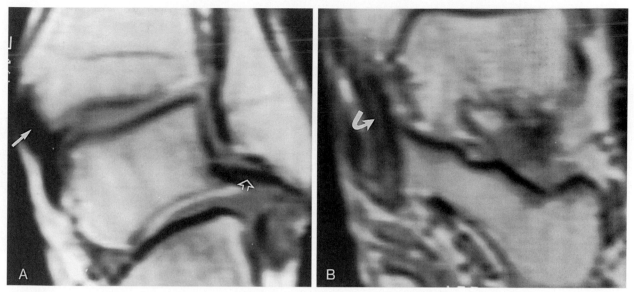

Figure 17–58
Normal ligaments of the ankle: MR imaging—deltoid ligament. Two coronal T1-weighted (TR/TE, 600/20) spin echo MR images show portions of the tibiotalar (solid straight arrow) and tibiocalcaneal (solid curved arrow) ligaments. In **A**, note visualization of the posterior talofibular (open arrow) ligament.

and the synovial sheath of the peroneal tendons is attached to this ligament.

The deltoid ligament is seen regularly and often in its entirety in coronal MR images (Fig. 17–58), particularly those obtained with 20 to 40 degrees of plantar flexion of the foot. In the coronal plane, however, inhomogeneity of signal intensity within some portions of the deltoid ligament may be encountered normally, perhaps related to partial volume artifact created by periligamentous collections of fatty or fibrocartilaginous tissue.[233] Transaxial MR images also are useful in studying both the superficial and deep portions of the deltoid ligament at any single level. Furthermore, the transaxial MR images show the relationship of the deltoid ligament to nearby tendons and neurovascular structures.

The tibiofibular ligaments are best evaluated in the transaxial plane, particularly in images located within 1 cm of the tibial plafond.[224] Both the anterior and posterior tibiofibular ligaments are identifiable (Fig. 17–59),

although analysis of several consecutive transaxial images often is required. Mink[234] has emphasized the difficulty that may be encountered in proper identification of the tibiofibular and talofibular ligaments in the transaxial MR images, owing in part to the oblique course of the anterior tibiofibular ligament and the tibial attachment site of the posterior tibiofibular ligament, which may be seen in transaxial images in which the remaining portion of the tibia no longer is visible. This investigator noted the importance of two osseous landmarks, the talus and the fibula, that can be used to allow correct identification of each of the talofibular and tibiofibular ligaments in the transaxial plane[234]:

1. Talus. At the level of its dome, the talus is nearly rectangular; this is the level at which the tibiofibular ligaments are observed. More distally, the talus is more elongated, and a portion of the sinus tarsi usually is visible; this is the level at which the talofibular ligaments are observed.

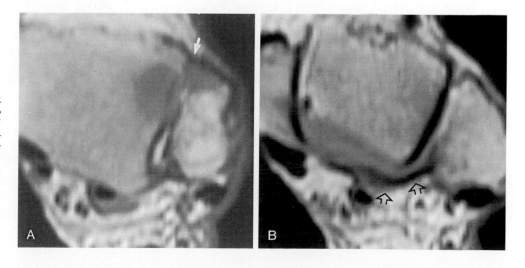

Figure 17–59
Normal ligaments of the ankle: MR imaging—tibiofibular ligaments. Two transaxial T1-weighted (TR/TE, 600/20) spin echo MR images, with **A** located at a level slightly above **B**, show the anterior tibiofibular (solid arrow) and posterior tibiofibular (open arrows) ligaments.

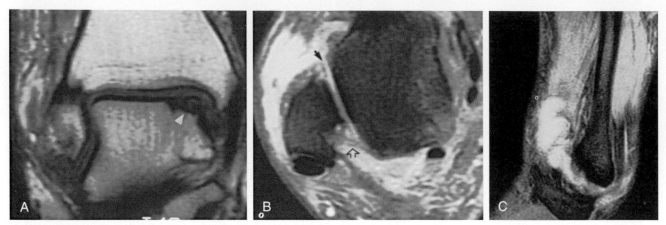

Figure 17–60
Injuries of the talofibular ligaments: MR imaging—acute complete tear of the anterior talofibular ligament and acute partial tear of the posterior talofibular ligament.

A A coronal T1-weighted (TR/TE, 600/20) spin echo MR image reveals subcutaneous edema laterally and an osteochondral fracture of the talus (arrowhead).

B A transaxial proton density–weighted (TR/TE, 2000/20) spin echo MR image obtained with chemical presaturation of fat (ChemSat) at a level just below the ankle shows soft tissue edema and hemorrhage (of high signal intensity), complete disruption of the anterior talofibular ligament (solid arrow), and attenuation of the posterior talofibular ligament (open arrow).

C A sagittal multiplanar gradient recalled (MPGR) (TR/TE, 500/11; flip angle, 15 degrees) MR image shows hemorrhage extending in front of the distal portion of the fibula.

(**A, B**, Courtesy of C. Sebrechts, M.D., San Diego, California; **C**, Courtesy of S. K. Brahme, M.D., San Diego, California.)

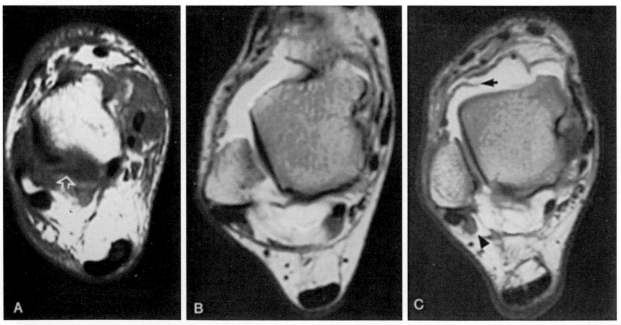

Figure 17–61
Injuries of the talofibular and calcaneofibular ligaments: MR imaging and MR arthrography.

A Acute complete tear of the anterior talofibular ligament. In a transaxial T1-weighted (TR/TE, 650/20) spin echo MR image, the anterior talofibular ligament is not seen, although some of the fibers of the posterior talofibular ligament are identified (open arrow).

B Acute complete tear of the anterior talofibular ligament. A transaxial T1-weighted (TR/TE, 600/16) spin echo MR image, obtained after the injection of a gadolinium compound into the ankle, reveals failure to visualize the anterior talofibular ligament and anterolateral extravasation of fluid.

C Acute complete tears of the anterior talofibular and calcaneofibular ligaments. In a transaxial MR arthrographic image with parameters identical to those in **B**, findings include a torn anterior talofibular ligament (arrow) and fluid in the peroneal tendon sheath (arrowhead), evidence of a tear of the calcaneofibular ligament.

(**A**, Courtesy of J. Beltran, M.D., New York, New York; **B, C**, Courtesy of V. Chandnani, M.D., Honolulu, Hawaii.)

2. Fibula. At the level of the distal portion of the fibular shaft, the fibula has a flattened medial border; the tibiofibular ligaments are observed at this level. At the level of the malleolar fossa (appearing as a deep indentation along the medial border of the lateral malleolus), the talofibular ligaments are seen.

The MR imaging findings associated with disruption of the ligaments about the ankle include interruption of a portion or an entire ligament, ligament laxity or waviness, thickening and irregularity of the ligament, surrounding hemorrhage and edema (in acute injuries), and accumulation of abnormal amounts of fluid in adjacent joints and tendon sheaths (Figs. 17–60, 17–61, 17–62, 17–63, and 17–64).[225, 227, 234] The abnormalities of the ligament itself are the most important diagnostic findings; the presence of a joint effusion or fluid in a tendon sheath is not specific for the diagnosis of ligamentous disruption. Inability to visualize a ligament may indicate a tear, but the reliability of this finding depends on the ligament under consideration and the technical aspects of the MR imaging examination. For example, the anterior tibiofibular and calcaneofibular ligaments are not identified universally in MR imaging examinations of the ankle, so that their nonvisualization cannot be used as a reliable sign of injury.[234] Inability to visualize the deltoid ligament, however, indicates a strong likelihood of its disruption.

Additional diagnostic problems related to assessment of ligamentous integrity with MR imaging include heterogeneous signal intensity, creating a striated appearance in normal ligaments (particularly the posterior talofibular and posterior tibiofibular ligaments and the deep portion of the deltoid ligament); the appearance

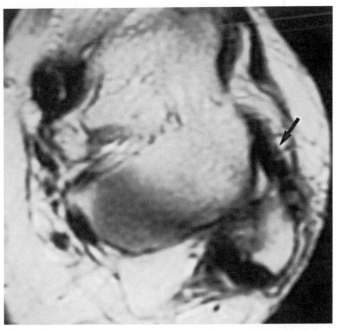

Figure 17–63
Injuries of the talofibular ligaments: MR imaging. A transverse proton density (TR/TE, 4000/14) spin echo MR image shows a thickened anterior talofibular ligament (arrow), indicative of a chronic injury.

of the normal posterior talofibular and posterior tibiofibular ligaments in the sagittal MR images, which may resemble that of intra-articular bodies; and an irregular and frayed superior edge of the normal posterior talofibular ligament, which may simulate a tear.[233–235]

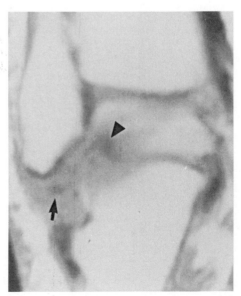

Figure 17–62
Injuries of the calcaneofibular ligament: MR imaging. Acute complete tear of the calcaneofibular ligament. A coronal T1-weighted (TR/TE, 550/20) spin echo MR image reveals a few residual fibers of the calcaneofibular ligament (arrow). Note the soft tissue mass of intermediate signal intensity about the torn ligament. Some of the fibers of the posterior talofibular ligament (arrowhead) are seen. (Courtesy of J. Beltran, M.D., New York, New York.)

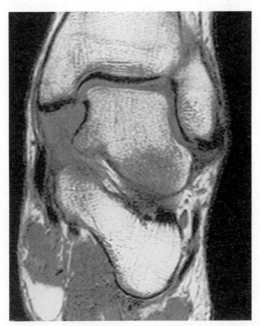

Figure 17–64
Injuries of the deltoid ligament: MR imaging. In this coronal T1-weighted (TR/TE, 717/20) spin echo MR image, both the superficial and deep portions of the deltoid ligament are torn. No ligamentous fibers on the medial side of the ankle can be identified. Rather edema, hemorrhage, and granulation tissue have led to a masslike appearance. (Courtesy of S. Eilenberg, M.D., San Diego, California.)

A potential role exists for MR arthrography employing intra-articular (talocrural joint) injection of a gadolinium compound or saline solution as a means to assess ligamentous injuries about the ankle (Fig. 17–65), although this role has yet to be proved (see Fig. 17–61).[230] In one study, MR arthrography accomplished with intra-articular injection of a gadolinium compound proved more accurate and sensitive in the detection of tears of the anterior talofibular ligament than was standard MR imaging or stress radiography.[230]

Therapy Considerations

The great majority of acute injuries to the lateral ligamentous complex of the ankle (Fig. 17–66A) are treated conservatively with aggressive and early rehabilitation. Certainly, nonoperative management is recommended for grade I and grade II injuries. Although the choice of treatment of grade III injuries is more controversial, most such injuries are treated conservatively. Surgical procedures are employed most often when there are large bone avulsions, associated osteochondral fractures

of the talus, or severe ligamentous damage on the medial side of the joint.[187]

Chronic sequelae after injuries to the lateral ligaments of the ankle are common, and mechanical instability of the joint may require operative intervention. The large number of surgical procedures that have been described to correct this instability is evidence that an ideal technique does not exist. One surgical approach is anatomic reconstruction or restoration of the lateral ligaments, which involves shortening the involved structures (usually both the anterior talofibular and calcaneofibular ligaments) and reattaching them.[185, 187, 236] This approach is exemplified by the Broström procedure (with suturing of the affected ligaments) (Fig. 17–66B) and its modifications (e.g., additional reinforcement provided by a portion of the lateral talocalcaneal ligament and plication of the inferior extensor retinaculum with or without lateral capsular advancement) (Fig. 17–66C). Another approach relates to tenodesis of the peroneus brevis tendon, as exemplified by the Evans, Chrisman-Snook (Fig. 17–66D), and Watson-Jones procedures (Fig. 17–66E).[185, 237] The Evans procedure involves re-

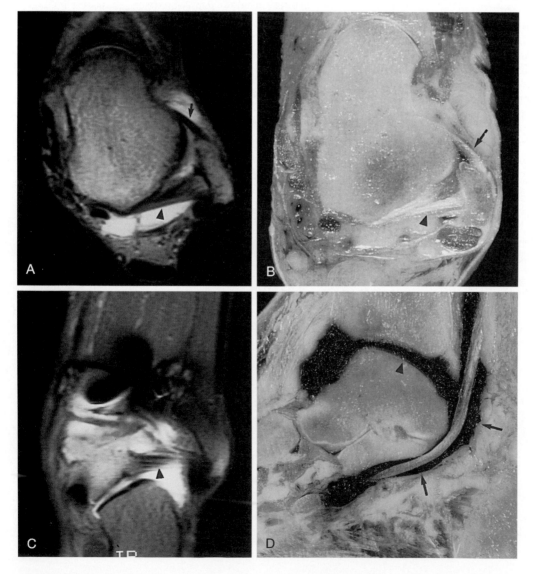

Figure 17–65
Ligaments of the ankle: MR arthrography.

A, B A transverse fat-suppressed T1-weighted spin echo MR image obtained after the intra-articular injection of a gadolinium-containing compound (**A**) and a transverse section of a cadaveric ankle at a similar level (**B**) show the features of the anterior (arrows) and posterior (arrowheads) talofibular ligaments. Contrast agent superficial to the ligaments in **A** is related to normal recesses of the ankle.

C A coronal fat-suppressed T1-weighted spin echo MR image obtained after the intra-articular injection of a gadolinium-containing compound shows the posterior talofibular ligament (arrowhead).

D This photograph of a sagittal section of a cadaveric ankle demonstrates normal communication of the joint (arrowhead) with the tendon sheath (arrows) of the flexor hallucis muscle, as evidenced by the distribution of latex.

(Courtesy of S. Lee, M.D., Los Angeles, California.)

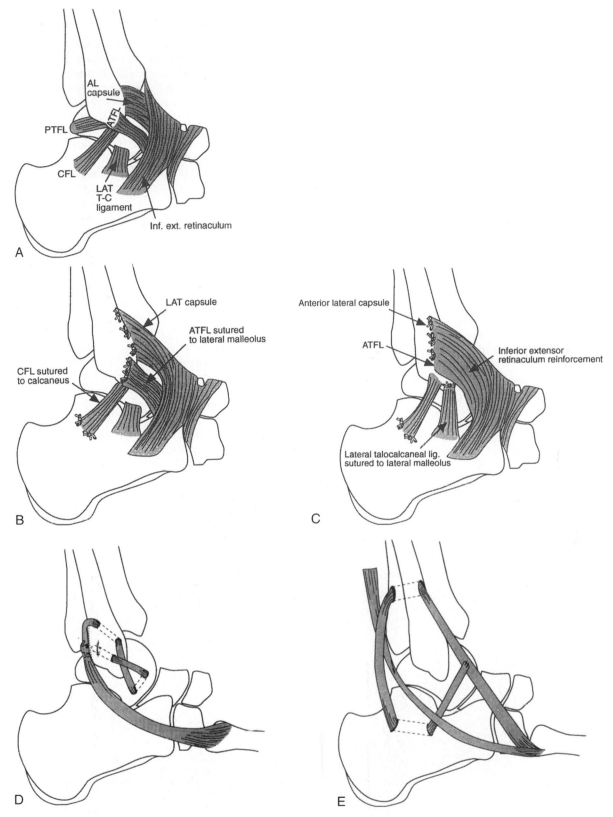

Figure 17–66

Injuries of the lateral ligamentous complex: Therapy considerations.

   A Anatomy of the lateral ankle ligamentous complex.

   B The Broström procedure.

   C The modified Broström-capsular shift procedure.

   D The Chrisman-Snook procedure.

   E The Watson-Jones procedure.

   AL, anterolateral; ATFL, anterior talofibular ligament; CFL, calcaneofibular ligament; LAT, lateral; PTFL, posterior talofibular ligament; T-C, talocalcaneal.

   (From Liu SH, Jason WJ: Clin Sports Med *4*:793, 1994.)

routing of the peroneus brevis tendon through the lateral malleolus and reattaching the tendon under tension to resist inversion; the torn ligaments are not reconstructed. The Chrisman-Snook procedure involves reconstruction of the anterior talofibular and calcaneofibular ligaments through drill holes with a half-split of the peroneus brevis tendon left attached distally.[185] Basically, this procedure uses a split peroneus brevis tendon graft. The graft is brought through the fibula from anterior to posterior to reconstruct the anterior talofibular ligament and is then brought posteriorly and inferiorly to the calcaneus to reconstruct the calcaneofibular ligament.[236] In the Watson-Jones procedure, in addition to tenodesis of the peroneus brevis tendon to the fibula, the graft is routed anteriorly through the talar neck to reconstruct the anterior talofibular ligament.[236]

With regard to acute injuries of the deltoid ligament, partial tears are treated conservatively. Complete tears may be treated conservatively or surgically. Favorable long-term results of either mode of treatment are dependent on precise anatomic reduction of the ankle mortise.

With regard to syndesmotic injuries, complete ruptures generally are treated surgically and partial tears (usually involving the anterior tibiofibular ligament) are treated conservatively.

Sinus Tarsi Syndrome

Between the two subtalar joints, the posterior subtalar and talocalcaneonavicular joints, a cone-shaped region is found, designated the tarsal sinus and tarsal canal (Fig. 17–67). The apex of the cone is located posteromedially, representing the tarsal canal, and the expanded anterolateral portion of the cone represents the tarsal sinus. The contents of the tarsal canal and sinus include fat, an arterial anastomosis with branches from the posterior tibial and peroneal arteries, joint capsules, nerve endings, and five ligaments. These ligaments are the medial, intermediate, and lateral roots of the inferior extensor retinaculum; the cervical ligament; and the ligament of the tarsal canal (talocalcaneal interosseous ligament).[238] Injury to these structures leads to a disorder termed the sinus tarsi syndrome, which is associated with lateral foot pain, tenderness, and hindfoot instability.

The ligaments of the tarsal sinus and canal, particularly the cervical and the talocalcaneal interosseous ligaments, limit inversion and maintain alignment between the talus and the calcaneus.[239] The cervical ligament is located at the lateral margin of the sinus tarsi. It originates from the superior surface of the calcaneus, medial to the origin of the extensor digitorum brevis muscle. From here, it extends in a superior and medial direction to attach to the tubercle on the inferior and lateral aspects of the talar neck. The cervical ligament is taut when the foot is inverted. The talocalcaneal interosseous ligament (ligament of the tarsal canal) extends from the sulcus tali to the sulcus calcanei. It is located just anterior to the posterior subtalar joint and is smaller than the cervical ligament. This ligament is taut when the foot is everted. The lateral root of the inferior extensor retinaculum attaches to the calcaneus at the external aspect of the tarsal sinus; the medial root of this retinaculum extends deep within the tarsal sinus, attaching to the calcaneus just anterior to the calcaneal attachment site of the ligament of the tarsal canal and to the talus in common with the ligament of the tarsal canal; and the intermediate root of the inferior extensor

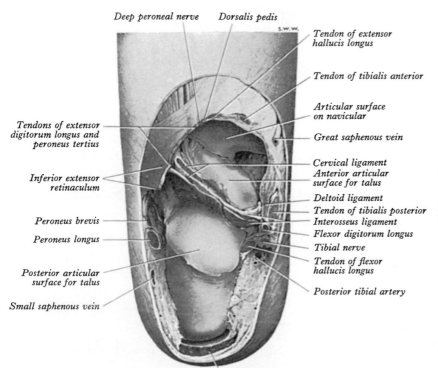

Labels on figure:
Deep peroneal nerve
Dorsalis pedis
Tendon of extensor hallucis longus
Tendon of tibialis anterior
Articular surface on navicular
Great saphenous vein
Tendons of extensor digitorum longus and peroneus tertius
Cervical ligament
Anterior articular surface for talus
Deltoid ligament
Tendon of tibialis posterior
Interosseus ligament
Flexor digitorum longus
Tibial nerve
Tendon of flexor hallucis longus
Posterior tibial artery
Inferior extensor retinaculum
Peroneus brevis
Peroneus longus
Posterior articular surface for talus
Small saphenous vein
Tendo calcaneus

Figure 17–67

Ligaments of the tarsal sinus and canal: Normal anatomy. A superior view of the calcaneus is provided by removal of the talus. See text for details. (From Williams PL, Warwick R [Eds]: Gray's Anatomy. 36th British edition. Edinburgh, Churchill Livingstone, 1980, p. 465.)

retinaculum attaches to the calcaneus within the tarsal sinus, just posterior to the attachment site of the cervical ligament.[238, 239] Experimentally induced tears of the cervical ligament and ligament of the tarsal canal produce minor degrees of instability of the hindfoot.[240]

The sinus tarsi syndrome leads to pain and tenderness, particularly in the lateral side of the foot, and a sensation of hindfoot weakness and instability.[240] In approximately 70 per cent of affected persons, an inversion injury to the ankle occurs which, in some cases, results in tears of various components of the lateral ligamentous complex of the ankle.[241, 242] The high association of injuries to the tarsal sinus and canal and injuries to the lateral ligaments of the ankle requires careful analysis of the sinus tarsi in all patients in whom inversion injuries of the ankle have occurred. Such analysis may be difficult, owing to the lack of clinical and routine radiographic findings that are sensitive to subtalar injury. In patients with a clinically serious ankle injury, negative results from stress tests (such as the anterior drawer and inversion stress tests) should arouse suspicion of an underlying subtalar sprain. Arthrography and MR imaging allow more direct assessment of the subtalar joints and the tarsal sinus and canal.

Arthrographic analysis of the tarsal sinus and canal requires contrast opacification of the posterior subtalar joint.[242–245] The basis of a positive arthrographic examination is the obliteration of the normal synovial recesses present about the talocalcaneal interosseous ligament. The changes apparently relate to synovial hyperplasia and may not be present immediately after trauma. Another arthrographic finding is leakage of contrast material into the sinus tarsi.[242] This abnormality apparently reflects disruption of fibers of the talocalcaneal interosseous ligament and possibly the cervical ligament as well. Further arthrographic findings include retraction of normal joint recesses, limited articular distention, lateral capsular leakage of contrast material, ganglion cysts, and abnormalities indicative of tears of the anterior talofibular and calcaneofibular ligaments.[242, 245] In one study, approximately 70 per cent of cases of chronic sinus tarsi syndrome had abnormal arthrograms.[246]

MR imaging has been employed to study the normal contents of the tarsal sinus and canal and to investigate patients with the sinus tarsi syndrome (Fig. 17–68).[222, 234, 238, 247] The sagittal, coronal, and transaxial MR images all are important in analyzing the sinus tarsi. The cervical ligament and portions of the inferior extensor retinaculum are seen in all normal ankles, and the interosseous ligament is evident in most normal ankles. Fluid collections with increased signal intensity in T2-weighted spin echo MR images normally are evident in the recesses about the talocalcaneal interosseous ligament, although the absence of these recesses with MR imaging (as opposed to arthrography) does not allow a diagnosis of the sinus tarsi syndrome.[238] MR imaging findings of this syndrome include poor definition of soft tissue structures (including the cervical and talocalcaneal interosseous ligaments), edema or fibrosis, and abnormal fluid collections (Figs. 17–69, 17–70, and 17–71).[234, 238] Abnormalities of adjacent structures, such as the anterior talofibular ligament, calcaneofibular ligament, and tibialis posterior tendon, also may be evident.[238] The MR imaging appearance of the abnormal tarsal sinus and canal are consistent with the known pathologic findings.[238] Chronic synovitis, inflammation, fibrosis, and synovial cysts are recognized pathologic abnormalities in the sinus tarsi syndrome.[241]

Subtalar Joint Instability

Normal stability of the subtalar joints (i.e., posterior subtalar and talocalcaneonavicular joints) is provided by the apposing, undulating articular surfaces and surrounding ligaments.[248] The cervical and interosseous ligaments hold the calcaneus and talus together, the deltoid ligament provides medial stability, and the calcaneofibular and lateral talocalcaneal ligaments provide lateral stability. Dysfunction of one or more of these ligaments can lead to increased mobility of the subtalar

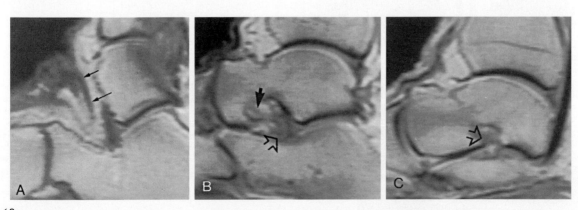

Figure 17–68

Normal tarsal sinus and canal: MR imaging. Three sagittal T1-weighted (TR/TE, 600/20) spin echo MR images are shown, with **A** being the most lateral, **B** being intermediate in position, and **C** being the most medial.

A The medial root of the inferior extensor retinaculum (solid arrows) extends from the extensor tendons to its insertion in the tarsal sinus.

B Just medial to **A**, the cervical ligament (solid arrow) extends from the talus to the calcaneus. A portion of the talocalcaneal interosseous ligament (open arrow) also is seen.

C Just medial to **B**, a portion of the talocalcaneal interosseous ligament (open arrow) is noted.

(Courtesy of D. Goodwin, M.D., and D. Salonen, M.D., San Diego, California.)

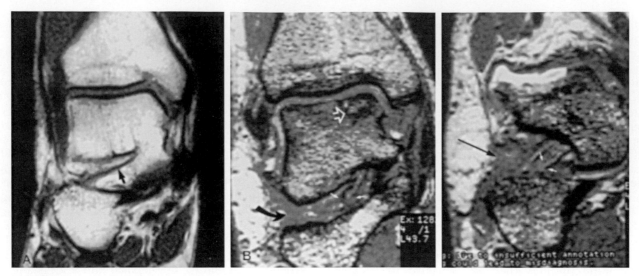

Figure 17–69
Sinus tarsi syndrome: MR imaging.

A Normal appearance. A coronal T1-weighted (TR/TE, 500/18) spin echo MR image reveals the normal talocalcaneal interosseous ligament (arrow), which is surrounded by fat.

B, C Sinus tarsi syndrome. Coronal reconstructions from a three-dimensional gradient recalled acquisition in the steady state (GRASS) MR image (TR/TE, 30/10; flip angle, 70 degrees), with **B** being slightly more posterior than **C**, show diffuse infiltration of the tarsal sinus (black arrows). In **B**, partial disruption of the talocalcaneal interosseous ligament has led to a wavy, discontinuous appearance (solid white arrows). A small osteochondral fracture of the medial talar dome (open white arrow) is seen. In **C** partial disruption of the cervical ligament (white arrows) is evident.

(From Klein MA, Spreitzer AM: Radiology *186*:233, 1993.)

joints, which if extreme may be manifested as subluxation or dislocation.

As many as 40 per cent of patients with an injury to the lateral ligamentous complex of the ankle develop chronic symtpoms, which may include a sensation of giving-way of the ankle (functional instability). In such patients, subtalar joint instability should be considered as a cause of these clinical manifestations, particularly if other causes of instability have been excluded.[249, 250] In cadavers, when inversion stress is applied to the foot, rupture of the interosseous talocalcaneal ligament occurs only after that of the anterior talofibular and calca-

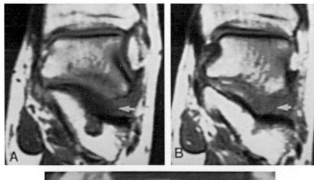

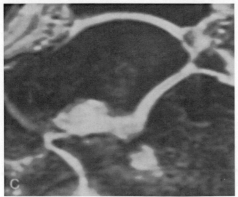

Figure 17–70
Sinus tarsi syndrome: MR imaging.

A, B Two coronal T1-weighted (TR/TE, 500/20) spin echo MR images show diffuse infiltration of the tarsal sinus with tissue of intermediate signal intensity (arrows) and loss of definition of the talocalcaneal interosseous ligament. A cystic lesion of the calcaneus is evident in **A**.

C In the same patient, a sagittal MPGR MR image (TR/TE, 1000/20; flip angle, 40 degrees) shows high signal intensity in the tarsal sinus and a calcaneal cyst and absence of visualization of the ligaments of the tarsal canal and sinus.

(Courtesy of J. Beltran, M.D., New York, New York.)

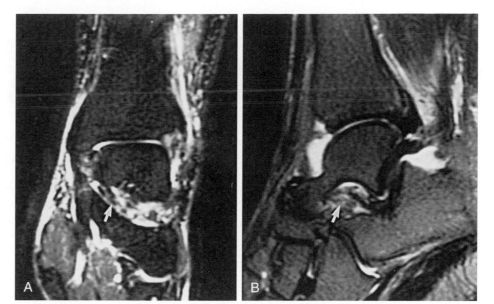

Figure 17–71
Sinus tarsi syndrome: MR imaging. Both the coronal fast spin echo STIR MR image (TR/TE, 5000/42; inversion time, 150 msec) **(A)** and the sagittal fat-suppressed fast spin echo MR image (TR/TE, 4600/126) **(B)** show abnormal high signal intensity in the tarsal canal, about the cervical and interosseous ligaments (arrows). Muscle and soft tissue edema reflect the presence of more extensive injury.

neofibular ligaments. Total rupture of the interosseous talocalcaneal and cervical ligaments results in dislocation of the subtalar joint.

Subtalar joint sprains may be divided into acute and chronic stages. Acute symptoms often are combined with those related to the coexistent ankle sprain. Chronic symptoms, including the functional instability noted previously, are similar to those accompanying chronic lateral ligamentous instability of the ankle and, in some cases, indicate the presence of the sinus tarsi syndrome (see previous discussion). Meyer and colleagues[242] divide subtalar sprains into four categories: Forced supination of the hindfoot with the ankle in

plantar flexion leads to disruption of the anterior talofibular ligament (and, possibly, the cervical ligament), followed by either disruption of the calcaneofibular ligament and lateral capsule (type 1) or tearing of the talocalcaneal interosseous ligament (type 2); forced supination of the hindfoot with the ankle in dorsiflexion leads to severe soft tissue abnormalities with rupture of the calcaneofibular, cervical, and talocalcaneal interosseous ligaments and an intact anterior talofibular ligament (type 3); and a combination of severe ankle and subtalar joint sprains may lead to subtalar dislocation with rupture of all lateral and medial capsuloligamentous components of the posterior tarsus (type 4) (Fig. 17–72).[187]

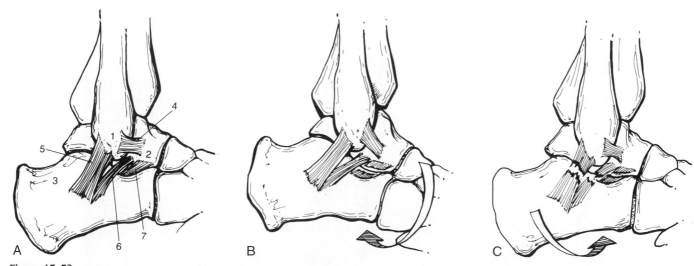

Figure 17–72
Subtalar joint sprains.

A Anterolateral and inferior ligamentous structures of the subtalar joint. 1, lateral malleolus; 2, talus; 3, calcaneus; 4, anterior talofibular ligament; 5, calcaneofibular ligament; 6, cervical ligament; 7, interosseous talocalcaneal ligament.

B Forceful inversion of the hindfoot with a plantar flexed ankle, possibly tearing the anterior talofibular ligament and the interosseous talocalcaneal ligament.

C Forceful inversion of the hindfoot with a dorsiflexed ankle, possibly tearing the calcaneofibular ligament, cervical ligament, and interosseous talocalcaneal ligament.

(From Meyer JM, Garcia J, Hoffmeyer P, et al: Clin Orthop *226*:169, 1988.)

Table 17–3. IMPINGEMENT SYNDROMES OF THE ANKLE

Location	Pathologic Findings
Anterior	Osteoarthritis of the ankle, osteophytes of anterior portions of the talus and tibia
Anterolateral	Injuries to the lateral capsule, anterior tibiofibular ligament, anterior talofibular ligament, or combinations of these, with formation of scar tissue
Posterior	Entrapment of the os trigonum or posterior process of the talus
Posterolateral	Injuries to the posterior tibiofibular ligament, including transverse ligament and intermalleolar slip, and capsule
Syndesmotic	Injuries to the anterior tibiofibular ligament and capsule
Medial	Cartilage abnormalities at the tip or anterior distal portion of the medial malleolus and the medial facet of the talus

Assessment of sprains of the subtalar joints requires clinical evaluation, routine radiography, and ankle and subtalar joint stress radiography.[248, 250] Stress radiographs of the subtalar joints usually are accomplished with an inversion load applied to the calcaneus.[250] Additional diagnostic methods include subtalar joint arthrography, CT scanning, and MR imaging (see discussion of sinus tarsi syndrome). Although conservative therapy may be adequate for less severe injuries, operative intervention with repair of ankle ligaments may be necessary when the injuries are severe.

Impingement Syndromes

Several impingement syndromes may lead to restricted motion of the ankle joint and, in some cases, may simulate an ankle sprain (Table 17–3). Impingement syndromes can be divided into five types: anterior, posterior, anterolateral, syndesmotic, and medial.

Anterior Impingement Syndrome

The anterior impingement syndrome results from impingement of the anterior aspect of the tibia against the superior portion of the neck of the talus.[251] The condition was described first in 1943 by Morris,[252] who used

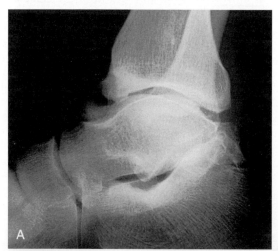
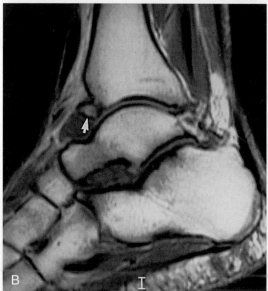
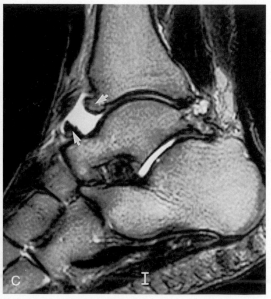

Figure 17–73
Anterior impingement syndrome: MR imaging.

A The routine radiograph shows anterior osteophytes involving the talus and tibia.

B, C Sagittal T1-weighted (TR/TE, 800/15) spin echo **(B)** and fast spin echo (TR/TE, 3650/120) **(C)** MR images reveal these osteophytes (arrows) and fluid in the ankle and posterior subtalar joints.

(Courtesy of J. Healy, M.D., San Diego, California.)

the term athlete's ankle. It commonly is observed in young athletic persons, particularly baseball, soccer and (American) football players, and professional dancers.[253-258] Any athlete who uses repetitive and forceful dorsiflexion in movements of the ankle may be susceptible to this syndrome. Other predisposing factors include an equinus foot and laxity of the lateral ligaments of the ankle, the latter allowing anterior subluxation of the tibia.[258] Clinical findings include pain and tenderness in the anterior region of the ankle, findings accentuated with dorsiflexion of the joint. Restricted motion may be an accompanying clinical manifestation. Affected patients may pronate the foot excessively to increase the range of ankle motion, and such pronation eventually may lead to other ankle problems. Routine radiography reveals osteophytes in the anterior surface of the tibia or the neck of the talus, or in both sites (Fig. 17–73A).[251] MR imaging shows similar features (Fig. 17–73B, C). Arthroscopic resection of the osteophytes may lead to symptomatic relief and increased ankle motion.[251, 259]

Posterior Impingement Syndrome

The posterior impingement syndrome may result from the presence of an os trigonum (Fig. 17–74) or a prominent process, termed Stieda's process, in the posterior surface of the talus (also see later discussion of abnormalities of the flexor hallucis longus tendon); alternatively, it may result from soft tissue injury. The first of these two types of posterior impingement often is referred to as the os trigonum or talar compression syndrome; the second type sometimes is designated posterior soft tissue impingement. With regard to the talar compression syndrome, symptoms are common, owing to limitation of plantar flexion at the ankle, and for athletes such as professional ballet dancers, the condition may be disabling, requiring excision of the os trigonum or the prominent posterior process of the talus (which may be intact or fractured). Accompanying inflammation in the sheath about the flexor hallucis longus tendon may be evident. Findings may be unilateral or bilateral in distribution. This syndrome is discussed later in this chapter.

Posterior (or posterolateral) soft tissue impingement, which may occur alone or in combination with anterolateral impingement, has several causes[260]: hypertrophy or tearing of the inferior portion of the posterior tibiofibular ligament, of the transverse tibiofibular ligament, or of the posterior intermalleolar ligament, or combinations of these injuries. Furthermore, a labrum on the posterior lip of the tibia may lead to such impingement.[505] The occurrence of entrapment and bucket handle tears of the posterior intermalleolar ligament has been emphasized as a cause of posterior impingement in ballet dancers.[505]

Anterolateral Impingement Syndrome

The anterolateral impingement syndrome generally occurs in young persons who have sustained an injury to the lateral ligaments of the ankle.[260-265] A complete or partial tear of the anterior talofibular ligament (or other lateral ligaments) is associated with intra-articular hemorrhage and hyperplasia of the synovial membrane that extends into the articular gutter in the lateral aspect of the ankle. Entrapment of the synovial membrane or reactive hyalinized connective or scar tissue between the talus and fibula or tibia may lead to cartilage erosion in the anterolateral portion of the talar dome.[234] MR imaging reveals the mass, which commonly is of intermediate signal intensity in both T1-weighted and T2-weighted spin echo MR images (Fig. 17–75). At arthroscopy, the hyalinized mass usually is associated with lesions of either the anterior talofibular ligament or the anterior tibiofibular syndesmotic ligament. Chondromalacia of the lateral portion of the talus or fibula also may be noted.[260] Resection of the meniscus-like tissue may be curative.[259, 260, 264-266] Additional causes of soft tissue lesions in this or other portions of the ankle include localized nodular synovitis, diffuse pigmented villonodular synovitis, idiopathic synovial (osteo)chondromatosis, ganglion cysts, and idiopathic arthrofibrosis.[259]

Syndesmotic Impingement Syndrome

Syndesmotic impingement usually results from injuries to the anterior tibiofibular ligament, with or without associated injuries to the interosseous membrane and posterior tibiofibular ligament. Synovitis and scar tissue lead to progressive pain and instability.[260] In one report, a separate fascicle of the anterior tibiofibular ligament led to this type of impingement.[267] This fascicle, which appears to be common, may be developmental or traumatic in pathogenesis.[268] Excisions of the fascicle and

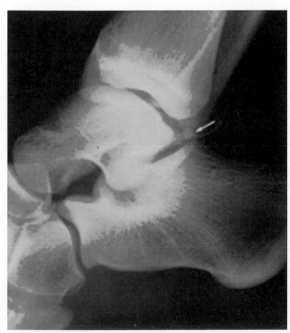

Figure 17–74

Posterior impingement syndrome: Routine radiography. In a 14 year old ballet student with pain during plantar flexion of the foot, a lateral radiograph of the foot in plantar flexion shows approximation of the surfaces of the tibia and calcaneus with an adjacent os trigonum (arrow). The os trigonum was excised with relief of pain. (Courtesy of G. Greenway, M.D., Dallas, Texas.)

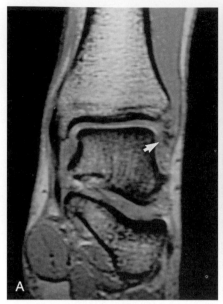 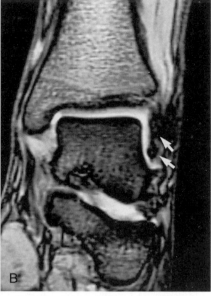

Figure 17–75

Anterolateral impingement syndrome: MR imaging. In this patient with persistent symptoms after a lateral ankle sprain, a coronal spoiled gradient echo (SPGR) MR image (TR/TE, 173/4; flip angle, 60 degrees) **(A)** and a coronal MPGR (TR/TE, 600/7; flip angle, 30 degrees) MR image **(B)** show scar tissue (arrows) of low signal intensity anterior to the fibula.

débridement of the ankle joint and anterior tibiofibular ligament, which can be accomplished arthroscopically, may be curative.[260]

Medial Impingement Syndrome

Inversion injuries resulting in rupture of one or more lateral ankle ligaments may be accompanied by residual complaints on the medial side of the joint. One cause of this is impingement between the medial malleolus and the medial facet of the talus.[506] Chondral abnormalities are detected arthroscopically at these points of abnormal contact, differing in location from cartilage lesions of the dome of the talus that are well recognized after a supination injury of the ankle. Other causes of medial ankle pain occurring after inversion injuries of the ankle are partial or complete ruptures of the deltoid ligament, chronic synovitis, osteophytes, and scar tissue.

Tendon Abnormalities

Anatomic Considerations

Numerous tendons extend from the lower portion of the leg into the foot, across the ankle. These include the peroneus longus and peroneus brevis tendons laterally; the Achilles tendon posteriorly; the posterior tibialis, flexor hallucis longus, and flexor digitorum longus tendons medially; and the anterior tibialis, extensor hallucis longus, extensor digitorum longus, and peroneus tertius tendons anteriorly. With the exception of the Achilles tendon, all of these tendons change from a vertical orientation in the lower leg to a horizontal orientation in the foot at or near the level of the ankle, a modification in direction that is accomplished by means of a pulley system consisting either of bone (i.e., the malleoli) or of retinacula.[44] To promote smooth movement at their sites of angulation, tendons are surrounded by either (1) a sheath of parietal synovium and

tenosynovial fluid in fibro-osseous tunnels (e.g., flexor hallucis longus tendon), under a bone pulley (e.g., peroneal tendons under the lateral malleolus), or under a fascial sling (e.g., anterior tibialis tendon under the extensor retinaculum), or (2) loose connective tissue, termed a peritenon (e.g., Achilles tendon).[44] Where tendons are applied to the surface of a bone, a groove or sulcus is present to promote angular deviations in their course that occur about the ankle. Examples include a groove in the posterior portion of the tibia for the tibialis posterior and flexor digitorum longus tendons, grooves in the posterior surface of the tibia and the talus and the inferior surface of the sustentaculum tali of the calcaneus for the flexor hallucis longus tendon, and a groove in the posterior surface of the fibula that houses the peroneus brevis tendon (and, to a lesser extent, the peroneus longus tendon). These grooves vary in size and in depth. The groove behind the fibula, through which pass the tendons of the peroneus brevis and peroneus longus muscles, is the smallest and most shallow, perhaps explaining the occurrence of subluxation of these tendons (see later discussion).

The movements of the ankle and foot are intimately related and complex. These movements lead to the development of dynamic forces in the many regional tendons whose magnitude is related to the osseous anatomy (which varies somewhat from one person to another), the volume of the contracting muscles, and the rapidity and type of movement. As the tendons of the ankle and foot are subjected to tremendous functional demands, not only during physical exertion but also as a response to routine activities such as walking, it is not surprising that a variety of tendon and tendon sheath abnormalities are encountered.

Pathologic Considerations

Jahss[269] has classified disorders of the tendons about the ankle and in the foot according to the following general categories: tenosynovitis, tethering, tears, dislocations, tumors and pseudotumors, ossification, congenital anomalies, contractures, and iatrogenic injuries. Inflammatory changes in or about a tendon, often designated tenosynovitis, can be defined more precisely according to which type of tissue is affected (Table 17–4). Such inflammation can affect a tendon sheath, the surrounding tissues, the region between the sheath and the tendon, or the tendon substance. If the tendon sheath itself is involved, the term tenosynovitis is most appropriate. Paratenosynovitis refers to inflammation of tissues about a tendon sheath, and paratendinitis refers to inflammation about a tendon that has no sheath. Peritendinitis is defined as inflammation of a peritenon. Tendinitis indicates inflammation within the substance of the tendon. Although such terminology is anatomically correct, inflammation commonly involves more than one of these structures, such that paratenosynovitis, tenosynovitis, and tendinitis can occur simultaneously. Inflammation of any or all of these structures may relate to direct or indirect injury, occupational stress and overuse syndromes, misuse syndromes related to anomalies of the foot or other structures, and local or systemic rheumatic diseases.[21] Although paratenosynovitis, paratendinitis, peritendinitis, tenosynovitis, and tendinitis occur in many different anatomic sites, inflammation leads to increased regional vascularity and cellular infiltration. When synovitis is a component of the inflammatory process, an increase in synovial fluid is apparent. Adhesions may develop between the sheath and the tendon (i.e., stenosing or constrictive tenosynovitis), leading to altered or restricted movement in a tendon sheath—tendon unit, which normally requires smooth, almost frictionless function. The wall of the sheath may thicken and become irregular, producing narrowing of the avenue through which the tendon or tendons pass. The pathologic findings that produce narrowing or constriction of the tendon sheath appear to be more common in locations in which more than one tendon occupies a single sheath, such as the sheath that surrounds the peroneus longus and peroneus brevis tendons.[44, 269]

Tenosynovitis in the ankle and foot relates primarily to a systemic rheumatic disease, an infection, or local mechanical factors. Rheumatoid arthritis, the seronegative spondyloarthropathies, and gout are among the rheumatic diseases that lead to such tenosynovitis. Infective tenosynovitis can be caused by a variety of microorganisms, although gonococcal or atypical mycobacterial infections deserve emphasis. Mechanical tenosynovitis is the most common type of disease, however. Causes of mechanical tenosynovitis include overuse syndromes in athletes, improper footwear, and bone anomalies (such as pes planus, an accessory navicular bone, and an enlarged peroneal tubercle).[269]

Paratenosynovitis may result from any inflammatory process that originates in the soft tissues and extends to the vicinity of a tendon sheath. Tendinitis, or inflammation in the substance of the tendon itself, may result from an injury leading to disruption of some of the tendinous fibers, xanthomatosis, gouty or rheumatoid involvement of the tendon, or irritation by enlargement or irregularity of an adjacent bone (e.g., flexor hallucis

Table 17–4. INFLAMMATION OF TENDONS AND SURROUNDING TISSUES

Tissue	Terminology
Tendon sheath	Tenosynovitis
Tissues about tendon sheath	Paratenosynovitis
Tissues about tendon that has no sheath	Paratendinitis
Peritenon	Peritendinitis
Tendon	Tendinitis

longus tendinitis produced by an enlarged os trigonum).[269] Peritendinitis also may occur secondary to a systemic process, such as rheumatoid arthritis, or spontaneously, particularly in the Achilles tendon and the tendon of the tibialis posterior muscle. Relative avascularity of these two tendons may make them more susceptible to this condition, which can lead to their attrition and eventual rupture.

By definition, a tethered tendon is one whose range of movement is limited, owing to its abnormal fixation to an adjacent structure. Causes of such tethering include anatomic anomalies (such as a single tendon sheath surrounding two tendons that normally have separate sheaths, or an accessory tendon that increases the volume of tissue within a single sheath), fractures with resulting deformities that lead to abnormal fixation or displacement of the tendon or its sheath (e.g., tethering of the peroneal tendons as a result of lateral extrusion of fragments of the calcaneus), a hypertrophied os trigonum that leads to constriction and displacement of the flexor hallucis longus tendon within its sheath, fracture-dislocations of the ankle that may cause tethering or even incarceration of one or more regional tendons, and checkrein deformities resulting from abnormal fixation of the flexor hallucis longus tendon under or just proximal to the flexor retinaculum (usually related to a fracture of the lower portion of the tibia) or under the annular ligament (which may occur secondary to a fracture, infection, or tumor).[269]

Partial or complete tears of the tendons of the foot and ankle may result from a laceration, especially in the sole of the foot or, more commonly, they may occur spontaneously. Spontaneous ruptures of these tendons (as well as those at other sites) usually imply some type of intrinsic pathologic process, as normal tendons rarely rupture in this fashion. Tendon degeneration in older persons or chronic inflammation in younger persons, particularly athletes, may predispose to spontaneous rupture. Although virtually any tendon of the foot or ankle may be affected, spontaneous disruptions of the tibialis posterior tendon and the Achilles tendon are encountered most frequently. Those of the tibialis anterior tendon, flexor hallucis longus tendon, and tendons of the peroneus longus and peroneus brevis muscles are far less common.

Additional lesions of tendons and their sheaths in the foot and ankle include tumors and tumor-like disorders (e.g., lipomas, xanthomas, gouty tophi, rheumatoid nodules, chondromas, pigmented villonodular tenosynovitis, idiopathic tenosynovial osteochondromatosis), anomalies (e.g., accessory or duplicated tendons and aberrant tendon insertions), contractures related to neuromuscular disease, infections, and ossification (e.g., ossification of the Achilles tendon). Many of these conditions are discussed elsewhere in this book.

Imaging Considerations

The assessment of tendon and tendon sheath abnormalities can be accomplished with a number of different imaging techniques. Routine radiography and bone scintigraphy lack sensitivity, ultrasonography is applicable to analysis of only those tendons accessible to a probe placed on the skin, and tenography provides indirect evidence of tendon abnormality and requires a needle puncture. CT and MR imaging are the two most commonly employed techniques for evaluation of the tendons of the foot and ankle. At this time, MR imaging generally is considered the best available imaging method in the detection of tendinitis, tenosynovitis, and partial and complete tendon ruptures; CT is superior to MR imaging in the delineation of tendon calcification and retinacular avulsions of bone; and CT and MR imaging are of approximately equal value in the analysis of tendon dislocations.

Routine Radiography. Routine radiographic findings associated with abnormalities of the tendons and tendon sheaths of the foot and ankle include soft tissue swelling, a change in contour, calcification or ossification of a tendon, bone proliferation, fracture fragments, and sesamoid displacement. Soft tissue swelling or fullness may accompany tenosynovitis, but the finding is not specific. A change in contour of an inflamed or torn tendon is best appreciated in locations where the tendon is surrounded by abundant fat (e.g., Achilles tendon), but the finding may be subtle unless low kilovolt radiography or xeroradiography is employed. Achilles tendinitis or a rupture of the Achilles tendon may be accompanied by edema or hemorrhage, with obscuration of portions of the preachilles fat body, and associated retrocalcaneal bursitis (which may occur in systemic rheumatic disorders and in Haglund's syndrome) leads to obliteration of the normal radiolucent retrocalcaneal recess between the Achilles tendon and the posterosuperior portion of the calcaneus. Calcific tendinitis in the foot is rare; ossification of the Achilles tendon is seen, however, and is detected readily by routine radiography (see later discussion).

Osseous proliferation or erosion is a recognized manifestation of inflammation of tendons and tendon sheaths that are located close or applied directly to the surface of a bone (Fig. 17–76). In the foot and ankle, this finding is observed most commonly in the posteromedial portion of the tibia in patients with rheumatoid arthritis or a seronegative spondyloarthropathy who have involvement of the tibialis posterior tendon and sheath. Infections of tendons and tendon sheaths also can lead to infective or reactive periostitis in the subjacent bone.

Avulsion fractures at sites of retinacular attachment may occur as a response to tendon subluxation or dislocation. An elongated bone fragment located lateral to the distal portion of the fibula is characteristic of a dislocation of the peroneal tendons (see later discussion) and may be seen as an isolated finding or in association with complex fracture-dislocations about the ankle.[270, 271] Displacement of the os peroneum may occur in patients with rupture of the tendon of the peroneus longus muscle.[272] This sesamoid bone ossifies in approximately 5 to 20 per cent of persons and normally is located adjacent to the lower border of the cuboid bone or at the level of the calcaneocuboid joint. Proximal migration with or without fragmentation of the os peroneum is consistent with attrition and rupture of the peroneus longus tendon just distal to the location of the sesamoid bone.

Ultrasonography. High resolution ultrasonography is an inexpensive and noninvasive technique that can be applied to the assessment of tendon abnormalities.[273] In the foot and ankle, the Achilles tendon is evaluated most easily and accurately with ultrasonography.[520] The normal Achilles tendon shows an internal network of fine parallel and linear fibrillar echoes that become more numerous and thinner as the ultrasonic frequency is increased.[274] Sonographic abnormalities of the Achilles tendon include increased thickness, interruption, fragmentation, or disappearance of the tendon fibrils.[274] With ultrasonography, complete tears of the tendon are accompanied by retraction of the fragments and a tendinous gap that may be filled with a hematoma.[273] Ultrasonographic examinations that are performed meticulously and interpreted by experienced observers are most likely to be beneficial in the evaluation of the Achilles tendon and other tendons in the foot and ankle.

Computed Tomography. CT can be used effectively to study the tendons of the foot and ankle.[273, 275–278] Transaxial CT images are the easiest to acquire and provide the most useful information, although reformatted transaxial data in the coronal or sagittal plane occasionally are required. The CT features of a normal tendon include a smooth contour, a size similar to that on the opposite side, a well-defined margin, and attenuation values (75 to 115 Hounsfield units) higher than those of the respective muscles.[273] Tenosynovitis is manifested as an enlarged tendon with an inhomogeneous appearance. The surrounding swollen, fluid-containing tendon sheath has a lower attenuation value than the tendon itself.[278] Tendon displacement, tethering, or rupture may be evident, and the relationship of the tendon to the adjacent bone is identified readily. Tendon ruptures are associated with partial or complete discontinuity of the fibers and a decrease in attenuation values (30 to 50 Hounsfield units). Diagnostic difficulties are encountered with CT, owing to beam-hardening artifacts, which cause inaccurate assessment of attenuation values, and to the presence of surrounding inflammation, which obscures the contour of the tendon and the tendon sheath. MR imaging is superior to CT in delineating small amounts of fluid around the tendon and allowing differentiation of scar tissue from edema and fluid.[273] CT is superior to MR imaging in demonstra-

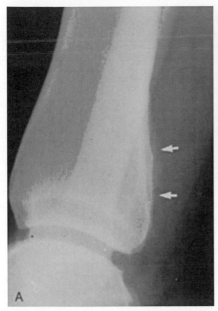
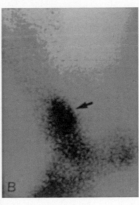
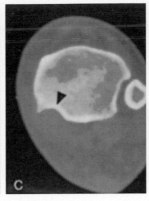
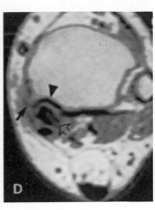

Figure 17–76

Tibialis posterior tendinitis and tenosynovitis: Bone proliferation and erosion displayed by routine radiography, bone scintigraphy, CT scanning, and MR imaging.

A A lateral radiograph shows soft tissue swelling and bone proliferation involving the posterior surface of the tibia (arrows).

B Bone scintigraphy shows increased accumulation (arrow) of the radiopharmaceutical agent in the distal portion of the tibia.

C A transaxial CT scan reveals bone erosion (arrowhead) of the tibia subjacent to the tibialis posterior tendon.

D A transaxial T1-weighted (TR/TE, 900/20) spin echo MR image confirms the presence of tibial erosion (arrowhead) and bone proliferation (solid arrow) adjacent to the tibialis posterior tendon (open arrow).

(Courtesy of T. Broderick, M.D., Orange, California.)

ting regions of tendon calcification and avulsion fractures related to the retinacula.

Tenography. Tenography is a procedure in which tendon sheaths are opacified directly with contrast medium. Initially used as a diagnostic method, tenography now is performed less commonly for this purpose because CT and MR imaging seem more efficient in the assessment of tendon disorders. Tenography still can be employed for therapeutic purposes, however.[279]

The peroneal tendon sheath was the first to be studied with tenography.[23, 280–282] The normal peroneal tenogram outlines the common sheath of the peroneus longus and peroneus brevis muscles and the point of bifurcation of this sheath into separate sheaths enclosing either tendon (Fig. 17–77). These sheaths can be

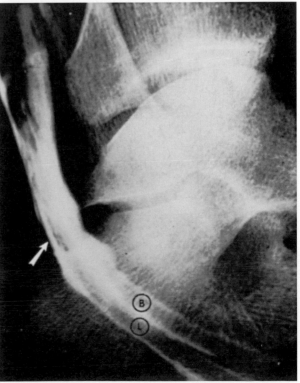

Figure 17–77

Peroneal tenography: Normal tenogram. The normal peroneal tenogram reveals a smooth synovial sheath (arrow) separating into sheaths enclosing the peroneus brevis (B) and peroneus longus (L) tendons. No impingement or deviation of the contrast-filled sheaths can be seen. (From Resnick D, Georgen TG: Radiology *115*:211, 1975.)

traced for variable distances in the foot, appearing smooth in outline and containing a radiolucent tendon without displacement. The peroneal tenogram may be abnormal after calcaneal fractures (see later discussion). Abnormal findings include extrinsic compression and irregularity of the sheath, lateral or anterior displacement of the tendons and sheath, complete obstruction of contrast flow, and tendon rupture. Peroneal tenography (and subtalar arthrography) also can be accompanied by lidocaine injection to localize the source of obscure pain in patients with previous calcaneal fractures.[23]

Contrast opacification of additional tendon sheaths about the ankle has been accomplished.[21, 273, 283, 284] Irregularity or nonvisualization of the injected tendon sheath is consistent with the diagnosis of stenosing tenosynovitis. More important, proper placement of the needle within the tendon sheath can be confirmed during the tenographic procedure, allowing accurate intrasynovial instillation of local anesthetic agents or corticosteroid preparations.

MR Imaging. MR imaging has been applied to the assessment of the tendons and other structures in the ankle and foot.[42, 228, 229, 273, 285–293] The tibialis posterior tendon[294–296] and the Achilles tendon[297–300] have received the greatest attention. The most commonly employed MR imaging sequences used in the ankle and foot are standard spin echo, multiplanar gradient recalled echo, and short tau inversion recovery (STIR) sequences. The use of three-dimensional Fourier transform (3DFT) gradient recalled images allows the rapid acquisition of thin, contiguous sections of the foot and ankle and reformatting of image data in oblique planes parallel to the long axis of the tendons,[291] although this method is not used routinely. MR images can be obtained in the sagittal, coronal, or transaxial (plantar) plane, or in combinations of these planes. The specific planes selected depend on the particular anatomic regions and structures to be evaluated and the clinical questions involved. Similarly, the position of the patient (supine versus prone), the inclusion of one foot and ankle or both feet and ankles, and the need for flexion of the knee or for flexion, extension, or a neutral position of the foot are influenced by the specific indications for the MR imaging examination.[44] With regard to the assessment of the tendons of the ankle and foot, at least two different imaging planes are required (the transaxial and sagittal imaging planes provide most of the information necessary to assess these tendons), T2-weighted spin echo (or some type of gradient recalled echo) images should be obtained in at least one plane, and both feet and ankles should be included in at least one plane (usually the transaxial plane), providing a means to compare the findings in the symptomatic side with those in the asymptomatic side. Standard T1-weighted spin echo MR images are useful for anatomic delineation of the tendons, and T2-weighted spin echo MR images are valuable for the detection of fluid, edema, hemorrhage, or scar formation in or about the tendons.[276] The presence of adjacent fat, as occurs about the Achilles tendon, aids in the MR imaging assessment of some tendons.

With minor exceptions, the normal tendons in the ankle and foot are homogeneous and of low signal intensity with all MR imaging sequences. They generally are equal in size in the two sides of the body and have a smooth contour. There are some exceptions to these general rules, however.

1. *Magic angle effect.* An increased signal intensity may be seen in normal tendons oriented obliquely with respect to the main magnetic field, an effect that is greatest when this orientation is at 55 degrees to that of the magnetic field (Fig. 17–78). This effect is greater when

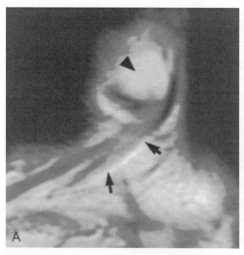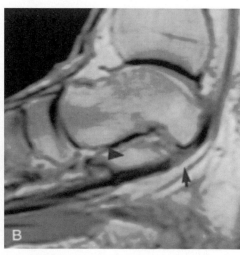

Figure 17–78
Tendons about the ankle: MR imaging, normal variations—magic angle phenomenon.
   A Peroneus longus and brevis tendons. A sagittal T1-weighted (TR/TE, 600/20) spin echo MR image reveals a slight increase in signal intensity (arrows) of the peroneus tendons as they course about the distal portion of the fibula (arrowhead). This alteration in signal intensity relates to the magic angle phenomenon.
   B Flexor hallucis longus tendon. A sagittal T1-weighted (TR/TE, 600/20) spin echo MR image shows a slight increase in signal intensity (arrow) in the flexor hallucis longus tendon near the sustentaculum tali (arrowhead) related to the magic angle phenomenon.
   (Courtesy of D. Goodwin, M.D., and D. Salonen, M.D., San Diego, California.)

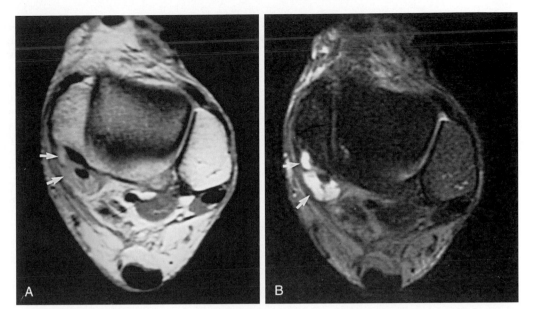

Figure 17–79
Tendons about the ankle: MR imaging—tenosynovial fluid. Transaxial proton density–weighted (TR/TE, 2200/19) **(A)** and T2-weighted (TR/TE, 4000/95) **(B)** fast spin echo MR images, the latter obtained with fat suppression, show fluid in the sheaths of the tibialis posterior and flexor digitorum longus tendons (arrows). (Courtesy of S. K. Brahme, M.D., La Jolla, California.)

the MR imaging examination employs spin echo techniques with short echo times or gradient echo techniques. The tibialis posterior tendon approximates this orientation at its site of attachment to the navicular bone, resulting in a normal appearance of increased signal intensity or heterogeneous signal intensity in this area. This alteration in signal intensity may be accentuated by volume averaging of different signal intensities derived from the joint capsule and fat in this region.[233] Although the change in signal intensity has a typical appearance that allows its distinction from a tear, the absence of abnormal findings on T2-weighted spin echo images is useful in eliminating the diagnosis of a pathologic condition of the tendon.[235] Furthermore, repeating the MR imaging examination with a foot in plantar flexion will diminish or eliminate this magic angle phenomenon.[291]

2. *Tenosynovial fluid.* The differentiation of a thickened tendon from one surrounded by a fluid-filled synovial sheath is difficult on T1-weighted spin echo MR images. Furthermore, the presence of small or even moderate amounts of fluid within a tendon sheath, by itself, is not diagnostic of an abnormality, as such fluid is seen in asymptomatic persons as well.[235] Tenosynovial fluid is more frequent in flexor tendons (as compared to extensor tendons) and may be particularly prominent about the flexor hallucis longus tendon (Figs. 17–79 and 17–80).[301] The precise amount of fluid that defines an abnormality of the tendon or tendon sheath has not been determined.

3. *Bulbous tendon insertion sites.* Insertion sites of tendons may appear bulbous (Fig. 17–81), perhaps related to volume averaging of their signal intensity with that of adjacent cortical bone. This appearance can simulate that of a tendon disruption, particularly of the tibialis posterior tendon.[295]

4. *Tendon striations.* When three-dimensional gradient recalled MR images are obtained, longitudinal lines of intermediate signal intensity in the distal portion of the tibialis posterior tendon may be noted.[291] These lines probably represent branches of the tendon, although their appearance may simulate that of a tendon tear.

In common with the findings derived by ultrasonography and CT, the major MR imaging finding of tenosynovitis is abnormal accumulation of fluid within the tendon sheath. This fluid is of low signal intensity on T1-weighted spin echo MR images and of high signal intensity on T2-weighted spin echo images. Pannus and scar formation about a tendon are characterized by intermediate signal intensity on T1-weighted spin echo MR images and intermediate to high signal intensity on T2-weighted spin echo MR images. Tendinitis is accompanied by focal areas of high signal intensity within the

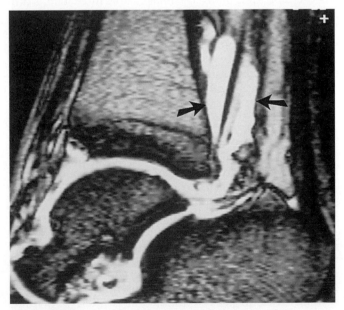

Figure 17–80
Tendons about the ankle: MR imaging—tenosynovial fluid. A sagittal fast low angle shot (FLASH) MR image (TR/TE, 600/18; flip angle, 20 degrees) shows fluid (arrows) in the sheath of the flexor hallucis longus tendon.

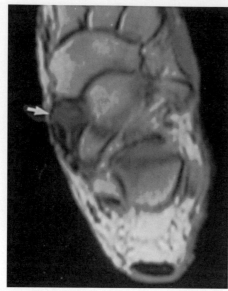

Figure 17–81

Tendons about the ankle: MR imaging, normal variations—bulbous tendon insertion sites. As shown in this transaxial T1-weighted (TR/TE, 600/20) spin echo MR image, the navicular insertion site (arrow) of the tibialis posterior tendon normally may appear bulbous and of increased signal intensity. (Courtesy of D. Goodwin, M.D., and D. Salonen, M.D., San Diego, California.)

substance of the tendon on proton density and T2-weighted spin echo MR images.[273] With chronic tendinitis, the tendon is enlarged and of low signal intensity in both T1-weighted and T2-weighted spin echo MR images.[273]

Tendon ruptures may be acute or chronic and partial or complete. With MR imaging, recent tendon tears frequently reveal regions of increased signal intensity in T2-weighted spin echo MR images and in certain gradient echo images, owing to the presence of edema and hemorrhage. Remote tendon tears generally do not have these high signal intensity characteristics, owing to the presence of scar tissue. With regard to the extent of the tendon tear, three MR imaging patterns have been described (Fig. 17–82)[273, 294]:

Type 1: Partial tendon rupture with tendon hypertrophy. The involved tendon appears hypertrophied or bulbous, and it reveals heterogeneous signal intensity. Focal areas of increased signal intensity are noted within its substance. The MR imaging pattern corresponds to a surgically evident, partially torn tendon possessing vertical splits and defects.

Type 2: Partial tendon rupture with tendon attenuation. The involved tendon is stretched and attenuated in size, MR imaging findings that correspond to those found at surgery.

Type 3: Complete tendon rupture with tendon retraction. The involved tendon is discontinuous and, in some cases, a gap is evident that is filled with fluid, fat, or scar tissue depending upon the age of the tear. The size of the gap, reflecting the degree of tendon retraction, is variable, both with MR imaging and at surgery.

The extent of the tendon tear, as well as its location, influences the type of surgical repair that may be attempted.[294] A small focal area of tendon rupture may be treated with surgical resection and end-to-end tendon anastomosis; a large area of tendon rupture may require side-to-side tendon anastomosis; and a large tendon rupture with tendon retraction may preclude direct anastomosis of the torn ends of the tendon, requiring arthrodesis in some cases in order to prevent further foot deformities.[302–304]

Tendon subluxation or dislocation is detected easily with MR imaging, as it is with CT, owing to an abnormal relationship of the tendon with the adjacent tissues. The tendon itself may be enlarged or partially torn, and associated soft tissue and bone injury may be evident.

Abnormalities of the Achilles Tendon

The Achilles tendon, which serves to plantar flex the foot at the ankle, is the strongest tendon and one of the longest tendons in the lower leg and, along with the tibialis posterior tendon, is one of the most commonly injured tendons in the foot.

Anatomy. The Achilles tendon, formed by the confluence of the gastrocnemius and soleus tendons, courses along the posterior surface of the ankle and is separated from the ankle joint by the preachilles fat

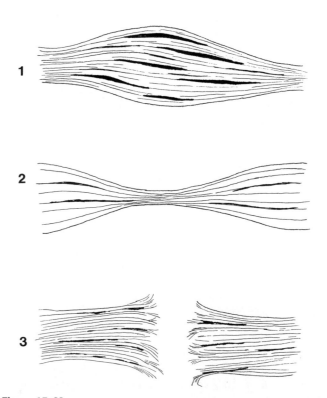

Figure 17–82

Tendons about the ankle: MR imaging—Types of tendon tears. Type 1 tears are characterized by partial disruption of the tendon with vertical splits and a bulbous or hypertrophied appearance. Type 2 tears are characterized by partial disruption of the tendon, which appears attenuated. Type 3 tears are characterized by complete disruption of the tendon and retraction of the torn ends. (Modified from Rosenberg ZS, et al: Radiology *169*:229, 1988.)

body. Although the tendon begins at the point of termination of the muscle belly of the gastrocnemius, it continues to receive muscle fibers on its anterior surface from the soleus almost to the malleolar level.[305] The precise contributions of the gastrocnemius and soleus tendons to the Achilles tendon vary; the gastrocnemius tendon usually contributes more tendinous fibers to the Achilles tendon than does the soleus tendon.[44] The soleus and gastrocnemius components of the tendon can be separated and identified almost to the tendon's insertion at the calcaneus.

Between its origin and insertion, the tendon twists laterally (approximately 90 degrees) so that the tendinous fibers from the gastrocnemius muscle insert into the posterolateral aspect and those from the soleus muscle insert into the posteromedial aspect of the calcaneus.[305] The plantaris muscle arises in close association with the lateral head of the gastrocnemius muscle. The plantaris muscle is flat and forms a slender, long tendon that courses obliquely downward and medially between the soleus and gastrocnemius muscles.[1] The tendon of the plantaris muscle is located along the medial border of the Achilles tendon and has a variable insertion site on the calcaneus.[1] The plantaris muscle and tendon are absent in about 7 per cent of persons, however.

In adults, the Achilles tendon is about 10 to 15 cm long.[183] Throughout its length, the tendon is separated from the deep muscles by areolar and adipose tissue and, distally, it is separated from the posterosuperior aspect of the calcaneus by the retrocalcaneal bursa. Superiorly, the Achilles tendon is a flattened band of tissue. As it descends, it becomes rounded, assuming a cordlike shape.[183] It then fans out as it approaches the tubercle of the calcaneus. Close to the point of attachment of the tendinous fibers to the calcaneus, the fibers take a spiral twist; the posterior strands swing from the medial to the lateral side and capture the outer rim of the posterior surface of the calcaneus, while the anterior fibers run from the lateral to the medial side and insert into the inner border of these same structures.[183] The vulnerable region of the Achilles tendon is just proximal to the inception of this spiral twist, involving a segment between 2 and 6 cm from its insertion into the calcaneus.[183] The normal blood supply in this region is tenuous,[306] a situation reminiscent of that in the distal portion of the supraspinatus tendon and one that may be responsible for tendinous disruption. Some studies have indicated, however, that another area of diminished blood supply in the Achilles tendon occurs just above its bone insertion,[307] a site that rarely ruptures, suggesting that factors other than vascular supply are important in the pathogenesis of Achilles tendon disruption.[308] The Achilles tendon does not possess a tendon sheath. Rather, it is covered by a peritenon whose system of vessels extends within and outside the Achilles tendon.

The distal portion of the Achilles tendon is approximately 4 to 7 mm thick and 12 to 25 mm wide. It has a flat to slightly concave anterior margin and rounded medial, posterior, and lateral aspects that give the tendon a crescent shape.[44] Just prior to its insertion into the calcaneus, the Achilles tendon assumes a more ovoid

shape with a flattened anterior margin.[44] These features are best displayed in sagittal and transaxial MR images (Fig. 17–83).

Tendinitis, Paratendinitis, and Peritendinitis. As the Achilles tendon does not possess a tendon sheath, inflammatory disorders are best classified as tendinitis (inflammation of the Achilles tendon itself), paratendinitis (inflammation about the Achilles tendon), and peritendinitis (inflammation of its peritenon). Any of the inflammatory processes may be acute or chronic, and acute episodes of inflammation may occur in or about a tendon that reveals chronic inflammatory changes as well. Inflammatory disease of the Achilles tendon may result from a systemic rheumatic disorder (such as rheumatoid arthritis) or relate to a local response to overuse or misuse of the foot and ankle. Older, sedentary people or young athletes may be affected. An increase in the level of training or a change in training protocol (e.g., running on hills as opposed to flat terrain), tibia vara, excessive pronation of the foot, or a cavus foot may

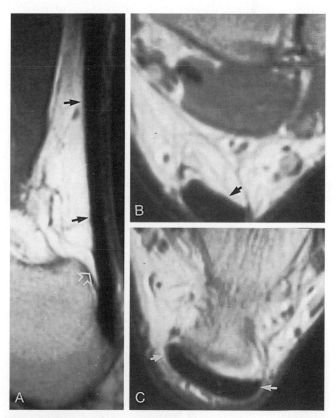

Figure 17–83
Normal Achilles tendon: MR imaging.
A A sagittal T1-weighted (TR/TE, 650/20) spin echo MR image shows the smooth straight contour of the Achilles tendon (solid arrows) and its sharp interface with the preachilles fat pad. Note the triangular region of fat (open arrow) that separates the Achilles tendon and the posterosuperior portion of the calcaneus.
B, C Transaxial T1-weighted (TR/TE, 650/20) spin echo MR images at the level of the ankle joint (**B**) and just above the calcaneal attachment of the Achilles tendon (**C**) show the changing shape of the Achilles tendon (arrows). In **B**, the anterior margin of the Achilles tendon is flat or slightly concave; in **C**, a wider structure with a flat anterior margin is evident.

cause acute and chronic tendinitis, paratendinitis, or peritendinitis.[44]

Chronic tendinitis leads to thickening of the Achilles tendon. One or both feet may be involved. The tendon is enlarged and slightly tender, and crepitation may be palpated when the foot is flexed and extended repeatedly. Chronic peritendinitis is associated with adhesions between the peritenon and adjacent Achilles tendon. The involved tendon feels thickened, fibrotic, and nodular on physical examination, and it may be tender to palpation.

Morphologically, in cases of chronic inflammation, the tendon reveals a loss in its normal luster, nodular thickening, and areas of calcification. Histologically, mucoid degeneration and fibrinoid necrosis may be apparent. The pathologic changes usually involve both the peritenon and the Achilles tendon to a variable extent, although in some cases, the peritenon alone is involved. Some investigators view these inflammatory conditions as separate and distinct, whereas others consider them stages of a single process.[305, 309] The common occurrence of microscopic evidence of tendon fiber disruption in cases of Achilles tendinitis indicates also that partial and complete tendon rupture is the final stage of Achilles tendinitis and peritendinitis (see later discussion). Furthermore, in common with the rotator cuff tendons of the shoulder, the absence of a significant inflammatory response on microscopic evaluation of the Achilles tendon in cases of tendinitis has led to the designations of tendinosis and tendinopathy to describe the alterations.

Routine radiography, CT scanning, and ultrasonography all are able to document the enlarged Achilles tendon that characterizes chronic tendinitis or tendinopathy. In general, however, the information provided by MR imaging in this condition is more complete, leading to its being considered the diagnostic method of choice. The classic MR imaging feature of chronic Achilles tendinitis with or without surrounding peritendinitis and paratendinitis is a diffusely or focally enlarged or thickened tendon (Fig. 17–84).[297, 298, 310] The signal intensity in the involved portion of the Achilles

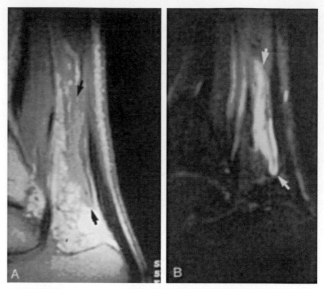

Figure 17–85
Achilles peritendinitis and paratendinitis: MR imaging. In a soccer player, a sagittal T1-weighted (TR/TE, 700/15) spin echo MR image **(A)** shows an irregular region of intermediate signal intensity (arrows) within the preachilles fat body. A sagittal fast spin echo STIR MR image (TR/TE, 5000/22; inversion time, 150 msec) **(B)** shows high signal intensity (arrows) anterior to the Achilles tendon. (Courtesy of C. Wakeley, M.D., Bristol, England.)

tendon generally is low; when intratendinous foci of increased signal intensity are observed in T2-weighted spin echo MR images, an accompanying partial tear of the Achilles tendon is likely. Peritendinitis or paratendinitis alone may lead to changes in the preachilles fat body with a normal-appearing Achilles tendon (Fig. 17–85).

Partial and Complete Tendon Ruptures. Achilles tendinitis or tendinosis generally is regarded as a chronic overuse syndrome, which may be associated with histologic evidence of disruption of some of the tendon fibers. This syndrome should be differentiated from more acute problems involving the Achilles tendon, which include complete tears of the tendon and some partial tears of the tendon, as well as from acute muscle strains. Although acute complete rupture of the Achilles tendon often is a catastrophic event, such rupture may be relatively asymptomatic or misdiagnosed as an ankle sprain. Complete disruption of the Achilles tendon by indirect violence is five to six times more common in men than in women, and the left side is affected more often than the right.[183] Although athletes of any age may develop Achilles tendon disruption, complete rupture of this tendon usually occurs in persons between the ages of 30 and 50 years. The typical patient is a middle-aged sedentary man who partakes in strenuous activity requiring sudden or forceful dorsiflexion or push-off of the plantar flexed foot.[269] Clinical findings include severe pain, local soft tissue swelling and hemorrhage, and a positive Thompson test, in which the patient is unable to stand tiptoe on the affected leg[269] and in which manually squeezing the calf results in a less vigorous response of plantar flexion of the foot than is seen

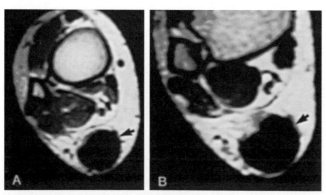

Figure 17–84
Chronic Achilles tendinitis: MR imaging. A transaxial proton density–weighted (TR/TE, 2500/20) spin echo MR image at the level of the distal portions of the tibia and fibula **(A)** and a transaxial T2-weighted (TR/TE, 2500/70) spin echo MR image at a slightly lower level **(B)** show a markedly enlarged Achilles tendon (arrows), which is of low signal intensity in both images.

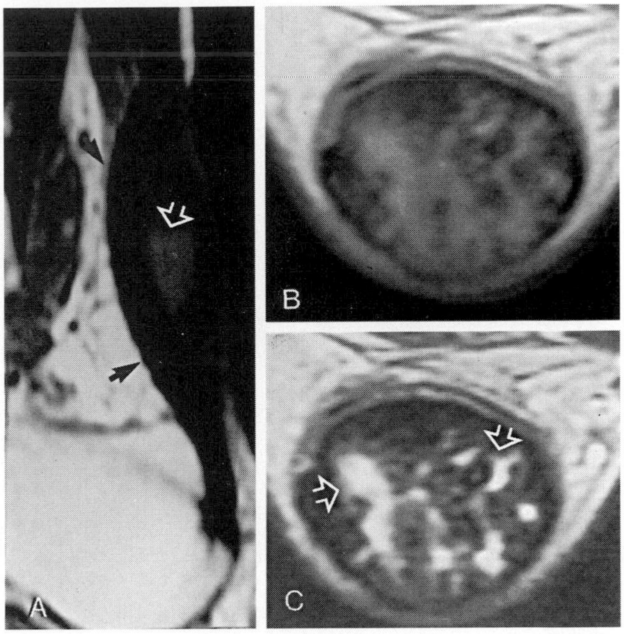

Figure 17–86

Chronic Achilles tendinitis with partial tear: MR imaging.

A A sagittal T1-weighted (TR/TE, 600/25) spin echo MR image shows a massively enlarged Achilles tendon (solid arrows) containing a region of intermediate signal intensity (open arrow).

B, C Transaxial proton density–weighted (TR/TE, 2000/20) **(B)** and T2-weighted (TR/TE, 2000/80) **(C)** spin echo MR images through the enlarged segment of the Achilles tendon show its inhomogeneous signal intensity, with regions of high signal intensity (open arrows) in **C**.

normally.[305] The Thompson test may be falsely positive, however, when the gastrocnemius aponeurosis alone is torn and is no longer connected to that of the soleus muscle.[305] A needle test has been advocated as a means to diagnose acute ruptures of the Achilles tendon; after insertion of a needle into the calf approximately 10 cm proximal to the superior border of the calcaneus, movement of the hub of the needle during passive dorsiflexion and plantar flexion of the foot provides information regarding the integrity of the Achilles tendon.[305]

Predisposing factors in cases of acute complete disruption include chronic tendinitis, partial tears of the Achilles tendon, tendon ossification or calcification, rheumatoid arthritis, systemic lupus erythematosus, and local injection or systemic administration of corticosteroid preparations. Local causative factors also may include tendon ischemia and anatomic variations. It has been proposed that inadequately interwoven collagen bundles of the soleus and the gastrocnemius muscles lead to asynchronous rubbing of tendinous fibers at the vulnerable level of the Achilles tendon, 2 to 6 cm proximal to the calcaneus.[311] Ruptures also may occur due to incongruity between the tones of muscle and tendon fibers, alignment abnormalities such as exaggerated pronation of the foot, or ineffective or poorly designed footwear.[298] The most common site of tendon disruption is 3 or 4 cm proximal to the insertion in the calcaneus; disruption at the musculotendinous junction also is encountered but is rare.

The MR imaging findings of a partial or complete tear of the Achilles tendon (Figs. 17–86, 17–87, 17–88, and 17–89) include discontinuity of some or all of its fibers, intratendinous regions of increased signal intensity in T2-weighted spin echo MR images and STIR images, and, in the case of total disruption of the Achilles tendon, a tendinous gap that is filled with blood and edema of increased signal intensity in these images.

The tendon often is enlarged, sometimes grossly so. Diagnostic difficulty arises in the differentiation of partial tears and those complete tears in which tendon retraction is not a prominent feature. Differentiating chronic tendinitis without tendon disruption from such tendinitis accompanied by a partial tear of the Achilles tendon also is difficult. As even normal Achilles tendons may reveal minor inhomogeneity in signal intensity, perhaps related to infolding of the peritenon,[507] other diagnostic problems arise occasionally. In general, however, MR imaging appears more accurate than CT and ultrasonography (Figs. 17–90, 17–91, 17–92, and 17–93) in allowing identification of partial and complete tears of the Achilles tendon.[297, 312–314]

The best method of treatment for acute complete ruptures of the Achilles tendon is controversial. Although conservative measures (i.e., casting of the leg) for Achilles tendon ruptures may be sufficient in older and sedentary patients, surgical repair often is required, particularly in athletes who wish to resume their previous level of physical activity. Nonoperative treatment is associated with a higher rate of recurrent rupture of the tendon. Furthermore, it is impossible to restore the correct anatomic length of the Achilles tendon without surgery.[315] Elongation of the muscle-tendon unit during healing weakens push-off strength and power. Scar tissue forms in the tendinous gap, but this tissue lacks the functional characteristics of a tendon. Numerous surgical techniques of tendinous repair have been advocated. Suturing alone or suturing reinforced with tendinous or fascial grafts (e.g., flexor hallucis, flexor digitorum longus, peroneus brevis, or plantaris tendon; fascia lata) or synthetic materials may be used.[299, 316–319] Surgery for partial ruptures of the Achilles tendon generally is indicated only when conservative treatment fails. In cases of chronic complete ruptures of the Achilles tendon, direct surgical repair may not be possible, and any number of augmentation procedures may be used.[319]

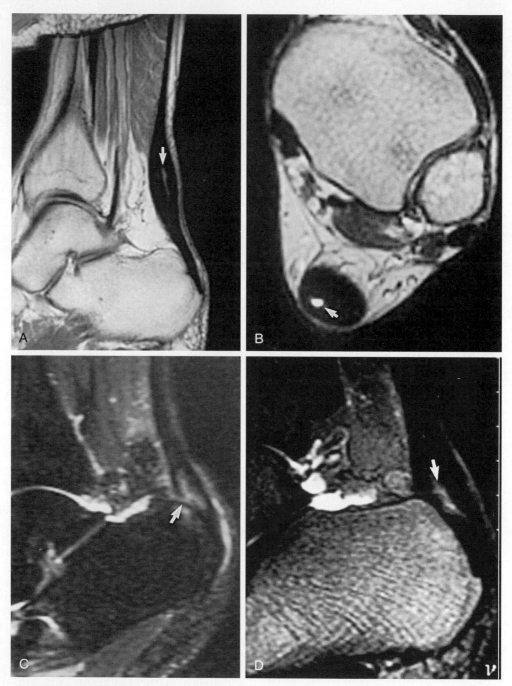

Figure 17–87
Chronic Achilles tendinitis with partial tear: MR imaging.

A, B On sagittal proton density–weighted (TR/TE, 2116/28) **(A)** and transverse T2-weighted (TR/TE, 4500/84) **(B)** spin echo MR images, note the thickened Achilles tendon and intratendinous region of altered signal intensity (arrows) representing a partial tear. (Courtesy of D. Goodwin, M.D., Hanover, New Hampshire.)

C, D In a professional baseball player, a sagittal fast spin echo STIR (TR/TE, 5000/39; inversion time, 160 msec) MR image **(C)** reveals the partial tendon tear (arrow) of high signal intensity. Also note evidence of retrocalcaneal and superficial bursitis. Four weeks later, after conservative treatment and despite marked clinical improvement, a sagittal fat-suppressed fast spin echo (TR/TE, 6000/105) MR image **(D)** reveals a persistent region of high signal intensity (arrow). This indicates the difficulty that may be encountered in judging clinical status using MR imaging.

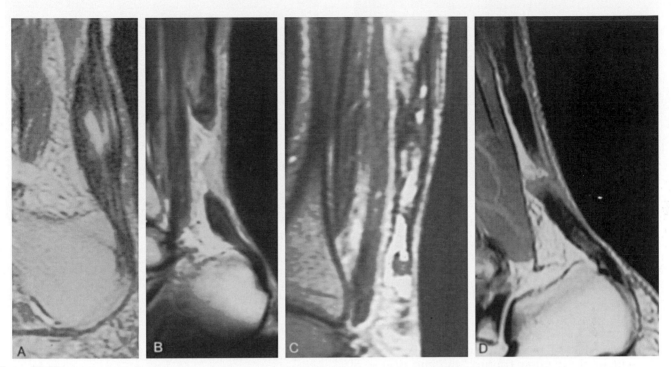

Figure 17–88
Chronic Achilles tendinitis with partial or complete tear: MR imaging.

A Partial tear. A sagittal T2-weighted (TR/TE, 2000/70) spin echo MR image shows an enlarged Achilles tendon containing irregular regions of high signal intensity.

B Complete tear. A sagittal proton density–weighted (TR/TE, 3000/30) spin echo MR image shows complete disruption of the Achilles tendon and a proximal segment that is inhomogeneous in signal intensity. Note edema and hemorrhage of high signal intensity about the acutely torn tendon.

C Complete tear. A sagittal T2-weighted (TR/TE, 1800/80) fat-suppressed spin echo MR image reveals an acute and complete tear of the Achilles tendon with multiple regions of high signal intensity. (Courtesy of D. Levey, M.D., Corpus Christi, Texas.)

D Complete tear. A sagittal proton density–weighted (TR/TE, 2000/20) spin echo MR image reveals a chronic tear characterized by complete disruption of the Achilles tendon.

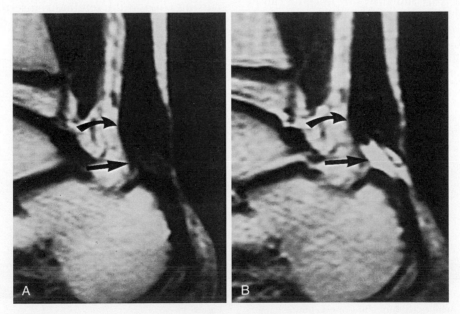

Figure 17–89
Chronic Achilles tendinitis with tendon avulsion from calcaneus: MR imaging. In an 11 year old boy, sagittal T1-weighted (TR/TE, 500/30) **(A)** and T2-weighted (TR/TE, 2000/60) **(B)** spin echo MR images show a thickened Achilles tendon (curved arrows) with tendinous avulsion (straight arrows) from the calcaneus.

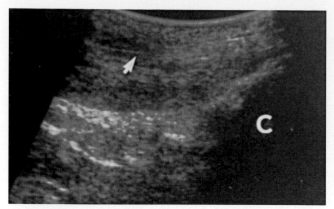

Figure 17–90
Chronic Achilles tendinitis with partial tear: Ultrasonography. A longitudinal scan of the ankle (with the cephalad aspect to the reader's left and the posterior aspect at the top of the image) shows a thickened Achilles tendon with coarse sonographic features (arrow) consistent with a partial tear (C, calcaneus). (Courtesy of T. Broderick, M.D., Orange, California.)

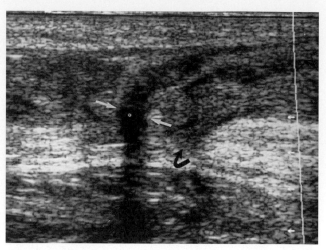

Figure 17–92
Chronic Achilles tendinitis with complete tear: Ultrasonography. A longitudinal scan demonstrates an anechoic cleft (straight arrows) filled with fluid representing the tear. The distal tendon stump is displaced anteriorly (curved arrow). (Courtesy of M. van Holsbeeck, M.D., Detroit, Michigan, and J. Jacobson, M.D., San Diego, California.)

The role of MR imaging (as well as ultrasonography) in the selection of patients who will derive the greatest benefit from surgery involves identification of the site and extent of the tendon rupture and the degree of separation of the torn ends of the tendon.[44] Assessment of the position of the tendon fragments in MR images obtained with the foot in a plantar flexed position may have some value.[313] After surgical repair, MR imaging can be used to evaluate the healing response of the Achilles tendon (Fig. 17–94).[44] A decrease in signal intensity within the Achilles tendon and an increase in its size, owing to the formation of scar tissue, are observed, although these findings occur gradually over a period of months or even a year. Similarly, MR imaging can be used to monitor the healing response within torn Achilles tendons that are treated conservatively.[310, 312, 314] Preliminary data also suggest that this method allows assessment of the Achilles tendon after its repair with prosthetic implants.[299]

Recurrent rupture of the Achilles tendon may occur after conservative (approximately 10 to 30 per cent of cases) or surgical treatment (approximately 5 per cent of cases) of the initial tendinous tear.[300] These retears may appear weeks or even months after the initiation of therapy.[269]

Calcification and Ossification. Calcification within the substance of the Achilles tendon relates to calcium hydroxyapatite or calcium pyrophosphate dihydrate crystal deposition. The calcific deposits are linear, occurring close to the tendinous insertion into bone, and they are well shown with routine radiography. Indeed,

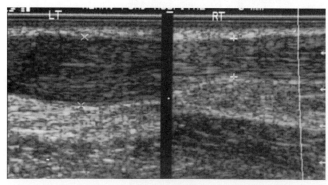

Figure 17–91
Acute partial tear of the Achilles tendon: Ultrasonography. A longitudinal scan of the injured left side (LT) demonstrates fusiform swelling (between the X markers) of the Achilles tendon with minimal interruption of the tendon fibers. The scan of the right side (RT) shows a normal tendon (between the + markers). (Courtesy of M. van Holsbeeck, M.D., Detroit, Michigan, and J. Jacobson, M.D., San Diego, California.)

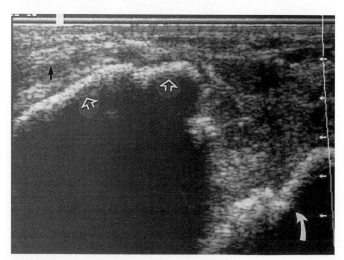

Figure 17–93
Calcaneal avulsion fracture with intact Achilles tendon: Ultrasonography. A sagittal scan reveals a posteriorly displaced fragment of bone (open arrows) that arose from the posterosuperior aspect of the calcaneus (curved arrow). The Achilles tendon (solid straight arrow) is intact. (Courtesy of M. van Holsbeeck, M.D., Detroit, Michigan, and J. Jacobson, M.D., San Diego, California.)

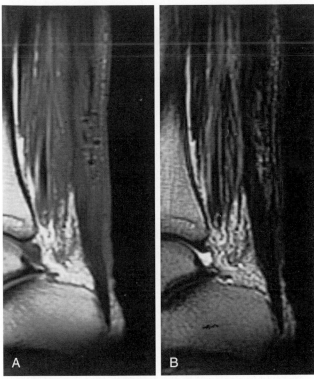

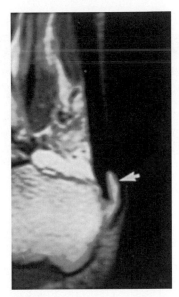

Figure 17–95
Calcaneal enthesophyte: MR imaging. A sagittal T1-weighted (TR/TE, 800/12) spin echo MR image shows a large calcaneal enthesophyte (arrow) containing marrow that arises at the site of insertion of the Achilles tendon.

Figure 17–94
Surgical repair of the Achilles tendon: MR imaging. Six months after successful repair of a tear of the Achilles tendon (in which direct suturing of the torn ends was accomplished), sagittal T1-weighted (TR/TE, 600/11) **(A)** and T2-weighted (TR/TE, 3000/112) **(B)** spin echo MR images show a thickened Achilles tendon containing sutures, with a slight increase in signal intensity in **B**.

such calcification may be overlooked during evaluation of MR images. The relationship of calcification in the Achilles tendon to chronic tendinitis and to clinical manifestations is not clear.

Ossification in the Achilles tendon takes two forms. More commonly, an enthesophyte develops at the calcaneal site of insertion of the tendon, and it appears to have little clinical significance (Fig. 17–95). Less commonly, a discrete ossicle of variable size or diffuse ossification occurs within the tendon several centimeters from its calcaneal attachment site. The process may be unilateral or bilateral, is often associated with a history of injury, and frequently is accompanied by evidence of tendon thickening (Fig. 17–96).

Urate Tophi, Rheumatoid Nodules, and Xanthomas. Involvement of the Achilles tendon in gout, rheumatoid arthritis, and various hypercholesterolemic conditions may lead to intratendinous nodules or diffuse thickening of the tendon. On palpation, the Achilles tendon may be nodular and enlarged. Ultrasonography, CT, and MR imaging (Figs. 17–97 and 17–98) represent effective methods for evaluation of these tendinous changes.[320–323]

The signal intensity of xanthomas, when studied with MR imaging, is variable, depending in part on the chemical constituents of the lesions. In vitro studies have documented that triglycerides may lead to high signal

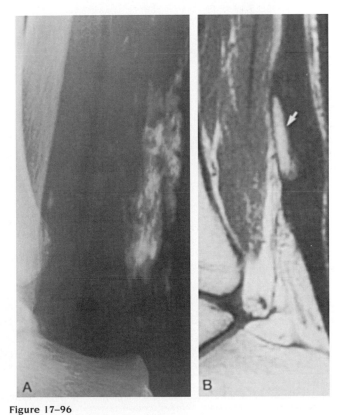

Figure 17–96
Achilles tendon ossification: Routine radiography and MR imaging.
 A Note diffuse plaquelike ossification in the Achilles tendon.
 B In a second patient, an elongated ossicle (arrow) containing marrow is located in a thickened portion of the Achilles tendon, as shown in a sagittal T1-weighted (TR/TE, 800/20) spin echo MR image.
 (Courtesy of J. Yu, M.D., Columbus, Ohio.)

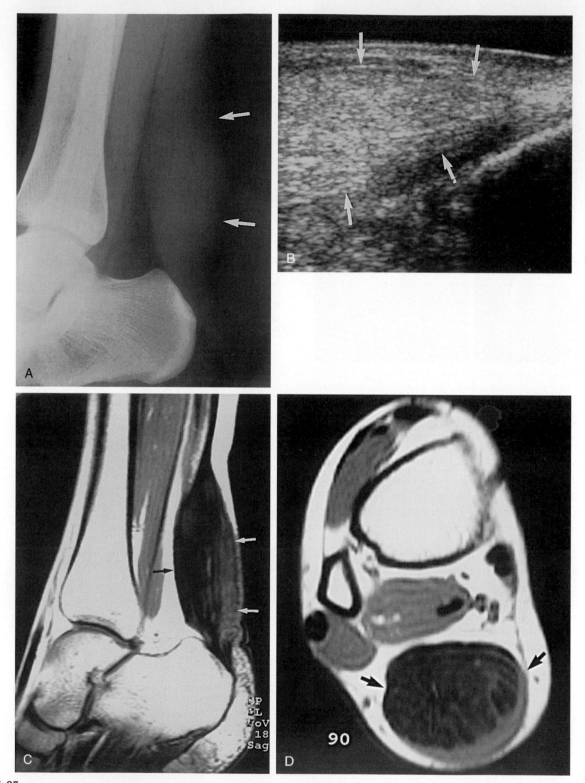

Figure 17–97

Xanthomas of the Achilles tendon: Ultrasonography and MR imaging.

A Note markedly enlarged Achilles tendon (arrows).

B During ultrasonography, a longitudinal scan shows a homogeneous echogenic mass (arrows) in the Achilles tendon.

C On a sagittal T1-weighted (TR/TE, 680/15) spin echo MR image, the Achilles tendon is enlarged (arrows) and inhomogeneous in signal intensity. Longitudinal columns of tissue with signal intensity similar to that of muscle can be seen within the tendon.

D A transaxial T1-weighted (TR/TE, 600/15) spin echo MR image reveals a markedly enlarged Achilles tendon (arrows). Regions of low signal intensity and of signal intensity similar to that of muscle are evident.

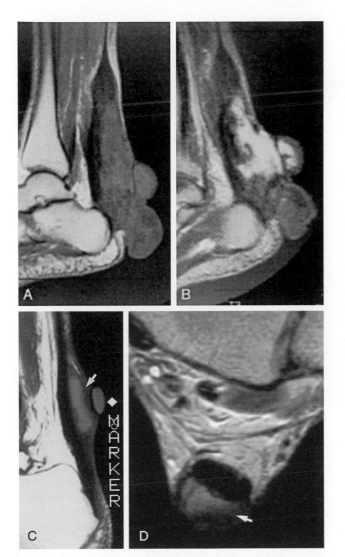

Figure 17–98

Xanthomas and tophi of the Achilles tendon: MR imaging.

A, B Xanthomas. Sagittal T1-weighted (TR/TE, 800/30) **(A)** and T2-weighted (TR/TE, 2000/80) **(B)** spin echo MR images show a large mass infiltrating the Achilles tendon. Note the high signal intensity within the mass in **B**. The Achilles tendon is partially torn. The opposite side was involved similarly. (From Tehranzadeh J, et al: Skel Radiol *21*:79, 1992.)

C, D Tophi. Sagittal T1-weighted (TR/TE, 450/15) **(C)** and transaxial T2-weighted (TR/TE, 2350/70) **(D)** spin echo MR images show a tophus (arrow) of persistent intermediate signal intensity.

intensity on some MR imaging sequences, whereas cholesterols do not. Although tendinous xanthomas may contain both triglycerides and cholesterols, most reports of MR imaging features of such lesions have documented persistent low to intermediate signal intensity on T1-weighted and T2-weighted spin echo MR images and signal inhomogeneity. Focal areas of high signal intensity occasionally may be encountered on T2-weighted images, however, perhaps indicating a high percentage of triglyceride deposition. Alternatively, such high signal intensity may relate to inflammatory changes in the tendon. A diffuse speckled or reticulated pattern of intratendinous signal intensity, most obvious on transaxial images and fat-suppressed T1-weighted im-

ages, is evident in some cases and may have diagnostic significance. This appearance differs from the typical features of acute or chronic tendinitis and partial tears, although diagnostic problems are encountered in some cases. In cases of xanthomatosis, the involved tendon may not be enlarged.

Abnormalities of the Tibialis Posterior Tendon

Anatomy. The tibialis posterior muscle plays a critical role in stabilizing the hindfoot, including the talus and subtalar joints, preventing valgus deformity of the hindfoot and excessive pronation of the forefoot. This muscle is involved in inversion and plantar flexion of the foot. As the flexor digitorum longus muscle acts in a fashion similar to that of the tibialis posterior muscle, incompetence of the latter muscle related to inflammation or rupture may be occult clinically.

The tibialis posterior muscle is the deepest of the flexor muscles of the foot. Its origin commonly is divided into two parts: the medial part of the muscle originates from the posterior surface of the interosseous membrane and from the posterior surface of the tibia; the lateral part of the muscle arises mainly from the posterior surface of the fibula. As it descends in the lower portion of the leg, the tendon of the tibialis posterior muscle is deep to that of the flexor digitorum longus muscle and lies within a groove behind the medial malleolus of the tibia (Figs. 17–99, 17–100, and 17–101). From here, the tendon of the tibialis posterior muscle enters the foot by passing deep to the flexor retinaculum and superficial to the tibiotalar and tibiocalcaneal components of the deltoid ligament. Its course is transtalar as it parallels the talocalcaneal portions of the talocalcaneonavicular joint, above the sustentaculum tali. The superficial and deep layers of the flexor retinaculum are intimate with the fibrous sheaths of the tibialis posterior, flexor digitorum longus, and flexor hallucis longus tendons, and between the first two fibrous tunnels and that of the flexor hallucis longus tendon lies a deep aponeurosis creating a compartment that houses the posterior tibial neurovascular bundle.[1] Distally, the tibialis posterior tendon divides into three components: anterior, middle, and posterior. The anterior component inserts into the tuberosity of the navicular bone, the inferior capsule of the cuneonavicular joint, and the medial cuneiform bone. The middle component continues distally as a tarsometatarsal extension, inserting on the second and third cuneiform and cuboid bones. Beyond this point, a metatarsal extension provides fibers that extend deep and dorsal to the peroneus longus tendon, forming three tendinous slips that attach to the bases of the second, third, fourth, and (sometimes) fifth metatarsal bone.[1] That tarsometatarsal extension also provides an attachment to the Y-shaped origin of the tendon of the flexor hallucis brevis muscle, explaining the functional connection between this latter muscle and the tibialis posterior muscle.[1] The posterior component originates from the main tendon prior to the insertion on the navicular bone, extends laterally and posteriorly, and inserts as a band on the anterior

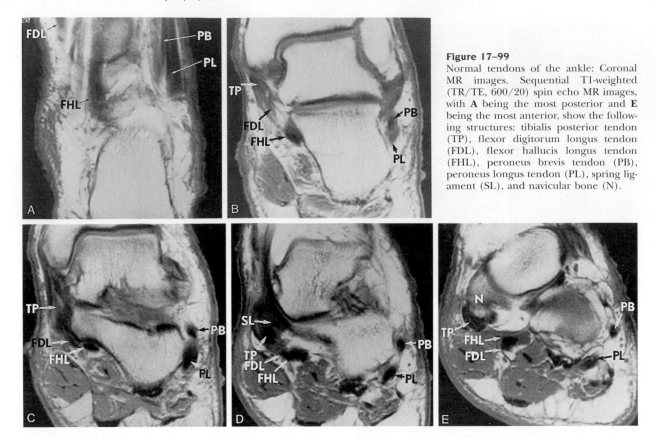

Figure 17–99

Normal tendons of the ankle: Coronal MR images. Sequential T1-weighted (TR/TE, 600/20) spin echo MR images, with **A** being the most posterior and **E** being the most anterior, show the following structures: tibialis posterior tendon (TP), flexor digitorum longus tendon (FDL), flexor hallucis longus tendon (FHL), peroneus brevis tendon (PB), peroneus longus tendon (PL), spring ligament (SL), and navicular bone (N).

aspect of the sustentaculum tali. These insertion sites in the cuneiform and metatarsal bones underscore the contribution of the muscle to maintenance of the longitudinal arch of the foot. Disruption of the tibialis posterior tendon, which is being recognized increasingly, is associated with inability to supinate and invert the foot while the toes are being wiggled and with progressive and painful planovalgus deformity of the foot.[324]

Tendinitis, Tenosynovitis, and Rupture. Inflammatory changes in the tendon and tendon sheath of the tibialis posterior muscle are encountered as a result of altered mechanics of the foot or as a response to a systemic articular disease such as rheumatoid arthritis or a seronegative spondyloarthropathy. Spontaneous rupture of the tibialis posterior tendon (i.e., occurring in the absence of a systemic rheumatic disease) classically is seen in patients in the fifth and sixth decades of life (average age, 55 years), with two thirds of cases occurring in women.[269, 303, 304, 325, 326] Unilateral involvement occurs in approximately 90 per cent of cases, with a left-sided predominance. Bilateral abnormalities of the tibialis posterior tendon are more frequent in cases associated with an underlying rheumatic disease. A spectrum of

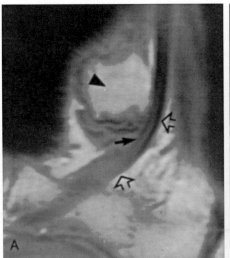
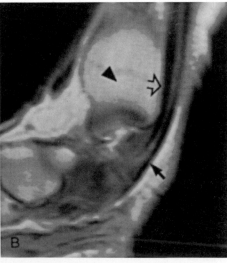

Figure 17–100

Normal tendons of the ankle: Sagittal MR images.

A A sagittal T1-weighted (TR/TE, 600/20) spin echo MR image through the lateral malleolus (arrowhead) shows portions of the peroneus longus (open arrows) and peroneus brevis (solid arrow) tendons.

B A sagittal T1-weighted (TR/TE, 600/20) spin echo MR image through the medial malleolus (arrowhead) reveals the tibialis posterior (open arrow) and flexor digitorum longus (solid arrow) tendons.

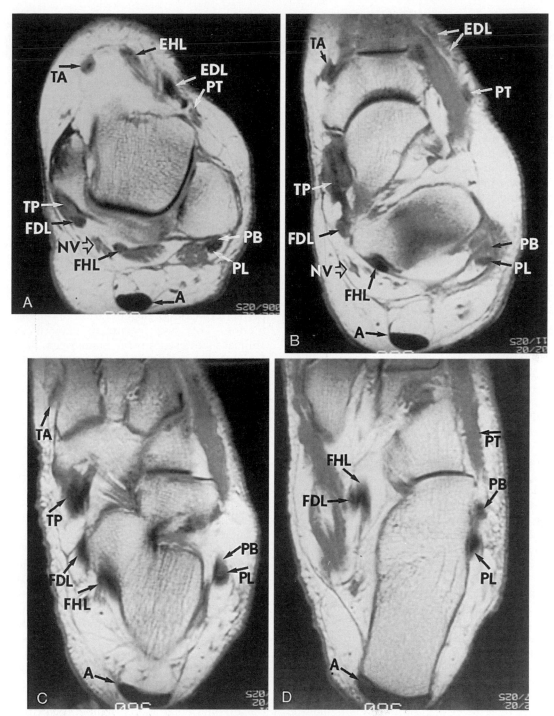

Figure 17–101

Normal tendons of the ankle: Transaxial MR images. Sequential T1-weighted (TR/TE, 600/20) spin echo MR images, with **A** being the most superior (at the level of the ankle joint) and **D** being the most inferior, show the following structures: tibialis posterior tendon (TP), flexor digitorum longus tendon (FDL), flexor hallucis longus tendon (FHL), posterior tibial artery and tibial nerve (NV), Achilles tendon (A), tibialis anterior tendon (TA), extensor hallucis longus tendon (EHL), extensor digitorum longus tendon (EDL), peroneus tertius tendon (PT), peroneus longus tendon (PL), and peroneus brevis tendon (PB).

clinical alterations is encountered, depending on the extent and chronicity of the changes. Initial manifestations include pain, swelling, and tenderness to palpation of the affected tendon. Progressive involvement results in weakness of inversion of the foot and flattening of the medial longitudinal arch of the foot, with the eventual appearance of severe pes planus deformity. Such dys-

function of the tibialis posterior tendon is characterized by eversion of the subtalar joint, a valgus alignment of the heel, and abduction of the foot at the talonavicular joint.[508] Associated alterations that accompany these changes in alignment include stretching of the spring ligament and loss of soft tissue supportive structures, including the deltoid ligament and capsule of the talonavicular joint.[508] Similar abnormalities also are identified in young athletic persons involved in tennis, soccer, ice hockey, basketball, volleyball, and ballet dancing[44, 327, 328] and in children.[329]

The cause of spontaneous rupture of the tibialis posterior tendon unrelated to a systemic rheumatic disease appears to result from local mechanical factors. The tibialis posterior tendon is the thickest of the medial group of tendons in the foot and resists the considerable weight-bearing forces that otherwise would lead to collapse of the longitudinal arch. The tendon is the main dynamic stabilizer of the hindfoot against valgus, or eversion, forces, and it serves to decelerate subtalar joint pronation after heel contact. The medial malleolus acts as a pulley that establishes an effective angle of pull on the ankle and subtalar joints, and the insertion of the tendon into the navicular tuberosity provides a second pulley, resulting in an effective angle of pull on the midtarsal joints in the direction of supination.[330] The tibialis posterior muscle may fatigue as it continuously serves to resist pronation forces. Acute angulation of the tendon behind the medial malleolus and, perhaps, a vulnerable blood supply make it susceptible to injury.[269, 331] Pes planovalgus occurring as a developmental abnormality or as a result of initial weakening of the tibialis posterior tendon accentuates the forces placed on this tendon, leading to progressive tendinous alterations and eventual tendon rupture. Acute fractures about the ankle may be responsible for some cases of rupture of the tibialis posterior tendon.[332] Furthermore, an accessory ossicle of the navicular bone may provide the site of attachment of some of the fibers of the tibialis posterior tendon (see later discussion), also predisposing to tendon failure.

Jahss[269] has classified abnormalities (i.e., degeneration) within the tibialis posterior tendon and surrounding structures according to the severity of involvement (Fig. 17–102). Stage IA disease, representing approximately 13 per cent of all such abnormalities, is mild or clinically occult. Manifestations, which usually have been present for approximately 4 to 12 months, include minimal swelling, mild tenderness, slight weakness during inversion of the foot, and minimal valgus deformity of the hindfoot during weight-bearing. Pathologic findings include longitudinal splits in the deep surface of the tendon with a normal outer surface and sheath. Stage IB disease, representing approximately 44 per cent of cases of tendon degeneration, is moderate in extent. Clinical abnormalities usually have been manifest for a period of 12 to 18 months and are associated with CT and MR imaging findings (see later discussion). Pathologic alterations include more extensive deep splitting of the tibialis posterior tendon, intramural degeneration, tendon laxity, and irregularity of the external surface of the tendon and adhesions among this tendon, the sheath, and the flexor retinaculum. Stage II or advanced disease represents 17 per cent of all cases of tibialis posterior tendon degeneration. Symptoms have been present for a period of approximately 18 to 30 months, and pes planus and heel valgus deformities and medial prominence of the head of the talus are observed. Pathologic findings include an elongated and fibrotic tendon, which is adherent to the medial malleolus. Bone proliferation in the medial malleolus is observed. The tendon is significantly degenerated, and its sheath is atrophic with scar formation. Multiple longitudinal tears of the tendon may be evident, and migration of the flexor digitorum longus tendon into the space previously occupied by the tibialis posterior tendon is seen, accounting for the failure to opacify the latter during tenography. Stage IIIA disease, present in approximately 15 per cent of patients with degeneration of the tibialis posterior tendon, represents complete rupture of the tendon. Symptoms usually have been present for 30 months to 4 years, and increasing peritalar subluxation, particularly during weight-bearing, is evident. In addition to tendon rupture, pathologic findings include separation of the scarred and frayed proximal and distal portions of the tendon with adherence of these portions to subjacent bone. The final stage, stage IIIB, is associated with complete tendon rupture and peritalar dislocation. It represents approximately 11 per cent of cases of degeneration of the tibialis posterior tendon. This stage occurs in patients who have had clinical manifestations for many years. Severe valgus deformity and medial dislocation of the talar head are observed on radiographic examination. The superior portion of the calcaneus abuts on the undersurface of the talar neck in the sinus tarsi. With weight-bearing, valgus rotation and superior displacement of the calcaneus obliterate the sinus tarsi. Secondary osteoarthritis in the subtalar joints is evident. The pathologic findings are similar to but more severe than those occurring in stage IIIA disease. The value of this staging system relates to the choice of appropriate therapy. Although conservative treatment, including orthoses, casting, and anti-inflammatory medications, may be an option in lesser degrees of degeneration of the tibialis posterior tendon,[44] surgery often is required. Jahss[269] recommends repair of tendon tears and plication of the tendon (if it is elongated) in stages IA and IB disease. More extensive surgical procedures, including triple arthrodesis, may be necessary for more severe involvement.

Although routine radiographs and those obtained during weight-bearing allow the diagnosis of long-standing disruption of the tibialis posterior tendon (Fig. 17–103), owing to the presence of a number of deformities (e.g., an increase in the angle between the long axis of the talus and that of the calcaneus, a sag at the calcaneonavicular and naviculocuneiform joints, and lateral subluxation of the navicular bone with respect to the talus),[333] these methods are less useful in the early diagnosis of such disruption. CT and MR imaging appear to be more valuable than ultrasonography and tenography in the evaluation of degeneration, inflammation, and disruption of the tibialis posterior tendon, although ultrasonography is effective as a diagnostic tool in some of these situations (Figs. 17–104 and 17–105). Rosenberg and coworkers[294] used a classification system of tibialis posterior tendon rupture in which three categories based on surgical findings were defined: type 1 lesions represented partially torn, bulbous, or hypertrophied tendons with vertical splits and defects; type 2 tears represented partially torn, attenuated tendons; and

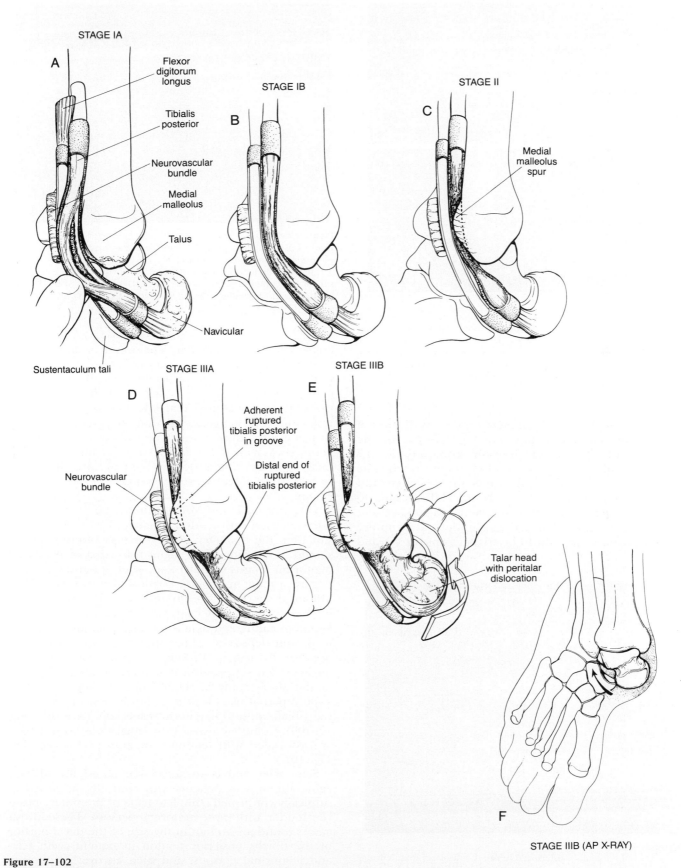

Figure 17–102

Tibialis posterior tendon abnormalities: Classification system. See text for details. (From Jahss MH: Disorders of the Foot and Ankle. 2nd Ed. Philadelphia, WB Saunders Co, 1991, p. 1485.)

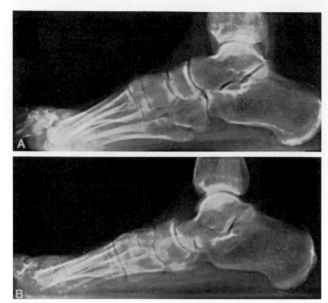

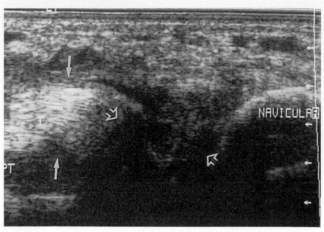

Figure 17–105

Injuries of the tibialis posterior tendon: Ultrasonography, acute complete tear. A longitudinal scan of the tibialis posterior tendon (solid arrows) reveals tendon discontinuity (open arrows) at the navicular site of attachment. (Courtesy of M. van Holsbeeck, M.D., Detroit, Michigan, and J. Jacobson, M.D., San Diego, California.)

Figure 17–103

Injuries of the tibialis posterior tendon: Routine and weight-bearing radiography. Complete tears. Although a lateral radiograph obtained without weight-bearing (**A**) appears normal, a lateral radiograph obtained with weight-bearing (**B**) shows plantar flexion of the distal portion of the talus with malalignment at the talonavicular joint. (From Myerson M, et al: Foot Ankle 9:219, 1989.)

type 3 tears represented complete tendinous disruption with an intratendinous gap (see Fig. 17–82). In the evaluation of 32 cases of clinically suspected chronic tears of the tibialis posterior tendon, these investigators found CT to be sensitive and specific in 90 per cent and 100 per cent of cases, respectively, and MR imaging to be sensitive and specific in 95 per cent and 100 per cent of cases, respectively. The accuracy in detecting rupture of this tendon was found to be 91 per cent for CT and

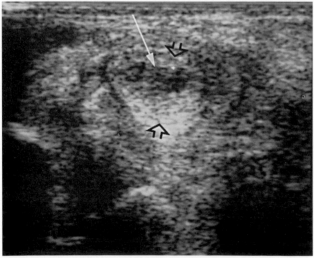

Figure 17–104

Injuries of the tibialis posterior tendon: Ultrasonography, chronic partial tear. A transverse scan shows a hypoechoic region (solid arrow) representing fluid within an enlarged hyperechoic tibialis posterior tendon (open arrows). (Courtesy of M. van Holsbeeck, M.D., Detroit, Michigan, and J. Jacobson, M.D., San Diego, California.)

96 per cent for MR imaging. The overall accuracy, which reflected the percentage of cases diagnosed correctly as well as those that were classified correctly, was 59 per cent for CT and 73 per cent for MR imaging. These investigators concluded that MR imaging was superior to CT in providing greater definition of tendon outline, vertical splits, synovial fluid, edema, and tissue degeneration; conversely, CT was judged to be superior to MR imaging in showing associated bone abnormalities such as periostitis, subtalar osteoarthritis, and subtalar dislocation.

With both CT and MR imaging, type 1 partial tears are associated with tendon hypertrophy (in the normal situation, the diameter of the tibialis posterior tendon should be no more than about twice that of the flexor digitorum longus tendon) and, when longitudinal splitting is prominent, tendon division into two parts. With MR imaging (Figs. 17–106 and 17–107), an abnormal increase in signal intensity may be seen within the enlarged or bifurcated tibialis posterior tendon, especially in proton density–weighted spin echo MR images, but occasionally also in T2-weighted spin echo and STIR images.[44] Fat suppression may increase the conspicuity of the abnormality in signal intensity (Fig. 17–108).[43] Type 2 partial tears lead to a diminution in the size of the tibialis posterior tendon, especially its width (Fig. 17–109). Complete tears of the tibialis posterior tendon are associated with tendon retraction and a gap (Fig. 17–110).[44]

Schweitzer and coworkers[295] compared the MR imaging findings in patients with clinically suspected or surgically confirmed complete tears of the tibialis posterior tendon with those in normal persons. These investigators found an overlap in the size of the distal portion of the tibialis posterior tendon in patients with tears and in normal persons, and such an overlap also was evident with regard to alterations in intratendinous signal intensity (i.e., increased signal intensity in T1-weighted and, to a lesser extent, T2-weighted spin echo

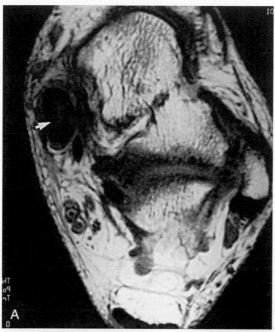

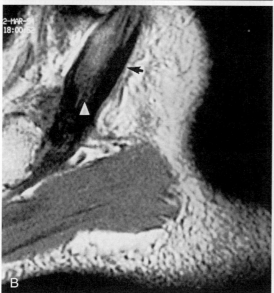

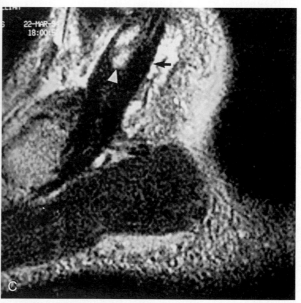

Figure 17–106

Injuries of the tibialis posterior tendon: MR imaging, chronic partial tear.

A In a 47 year old male runner, a transverse T1-weighted (TR/TE, 650/15) spin echo MR image demonstrates an enlarged tibialis posterior tendon (arrow).

B, C Sagittal proton density–weighted (TR/TE, 2000/20) **(B)** and T2-weighted (TR/TE, 2000/90) **(C)** spin echo MR images show the thickened tendon (arrows) and intrasubstance tear (arrowheads).

(Courtesy of D. Wilcox, M.D., Kansas City, Missouri.)

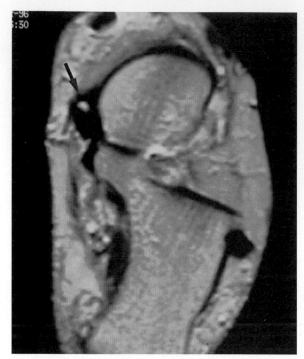

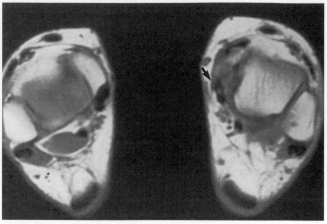

Figure 17–109
Injuries of the tibialis posterior tendon: MR imaging, chronic partial tear. As shown in this transverse T1-weighted spin echo MR image, the tibialis posterior tendon in the left ankle is attenuated, with a split appearance and abnormal internal signal intensity (arrow). Compare this appearance with that in the opposite (normal) ankle. (Courtesy of J. Kingsley, M.D., Phoenix, Arizona.)

Figure 17–107
Injuries of the tibialis posterior tendon: MR imaging, chronic partial tear. A transverse fast spin echo (TR/TE, 4500/95) MR image demonstrates an enlarged tendon (arrow) with a focus of high signal intensity.

MR images). Schweitzer and colleagues found that MR imaging abnormalities such as changes in the alignment of the talus and navicular bone, prominence of the medial tubercle of the navicular bone, and an accessory ossicle in the navicular bone were useful findings in predicting a tear of the tibialis posterior tendon. These latter abnormalities, however, also can be seen on routine radiographs, conventional tomograms, and CT scans.

The value of MR imaging in the assessment of the degenerated or torn tibialis posterior tendon requires further analysis.[509] Similarly, any role for MR imaging in the evaluation of this tendon after surgical repair awaits the results of additional studies.[44] The intravenous administration of a gadolinium contrast agent and the application of reformatted 3DFT gradient recalled MR imaging to the analysis of this and other tendons in the foot and ankle may lead to more accurate diagnosis of tendon injury,[291] although the value of these methods likewise is not yet proved.

Nonoperative treatment of ruptures of the tibialis posterior tendon is appropriate in the elderly, in those who have low levels of physical activity, and in relatively asymptomatic patients. Although the choice of a specific surgical technique in appropriate candidates with such tendinous ruptures is influenced by the site and extent of injury and flexibility and duration of the foot defor-

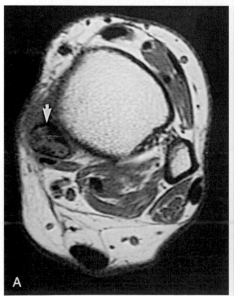
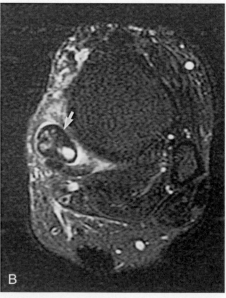

Figure 17–108
Injuries of the tibialis posterior tendon: MR imaging, chronic partial tear.

A A transaxial T1-weighted (TR/TE, 500/17) spin echo MR image shows an enlarged tibialis posterior tendon (arrow), which is inhomogeneous in signal intensity.

B A transaxial fat-suppressed fast spin echo MR image (TR/TE, 4500/114) reveals the hypertrophied tendon (arrow) containing longitudinal splits. Fluid is present in the surrounding tendon sheath, and soft tissue edema also is evident.

(Courtesy of D. Goodwin, M.D., Hanover, New Hampshire.)

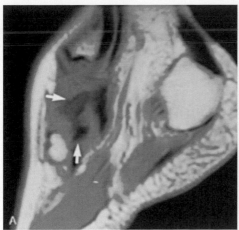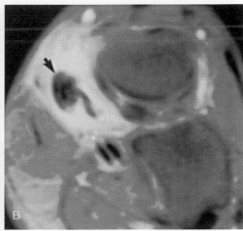

Figure 17–110

Injuries of the tibialis posterior tendon: MR imaging, acute complete tear.

A A sagittal T1-weighted (TR/TE, 800/12) spin echo MR image shows disorganization of the tibialis posterior tendon (arrows) near its navicular site of insertion. Note a mass of intermediate signal intensity about the tendon.

B A coronal T1-weighted (TR/TE, 650/20) spin echo MR image obtained with chemical presaturation of fat (ChemSat) after the intravenous administration of a gadolinium compound reveals the torn tibialis posterior tendon (arrow). Note enhancement of signal intensity about the torn tendon.

mity, four basic surgical procedures are used[305]: end-to-end suture, reattachment or advancement of the tendon to its insertion site on the navicular bone, reconstruction of the tendon, and a limited or triple arthrodesis.

Abnormalities of the Flexor Hallucis Longus Tendon

Anatomy. The flexor hallucis longus muscle arises from the lower two thirds of the posterior surface of the shaft of the fibula. In common with the tibialis posterior and flexor digitorum longus tendons, the flexor hallucis longus tendon is contained in a fibrous tunnel behind the medial malleolus, beneath the flexor retinaculum. The tendon descends into the foot by crossing the posterior subtalar joint and passing under the inferior surface of the sustentaculum tali. As it descends, it converges medially, approaching the tendon of the flexor digitorum longus muscle. In the middle plantar compartment, these two tendons cross, with the flexor digitorum longus tendon being more superficial (or plantar). In the sole of the foot, a tendinous slip extends from the lateral border of the flexor hallucis longus tendon to anastomose with the flexor digitorum longus tendon.[1] This slip tethers the flexor hallucis longus tendon and prevents excessive retraction of the proximal segment when the tendon is severed.[305] Farther distally, the flexor hallucis longus tendon passes through the medial septum, entering the medial plantar compartment. It crosses the lateral belly of the flexor hallucis brevis muscle in an oblique fashion and reaches the intersesamoid interval.[1] In the great toe, the flexor hallucis longus tendon lies superficial to and between the two heads of the flexor hallucis brevis muscle,[305] and it inserts in a transverse fashion into the base of the distal phalanx of the great toe.

Tendinitis and Rupture. Abnormalities of the flexor hallucis longus tendon are encountered less commonly than those of the Achilles and tibialis posterior tendons. Such abnormalities include tendinitis and partial or complete disruption, partial tethering (i.e., os trigonum syndrome), and complete tethering (i.e., checkrein deformity).[269]

Injuries of the tendon of the flexor hallucis longus muscle at the level of the medial malleolus are observed in athletes, particularly dancers, who actively plantar flex their feet.[521, 522] Indeed, this tendon often is considered the "Achilles tendon" of the foot in dancers, and inflammation of the flexor hallucis longus tendon in dancers frequently is referred to as dancer's tendinitis.[258, 334] The flexor hallucis longus tendon extends through a fibro-osseous tunnel from the posterior aspect of the talus to the level of the sustentaculum tali, much like a rope through a pulley.[334] Irritation and swelling of the tendon in this area may lead to triggering of the great toe,[269] a condition known as hallux saltans.[334] Such inflammation may result not only from the trauma associated with ballet dancing or other sports requiring repetitive push-off maneuvers from the forefoot but also from systemic rheumatic diseases (such as rheumatoid arthritis) or acute trauma (e.g., comminuted calcaneal fractures).[44] The tendon eventually may rupture with loss of plantar flexion of the interphalangeal joint of the hallux.[335, 336]

Flexor hallucis longus tendinitis usually occurs behind the medial malleolus, but it occasionally can be found at Henry's knot, under the base of the first metatarsal bone, where the flexor digitorum longus tendon crosses over the flexor hallucis longus tendon or at the level of the head of the first metatarsal bone where the tendon of the flexor hallucis longus muscle passes between the sesamoid bones.[334, 337]

MR imaging can be used to assess inflammation or rupture of the flexor hallucis longus tendon (Fig. 17–111), although fluid in the sheath of this tendon may be a normal finding in patients with large ankle effusions, owing to communication of the sheath with the ankle in approximately 20 per cent of normal persons.[44]

Os Trigonum Syndrome. Partial tethering of the tendon of the flexor hallucis longus muscle may result from hypertrophy of the os trigonum, a condition designated the os trigonum syndrome.[510] The posterior aspect of the talus normally has two tubercles, the medial tubercle and the lateral tubercle, between which is found the fibro-osseous tunnel of the flexor hallucis longus tendon.[334] The normal ossification process of the body

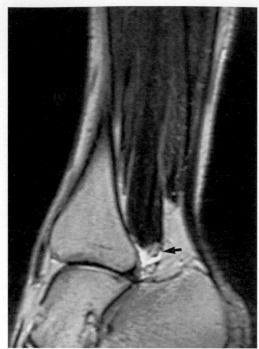

Figure 17–111
Injuries of the flexor hallucis longus tendon: MR imaging, acute partial tear. This 43 year old man heard a pop while running, which was followed immediately by severe pain. A sagittal T2-weighted (TR/TE, 3500/102) fast spin echo MR image shows the site of tendon tear (arrow), which is associated with high signal intensity. Other images showed that some of the tendinous fibers were intact.

of the talus progresses posteriorly. A separate ossification center in the posterior border of the talar body may occur, however, appearing between the ages of 8 and 10 years in girls and 11 and 13 years in boys. This center usually fuses with the remainder of the bone within a year of its appearance. If it persists after skeleton maturation, it is designated an os trigonum. The os trigonum is the ununited lateral tubercle of the talus, is present in approximately 10 per cent of persons, and is bilateral in 50 per cent of persons. The medial edge of this bone (or trigonal process of the talus) lies under the flexor hallucis longus tendon, on the lateral side of the flexor hallucis longus tunnel, and it may lead to compression of the tendon in this area. Resulting symptoms often are designated the talar compression syndrome or posterior impingement syndrome of the ankle,[338, 339] and they are common in activities such as those occurring during ballet dancing (e.g., demi-pointe, full pointe, tendu, the frappé, the relevé, or leaving the ground in a jump), in which full weight-bearing occurs with maximum plantar flexion at the ankle.[334] These maneuvers decrease the space between the superior border of the os calcis and the posterior lip of the tibia, in which the os trigonum (or trigonal process) is found. Laxity of the lateral ligaments of the ankle may predispose to or accentuate this syndrome. Pain and tenderness are apparent in the posterolateral region of the ankle, findings that may simulate those of peroneal or Achilles tendinitis.[334] Although radiographs will reveal an os trigonum in many patients with a poste-

rior impingement syndrome (Fig. 17–112), the size of the os is a poor indicator of the severity of the clinical manifestations. Furthermore, this syndrome may occur in the absence of an os trigonum, and a prominent os trigonum can occur in the absence of this syndrome. Soft tissue entrapment between the calcaneus and talus or a plica in the posterior region of the ankle (with or without an os trigonum) also may lead to the posterior impingement syndrome.[334, 340] CT or MR imaging is useful in defining the relationship between the os trigonum and flexor hallucis longus tendon in some patients with this syndrome.[269] Removal of the accessory ossification center generally is curative.

Checkrein Deformity. The checkrein deformity consists of a fixed tethering of the flexor hallucis longus tendon under, or just proximal to, the flexor retinaculum (internal annular ligament) of the ankle, which leads to unexplained flexion contracture of the interphalangeal joint of the hallux with a mild extension contracture of the first metatarsophalangeal joint (claw hallux).[269] A healing fracture of the lower portion of the tibia may lead to this deformity, related to posttraumatic adhesions.

Abnormalities of the Tibialis Anterior Tendon

The tendon of the tibialis anterior muscle is invested by a synovial sheath and traverses three retinacular tunnels.

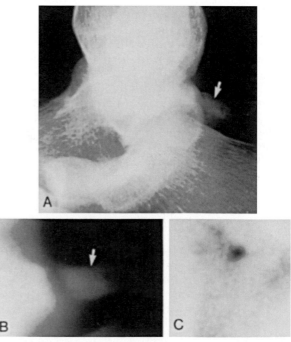

Figure 17–112
Os trigonum syndrome. A 16 year old girl complained of pain and tenderness in the posterior region of the ankle. Routine radiograph **(A)** and conventional tomogram **(B)** reveal a prominent os trigonum (arrows) with an irregular gap between it and the posterior margin of the talus. Bone scintigraphy **(C)**, accomplished in the lateral projection, shows uptake of the radionuclide in the area of the os trigonum. Surgery confirmed the presence of fibrous tissue between the talus and the os trigonum, and symptoms disappeared after excision of the latter. (Courtesy of G. Greenway, M.D., Dallas, Texas.)

This tendon begins near the junction of the lower and middle thirds of the tibia and slightly below this level acquires a tendon sheath with which it descends further into the ankle and foot.[183] The three retinacular tunnels are contributed to by the superior extensor retinaculum and the bifurcating limbs of the inferior extensor retinaculum.[183] After crossing the ankle joint, the tibialis anterior tendon inserts into the medial and plantar aspects of the medial cuneiform bone and the adjacent base of the first metatarsal bone.[305] The tibialis anterior muscle is the primary dorsiflexor of the foot and, because of the tendon's medial site of insertion, also adducts and supinates the foot.[305] The blood supply both to the muscle and to the tendon is derived solely from the anterior tibial artery, perhaps making these structures more susceptible to ischemia than the other muscles of the anterior compartment (i.e., extensor hallucis longus, extensor digitorum longus, and peroneus tertius) that have further sources of vascularity.[305]

Spontaneous rupture of the tibialis anterior tendon is rare.[341-344] Ruptures may occur at various levels of the tendon, although those appearing between the superior and inferior extensor retinacula are most common.[183] Rupture also may occur at the level of the medial tarsometatarsal joint, perhaps related to a dorsal osteophyte.[269] Spontaneous ruptures appear most typically in patients over the age of 45 or 50 years, and they may be complete or partial.[511] Athletes, such as runners, soccer players, and hikers, also may develop ruptures of the tibialis anterior tendon.[44] Injuries relate to forced plantar flexion of the foot and eversion of the ankle.[183] Footdrop results from these injuries, which create difficulty in walking, although women who wear high-heeled shoes may experience only minor difficulty during walking.[183] Thus, accurate diagnosis may be delayed. On clinical examination, a mass related to protrusion of the proximal portion of the torn tendon above the inferior retinaculum may be noted.[269] Retraction of the torn end beneath the superior retinaculum also may be seen. Inflammation of the adjacent tendon sheaths frequently is apparent. MR imaging (Figs. 17–113 and 17–114) and CT allow accurate diagnosis in most cases.

Abnormalities of the Peroneal Tendons

Anatomy. The peroneus longus and brevis muscles are important lateral stabilizers of the ankle joint (see Fig. 17–11). The peroneus longus muscle serves to evert and dorsiflex the foot, the contribution to eversion being far more apparent when the foot is off the ground. Along with the peroneus brevis muscle, the peroneus longus muscle acts to maintain the concavity of the foot in takeoff of the foot from the ground during walking and when tiptoeing. The peroneus brevis muscle contributes to eversion of the foot.

In their course from the ankle to the foot, the tendons of these two muscles come to lie together behind the lateral malleolus in a common synovial sheath (Fig. 17–115). Here, the tendon of the peroneus longus muscle lies in a retrofibular groove that is shared by the tendon of the peroneus brevis muscle. Indeed, the peroneus brevis tendon lies more securely within this groove

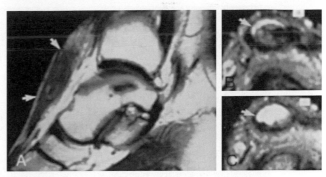

Figure 17–113

Injuries of the tibialis anterior tendon: MR imaging, acute complete tear. This 22 year old man twisted his ankle while running and developed pain and swelling in front of the ankle.

A A sagittal T1-weighted (TR/TE, 450/15) spin echo MR image shows an enlarged tibialis anterior tendon and sheath (arrows) containing foci of increased signal intensity.

B, C Two transaxial T2-weighted (TR/TE, 1800/90) spin echo MR images obtained near the ankle joint are shown. At the higher level (**B**), fluid of high signal intensity (arrow) is evident within the sheath and surrounds the tendon. At the lower level (**C**), the fluid-filled sheath (arrow) is seen, but the tibialis anterior tendon is not visible.

than the posteriorly located peroneus longus tendon.[183] The tendons and their sheath are kept in place and supported within the groove by the superior peroneal retinaculum, a structure that inserts into the medial and lateral ridges of the sulcus, converting the groove into a tunnel. More distally, the peroneus longus tendon is applied to the lateral surface of the calcaneus, inferior to the tendon of the peroneus brevis muscle and the peroneal trochlea, or tubercle (an elevation in the lateral surface of the calcaneus), and above the calcaneal tubercle that serves as the insertion site for the calcaneofibular ligament (see Fig. 17–115). In this area, the peroneus longus tendon passes beneath a tunnel created by the inferior peroneal retinaculum. Further distally, the tendon of the peroneus longus muscle is intimate, first with the lateral side, and then with the inferior surface of the cuboid bone. Beneath the cuboid bone, this tendon lies within a groove that is converted to a tunnel by the long plantar ligament. The tendon then inserts into the lateral side of the base of the first metatarsal bone and the medial cuneiform bone. During its course, the peroneus longus tendon undergoes an abrupt change in direction at two points[305]: at the tip of the lateral malleolus and at the distal (lateral) edge of the cuboid bone. In both of these locations, the tendon is thickened, and at the point of contact with the smooth surface of the edge of the cuboid bone, a sesamoid within the tendon composed of fibrocartilage or bone may be found.[305] Rarely, a sesamoid bone also is found in the retromalleolar portion of the tendon or, very exceptionally, in the calcaneal portion of the tendon.[1] Additional anatomic variations of this tendon include a fibrous connection between the tendon and the base of the fifth metatarsal bone at the level of the cuboid bone, a tendinous slip extending to the peroneus longus tendon from the tibialis posterior tendon and a posterior frenular ligament extending from the peroneal sesamoid to the cuboid bone.[1]

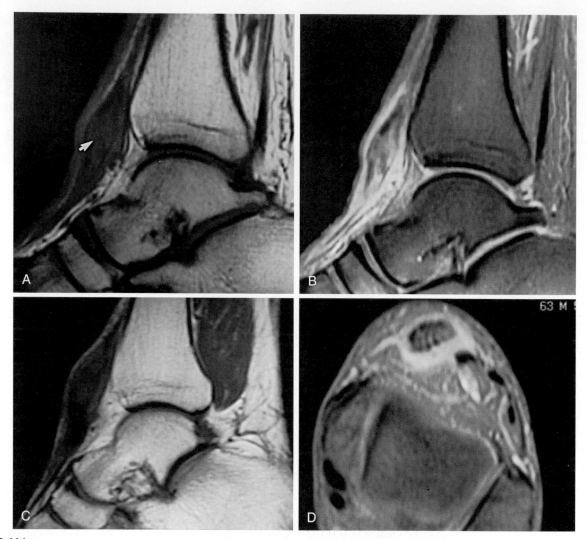

Figure 17–114

Injuries of the tibialis anterior tendon: MR imaging, chronic partial tear.

A, B The sagittal T1-weighted (TR/TE, 750/15) spin echo MR image **(A)** shows an enlarged tendon (arrow), which is inhomogeneous in signal intensity. After intravenous injection of a gadolinium compound, a sagittal fat-suppressed T1-weighted (TR/TE, 550/15) spin echo MR image **(B)** reveals enhancement of signal intensity in the torn tendon and surrounding tissues.

C, D In a second patient, a sagittal T1-weighted (TR/TE, 633/16) spin echo MR image **(C)** shows findings almost identical to those of **A**. After intravenous administration of a gadolinium compound, a transverse fat-suppressed T1-weighted (TR/TE, 600/13) spin echo MR image **(D)** reveals enhancement of signal intensity within and around the abnormal tendon.

The tendon of the peroneus brevis muscle, after passing behind the fibula, runs forward on the lateral surface of the calcaneus, above the peroneus longus tendon. Here, it lies close to but above the peroneal trochlea (i.e., tubercle) in an osteoaponeurotic canal created by the inferior peroneal retinaculum. The peroneus brevis tendon inserts into the tuberosity of the lateral aspect of the base of the fifth metatarsal bone. Numerous anatomic variations may be encountered, including the presence of a tendinous slip (peroneus digiti quinti) extending from the peroneus brevis tendon through the tendon of the peroneus tertius muscle to the proximal phalanx of the fifth toe, the existence of a peroneus quartus muscle extending from the fibula to the calcaneus, and the occurrence of a lateral peroneocalcaneus muscle that may originate from the peroneus longus and brevis muscle mass.[1]

Two distal extensions of the common synovial sheath individually surround the peroneus longus and peroneus brevis tendons. The intimate relationship of the common peroneal tendon sheath and the calcaneofibular ligament explains the arthrographic finding of opacification of the sheath after injuries to the ankle joint. Tears of the calcaneofibular ligament allow the synovial sheath to become apposed to the ankle joint, explaining its opacification during arthrography. Isolated tears of the anterior talofibular ligament are not associated with this pattern of communication.

The superior peroneal retinaculum is believed to be the primary restraint to subluxation or dislocation of the peroneal tendons in the fibular groove. Most commonly, this retinaculum consists of a fibrous band originating from the posterior ridge of the distal portion of the fibula that extends posteriorly and inferiorly to insert as a single band on the lateral wall of the calcaneus, although numerous anatomic variations are encoun-

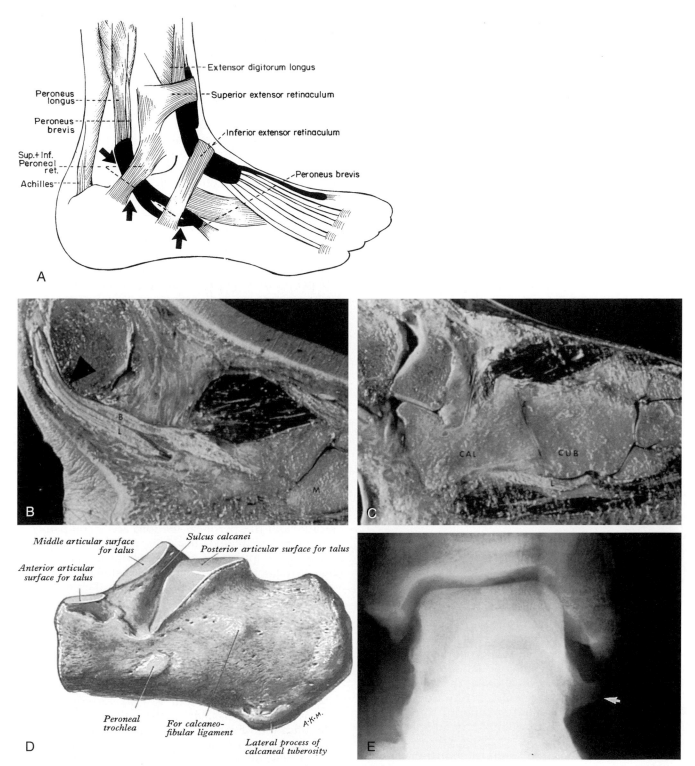

Figure 17–115

Peroneal tendons and tendon sheath: Normal anatomy.

A A drawing depicts the peroneus longus and brevis tendons and their sheath.

B A lateral sagittal section of the foot and ankle demonstrates the peroneus brevis (B) and peroneus longus (L) tendons passing around the lateral malleolus (arrowhead). The peroneus brevis can be followed close to the base of the fifth metatarsal bone (M).

C A slightly more medial sagittal section through the calcaneus (CAL) and cuboid (CUB) bone outlines the peroneus longus (L) tendon as it crosses underneath the foot.

(A, From Gilula LA, et al: Radiology *151*:581, 1984. **B, C,** From Resnick D, Goergen TG: Radiology *115*:211, 1975.)

D The lateral aspect of the calcaneus is shown. Note the position of the peroneal trochlea, or tubercle. (From Gray's Anatomy, Edited by R. Warwick and PL Williams. 35th British edition. Philadelphia, W.B. Saunders Company, 1973, p. 378.)

E A frontal radiograph of the ankle shows an enlarged peroneal tubercle (arrow). Such enlargements may be associated with stenosing tenosynovitis of the peroneal tendon sheath.

tered.[345] Dissections generally confirm the existence of retinacular insertions on both the calcaneus and the Achilles tendon, with the sural nerve and the lateral calcaneal nerve and vessels located beneath the retinaculum. The calcaneal attachment site of the superior peroneal retinaculum may have one or two bands and is intimate with the calcaneal insertion of the calcaneofibular ligament. Indeed, both this ligament and the retinaculum are at maximum length in ankle dorsiflexion, and stretching or rupture of the calcaneofibular ligament after inversion injury of the ankle may be associated with injury to the superior retinaculum as well.[345, 512] Less commonly, this retinaculum attaches not to the calcaneus but to the Achilles tendon, and the frequency of tears of the peroneus brevis tendon in such cases may be less.[345]

The inferior peroneal retinaculum is in continuity with the lateral root of the inferior extensor retinaculum. It originates from the posterior segment of the lateral rim of the sinus tarsi and consists of two layers[1]: The superficial fibers pass downward and posteriorly, cross the trochlear process, and insert on the lateral surface of the calcaneus just above the posterolateral tubercle; the deep fibers attach on the apex of the trochlear process. This arrangement creates two fibrous tunnels; the peroneus brevis tendon is located in the upper tunnel and the peroneus longus tendon is located in the lower tunnel.

Subluxation and Dislocation. Subluxation and dislocation of the peroneal tendons often are classified as habitual (i.e., voluntary) and traumatic.[183, 346–350] Habitual subluxations commonly are bilateral and are reproduced by voluntary maneuvers involving the ankle and foot, often leading to a snapping sensation or sound. Such snapping relates to anterior movement of the peroneus brevis tendon, which carries with it the tendon of the peroneus longus muscle, enclosed within the common tendon sheath, although the two never lie in front of the lateral malleolus.[183]

Traumatic dislocations of the peroneal tendons are associated with disruption of the superior retinaculum or stripping of the periosteal membrane in the distal portion of the fibula at the sites of attachment of this retinaculum. In either situation, the retinaculum becomes functionally deficient, allowing the peroneal tendons to subluxate in a lateral or forward direction. Rarely do they assume a position anterior to the fibula, however. These injuries are common in athletes, particularly those involved in hockey, skiing, soccer, and basketball. The mechanism of injury is controversial; one school of thought implicates inversion at the ankle with the foot in a position of plantar flexion, a mechanism that also can lead to injury to the lateral ligaments of the ankle. Another school implicates sudden forceful, passive dorsiflexion of the ankle with the foot in slight eversion,[305] resulting in a powerful reflex contraction of the peroneal muscles. Eversion of the ankle tenses both of these tendons and the calcaneofibular ligament, forcing the tendons against the superior retinaculum. Dorsiflexion causes a maximal change in the direction of the peroneal tendons at the lateral malleolus, also pressing them against the retinaculum. Congenital variations of the shape of the retrofibular groove or the strength of the superior peroneal retinaculum can predispose to subluxation or dislocation of the peroneal tendons.

In a study of 73 cases of acute dislocation of the peroneal tendons, Eckert and Davis[347] concluded that true rupture of the superior retinaculum was rare, but instead the retinaculum is elevated, leading to either periosteal stripping or bone avulsion involving the lateral malleolus. Three grades of injury were defined: grade I, in which the periosteum and retinaculum are elevated from the lateral malleolus and the tendons lie between the periosteum and bone; grade II, in which the distal 1 or 2 cm of a fibrous ridge in the posterior lip of the lateral malleolus is elevated along with the retinaculum; and grade III, in which avulsion of a rim of bone, the fibrous ridge, periosteum, and retinaculum occurs. In grade I injuries, which were evident in about 50 per cent of patients, the peroneal tendons, once reduced, were unstable only when placed under tension; in grade II injuries (about 33 per cent of patients) and grade III injuries (about 15 per cent of patients), the tendons remained unstable after reduction of the dislocation.

Traumatic peroneal tendon dislocations may be acute or chronic, the latter type often related to misdiagnosis of the initial injury with the subsequent development of recurrent dislocations. Acute injuries often are associated with a snapping sensation, edema, and ecchymoses involving the posterolateral aspect of the ankle. The clinical findings simulate those of a sprain of the lateral ligaments of the ankle, although the anterior talofibular, calcaneofibular, and anterior tibiofibular ligaments usually are intact. A fracture of the lateral malleolus may be an associated finding. Chronic subluxations and dislocations of the peroneal tendons are accompanied by a sense of lateral ankle instability and, in some cases, by recurrent snapping or popping about the ankle. Fluid may be palpated in the peroneal tendon sheath.[351] Provocative testing of the ankle by having the patient contract the peroneal muscles in the foot in eversion may lead to subluxation of the tendons, although the results of this test also may be inconclusive.[305] Routine radiography may disclose a small avulsion fracture adjacent to the lateral surface of the lateral malleolus, an important and often diagnostic observation (Fig. 17–116). This finding, however, is observed only in cases of grade III injury. The bone fragment is 1 to 1.5 cm in length and is best appreciated on the ankle mortise view.[305] Identification of subluxation or dislocation of the peroneal tendons also can be accomplished with peroneal tenography, ultrasonography, CT scanning, and MR imaging (Fig. 17–117).[44, 349, 352] With regard to MR imaging, volumetric gradient echo sequences (with reconstruction of imaging data in nonorthogonal planes) may be useful. Accurate diagnosis is important as, if left untreated, chronic recurrent subluxation, tendon tears, and stenosing tenosynovitis may develop.[353]

With regard to treatment, chronic dislocations of the peroneal tendons generally are managed operatively. Acute dislocations may be treated with or without surgical intervention. Grades I or II injuries may be repaired by suturing the retinaculum to the fibrous ridge and

Figure 17–116
Injuries of the peroneal tendons and sheath: Peroneal tendon dislocation. In this patient with a comminuted calcaneal fracture, a routine radiograph (**A**) reveals the avulsed fibular bone fragment (arrow) that is characteristic of a peroneal tendon dislocation. A coronal CT scan (**B**) confirms the bone avulsion (arrow). Note its relationship to the peroneal tendons (arrowhead) and the fracture of the calcaneus.

bone of the lateral malleolus, whereas grade III injuries may require open reduction and wire fixation of the bone fragment. With regard to the operative treatment of recurrent dislocations, five basic types of procedure are used[305]: bone block procedures, tendon rerouting procedures, periosteal flaps, tendon slings, and procedures that deepen the peroneal groove of the fibula. Although these operative procedures often are successful, unusual types of peroneal tendon dislocation may not respond to standard surgical techniques. As one example of this, subluxation of the peroneal tendons within their sheath may be encountered.[354] In this situation, posterolateral displacement of the peroneus brevis tendon from its normal position anterior to the peroneus longus tendon becomes evident.

Entrapment or Impingement. Fractures of the calcaneus may be associated with lateral displacement of the lateral wall of the bone, resulting in narrowing of the fibulocalcaneal space. Entrapment of the peroneal tendons between the fibula, calcaneus, and talus or subluxation or dislocation of the peroneal tendons, or a combination of the two, may result.[355] Clinical manifestations of peroneal tendon entrapment include findings of tenosynovitis, limited subtalar motion, local tenderness, and an antalgic gait. Once again, diagnostic information is provided by routine radiography, supplemented with ultrasonography, peroneal tenography (Fig. 17–118), or MR imaging.

Tendinitis and Tenosynovitis. Inflammatory changes in the peroneal tendons or their sheaths usually result from acute injury or chronic stress. Typical causes include calcaneal fractures with peroneal tendon entrapment, systemic rheumatic disorders, tarsal coalition, developmental variations and anomalies of the peroneal tendons, congenital or acquired hypertrophy of the pe-

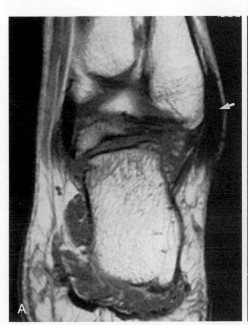
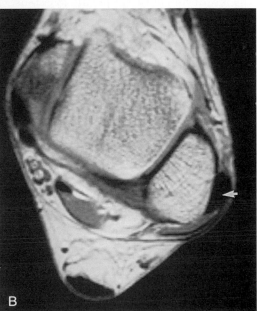

Figure 17–117
Injuries of the peroneal tendons and sheath: Peroneal tendon dislocation. In a 28 year old woman who had suffered a talar fracture several months previously, a coronal T1-weighted (TR/TE, 600/15) spin echo MR image (**A**) and a transaxial proton density–weighted (TR/TE, 2000/20) spin echo MR image (**B**) document anterolateral dislocation of the peroneal tendons (arrows). (Courtesy of D. Wilcox, M.D., Kansas City, Missouri.)

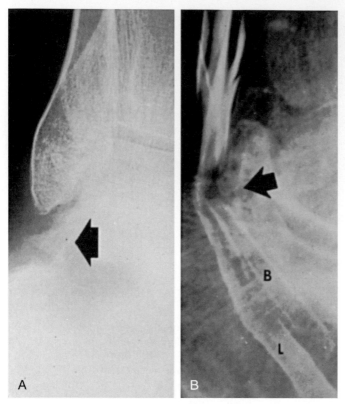

Figure 17–118
Injuries of the peroneal tendons and sheath: Entrapment or impingement. In a patient with a previous calcaneal fracture, the routine radiograph **(A)** reveals a lateral calcaneal spicule (arrow) beneath the fibula. The peroneal tenogram **(B)** outlines impingement and compression of the sheath as it passes around the lateral malleolus (arrow) associated with incomplete filling of the peroneus brevis (B) and peroneus longus (L) sheaths. **(B**, From Resnick D, Georgen TG: Radiology *115*:211, 1975.)

roneal tubercle, altered foot mechanics, and improper footwear.[21, 349, 513] Pain, tenderness, and swelling are common clinical manifestations.

Stenosing tenosynovitis of the peroneal tendon sheath typically occurs in three specific locations[356]: posterior to the lateral malleolus (peroneal sulcus), at the peroneal trochlea, and at the plantar surface of the calcaneus.[305] This condition appears more common when the peroneal tubercle is well developed. The sheath is thickened and stenotic, the retinaculum may be thickened, and the tendons themselves generally are intact.[356]

Ultrasonography, tenography (Fig. 17–119), and MR imaging (Fig. 17–120) can be applied to the diagnosis of inflammation of the peroneal tendons and sheath. MR imaging reveals significant fluid within the sheath of the peroneal tendons and, possibly, altered tendon size and intratendinous signal intensity.[44] Differentiation of physiologic versus pathologic collections of fluid in the peroneal tendon sheath, however, is difficult. Furthermore, tears of the calcaneofibular ligament allow communication of the ankle and the peroneal tendon sheath, accounting for fluid in the sheath in some patients who have had ankle trauma.

Rupture. Partial or complete disruption of one or both peroneal tendons can accompany an acute injury (e.g., calcaneal fracture) or may occur spontaneously.[357–361]

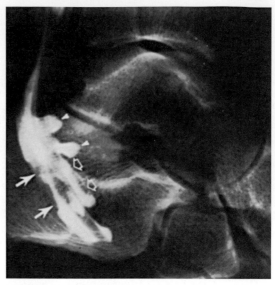

Figure 17–119
Injuries of the peroneal tendons and sheath: Stenosing and nodular tenosynovitis, peroneal tenography. The margins of the peroneus longus (solid arrows) and peroneus brevis (open arrows) tendon sheaths are markedly irregular, with pseudodiverticula (arrowheads) of the peroneus brevis tendon sheath.
(From Gilula LA, et al: Radiology *151*:581, 1984.)

Spontaneous ruptures of these tendons are rare, usually occurring in young adults and involving the peroneus brevis tendon.[269] Partial tears are more common than complete disruptions of the peroneal tendons.

In the usual situation, longitudinal splits and hypertrophy of the peroneus brevis tendon are evident pathologically. Typically, these longitudinal tears are 2.5 to 5.0 cm in length, beginning near the tip of the lateral malleolus and propagating distally or proximally, or in both directions.[514] In some situations, longitudinal splits divide the peroneus brevis tendon into two parts (peroneal split syndrome). The precise pathogenesis of these

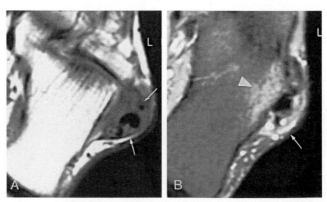

Figure 17–120
Injuries of the peroneal tendons and sheath: Peroneal tendinitis and tenosynovitis. A transaxial T1-weighted (TR/TE, 400/17) spin echo MR image **(A)** and a transaxial T2-weighted (TR/TE, 3300/100) fast spin echo fat-suppressed MR image **(B)** obtained at a slightly more inferior level than **A** show a fluid-filled mass (arrows) about the peroneus longus and peroneus brevis tendons. Note the reactive edema of the marrow of the calcaneus (arrowhead) in **B**. (Courtesy of S. Eilenberg, M.D., San Diego, California.)

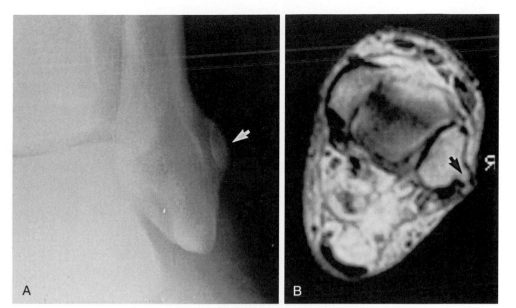

Figure 17–121
Injuries of the peroneal tendons and sheath: Chronic subluxations of the peroneal tendons. Bone proliferation (arrows) involving the posterolateral surface of the fibula, as shown with routine radiography (**A**) and on a transaxial MR image (**B**), is characteristic of chronic, recurrent tendon subluxation, often associated with the peroneal split syndrome.

splits may relate to contraction of the peroneus longus muscle causing compression and splaying of the peroneus brevis tendon over the fibula.[514] With inversion of the ankle, the peroneus longus tendon may then become situated between the two halves of the peroneus brevis tendon, preventing its healing.[305, 356] A similar situation may become evident in patients with chronic, recurrent subluxations of the peroneal tendons associated with laxity of the superior peroneal retinaculum. Bone proliferation on the posterolateral surface of the fibula and alterations in the fibular groove are helpful diagnostic clues in some cases (Fig. 17–121).

Tears of the peroneus longus tendon often are found distally as the tendon enters the cuboid groove.[357] Complete ruptures may be associated with a change in position of the os peroneum, which may be retracted proximally, even as far as the level of the lateral malleolus. Fractures of the os peroneum also may lead to disruptions of this tendon (Fig. 17–122).[362] When the os peroneum is present, tendon rupture usually is related to an avulsion fracture, with diastasis and retraction of the proximal fragment; rarely the rupture occurs proximal or distal to the os peroneum.[514] Chronic tears of the peroneus longus tendon often are longitudinal splits beginning at the tip of the lateral malleolus or at the peroneal tubercle and extending distally to the cuboid groove.[514]

MR imaging allows assessment of the location and extent of the peroneal tendon disruption (Fig. 17–123). This technique permits the identification of abnormal signal intensity or size of the tendon (see Fig. 17–123). A multipartite appearance of the tendon is consistent with the presence of longitudinal splits (Fig. 17–124).[358] Diagnostic pitfalls relate to the existence of accessory tendons (e.g., peroneus quartus tendon) and to the occurrence of a normal variation leading to bifurcated insertions of this tendon.[44, 358] In cases of complete disruption of either the peroneus longus or peroneus brevis tendon, analysis of serial MR images in one or more imaging planes (typically transaxial and sagittal planes)

will document the absence of a normal tendon structure. Retraction of the torn tendon is less common in cases of peroneal tendon disruption than in those of disruption of the Achilles tendon.[44]

Developmental Abnormalities

In addition to the os trigonum, which is considered earlier in this chapter, several developmental abnormalities of the ankle and foot deserve emphasis.

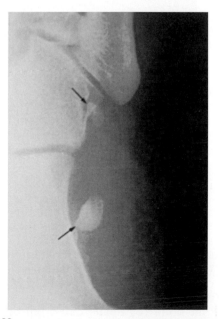

Figure 17–122
Injuries of the peroneal tendons and sheath: Complete tear of the peroneus longus tendon with fracture of the os peroneum. Note wide separation of the fracture fragments (arrows) and adjacent soft tissue swelling. (Courtesy of M. Pathria, M.D., San Diego, California.)

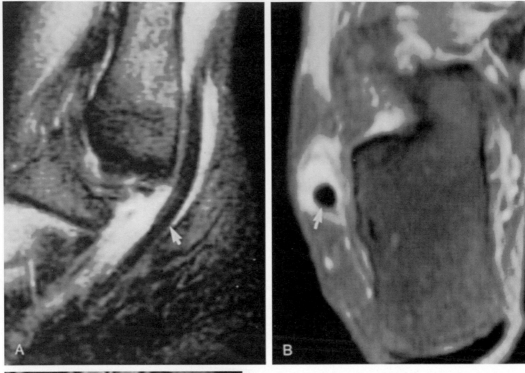

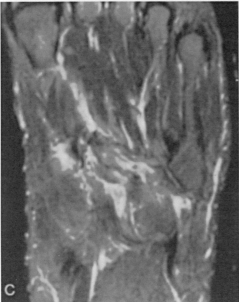

Figure 17–123

Injuries of the peroneal tendons and sheath: MR imaging.

A Complete tear of the peroneus brevis tendon. A sagittal MPGR MR image (TR/TE, 500/11; flip angle, 25 degrees) shows the peroneus longus tendon (arrow) with a fluid-filled sheath. The peroneus brevis is not visualized. (Courtesy of C. Sebrechts, M.D., San Diego, California.)

B Complete tear of the peroneus brevis tendon. In a second patient, a transaxial proton density–weighted (TR/TE, 2000/20) spin echo MR image obtained with chemical presaturation of fat (ChemSat) shows fluid of high signal intensity about the peroneus longus tendon (arrow) with nonvisualization of the peroneus brevis tendon. (Courtesy of C. Sebrechts, M.D., San Diego, California.)

C Complete tear of the peroneus longus tendon. A transaxial T2-weighted (TR/TE, 3000/80) fat-suppressed fast spin echo MR image shows nonvisualization of the distal portion of the peroneus longus tendon, with high signal intensity in the plantar soft tissues. (Courtesy of S. Eilenberg, M.D., San Diego, California.)

Accessory Ossicles

Some accessory ossicles or ossification centers about the ankle and foot may have clinical significance. The os vesalianum adjacent to the cuboid and the base of the fifth metatarsal[363] and the os intermetatarseum between the bases of the first and second metatarsals are examples of accessory ossicles that reportedly have been accompanied by pain. The clinical significance of an accessory navicular bone (os tibiale externum or naviculare secundarium), however, has received the greatest attention.

Two distinct types of accessory navicular bone have been described: A separate ossicle may occur as a sesamoid bone in the posterior tibial tendon (type I), and an accessory ossification center may appear in the tubercle of the navicular bone (type II).[364] Type I ossicles account for approximately 30 per cent of cases, generally are well defined, are round or oval, measure 2 to 6 mm in diameter, and are situated up to 5 mm medial and posterior to the medial aspect of the navicular. Type II accessory ossification centers represent approximately 70 per cent of cases, are triangular or heart-shaped, measure 9 to 12 mm in size, and are located within 1 to 2 mm from the medial and posterior aspect of the navicular.[365] An anomaly termed a cornuate navicular involves the medial aspect of the navicular bone and is related to the presence of an osseous bridge connecting

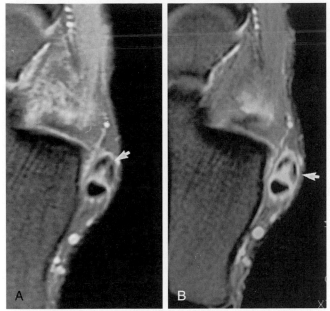

Figure 17–124
Injuries of the peroneal tendons and sheath: Peroneal split syndrome. Observe the longitudinal splitting of the peroneus brevis tendon (arrows) as demonstrated on a transaxial fat-suppressed fast spin echo MR image (TR/TE, 4700/14) **(A)** and a transaxial fat-suppressed T1-weighted (TR/TE, 600/12) spin echo MR image obtained after intravenous administration of a gadolinium compound **(B)**.

an accessory bone with the medial aspect of the navicular.

Of these three patterns, it is the type II ossification center and the cornuate navicular that have been associated with clinical manifestations, particularly pain, which usually becomes evident in the second decade of life. Increased accumulation of a bone-seeking radionuclide during scintigraphy represents a sensitive (but not entirely specific) finding of a painful accessory navicular bone.[366] With MR imaging, marrow edema in the accessory ossification center and adjacent navicular bone has been reported to be associated with pain (Fig. 17–125).[367] Histologic analysis has revealed inflammatory chondro-osseous changes compatible with chronic stress-related injury.[365, 368]

With regard to the sesamoid bone that characterizes the type I anomaly, a relationship with pes planus, due to the abnormal insertion of the tibialis posterior tendon into the accessory ossicle, has been proposed but is unproved.[369, 370]

Tarsal Fusion (Coalition)

Tarsal coalition represents an abnormal fusion of one or more of the tarsalia. The union may be fibrous, cartilaginous, or osseous and can be congenital (developmental) or acquired in response to infection, trauma, articular disorders, or surgery.[371] Congenital, or developmental, tarsal coalition is of unknown cause.[372] Although in 1896 Pfitzner[373] proposed that tarsal coalitions were caused by the gradual incorporation of accessory ossicles into the adjacent tarsal bones, a suggestion that was supported at least in part by later investigators,[374–377] the

observation of tarsal fusion in fetuses discounts such a proposal. In some cases, a familial history of identical abnormalities is obtained.[378–381]

Despite an early description of peroneal spastic flatfoot by Sir Robert Jones in 1897,[382] it was not until 1921 that a relationship of this clinical entity and tarsal coalition was documented.[374] This association now is well recognized,[375, 383] although it is not uniform in all cases of peroneal spastic flatfoot; other conditions, such as juvenile chronic arthritis, tuberculosis, osteoarthritis, and fracture can cause a similar clinical problem. Typically, symptoms and signs of tarsal coalition appear in the second or third decade of life; an earlier age of onset is rare, perhaps owing to the fact that the fusion is fibrous or cartilaginous in the young child or adolescent, and only with the appearance of ossification do pain and restricted motion become evident. After minor trauma or unusual activity, the affected person complains of vague pain in the foot, aggravated by prolonged standing or athletic endeavor.[384] Limited subtalar motion, pes planus, and shortening with persistent or intermittent spasm of the peroneal muscles are seen on physical examination. The rigid foot may be held in a valgus attitude, although anterior tibial spasm can lead to varus deformity.[385, 386] Coalition also can be manifested as a cavus foot[387, 388] or as an incidental finding in an asymptomatic person.

Isolated partial coalitions can be classified according to the bones that are affected; calcaneonavicular, talocalcaneal, talonavicular, and calcaneocuboid fusions, in order of decreasing frequency, can be detected. Tarsal fusions accompanying multiple malformation syndromes may have "atypical" patterns or may involve the

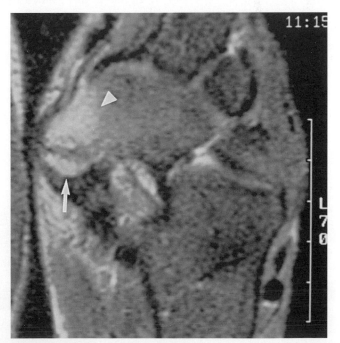

Figure 17–125
Accessory navicular bone: MR imaging. A transaxial fat-suppressed fast spin echo MR image (TR/TE, 5300/54) shows high signal intensity in a type II accessory navicular bone (arrow) and navicular tuberosity (arrowhead). (From Miller TT, et al: Radiology *195*:849, 1995.)

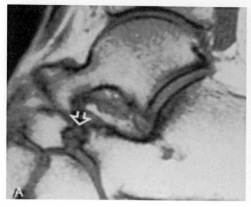

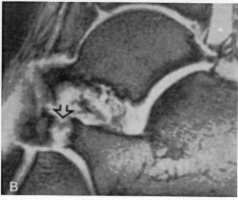

Figure 17–126

Calcaneonavicular tarsal coalition.

A A sagittal T1-weighted (TR/TE, 400/20) spin echo MR image reveals a nonosseous coalition (arrow) between the calcaneus and navicular bones. Its signal characteristics are compatible with the presence of fibrocartilaginous tissue.

B A sagittal gradient echo (MPGR) image (TR/TE, 500/20; flip angle, 25 degrees) also shows the coalition (arrow) and confirms the cartilaginous nature of the abnormal union.

entire tarsus.[389] Identification of the nature and extent of a coalition frequently requires routine radiography that in some instances can be supplemented with special views, conventional tomography, CT scanning, MR imaging, scintigraphy, and even arthrography.[384, 390–397]

Calcaneonavicular coalition is one of the most frequent,[398–401] is sometimes bilateral,[402] and can be asymptomatic or associated with rigid flatfoot.[403] In general, symptoms and signs are less severe than those accompanying talocalcaneal coalitions, and "secondary" radiographic abnormalities may be less marked. Coalition is identified optimally on a 45 degree medial oblique view of the foot.[404] The diagnosis is simplified by the presence of a solid bony bar extending between the calcaneus and the navicular bone but is more difficult in cases of cartilaginous or fibrous coalition. Elongation of the anterosuperior portion of the calcaneus suggests the diagnosis, and such elongation, when viewed on the lateral radiograph, has been designated the "anteater nose" sign.[405] A secondary radiographic sign of calcaneonavicular coalition is hypoplasia of the head of the talus.[407] Talar "beaking" is uncommon. Rarely, a fracture of the abnormal calcaneonavicular osseous bridge is identified.[401] Although other diagnostic techniques such as scintigraphy, CT, and MR imaging have been used to evaluate patients with this common type of coalition,[393, 407] generally they are not required (Figs. 17–126 and 17–127).

The talocalcaneal fusion represents the other common type of tarsal coalition. Almost all such fusions occur at the middle facet, between the talus and susten-

taculum tali; ankylosis of the posterior subtalar joint or of the anterior facets is far less frequent. The condition is more common in boys than in girls and is bilateral in 20 to 25 per cent of patients. Cartilaginous, fibrous, or bony bridges may be identified, although radiographic evaluation often requires special views in addition to standard anteroposterior and lateral projections. A penetrated axial radiograph (Harris-Beath view) obtained with varying degrees of beam angulation, oblique radiographs, and anterior and lateral conventional tomograms may be necessary. These techniques may identify the actual site of osseous fusion, although closely apposed and irregular bony articular surfaces can indicate the presence of bridging fibrous or cartilaginous tissue.[408] Cartilaginous coalitions usually are associated with marked narrowing of the joint, whereas fibrous coalitions, which typically involve the most posterior part of the sustentaculum tali, may lead only to subtle diminution of the interosseous space,[408] although hypoplasia of the sustentaculum tali also may be apparent.[409] In both fibrous and cartilaginous coalitions, CT alone, arthrography alone, or CT and arthrography together may be helpful. Contrast medium introduced into the talonavicular space of this joint will fail to flow beneath the anterior aspect of the talus and over the sustentaculum tali owing to the abnormal tissue elements.[410]

Fortunately, a number of secondary radiographic signs have been described in association with talocalcaneal coalition.[384, 390] These include the following: talar beaking, broadening of the lateral process of the talus, narrowing of the posterior subtalar joint, concave under-

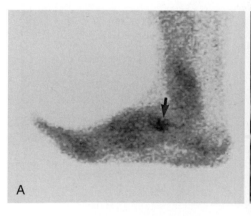

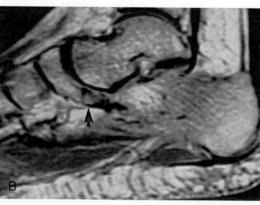

Figure 17–127

Calcaneonavicular tarsal coalition.

A In a 39 year old woman, a bone scan shows abnormal accumulation of the radionuclide in the midfoot (arrow).

B A sagittal proton density–weighted (TR/TE, 3000/14) spin echo MR image shows a calcaneonavicular coalition (arrow).

(Courtesy of V. Lim, M.D., San Diego, California.)

surface of the talar neck and asymmetry of the talocalcaneonavicular joint, failure of visualization of the "middle" subtalar joint, a C-shaped curvilinear radiodense shadow extending from the ankle beneath the posterior subtalar joint, and a ball-and-socket ankle joint.[411-420]

Although direct visualization of the bone bridge or identification of one or more of these secondary signs ensures accurate radiographic diagnosis of talocalcaneal coalition in many instances, the importance of bone scintigraphy as a screening examination[395, 396] and of CT as a definitive examination[393-395, 407, 421-425] should be understood. With regard to scintigraphy, abnormal uptake of the bone-seeking radionuclide occurs about the subtalar joints and in the dorsum of the foot; with regard to CT scanning, a coronal scanning plane, with or without slight angulation of the x-ray beam, appears to be best, and the technique allows assessment of both feet at the same time (Figs. 17–128, 17–129, and 17–130). Plantar plane images as well as those obtained in

a modified sagittal plane also may be useful.[423] The technique can be applied successfully to the assessment of fibrous and cartilaginous coalitions.[408, 409] MR imaging provides information similar to that of CT scanning, although regions of bone marrow edema also may be identified (Figs. 17–130 and 17–131).

Other types of tarsal coalition, including talonavicular and calcaneocuboid coalitions, are uncommon.[426-435]

Synovial and Capsular Abnormalities

Joint Effusion

Noninflammatory or inflammatory fluid may accumulate in the ankle joint or in any of the joints of the foot. Detection of such fluid with routine radiography often is difficult unless the effusion is large. In the ankle, however, as little as 5 ml of joint fluid can be detected

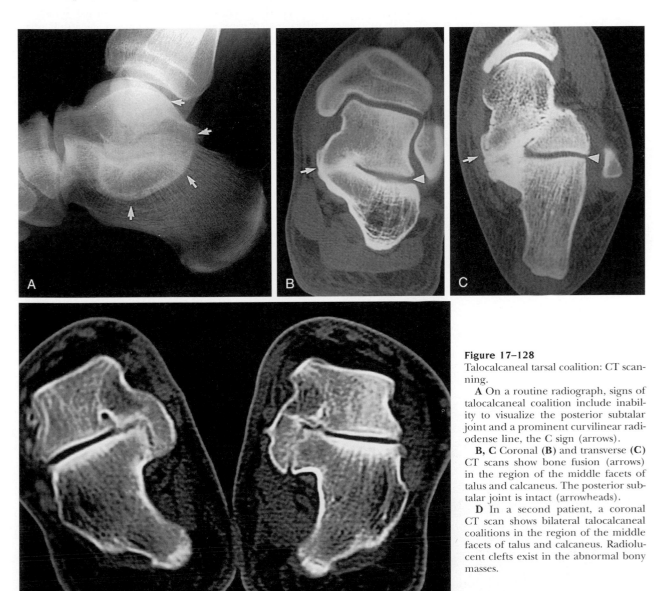

Figure 17–128

Talocalcaneal tarsal coalition: CT scanning.

A On a routine radiograph, signs of talocalcaneal coalition include inability to visualize the posterior subtalar joint and a prominent curvilinear radiodense line, the C sign (arrows).

B, C Coronal (**B**) and transverse (**C**) CT scans show bone fusion (arrows) in the region of the middle facets of talus and calcaneus. The posterior subtalar joint is intact (arrowheads).

D In a second patient, a coronal CT scan shows bilateral talocalcaneal coalitions in the region of the middle facets of talus and calcaneus. Radiolucent clefts exist in the abnormal bony masses.

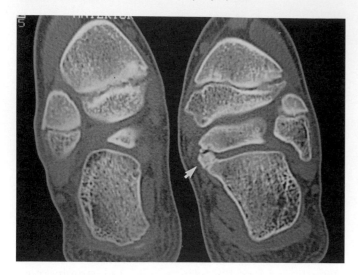

Figure 17–129
Talocalcaneal tarsal coalition: CT scanning. A coronal CT scan of both ankles reveals a nearly complete osseous coalition (arrow) of the left posterior subtalar joint. This is an unusual site of such coalition. (Courtesy of G. Bock, M.D., Winnipeg, Manitoba, Canada.)

on a lateral radiograph owing to the presence of a radiodense shadow in front of or behind the joint, or at both sites. Ultrasonography is more sensitive than routine radiography in the detection of a joint effusion in the ankle (as well as the joints of the foot),[436] although the presence of a small amount of such fluid can be evident in asymptomatic persons.[437] With ultrasonography, plantar flexion of the foot may improve the sensitivity to detection of fluid in the anterior portion of the ankle. MR imaging appears to be more sensitive than ultrasonography in the delineation of joint effusions, however.

Adhesive Capsulitis

Although it is far better known in the glenohumeral joint, posttraumatic adhesive capsulitis is encountered

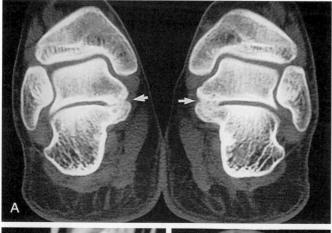

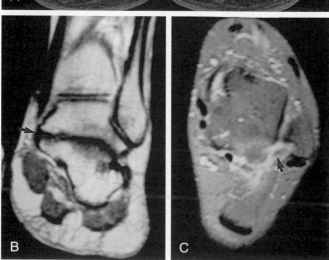

Figure 17–130
Talocalcaneal tarsal coalition: CT scanning and MR imaging. This 26 year old woman developed ankle pain after a fall.

A The coronal CT scan shows bilateral, almost complete osseous coalition involving the middle facets of the talus and calcaneus (arrows).

B The region of the tarsal coalition (arrow) is evident on this coronal fast spin echo MR image (TR/TE, 5150/14) of the left ankle, although the diagnosis is not so apparent as in **A.**

C A transverse T1-weighted (TR/TE, 633/12) spin echo MR image of the left ankle, obtained with fat suppression and after intravenous administration of a gadolinium compound, shows enhancement of signal intensity (arrowhead) about a torn posterior talofibular ligament.

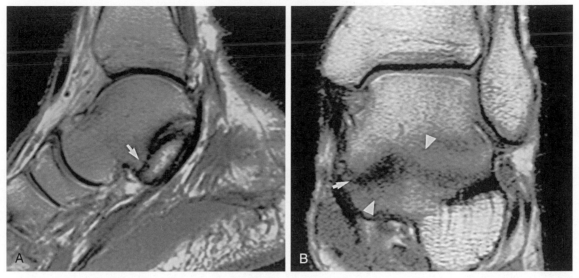

Figure 17–131
Talocalcaneal tarsal coalition: MR imaging. Sagittal T1-weighted (TR/TE, 600/20) **(A)** and coronal T1-weighted (TR/TE, 717/20) **(B)** spin echo MR images show an incomplete coalition (arrows) between the middle facets of talus and calcaneus and adjacent bone marrow edema (arrowheads). (Courtesy of S. Eilenberg, M.D., San Diego, California.)

in the ankle. Restriction of ankle motion is detected on clinical examination. Arthrography delineates a decrease in the articular capacity, with resistance to injection of contrast material, obliteration of the normal anterior and posterior recesses or the tibiofibular syndesmosis, opacification of lymphatic vessels, and extravasation of contrast material along the needle tract (Fig. 17–132). The relationship of this condition to posttraumatic arthrofibrosis of the ankle and to causes of the anterolateral impingement syndrome is not clear.

Synovitis

In common with other joints, the ankle may be affected in a variety of systemic rheumatic diseases and local processes. Rheumatoid arthritis, juvenile chronic arthritis (Fig. 17–133), the seronegative spondyloarthropathies, hemophilia, gout, and calcium pyrophosphate dihydrate crystal deposition disease are among the systemic disorders that may involve the ankle. Pigmented villonodular synovitis (Fig. 17–134), idiopathic synovial (osteo)chondromatosis, and infection are among the monoarticular processes that may localize to the ankle.[428–440] Because of the proximity of the ankle joint and adjacent tendon sheaths, a variety of processes involving such sheaths can extend into the ankle. These processes include tenosynovial (osteo)chondromatosis, pigmented villonodular tenosynovitis, localized nodular synovitis, giant cell tumors of the tendon sheath, and septic tenosynovitis (Fig. 17–135). Gi-

Figure 17–132
Adhesive capsulitis: Arthrography. On the lateral view, there is no filling of normal anterior and posterior recesses, and extravasation of contrast material is seen along the needle track (arrowhead).

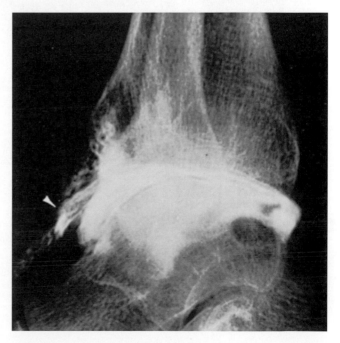

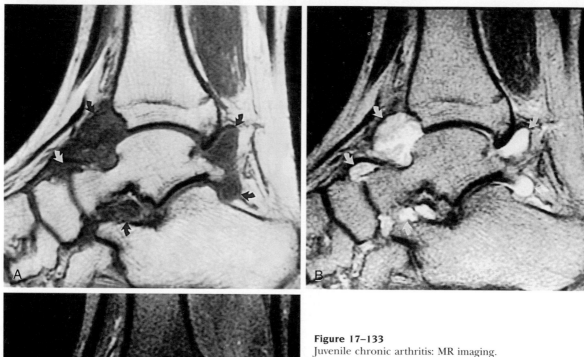

Figure 17–133

Juvenile chronic arthritis: MR imaging.

A A sagittal T1-weighted (TR/TE, 600/20) spin echo MR image reveals fluid or pannus, or both, distending the anterior and posterior recesses of the ankle joint and posterior recess of the posterior subtalar joint (black arrows) and the anterior talocalcaneonavicular joint (white arrow). Abnormal signal intensity also is present beneath the anterior portion of the talus (lower black arrow).

B With T2 weighting (TR/TE, 2000/80), these areas show mainly high signal intensity (arrows).

C Immediately after the intravenous injection of a gadolinium compound, a sagittal T1-weighted (TR/TE, 600/20) spin echo MR image obtained with fat suppression shows pannus of high signal intensity (arrows), as well as fluid of low signal intensity.

(Courtesy of J.S. Suh, M.D., Seoul, Korea.)

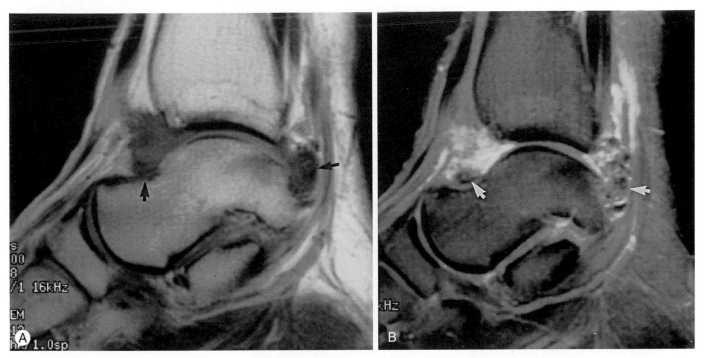

Figure 17–134

Diffuse (intra-articular) pigmented villonodular synovitis: MR imaging.

A A sagittal T1-weighted (TR/TE, 700/18) spin echo MR image shows distention of the ankle. Note foci of low signal intensity (arrows), representing hemosiderin deposits.

B Immediately after the intravenous administration of a gadolinium compound, a sagittal T1-weighted (TR/TE, 700/18) spin echo MR image obtained with fat suppression reveals inflamed synovium of high signal intensity in the ankle and posterior tendon sheaths and hemosiderin deposits (arrows), which remain of low signal intensity.

(Courtesy of C. Neumann, M.D., Palm Springs, California.)

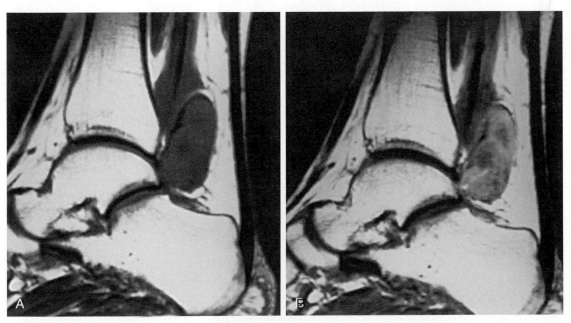

Figure 17–135

Localized nodular synovitis: MR imaging. Sagittal T1-weighted (TR/TE, 500/15) spin echo MR images obtained before **(A)** and after **(B)** intravenous administration of a gadolinium compound reveal a well-defined posterior mass at the level of the ankle joint intimate with the flexor hallucis longus muscle and tendon. It is of low signal intensity in **A,** with irregular enhancement of signal intensity in **B.**

ant cell tumors of a tendon sheath can also occur as a mass involving any of the toes (Fig. 17–136).

Synovial and Ganglion Cysts

Synovial and ganglion cysts are encountered about the ankle and, less commonly, in the foot.[441] These may communicate with an adjacent joint or tendon sheath, or (in the case of a ganglion cyst) bone. The MR imaging features are characteristic and, in some instances, specific (Figs. 17–137 and 17–138).

Bursitis

Any of the bursae in the foot and ankle may become involved as a manifestation of rheumatoid arthritis or other synovial inflammatory processes. Of these, involvement of the retrocalcaneal bursa should be emphasized. As indicated earlier in this chapter, this bursa is located between the Achilles tendon and posterosuperior aspect of the calcaneus. It is distinct from an acquired bursa, the superficial tendo Achillis bursa, that is posterior to the attachment site of the Achilles tendon.

The constellation of retrocalcaneal bursitis, superficial tendo Achillis bursitis, and thickening of the Achilles tendon at its site of insertion is termed Haglund's syndrome (Fig. 17–139).[442–444] This syndrome may be seen in certain athletes, such as hockey players and golfers, related to the type of footwear used in these sports. It also has been associated with a prominent, convex superior tuberosity of the calcaneus, the bursal

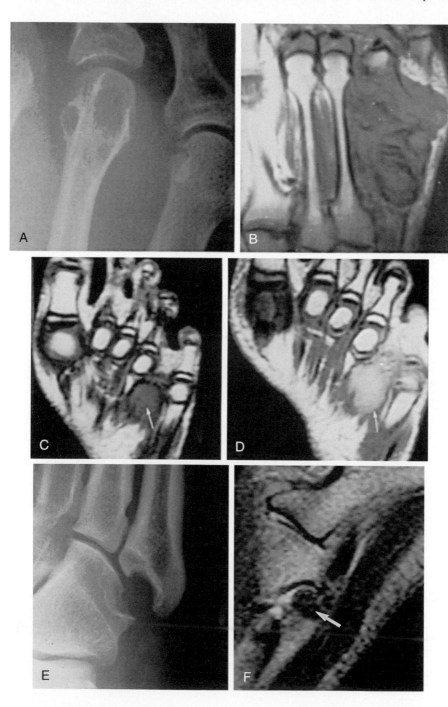

Figure 17–136

Giant cell tumor of tendon sheath: Routine radiography and MR imaging.

A, B In a 63 year old man, a routine radiograph (**A**) reveals erosion of the fourth metatarsal head. A transverse T1-weighted (TR/TE, 588/34) spin echo MR image (**B**) shows the extent of the mass, which is of low signal intensity.

C, D In a 7 year old girl, a transverse T1-weighted (TR/TE, 600/11) spin echo MR image (**C**) reveals a mass (arrow) of low signal intensity between the fourth and fifth metatarsal bones. A transverse T1-weighted (TR/TE, 600/12) spin echo MR image obtained after the intravenous administration of a gadolinium compound (**D**) shows an increase in signal intensity in the mass (arrow).

E, F In a 16 year old girl, routine radiography (**E**) shows bone erosion involving apposing portions of the cuboid bone and fifth metatarsal base. A mass (arrow) of low signal intensity is seen on a sagittal T2-weighted (TR/TE, 1400/80) spin echo MR image (**F**).

(**A, B,** Courtesy of G. Greenway, M.D., Dallas, Texas.)

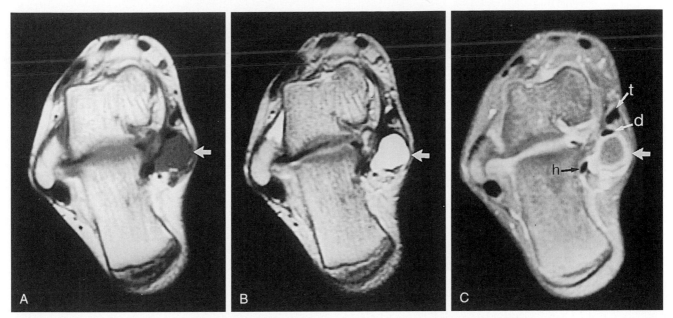

Figure 17–137

Ganglion cyst: MR imaging. Transverse T1-weighted (TR/TE, 600/20) (**A**), transverse T2-weighted (TR/TE, 200/80) (**B**), and transverse T1-weighted (TR/TE, 600/20) (**C**) spin echo MR images, the last obtained with fat suppression after intravenous administration of a gadolinium compound, show a ganglion cyst (arrows) in the region of the tarsal tunnel in an 11 year old girl. t, Tibialis posterior tendon; d, flexor digitorum longus tendon; h, flexor hallucis longus tendon. (Courtesy of J. Aoki, M.D., and F. Fujioka, M.D., Matsumoto, Japan.)

projection. A similar condition also associated with bursitis about the Achilles tendon insertion is designated a pump bump because of its association with a specific type of shoe worn by women.

Ultrasonography (Fig. 17–140) and MR imaging (Fig. 17–141) can be applied to the assessment of retrocalcaneal and superficial tendo Achillis bursitis. Fluid within the retrocalcaneal bursa may be seen in asymptomatic persons, however.

Cartilage Abnormalities

Cartilage Degeneration

Although extensive degeneration of articular cartilage becomes evident on routine radiographs as loss of joint space, the inadequacies of this imaging method in detecting cartilage degeneration at an early stage are well recognized. Among the other diagnostic techniques that

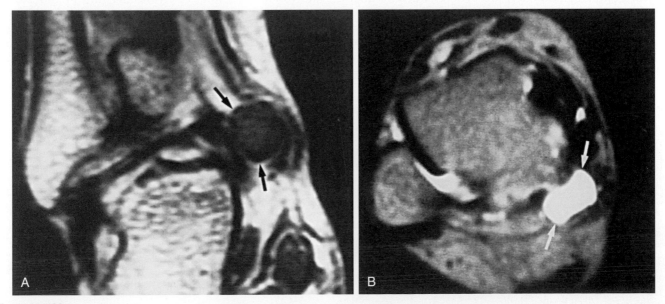

Figure 17–138

Ganglion cyst: MR imaging. In this 33 year old woman, observe the well-defined cystic lesion (arrows) in the posteromedial aspect of the ankle, as displayed on coronal T1-weighted (TR/TE, 450/25) (**A**) and transverse T2-weighted (TR/TE, 2000/90) (**B**) spin echo MR images. In **B**, the ganglion cyst has high signal intensity and appears to be communicating with the joint.

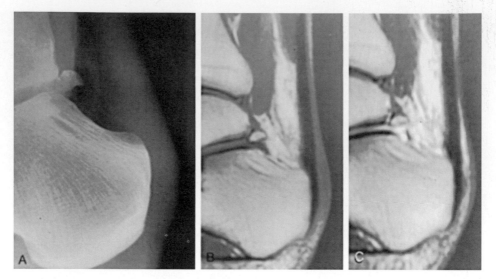

Figure 17–139
Haglund's syndrome.
 A On the routine lateral view of the foot, a superficial soft tissue swelling is seen at the insertion of the Achilles tendon (superficial tendo Achillis bursitis), the Achilles tendon is poorly defined and thickened (tendinitis), and loss of the normal lucent retrocalcaneal recess between the Achilles tendon and the extreme superior aspect of the bone (retrocalcaneal bursitis) is observed.
 B Sagittal T1-weighted spin echo MR image (TR/TE, 500/16) demonstrates soft tissue thickening posterior to the Achilles tendon. Fat does not extend between the calcaneus and the tendon. The Achilles tendon has normal low signal intensity.
 C Sagittal T2-weighted spin echo MR image (TR/TE, 2000/70) demonstrates high signal intensity posterior to the Achilles tendon, consistent with superficial tendo Achillis bursitis.
 (Courtesy of H. Pavlov, M.D., New York, New York.)

have been applied to cartilage analysis, MR imaging appears to hold the greatest promise. As indicated in Chapter 16, numerous modifications in MR imaging protocols have been introduced with the common goal of improving the sensitivity of the imaging method. When applied to the knee and, particularly, to the patellofemoral joint, 3DFT gradient echo sequences, magnetization transfer contrast, and MR arthrography (using direct intra-articular instillation of a gadolinium compound) generally have been most successful. The value of these techniques in the analysis of the articular cartilage of the ankle joint has not received great attention, however. Although it is likely that these same MR imaging methods are the best currently available to study the apposing cartilaginous surfaces of the tibia and talus

(Fig. 17–142), the thinness of these surfaces, when compared to the patellofemoral (and femorotibial) surfaces in the knee, certainly makes the study of articular cartilage of the ankle with MR imaging more challenging.

Cartilage Injury

The subjects of osteochondral fractures and osteochondritis dissecans, including involvement of the talus, are addressed in Chapter 8. Of the imaging methods used to assess these lesions, CT scanning, CT arthrography, MR imaging, and MR arthrography appear best (Figs. 17–143 and 17–144), although the superiority of any one of these techniques is not clear. With MR imaging, the size of the lesion can be determined, and if fluid is

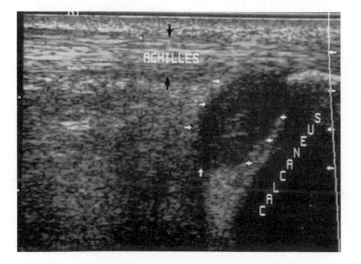

Figure 17–140
Retrocalcaneal bursitis: Ultrasonography. A sagittal scan of the posterior aspect of the ankle demonstrates anechoic bursal fluid (white arrows) and an intact Achilles tendon (black arrows). (Courtesy of M. van Holsbeeck, M.D., Detroit, Michigan, and J. Jacobson, M.D., San Diego, California.)

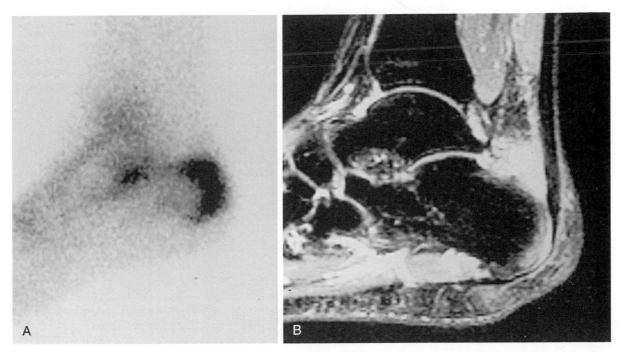

Figure 17–141
Retrocalcaneal bursitis: Scintigraphy and MR imaging, Reiter's syndrome.
 A A bone scan shows increased accumulation of the radionuclide in the calcaneus and about the posterior subtalar joint.
 B A sagittal STIR (TR/TE, 1500/30; inversion time, 120 msec) MR image reveals fluid of high signal intensity (as well as pannus of high signal intensity) in the retrocalcaneal bursa, marrow edema in the posterior portion of the calcaneus, and inflammatory changes in the plantar soft tissues.
 (Courtesy of E. Bosch, M.D., Santiago, Chile.)

present in the joint (i.e., a native effusion or a contrast agent injected intra-articularly), the status of the overlying articular cartilage may be judged. Although the findings of osteochondritis dissecans of the talus generally are diagnostic, posttraumatic intraosseous cysts, osteonecrosis, certain tumors, and even osteomyelitis occasionally present diagnostic difficulties (Fig. 17–145).

Arthroscopy can be used both as a diagnostic and as a therapeutic method in cases of chondral or osteochondral lesions of the talus. Débridement of fibrillated or partially detached pieces of cartilage and drilling of subchondral bone to establish vascular channels may be accomplished.[259]

Osteochondral Bodies

On the basis of data derived from analysis of other joints, especially the knee, the best imaging methods for the detection of intra-articular bodies in the ankle are CT arthrography and MR imaging, particularly that employing an intra-articular contrast agent (Fig. 17–146). The success of any technique is dependent on the size of the fragment (or fragments), its composition (chondral, osteochondral, or osseous), and its location. In the ankle, free intra-articular bodies often migrate to anterior and posterior recesses of the joint, where they may become embedded in the synovial membrane.

Arthroscopy offers both diagnostic and therapeutic capabilities in cases of intra-articular bodies in the ankle. Although arthroscopy can be performed without the benefit of information derived from CT scans or MR

images, such information regarding the number and location of bodies in the ankle joint may influence the manner in which arthroscopy is performed.

Muscle Abnormalities

Muscle abnormalities occurring about the ankle and foot are similar to those observed in other anatomic regions. Inflammatory, infectious, and traumatic disorders (Fig. 17–147) may involve the muscles of the foot and ankle, either in isolation or in combination with changes elsewhere.

Accessory and Anomalous Muscles

Although accessory and anomalous muscles occur elsewhere in the body, those in the foot and ankle have received the greatest attention.

An accessory soleus muscle appears to represent a frequent finding, especially on MR imaging examinations. Affected persons commonly are asymptomatic, although soft tissue fullness or a mass and occasionally pain and swelling after exercise may be seen, especially in teenagers and young adults.[445–450] Accentuation of foot deformity has been noted in patients with equinovarus conditions who also have an accessory soleus muscle.[449]

The origin and insertion sites of an accessory soleus muscle vary.[450] The muscle may arise from the proximal third of the fibula, the oblique soleal line of the tibia,

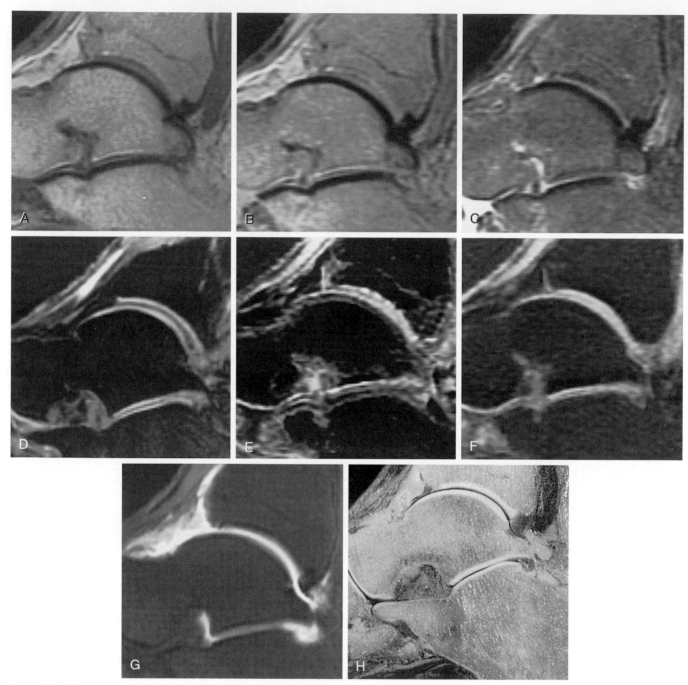

Figure 17–142

Analysis of tibiotalar cartilage: MR imaging. Sagittal MR images of a cadaveric ankle using different techniques are displayed. **A,** T1-weighted (TR/TE, 500/20) spin echo; **B,** proton density–weighted (TR/TE, 2000/20) spin echo; **C,** T2-weighted (TR/TE, 2000/80) spin echo; **D,** fat-suppressed, 3DFT spoiled gradient recalled acquisition in the steady state (SPGR) (TR/TE, 50/10; flip angle, 60 degrees); **E,** pulsed saturation transfer subtraction (STS) (TR/TE, 800/6; flip angle, 45 degrees); **F,** fat-suppressed STS (TR/TE, 800/6; flip angle, 45 degrees); **G,** MR arthrography with intra-articular injection of a gadolinium compound combined with fat-suppressed T1-weighted (TR/TE, 500/20) spin echo MR image; **H,** cadaveric section. Owing to the thinness of the articular cartilage, significant errors are introduced with any of these imaging methods when measurement of cartilage thickness is attempted. The fat-suppressed SPGR image **(D)** appears to be superior to the others, however.

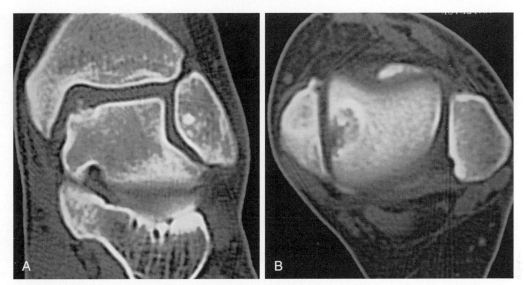

Figure 17-143
Osteochondritis dissecans: Talus, CT scanning. Direct coronal (**A**) and transverse (**B**) CT scans show the medial talar lesion containing multiple bone fragments.

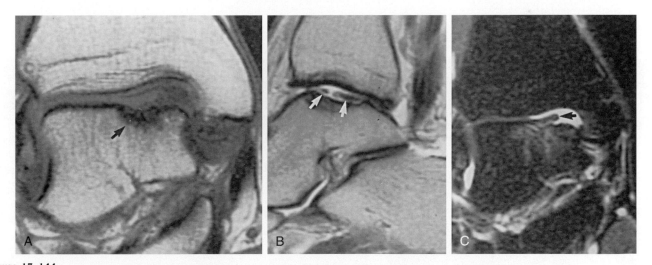

Figure 17-144
Osteochondritis dissecans: Talus, MR imaging.
  A A coronal T1-weighted (TR/TE, 450/15) spin echo MR image shows a medial talar lesion (arrow) with an irregular osseous surface. The cartilage overlying the lesion appears thickened.
  B A sagittal T2-weighted (TR/TE, 3800/98) fast spin echo MR image reveals partially displaced osteochondral fragments (arrows).
  C A coronal fast spin echo STIR MR image (TR/TE, 4000/42; inversion time, 150 msec) shows a partially displaced osteochondral fragment (arrow). Note a joint effusion and slightly altered signal intensity in the talus.

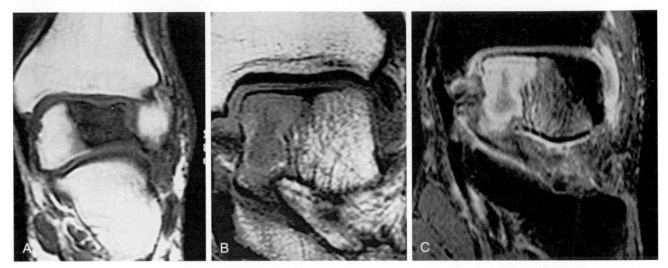

Figure 17–145

Talar lesions simulating osteochondritis dissecans: MR imaging.

A Osteonecrosis. Observe the well-defined lesion of the talus and associated collapse of the articular surface on a coronal T1-weighted (TR/TE, 700/16) spin echo MR image.

B, C Osteomyelitis. A fluid-filled infective lesion (related to coccidioidomycosis) involving the talus and associated with a joint effusion is shown on T1-weighted (TR/TE, 767/20) spin echo **(B)** and T1-weighted (TR/TE, 867/20) fat-suppressed spin echo **(C)** MR images, the latter image being obtained after the intravenous administration of a gadolinium compound.

B, C, Courtesy of R. Kerr, M.D., Los Angeles, California.)

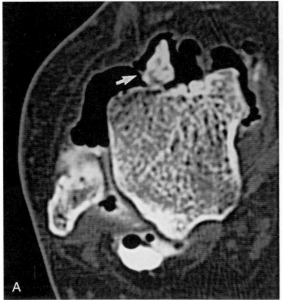

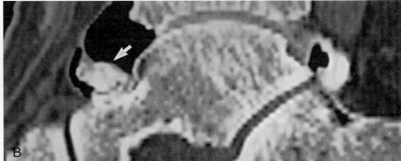

Figure 17–146

Intra-articular osteochondral bodies: CT arthrography. After the introduction of 10 ml of air and 1 ml of iodinated contrast material into the ankle, a transaxial CT scan **(A)** and a reformatted sagittal CT scan **(B)** show an osteochondral body (arrows) attached to the synovium in the anterior portion of the joint.

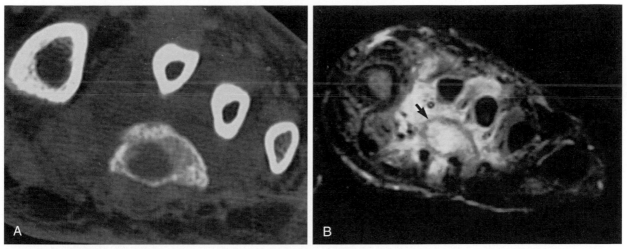

Figure 17–147
Posttraumatic heterotopic bone formation (myositis ossificans): CT scanning and MR imaging. In this patient who had had a recent injury to the foot, a coronal CT scan **(A)** shows a plantar soft tissue mass containing ossification. Note the ring-like pattern of bone formation. A coronal STIR (TR/TE, 1600/30; inversion time, 120 msec) MR image **(B)** reveals the extent of this mass and surrounding edema. Note that the ossific shell (arrow) has low signal intensity.

the aponeurosis of the flexor digitorum longus muscle, the anterior portion of the normal soleus muscle, or combinations of these structures.[447, 451, 452] The insertion sites of the accessory soleus muscle include the Achilles tendon and the superior and medial surfaces of the calcaneus.[453] The diagnosis of this accessory muscle can be provided by routine radiography (Fig. 17–148), CT (see Fig. 17–148), and MR imaging (Figs. 17–148, 17–149, and 17–150). Of these techniques, MR imaging appears to be best.[450] MR imaging confirms that the abnormal tissue has signal intensity characteristics identical to those of normal muscle, unless intramuscular hemorrhage or a hematoma is present. Treatment of symptomatic patients with an accessory soleus muscle includes fasciotomy of the muscle sheath or excision of the muscle, owing to the belief that the condition may predispose to a localized compartment syndrome.[451]

The peroneus quartus muscle, also designated the peroneus accessorius, peroneus externus, and peroneus calcaneus externus muscle, has been associated with chronic pain and swelling about the ankle.[450, 454–456] Its reported frequency, on the basis of results of cadaveric dissections, has varied from approximately 12 to 22 per cent.[457] Its site of origin may include the distal lateral portion of the fibula and the peroneus brevis or longus muscle, and its site of insertion may include the phalanges or metatarsal bone of the fifth toe, the calcaneus, the cuboid bone, and the lateral retinaculum of the ankle.[450] Accurate diagnosis again is provided by MR imaging.[450]

The flexor digitorum longus accessorius is a third anomalous muscle with variable sites of origin and insertion.[450] It may arise from the tibia, fibula, or interosseous membrane, or combinations of these structures, and it may insert into the flexor digitorum longus tendon at various levels. Clinical manifestations usually are absent. An anomalous flexor hallucis longus muscle also has been described.[458]

The tensor fasciae suralis is an anomalous muscle and tendon that originates from the semitendinosus muscle and contributes to the Achilles tendon.[459] This structure, which may lead to a clinically evident mass, can be diagnosed on the basis of MR imaging findings.

Muscle Hernias

Herniation of portions of a muscle through its fascial sheath is encountered most often in the leg. Although the tibial anterior muscle is the typical site of involvement, other muscles, such as the peroneus longus, may be affected.[515] Most persons with muscle hernias are asymptomatic, and multiple hernias with bilateral involvement are not uncommon. Although muscle hernias can result from traumatic rupture of the adjacent fascial sheath, appearing slowly or rapidly after penetrating wounds or open fractures of the tibia or fibula, most develop spontaneously, perhaps related to developmental defects in the fascia. Their precise sites of involvement may correspond to the points of entrance of nerves and vessels in the fascia.[515] Strong muscle contraction or rapid muscle hypertrophy, as seen in athletes, may predispose to muscle hernias.

Accurate diagnosis can be accomplished clinically in many persons. Indeed, the symmetry of bilateral lesions is an important diagnostic clue. MR imaging allows correct diagnosis in most cases, as the subcutaneous masses are seen to be portions of the muscle that have extended through defects in the overlying fascia.

Abnormalities of the Plantar Soft Tissues

Plantar Fasciitis

The plantar aponeurosis is the strong, fibrous, investing layer of the sole of the foot,[1] subcutaneous in location and extending as a thick, strong band of tissue from the

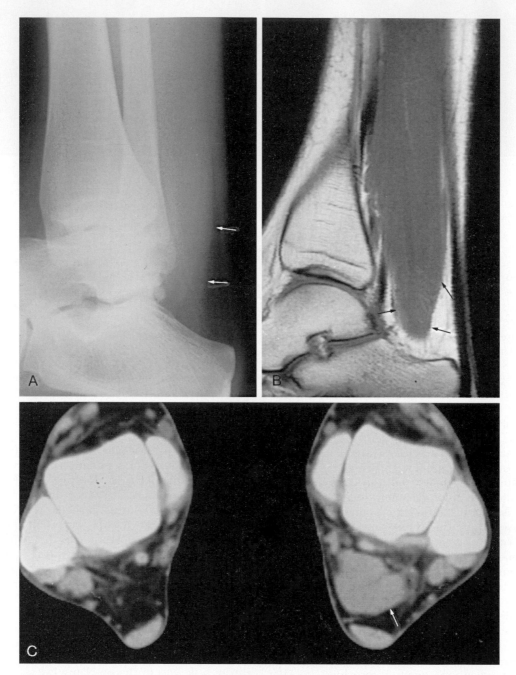

Figure 17–148

Accessory soleus muscle: Routine radiography, CT scanning, and MR imaging.

A, B A lateral radiograph **(A)** and a sagittal T1-weighted (TR/TE, 600/16) spin echo MR image **(B)** show the accessory muscle (arrows). (Courtesy of G. Greenway, M.D., Dallas, Texas.)

C In a second patient, a transaxial CT scan reveals the accessory soleus muscle (arrow). Compare with the opposite side. (Courtesy of A. Newberg, M.D., Boston, Massachusetts.)

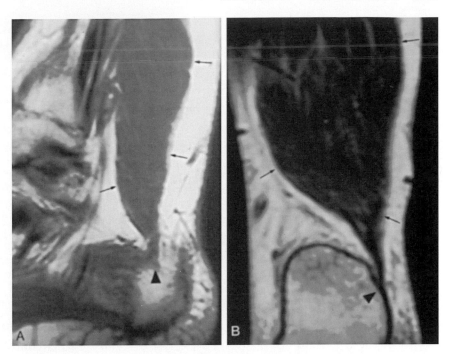

Figure 17–149
Accessory soleus muscle: MR imaging. A sagittal T1-weighted (TR/TE, 600/20) spin echo MR image **(A)** and a coronal T1-weighted (TR/TE, 800/25) spin echo MR image **(B)** show the accessory soleus muscle (arrows), which is attaching to the medial aspect of the calcaneus (arrowheads). (Courtesy of V. Chandnani, M.D., San Antonio, Texas.)

calcaneus posteriorly to the region of the metatarsal heads and beyond. It is composed of a prominent central part and lateral and medial parts (Fig. 71–151). The central part of the plantar aponeurosis is triangular and originates as a narrow tissue attaching to the medial process of the tuberosity of the calcaneus. The central part of the plantar aponeurosis may receive contributions from the plantaris and Achilles tendons. As it

extends distally, it broadens and, near the metatarsal heads, divides into five processes, each with superficial and deep components, and each extending into one toe. The lateral part of the plantar aponeurosis, which is inferior to the abductor digiti minimi muscle, has a thick proximal portion that extends between the lateral process of the calcaneal tuberosity and the base of the fifth metatarsal bone. It is thinner distally, with bands that extend to the plantar plate of the fourth and fifth toes. The medial part of the plantar aponeurosis is located inferior to the abductor hallucis muscle. It is thin and continuous proximally with the flexor retinaculum, laterally with the central part of the plantar aponeurosis, and medially with the fascia dorsalis pedis.

Plantar fasciitis represents inflammation of the plantar fascia and the perifascial structures.[460] Its causes may be divided into three categories[461–463]: mechanical, degenerative, and systemic. Mechanical factors associated with plantar fasciitis include pes cavus, a pronated foot, and an externally rotated lower extremity.[464] Such factors, particularly when present in active persons, may predispose to inflammation of the plantar fascia. Degenerative causes of plantar fasciitis include atrophy of the heel pad and age-related increases in foot pronation. Systemic causes include a wide variety of rheumatic disorders, especially rheumatoid arthritis and the seronegative spondyloarthropathies.[465] As the factors responsible for plantar fasciitis vary, the pathologic findings also are variable. In the setting of predisposing mechanical factors and overuse syndromes (cases associated with participation in competitive sports), tearing of some of the fibers of the plantar fascia may occur.[466–468] These abnormalities initially predominate at the site of origin of the plantar fascia and are accompanied by a local inflammatory reaction. Histologic findings include angiofibroblastic hyperplasia, collagen degeneration and necrosis, and matrix calcification.[469, 470] With chronicity,

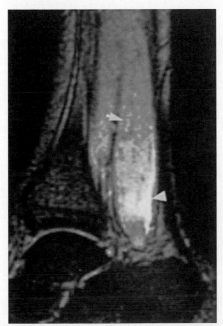

Figure 17–150
Accessory soleus muscle: MR imaging. A sagittal MPGR MR image (TR/TE, 517/11; flip angle, 15 degrees) reveals an accessory soleus muscle (arrow) with distal high signal intensity (arrowhead) related to hemorrhage after an injury. (Courtesy of S. Moreland, M.D., San Diego, California.)

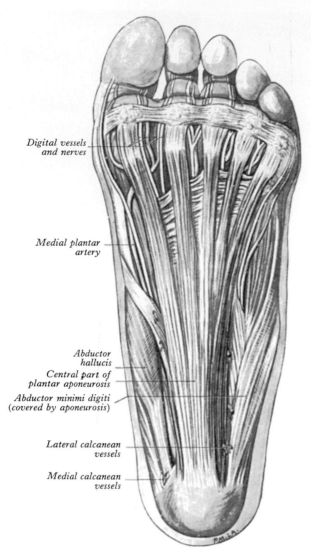

Figure 17–151

Plantar aponeurosis and related structures: Normal anatomy. See text for details. (From Williams PL, Warwick R [Eds]: Gray's Anatomy. 36th British edition. Edinburgh, Churchill Livingstone, 1980, p 579.)

the entire course of the plantar aponeurosis may be affected, with thickening and nodularity. Clinical findings include pain and tenderness localized to the regions of inflammation. Dorsiflexion of the toes may lead to an exacerbation of the findings, owing to stretching of the fibers of the plantar fascia. Conservative therapy is the preferred treatment in the early stages of plantar fasciitis; in chronic cases or in those that do not respond to conservative measures, surgical therapy, consisting of release of the origin of the plantar fascia with decompression of the lateral plantar nerve, may be required.[467]

Although bone scintigraphy may reveal regions of increased accumulation of the radiopharmaceutical agent at the site of inflammation, the increased scintigraphic activity may be more widespread, producing a nonspecific pattern. MR imaging, however, appears to be both sensitive and specific in the diagnosis of plantar fasciitis (Figs. 17–152, 17–153, 17–154, and 17–155), and it may be useful in cases in which the clinical diagnosis

is in doubt. MR imaging abnormalities of plantar fasciitis include thickening of the plantar fascia (which may grow to a thickness of 7 or 8 mm, in comparison to the 3 or 4 mm thickness that characterizes normal plantar fascia) and intrafascial alterations in signal intensity.[471–473] In T1-weighted spin echo MR images, foci of intermediate signal intensity may be seen within the plantar fascia, which normally is of uniform low signal intensity. In T2-weighted spin echo and STIR MR images, areas of high signal intensity may be evident in the plantar fascia and subcutaneous tissue. Alterations in the signal intensity in the marrow of the calcaneus, reflecting edema, also may be apparent.

Plantar fasciitis is but one of the many causes of plantar heel pain. Other causes of plantar pain include enthesophytes, trauma to the heel pad, rupture of the plantar fascia, nerve entrapment syndromes, atrophy or inflammation of the fat pad, tendinitis and tenosynovitis, calcaneal stress fractures, infections, foreign bodies, and tumors (Figs. 17–156, 17–157, and 17–158).[474, 475]

Plantar Fibromatosis

Plantar fibromatosis is a common condition associated with fibrous proliferation and replacement of portions

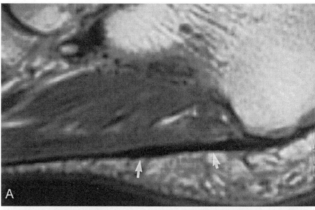

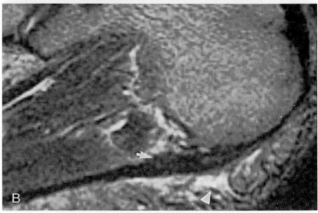

Figure 17–152

Plantar fasciitis: MR imaging.

A Normal plantar fascia. A sagittal proton density–weighted (TR/TE, 2000/20) spin echo MR image shows the normal thin plantar fascia (arrows) and overlying subcutaneous fibrous septa.

B Plantar fasciitis. A sagittal T2-weighted (TR/TE, 2000/80) spin echo MR image reveals subcutaneous edema (arrowhead) and focally thickened plantar fascia (arrow). A plantar calcaneal enthesophyte also is present.

(From Berkowitz JF, et al: Radiology *179*:665, 1991.)

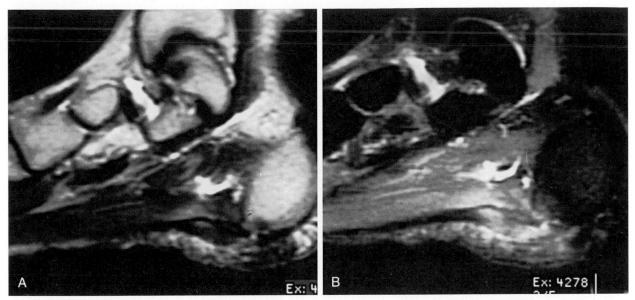

Figure 17–153
Plantar fasciitis: MR imaging. Evidence of edema both deep and superficial to a thickened plantar fascia appears as regions of high signal intensity in sagittal fast spin echo (TR/TE, 3766/90) **(A)** and STIR (TR/TE, 3200/19; inversion time, 150 msec) **(B)** MR images. (Courtesy of D. Levey, M.D., Corpus Christi, Texas.)

of the plantar aponeurosis. The disorder is seen in persons of all ages and is more common in men. Lesions may be solitary or multiple and unilateral or bilateral.[176, 177] Affected persons usually are asymptomatic, the nodules being discovered by palpation. Mild pain and discomfort in the plantar aspect of the foot after walking or prolonged standing may be evident, however. An association of plantar fibromatosis with other conditions associated with proliferation of fibrous tissue, such as Dupuytren's contractures of the hand, Peyronie's disease of the penis, and keloids, has been suggested but is not proved.[478] Plantar fibromatosis may become more extensive over a number of years, with gradual enlargement of the nodules and an increased number of nodules, although contractures of the toes generally do not occur.[479] On physical examination, the masses are firm and fixed to the plantar fascia. They may be treated conservatively or removed surgically. Incomplete excision may be followed by local recurrence of the lesions.

Histologically, the lesions are composed of fibroblasts separated by variable amounts of collagen tissue. They are not encapsulated and may infiltrate surrounding structures, leading to difficulty in defining the full extent of the lesions, but plantar fibromatosis does not undergo malignant transformation. Three phases of the disorder have been defined[478]: an initial proliferative phase is associated with increased fibroblastic activity and cellular proliferation; an involutional (active) phase is associated with the formation of nodules; and a residual phase is accompanied by reduced fibroblastic activity, maturation of collagen, and tissue contracture.

With MR imaging, single or multiple nodules in the plantar fascia and subcutaneous tissue are observed. The lesions are of low signal intensity (similar to that of muscle) in T1-weighted spin echo images (Fig. 17–159 and 17–160) and of low to intermediate signal intensity on T2-weighted spin echo MR images. In some cases, regions of high signal intensity are seen in T2-weighted

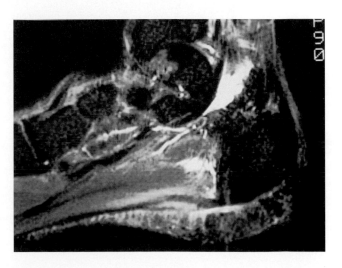

Figure 17–154
Plantar fasciitis: MR imaging. Intravenous administration of a gadolinium compound, when combined with fat suppression, can accentuate the signal intensity abnormalities of plantar fasciitis, as shown in this sagittal MR image. (Courtesy of R. Kerr, M.D., Los Angeles, California.)

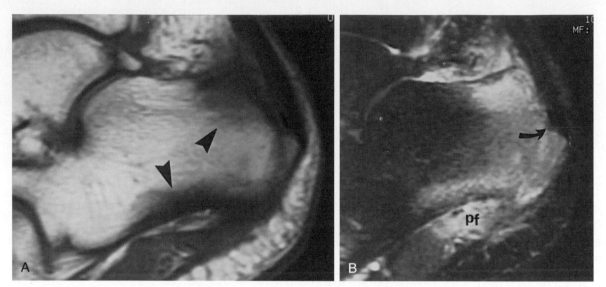

Figure 17–155

Plantar fasciitis: MR imaging. Juvenile-onset seronegative enthesopathy—arthropathy (SEA) syndrome. In this 17 year old man, a routine radiograph (not shown) revealed erosions and proliferation in the plantar and posterior surfaces of the calcaneus.

A A sagittal T1-weighted (TR/TE, 600/13) spin echo MR image shows loss of signal intensity in the plantar and posterior portions of the calcaneus (arrowheads), related to edema caused by inflammation.

B A sagittal STIR MR image (TR/TE, 4000/40; inversion time, 160 msec) shows marrow edema, an erosion of the calcaneus (curved arrow), and inflammation in the plantar muscles and fascia (pf).

(From Azouz EM, et al: Skel Radiol *24*:399, 1995.)

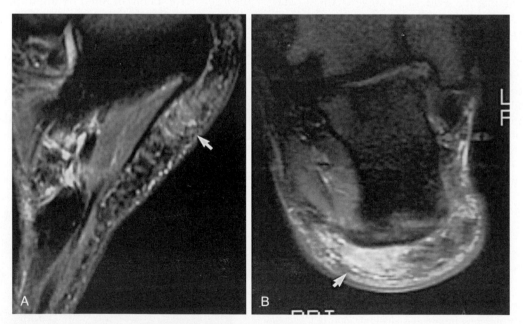

Figure 17–156

Heel pad injury: MR imaging. Sagittal (TR/TE, 3550/40; inversion time, 150 msec) **(A)** and coronal (TR/TE, 3316/21; inversion time, 150 msec) **(B)** STIR MR images show edema (arrows) of the heel pad, which was related to a malfunctioning clutch pedal of an automobile. The plantar fascia is intact. (Courtesy of J. Healy, M.D., San Diego, California.)

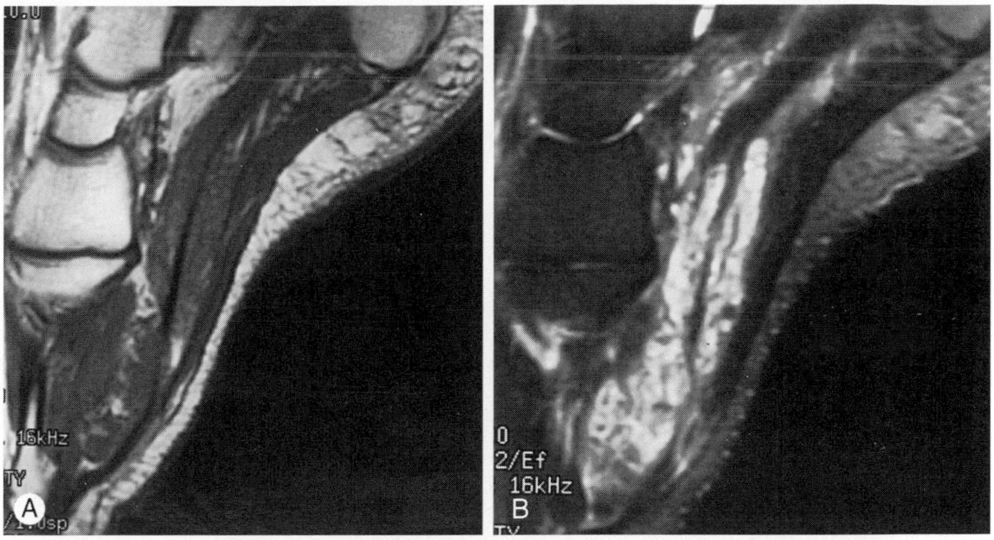

Figure 17–157
Hemangioma: MR imaging. Sagittal T1-weighted (TR/TE, 600/17) **(A)** and T2-weighted (TR/TE, 3000/85) **(B)** spin echo MR images, the latter obtained with fat suppression, show a hemangioma in the plantar musculature. Note the tubular regions of high signal intensity in **B**. (Courtesy of D. Witte, M.D., Memphis, Tennessee.)

spin echo or STIR MR images.[478] Enhancement of signal intensity is variable after intravenous administration of a gadolinium compound, although marked enhancement may be encountered (see Figs. 17–159 and 17–160).[480] In general, correct diagnosis is provided by the location of the lesion and, in some cases, the low signal intensity apparent on the T2-weighted images, although the latter feature may be apparent in other lesions, such as clear cell sarcoma.[480] Furthermore, fibrosis (unlike plantar fibromatosis) in the subcalcaneal fat may lead to focal hypointensity in this region.[480]

Plantar Infections

The plantar aspect of the foot is especially vulnerable to soft tissue infection. Foreign bodies, puncture wounds, or skin ulceration from weight-bearing can represent the portal of entry for various organisms. In a diabetic patient, soft tissue breakdown over certain pressure points (such as the metatarsal heads and calcaneus) leads to infection that is combined with vascular and neurologic abnormalities.

There are three plantar muscle compartments—medial, intermediate, and lateral (Fig. 17–161).[481–483] These compartments are separated from each other by two intermuscular septa extending from the plantar fascia to the overlying osseous structures. The medial compartment contains the abductor hallucis and flexor hallucis brevis muscles and the flexor hallucis longus tendon. The lateral compartment contains the abductor and short flexor muscle and, when present, opponens muscle of the fifth toe. The intermediate, or central, compartment contains the flexor digitorum brevis muscle, the flexor digitorum longus tendon, the quadratus plantar muscle, the lumbrical muscles, and the adductor hallucis muscle. The flexor hallucis longus tendon passes through the proximal aspect of this compartment before entering the medial compartment.[483] Cadaveric injection studies[481] have emphasized that (1) the intermediate compartment contains the greatest amount of

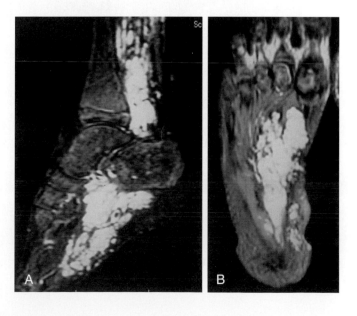

Figure 17–158
Venous malformation: MR imaging. The extent of the malformation is well shown in a sagittal STIR (TR/TE, 3700/51; inversion time, 150 msec) MR image **(A)** and a transverse fat-suppressed fast spin echo (TR/TE, 3000/19) MR image **(B)**. (Courtesy of W. Tam, M.D., Oklahoma City, Oklahoma.)

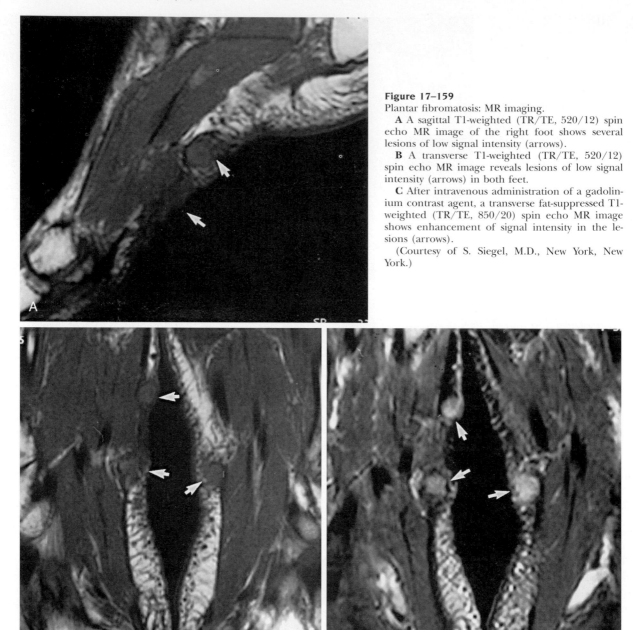

potential space; when this compartment becomes filled, continued infusion of fluid will produce extravasation either into the medial compartment or more importantly along the flexor hallucis longus tendon into the lower leg; (2) the lateral compartment has the least amount of potential space; extravasation from this area occurs into the dorsal compartment or plantar fat of the foot; and (3) the medial compartment has a potential space somewhat greater than that of the lateral compartment and less than that of the intermediate compartment; extravasation from this area commonly occurs into the intermediate compartment.

These experimental observations can be applied to the evaluation of soft tissue infections in the plantar aspect of the foot (Fig. 17–162). Soft tissue dissemination of infection can occur via the medial, lateral, or intermediate compartment; in these instances, osteomyelitis and septic arthritis can be seen to be remote from the initial site of soft tissue contamination. Furthermore, the intermediate compartment provides a pathway by which infection can spread from the plantar aspect of the foot into the lower leg (Fig. 17–163). The existence of these avenues within the soft tissues in the foot that allow dissemination of localized infection underscores the need for early diagnosis in the treatment of such infection, especially in a vulnerable person, such as the patient with diabetes mellitus. Plain film radiography often is insensitive and inadequate in this regard, stimu-

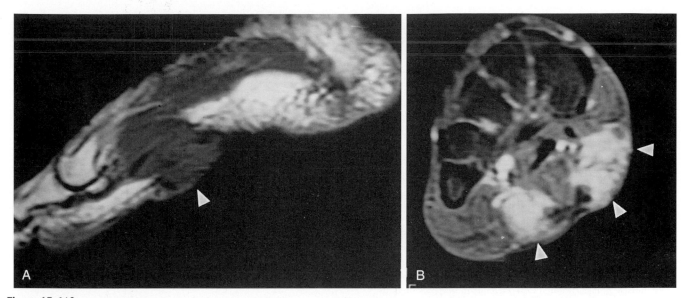

Figure 17–160

Plantar fibromatosis: MR imaging.

A A sagittal T1-weighted (TR/TE, 500/11) spin echo MR image shows a lesion (arrowhead) of low signal intensity in the plantar soft tissues.

B After intravenous administration of a gadolinium compound, a coronal fat-suppressed T1-weighted (TR/TE, 600/14) spin echo MR image shows enhancement of signal intensity in several lesions (arrowheads).

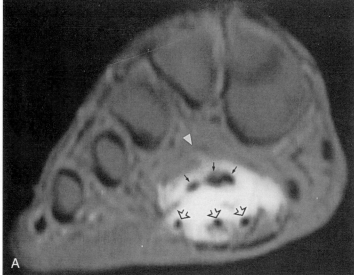

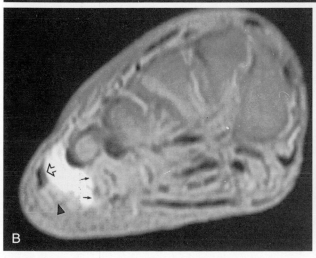

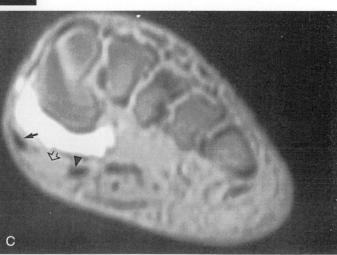

Figure 17–161

Plantar muscle compartments: Anatomy. These coronal fat-suppressed T1-weighted (TR/TE, 600/20) spin echo MR images were obtained after injection of a gadolinium-containing contrast agent into various plantar compartments.

A Intermediate (central) compartment. Note contrast material surrounding the flexor digitorus longus (solid arrows) and flexor digitorum brevis (open arrows) tendons. Also note lack of contrast material surrounding the adductor hallucis muscle (arrowhead) in the deep subcompartment.

B Lateral compartment. Contrast material in the lateral compartment outlines lateral aponeurotic septum (solid arrows) and displaces the abductor digiti minimi (open arrow) and flexor digiti minimi (arrowhead) muscles lateral to the fifth metatarsal bone.

C Medial compartment. Contrast material in the medial compartment displaces the abductor hallucis muscle (solid arrow), the flexor hallucis brevis muscle (open arrow), and the flexor hallucis longus tendon (arrowhead).

(**A, B,** From Goodwin DW, et al: Radiology *196*:623, 1995.)

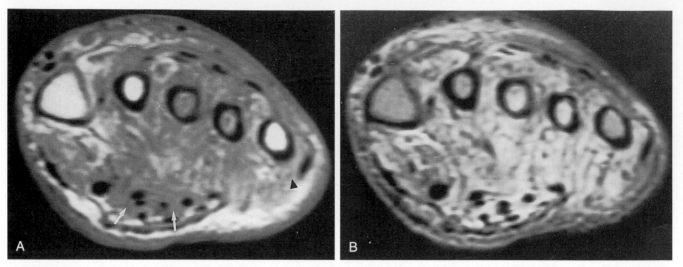

Figure 17–162

Plantar muscle compartments: Osteomyelitis in diabetes mellitus.

   A A coronal T1-weighted (TR/TE, 983/13) spin echo MR image shows abnormal low signal intensity in the marrow of the third and fourth metatarsal bones. Fluid is present in the central (arrows) and lateral (arrowhead) compartments.

   B On a coronal T2-weighted (TR/TE, 2500/80) spin echo MR image, the involved bone and soft tissues show high signal intensity.

   (From Goodwin D, et al: Radiology *196*:623, 1995.)

lating a search for other diagnostic techniques. Scintigraphy using a variety of radiopharmaceutical agents, CT, and MR imaging are three methods that provide information regarding the presence of soft tissue infection. With scintigraphy, problems arise in differentiating infection confined to soft tissue and that affecting adjacent bones or joints or both. With CT, the separation of suppuration, edema, and fibrosis in the soft tissue is difficult. MR imaging may represent the most sensitive and specific imaging technique, although diagnostic problems and pitfalls may be encountered.

   Puncture wounds of the plantar aspect of the foot can lead to osteomyelitis and septic arthritis. These injuries are especially prominent in children who walk barefoot, exposing the unprotected foot to nails, glass, splinters, thorns, and other sharp objects. The infective organisms

can vary, but gram-negative agents such as *Pseudomonas aeruginosa* frequently are implicated. Ultrasonography, CT scanning, and MR imaging may provide useful information in these cases (Figs. 17–164, 17–165, and 17–166).

Abnormalities of Nerves

Entrapment Neuropathies

Entrapment neuropathies occurring in the foot and ankle are described in Chapter 11. The most important of these relate to compression of the posterior tibial nerve in the medial aspect of the ankle (i.e., the tarsal

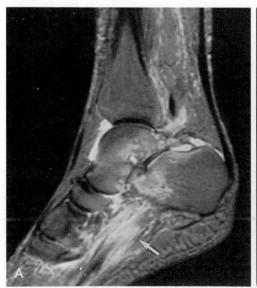
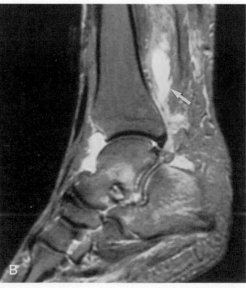

Figure 17–163

Plantar muscle compartments: Osteomyelitis in diabetes mellitus. As shown on sagittal fat-suppressed fast spin echo MR images (TR/TE, 4000/34), infection in the soft tissues in the plantar aspect of the foot (arrow, **A**), in this case in the intermediate compartment, can spread into the calf (arrow, **B**). Note osteomyelitis with high signal intensity in the talus and calcaneus. (Courtesy of D. Goodwin, M.D., Hanover, New Hampshire.)

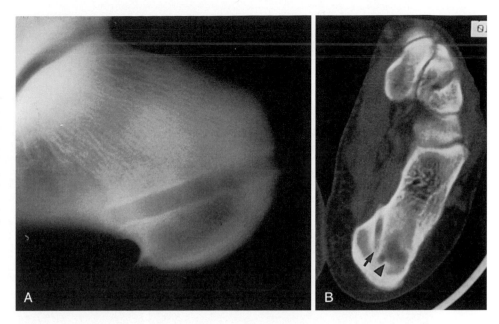

Figure 17–164

Puncture wounds: CT scanning. This 43 year old woman had a 1 year history of heel pain. She could not recall any injury.

A Conventional tomogram shows a channel-like radiolucent area extending obliquely through the calcaneus.

B A transverse CT scan shows the channel (arrow) and an area of osteolysis (arrowhead). At surgery, a toothpick, 5 cm long and surrounded by granulation tissue, was found, protruding from the posterior aspect of the calcaneus.

(Courtesy of D.E. Freedman, M.D., Nashua, New Hampshire.)

tunnel syndrome) and entrapment of the deep peroneal nerve.

The tarsal tunnel is located behind and below the medial malleolus; its floor is bony and its roof is formed by the flexor retinaculum. The resulting fibro-osseous channel allows passage of the tendons of the tibialis posterior, flexor digitorum longus, and flexor hallucis longus muscles, the posterior tibial artery and vein, and the posterior tibial nerve. Causes of compression of the posterior tibial nerve within the tarsal tunnel include tumors of nerves and other structures (Fig. 17–167), tenosynovitis, ganglion cysts (Figs. 17–168 and 17–169), posttraumatic fibrosis, and dilated or tortuous veins. Many of the causes can be defined with CT or MR imaging.[484–487]

Entrapment of the deep peroneal nerve in the ankle and foot may occur in several different locations. The most common site of compression is beneath the infe-

rior extensor retinaculum, a condition referred to as the anterior tarsal tunnel syndrome.[488, 489] The typical site of involvement is subjacent to the superior edge of this retinaculum, close to the extensor hallucis longus tendon. Entrapment of the nerve in a more distal location may relate to osteophytes that form at the talonavicular, naviculocuneiform, or tarsometatarsal joints or to an os intermetatarseum.[490, 516] Deep peroneal nerve entrapment may occur in skiers, owing to tight-fitting ski boots, or in soccer players who kick the ball with the dorsum of the foot.[489, 490] Clinical findings vary according to the site of entrapment but may include pain, numbness, muscle weakness, and paresthesia.

Sural nerve entrapment may occur in the ankle, generally related to fibrosis occurring as a response to an ankle sprain, fracture (e.g., calcaneal or fifth metatarsal fracture), Achilles tendon rupture, or a ganglion cyst.[490–492] Entrapment of the superficial peroneal nerve, particu-

Figure 17–165

Puncture wounds: MR imaging. This 5 year old boy stepped on a nail, which penetrated his sandals. Fever and pain developed over a 3 week period.

A A sagittal T1-weighted (TR/TE, 400/16) spin echo MR image shows abnormal signal intensity in the cuboid bone and plantar soft tissues.

B On the sagittal STIR MR image (TR/TE, 2383/40; inversion time, 165 msec), note the high signal intensity in the cuboid bone, representing osteomyelitis, as well as in the plantar soft tissues (arrows). *Pseudomonas aeruginosa* was cultured from a bone specimen.

(Courtesy of R. Kerr, M.D., Los Angeles, California.)

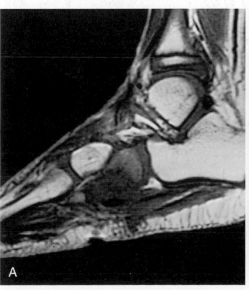
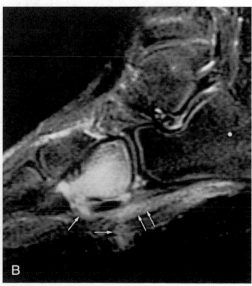

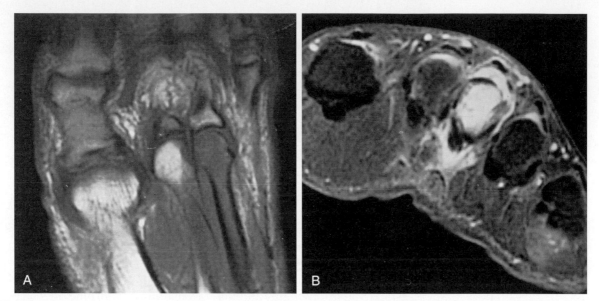

Figure 17–166
Puncture wounds: MR imaging. After a puncture wound occurred in the plantar soft tissues, this 55 year old man developed signs of local infection.
   A A transverse T1-weighted (TR/TE, 600/14) spin echo MR image shows low signal intensity in the marrow of the third metatarsal bone.
   B A coronal fat-suppressed T1-weighted (TR/TE, 750/14) spin echo image obtained after intravenous gadolinium injection shows enhancement of signal intensity in the involved metatarsal bone and adjacent plantar soft tissues.
   (Courtesy of S. K. Brahme, M.D., La Jolla, California.)

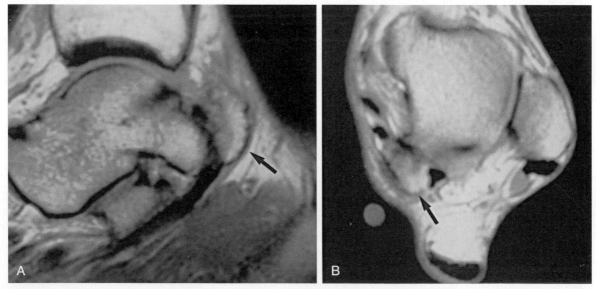

Figure 17–167
Dysplasia epiphysealis hemimelica (Trevor's disease): MR imaging. As shown in sagittal proton density (TR/TE, 1800/20) **(A)** and transaxial proton density (TR/TE, 2000/20) **(B)** spin echo MR images, an osteochondroma (arrows) arising from the posteromedial surface of the talus can lead to compression of the posterior tibial nerve. (Courtesy of S. Kingston, M.D. and R. Kerr, M.D., Los Angeles, California.)

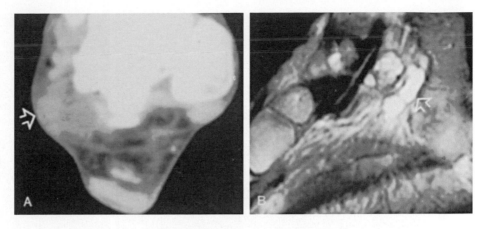

Figure 17–168
Ganglion cysts: CT scanning and MR imaging. Both of these ganglion cysts, which developed in the medial aspect of the ankle, led to compression of the posterior tibial nerve. A transaxial CT scan (**A**) in one patient and a sagittal T2-weighted (TR/TE, 2000/75) spin echo MR image (**B**) in a second patient show the location of the ganglion cysts (open arrows). (**A**, Courtesy of C. Chen, M.D., Kaohsiung, Taiwan; **B**, Courtesy of S. Eilenberg, M.D., San Diego, California.)

larly in the distal portion of the leg and ankle, also occurs, especially as a result of fibrosis secondary to ankle injuries.[490]

Interdigital Neuromas

Interdigital neuromas, or Morton's neuromas, are not true tumors but rather represent a fibrotic response that occurs in and about the plantar digital nerves.[493–495] Interdigital neuromas are encountered most frequently in young and middle-aged persons, especially women. A unilateral distribution predominates but is not universal. The interspace between the third and fourth toes is affected most commonly (Fig. 17–170). The third plantar digital nerve may be most vulnerable, owing to its large size and relatively fixed position.[490] Clinical findings include pain at the level of the metatarsophalangeal joint that may radiate into the adjacent toes. Trauma

with resulting fibrosis appears to be important in the pathogenesis of this condition. Because of its persistently low signal intensity in both T1-weighted and T2-weighted spin echo MR images (see Chapter 11), interdigital neuromas generally can be differentiated from true neuromas, as well as other lesions of nerves, which show high signal intensity in T2-weighted spin echo MR images (Fig. 17–171 and 17–172).

Bone Abnormalities

Many abnormalities affect the bones about the ankle and in the foot. These include occult fractures (Figs. 17–173 and 17–174) (see Chapter 8),[517, 518] transient or migratory bone marrow edema or osteoporosis, osteonecrosis, osteomyelitis, and tumors and tumor-like conditions. Imaging evaluation of these conditions usu-

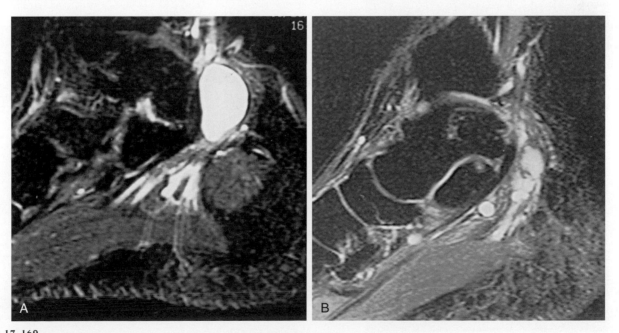

Figure 17–169
Ganglion cysts: MR imaging.
  A An example of one classic location of a ganglion cyst (adjacent to the flexor tendons and neurovascular bundle) is shown on a sagittal fast spin echo STIR MR image (TR/TE, 4500/42; inversion time, 150 msec).
  B In a second patient, a smaller ganglion cyst in a similar location is shown on a sagittal STIR MR image (TR/TE, 2117/30; inversion time, 160 msec). (Courtesy of S. Eilenberg, M.D., San Diego, California.)

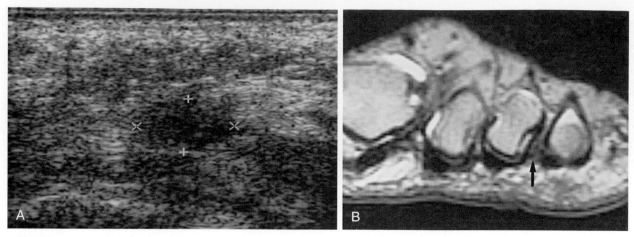

Figure 17–170

Interdigital (Morton's) neuromas.

A Ultrasonography. A plantar sonogram demonstrates a hypoechoic mass (outlined by markers) between the third and fourth metatarsal bones. (Courtesy of M. van Holsbeeck, M.D., Detroit, Michigan, and J. Jacobson, M.D., San Diego, California.)

B MR imaging. A coronal T2-weighted (TR/TE, 2000/70) spin echo MR image shows a lesion (arrow) of low signal intensity between the third and fourth metatarsal heads. (Courtesy of D. Berthoty, M.D., Las Vegas, Nevada.)

ally begins with routine radiography. Bone scintigraphy provides a sensitive but nonspecific means of further evaluation of these processes, particularly if they are radiographically occult. CT allows more specific assessment of most lesions, and MR imaging provides both sensitivity and specificity in their analysis.

Osteonecrosis

Osteonecrosis involving the bones about the ankle and in the foot is uncommon. Occasionally, however, widespread osteonecrosis in these sites may be seen, particularly in association with administration of corticosteroid medications or in patients with hemoglobinopathies or systemic lupus erythematosus (Figs. 17–175 and 17–176). Typical MR imaging features are encountered, allowing specific diagnosis.

Spontaneous osteonecrosis of the tarsal navicular bone in adults is termed Mueller-Weiss syndrome. Bilat-

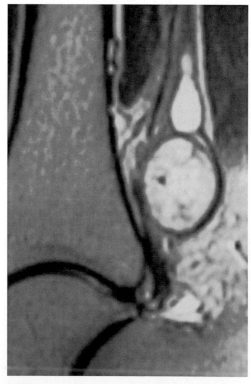

Figure 17–171

Neurilemoma of tibial nerve: MR imaging. A sagittal T2-weighted (TR/TE, 3000/100) fast spin echo MR image shows the large tumor of high signal intensity. (Courtesy of P. Kindynis, M.D., Geneva, Switzerland.)

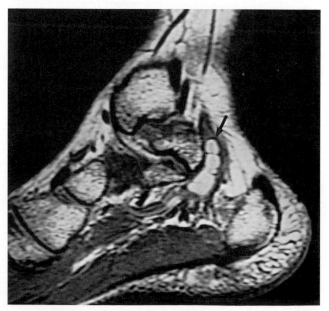

Figure 17–172

Intraneural ganglion cyst: MR imaging. A sagittal gradient echo MR image shows a lobulated mass (arrow) of high signal intensity behind the medial malleolus, which at the time of surgery proved to be a ganglion cyst within the posterior tibial nerve. (Courtesy of G. Greenway, M.D., Dallas, Texas.)

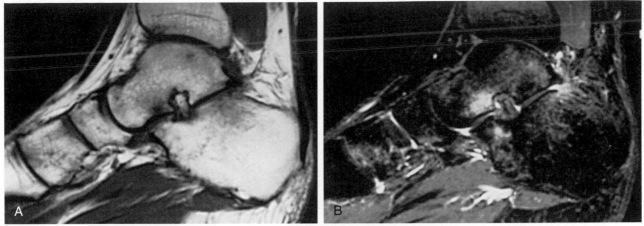

Figure 17–173
Occult bone injuries: MR imaging, chronic overuse syndrome. In this 24 year old soldier, diffuse abnormalities in the marrow of the tarsal bones, shown in a sagittal T1-weighted (TR/TE, 580/15) spin echo MR image **(A)** and in a sagittal STIR (TR/TE, 3500/19; inversion time, 140 msec) MR image **(B)**, are consistent with trabecular microfractures, or bone bruises.

Figure 17–174
Occult fractures: MR imaging.

A, B Insufficiency fracture of fibula. A fracture line (arrows) and adjacent marrow and soft tissue edema are evident on a sagittal fast spin echo STIR MR image (TR/TE, 3200/39; inversion time, 120 msec) **(A)** and a coronal fat-suppressed T1-weighted (TR/TE, 600/11) spin echo MR image obtained after intravenous gadolinium administration **(B)**. (Courtesy of D. Goodwin, M.D., Hanover, New Hampshire.)

C Insufficiency fractures of calcaneus and cuboid bone. This sagittal T1-weighted (TR/TE, 600/20) spin echo MR image shows irregular fracture lines (arrows) and, in the cuboid bone, adjacent marrow edema. (Courtesy of S. Eilenberg, M.D., San Diego, California.)

D Fatigue fracture of medial malleolus. Observe bone marrow edema (arrow) in the malleolus on a transaxial fat-suppressed fast spin echo MR image (TR/TE, 4000/80).

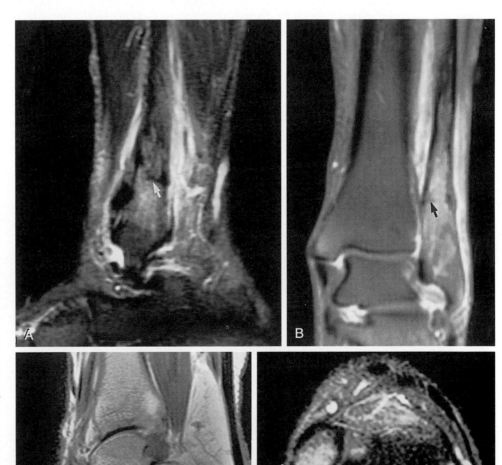

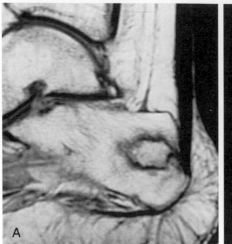

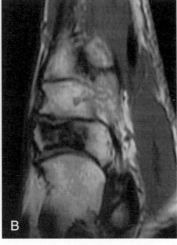

Figure 17–175
Osteonecrosis: MR imaging.
   A Steroid-induced osteonecrosis of the calcaneus. A sagittal T1-weighted (TR/TE, 500/16) spin echo MR image reveals the classic appearance of osteonecrosis involving the calcaneus. (Courtesy of R. Abrahim-Zadeh, M.D., Valhalla, New York.)
   B Posttraumatic osteonecrosis of the navicular bone. A transverse T1-weighted (TR/TE, 550/15) spin echo MR image shows involvement of the medial portion of the navicular bone.

eral abnormalities are more common than unilateral disease. Women are affected more frequently than men, and pes planus and valgus deformity of the ankle are associated features. Initial radiographic alterations (Fig. 17–177) include a loss of volume and an increase in radiodensity in the lateral aspect of the tarsal navicular bone. The tarsal navicular assumes a comma-like shape because of lateral compression. Subsequently, dorsal protrusion and fragmentation of the bone may become evident. CT allows precise delineation of the sites of fracture and fragmentation. MR imaging shows a homogeneous decrease in the signal intensity of the navicular bone on T1-weighted spin echo images (see Fig. 17–177). The changes in signal intensity are more variable on T2-weighted images. Effusions in neighboring joints may be observed.

The Mueller-Weiss syndrome certainly is distinct from the well-recognized osteochondrosis of the tarsal navicular bone occurring in children (Köhler's disease). The precise cause of the Mueller-Weiss syndrome is not clear,

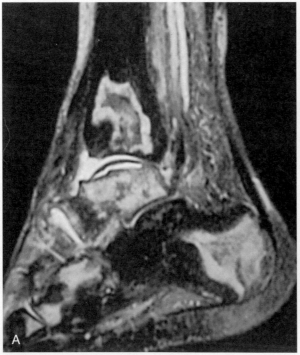

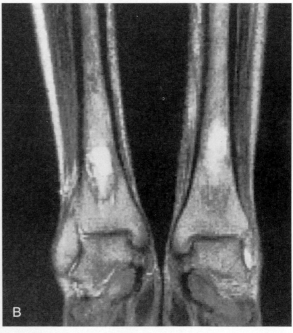

Figure 17–176
Osteonecrosis: MR imaging.
   A This sagittal fast spin echo STIR (TR/TE, 3000/32; inversion time, 150 msec) MR image shows classic features of osteonecrosis involving the distal portion of the tibia, the talus, the calcaneus, and the cuboid bone. Note the crescent-like lesion in the dome of the talus. (Courtesy of D. Goodwin, M.D., Hanover, New Hampshire.)
   B Marrow ischemia in the distal tibial metaphyses in a patient with sickle cell anemia is shown as regions of high signal intensity in a coronal T2-weighted spin echo MR image. Note the extended pattern of hematopoietic marrow in this patient. (From Moore SG, et al: Radiology 179:345, 1991.)

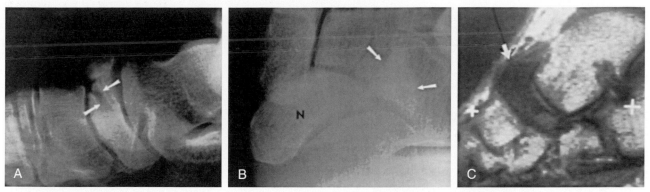

Figure 17–177

Spontaneous osteonecrosis of the tarsal navicular bone (Mueller-Weiss syndrome): MR imaging. This 49 year old obese woman had tarsal pain. No evidence of underlying systemic disease was present.

A A lateral radiograph shows an oblique cleft (arrows), presumably a stress fracture, in the navicular bone. The radiodensity of the bone is increased, with dorsal displacement of the lateral fragment.

B The frontal radiograph shows medial displacement of a comma-shaped navicular bone (N). The lateral fracture fragment overlies the cuboid and lateral cuneiform bones (arrows).

C A sagittal T1-weighted (TR/TE, 600/20) spin echo MR image reveals loss of signal intensity in the marrow of a dorsally displaced navicular bone (arrow).

(From Haller J, et al: AJR *151*:355, 1988. Copyright 1988, American Roentgen Ray Society.)

however. Osteonecrosis of the tarsal navicular bone also may accompany systemic diseases, such as systemic lupus erythematosus, and may complicate corticosteroid administration. Insufficiency fractures of this bone may be evident in patients with rheumatoid arthritis, chronic renal disease, and diabetes mellitus.

Osteomyelitis

Although hematogenous osteomyelitis may involve the bones in the ankle and foot (Fig. 17–178), osteomyelitis in these locations is encountered far more commonly in the patient with diabetes mellitus, in whom soft tissue

Figure 17–178

Hematogenous osteomyelitis: MR imaging.

A A coronal oblique CT scan in this 11 year old boy shows an osteolytic focus in a metaphyseal-equivalent area of the left calcaneus. The adjacent apophyseal cartilaginous plate is minimally irregular.

B The transverse T1-weighted (TR/TE, 766/13) spin echo MR image reveals the focus of osteomyelitis with surrounding marrow edema.

C Involvement of the adjacent apophyseal cartilaginous plate, apophysis, and posterior soft tissues, as well as the extent of marrow edema, is more readily apparent on a transverse fat-suppressed fast spin echo MR image (TR/TE, 3633/108).

(Courtesy of P. Fenton, M.D., Kingston, Ontario, Canada.)

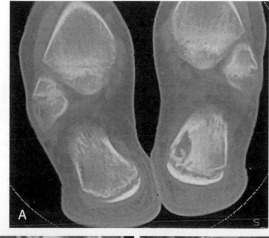

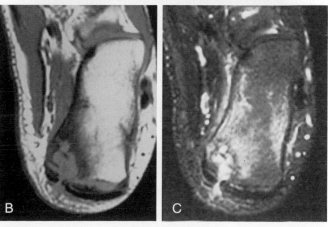

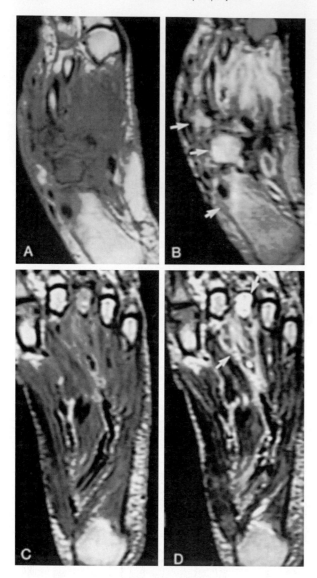

Figure 17–179

Diabetic foot infection: MR imaging.

A, B Transverse T1-weighted (TR/TE, 700/12) **(A)** and T2-weighted (TR/TE, 2000/80) **(B)** spin echo MR images show the extent of soft tissue and bone involvement in the plantar aspect of the foot. The process is of low signal intensity in **A** and of high signal intensity in **B** and affects the fifth metatarsal base, cuboid bone, and calcaneus, better seen in **B** (arrows).

C, D In a different patient, proton density (TR/TE, 2000/30) **(C)** and T2-weighted (TR/TE, 2000/70) **(D)** spin echo MR images in the transverse plane show changes in signal intensity within areas of soft tissue and bone infection similar to those in **A** and **B.** Note the high signal intensity in the infected soft tissues and head of the third metatarsal bone in **D** (arrows).

infection can lead to contamination of nearby bones (and joints). The assessment of infection in the feet of diabetic patients provides unique challenges. Although reported data indicate the value of scintigraphic methods, particularly ^{111}In-labeled leukocyte imaging with or without bone scintigraphy in this assessment, the day-to-day clinical experience of many physicians suggests otherwise. A normal bone scan virtually excludes the presence of osteomyelitis, but this is relatively uncommon in diabetic patients whose routine radiographs of the feet reveal changes of soft tissue infection, neuropathic osteoarthropathy, or both. The hyperemia associated with either process can lead to positive results with three-phase bone scintigraphy. Although ^{67}Ga-citrate scintigraphy may increase the specificity for diagnosing osteomyelitis, uptake of this agent in neuropathic osteoarthropathic sites is encountered. Decreased blood flow and possible impaired leukocyte responsiveness limit the sensitivity achievable with ^{111}In-labeled leukocyte scintigraphy in diabetic foot infections, although specificity may be increased. Reports indicate that the finding of a definitely increased uptake on leukocyte

scans has a high positive predictive value but a somewhat lower sensitivity in the diagnosis of osteomyelitis complicating soft tissue infection, whereas absence of increased leukocyte uptake in or near bone makes the diagnosis of osteomyelitis very unlikely. When increased leukocyte uptake is subtle or cannot be localized exclusively to soft tissue, other imaging techniques may be necessary.

It is not surprising, therefore, that MR imaging has been applied to the analysis of infections in the feet of diabetic patients. Although high signal intensity in the bone marrow on T2-weighted spin echo and STIR images and on T1-weighted spin echo MR images (with or without fat saturation) after the intravenous administration of gadolinium contrast agent is compatible with the diagnosis of osteomyelitis (Fig. 17–179 and 17–180), it is not a specific finding (Figs. 17–181 and 17–182). Some investigators indicate that neuropathic osteoarthropathy in the absence of coexistent infection is accompanied by persistent low signal intensity in the bone marrow on T2-weighted spin echo MR images, although this is not a constant finding. Furthermore, sympathetic joint effusions in the feet of diabetic pa-

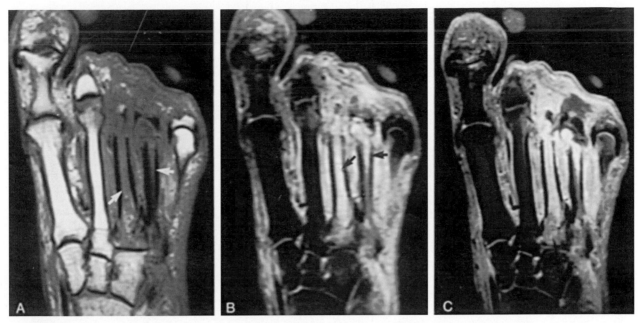

Figure 17–180
Diabetic foot infection: MR imaging. This 63 year old man had required amputation of the third toe at the level of the metatarsophalangeal joint for control of infection. He later developed clinical manifestations of recurrent infection.

A Transverse T1-weighted (TR/TE, 700/15) spin echo MR image shows abnormally low signal intensity in the third and fourth metatarsal bones (arrows) and in the adjacent soft tissues. The head of the second metatarsal bone also appears to be involved.

B Transverse short tau inversion recovery (STIR) image (TR/TE, 1800/25; inversion time, 160 msec) reveals high signal intensity in these metatarsal bones (arrows) and soft tissues.

C Transverse T1-weighted (TR/TE, 900/13) fat suppressed (ChemSat) image obtained in conjunction with intravenous administration of gadolinium contrast agent gives information similar to that in **B**. A third and fourth ray resection confirmed the presence of osteomyelitis.

tients produce findings on MR imaging that are very similar to those of septic arthritis, and differentiation of soft tissue edema and soft tissue infection with MR imaging in this clinical setting is a problem.

The differentiation of osteomyelitis (with or without neuropathic osteoarthropathy) and neuropathic osteoarthropathy alone in the diabetic foot using MR imaging is improved if associated findings of infection are sought. These findings include cortical interruption, enhancement of signal intensity in the rim of an abscess within the marrow cavity, sequestrum formation, extension of a sinus tract from the bone to the skin surface, and cellulitis adjacent to an osseous abnormality (Fig. 17–183).

MR imaging is extremely valuable in excluding the diagnosis of osteomyelitis. If no abnormalities in the

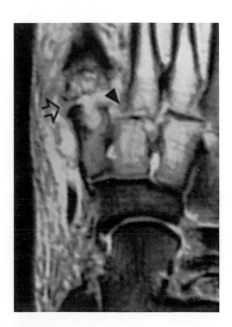

Figure 17–181
Diabetic neuropathic osteoarthropathy and osteomyelitis: MR imaging. A transverse short tau inversion recovery (STIR) image (TR/TE, 1800/20; inversion time, 125 msec) shows high signal intensity in the marrow of the second and third metatarsal bones, in the intermediate and lateral cuneiforms, and in the soft tissues. Note the neuropathic changes about the first tarsometatarsal joint (arrow) and a Lisfranc pattern of subluxation (arrowhead). Differentiating sites of osteomyelitis and of neuropathic disease with marrow edema in such cases is difficult.

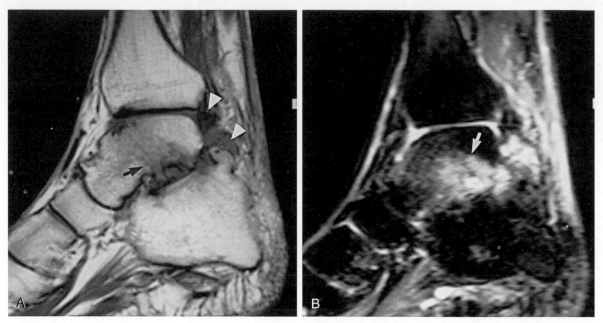

Figure 17–182

Diabetic neuropathic osteoarthropathy and osteomyelitis: MR imaging. This 71 year old man with diabetes mellitus and peripheral neuropathy had documented septic arthritis of the ankle and posterior subtalar joint. Routine radiography (not shown) revealed joint effusions and bone destruction with indistinct margins.

A A sagittal T1-weighted (TR/TE, 700/15) spin echo MR image shows fluid (arrowheads) in both the ankle and the posterior subtalar joint and abnormally low signal intensity in the marrow, especially in the talus (arrow). Subcutaneous edema about the Achilles tendon and posterior surface of the calcaneus is evident.

B On a sagittal short tau inversion recovery (STIR) MR image (TR/TE, 4132/19; inversion time, 140 msec), note the high signal intensity in the talus (arrow), in the subcutaneous tissue, and of the joint fluid.

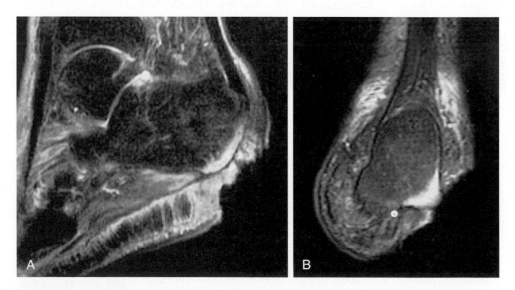

Figure 17–183

Diabetic osteomyelitis: MR imaging.

A A sagittal fast spin echo STIR MR image (TR/TE, 3800/17; inversion time, 150 msec) demonstrates a large skin ulceration of the heel and abnormally high signal intensity in the adjacent soft tissues and posterior surface of the calcaneus.

B On a coronal fat-suppressed fast spin echo MR image (TR/TE, 4400/120), note the involvement of the calcaneus.

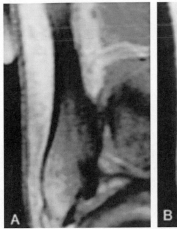
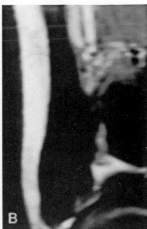

Figure 17–184
Cellulitis: MR imaging.
   A Coronal gadolinium-enhanced, fat suppressed T1-weighted (TR/TE, 517/12) spin echo MR image shows high signal intensity in the inflamed soft tissues but no marrow abnormalities in the adjacent fibula.
   B Coronal STIR MR image (TR/TE, 2100/35; inversion time, 160 msec) demonstrates similar findings.
   (Courtesy of M. Pathria, M.D., and D. Bates, M.D., San Diego, California.)

signal intensity of the marrow are encountered when sensitive MR imaging protocols are used (Fig. 17–184), the diagnosis of osteomyelitis is very unlikely.

Bone Tumors and Tumor-like Lesions

Although a great variety of tumors and tumor-like lesions may involve the bones about the ankle and in the foot (Table 17–5), MR imaging in most cases provides a sensitive technique that lacks specificity. Exceptions to this include intraosseous lipomas (which predominate in the calcaneous and may contain tissue with signal intensity characteristics identical to those of fat) (Fig. 17–185) and aneurysmal bone cysts (which may reveal fluid levels) (Fig. 17–186). Metastatic disease involving

Table 17–5. TUMORS AND TUMOR-LIKE LESIONS OF BONE: FREQUENCY OF INVOLVEMENT OF BONES IN THE FOOT AND ANKLE

Lesion	Frequency %*
Enostosis	5
Osteoid osteoma	11
Osteoblastoma	8
Osteosarcoma	1
Enchondroma	7
Periosteal chondroma	5
Chondroblastoma	10
Chondromyxoid fibroma	16
Osteochondroma	6
Chondrosarcoma	3
Nonossifying fibroma	1
Desmoplastic fibroma	2
Fibrosarcoma	2
Giant cell tumor	2
Malignant fibrous histiocytoma	2
Lipoma	15
Hemangioma	5
Hemangiopericytoma	4
Hemangioendothelioma	6
Neurofibroma/neurilemoma	3
Simple bone cyst	1
Aneurysmal bone cyst	8
Adamantinoma	1
Ewing's sarcoma	3

*Approximate figures based on analysis of major reports containing the greatest number of cases.

the bones in the ankle and foot arises most often from carcinomas of the lung and kidney, although exceptions to this rule are encountered (Figs. 17–187 and 17–188).

The nonspecificity of findings on MR images in patients with benign and malignant bone tumors about the ankle and in the foot deserves emphasis (Figs. 17–189 and 17–190). Often, it is the routine radiographic abnormalities that allow correct diagnosis.

Miscellaneous Abnormalities

Metatarsalgia

Pain involving the metatarsal region of the foot is an extremely common complaint. Such pain occurring after a physical injury can relate to a variety of fractures or dislocations or to capsular disruption (turf toe), as described earlier in this chapter. Additional causes of metatarsalgia include biomechanical disturbances of the forefoot related to variations in length of the metatarsal bones, chronic instability of the metatarsophalangeal joints (especially the second) often related to participation in sports,[496] Morton's interdigital neuromas, synovitis, stress fractures, and Freiberg's infraction (Figs. 17–191 and 17–192). In addition to routine radiography scintigraphy, ultrasonography, CT scanning, or MR imaging may be diagnostically helpful in some cases (Figs. 17–193 and 17–194).

Sesamoid Dysfunction

Pain in the plantar aspect of the first metatarsophalangeal joint may relate to abnormalities of the two sesamoid bones that are located in the tendons of the flexor hallucis brevis muscle. Such abnormalities include fractures, dislocations, osteomyelitis, osteochondritis (which may be secondary to osteonecrosis), and sesamoiditis (a diagnosis of exclusion which may be secondary to cartilage or bone injury). Routine or advanced imaging methods may be used to investigate these conditions (Fig. 17–195).

Text continued on page 918

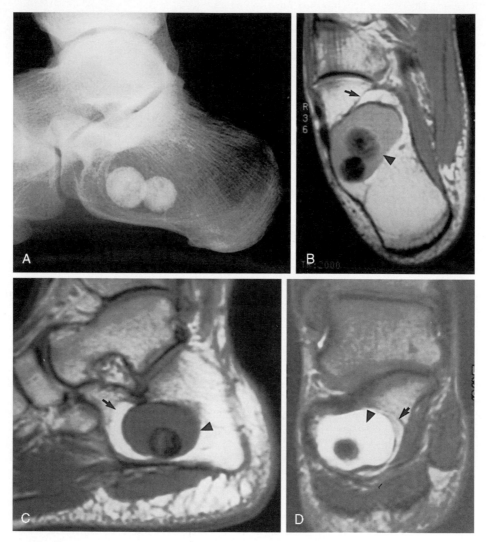

Figure 17–185

Intraosseous lipoma: MR imaging.

A A routine radiograph reveals a cyst-like lesion of the calcaneus containing two foci of calcification.

B A transverse proton density–weighted (TR/TE, 2000/16) spin echo MR image shows the calcaneal lesion with its regions of calcification. Portions of the lesion (arrow) reveal signal intensity characteristics of fat; others demonstrate signal intensity characteristics of fluid (arrowhead).

C A sagittal T1-weighted (TR/TE, 566/15) spin echo MR image again reveals the fluid (arrowhead) and fatty (arrow) components of the lesion and one area of calcification.

D A coronal T2-weighted (TR/TE, 2000/80) spin echo MR image documents fluid (arrowhead) and fat (arrow) in the lesion.

(Courtesy of T. Armbuster, M.D., Fort Wayne, Indiana.)

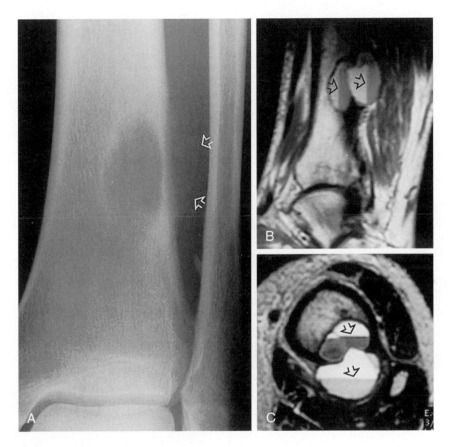

Figure 17–186

Aneurysmal bone cyst: MR imaging.

A In a 42 year old man, a routine radiograph reveals an osteolytic lesion in the distal portion of the tibia. Although its features are not entirely specific, the presence of an osseous shell (arrows) at the margin of the lesion is suggestive of the diagnosis of an aneurysmal bone cyst.

B, C Sagittal T1-weighted (TR/TE, 600/15) spin echo **(B)** and transaxial fast spin echo (TR/TE, 5500/90) **(C)** MR images confirm the intraosseous and extraosseous components of this well-marginated lesion. Note the highly characteristic fluid levels (arrows).

(Courtesy of L. Vaughn, M.D., San Diego, California.)

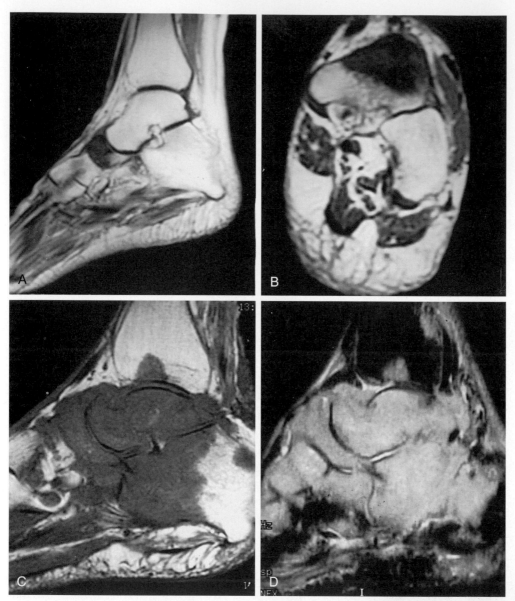

Figure 17–187
Skeletal metastasis: MR imaging.

A, B Skeletal metastasis (carcinoma of the breast). Sagittal (TR/TE, 749/16) **(A)** and coronal (TR/TE, 543/13) **(B)** T1-weighted spin echo MR images show the metastatic lesion of low signal intensity involving the dorsal portion of the navicular bone.

C, D Skeletal metastasis (endometrial carcinoma). Sagittal T1-weighted (TR/TE, 600/17) spin echo **(C)** and fast spin echo STIR (TR/TE, 4000/46; inversion time, 150 msec) **(D)** MR images show involvement of most of the tarsal bones and a metastatic lesion also in the tibia.

(Courtesy of D. Witte, M.D., Memphis, Tennessee.)

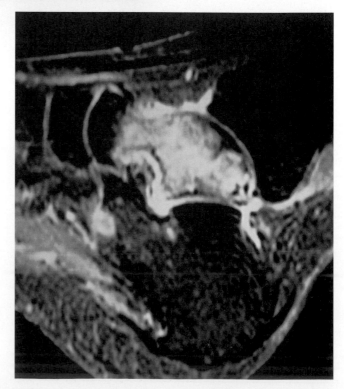

Figure 17–188
Skeletal metastasis: MR imaging. Renal cell carcinoma metastatic to the talus is vividly displayed as regions of high signal intensity on this sagittal fat-suppressed T1-weighted (TR/TE, 500/11) spin echo MR image obtained after intravenous administration of gadolinium contrast agent. (Courtesy of D. Levey, M.D., Corpus Christi, Texas.)

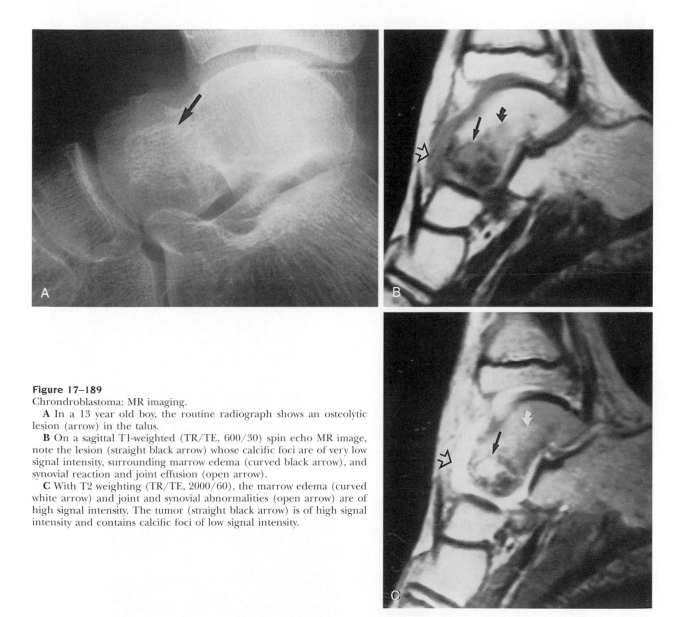

Figure 17–189
Chrondroblastoma: MR imaging.
A In a 13 year old boy, the routine radiograph shows an osteolytic lesion (arrow) in the talus.
B On a sagittal T1-weighted (TR/TE, 600/30) spin echo MR image, note the lesion (straight black arrow) whose calcific foci are of very low signal intensity, surrounding marrow edema (curved black arrow), and synovial reaction and joint effusion (open arrow).
C With T2 weighting (TR/TE, 2000/60), the marrow edema (curved white arrow) and joint and synovial abnormalities (open arrow) are of high signal intensity. The tumor (straight black arrow) is of high signal intensity and contains calcific foci of low signal intensity.

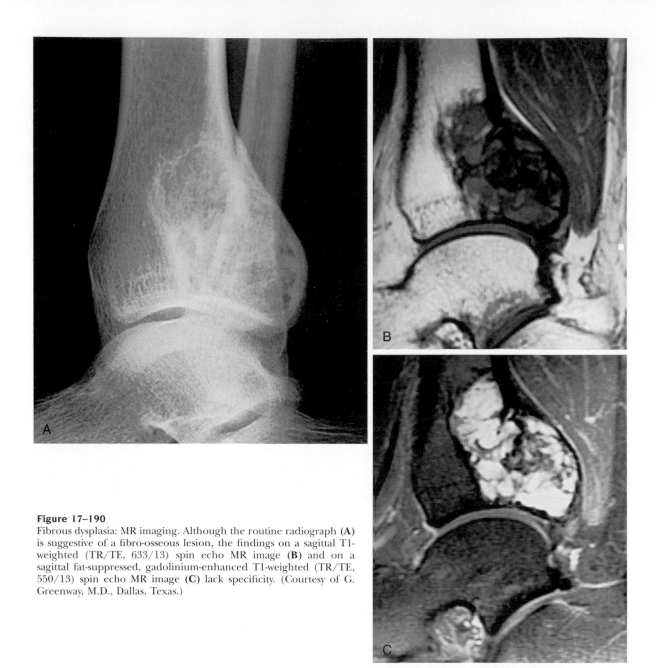

Figure 17–190

Fibrous dysplasia: MR imaging. Although the routine radiograph **(A)** is suggestive of a fibro-osseous lesion, the findings on a sagittal T1-weighted (TR/TE, 633/13) spin echo MR image **(B)** and on a sagittal fat-suppressed, gadolinium-enhanced T1-weighted (TR/TE, 550/13) spin echo MR image **(C)** lack specificity. (Courtesy of G. Greenway, M.D., Dallas, Texas.)

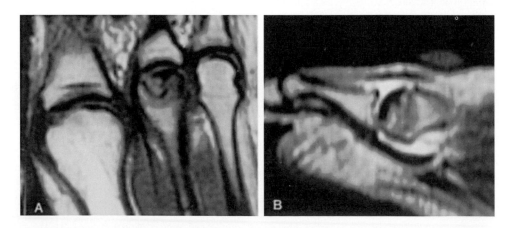

Figure 17–191

Freiberg's infraction: MR imaging. A 14 year old girl had pain and tenderness about the second metatarsophalangeal joint of the left foot.

A On this T1-weighted (TR/TE, 600/20) spin echo MR image obtained in the plantar plane, abnormal signal intensity in the head of the second metatarsal bone is observed. A serpentine region of low signal intensity outlines the area of necrosis, which contains tissue of signal intensity identical to that of marrow fat. Surrounding bone marrow edema is characterized by intermediate signal intensity, and an effusion has led to distention of the joint capsule.

B A sagittal T2-weighted (TR/TE, 2000/80) spin echo MR image again shows the marrow abnormalities, flat metatarsal head, and joint effusion.

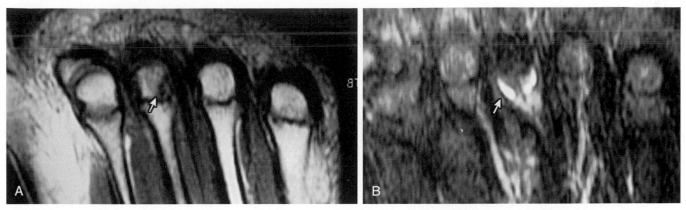

Figure 17–192
Freiberg's infraction: MR imaging. A 13 year old girl developed pain and swelling about the third metatarsophalangeal joint.

A A transverse T1-weighted (TR/TE, 300/20) spin echo MR image shows abnormal signal intensity (arrow) in the lateral aspect of the epiphysis of the third metatarsal bone.

B A transverse fat-suppressed fast spin echo MR image (TR/TE, 4000/92) reveals fluid (arrow) in the third metatarsophalangeal joint and low signal intensity of the bone marrow in the involved epiphysis.

(Courtesy of P. Kindynis, M.D., Geneva, Switzerland.)

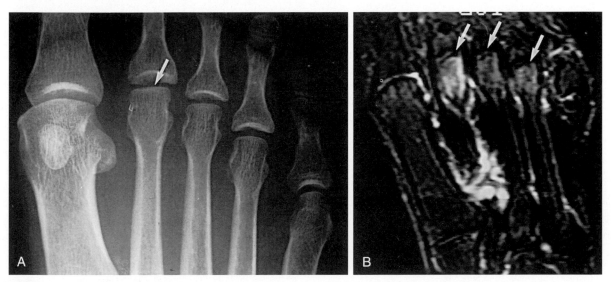

Figure 17–193
Metatarsalgia: Fatigue fractures of the metatarsal heads.

A A routine radiograph in this 51 year old man who is an avid runner shows subtle sclerosis of the second metatarsal head (arrow).

B A transverse fat-suppressed fast spin echo MR image (TR/TE, 4000/119) shows marrow edema in the heads of the second, third, and fourth metatarsal bones (arrows). An effusion in the first metatarsophalangeal joint also is evident.

Figure 17–194
Metatarsalgia: Gouty synovitis of the first metatarsophalangeal joint (I MTP). A sagittal sonogram shows an anechoic effusion (x markers) of the joint. (Courtesy of M. van Holsbeeck, M.D., Detroit, Michigan, and J. Jacobson, M.D., San Diego, California.)

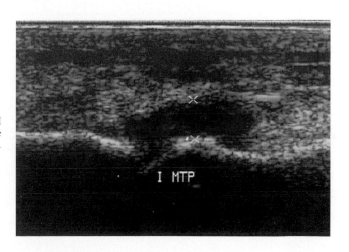

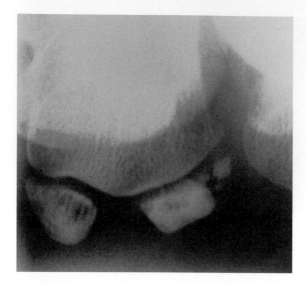

Figure 17–195
Osteonecrosis (osteochondritis) of a sesamoid bone. The sclerosis and fragmentation of the lateral sesamoid bone of the first metatarsophalangeal joint was related to osteonecrosis, probably secondary to an injury.

SUMMARY

This survey of some of the more important conditions that involve the ankle and foot stresses anatomic and biomechanical principles and the diagnostic role of newer imaging methods, especially MR imaging. MR imaging has assumed clinical importance in the analysis of abnormalities of tendons, muscles, ligaments, bones, joints, nerves, and other soft tissues.

REFERENCES

1. Sarrafian SK: Anatomy of the Foot and Ankle: Descriptive, Topographic, Functional. 2nd Ed. Philadelphia, JB Lippincott Co, 1993.
2. Ramsey PL, Hamilton W: Changes in tibiotalar area of contact caused by lateral talar shift. J Bone Joint Surg [Am] 58:356, 1976.
3. Skinner EH: The mathematical calculation of progress in fractures at the ankle and wrist. Surg Gynecol Obstet 18:238, 1914.
4. Joy G, Patzakis MJ, Harvey JP Jr: Precise evaluation of the reduction of severe ankle fractures: Technique and correlation with end results. J Bone Joint Surg [Am] 56:979, 1974.
5. Hutter CG Jr, Scott W: Tibial torsion. J Bone Joint Surg [Am] 31:511, 1949.
6. Goergen TG, Danzig LA, Resnick D, et al: Roentgenographic evaluation of the tibiotalar joint. J Bone Joint Surg [Am] 59:874, 1977.
7. Jonsson K, Fredin HO, Cederlund CG, et al: Width of the normal ankle joint. Acta Radiol Diagn 25:147, 1984.
8. Kaye JJ, Bohne WHO: A radiographic study of the ligamentous anatomy of the ankle. Radiology 125:659, 1977.
9. Towbin R, Dunbar JS, Towbin J, et al: Teardrop sign: Plain film recognition of ankle effusion. AJR 134:985, 1980.
10. Hall FM: Pitfalls in the diagnosis of ankle joint effusion. AJR 136:637, 1981.
11. Resnick D: Radiology of the talocalcaneal articulations: Anatomic considerations and arthrography. Radiology 111:581, 1974.
12. Rhea JT, De Luca SA, Sheehan J: Radiographic anatomy of the tarsal bones. Med Radiogr Photogr 59:2, 1983.
13. Mehrez M, el-Geneidy S: Arthrography of the ankle. J Bone Joint Surg [Br] 52:308, 1970.
14. Olson RW: Arthrography of the ankle: Its use in the evaluation of ankle sprains. Radiology 92:1439, 1969.
15. Faure C: The skeleton of the anterior foot. Anat Clin 3:49, 1981.
16. de Britto SR: The first metatarso-sesamoid joint. Int Orthop (SICOT) 6:61, 1982.
17. Scranton PE Jr, Rutkowski R: Anatomic variations in the first ray. II. Disorders of the sesamoids. Clin Orthop 151:256, 1980.
18. McCarthy DJ: The surgical anatomy of the first ray. I. The distal segment. J Am Podiatr Assoc 73:111, 1983.
19. Palmer DG: Tendon sheaths and bursae involved by rheumatoid disease at the foot and ankle. Australas Radiol 14:419, 1970.
20. Teng MMH, Destouet JM, Gilula LA, et al: Ankle tenography: A key to unexplained symptomatology. I. Normal tenographic anatomy. Radiology 151:575, 1984.
21. Gilula LA, Oloff L, Caputi R, et al: Ankle tenography: A key to unexplained symptomatology. II. Diagnosis of chronic tendon disabilities. Radiology 151:581, 1984.
22. Meurman KOA: Bursa tendinis musculi flexoris hallucis longi. ROFO 136:27, 1982.
23. Resnick D, Goergen TG: Peroneal tenography in previous calcaneal fractures. Radiology 115:211, 1975.
24. Sutro CJ: The os calcis, the tendo-achillis and the local bursae. Bull Hosp Joint Dis 27:76, 1966.
25. Weston WJ: The bursa deep to the tendo achillis. Australas Radiol 14:327, 1970.
26. Lieber GA, Lemont H: The posterior triangle of the ankle: Determination of its true anatomical boundary. J Am Podiatr Assoc 72:363, 1982.
27. Goodman LR, Shanser JD: The pre-Achilles fat pad: An aid to early diagnosis of local systemic disease. Skel Radiol 2:81, 1977.
28. Minns RJ, Hunter JAA: The mechanical and structural characteristics of the tibiofibular interosseous membrane. Acta Orthop Scand 47:236, 1976.
29. Schweitzer ME, Resnick D: Normal anatomy of the foot and ankle. In AL Deutsch, JH Mink, R Kerr (Eds): MRI of the Foot and Ankle. New York, Raven Press, 1992, p. 33.
30. Jaffe WL, Gannon PJ, Laitman JT: Paleontology, embryology, and anatomy of the foot. In MH Jahss (Ed): Disorders of the Foot and Ankle. 2nd Ed. Philadelphia, WB Saunders Co, 1991, p. 3.
31. Mann RA: Biomechanics of the foot and ankle linkage. In JC DeLee, D Drez Jr (Eds): Orthopaedic Sports Medicine: Principles and Practice. Philadelphia, WB Saunders Co, 1994, p. 1632.
32. Bremer SW: The unstable ankle mortise—functional ankle varus. J Foot Surg 24:313, 1985.
33. Lambert KL: The weight-bearing function of the fibula: A strain gauge study. J Bone Joint Surg [Am] 53:507, 1971.
34. Close JR: Some applications of the functional anatomy of the ankle joint. J Bone Joint Surg [Am] 38:761, 1956.
35. Weinert CR Jr, McMaster JH, Ferguson RJ: Dynamic function of the human fibula. Am J Anat 138:145, 1973.
36. Scranton PE, McMaster JH, Kelly E: Dynamic fibular function. A new concept. Clin Orthop 118:76, 1976.
37. Olson RW: Arthrography of the ankle: Its use in the evaluation of ankle sprains. Radiology 92:1439, 1969.
38. Haller J, Resnick D, Sartoris D, et al: Arthrography, tenography, and bursography of the ankle and foot. Clin Podiatr Med Surg 5:893, 1988.
39. Arner O, Ekengren K, Hulting B, et al: Arthrography of the talocrural joint: Anatomic, roentgenographic and clinical aspects. Acta Chir Scand 113:253, 1957.
40. Resnick D: Radiology of the talocalcaneal articulations: Anatomic considerations and arthrography. Radiology 111:581, 1974.
41. Goossens M, De Stoop N, Claessens H, et al: Posterior subtalar joint arthrography: A useful tool in the diagnosis of hindfoot disorders. Clin Orthop 249:248, 1989.
42. Terk MR, Kwong PK: Magnetic resonance imaging of the foot and ankle. Clin Sports Med 13:883, 1994.
43. Kneeland JB: Technical considerations for magnetic resonance imaging of the ankle and foot. MRI Clin North Am 2:23, 1994.
44. Mink JH: Tendons. In AL Deutsch, JH Mink, R Kerr (Eds): MRI of the Foot and Ankle. New York, Raven Press, 1992, p. 135.
45. Unger EC, Schilling JD, Awad AN, et al: MR angiography of the foot and ankle. J Magn Reson Imaging 5:1, 1995.
46. Rogers LF: Radiology of Skeletal Trauma. 2nd Ed. New York, Churchill Livingstone, 1992.
47. Gershuni DH, Skyhar MJ, Thompson B, et al: A comparison of conventional radiography and computed tomography in the evaluation of spiral fractures of the tibia. J Bone Joint Surg [Am] 67:1388, 1985.

48. Sarmiento A: A functional below-the-knee brace for tibial fractures. J Bone Joint Surg [Am] *52*:295, 1970.

49. Sarmuento A, Gersten LM, Sobol PA, et al: Tibial shaft fractures treated with functional brace: Experience with 780 fractures. J Bone Joint Surg [Br] *71*:602, 1989.

50. Skak SV, Jensen TT, Poulsen TD: Fracture of the proximal metaphysis of the tibia in children. Injury *18*:149, 1987.

51. Zionts LE, Harcke HT, Brooks KM, et al: Posttraumatic tibia valga: A case demonstrating asymmetric activity at the proximal growth plate on technetium bone scan. J Pediatr Orthop *7*:458, 1987.

52. Robert M, Khouri N, Carlioz H, et al: Fractures of the proximal tibial metaphysis in children: Review of a series of 25 cases. J Pediatr Orthop *7*:444, 1987.

53. Brougham DI, Nicol RO: Valgus deformity after proximal tibial fractures in children. J Bone Joint Surg [Br] *69*:482, 1987.

54. Wood KB, Bradley JP, Ward WT: Pes anserinus interposition in a proximal tibial physeal fracture: A case report. Clin Orthop *264*:239, 1991.

55. Michelson JD: Fractures about the ankle. J Bone Joint Surg [Am] *77*:142, 1995.

56. Neer CS: Injuries of the ankle joint—evaluation. Conn St Med J *17*:580, 1953.

57. Karlsson J, Lansinger O: Lateral instability of the ankle joint. Clin Orthop *276*:253, 1992.

58. Rijke AM, Jones B, Vierhout PAM: Stress examination of traumatized lateral ligaments of the ankle. Clin Orthop *210*:143, 1986.

59. Larsen E: Experimental instability of the ankle. A radiographic investigation. Clin Orthop *204*:193, 1986.

60. Ashhurst APC, Brumer RS: Classification and mechanism of fractures of the leg bones involving the ankle: Based on a study of three hundred cases from the Episcopal Hospital. Arch Surg *4*:51, 1922.

61. Lauge-Hansen N: Fractures of the ankle: Genetic roentgenologic diagnosis of fractures of the ankle. AJR *71*:456, 1954.

62. Lauge-Hansen N: Fractures of the ankle: Clinical use of genetic roentgen diagnosis and genetic reduction. Arch Surg *64*:488, 1952.

63. Nielsen J, Dons-Jenson H, Sørensen HT: Lauge-Hansen classification of malleolar fractures: An assessment of the reproducibility in 118 cases. Acta Orthop Scand *61*:385, 1990.

64. Thomsen NOB, Overgaard S, Olsen LH, et al: Observer variation in the radiographic classification of ankle fractures. J Bone Joint Surg [Br] *73*:676, 1991.

65. Daffner RH: Ankle trauma. Semin Roentgenol *29*:134, 1994.

66. Michelson J, Curtis M, Magid D: Controversies in ankle fractures. Foot Ankle *14*:170, 1993.

67. Kristensen TB: Treatment of malleolar fractures according to Lauge-Hansen's method. Acta Chir Scand *97*:362, 1949.

68. Protas JM, Kornblatt BA: Fractures of the lateral margin of the distal tibia: The Tillaux fracture. Radiology *138*:55, 1981.

69. Berg EE: The symptomatic os subfibulare: Avulsion fracture of the fibula associated with recurrent instability of the ankle. J Bone Joint Surg [Am] *73*:1251, 1991.

70. Pankovich AM: Maisonneuve fracture of the fibula. J Bone Joint Surg [Am] *58*:337, 1976.

71. Lock TR, Schaffer JJ, Manoli A II: Maisonneuve fracture: Case report of a missed diagnosis. Ann Emerg Med *16*:805, 1987.

72. Lauge-Hansen N: Fractures of the ankle. V. Pronation-dorsiflexion fracture. Arch Surg *67*:813, 1953.

73. Ayeni JP: Pilon fractures of the tibia: A study based on 19 cases. Injury *19*:109, 1988.

74. Bourne RB: Pylon fractures of the distal tibia. Clin Orthop *240*:42, 1989.

75. Mast JW, Spiegel PG, Pappas JN: Fractures of the tibial pilon. Clin Orthop *230*:68, 1988.

76. Giachino AA, Hammond DI: The relationship between oblique fractures of the medial malleolus and concomitant fractures of the anterolateral aspect of the tibial plafond. J Bone Joint Surg [Am] *69*:381, 1987.

77. Mainwaring BL, Daffner RH, Riemer BL: Pylon fractures of the ankle: A distinct clinical and radiologic entity. Radiology *168*:215, 1988.

78. Yde J: The Lauge-Hansen classification of malleolar fractures. Acta Orthop Scand *51*:181, 1980.

79. Mandell J: Isolated fractures of the posterior tibial lip at the ankle as demonstrated by an additional projection, the "poor" lateral view. Radiology *101*:319, 1971.

80. Auletta AG, Conway WF, Hayes CW, et al: Indications for radiography in patients with acute ankle injuries: Role of the physical examination. AJR *157*:789, 1991.

81. Magid D, Michelson JD, Ney DR, et al: Adult ankle fractures: Comparison of plain films and interactive two- and three-dimensional CT scans. AJR *154*:1017, 1990.

82. Maurice H, Watt I: Technetium-99m hydroxymethylene diphosphonate scanning of acute injuries to the lateral ligaments of the ankle. Br J Radiol *62*:31, 1989.

83. Toohey JS, Worsing RA Jr: A long-term follow-up study of tibiotalar dislocations without associated fractures. Clin Orthop *239*:207, 1989.

84. Colville MR, Colville JM, Manoli A II: Posteromedial dislocation of the ankle without fracture. J Bone Joint Surg [Am] *69*:706, 1987.

85. Segal LS, Lynch CJ, Stauffer ES: Anterior ankle dislocation with associated trigonal process fracture: A case report and literature review. Clin Orthop *278*:171, 1992.

86. Hoblitzell RM, Ebraheim NA, Merritt T, et al: Bosworth fracture-dislocation of the ankle: A case report and review of the literature. Clin Orthop *255*:257, 1990.

87. Molinari M, Bertoldi L, De March L: Fracture dislocation of the ankle with the fibula trapped behind the tibia: A case report. Acta Orthop Scand *61*:471, 1990.

88. Bosworth DM: Fracture-dislocation of the ankle with fixed displacement of the fibula behind the tibia. J Bone Joint Surg [Am] *29*:130, 1947.

89. Schatzker J, Johnson RG: Fracture dislocation of the ankle with anterior dislocation of the fibula. J Trauma *23*:420, 1983.

90. Rogers LF, Campbell RE: Fractures and dislocations of the foot. Semin Roentgenol *13*:157, 1978.

91. Anderson HG: The Medical and Surgical Aspects of Aviation. London, Oxford University Press, 1919.

92. Kenwright J, Taylor RG: Major injuries of the talus. J Bone Joint Surg [Br] *52*:36, 1970.

93. Dimon JH: Isolated displaced fracture of the posterior facet of the talus. J Bone Joint Surg [Am] *43*:275, 1961.

94. Coltart WD: "Aviator's astralagus." J Bone Joint Surg [Br] *34*:545, 1952.

95. Hawkins LG: Fractures of the neck of the talus. J Bone Joint Surg [Am] *52*:991, 1970.

96. Canale ST, Kelly FB Jr: Fractures of the neck of the talus: Long-term evaluation of seventy-one cases. J Bone Joint Surg [Am] *60*:143, 1978.

97. Lorentzen JE, Christensen SB, Krogsoe O, et al: Fractures of the neck of the talus. Acta Orthop Scand *48*:115, 1977.

98. Canale ST: Fractures of the neck of the talus. Orthopedics *13*:1105, 1990.

99. Bodamer WJ, Torre RJ, Cotch MT, et al: Avascular necrosis of the talar head: A complication of group 4 fracture of the talar neck. J Am Podiatr Assoc *77*:217, 1987.

100. Lieberg OU, Henke JA, Bailey RW: Avascular necrosis of the head of the talus without death of the body: Report of an unusual case. J Trauma *15*:926, 1975.

101. Sneppen O, Christensen SB, Krogsoe O, Lorentzen J: Fracture of the body of the talus. Acta Orthop Scand *48*:317, 1977.

102. Heckman JD, McLean MR: Fractures of the lateral process of the talus. Clin Orthop *199*:108, 1985.

103. El-Khoury GY, Yousefzadeh DK, Mulligan GM, Moore TE: Subtalar dislocation. Skel Radiol *8*:99, 1982.

104. Monson ST, Ryan JR: Subtalar dislocation. J Bone Joint Surg [Am] *63*:1156, 1981.

105. St Pierre RK, Velazco A, Fleming LL, et al: Medial subtalar dislocation in an athlete: A case report. Am J Sports Med *10*:240, 1982.

106. Mattingly DA, Stern PJ: Bilateral subtalar dislocations: A case report. Clin Orthop *177*:122, 1983.

107. Goldner JL, Poletti SC, Gates HS III, et al: Severe open subtalar dislocations: Long-term results. J Bone Joint Surg [Am] *77*:1075, 1995.

108. Zimmer TJ, Johnson KA: Subtalar dislocations. Clin Orthop *238*:190, 1989.

109. Buckingham WW Jr: Subtalar dislocation of the foot. J Trauma *13*:753, 1973.

110. Grantham SA: Medial subtalar dislocation: Five cases with a common etiology. J Trauma *4*:845, 1964.

111. Detenbeck LC, Kelly PJ: Total dislocation of the talus. J Bone Joint Surg [Am] *51*:283, 1969.

112. Ritsema GH: Total talar dislocation. J Trauma *28*:692, 1988.

113. Heger L, Wulff K: Computed tomography of the calcaneus: Normal anatomy. AJR *145*:123, 1985.

114. Heger L, Wulff K, Seddiqi MSA: Computed tomography of calcaneal fractures. AJR *145*:131, 1985.

115. Pablot SM, Daneman A, Stringer DA, et al: The value of computed tomography in the early assessment of comminuted fractures of the calcaneus: A review of three patients. J Pediatr Orthop *5*:435, 1985.

116. Gilmer PW, Herzenberg J, Frank JL, Silverman P, Martinez S, Goldner JL: Computerized tomographic analysis of acute calcaneal fractures. Foot Ankle *6*:184, 1986.

117. Crosby LA, Fitzgibbons T: Computerized tomography scanning of acute intra-articular fractures of the calcaneus: A new classification system. J Bone Joint Surg [Am] *72*:852, 1990.

118. Rosenberg ZS, Feldman F, Singson RD: Intra-articular calcaneal fractures: Computed tomographic analysis. Skel Radiol *16*:105, 1987.

119. Bradley SA, Davies AM: Computed tomographic assessment of old calcaneal fractures. Br J Radiol *63*:926, 1990.

120. Janzen DL, Connell DG, Munk PL, et al: Intraarticular fractures of the calcaneus: Value of CT findings in determining prognosis. AJR *158*:1271, 1992.

121. Richardson ML, Vu MV, Vincent LM, et al: CT measurement of the calcaneal varus angle in the normal and fractured hindfoot. J Comput Assist Tomogr *16*:261, 1992.

122. Eastwood DM, Gregg PJ, Atkins RM: Intra-articular fractures of the calcaneum. I. Pathological anatomy and classification. J Bone Joint Surg [Br] *75*:183, 1993.

123. Essex-Lopresti P: The mechanism, reduction technique, and results in fractures of the os calcis. Br J Surg *39*:395, 1952.

124. Paley D, Hall H: Intra-articular fractures of the calcaneus: A critical analysis of results and prognostic factors. J Bone Joint Surg [Am] *75*:342, 1993.

125. Giachino AA, Uhthoff HK: Intra-articular fractures of the calcaneus. J Bone Joint Surg [Am] *71*:784, 1989.

126. Palmer I: The mechanism and treatment of fractures of the calcaneus. J Bone Joint Surg [Am] *30*:2, 1948.

127. Norfray JF, Rogers LF, Adamo GP, et al: Common calcaneal avulsion fracture. AJR *134*:119, 1980.

128. Brijs S, Brijs A: Calcaneal avulsion: a frequent traumatic foot lesion. ROFO *156*:495, 1992.

129. Nielsen S, Agnhold J, Christensen H: Radiologic findings in lesions of the ligamentum bifurcatum of the midfoot. Skel Radiol *16*:114, 1987.

130. Renfrew DL, El-Khoury GY: Anterior process fractures of the calcaneus. Skel Radiol *14*:121, 1985.

131. Schantz K, Rasmussen F: Calcaneus fracture in the child. Acta Orthop Scand *58*:507, 1987.

132. Starshak RJ, Simons GW, Sty JR: Occult fracture of the calcaneus—another toddler's fracture. Pediatr Radiol *14*:37, 1984.

133. Soeur R, Remy R: Fractures of the calcaneus with displacement of the thalamic portion. J Bone Joint Surg [Br] *57*:413, 1975.

134. Stephenson JR: Displaced fractures of the os calcis involving the subtalar joint: The key role of the superomedial fragment. Foot Ankle *4*:91, 1983.

135. Champetier J, Laborde Y, Letoublon Ch, et al: Fractures articulaires du calcanéum. J Radiol *61*:269, 1980.

136. Mains DB, Sullivan RC: Fracture of the os peroneum: A case report. J Bone Joint Surg [Am] *55*:1529, 1973.

137. Mikami M, Azuma H: Fracture of the os tibiale externum: A case report. J Bone Joint Surg [Am] *60*:556, 1978.

138. Thompson FM, Patterson AH: Rupture of the peroneus longus tendon: Report of three cases. J Bone Joint Surg [Am] *71*:293, 1989.

139. Main BJ, Jowett RL: Injuries of the midtarsal joint. J Bone Joint Surg [Br] *57*:89, 1975.

140. Dewar FP, Evans DC: Occult fracture-subluxation of the midtarsal joint. J Bone Joint Surg [Br] *50*:386, 1968.

141. Brantigan JW, Pedegana LR, Lippert FG: Instability of the subtalar joint: Diagnosis by stress tomography in three cases. J Bone Joint Surg [Am] *59*:321, 1977.

142. Vuori J-P, Aro HT: Lisfranc joint injuries: Trauma mechanisms and associated injuries. J Trauma *35*:40, 1993.

143. Cássebaum WH: Lisfranc-fracture-dislocations. Clin Orthop *30*:116, 1963.

144. Foster SC, Foster RR: Lisfranc's tarsometatarsal fracture-dislocation. Radiology *120*:79, 1976.

145. Wiley JJ: The mechanism of tarso-metatarsal joint injuries. J Bone Joint Surg [Br] *53*:474, 1971.

146. Wilson DW: Injuries of the tarso-metatarsal joints: Etiology, classification and results of treatment. J Bone Joint Surg [Br] *54*:677, 1972.

147. Goossens M, DeStoop N: Lisfranc's fracture-dislocations: Etiology, radiology, and results of treatment. A review of 20 cases. Clin Orthop *176*:154, 1983.

148. Blouet JM, Rebaud C, Marquer Y, et al: Anatomy of the tarsometatarsal joint and its applications to dislocation of this articular surface. Anat Clin *5*:9, 1983.

149. Ashhurst APC: Divergent dislocation of the metatarsus. Ann Surg *83*:132, 1926.

150. Aitken AP, Poulson D: Dislocations of the tarsometatarsal joint. J Bone Joint Surg [Am] *45*:246, 1963.

151. Faciszewski T, Burks RT, Manaster BJ: Subtle injuries of the Lisfranc joint. J Bone Joint Surg [Am] *72*:1519, 1990.

152. Goiney RC, Connell DG, Nichols DM: CT evaluation of tarsometatarsal fracture-dislocation injuries. AJR *144*:985, 1985.

153. Fagel VL, Ocon E, Cantarella JC, et al: Case report 183. Skel Radiol *7*:287, 1982.

154. Dines DM, Hershon SJ, Smith N, et al: Isolated dorsomedial dislocation of the first ray at the medial cuneonavicular joint of the foot: A rare injury to the tarsus. Clin Orthop *186*:162, 1984.

155. Macy NJ, DeBoer P: Mid-tarsal dislocation of the first ray: A case report. J Bone Joint Surg [Am] *65*:265, 1983.

156. Tountas AA: Occult fracture-subluxation of the midtarsal joint. Clin Orthop *243*:195, 1989.

157. Kollmannsberger A, DeBoer P: Isolated calcaneo-cuboid dislocation: Brief report. J Bone Joint Surg [Br] *71*:323, 1989.

158. Yamashita F, Sakakida K, Hara K, et al: Diastasis between the medial and the intermediate cuneiforms. J Bone Joint Surg [Br] *75*:156, 1993.

159. Main BJ, Jowett RL: Injuries of the midtarsal joint. J Bone Joint Surg [Br] *57*:89, 1975.

160. Salamon PB, Gelberman RH, Huffer JM: Dorsal dislocation of the metatarsophalangeal joint of the great toe: A case report. J Bone Joint Surg [Am] *56*:1073, 1974.

161. Barnett JC, Crespo A, Daniels VC: Intra-articular accessory sesamoid dislocation of the great toe: Report of a case. J Fla Med Assoc *66*:613, 1979.

162. Szues R, Hurwitz J: Traumatic subluxation of the interphalangeal joint of the hallux with interposition of the sesamoid bone. AJR *152*:652, 1989.

163. Meaney JFM, Desmond JM: Case report 721. Skel Radiol *21*:319, 1992.

164. Miki T, Yamamuro T, Kitai T: An irreducible dislocation of the great toe: Report of two cases and review of the literature. Clin Orthop *230*:200, 1988.

165. Katayama M, Murakami Y, Takahashi H: Irreducible dorsal dislocation of the toe: Report of three cases. J Bone Joint Surg [Am] *70*:769, 1988.

166. Rodeo SA, O'Brien S, Warren RF, et al: Turf-toe: An analysis of metatarsophalangeal joint sprains in professional football players. Am J Sports Med *18*:280, 1990.

167. Bowers KD Jr, Martin RB: Turf toe: A shoe surface related football injury. Med Sci Sports *8*:81, 1976.

168. Clanton TO, Butler JE, Eggert A: Injuries to the metatarsophalangeal joints in athletes. Foot Ankle *7*:162, 1986.

169. Coughlin MJ: Conditions of the forefoot. *In* JC DeLee, D Drez Jr (Eds): Orthopaedic Sports Medicine: Principles and Practice. Philadelphia, WB Saunders Co, 1994, p. 1842.

170. Graves SC, Prieskorn D, Mann RA: Posttraumatic proximal migration of the first metatarsophalangeal joint sesamoids: A report of four cases. Foot Ankle *12*:117, 1991.

171. Potter HG, Pavlov H, Abrahams TG: The hallux sesamoids revisited. Skel Radiol *21*:437, 1992.

172. Joseph J: Range of movement of the great toe in men. J Bone Joint Surg [Br] *36*:450, 1954.

173. Yao L, Do HM, Cracchiolo A, et al: Plantar plate of the foot: Findings on conventional arthrography and MR imaging. AJR *163*:641, 1994.

174. Tewes DP, Fischer DA, Fritts HM, et al: MRI findings of acute turf toe: A case report and review of anatomy. Clin Orthop *304*:200, 1994.

175. Munro TG: Fractures of the base of the fifth metatarsal. Can Assoc Radiol J *40*:260, 1989.

176. Dameron TB Jr: Fractures and anatomic variations of the proximal portion of the fifth metatarsal. J Bone Joint Surg [Am] *57*:788, 1975.

177. Torg JS, Balduini FC, Zelko RR, et al: Fractures of the base of the fifth metatarsal distal to the tuberosity: Classification and guidelines for nonsurgical and surgical management. J Bone Joint Surg [Am] *66*:209, 1984.

178. Richli WR, Rosenthal DI: Avulsion fracture of the fifth metatarsal: Experimental study of pathomechanics. AJR *143*:889, 1984.

179. Jones R: Fractures of the base of the fifth metatarsal bone by indirect violence. Ann Surg *35*:697, 1902.

180. Galant JM, Spinosa FA: Digital fractures: A comprehensive review. J Am Podiatr Assoc *81*:593, 1991.

181. Pinckney LE, Currarino G, Kennedy LA: The stubbed great toe: A cause of occult compound fracture and infection. Radiology *138*:375, 1981.

182. Schon LC, Ouzounian TJ: The ankle. *In* MH Jahss (Ed): Disorders of the Foot and Ankle. 2nd Ed. Philadelphia, WB Saunders Co, 1991, p. 1417.

183. Kelikian H, Kelikian AS: Disorders of the Ankle. Philadelphia, WB Saunders Co, 1985.

184. Kannus P, Renstrom P: Treatment for acute tears of the lateral ligaments of the ankle. J Bone Joint Surg [Am] *73*:305, 1991.

185. Liu SH, Jason WJ: Lateral ankle sprains and instability problems. Clin Sports Med *13*:793, 1994.

186. Marder RA: Current methods for evaluation of ankle ligament injuries. J Bone Joint Surg [Am] *76*:1103, 1994.

187. Renstrom PAFH, Kannus P: Injuries of the foot and ankle. *In* JC DeLee, D Drez Jr (Eds): Orthopaedic Sports Medicine: Principles and Practice. Philadelphia, WB Saunders Co, 1994, p. 1705.

188. Siegler S, Block J, Schneck CD: The mechanical characteristics of the collateral ligaments of the human ankle joint. Foot Ankle *8*:234, 1988.

189. Frost HM, Hanson CA: Technique for testing the drawer sign in the ankle. Clin Orthop *123*:49, 1977.

190. Raatikainen T, Putkonen M, Puranen J: Arthrography, clinical examination, and stress radiograph in the diagnosis of acute injury to the lateral ligaments of the ankle. Am J Sports Med *20*:2, 1992.

191. Tohyama H, Beynnon BD, Renstrom PA, et al: Biomechanical analysis of the ankle anterior drawer test for anterior talofibular ligament injuries. J Orthop Res *13*:609, 1995.

192. Gaston SR, McLaughlin HL: Complex fractures of the lateral malleolus. J Trauma *1*:69, 1961.

193. Staples OS: Injuries to the medial ligaments of the ankle. J Bone Joint Surg [Am] *42*:1287, 1960.

194. Pankovich AM, Shivaram MS: Anatomical basis of variability in injuries of the medial malleolus and the deltoid ligament. I. Anatomical studies. Acta Orthop Scand *50*:217, 1979.

195. Pankovich AM, Shivaram MS: Anatomical basis of variability in injuries of the medial malleolus and the deltoid ligament. II. Clinical studies. Acta Orthop Scand *50*:225, 1979.

196. Fritschy D: An unusual ankle injury in top skiers. Am J Sports Med *17*:282, 1989.

197. Stiehl JB: Complex ankle fracture dislocations with syndesmotic diastasis. Orthop Rev *14*:499, 1990.

198. Hocker K: The skeletal radiology of the distal tibiofibular joint. Arch Orthop Trauma Surg *113*:345, 1994.

199. Xenos JS, Hopkinson WJ, Mulligan ME, et al: The tibiofibular syndesmosis: Evaluation of the ligamentous structures, methods of fixation, and radiographic assessment. J Bone Joint Surg [Am] *77*:847, 1995.

200. Ostrum RF, DeMeo P, Subramanian RS: A critical analysis of the anterior-posterior radiographic anatomy of the ankle syndesmosis. Foot Ankle *16*:128, 1995.

201. Veltri DM, Pagnani MJ, O'Brien SJ, et al: Symptomatic ossification of the tibiofibular syndesmosis in professional football players: A sequela of the syndesmotic ankle sprain. Foot Ankle *16*:285, 1995.

202. Broström L, Liljedahl SO, Lindvall N: Sprained ankles. II. Arthrographic diagnosis of recent ligament ruptures. Acta Chir Scand *129*:485, 1965.

203. Spiegel PK, Staples OS: Arthrography of the ankle joint: Problems in diagnosis of acute lateral ligament injuries. Radiology 114:587, 1975.

204. Fordyce AJW, Horn CV: Arthrography in recent injuries of the ligament of the ankle. J Bone Joint Surg [Br] 54:116, 1972.

205. Ala-Ketola L, Puranen J, Koivisto E, et al: Arthrography in the diagnosis of ligament injuries and classification of ankle injuries. Radiology 125:63, 1977.

206. Mehrez M, El Geneidy S: Arthrography of the ankle. J Bone Joint Surg [Br] 52:308, 1970.

207. Fussell ME, Godley DR: Ankle arthrography in acute sprains. Clin Orthop 93:278, 1973.

208. Sanders HWA: Ankle arthrography and ankle distortion. Radiol Clin Biol 46:1, 1977.

209. Gordon RB: Arthrography of the ankle joint: Experience in 107 studies. J Bone Joint Surg [Am] 52:1623, 1970.

210. Percy EC, Hill RO, Callaghan JE: The "sprained" ankle. J Trauma 9:972, 1969.

211. Sauser DD, Nelson RC, Lavine MH, et al: Acute injuries of the lateral ligaments of the ankle: Comparison of stress radiography and arthrography. Radiology 148:653, 1983.

212. Haller J, Resnick D, Sartoris D, et al: Arthrography, tenography, and bursography of the ankle and foot. Clin Podiatr Med Surg 5:893, 1988.

213. Bleichrodt RP, Kingma LM, Binnendijk B, et al: Injuries of the lateral ankle ligaments: Classification with tenography and arthrography. Radiology 173:347, 1989.

214. van Moppes FI, van den Hoogenband CR, van Engelshoven JMA, et al: Arthrography, talar tilt and surgical findings after inversion trauma of the ankle. ROFO 134:413, 1981.

215. van Moppes FI, van den Hoogenband CR: The significance of the peroneus tendon sheath in ankle arthrography. ROFO 132:573, 1980.

216. Vuust M: Arthrographic diagnosis of ruptured calcaneofibular ligament. I. A new projection tested on experimental injury post mortem. Acta Radiol Diagn 21:123, 1980.

217. Vuust M, Niedermann B: Arthrographic diagnosis of ruptured calcaneofibular ligament. II. Clinical evaluation of a new method. Acta Radiol Diagn 21:231, 1980.

218. Lindholmer E, Andersen A, Andersen SB, et al: Arthrography of the ankle: Value in diagnosis of rupture of the calcaneofibular ligament. Acta Radiol Diagn 24:217, 1983.

219. van Moppes FI, Meijer F, van den Hoogenband CR: Arthrographic differential diagnosis between ruptures of the anterior talofibular ligament, the joint capsule and the anterior tibiofibular ligament. ROFO 133:534, 1980.

220. Brasseur JL, Luzzati A, Lazennec JY, et al: Ultrasono-anatomy of the ankle ligaments. Surg Radiol Anat 16:87, 1994.

221. Brasseur JL, Richard O, Tardieu M, et al: Echographie des ligaments de la cheville. J Traumatol Sport 11:45, 1994.

222. Beltran J, Munchow AM, Khabiri H, et al: Ligaments of the lateral aspect of the ankle and sinus tarsi: An MR imaging study. Radiology 177:455, 1990.

223. Erickson SJ, Smith JW, Ruiz ME, et al: MR imaging of the lateral collateral ligament of the ankle. AJR 156:131, 1991.

224. Schneck CD, Mesgarzadeh M, Bonakdarpour A, et al: MR imaging of the most commonly injured ankle ligaments. I. Normal anatomy. Radiology 184:499, 1992.

225. Schneck CD, Mesgarzadeh M, Bonakdarpour A: MR imaging of the most commonly injured ankle ligaments. II. Ligament injuries. Radiology 184:507, 1992.

226. Oloff LM, Sullivan BT, Heard GS, et al: Magnetic resonance imaging of traumatized ligaments of the ankle. J Am Podiatr Med Assoc 82:25, 1992.

227. Cardone BW, Erickson SJ, Den Hartog BD, et al: MRI of injury to the lateral collateral ligamentous complex of the ankle. J Comput Assist Tomogr 17:102, 1993.

228. Ho CP: Magnetic resonance imaging of the ankle and foot. Semin Roentgenol 30:294, 1995.

229. Beltrab J: Magnetic resonance imaging of the ankle and foot. Orthopedics 17:1075, 1994.

230. Chandnani VP, Harper MT, Ficke JR, et al: Chronic ankle instability: Evaluation with MR arthrography, MR imaging, and stress radiography. Radiology 192:189, 1994.

231. Mesgarzadeh M, Schneck CD, Tehranzadeh J, et al: Magnetic resonance imaging of ankle ligaments: Emphasis on anatomy and injuries to lateral collateral ligament. MRI Clin North Am 2:39, 1994.

232. Klein MA: MR imaging of the ankle: Normal and abnormal findings in the medial collateral ligament. AJR 162:377, 1994.

233. Noto AM, Cheung Y, Rosenberg ZS, et al: MR imaging of the ankle: Normal variants. Radiology 170:121, 1989.

234. Mink JH: Ligaments of the ankle. In AL Deutsch, JH Mink, R Kerr (Eds): MRI of the Foot and Ankle. New York, Raven Press, 1992, p. 173.

235. Mink SC, Erickson SJ, Timins ME: MR imaging of the ankle and foot: Normal structures and anatomic variants that may simulate disease. AJR 161:607, 1993.

236. Colville MR: Reconstruction of the lateral ankle ligaments. J Bone Joint Surg [Am] 76:1092, 1994.

237. Hoy GA, Henderson IJP: Results of Watson-Jones ankle reconstruction for instability. J Bone Joint Surg [Br] 76:610, 1994.

238. Klein MA, Spreitzer AM: MR imaging of the tarsal sinus and canal: Normal

239. anatomy, pathologic findings, and features of the sinus tarsi syndrome. Radiology 186:233, 1993.

239. Cahill DR: The anatomy and function of the contents of the human tarsal sinus and canal. Anat Rec 153:1, 1965.

240. Kjaersgaard-Anderson P, Wethelund JO, Helmig P, et al: The stabilizing effect of the ligamentous structures in the sinus and canalus tarsi on movements in the hind foot: An experimental study. Am J Sports Med 16:512, 1988.

241. Lowe A, Schilero J, Kanat IO: Sinus tarsi syndrome: A postoperative analysis. J Foot Surg 24:108, 1985.

242. Meyer J-M, Garcia J, Hoffmeyer P, et al: The subtalar sprain. A roentgenographic study. Clin Orthop 226:169, 1988.

243. Meyer JM: L'arthrographie de l'articulation sous-astragalienne postérieure et de l'articulation de Chopart. Thèse Méd Genève, No 3318, 1973.

244. Meyer JM, Lagier R: Post-traumatic sinus tarsi syndrome: An anatomical and radiological study. Acta Orthop Scand 48:121, 1977.

245. Goosens M, De Stoop N, Claessens H, et al: Posterior subtalar joint arthrography: A useful tool in the diagnosis of hindfoot disorders. Clin Orthop 249:248, 1989.

246. Taillard W, Meyer JM, Garcia J, et al: The sinus tarsi syndrome. Int Orthop 5:117, 1981.

247. Rule J, Yao L, Seeger LL: Spring ligament of the ankle: Normal MR anatomy. AJR 161:1241, 1993.

248. Kato T: The diagnosis and treatment of instability of the subtalar joint. J Bone Joint Surg [Br] 77:400, 1995.

249. Clanton TO: Instability of the subtalar joint. Orthop Clin North Am 20:583, 1989.

250. Louwerens JWK, Ginai AZ, van Linge B, et al: Stress radiography of the talocrural and subtalar joints. Foot Ankle 16:148, 1995.

251. Ogilvie-Harris DJ, Mahomed N, Demazière A: Anterior impingement of the ankle treated by arthroscopic removal of bony spurs. J Bone Joint Surg [Br] 75:437, 1993.

252. Morris LH: Athlete's ankle. J Bone Joint Surg 25:220, 1943.

253. McMurray TP: Footballer's ankle. J Bone Joint Surg [Br] 32:68, 1950.

254. King JW, Tullos H, Stanley R, et al: Lesions of the feet in athletes. South Med J 64:45, 1971.

255. Brodelius A: Osteoarthritis of the talar joints in footballers and ballet dancers. Acta Orthop Scand 30:309, 1960.

256. O'Donoghue DH: Impingement exostoses of the talus and tibia. J Bone Joint Surg [Am] 39:835, 1957.

257. Hardaker WT Jr, Margello S, Goldner JL: Foot and ankle injuries in theatrical dancers. Foot Ankle 6:59, 1985.

258. Khan K, Brown J, Way S, et al: Overuse injuries in classical ballet. Sports Med 19:341, 1995.

259. Ferkel RD, Scranton PE Jr: Arthroscopy of the ankle and foot. J Bone Joint Surg [Am] 75:1233, 1993.

260. Jaivin JS, Ferkel RD: Arthroscopy of the foot and ankle. Clin Sports Med 13:761, 1994.

261. Bassett F, Gates H, Billys J, et al: Talar impingement by the anteroinferior tibiofibular ligament. J Bone Joint Surg [Am] 72:55, 1990.

262. Ferkel R, Fischer S: Progress in ankle arthroscopy. Clin Orthop 240:210, 1988.

263. McCarroll J, Schrader J, Shelbourne K, et al: Meniscoid lesions of the ankle in soccer players. Am J Sports Med 15:255, 1987.

264. Martin D, Curl W, Baker C: Arthroscopic treatment of chronic synovitis of the ankle. Arthroscopy 5:110, 1989.

265. Wolin I, Glassman F, Sideman S, et al: Internal derangement of the talofibular component of the ankle. Surg Gynecol Obstet 91:193, 1950.

266. Liu SH, Raskin A, Osti L, et al: Arthroscopic treatment of anterolateral ankle impingement. J Arthrosc Rel Surg 10:215, 1994.

267. Bassett FH III, Gates HS III, Billys TE: Talar impingement by anteroinferior tibiofibular ligament. J Bone Joint Surg [Am] 72:55, 1990.

268. Ferkel RD, Fasulo GJ: Arthroscopic treatment of ankle injuries. Orthop Clin North Am 25:17, 1994.

269. Jahss MH: Tendon disorders of the foot and ankle. In MH Jahss (Ed): Disorders of the Foot and Ankle. 2nd Ed. Philadelphia, WB Saunders Co, 1991, p. 1461.

270. Morti R: Dislocation of the peroneal nerve. Am J Sports Med 5:19, 1977.

271. Murr S: Dislocation of the peroneal tendon with marginal fracture of the lateral malleolus. J Bone Joint Surg [Br] 43:563, 1965.

272. Thompson FM, Patterson AH: Rupture of the peroneus longus tendon: Report of three cases. J Bone Joint Surg [Am] 71:293, 1989.

273. Cheung Y, Rosenberg ZS, Magee T, et al: Normal anatomy and pathologic conditions of ankle tendons: Current imaging techniques. Radiographics 12:429, 1992.

274. Martinoli C, Derchi LE, Pastorino C, et al: Analysis of echotexture of tendons with US. Radiology 186:839, 1993.

275. Solomon MA, Gilula LA, Oloff LM, et al: CT scanning of the foot and ankle. 2. Clinical applications and review of the literature. AJR 146:1204, 1986.

276. Rosenberg ZS, Feldman F, Singson RD: Peroneal tendon injuries: CT analysis. Radiology 161:743, 1986.

277. Szczukowski M, St Pierre RK, Fleming LL, et al: Computerized tomography in the evaluation of peroneal tendon dislocation: A report of two cases. Am J Sports Med 11:444, 1983.

278. Keyser CK, Gilula LA, Hardy DC, et al: Soft-tissue abnormalities of the foot and ankle: CT diagnosis. AJR *150*:845, 1988.

279. Baker KS, Gilula LA: The current role of tenography and bursography. AJR *154*:129, 1990.

280. Deyerle WM: Long term follow-up of fractures of the os calcis: Diagnostic peroneal synoviagram. Orthop Clin North Am *4*:213, 1973.

281. Abraham E, Stirnaman JE: Neglected rupture of the peroneal tendons causing recurrent sprains of the ankle: Case report. J Bone Joint Surg [Am] *61*:1247, 1979.

282. Evans GA, Frenyo SK: The stress-tenogram in the diagnosis of ruptures of the lateral ligament of the ankle. J Bone Joint Surg [Br] *61*:347, l979.

283. Teng MMH, Destouet JM, Gilula LA, et al: Ankle tenography: A key to unexplained symptomatology. I. Normal tenographic anatomy. Radiology *151*:575, 1984.

284. Reinus WR, Gilula LA, Lesiak LF, et al: Tenography in unresolved ankle tenosynovitis. Orthopedics *10*:497, l987.

285. Beltran J, Noto AM, Mosure JC, et al: Ankle: Surface coil MR imaging at 1.5T. Radiology *161*:203, 1986.

286. Hajek PC, Baker LL, Bjorkengren A, et al: High-resolution magnetic resonance imaging of the ankle: Normal anatomy. Skel Radiol *15*:536, 1986.

287. Kneeland JB, Macrandar S, Middleton WD, et al: MR imaging of the normal ankle: Correlation with anatomic sections. AJR *151*:117, 1988.

288. Rosenberg ZS, Cheung Y, Jahss M: Computed tomography and magnetic resonance imaging of ankle tendons: An overview. Foot Ankle *8*:297, 1988.

289. Berquist TH: Magnetic resonance imaging of the foot and ankle. Semin Ultrasound CT MR *11*:327, 1990.

290. Kier R, McCarthy S, Dietz MJ, et al: MR appearance of painful conditions of the ankle. Radiographics *11*:401, 1991.

291. Klein MA: Reformatted three-dimensional Fourier transform gradient-recalled echo MR imaging of the ankle: Spectrum of normal and abnormal findings. AJR *161*:831, 1993.

292. Aerts P, Disler DG: Abnormalities of the foot and ankle: MR imaging findings. AJR *165*:119, 1995.

293. Smith DK: Imaging of sports injuries of the ankle and foot. Oper Tech Sports Med *3*:47, 1995.

294. Rosenberg ZS, Cheung Y, Jahss MH, et al: Rupture of posterior tibial tendon: CT and MR imaging with surgical correlation. Radiology *169*:229, 1988.

295. Schweitzer ME, Caccese R, Karasick D, et al: Posterior tibial tendon tears: Utility of secondary signs for MR imaging diagnosis. Radiology *188*:655, 1993.

296. Rosenberg ZS: Chronic rupture of the posterior tibial tendon. MRI Clin North Am *2*:79, 1994.

297. Weinstabl R, Stiskal M, Neuhold A, et al: Classifying calcaneal tendon injury according to MRI findings. J Bone Joint Surg [Br] *73*:683, 1991.

298. Neuhold A, Stiskal M, Kainberger F, et al: Degenerative Achilles tendon disease: Assessment by magnetic resonance and ultrasonography. Eur J Radiol *14*:213, 1992.

299. Liem MD, Zegel HG, Balduini FC, et al: Repair of Achilles tendon ruptures with a polylactic acid implant: Assessment with MR imaging. AJR *156*:769, 1991.

300. Chandnani VP, Bradley YC: Achilles tendon and miscellaneous tendon lesions. MRI Clin North Am *2*:89, 1994.

301. Schweitzer ME, van Leersum M, Ehrlich SS, et al: Fluid in normal and abnormal ankle joints: Amount and distribution as seen on MR images. AJR *162*:111, 1994.

302. Kettlekamp DB, Alexander HH: Spontaneous rupture of the posterior tibial tendon. J Bone Joint Surg [Am] *51*:759, 1969.

303. Jahss MH: Spontaneous rupture of the tibialis posterior tendon: Clinical findings, tenographic studies, and a new technique of repair. Foot Ankle *3*:158, 1982.

304. Johnson KA: Tibialis posterior tendon rupture. Clin Orthop *177*:140, 1983.

305. Keene JS: Tendon injuries of the foot and ankle. *In* JC DeLee, D Drez Jr (Eds): Orthopaedic Sports Medicine: Principles and Practice. Philadelphia, WB Saunders Co, 1994, p. 1768.

306. Lagergren C, Lindholm A: Vascular disruption in the achilles tendon and angiographic and microangiographic study. Acta Chir Scand *116*:481, 1985.

307. Astrom M, Westlin N: Blood flow in the human Achilles tendon assessed by laser Doppler flowmetry. J Orthop Surg *12*:246, 1994.

308. Schmidt-Rohlfing B, Graf J, Schneider U, et al: The blood supply of the Achilles tendon. Int Orthop (SICOT) *16*:29, 1992.

309. DeMaio M, Paine R, Drez DJ Jr: Achilles tendonitis. Orthopedics *18*:195, 1995.

310. Quinn SF, Murray WT, Clark RA, et al: Achilles tendon: MR imaging at 1.5T. Radiology *164*:767, 1987.

311. Christensen IB: Rupture of the Achilles tendon: Analysis of 57 cases. Acta Chir Scand *106*:50, 1953.

312. Marcus DS, Reicher MA, Kellerhouse LE: Achilles tendon injuries: The role of MR imaging. J Comput Assist Tomogr *13*:480, 1989.

313. Keene JS, Lash EG, Fisher DR, et al: Magnetic resonance imaging of achilles tendon ruptures. Am J Sports Med *17*:333, 1989.

314. Reinig JW, Dorwart RH, Roden WC: MR imaging of a ruptured Achilles tendon. J Comput Assist Tomogr *9*:1131, 1985.

315. Soma CA, Mandelbaum BR: Repair of acute Achilles tendon ruptures. Orthop Clin North Am *26*:239, 1995.

316. Kellam JF, Hunter GA, McElwain JP: Review of the operative treatment of Achilles tendon rupture. Clin Orthop *201*:80, 1985.

317. Beskin JL, Sanders RA, Hunter SC, et al: Surgical repair of Achilles tendon ruptures. Am J Sports Med *15*:1, 1987.

318. Inglis AE, Sculco TP: Surgical repair of ruptures of the tendo Achilles. Clin Orthop *156*:160, 1981.

319. Greenfield G, Stanish WD: Tendinitis and tendon ruptures. Oper Techniques Sports Med *2*:9, 1994.

320. Bude RO, Adler RS, Bassett DR, et al: Heterozygous familial hypercholesterolemia: Detection of xanthomas in the Achilles tendon with US. Radiology *188*:567, 1993.

321. Bude RO, Adler RS, Bassett DR: Diagnosis of Achilles tendon xanthoma in patients with heterozygous familial hypercholesterolemia: MR vs sonography. AJR *162*:913, 1994.

322. Dussault RG, Kaplan PA, Roederer GA: MR imaging of Achilles tendon in patients with familial hyperlipidemia: Comparison with plain films, physical examination, and patients with traumatic tendon lesions. AJR *164*:403, 1995.

323. Koivunen-Niemela T, Komu M, Viikari J, et al: Magnetic resonance imaging of Achilles tendon xanthomas using a fat-water discrimination technique at 0.1 T. Acad Radiol *2*:319, 1995.

324. Rooks MD: Tendon, vascular, nerve, and skin injuries. *In* JS Gould (Ed): Operative Foot Surgery. Philadelphia, WB Saunders Co, 1994, p. 515.

325. Funk DA, Cass JR, Johnson KA: Acquired adult flat foot secondary to posterior tibial tendon pathology. J Bone Joint Surg [Am] *68*:95, 1986.

326. Goldner JL, Keats PK, Bassett FH III: Progressive talipes equinovalgus due to trauma or degeneration of the posterior tibial tendon and medial plantar ligaments. Orthop Clin North Am *15*:39, 1974.

327. Scheller AD, Kasser JR, Quigley TB: Tendon injuries about the ankle. Orthop Clin North Am *11*:801, 1980.

328. Marcus RE, Goodfellow DB, Pfister ME: The difficult diagnosis of posterior tibialis tendon rupture in sports injuries. Orthopedics *18*:715, 1995.

329. Masterson E, Jagannathan S, Borton D, et al: Pes planus in childhood due to tibialis posterior tendon injuries. J Bone Joint Surg [Br] *76*:444, 1994.

330. Blake RL, Anderson K, Ferguson H: Posterior tibial tendinitis. A literature review with case reports. J Am Podiatr Med Assoc *84*:141, 1994.

331. Frey C, Shereff M, Greenridge N: Vascularity of the posterior tibial tendon. J Bone Joint Surg [Am] *72*:884, 1990.

332. Stein R: Rupture of the posterior tibial tendon in closed ankle fractures: Possible prognostic value of a medial bone flake. Report of two cases. J Bone Joint Surg [Am] *67*:493, 1985.

333. Karasick D, Schweitzer ME: Tear of the posterior tibial tendon causing asymptomatic flatfoot: Radiologic findings. AJR *161*:1237, 1993.

334. Hamilton WG: Conditions seen in classical ballet and modern dance. *In* JS Gould (Ed): Operative Foot Surgery. Philadelphia, WB Saunders Co, 1994, p. 954.

335. Gould N: Stenosing tenosynovitis of the flexor hallucis longus tendon at the great toe. Foot Ankle *2*:46, 1981.

336. Sammarco GJ, Miller ED: Partial rupture of the flexor hallucis longus tendon in classical ballet dancers. J Bone Joint Surg [Am] *61*:149, 1979.

337. Romash MM: Closed rupture of the flexor hallucis longus tendon in a long distance runner: Report of a case and review of the literature. Foot Ankle *15*:433, 1994.

338. Howse AJG: Posterior block of the ankle joint in dancers. Foot Ankle *3*:81, 1982.

339. Hamilton WG: Stenosing tenosynovitis of the flexor hallucis longus tendon and posterior impingement upon the os trigonum in ballet dancers. Foot Ankle *3*:74, 1982.

340. Hamilton WG: Foot and ankle injuries in dancers. Clin Sports Med *7*:143, 1988.

341. Lapidus PW: Indirect subcutaneous rupture of the anterior tibial tendon: Report of two cases. Bull Hosp Joint Dis *2*:119, 1941.

342. Moberg E: Subcutaneous rupture of the tendon of the tibialis anterior muscle. Acta Chir Scand *95*:455, 1947.

343. Mensor MC, Ordway GI. Traumatic subcutaneous rupture of the tibialis anterior tendon. J Bone Joint Surg [Am] *35*:675, 1953.

344. Ouzounian TJ, Anderson R: Anterior tibial tendon rupture. Foot Ankle *16*:406, 1995.

345. Davis WH, Sobel M, Deland J, et al: The superior peroneal retinaculum: An anatomic study. Foot Ankle *15*:271, 1994.

346. Kojima Y, Kataoka Y, Suzuki S: Dislocations of the peroneal tendons in neonates and infants. Clin Orthop *266*:180, 1991.

347. Eckert WR, Davis EA: Acute rupture of the peroneal retinaculum. J Bone Joint Surg [Am] *58*:670, 1976.

348. Oden R: Tendon injuries about the ankle resulting from skiing. Clin Orthop *216*:63, 1987.

349. Rosenberg Z, Feldman F, Singson R: Peroneal tendon injuries: CT analysis. Radiology *161*:743, 1986.

350. Tourne Y, Saragaglia D, Benzakour D, et al: La Luxation traumatique des tendons peroniers: A propos de 36 cas. Int Orthop (SICOT) *19*:197, 1995.

351. Hutchinson BL, Gustafson LS: Chronic peroneal tendon subluxation: New surgical technique and retrospective analysis. J Am Podiatr Med Assoc *84*:511, 1994.

352. Zeiss J, Saddemi SR, Ebraheim NA: MR imaging of the peroneal tunnel. J Comput Assist Tomogr *13*:840, 1989.

353. Trevino S, Gould N, Korson R: Surgical treatment of stenosing tenosynovitis at the ankle. Foot Ankle 2:37, 1981.

354. McConkey JP, Favero KJ: Subluxation of the peroneal tendons within the peroneal sheath: A case report. Am J Sports Med 15:511, 1987.

355. Deyerle WM: Long term follow-up of fractures of the os calcis. Orthop Clin North Am 4:213, 1973.

356. Burman M: Stenosing tendovaginitis of the foot and ankle. Arch Surg 67:686, 1953.

357. Sammarco GJ: Peroneus longus tendon tears: Acute and chronic. Foot Ankle 16:245, 1995.

358. Yao L, Tong DJF, Cracchiolo A, et al: MR findings in peroneal tendonopathy. J Comput Assist Tomogr 19:460, 1995.

359. Thompson F, Patterson A: Rupture of the peroneus longus tendon: Report of three cases. J Bone Joint Surg [Am] 71:293, 1989.

360. Munk RL, Davis PH: Longitudinal rupture of the peroneus brevis tendon. J Trauma 16:803, 1976.

361. Peacock KC, Resnick EJ, Thoder JJ: Fracture of the os peroneum with rupture of the peroneus longus tendon. Clin Orthop 202:223, 1984.

362. Sobel M, Pavlov H, Geppert MJ, et al: Painful os peroneum syndrome: A spectrum of conditions responsible for painful lateral foot pain. Foot Ankle 15:112, 1994.

363. Smith AD, Carter JR, Marcus RE: The os vesalianum: An unusual cause of lateral foot pain: A case report and review of the literature. Orthopedics 7:86, 1984.

364. Sella EJ, Lawson JP, Ogden JA: The accessory navicular synchondrosis. Clin Orthop 209:280, 1986.

365. Lawson JP, Ogden JA, Sella E, et al: The painful accessory navicular. Skel Radiol 12:250, 1984.

366. Romanowski CAJ, Barrington NA: The accessory navicular—an important cause of medial foot pain. Clin Radiol 46:261, 1992.

367. Miller TT, Staron RB, Feldman F, et al: The symptomatic accessory tarsal navicular bone: Assessment with MR imaging. Radiology 195:849, 1995.

368. Grogan DP, Gasser SI, Ogden JA: The painful accessory navicular: A clinical and histopathological study. Foot Ankle 10:164, 1989.

369. Kidner FC: The prehallux (accessory scaphoid) in its relation to flatfoot. J Bone Joint Surg 11:831, 1929.

370. Sullivan JA, Miller WA: The relationship of the accessory navicular to the development of the flat foot. Clin Orthop 144:233, 1979.

371. Bower BL, Keyser CK, Gilula LA: Rigid subtalar joint—a radiographic spectrum. Skel Radiol 17:583, 1989.

372. Harris BJ: Anomalous structures in the developing human foot. Anat Rec 121:399, 1955.

373. Pfitzner W: Die Variationen im Aufbau des Fussskelets. Morphol Arb 6:245, 1896.

374. Slomann HC: On coalition calcaneo-navicularis. J Orthop Surg 3:586, 1921.

375. Harris RI, Beath T: Etiology of peroneal spastic flat foot. J Bone Joint Surg [Br] 30:624, 1948.

376. Chambers CH: Congenital anomalies of the tarsal navicular with particular reference to calcaneo-navicular coalition. Br J Radiol 23:580, 1950.

377. Hark FW: Congenital anomalies of the tarsal bones. Clin Orthop 16:21, 1960.

378. Rothberg AS, Feldman JW, Schuster OF: Congenital fusion of astragalus and scaphoid: Bilateral, inherited. NY State Med J 35:29, 1935.

379. Webster FS, Roberts WM: Tarsal anomalies and peroneal spastic flatfoot. JAMA 146:1099, 1951.

380. Bersani FA, Samilson RL: Massive familial tarsal synostosis. J Bone Joint Surg [Am] 39:1187, 1957.

381. Leonard MA: The inheritance of tarsal coalition and its relationship to spastic flat foot. J Bone Joint Surg [Br] 56:520, 1974.

382. Jones Sir R: Peroneal spasm and its treatment: Report of a meeting of the Liverpool Medical Institution. Liverpool Med Chir J 17:442, 1897.

383. Badgley CE: Coalition of the calcaneus and the navicular. Arch Surg 15:75, 1927.

384. Conway JJ, Cowell HR: Tarsal coalition: Clinical significance and roentgenographic demonstration. Radiology 92:799, 1969.

385. Kendrick JI: Treatment of calcaneonavicular bar. JAMA 172:1242, 1960.

386. Simmons EH: Tibialis spastic varus foot with tarsal coalition. J Bone Joint Surg [Br] 47:533, 1965.

387. Schmidt F: Über eine symmetrische Synostosis calcaneo-navicularis bei gleichzeitigem Klumphohlfuss. Arch Orthop Unfallchir 30:289, 1931.

388. Lapidus PW: Spastic flat foot. J Bone Joint Surg 28:126, 1946.

389. Poznanski AK: Foot manifestations of the congenital malformation syndromes. Semin Roentgenol 5:354, 1970.

390. Beckly DE, Anderson PW, Pedegana LR: The radiology of the subtalar joint with special reference to talo-calcaneal coalition. Clin Radiol 26:333, 1975.

391. Jack EA: Bone anomalies of the tarsus in relation to "peroneal spastic flat foot." J Bone Joint Surg [Br] 36:530, 1954.

392. Feist JH, Mankin JH: The tarsus. I. Basic relationships and motions in the adult and definition of optimal recumbent oblique projection. Radiology 79:250, 1962.

393. Sarno RC, Carter BL, Bankoff MS, et al: Computed tomography in tarsal coalition. J Comput Assist Tomogr 8:1155, 1984.

394. Sartoris DJ, Resnick DL: Tarsal coalition. Arthritis Rheum 28:331, 1985.

395. Deutsch AL, Resnick D, Campbell G: Computed tomography and bone scintigraphy in the evaluation of tarsal coalition. Radiology 144:137, 1982.

396. Goldman AB, Pavlov H, Schneider R: Radionuclide bone scanning in subtalar coalitions: Differential considerations. AJR 138:427, 1982.

397. Pineda C, Resnick D, Greenway G: Diagnosis of tarsal coalition with computed tomography. Clin Orthop 208:282, 1986.

398. Stormont DM, Peterson HA: The relative incidence of tarsal coalition. Clin Orthop 181:28, 1983.

399. Mosier KM, Asher M: Tarsal coalitions and peroneal spastic flat foot: A review. J Bone Joint Surg [Am] 66:976, 1984.

400. Rosen JS: Tarsal coalitions: Rare or not. J Am Podiatry Assoc 74:572, 1984.

401. Richards RR, Evans JG, McGoey PF: Fracture of a calcaneonavicular bar: A complication of tarsal coalition. A case report. Clin Orthop 185:220, 1984.

402. Wheeler R, Guevara A, Bleck EE: Tarsal coalitions: A review of the literature and case report of bilateral dual calcaneonavicular and talocalcaneal coalitions. Clin Orthop 156:175, 1981.

403. Inglis G, Buxton RA, Macnicol MF: Symptomatic calcaneonavicular bars: The results 20 years after surgical excision. J Bone Joint Surg [Br] 68:128, 1986.

404. Herschel H, von Ronnen JR: The occurrence of calcaneonavicular synosteosis in pes valgus contractus. J Bone Joint Surg [Am] 32:280, 1950.

405. Oestreich AE, Mize WA, Crawford AH, et al: The "anterior nose": A direct sign of calcaneonavicular coalition on the lateral radiograph. J Pediatr Orthop 7:709, 1987.

406. Braddock GTF: A prolonged follow-up of peroneal spastic flat foot. J Bone Joint Surg [Br] 43:734, 1961.

407. Warren MJ, Jeffree MA, Wilson DJ, et al: Computed tomography in suspected tarsal coalition: Examination of 26 cases. Acta Orthop Scand 61:554, 1990.

408. Kumar SJ, Guille JT, Lee MS, et al: Osseous and non-osseous coalition of the middle facet of the talocalcaneal joint. J Bone Joint Surg [Am] 74:529, 1992.

409. Lee MS, Harcke HT, Kumar SJ, et al: Subtalar joint coalition in children: New observations. Radiology 172:635, 1989.

410. Kaye JJ, Ghelman B, Schneider R: Talocalcaneonavicular joint arthrography for sustentacular-talar tarsal coalitions. Radiology 115:730, 1975.

411. Resnick D: Talar ridges, osteophytes, and beaks: A radiologic commentary. Radiology 151:329, 1984.

412. Shaffer HA Jr, Harrison RB: Tarsal pseudo-coalition—a positional artifact. Can Assoc Radiol J 31:236, 1980.

413. Brahme F: Upper talar enarthrosis. Acta Radiol 55:221, 1961.

414. Schrieber RR: Congenital and acquired ball-and-socket ankle joint. Radiology 84:940, 1965.

415. Lamb D: The ball and socket ankle joint—a congenital abnormality. J Bone Joint Surg [Br] 40:240, 1958.

416. Channon GM, Brotherton BJ: The ball and socket ankle joint. J Bone Joint Surg [Br] 61:85, 1979.

417. Takakura Y, Tamai S, Masuhara K: Genesis of the ball-and-socket ankle. J Bone Joint Surg [Br] 68:834, 1986.

418. Pistoia F, Ozonoff MB, Wintz P: Ball-and-socket ankle joint. Skel Radiol 16:447, 1987.

419. Dennis DA, Clayton ML, Ferlic DC: Osteoarthritis associated with a ball-and-socket ankle joint: A case report. Clin Orthop 215:196, 1987.

420. Lateur LM, Van Hoe LR, Van Ghillewe KV, et al: Subtalar coalition: Diagnosis with the C sign on lateral radiographs of the ankle. Radiology 193:847, 1994.

421. Scranton PE Jr: Treatment of symptomatic talocalcaneal coalition. J Bone Joint Surg [Am] 69:533, 1987.

422. Takakura Y, Sugimoto K, Tanaka Y, et al: Symptomatic talocalcaneal coalition: Its clinical significance and treatment. Clin Orthop 269:249, 1991.

423. Wechsler RJ, Karasick D, Schweitzer ME: Computed tomography of talocalcaneal coalition: Imaging techniques. Skel Radiol 21:353, 1992.

424. Herzenberg JE, Goldner JL, Martinez S, et al: Computerized tomography of talocalcaneal tarsal coalition: A clinical and anatomic study. Foot Ankle 6:273, 1986.

425. Percy EC, Mann DL: Tarsal coalition: A review of the literature and presentation of 13 cases. Foot Ankle 9:40, 1988.

426. Boyd HB: Congenital talonavicular synostosis. J Bone Joint Surg 26:682, 1944.

427. Challis J: Hereditary transmission of talonavicular coalition in association with anomaly of the little finger. J Bone Joint Surg [Am] 56:1273, 1974.

428. Zeide MS, Wiesel SW, Terry RL: Talonavicular coalition. Clin Orthop 126:225, 1977.

429. Cowell HR, Elener V: Rigid painful flatfoot secondary to tarsal coalition. Clin Orthop 177:54, 1983.

430. Mahaffey HW: Bilateral congenital calcaneocuboid synostosis, a case report. J Bone Joint Surg 27:164, 1945.

431. Veneruso LC: Unilateral congenital calcaneocuboid synostosis with complete absence of a metatarsal and toe, a case report. J Bone Joint Surg 27:718, 1945.

432. Outland T, Murphy ID: Relation of tarsal anomalies to spastic and rigid flatfeet. Clin Orthop 1:217, 1953.

433. Waugh W: Partial cubo-navicular coalition as a cause of peroneal spastic flat foot. J Bone Joint Surg [Br] 39:520, 1957.

434. Lusby HLJ: Naviculo-cuneiform synostosis. J Bone Joint Surg [Br] 41:150, 1959.

435. Gregersen HN: Naviculocuneiform coalition. J Bone Joint Surg [Am] 59:128, 1977.

436. Koski JM: Ultrasonography of the metatarsophalangeal and talocrural joints. Clin Exper Rheumatol 2:347, 1990.

437. Nazarian LN, Rawool NM, Martin CE, et al: Synovial fluid in the hindfoot and ankle: Detection of amount and distribution with US. Radiology 197:275, 1995.

438. Friscia DA: Pigmented villonodular synovitis of the ankle: A case report and review of the literature. Foot Ankle 15:674, 1994.

439. Cheung KMC, Chow SP: Pigmented villonodular synovitis of the ankle: Correlation of MRI and operative findings. J Orthop Rheumatol 7:117, 1994.

440. Ontell F, Greenspan A: Chondrosarcoma complicating synovial chondromatosis: Findings with magnetic resonance imaging. Can Assoc Rad J 45:318, 1994.

441. Bergman AG: Magnetic resonance imaging manifestations of synovial lesions of the ankle and foot. MRI Clin N Amer 2:131, 1994.

442. Haglund P: Beitrag zur Klinik der Achillessechne. Z Orthop Chir 49:49, 1927.

443. Pavlov H, Henneghan MA, Hersh A, et al: Haglund's deformity: Diagnosis and differential diagnosis of posterior heel pain. Radiology 144:83, 1982.

444. Rufai A, Ralphs JR, Benjamin M: Structure and histopathology of the insertional region of the human Achilles tendon. J Orthop Res 13:585, 1995.

445. Dunn AW: Anomalous muscles simulating soft tissue tumors in the lower extremities: Report of three cases. J Bone Joint Surg [Am] 47:1397, 1965.

446. Ger E, Sedlin E: The accessory soleus muscle. Clin Orthop 116:200, 1976.

447. Gordon SL, Matheson DW: The accessory soleus. Clin Orthop 97:129, 1973.

448. Paul MA, Imanse J, Golding RP, et al: Accessory soleus muscle mimicking a soft tissue tumor: A report of 2 patients. Acta Orthop Scand 62:609, 1991.

449. Danielsson LG, El-Haddad I, Sabri T: Clubfoot with supernumerary soleus muscle: Report of 2 cases. Acta Orthop Scand 61:371, 1990.

450. Buschmann WR, Cheung Y, Jahss MH: Magnetic resonance imaging of anomalous leg muscles: Accessory soleus, peroneus quartus and the flexor digitorum longus accessorius. Foot Ankle 12:109, 1991.

451. Percy EC, Telep GN: Anomalous muscles in the leg: Soleus accessorium. Am J Sports Med 12:447, 1984.

452. Beasley AW: The accessory soleus. Aust N Zeal J Surg 49:86, 1979.

453. Lorentzon R, Wirell S: Anatomic variations of the accessory soleus muscle. Acta Radiol 28:627, 1987.

454. White AA, Johnson DJ, Griswold DM: Chronic ankle pain associated with the peroneus accessorius. Clin Orthop 103:53, 1974.

455. Wachter S, Beekman S: Peroneus quartus: A case report. J Am Podiatr Assoc 73:523, 1983.

456. Regan TP, Hughston JC: Chronic ankle "sprain" secondary to anomalous peroneal tendon. Clin Orthop 123:55, 1977.

457. Sobel M, Levy ME, Bohne WHO: Congenital variations of the peroneus quartus muscle: An anatomic study. Foot Ankle 11:81, 1990.

458. Moorman CT III, Monto RR, Bassett FH III: So-called trigger ankle due to an aberrant flexor hallucis longus muscle in a tennis player: A case report. J Bone Joint Surg [Am] 74:294, 1992.

459. Chason DP, Schultz SM, Fleckenstein JL: Tensor fasciae suralis: Depiction on MR images. AJR 165:120, 1995.

460. DeMaio M, Paine R, Mangine RE, et al: Plantar fasciitis. Orthopedics 16:1153, 1993.

461. McBryde AM: Plantar fasciitis. Instr Course Lect 33:278, 1984.

462. Bordelon RL: Subcalcaneal pain. Clin Orthop 177:49, 1983.

463. Leach RE, Dilorio E, Harney RA: Pathologic hindfoot conditions in the athlete. Clin Orthop 177:116, 1983.

464. Kwong PK, Kay D, Voner RT, et al: Plantar fasciitis: Mechanics and pathomechanics of treatment. Clin Sports Med 7:119, 1988.

465. Azouz EM, Duffy CM: Juvenile spondyloarthropathies: Clinical manifestations and medical imaging. Skel Radiol 24:399, 1995.

466. Graham CE: Painful heel syndrome: Rationale of diagnosis and treatment. Foot Ankle 3:261, 1983.

467. Baxter DE, Thigpen CM: Heel pain—operative results. Foot Ankle 5:16, 1984.

468. Furey JG: Plantar fasciitis: The painful heel syndrome. J Bone Joint Surg [Am] 57:672, 1975.

469. Clancy WG Jr: Tendinitis and plantar fasciitis in runners. Orthopedics 6:217, 1983.

470. Snider MP, Clancy WG Jr, McBeath AA: Plantar fascia release for chronic plantar fasciitis in runners. Am J Sports Med 11:215, 1983.

471. Berkowitz JF, Kier R, Rudicel S: Plantar fasciitis: MR imaging. Radiology 179:665, 1991.

472. Helie O, DuBayle P, Boyer B, et al: Imagerie par résonance magnétique de lésions de l'aponévrose plantaire superficielle. J Radiol 76:37, 1995.

473. Kier R: Magnetic resonance imaging of plantar fasciitis and other causes of heel pain. MRI Clin North Am 2:97, 1994.

474. Buschmann WR, Jahss MH, Kummer F, et al: Histology and histomorphometric analysis of the normal and atrophic heel fat pad. Foot and Ankle 16:254, 1995.

475. Prichasuk S, Subhadrabandhu T: The relationship of pes planus and calcaneal spur to plantar heel pain. Clin Orthop 306:192, 1994.

476. Aviles E, Arlen M, Miller T: Plantar fibromatosis. Surgery 69:117, 1971.

477. Allen RA, Woolner LB, Ghormley RK: Soft-tissue tumors of the sole: With special reference to plantar fibromatosis. J Bone Joint Surg [Am] 37:14, 1955.

478. Lee TH, Hecht PJ: Plantar fibromatosis. J Bone Joint Surg [Am] 75:1080, 1993.

479. Pickren JW, Smith AG, Stevenson TW Jr, et al: Fibromatosis of the plantar fascia. Cancer 4:846, 1951.

480. Morrison WB, Schweitzer ME, Wapner KL, et al: Plantar fibromatosis: A benign aggressive neoplasm with a characteristic appearance on MR images. Radiology 193:841, 1994.

481. Feingold ML, Resnick D, Niwayama G, et al: The plantar compartments of the foot: A roentgen approach. Invest Radiol 12:281, 1977.

482. Sartoris DJ, Devine S, Resnick D, et al: Plantar compartmental infection in the diabetic foot: The role of computed tomography. Invest Radiol 20:772, 1985.

483. Goodwin DW, Salonen DC, Yu JS, et al: Plantar compartments of the foot: MR appearance in cadavers and diabetic patients. Radiology 196:623, 1995.

484. Erickson SJ, Quinn SF, Kneeland JB, et al: MR imaging of the tarsal tunnel and related spaces: Normal and abnormal findings with anatomic correlation. AJR 155:323, 1990.

485. Kerr R, Frey C: MR imaging in tarsal tunnel syndrome. J Comput Assist Tomogr 15:280, 1991.

486. Zeiss J, Ebraheim N, Rusin J: Magnetic resonance imaging in the diagnosis of tarsal tunnel syndrome: Case report. Clin Imaging 14:123, 1990.

487. Zeiss J, Fenton P, Ebraheim N, et al: Normal magnetic resonance anatomy of the tarsal tunnel. Foot Ankle 10:214, 1990.

488. Dellon AL: Deep peroneal nerve entrapment on the dorsum of the foot. Foot Ankle 11:73, 1990.

489. Schon LC, Baxter DE: Neuropathies of the foot and ankles in athletes. Clin Sports Med 9:489, 1990.

490. Kerr R: Spectrum of disorders. In AL Deutsch, JH Mink, R Kerr (Eds): MRI of the Foot and Ankle. New York, Raven Press, 1992, p. 345.

491. Raynor KJ, Raczka EK, Stone PA, et al: Entrapment of the sural nerve. J Am Podiatr Med Assoc 76:401, 1986.

492. Pringle RM, Protheroe K, Mukherjee SK: Entrapment neuropathy of the sural nerve. J Bone Joint Surg [Br] 56:465, 1974.

493. Addante JB, Peicott PS, Wong KY, et al: Interdigital neuromas: Results of surgical excision of 152 neuromas. J Am Podiatr Med Assoc 76:493, 1986.

494. Reed RJ, Bliss BO: Morton's neuroma. Arch Pathol 95:123, 1973.

495. Mann RA, Reynolds JC: Interdigital neuroma—a critical clinical analysis. Foot Ankle 3:238, 1983.

496. Coughlin MJ: Second metatarsophalangeal joint instability in the athlete. Foot Ankle 14:309, 1993.

497. Rubin DA, Towers JD, Britton CA: MR imaging of the foot: Utility of complex oblique imaging planes. AJR 166:1079, 1996.

498. Morris JR, Lee J, Thordarson D, et al: Magnetic resonance imaging of acute Maisonneuve fractures. Foot Ankle 17:259, 1966.

499. Matsui Y, Myoui A, Nakahara H, et al: Prognostic significance of posterior subtalar joint arthrography following fractures of the calcaneus. Arch Orthop Trauma Surg 114:257, 1995.

500. Khoury NJ, El-Khoury GY, Saltzman CL, et al: Intraarticular foot and ankle injections to identify source of pain before arthrodesis. AJR 167:669, 1996.

501. Truong DT, Dussault RG, Kaplan PA: Fracture of the os peroneum and rupture of the peroneus longus tendon as a complication of diabetic neuropathy. Skeletal Radiol 24:626, 1995.

502. Yao L, Cracchiolo A, Farahani K, et al: Magnetic resonance imaging of plantar plate rupture. Foot Ankle 17:33, 1996.

503. Grebe P, Kreitner KF, Roeder W, et al: Außenbandrupturen des Sprunggelenkes—Darstellung mit der MRT vor und nach functioneller Therapie. Fortschr Röntgenstr 163:225, 1995.

504. Breitenseher MJ, Trattnig S, Kukla C, et al: Verletzungen des Außenbandapparates am oberen Sprunggelenk: Untersuchungstechnik und Nachweis mittels MRT. Fortschr Röntgenstr 164:226, 1996.

505. Rosenberg ZS, Cheung YY, Beltran J, et al: Posterior intermalleolar ligament of the ankle: Normal anatomy and MR imaging features. AJR 165:387, 1995.

506. van Duk CN, Bossuyt PMM, Marti RK: Medial ankle pain after lateral ligament rupture. J Bone Joint Surg [Br] 78:562, 1996.

507. Rollandi GA, Bertolotto M, Perrone R, et al: MRI of normal Achilles tendon. Eur Radiol 5:596, 1995.

508. Myerson MS: Adult acquired flatfoot deformity. Treatment of dysfunction of the posterior tibial tendon. J Bone Joint Surg [Am] 78:780, 1996.

509. Khoury NJ, El-Khoury GY, Saltzman CL, et al: MR imaging of posterior tibial tendon dysfunction. AJR 167:675, 1996.

510. Karasick D, Schweitzer ME: The os trigonum syndrome: Imaging features. AJR 166:125, 1996.

511. Khoury NJ, El-Khoury GY, Saltzman CL, et al: Rupture of the anterior tibial tendon: Diagnosis by MR imaging. AJR 167:351, 1996.

512. Geppert MJ, Sobel M, Bohne WHO: Lateral ankle instability as a cause of superior peroneal retinacular laxity: An anatomic and biomechanical study of cadaveric feet. Foot Ankle 14:330, 1993.

513. Pierson JL, Inglis AE: Stenosing tenosynovitis of the peroneus longus tendon associated with hypertrophy of the peroneal tubercle and an os peroneum. A case report. J Bone Joint Surg [Am] 74:440, 1992.

514. Khoury NJ, El-Khoury GY, Saltzman CL, et al: Peroneus longus and brevis tendon tears: MR imaging evaluation. Radiology 200:833, 1996.

515. Braunstein JT, Crues JV III: Magnetic resonance imaging of hereditary hernias of the peroneus longus muscle. Skeletal Radiol 24:601, 1995.

516. Lawrence SJ, Botte MJ: The deep peroneal nerve in the foot and ankle: An anatomic study. Foot Ankle 16:724, 1995.

517. Schweitzer ME, White LM: Does altered biomechanics cause marrow edema? Radiology 198:851, 1996.

518. Nishimura G, Yamato M, Togawa M: Trabecular trauma of the talus and medial malleolus concurrent with lateral collateral ligamentous injuries of the ankle: evaluation with MR imaging. Skeletal Radiol 25:49, 1996.

519. Martin DE, Kaplan PA, Kahler DM, et al: Retrospective evaluation of graded stress examination of the ankle. Clin Orthop Rel Res 328:165, 1996.

520. Aström M, Gentz C-F, Nilsson P, et al: Imaging in chronic achilles tendinopathy: A comparision of ultrasonography, magnetic resonance imaging and surgical findings in 27 histologically verified cases. Skeletal Radiol 25:615, 1996.

521. Hamilton WG, Geppert MJ, Thompson FM: Pain in the posterior aspect of the ankle in dancers: Differential diagnosis and operative treatment. J Bone Joint Surg [Am] 78:1491, 1996.

522. Kolettis GJ, Micheli LJ, Klein JD: Release of the flexor hallucis longus tendon in ballet dancers. J Bone Joint Surg [Am] 78:1386, 1996.

Tables of Disease Processes

Table I. SOME TUMORS AND TUMOR-LIKE LESIONS OF BONE

Lesion	Typical Age (Years)	Typical Location	MR Imaging Features
Bone-Forming Tumors			
Osteoma	15–35	Skull, sinuses, mandible	Well-defined, on surface of bone, low signal intensity
Enostosis	All ages	Pelvis, ribs, femur	Thorny radiations, low signal intensity
Osteoid osteoma	7–25	Long bones	Nidus of variable signal intensity, surrounding marrow and soft tissue edema, synovitis and joint effusion with intra-articular lesions
Osteoblastoma	10–30	Vertebrae, flat bones	Similar to osteoid osteoma
Osteosarcoma	10–25	Long bones, metaphyseal	Ill-defined, inhomogenous or homogenous appearance, low signal intensity in T1-weighted images and high signal intensity in T2-weighted images, soft tissue involvement, ± fluid levels in telangiectatic variety
Parosteal osteosarcoma	20–45	Long bones, especially posterior femur about knee, metaphyseal	Lobulated mass adjacent to bone, variable signal intensity, ± bone involvement
Cartilage-Forming Tumors			
Enchondroma	15–35	Phalanges of hand and foot, long bones, metaphyseal	Well-defined, lobulated, ± endosteal erosion, ± calcification, low signal intensity in T1-weighted images and high signal intensity in T2-weighted images
Chondroblastoma	10–25	Long bones, epiphyseal	Well- or ill-defined, ± joint involvement, low signal intensity in T1-weighted images and variable signal intensity in T2-weighted images, inflammatory response in adjacent metaphysis
Chondromyxoid fibroma	10–25	Long bones, metadiaphyseal	Variable
Osteochondroma	10–30	Long bones, metaphyseal, pelvis	Outgrowth extending from surface of bone, composed of cortical and medullary bone, cartilage cap of high signal intensity in T2-weighted images, complications including fracture, vascular or muscular injury, osseous deformity, bursitis, and malignant transformation
Chondrosarcoma	30–60	Long bones, metaphyseal, pelvis, ribs	Central or peripheral location, inhomogeneous signal intensity, ± soft tissue mass, ± calcification
Tumors Arising from or Forming Fibrous Connective Tissue			
Nonossifying fibroma and fibrous cortical defect	5–25	Long bones, metaphyseal	Single or multiple, eccentric location, well-defined, low signal intensity in T1-weighted images and variable signal intensity in T2-weighted images
Periosteal desmoid (avulsive cortical irregularity)	15–20	Femur, distal metaphyseal	Cortical proliferation or erosion, may be bilateral, low signal intensity in T1-weighted images and variable signal intensity in T2-weighted images
Fibrous dysplasia	Variable	Long and short tubular bones, skull, facial bones, ribs, pelvis	Monostotic or polyostotic, well-defined or ill-defined, low signal intensity in T1-weighted images and variable signal intensity in T2-weighted images
Fibrosarcoma	25–55	Long bones, metadiaphyseal	Ill-defined, ± soft tissue mass, low signal intensity in T1-weighted images and high signal intensity in T2-weighted images

Table 1. SOME TUMORS AND TUMOR-LIKE LESIONS OF BONE *Continued*

Lesion	Typical Age (Years)	Typical Location	MR Imaging Features
Histiocytic or Fibrohistiocytic Tumors			
Giant cell tumor	20–40	Long bones, metaepiphyseal, spine, pelvis	Eccentric, well- or ill-defined, low signal intensity in T1-weighted images and high signal intensity in T2-weighted images, ± fluid levels
Malignant fibrous histiocytoma	40–70	Long bones, metaphyseal, pelvis	Ill-defined, ± soft tissue mass, inhomogeneous signal intensity but mainly low signal intensity in T1-weighted images and high signal intensity in T2-weighted images
Tumors of Fatty Differentiation			
Lipoma	25–50	Femur, calcaneus, fibula, tibia	Intraosseous lesions are well-defined with signal intensity indicative of fat, ± fluid, ± ossification; parosteal lesions are well-defined with signal intensity indicative of fat, ± bone proliferation
Tumors of Vascular Differentiation			
Hemangioma	25–50	Spine, skull, facial bones	Well- or ill-defined, ± soft tissue mass, low or high signal intensity in T1-weighted images, generally high signal intensity in T2-weighted images
Glomus tumor	Variable	Fingertips or nail beds	Small mass, intermediate signal intensity in T1-weighted images and high signal intensity in T2-weighted images
Angiosarcoma	30–40	Long bones, metadiaphyseal, pelvis, ribs	Single or multifocal, variable and inhomogeneous signal intensity
Tumors and Tumor-Like Lesions of Miscellaneous Origin			
Simple bone cyst	5–25	Long bones, metadiaphyseal, pelvis, calcaneus	Well-defined, single intensity characteristics of fluid, rare fluid levels
Epidermoid cyst	15–35	Skull, phalanges of hand	Well-defined, low to high signal intensity in T1-weighted images and high signal intensity in T2-weighted images
Aneurysmal bone cyst	10–30	Long bones, metaphyseal, spine	Well- or ill-defined, ± soft tissue mass, internal septations, inhomogeneous signal intensity in T1-weighted and T2-weighted images, ± fluid levels
Intraosseous ganglion cyst	20–60	Long bones, epiphyscal, acetabulum, lunate bone	Well-defined, signal intensity characteristics of fluid, ± soft tissue ganglion
Adamantinoma	10–40	Tibia, diaphyseal	Well- or ill-defined, low signal intensity in T1- weighted images and high signal intensity in T2-weighed images
Ewing's sarcoma	10–25	Long bones, metadiaphyseal, pelvis, spine	Ill-defined, soft tissue mass and edema, low signal intensity in T1-weighted images and high signal intensity in T2-weighted images
Plasma cell myeloma	55–75	Spine, skull, pelvis	Multifocal or rarely solitary (plasmacytoma), well- or ill-defined, ± soft tissue mass, low signal intensity in T1-weighted images and variable signal intensity in T2-weighted images
Lymphomas and leukemias	Variable	Spine, pelvis, long bones	Solitary or multifocal, well- or ill-defined, ± soft tissue mass, low signal intensity in T1-weighted images and variable signal intensity in T2-weighted images
Skeletal metastasis	50–75	Spine, pelvis	Multiple, ill-defined, low signal intensity in T1-weighted images and high signal intensity in T2-weighted images

Table 2. SOME TUMORS AND TUMOR-LIKE LESIONS OF SOFT TISSUE

Lesion	Typical Age (Years)	Typical Location	MR Imaging Features T1 Signal Intensity	T2 Signal Intensity	Other Features
Tumors of Fat					
Lipoma	30–50	Variable	↑	→	Homogeneous or thin septations
Lipoma arborescens	Adults	Knee	↑	→	Diffuse infiltration of synovium
Lipomatosis	Children and adults	Variable, including shoulder girdle	↑	→	Unilateral or bilateral
Macrodystrophia lipomatosa	Children and adults	Hand, foot	↑	→	Macrodactyly
Fibrolipomatous hamartoma	Early adulthood	Carpal tunnel (median nerve)	↑	→	Tubular structures of low signal intensity may be observed
Liposarcoma	35–70	Variable	Variable	↑	Inhomogeneous, may contain fat, ± septations
Tumors of Fibrous Tissue					
Fibromatoses (see also Table 3)	Children and adults	Variable	↓	Variable	Entrapped fat may be seen in cases of elastofibroma
Fibrosarcoma	Children and adults	Peripheral soft tissues	↓	Variable	
Tumors of Muscle					
Rhabdomyosarcoma	2–6; 14–18	Variable	↓	Variable	
Myxomatoses					
Ganglion cyst	Adults	Hand, wrist, foot, knee	↓	↑	May cause nerve entrapment
Myxoma	40–70	Variable	↓	↑	Single or multiple, associated with fibrous dysplasia
Tumors of Histiocytic Origin					
Xanthomatoses	Adults	Variable, often arise from tendons	↓	Variable, often ↓	Often multiple
Giant cell tumor of tendon sheath	Adults	Hand, foot	↓	Variable, often ↓	
Angiomatoses					
Hemangioma	Children and adults	Variable	Variable, often ↑	↑	May contain fat, foci of low signal intensity represent calcifications or rapid blood flow, ± tubular structures
Glomus tumor	Adults	Fingernail	↓	↑	Nodular appearance
Hemangioendothelioma	Adults	Variable	↓	↑	
Cartilaginous and Osseous Tumors					
Chondroma	20–40	Hand, foot	↓	↑	May calcify, intracapsular tumors are seen in the knee
Tenosynovial chondromatosis	Adults	Hand, wrist, foot, ankle	↓	↑	May calcify or ossify and erode bone
Chondrosarcoma	Adults	Variable	↓	↑	May calcify, often lobulated
Osteoma	Adults	Head, thigh	↓	↑	May ossify
Osteosarcoma	40–70	Extremities	↓	↑	May ossify
Synovial Tumors					
Synovial sarcoma	Adults	Lower extremity	↓	↑	Inhomogeneous signal intensity, ± fluid levels
Tumors of Peripheral Nerves					
Neurofibroma	Variable	Variable	↓	↑	Solitary or multiple, ± neurofibromatosis, target appearance
Neurilemoma	20–50	Head, neck, extremities	↓	↑	Generally solitary, target appearance, ± associated with nearby nerve, ± muscle atrophy
Morton's neuroma	Adults	Foot	↓	↓	Generally in web space between third and fourth toes
Malignant schwannoma	Adults	Trunk, extremities	↓	↑	Inhomogeneous signal intensity, no target appearance
Miscellaneous Tumors					
Clear cell sarcoma	Adults	Extremities	↓	Variable	
Alveolar soft part sarcoma	Children and adults	Orbit, retroperitoneum, extremities	↑	↑	Signal void may be evident
Epithelioid sarcoma	Adults	Finger, hand, forearm	↓	Variable	May calcify or ossify
Metastasis	Adults	Variable	↓	↑	—

↑ = High signal intensity; → = Intermediate signal intensity; ↓ = Low signal intensity.

Table 3. BENIGN FIBROUS PROLIFERATIONS AND FIBROMATOSES

Diagnosis	Typical Age of Presentation	Typical Location	Miscellaneous Data
Fibrous Proliferations of Infancy and Childhood			
Fibrous hamartoma	Infancy	Axillary, inguinal regions	Solitary, rarely recur
Congenital generalized fibromatosis (infantile myofibromatosis)	Infancy	Soft tissue, viscera, bone	Solitary or multiple, may regress, rarely recur
Infantile digital fibromatosis	Infancy	Fingers and toes	Solitary or multiple, may regress, commonly recur
Fibromatosis colli	Infancy	Sternocleidomastoid muscle	Solitary, rarely bilateral, may regress, rarely recur, associated torticollis
Juvenile aponeurotic fibroma	Infancy, childhood, or adolescence	Hands and feet	Solitary, may regress, commonly recur, may calcify
Juvenile hyaline fibromatosis	Childhood	Dermis and subcutis	Multiple, do not regress or recur
Infantile desmoid type fibromatosis	Infancy and childhood	Musculature	Solitary, commonly recur, no regression
Fibrous Proliferations of Adulthood			
Nodular fasciitis (pseudosarcomatous fasciitis)	Adulthood	Extremities	Solitary, may regress, rarely recur
Proliferative fasciitis	Adulthood	Extremities	Solitary
Proliferative myositis	Late adulthood	Trunk, shoulder girdle	Solitary
Elastofibroma	Late adulthood	Chest wall, scapula	Unilateral > bilateral
Keloid	Adolescence or adulthood	Face, shoulders, forearms, hands	Solitary or multiple, do not regress, common in blacks
Fibromatoses			
Palmar fibromatosis	Late adulthood	Hands	Unilateral or bilateral, associated Dupuytren's contracture
Plantar fibromatosis	Childhood or adulthood	Feet	Unilateral or bilateral, associated palmar fibromatosis
Peyronie's disease	Adulthood	Penis	May regress, associated palmar and plantar fibromatosis
Extra-abdominal fibromatosis (desmoid tumors)	Adulthood	Musculature	Rarely regress, commonly recur
Abdominal fibromatosis (desmoid tumors)	Early adulthood	Musculature	Commonly recur, occur during or after pregnancy
Intra-abdominal fibromatosis (pelvic fibromatosis, mesenteric fibromatosis, Gardner's syndrome)	Adulthood	Musculature, mesentery	May recur

Taken in part from Enzinger FM, Weiss SW: *Soft Tissue Tumors*. St. Louis, CV Mosby, 1983, p 71.

Table 4. OSTEOCHONDROSES

Disorder	Site	Age (Years)	Probable Mechanism
Legg-Calvé-Perthes disease	Femoral head	4–8	Osteonecrosis, perhaps due to trauma
Freiberg's infarction	Metatarsal head	13–18	Osteonecrosis due to trauma
Kienböck's disease	Carpal lunate	20–40	Osteonecrosis due to trauma
Köhler's disease	Tarsal navicular	3–7	Osteonecrosis or altered sequence of ossification
Panner's disease	Capitulum of humerus	5–10	Osteonecrosis or altered sequence of ossification
Thiemann's disease	Phalanges of hand	11–19	Osteonecrosis, perhaps due to trauma
Osgood-Schlatter disease	Tibial tuberosity	11–15	Trauma
Blount's disease	Proximal tibial epiphysis	1–3 (infantile) 8–15 (adolescent)	Trauma
Scheuermann's disease	Discovertebral junction	13–17	Trauma
Sinding-Larsen-Johansson disease	Patella	10–14	Trauma
Sever's phenomenon	Calcaneus	9–11	Normal variation in ossification
Van Neck's phenomenon	Ischiopubic synchondrosis	4–11	Normal variation in ossification

Table 5. SOME USEFUL MR IMAGING PROTOCOLS IN ASSESSMENT OF MUSCULOSKELETAL INFECTIONS

Condition	Suggested Protocols
Osteomyelitis in red marrow	T2-weighted spin echo T1-weighted spin echo with gadolinium contrast enhancement STIR
Osteomyelitis in yellow marrow	T1-weighted spin echo T1-weighted spin echo with gadolinium contrast enhancement and fat suppression STIR
Septic arthritis	T1-weighted spin echo with gadolinium contrast enhancement with or without fat suppression
Soft tissue infection	T1-weighted spin echo with gadolinium contrast enhancement with or without fat suppression

Index

Note: Page numbers in *italics* refer to illustrations; page numbers followed by t refer to tables.